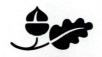

FETOLOGY

Diagnosis & Management
of the Fetal Patient

FETOLOGY

Diagnosis & Management of the Fetal Patient

Diana W. Bianchi, M.D.
Professor of Pediatrics and Obstetrics and Gynecology
Tufts University School of Medicine

Chief, Division of Genetics,
Department of Pediatrics
Chief of Perinatal Genetics,
Department of Obstetrics and Gynecology
New England Medical Center
Boston, Massachusetts

Timothy M. Crombleholme, M.D.
Assistant Professor of Surgery and Obstetrics and Gynecology
University of Pennsylvania School of Medicine

Fetal Surgeon, Center for Fetal Diagnosis and Therapy
Children's Hospital of Philadelphia
Philadelphia, Pennsylvania

Mary E. D'Alton, M.D.
Professor of Clinical Obstetrics and Gynecology
Columbia University College of Physicians and Surgeons

Director, Division of Maternal-Fetal Medicine
Department of Obstetrics and Gynecology
New York Presbyterian Hospital
New York, New York

McGraw-Hill
Medical Publishing Division

New York   St. Louis   San Francisco   Auckland   Bogotá   Caracas   Lisbon   London
Madrid   Mexico City   Milan   Montreal   New Delhi   San Juan
Singapore   Sydney   Tokyo   Toronto

McGraw-Hill

A Division of The McGraw·Hill Companies

Fetology: Diagnosis and Management of the Fetal Patient

Copyright © 2000 by The **McGraw-Hill Companies**, Inc. All rights reserved. Printed in the United States of America. Except as permitted under the United States Copyright Act of 1976, no part of this publication may be reproduced or distributed in any form or by any means, or stored in a data base or retrieval system, without the prior written permission of the publisher.

1234567890 QWK QWK 01234567890

ISBN 0-8385-2570-9

This book was set in Garamond by York Graphic Services, Inc.
The editor was Michael Medina.
The production supervisor was Phil Galea.
Project management was performed by York Production Services, Inc.
The designer was Mary Skudlarek.
Index prepared by Deborah K. Tourtlotte.
Quebecor World/Kingsport was printer and binder.

This book is printed on acid-free paper.

Cataloging-in-Publication Data is on file for this title at the Library of Congress.

TO:
John, Josh, and Elliott
Peg, Caitlin, Hayley, and Kye
Richard, Joseph, Conor, and Emer

CONTENTS

x   CONTENTS

A color insert falls between pages 506 and 507.

PREFACE

We wrote this book to provide a multidisciplinary approach to the full implications of a fetal sonographic or chromosomal diagnosis—from prenatal management to long-term outcome—for an affected child. We believed that what we, our colleagues, our trainees, and our patients needed was a compilation of available information to answer many of the questions that parents ask when a fetal anomaly is diagnosed.

In our experience, pregnant patients frequently receive conflicting information about the prognosis for the infant, depending on the sometimes narrow perspective of a subspecialist. The diagnosis and management of a fetus with an anomaly requires that an expertise be developed outside the traditional boundaries of the existing specialties of obstetrics, pediatrics, and surgery. These traditionally defined disciplines do not serve us well in addressing problems that exist outside our usual practice. By convention, pediatric care begins with the birth of an infant; however, we believe that pediatricians and pediatric surgeons can significantly contribute to the care of the fetus, their future patient. Similarly, obstetricians who do not generally provide medical care to the infant after delivery might enhance their antenatal care by being better informed about pediatric prognoses and outcomes. Pediatric surgeons who operate on fetuses or infants with congenital anomalies have more in common with perinatologists and neonatologists than with their other surgical colleagues. The problem-oriented multidisciplinary team approach has analogies in other specialties, such as cardiology, where the cardiologist, cardiac surgeon, and radiologist all focus on heart disease.

This book's intended audience consists of practitioners who care for fetuses or neonates with sonographically detected anomalies, and who seek prenatal and postnatal information regarding specific conditions. Included in this audience are general obstetricians, perinatologists, genetic counselors, neonatologists, pediatricians, pediatric subspecialists, and pediatric surgeons. We have also included information on some of the common chromosomal aneuploidies that may be detected when karyotyping is performed for a sonographic abnormality. Although the book is directed toward a medical audience, prospective parents were never far from our minds while we were writing. Most of the chapters were written by imagining that the prospective parents were in our offices seeking advice regarding the abnormal fetal finding. We have attempted to provide a balanced, scholarly, nondirective approach to management, which may differ significantly from what prospective parents may find on the Internet. Each chapter has a consistent format to facilitate locating specific kinds of information.

We have personally treated patients with most if not all of the conditions described within the following chapters as part of our collaborative work that began in the Fetal Diagnosis and Treatment Program at New England Medical Center and Tufts University School of Medicine in Boston in 1993. While the three of us brought to each case our individual approaches based on our different subspecialty training, we collectively recognized the need to present a coordinated and comprehensive plan to parents faced with a diagnosis of a fetal abnormality. Dr. Bianchi is a pediatrician, neonatologist, and medical geneticist who is interested in the correlation of pediatric outcome with prenatal sonographic findings; Dr. Crombleholme is a pediatric surgeon who has also trained in fetal surgical intervention. He writes extensively on the possibilities for surgical treatment of these diverse conditions and provides important information on long-term outcome. Dr. D'Alton is an obstetrician and perinatologist with expertise in antenatal sonographic diagnosis of anomalies.

Because our approach was unique, we felt that a multi-authored textbook would not specifically address the multiplicity of expertise necessary to care for the fetal patient. In establishing our Fetal Treatment Program we worked collaboratively to bring our individual training, experience, and knowledge base to each fetal patient on whom we consulted and whom we treated. We wanted this book to be more than a mere collation of facts; we wanted a cohesive approach to diagnosis, management, and in some cases, treatment of the fetal patient. We felt that in order for this book to reflect this approach it would be best for the three of us to have input into each chapter.

Finally, we must share with the reader that the most difficult aspect of writing this book was selecting a title. Although we, as the authors, were in complete agreement regarding the body of knowledge and clinical information we wanted to convey, it did not fit simply or neatly into a single existing medical specialty. While it is the general obstetrician or perinatologist who first suspects (and diagnoses) an abnormality in the fetus, it is the pediatric medical or surgical specialist who will ultimately treat the newborn infant. In many medical settings, however, prospective parents of a fetus with an abnormality never meet with any pediatric specialists, let alone members of a fetal treatment team. After much debate, we selected the title, *Fetology: Diagnosis & Management of the Fetal Patient* to indicate that the focus of this book is on the diagnosis and the overall management of the fetal patient. No one medical specialty is devoted to the care of the fetus. By definition, therefore, *fetology* requires a multidisciplinary team approach. We wrote this book as a summary of available information for ourselves, our colleagues, our trainees, and our patients to answer many of the questions that are asked when a fetal anomaly is diagnosed.

Fetology, however, is an evolving field. Many of the subtle prenatal sonographic findings in this book have only recently been described. We therefore await future clinical research to provide further information on the long-term clinical significance of many of the fetal findings reviewed here. We hope that this reference serves to increase recognition of the unique aspects of caring for the fetal patient. We hope that by viewing conditions from both the prenatal and postnatal perspective, we will foster collaboration between the existing medical specialties, and ultimately benefit the care of fetal patients and their families.

Diana W. Bianchi, M.D.

Timothy M. Crombleholme, M.D.

Mary E. D'Alton, M.D.

ACKNOWLEDGMENTS

Mary E. D'Alton, M.D.: The years that I spent working with Dr. Diana Bianchi and Dr. Tim Crombleholme were some of the most rewarding years of my academic life. During this time, we worked collectively to create a seamless, multidisciplinary approach to prenatal diagnosis and therapy for our patients. Our collaboration is reflected in this manuscript. I wish to acknowledge the support of my former fellows and residents. All of these individuals in their unique way helped shape the Division of Maternal Fetal Medicine, initially at Tufts University School of Medicine, and now at Columbia University College of Physicians and Surgeons. Some former fellows stayed on as faculty, initially at Tufts, and more recently at New York Presbyterian Hospital, and others are practicing in many other areas of the world. They include Drs. Achilles M. Athanassiou, Emily R. Baker, Juan Castaner, Sabrina D. Craigo, Annette Perez Delboy, Karen Davidson, Patricia Devine, Marla Eglowstein, Sara Garmel, Martin Gillieson, Laura Goetzel, Gary Kaufman, Fergal D. Malone, Teresa Marino, Lucie Morin, Jose A. Nores, Steven Ralston, Dale P. Reisner, Rebecca Elliot Rigsby, Lynn Simpson, Julia Elizabeth Solomon, and Theresa Stewart. Other faculty members at New England Medical Center who helped create a multidisciplinary team include Drs. John Fiascone, Ivan Frantz, Michael Goldberg, Karen Harvey Wilkes, Ziyad Hijazi, George Klauber, Michael Lewis, Gerald Marx, Heber Nielsen, N. Paul Rosman, Joseph Semple, and Ralph Yarnell. I owe an enormous gratitude to the obstetric sonographers, Jean Crowley, Rachel Duguay, Peg Meyers, and Pam Sullivan, and to the genetic counselors, Beth Berlin, Mona Inati, DeeDee Lafayette, Emily Lazar, and Michele Murray, for their excellence and devotion to patient care. I extend a special thank you to a model mentor, Dr. John Hobbins, who is widely considered to be the father of obstetric ultrasound. In the program he initially established at Yale University, ultrasound assumed an integral role in patient care. This program became a model for many perinatal units throughout the United States. He irreversibly changed the way in which I considered the practice of maternal fetal medicine. In particular, I wish to acknowledge the contributions of Drs. Richard Berkowitz, Fergal D. Malone, and Lynn Simpson, who critically read many of the chapters. The loyal support and personal and professional encouragement provided by Dr. Fergal Malone on an ongoing basis is deeply acknowledged and much appreciated. My part of this manuscript could not have been completed without the superb editorial skills of Star Poole, virtuoso word processor, who served as a medical editor in the Division of Maternal Fetal Medicine at Tufts University.

Timothy M. Crombleholme, M.D.: During the writing of this book, our understanding and approach to diagnosis and management of many fetal conditions has continued to evolve. Progress has only been possible through the supportive interactions of numerous professional colleagues in many disciplines who bring their unique expertise to bear on the fetus. I would like to acknowledge my research fellows and colleagues who have contributed to the development of the field of fetal surgery and fetology: at Tufts University, Sarah Garmel, Frank Robertson, Kevin Moriarty, and E. Kerry Gallivan, and at The Children's Hospital of Philadelphia, Darryl Cass, Karl Sylvester, Kenneth Liechty, Harold Lovvorn, Heung Bae Kim, Aimen Shaaban, Colette Pameijer, Danielle Walsh, Yoshihiro Kitano, Adina Knight, Ross Milner, Natalie Rintoul, Holly Hedrick, and Oluyinka Olutoye.

I wish to acknowledge the loyal support and guidance of Lori Howell, who has been instrumental in the development of fetal treatment programs, both at The University of California, San Francisco, and at The Children's Hospital of Philadelphia. The support and encouragement during the writing of this book of N. Scott Adzick and Alan Flake, my partners in fetal surgery at The Children's Hospital of Philadelphia, is gratefully acknowledged as is Michael R. Harrison, who as the father of fetal surgery was practicing fetology before it had a name. I would particularly like to thank my colleagues in other disciplines who have taught me so much and contributed to our understanding of the fetal patient, including Mark Johnson, Beverly Coleman, Stephen Horii, Jill Langer, Harvey Nisenbaum, and Mary King for their sonographic skill and enthusiastic support of fetal surgery; Anne Hubbard and Larissa Bilaniuk for their pioneering work on fetal MRI; Zhi-Yun Tien, Jack Rychik, Meryl Cohen, Marie Gleason, and Bill Mahle for their excellent echocardiographic support; and Elaine Zackai and Stefanie Kasperski for genetic evaluation and counseling at The Children's Hospital of Philadelphia. In the operating room at the Hospital of the University of Pennsylvania and The Children's Hospital of Philadelphia, I would like to acknowledge the contributions of Ted Cheek, Bob Gaiser, Dean Kurth, David Cohen, and Jeff Galinkin, who have done so much to advance the anesthetic management of fetal surgical patients. Also, acknowledged in the operating room are Joy Kerr, Marianne Daskalakis, and Helen Lewis and, most particularly, in the postnatal care and evaluation of our fetal patients, Kelli Burns and Sue Von Nessen. Lastly, for their ability to decipher my hieroglyphic writing and secretarial support, I give special thanks to Dee Caton and Noreen Mulholland.

Diana W. Bianchi, M.D.: In addition to the faculty and fellows in maternal–fetal medicine and neonatology listed by Dr. D'Alton, I would like to acknowledge the collaboration, support, and expertise of the medical genetics faculty at Tufts University, which during the past six years has included Janet Cowan, Patricia Wheeler, Rosemarie Smith, Janey Wiggs, and Mira Irons. I am enormously grateful to the genetic counselors listed by Dr. D'Alton, who not only provide outstanding and compassionate care when a fetal anomaly is diagnosed, but alerted us to the existence of cases that would present useful teaching examples for this book. I would also like to acknowledge the perinatal genetics fellows who worked in my research laboratory during this time period, who read chapter drafts and provided me with helpful feedback. They include Antonio Farina, JiYi Wang, Akihiko Sekizawa, Osamu Samura, Barbara Pertl, Satoshi Sohda, Kirby Johnson, Paula Farrell, Nancy Weinschenk, and Bharath Srivatsa.

I would also like to thank current or former Tufts faculty members who critically read sections of the manuscript, including Dr. Joseph Semple of Pathology, who supplied many photographs; Dr. Michael Lewis of Plastic Surgery; Dr. Michael Goldberg of Orthopedic Surgery; Drs. Gerald Marx, Ziyad Hijazi, and Jonathan Rhodes of Pediatric Cardiology; Dr. George Klauber of Urology; and Dr. N. Paul Rosman of Pediatric Neurology. In addition, I would like to thank Dr. Deborah Levine for her expertise in fetal MRI, Dr. Marjorie Treadwell for supplying additional illustrations, and Drs. Wolfgang Holzgreve and Roberto Romeo for both illustrations and helpful discussions. I would also like to thank my secretarial staff for their help and support in the writing and researching of the manuscript, including Lynne Aufiero, Maria McCarthy, and Glenn Christie. I would also like to thank Jane Licht, our orignal editor at Appleton & Lange, who guided me through the process of putting together a large textbook. I would like to give a special acknowledgment to Dr. Mary Ellen Avery, who not only provided moral support, but helpful information on the origin of the term *neonatology,* as background for selecting the title of this book. Last but by no means least, I would like to thank Dr. Alan Guttmacher, who originally suggested the title for this book: *Fetology.* Although we as authors initially did not *bond* to this term, in the end, we decided that it was the most appropriate way to describe the body of knowledge in what is arguably a new field of medicine.

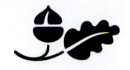

PART I

Introduction

CHAPTER 1

Prenatal Imaging

The development and practice of fetology has been dependent on advances in the field of prenatal imaging. Without the ability to accurately visualize the structure and well-being of the fetus within its own intrauterine environment, it would not be possible to diagnose or treat the huge range of abnormalities that are now addressed by the multidisciplinary fetal health care team. Rapid advances in the technologic basis of two imaging methods—ultrasonography and magnetic resonance imaging—have resulted in highly accurate visualization of all parts of the fetal anatomy.

▶ PRENATAL ULTRASONOGRAPHY

Development

Ultrasonography in obstetrics was first introduced in the late 1950s and has since become the method of choice for imaging the fetus. Gray-scale imaging became available in 1973 and resulted in an enhancement of the ability to differentiate the appearance of various organs and tissue interfaces. The advent of real-time sonographic scanning during the 1970s was vital for the accurate visualization of the constantly moving fetus. The subsequent development of higher-frequency transabdominal and transvaginal transducers in the late 1970s resulted in vast improvements in the resolution of fetal images and also pushed back the gestational age barrier for accurate prenatal diagnosis into the late first and early second trimesters (D'Alton 1998).

The 1980s saw innovations in obstetric sonographic technology, including the use of pulsed and color Doppler sonography, which allowed for detailed analysis of fetal perfusion and improvements in the visualization of fetal cardiac anatomy. More recent advances include the development of power Doppler, which displays the strength of a Doppler signal rather than the direction of flow. This technique is useful in fetal imaging for low-flow states and may aid in the definition of fetal tumors and assessing placental function (Ogle and Rodeck 1998). Three-dimensional ultrasonography is now also available for fetal imaging and has the potential to revolutionize the field of prenatal imaging by allowing simple sonographic acquisition of a "block" of fetal tissue. Post-acquisition computer processing allows reconstruction of any number of planes through the organ of interest. However, to date no adequate studies have been published to describe the potential advantage of three-dimensional sonographic visualization of fetal anomalies over views obtained by an expert using traditional two-dimensional imaging.

Controversies

Ultrasonographic imaging is an integral part of obstetric practice today. In the United States, it is performed in at least 70% of all pregnancies (Goncalves and Romero 1993; Horger and Tsai 1989). Sonography has been used routinely for accurate dating of pregnancy, confirmation of pregnancy location and number of gestations, prenatal diagnosis of congenital malformations, and assessment of fetal well-being. With the increasing availability of ultrasound equipment, the performance of obstetric ultrasonography has grown to the point that, in some countries, one or more ultrasound examinations are recommended during all pregnancies (Royal College of Obstetricians and Gynaecologists 1997).

Significant disagreement exists within the international obstetric community regarding the role of routine ultrasound evaluation during pregnancy. In 1984, the United States National Institutes of Health (NIH) published a consensus statement that concluded that there was no clinical benefit from routine obstetric ultrasonography (United States Department of Health and

Human Services, 1984). Subsequently the American College of Obstetricians and Gynecologists (ACOG) published a Technical Bulletin agreeing with the position of the NIH and concluding that, in the United States, the routine use of ultrasonography could not be supported from a cost-benefit standpoint (American College of Obstetricians and Gynecologists 1993). By contrast, the Royal College of Obstetricians and Gynaecologists in the United Kingdom has stated that, since 70% of the pregnant population has a recognized indication for the performance of an ultrasound examination, it would be wrong to deny the remaining 30% of the population a potentially valuable test (Royal College of Obstetricians and Gynaecologists 1994).

Studies evaluating the performance of ultrasonography in pregnancy have yielded conflicting results. During the past 7 years, at least nine studies have been published in which the performance of second-trimester ultrasonography for the detection of fetal anomalies has been evaluated. These studies have been summarized and are described in detail in Table 1-1 (Van Dorsten et al. 1998). Reported sensitivities of ultrasonography for the detection of fetal anomalies range from a low of 16.6% in the RADIUS Trial to a high of 84.3% in the study by Luck (Crane et al. 1994; Luck 1992). By contrast, almost all studies agree that the specificity of a normal prenatal ultrasound examination approaches 100%.

Apart from the detection of congenital abnormalities, obstetric ultrasonography can be expected to be beneficial in other aspects of pregnancy management. The routine use of obstetric ultrasonography has been shown to reduce the rate of postdated pregnancies and to reduce the use of tocolytic medications, both because of an improvement in the accuracy of pregnancy dating (LeFevre et al. 1993; Saari-Kemppainen et al. 1990). In addition, the routine use of obstetric ultrasonography has been shown to significantly increase the early detection of multiple gestations, which is essential if ap-

propriate modifications in pregnancy management are to be applied (LeFevre et al. 1993).

While the RADIUS Trial did not demonstrate any improvement in overall perinatal outcome from routine obstetric ultrasonography, this study has been criticized because of its poor performance in the detection of anomalies (Ewigman et al. 1993; Goncalves and Romero 1993). Other studies have demonstrated a significant reduction in perinatal mortality following routine obstetric ultrasonography, mostly because of an increase in the rate of pregnancy termination for congenital anomalies (Saari-Kemppainen et al. 1990). A meta-analysis of four randomized clinical trials of routine versus indicated ultrasonography also confirmed a significantly lower perinatal mortality rate in patients allocated to routine scanning (Bucher and Schmidt 1993).

Impact of Skill and Experience

Perhaps the most likely reason for the significant discrepancy in the sensitivities of ultrasonography for the detection of anomalies shown in Table 1-1 is the effect of the skill and experience of the sonographer. There is undoubtedly wide variation in the skill levels of sonographers between different centers that practice obstetric ultrasonography. In the RADIUS Trial, for example, there was a significant difference in the rates of anomaly detection between participating tertiary- and nontertiary-level centers (Crane et al. 1994). Nontertiary-level centers detected only 13% of congenital anomalies in the RADIUS Trial and were unable to detect any craniofacial, cardiac, gastrointestinal, or skeletal malformations. Tertiary-level centers performed significantly better, detecting 35% of anomalies (Goncalves and Romero 1993).

In a retrospective study from Vienna, the impact of sonographer experience was demonstrated by a wide variation in rates of anomaly detection between different centers with different skill levels (Bernaschek et al.

▶ **TABLE 1-1.** COMPARISON OF STUDIES OF PERFORMANCE OF SECOND-TRIMESTER SONOGRAPHY

Study	Years	No. of Fetuses	Gestation Age at Examination (wk)	Prevalence of Anomaly	Sensitivity	Specificity
Rosendahl and Kivinen 1989	91–93	3,098	18	1.03%	39.4%	99.9%
Saari-Kemppainen et al. 1990	86–87	4,691	16–20	0.43%	40.9%	99.8%
Levi et al. 1991	84–89	16,353	18–20	2.3%	20.8%	99.9%
Chitty et al. 1991	89–90	8,432	18–20	1.48%	74.4%	99.98%
Shirley et al. 1992	89–90	6,183	19	1.36%	60.7%	99.98%
Luck 1992	88–91	8,523	19	1.95%	84.3%	99.9%
Crane et al. 1994	87–91	7,685	15–22	2.4%	16.6%	99.9%
Anderson et al. 1995	91–93	7,880	16–20	1.98%	60.0%	—
Van Dorsten et al. 1998	93–96	2,031	15–22	3.0%	75.0%	99.9%
Boyd et al. 1998	91–96	33,376	18–22	2.2%	55%	—

Adapted, with permission, from Van Dorsten JP, Hulsey TC, Newman RB, et al. Fetal anomaly detection by second-trimester ultrasonography in a tertiary center. Am J Obstet Gynecol 1998;178:742–749.

1996). In that study, the overall anomaly detection rate was only 22% for obstetric ultrasonography performed in private obstetricians' offices, 40% in general hospitals, and 90% for ultrasonography performed by experts in fetal imaging.

Because of the clear association between the skill or experience of the sonographer and rates of anomaly detection, it has been suggested that obstetric ultrasonography should be performed only in tertiary-level centers, where up to four times as many fetuses with anomalies may be detected (DeVore 1994). However, it is not clear that all pregnant patients will have equal access to tertiary-level centers, which may be especially problematic in rural or other underserved areas.

Accreditation and Maintenance of Standards

Given the influence of the sonographer's skill and experience on the rate of anomaly detection for obstetric ultrasonography, it is logical to expect that basic standards and requirements for the performance of ultrasonography be delineated. However, in the United States there is no mandatory requirement for licensure or accreditation for practitioners who provide obstetric ultrasonography services. Minimum standards are described only in the form of suggested guidelines, and any form of accreditation is entirely voluntary in nature.

The American Institute of Ultrasound in Medicine (AIUM) has suggested minimum qualifications for all practitioners involved in obstetric ultrasonography (American Institute of Ultrasound in Medicine 1993). One of the key components of such qualification is the completion of an approved residency program, or the performance and interpretation of at least 500 obstetric ultrasound examinations. Furthermore, the AIUM now accredits obstetric ultrasonography practices, which involves evaluation of the credentials of sonographers, quality of fetal images, type of ultrasound equipment, methods of data storage, and presence of quality-control measures in place (American Institute of Ultrasound in Medicine 1995).

Even though such methods of accreditation and maintenance of standards are currently voluntary in the United States, it is likely that third-party payers, such as the U.S. Health Care Financing Administration and private insurance companies, will require proof of accreditation before releasing reimbursement for ultrasound services. If this practice becomes widespread, it will have the effect of mandating standardization and credentialing on obstetric ultrasonography practices within the United States. In addition, the increasing frequency of medical malpractice litigation will inevitably result in more obstetric ultrasound examinations being performed only by highly qualified practitioners.

Fetal Telemedicine

The emerging field of telemedicine seems to offer a solution to many of the problems associated with how to provide high-quality routine obstetric ultrasonography. Telemedicine involves the delivery of health care across distances by combining medical expertise with telecommunications technology (Goldberg 1996). *Fetal telemedicine* is a term used to describe the application of telemedicine principles to the provision of obstetric ultrasonography (Fisk et al. 1996).

Like videotape review, fetal telemedicine allows patients the convenience of remaining in their own communities rather than having to travel to an urban center or a tertiary-care facility for ultrasonography. In addition, it maintains quality ultrasonography, since images are both reviewed and interpreted by a specialist in fetal imaging. Because instantaneous feedback between physician and sonographer maximizes the quality of the images obtained, fetal telemedicine entails no dependence on couriers to transport images and is not as reliant on the skill of the sonographer as is videotape review. Fetal telemedicine systems make full use of computerization and modern telecommunications to efficiently provide an obstetric ultrasonography service.

Several studies have already validated the use of telemedicine for providing screening sonography during the first trimester (Nores et al. 1997a), as well as in the second and third trimesters (Malone et al. 1997). The technical requirements for telemedicine transmission of real-time obstetric sonography have also been described (Malone et al. 1998b; Nores et al. 1997a), and cost issues surrounding the use of obstetric telemedicine have been addressed (Malone et al. 1998a). Telemedicine transmission of obstetric ultrasonography may also be of use in providing additional tertiary-level opinions for complicated prenatal diagnosis cases. Telemedicine transmission of obstetric ultrasonography effectively provides a limitless number of second opinions in cases of diagnostic difficulty.

Safety

Theoretical safety risks from ultrasound energy include thermal damage or cavitation, with subsequent tissue injury. Most prenatal ultrasound examinations produce energies of 10 to 20 mW per square centimeter, which is well below the arbitrarily defined safe cut-off level of 100 mW per square centimeter (American College of Obstetricians and Gynecologists 1993). Newer prenatal imaging methods, such as those that use power Doppler, may be associated with higher energy outputs, which reinforces the need to continuously monitor power output during prenatal ultrasonography and to achieve the lowest possible energy exposure.

Randomized trials on the safety of diagnostic ultrasonography in pregnancy have demonstrated no significant differences in developmental, neurologic, or psychologic outcomes, with up to 12 years of follow-up (Stark et al. 1984). One study did demonstrate a nonsignificant increase in the frequency of dyslexia in the group exposed to ultrasound in utero, as compared with the group with no ultrasound exposure (Stark et al. 1984). A subsequent study evaluating school performance and dyslexia in groups exposed and not exposed to ultrasound in utero found no differences in any outcome measures, although there was an association between left-handedness and in utero ultrasound exposure (Salvesen et al. 1992, 1993). One study has also suggested an association between frequent ultrasound exposure in utero (five ultrasound examinations) and growth restriction, although this has not been confirmed by other investigators (Newnham et al. 1993).

Overall, it appears that routine ultrasonography in pregnancy is not associated with any adverse outcome for the fetus. Repeat ultrasound examinations should be performed only as indicated, when the benefits of the investigation clearly outweigh any theoretic risk of growth disturbance.

Current Role

The four main roles of prenatal ultrasonography in contemporary obstetric practice are

1. To confirm fetal gestational age and number
2. To search for fetal malformation
3. To confirm fetal well-being
4. To aid in the performance of invasive diagnostic and therapeutic fetal procedures.

The ability of prenatal ultrasonography to accurately confirm fetal gestational age and number of fetuses is self-evident. The RADIUS Trial demonstrated a significantly decreased chance of postdated induction of labor following accurate sonographic dating of pregnancy and a significant increase in the prenatal detection of multiple gestations (LeFevre et al. 1993).

The ability of prenatal ultrasonography to diagnose fetal malformations, both as a screening tool and for targeted examinations, has also been confirmed. In expert hands, screening ultrasonography can be expected to detect approximately 70% of all fetal malformations (Boyd et al. 1998; Van Dorsten et al. 1998). However, the detection rate for individual anomalies varies significantly. While almost all spinal, renal, and abdominal-wall malformations are detected by screening prenatal ultrasonography, the detection rate for isolated cardiac defects and Down syndrome is only 50% (Boyd et al. 1998). Efforts to increase the second-trimester detection rate of Down syndrome by including so-called soft markers for aneuploidy (such as short femur, short humerus, echogenic bowel, nuchal thickening, and choroid plexus cysts) may be successful, although it is likely that any such improvement will be accompanied by an increase in the false positive rate. This will inevitably lead to increased rates of fetal loss secondary to invasive diagnostic procedures, together with an increased risk of psychologic morbidity for parents (Boyd et al. 1998). A new approach to screening for Down syndrome using first-trimester sonographic measurement of fetal nuchal translucency thickness, in combination with biochemical markers, is currently being evaluated and may lead to a more efficient method of population screening.

Prenatal ultrasonography also plays a crucial role in the confirmation of fetal well-being, especially following the identification of a fetal abnormality or a condition associated with a high risk of adverse fetal outcome. Fetal biophysical profile and pulsed Doppler assessment of fetal arterial flow may be used for identifying fetuses with compromised reserve that may benefit from either intensive surveillance or elective premature delivery.

The ability to perform invasive prenatal diagnostic procedures safely, as well as fetal therapy, has been significantly improved by real-time ultrasonography. Diagnostic procedures during the first trimester, such as chorionic villus sampling and embryofetoscopy, are now commonly performed under ultrasound guidance. Amniocentesis, fetal blood sampling, vesicocentesis, thoracentesis, and fetal biopsies are also possible because of the availability of real-time ultrasonography. The ability to treat the fetus using blood transfusions, drug infusions, and shunt placement is now also possible as a result of advances in sonographic technology and availability.

▶ PRENATAL MAGNETIC RESONANCE IMAGING (MRI)

Development

Magnetic resonance imaging has been available for clinical use for over 15 years, but until recently it has rarely been applied in prenatal diagnosis. However, the potential for MRI in prenatal diagnosis was recognized early on, with reports of imaging of fetal abnormalities (Lowe et al. 1985; McCarthy et al. 1985; Weinreb et al. 1985). However, a serious limitation of these early attempts at prenatal MRI was the long acquisition times of standard spin-echo images. The amount of fetal movement that would occur during image acquisition degraded the images obtained. The noise associated with MRI scanning made the likelihood of a fetus sleeping motionless during the study very small. The quality of the images that were possible prompted the use of paralyzing agents administered either by intramuscular injection into the fetus or umbilical cord injection to obtain motion-free spin echo images (Daffos et al. 1988). The invasive nature of this approach dampened the initial enthusiasm for prenatal MRI.

During the early 1990s, ultrafast MRI sequences and fast scanners, such as echo-planar MRI, were developed (Johnson et al. 1990; Mansfield et al. 1990). By 1996, ultrafast MRI sequences, using half-Fourier acquisition single-shot turbo spin-echo (HASTE) technique were developed, which allowed a single T_2-weighted anatomic image to be acquired in less than 500 msec (Semelka et al. 1996). The ultrafast scanning technique eliminates, or significantly reduces, the artifacts caused by fetal movement, making fetal sedation or paralysis unnecessary for prenatal MRI (Hubbard and Harty 1999). These ultrafast sequences are now being successfully employed in imaging the human fetus (Garden et al. 1995; Hubbard and Harty 1999; Hubbard et al. 1997, 1998; Levine et al. 1996; Quinn et al. 1998; Yamashita et al. 1997). Fetal anatomy has been well described by MRI scanning in fetuses over 18 weeks of gestation and is increasingly being used as an adjunct to prenatal ultrasound examination in the evaluation of structural fetal anomalies, facilitating appropriate prenatal counseling, and guiding fetal therapy (Hubbard and Harty 1999; Levine et al. 1996; Quinn et al. 1998).

Safety

The safety of MRI in prenatal diagnosis remains a concern, but to date there are no known harmful effects in the developing fetus with the use of scanners at field strengths of 1.5 Tesla or less (Hubbard et al. 1999). Guidelines for patient safety were issued by the safety committee of the Society of Magnetic Resonance Imaging. The recommendations are that MRI may be used in a pregnant woman when other nonionizing forms of diagnostic imaging are inadequate (Shellock and Kanal 1991). Even though no deleterious effects of fetal MRI have been established, the safety of fetal MRI has not been proven, and the few centers using this technique limit its use to fetuses older than 18 weeks of gestation. By this time in gestation, organogenesis is complete and the risks of teratogenic effects are minimal.

MRI of the Fetal Central Nervous System

MRI had been used to characterize the developing brain as early as 1983 (Gilles et al. 1983). The use of the HASTE technique has provided excellent anatomic information about the fetal central nervous system (CNS) without the need for fetal paralysis (Levine et al. 1996, 1997; Yamashita et al. 1997). Ultrasound examination remains the primary method of prenatal imaging but, especially in the brain, MRI is becoming an invaluable adjunct, providing superior characterization of fetal brain maturation, and morphology. In most instances, MRI is used for fetuses in which a CNS abnormality has already been demonstrated or is suspected by ultrasonography (Bilaniuk 1999). The most common CNS abnormalities diagnosed by ultrasound examination and referred for evaluation by MRI include cysts, Dandy–Walker malformation or variant, agenesis of the corpus callosum, hydrocephalus, vein of Galen aneurysm, encephaloceles, and otherwise malformed brains.

Ventriculomegaly is a common indication for fetal MRI. T_2-weighted sequences provide excellent imaging of the size and configuration of the ventricles. Criteria for ventriculomegaly in fetal MRI is based on ultrasound data demonstrating ventricles of a width of at least 10 mm. However, the size of the ventricles tends to be slightly larger when obtained by MRI than the measurements obtained in the same fetus by ultrasound examination. Once ventriculomegaly is identified, a detailed examination of the entire fetus should be performed to detect associated anomalies. When ventricular enlargement is due to a myelomeningocele, MRI is particularly good for demonstrating the Chiari II malformation, the extent of the neural-tube defect, and the level of the sac (Bilaniuk 1999).

MRI provides excellent tissue discrimination in defining congenital CNS abnormalities such as calvarial defects, differentiating hemangioma or lymphangioma from encephalocele or meningocele, and demonstrating partial or complete agenesis of the corpus callosum. The finding of an abnormality of the corpus callosum is rarely isolated and often indicates the presence of other cerebral abnormalities (Atlas et al. 1986; Barkovich and Norman 1988). Occasionally, ultrasound examination may have difficulty in differentiating partial agenesis of the corpus callosum from normal anatomy. MRI can be helpful in further delineating the anatomy.

Vein of Galen aneurysm is a vascular malformation that may be misdiagnosed as a cyst or a mass if not examined using color Doppler on ultrasound. MRI can demonstrate not only the vascular anatomy, but also the condition of the brain, which is of concern because these lesions can be associated with encephalomalacia and macrocrania. The presence of encephalomalacia in cases of vein of Galen aneurysm indicates a poor prognosis (Bilaniuk 1999).

MRI of the Fetal Neck

Fetal MRI may be particularly useful in evaluating fetal neck masses. Distinguishing between lymphangioma and a cervical teratoma may be difficult based on ultrasound images alone (see Chapters 32 and 111). In addition, the risk of a compromised airway at birth is high with each of these lesions. MRI of cervical fetal masses allows for more global imaging of the mass than with ultrasound because of the larger field of view. In a report by Hubbard et al. (1998), fetal MRI was able to accurately diagnose the nature of the mass and define the anatomy of the airway. In each case, as compared with ultrasound examination, fetal MRI provided better detail about the size and position of the mass and its relationship to the airway. The HASTE sequence images provide the best anatomic definition of the normal fetal cranial structures and their relationship to the mass (Semelka et al. 1996).

Lymphangiomas appear to be complex masses with cystic and solid components that may compress or surround the airway (Benacerraf and Frigoletto 1987; Hubbard et al. 1998; Zadvinskis et al. 1992). Cervical teratomas arise from the anterolateral neck and tend to cross the midline (Sherer et al. 1993). These tumors can be solid and cystic with areas of calcification and hemorrhage (Rothschild et al. 1994). On more T_2-weighted fast sequences, cystic components can be evaluated. The oropharynx and trachea are filled with amniotic fluid, which is bright and can be differentiated from the tumor. Areas of acute hemorrhage can be identified by sequences that have more T_1-weighting, which helps delineate teratoma from lymphangioma (Hubbard et al. 1998). Hemorrhage and calcification can be identified on either gradient-echo or echo-planar images.

MRI of the Fetal Chest

The most common thoracic abnormalities identified on prenatal ultrasound examination include congenital diaphragmatic hernia (CDH), congenital cystic adenomatoid malformation of the lung (CCAM), bronchopulmonary sequestration (BPS), and fetal hydrothorax (Morin et al. 1994). CDH has been recognized by herniation of the stomach to the level of the four-chamber view of the heart and a shift of the mediastinum away from the hernia (Chinn et al. 1983). Although the sonographic features of CDH are well described, the diagnosis of CDH has been missed in a significant number of fetuses who have been studied by prenatal ultrasound (Lewis et al. 1997). Even in cases in which CDH is correctly diagnosed by ultrasound examination, determination of the presence or absence of liver herniation may be difficult. Herniation of the liver has been found to be a predictor of poor postnatal outcome in CDH (Metkus et al. 1996). Ultrasound examination relies on indirect indicators of liver herniation, such as kinking of the umbilical vein as it enters the sinus venosus (Bootstaylor et al. 1995). Fetal MRI can directly identify the position and degree of herniation of the liver in CDH (Hubbard et al. 1997a, 1997b). The fetal liver has high signal intensity on fast gradient-echo sequences with T_1-weighting, making it easily identifiable relative to the diaphragmatic ridge and the compressed ipsilateral lung. The lung is intermediate to high in signal intensity, which allows differentiation from mediastinal structures and herniated viscera (Hubbard et al. 1997). On HASTE sequence with T_2-weighting, the fluid filled stomach is high in signal intensity, equal to the signal intensity in amniotic fluid. The selection criteria for fetal surgery for CDH includes herniation of the liver, making accurate delineation of this anatomy all the more important (Shaaban et al. 1999).

MRIs in CCAM vary in appearance, depending on their size and number and size of cysts. The larger the size and number of cysts, the higher the signal intensity of the CCAM on sequences with T_2-weighting. MRI is able to distinguish CCAM from normal compressed lung and determine the lobe of the lung from which the tumor arises. BPS has very high signal intensity as compared with normal lung and is very homogeneous, with discrete margins (Hubbard et al. 1997). BPS in late gestation can become iso-echogenic with adjacent lung and may seem to disappear on ultrasound examination. These lesions show up distinctly from adjacent normal lung on MRI (Hubbard and Harty 1999). One disadvantage of fetal MRI in evaluating fetal chest masses has been the inability to demonstrate systemic feeding vessels to BPS. This is a distinct advantage of color flow Doppler over MRI in evaluating BPS or hybrid CCAM lesions, which also have a septicemic blood supply. Because of its larger field of view, fetal MRI may be especially helpful in evaluating unusual chest lesions such as neurenteric cysts, laryngotracheal or bronchial obstruction, or mediastinal masses (Hubbard et al. 1997).

MRI of the Fetal Abdomen and Pelvis

In most instances ultrasound examination is excellent to evaluate anomalies of the fetal abdomen and pelvis. There are instances, however, when MRI can be helpful. In fetuses with oligohydramnios, ultrasound evaluation can be extremely difficult, whereas fetal MRI imaging is unaffected by a lack of amniotic fluid. It is often difficult to distinguish proximal from distal small-bowel obstruction on prenatal ultrasound examination. There are different MRI signal characteristics that are helpful in these cases, distinguishing proximal from distal small bowel (Hubbard and Harty 1999). Proximal bowel will have high to intermediate signal intensity on T_2-weighted sequences, similar to amniotic fluid, while distal bowel has intermediate to low signal intensity. Conversely, distal bowel has a high signal intensity on T_1-weighted sequences because of meconium filling the bowel lumen. Using these sequences, dilated loops of bowel may be distinguished as either proximal or distal (Hubbard and Harty 1999). Because of the large field of view, complex anomalies such as persistent cloaca or cloacal exstrophy may be better imaged on MRI.

The imaging of the fetal urinary tract with ultrasound examination is excellent and rarely improved on by MRI. Exceptions to this include cases of obstructive uropathy complicated by oligohydramnios, polycystic kidneys, and renal tumors. This is also true of sacro-coccygeal teratomas (SCTs), which arise from Hensen's node at the tip of the coccyx. SCTs are most commonly exophytic, but can also extend into the pelvis or abdomen with compression of bladder and intestines.

Fetal MRI is not indicated as a primary imaging method in any fetal anomaly or condition. As discussed above, however, there are instances in which the information provided by fetal MRI complements that obtained by prenatal ultrasound examination. The role of MRI in prenatal diagnosis is still evolving. At present, MRI is best used selectively in cases in which prenatal sonography is unable to make a definitive diagnosis, where a larger field of view is required, or in acquiring specific information necessary for selection for fetal intervention. Real-time interventional MRI is currently available in a select few centers, and it is anticipated that reports of its use in fetal therapy will soon appear.

REFERENCES

American College of Obstetricians and Gynecologists. Ultrasonography in pregnancy. Washington, DC: Technical Bulletin no. 187. American College of Obstetricians and Gynecologists, December 1993.

American Institute of Ultrasound in Medicine. Standards for accreditation of obstetrical and gynecological ultrasound practices. Laurel, MD: American Institute of Ultrasound in Medicine, 1995.

American Institute of Ultrasound in Medicine. Training guidelines for physicians who evaluate and interpret diagnostic ultrasound examinations. Rockville, MD: American Institute of Ultrasound in Medicine, 1993.

Anderson N, Boswell O, Duff G. Prenatal sonography for the detection of fetal anomalies: results of a prospective study and comparison with prior series. AJR Am J Roentgenol 1995;165:943–950.

Atlas SW, Zimmerman RA, Bilaniuk LT, et al. Corpus callosum and limbic system: neuroanatomic MR evaluation of developmental anomalies. Radiology 1986;160:355–362.

Barkovich AJ, Norman D. Anomalies of the corpus callosum: correlation with further anomalies of the brain. AJNR Am J Neuroradiol 1988;9:493–501.

Benacerraf B, Frigoletto F. Prenatal sonographic diagnosis of isolated congenital cystic hygroma, unassociated with lymphedema or other morphologic abnormality. J Ultrasound Med 1987;6:63–66.

Bernaschek G, Stuempflen I, Deutinger J. The influence of the experience of the investigator on the rate of sonographic diagnosis of fetal malformations in Vienna. Prenat Diagn 1996;16:807–811.

Bilaniuk LT. Magnetic resonance imaging of the fetal brain. Semin Roentgenol 1999;34:48–61.

Bootstaylor B, Filly R, Harrison M, et al. Prenatal sonographic predictors of liver herniation in congenital diaphragmatic hernia. J Ultrasound Med 1995;14:515–520.

Boyd PA, Chamberlain P, Hicks NR. 6-year experience of prenatal diagnosis in an unselected population in Oxford, UK. Lancet 1998;352:1577–1581.

Bucher HC, Schmidt JG. Does routine ultrasound scanning improve outcome in pregnancy? Meta-analysis of various outcome measures. BMJ 1993;307:13–17.

Chinn D, Filly R, Callen P, et al. Congenital diaphragmatic hernia diagnosed prenatally by ultrasound. Radiology 1983;148:119–123.

Chitty LS, Hunt GH, Moore J, et al. Effectiveness of routine ultrasonography in detecting fetal structural abnormalities in a low risk population. BMJ 1991;303:1165–1169.

Crane JP, LeFevre ML, Winborn RC, et al. A randomized trial of prenatal ultrasonographic screening: impact on the detection, management, and outcome of anomalous fetuses. Am J Obstet Gynecol 1994;171:392–399.

D'Alton MD. Ultrasound in obstetrics and gynecology: an imaging revolution. Contemp Obstet Gynecol 1998;43: 67–84.

Daffos F, Forestier F, Aleese J, et al. Fetal curarization for prenatal magnetic resonance imaging in prenatal diagnoses. Prenat Diagn 1988;8:311–314.

DeVore GR. The routine antenatal diagnostic imaging with ultrasound study: another perspective. Obstet Gynecol 1994;84:622–626.

Ewigman BG, Crane JP, Frigoletto FD, et al. Effect of prenatal ultrasound screening on perinatal outcome. N Engl J Med 1993;329:821–827.

Fisk NM, Sepulveda W, Drysdale K, et al. Fetal telemedicine: six month pilot of real-time ultrasound and video consultation between the Isle of Wight and London. Br J Obstet Gynaecol 1996;103:1092–1095.

Garden A, Weindling A, Griffiths R, et al. Fast-scan magnetic resonance imaging of fetal anomalies. Br J Obstet Gynecol 1995;98:1217–1222.

Gilles FH, Shankle W, Dooling EC. Myelinatal tracts: growth patterns. In: Gilles FH, Leviton A, Dooling EC, eds. The developing human brain. Littleton, MA: John Wright PSG, 1983:117–174.

Goldberg MA. Teleradiology and telemedicine. Radiol Clin North Am 1996;34:647–665.

Goncalves LF, Romero R. A critical appraisal of the RADIUS study. Fetus 1993;3:7–18.

Horger EO, Tsai CC. Ultrasound and the prenatal diagnosis of congenital anomalies: a medicolegal perspective. Obstet Gynecol 1989;74:617–619.

Hubbard AM, Adzick NS, Crombleholme TM, et al. Left-sided congenital diaphragmatic hernia: value of prenatal MR imaging in preparation for fetal surgery. Radiology 1997a;203:636–640.

Hubbard AM, Adzick NS, Crombleholme TM, et al. Prenatal MRI imaging of congenital chest tumors. Presented at the meeting of the Radiology Society of North America, Chicago, December 1, 1997b.

Hubbard AM, Crombleholme TM, Adzick NS. Prenatal MRI evaluation of giant neck masses in preparation for the fetal EXIT procedure. Am J Perinatol 1998;15:253–257.

Hubbard AM, Harty P. Prenatal magnetic resonance imaging of fetal anomalies. Semin Roentgenol 1999;34:41–47.

Johnson I, Stehling M, Blamire A, et al. Study of internal structures of the human fetus in utero by echo-planar magnetic resonance imaging. Am J Obstet Gynecol 1990;163:601–607.

LeFevre ML, Bain RP, Ewigman BG, et al. A randomized trial of prenatal ultrasonographic screening: impact on maternal management and outcome. Am J Obstet Gynecol 1993;169:483–489.

Levi S, Jyjazi Y, Schapps JP, et al. Sensitivity and specificity of routine antenatal screening for congenital anomalies by ultrasound: the Belgian multicentric study. Ultrasound Obstet Gynecol 1991;1:102–110.

Levine D, Barnes PD, Madsen JR, et al. Fetal central nervous system anomalies: MR imaging augments sonographic diagnosis. Radiology 1997;204:635–642.

Levine D, Hataba H, Goa J, et al. Fetal anatomy revealed with fast MR sequences. AJR Am J Roentgenol 1996;167:905–908.

Lewis D, Reickert C, Bowerman R, et al. Prenatal ultrasonography fails to diagnose congenital diaphragmatic hernia. J Pediatr Surg 1997;32:352–356.

Lowe T, Weinreb J, Santos-Ramos R, et al. Magnetic resonance imaging in human pregnancy. Obstet Gynecol 1985;66:629–633.

Luck CA. Value of routine ultrasound screening at 19 weeks: a four year study of 8849 deliveries. BMJ 1992;304:1474–1478.

Malone FD, Athanassiou A, Craigo SD, et al. Cost issues surrounding the use of computerized telemedicine for obstetric ultrasonography. Ultrasound Obstet Gynecol 1998a;12:120–124.

Malone FD, Athanassiou A, Nores J, et al. Effect of ISDN bandwidth on image quality for telemedicine transmission of obstetric ultrasonography. Telemed J 1998b;4:161–165.

Malone FD, Nores JA, Athanassiou A, et al. Validation of fetal telemedicine as a new obstetric imaging technique. Am J Obstet Gynecol 1997;177:626–631.

Mansfield P, Stehling M, Ordidge R, et al. Echo planar imaging of the human fetus in utero at 0.5 T. Br J Radiol 1990;63:833–841.

McCarthy S, Filly R, Stark D, et al. Obstetric magnetic resonance imaging. Radiology 1985;154:427–432.

Metkus A, Filly R, Stinger M, et al. Sonographic predictors of survival in fetal diaphragmatic hernia. J Pediatr Surg 1996;31:148–152.

Morin L, Crombleholme TM, D'Alton M. Prenatal diagnosis and management of fetal thoracic lesions. Semin Perinatol 1994;18:228–253.

Newnham JP, Evans SF, Michael CA, et al. Effects of frequent ultrasound during pregnancy: a randomized controlled trial. Lancet 1993;342:887–891.

Nores J, Athanassiou A, Malone FD, et al. Technical dependability of obstetric ultrasound transmission via ISDN. Telemed J 1997a;3:191–195.

Nores J, Malone FD, Athanassiou A, et al. Validation of first-trimester telemedicine as an obstetric imaging technology: a feasibility study. Obstet Gynecol 1997b;90:353–356.

Ogle RF, Rodeck CH. Novel fetal imaging techniques. Curr Opin Obstet Gynecol 1998;10:109–115.

Quinn TM, Hubbard AM, Adzick NS. Prenatal magnetic resonance imaging enhances fetal diagnosis. J Pediatr Surg 1998;33:553–558.

Rosendahl H, Kivinen S. Antenatal detection of congenital malformations by routine ultrasonography. Obstet Gynecol 1989;73:947–951.

Rothschild M, Catalano P, Urben M, et al. Evaluation and management of congenital cervical teratoma: case report and review. Arch Otolaryngol Head Neck Surg 1994;120:444–448.

Royal College of Obstetricians and Gynaecologists. Ultrasound screening for fetal abnormalities: report of the RCOG working party. London: RCOG Press, October 1997.

Royal College of Obstetricians and Gynaecologists. The value of ultrasound in pregnancy: Royal College of Obstetricians and Gynaecologists Guidelines #4. London: RCOG Press, August 1994.

Saari-Kemppainen A, Karjalainen O, Ylostalo P, et al. Ultrasound screening and perinatal mortality: controlled trial of systematic one-stage screening in pregnancy. Lancet 1990;338:387–391.

Salvesen KA, Bakketeig LS, Eik-Nes SH, et al. Routine ultrasonography in utero and school performance at age 8–9 years. Lancet 1992;339:85–89.

Salvesen KA, Vatten LJ, Eik-Nes SH, et al. Routine ultrasonography in utero and subsequent handedness and neurological development. BMJ 1993;307:159–164.

Semelka R, Kelekis N, Thomasson D, et al. HASTE MR imaging: description of technique and preliminary results in the abdomen. J Magn Reson Imaging 1996;6:698–699.

Shaaban AF, Kim HB, Milner R, et al. The role of ultrasonography in fetal surgery and invasive fetal procedures. Semin Roentgenol 1999;34:62–79.

Shellock F, Kanal E. Policies guidelines and recommendations for MR imaging, safety, and patient management. J Magn Reson Imaging 1991;1:97–100.

Sherer P, Woods J, Abramowicz J, et al. Prenatal sonographic assessment of early, rapidly growing fetal cervical teratoma. Prental Diagn 1993;13:179–184.

Shirley IM, Bottomley F, Robinson VP. Routine radiographer screening for fetal abnormalities by ultrasound in an unselected low risk population. Br J Radiol 1992;65:565–569.

Stark CR, Orleans M, Haverkamp AD, et al. Short and long term risk after exposure to diagnostic ultrasound in utero. Obstet Gynecol 1984;63:194–200.

United States Department of Health and Human Services. Diagnostic ultrasound imaging in pregnancy. National Institutes of Health Consensus Statement, publication no. 84-667, Bethesda, MD, 5(1):1–16, February 1984.

Van Dorsten JP, Hulsey TC, Newman RB, et al. Fetal anomaly detection by second-trimester ultrasonography in a tertiary center. Am J Obstet Gynecol 1998;178:742–749.

Weinreb J, Lowe T, Santos-Ramos R, et al. Magnetic resonance imaging in human pregnancy. Radiology 1985;154:157–161.

Yamashita Y, Namimoto T, Abe Y, et al. MR imaging of the fetus by a HASTE sequence. AJR Am J Roentgenol 1997;168:513–519.

Zadvinskis D, Benson M, Kerr H, et al. Congenital malformations of the cervicothoracic lymphatic system: embryology and pathogenesis. Radiographers 1992;12:1175–1189.

CHAPTER 2

Prenatal Diagnostic Procedures

The overall objective of prenatal diagnostic procedures is to obtain genetic, biochemical, and physiologic information about the fetus. The techniques described in this chapter—amniocentesis, chorionic villus sampling, and percutaneous umbilical blood sampling (PUBS)—allow detection of an ever-expanding list of inherited conditions. Ideally, perinatal centers should have the technical expertise to perform all these procedures and to select the best procedure for each clinical situation. Of paramount importance is the ability to provide genetic counseling to patients about their various diagnostic options. These options and their risks and consequences should be communicated to patients in a nondirective, supportive way.

▶ AMNIOCENTESIS

Amniocentesis was first used during the 1880s for decompression of polyhydramnios (Lambl 1881; Schatz 199213). In 1930 placental localization was achieved after the intra-amniotic injection of contrast medium (Menees et al. 1930). Aburel (1937) described the termination of a pregnancy by the intra-amniotic injection of hypertonic saline. During the 1950s the role of amniocentesis and measurement of bilirubin concentrations in monitoring rhesus disease was reported (Bevis 1950; Walker 1957).

Amniocentesis for fetal chromosome analysis was also initiated in the 1950s. (The number of human chromosomes was not known until 1956.) The first reported application was for fetal sex determination (Fuchs and Riis, 1956). The feasibility of culturing and karyotyping amniotic fluid cells was demonstrated by Steele and Breg in 1966. The first prenatal diagnosis of an abnormal karyotype, a balanced translocation, was reported in 1967 by Jacobson and Barter. Trisomy 21 was first detected prenatally by Valenti et al. in 1968. During the same year the first diagnosis of the metabolic disorder galactosemia was reported by Nadler.

Indications

In the United States, it is considered standard practice to offer prenatal cytogenetic analysis to all women who will be 35 years of age or older at their expected time of delivery. The risk of numerical chromosomal abnormalities (aneuploidy) increases with advancing maternal age as a result of nondisjunction, which occurs during maternal meiosis. Age 35 is the cutoff because at this age the risk of miscarriage associated with amniocentesis is equal to the risk of a fetal chromosomal abnormality, approximately 1 in 200 (Hook 1983). The relationship between maternal age and the estimated risk of chromosomal abnormalities is shown in Table 2-1 (Hook 1981; Hook et al. 1983).

Amniocentesis or chorionic villus sampling is indicated when there is a need to obtain fetal material for cytogenetic, biochemical, or DNA studies. Increasingly, the DNA abnormalities responsible for the etiology of many disorders are being identified. A list of common genetic conditions for which DNA-based prenatal diagnosis is available is given in Table 2-2 (D'Alton 1994). Because this list changes frequently, it is best to check the most up-to-date data using the Internet. A free website, previously called Helix (http://www.genetest.org), is maintained by the University of Washington and funded by the National Library of Medicine, in which the currently available DNA tests and the laboratories that perform them are listed.

The established screening test for fetal open spina bifida (OSB) is measurement of maternal serum α-fetoprotein (MSAFP) levels followed by amniocentesis in patients with elevated results (UK Collaborative Study

▶ **TABLE 2-1.** RELATION BETWEEN MATERNAL AGE AND THE ESTIMATED RATE OF CHROMOSOMAL ABNORMALITIES*

Age	Risk of Down Syndrome	Risk of Chromosomal Abnormality
20	1/1667	1/526
25	1/1250	1/476
30	1/952	1/385
35	1/385	1/202
36	1/295	1/162
37	1/227	1/129
38	1/175	1/102
39	1/137	1/82
40	1/106	1/65
41	1/82	1/51
42	1/64	1/40
43	1/50	1/32
44	1/38	1/25
45	1/30	1/20
46	1/23	1/16
47	1/18	1/13
48	1/14	1/10
49	1/11	1/7

*Ages are at the expected time of delivery.
Data have been modified from Hook (1981) and Hook et al. (1983). Reprinted, with permission, from D'Alton ME, DeCherney AH. Prenatal diagnosis. N Engl J Med 1993;28:114–120.

▶ **TABLE 2-2.** LIST OF CONDITIONS AMENABLE TO DNA ANALYSIS

Disorder	Mode of Inheritance	Chromo- some
α_1-Antitrypsin deficiency	AR	14
α-Thalassemia	AR	16
Adult polycystic kidney disease (type 1)	AD	16
β-Thalassemia	AR	11
Congenital adrenal hyperplasia	AR	6
Cystic fibrosis	AR	7
DiGeorge syndrome	AD	22
Duchenne/Becker muscular dystrophy	XLR	X
Familial Alzheimer disease	AD	21
Familial hypercholesterolemia	AD	19
Familial polyposis coli	AD	5
Fragile X syndrome	XLR	X
Gardner syndrome	AD	5
Hemoglobin Sc	AR	11
Hemophilia A (factor IX deficiency)	XLR	X
Huntington disease	AD	4
Marfan syndrome	AD	15
Multiple endocrine neoplasia type I	AD	11
Multiple endocrine neoplasia type IIA	AD	10
Myotonic dystrophy	AD	19
Neurofibromatosis (type 1)	AD	17
Neurofibromatosis (type 2)	AD	22
Norrie disease	XLR	X
Ornithine transcarbamylase deficiency	XLR	X
Phenylketonuria	AR	12
Retinoblastoma	AD	13
Sickle cell anemia	AR	11
Spinal muscular atrophy	AR/AD	5
Tay–Sachs disease	AR	5
von Hippel–Lindau syndrome	AD	3
Wiskott–Aldrich syndrome	XLR	X

AR = autosomal recessive; AL = autosomal dominant; XLR = X-linked recessive.
Reprinted, with permission, from D'Alton ME. Prenatal diagnostic procedures. Part 1—Diagnosis and treatment of fetal disease. Semin Perinatol 1994;18:140–162.

1979). The ultrasound diagnosis of fetal OSB has been greatly enhanced by the recognition of associated abnormalities in the skull and brain. These abnormalities include cerebral ventriculomegaly, microcephaly, frontal bone scalloping (lemon sign), and obliteration of the cisterna magna with either an "absent" cerebellum or abnormal anterior curvature of the cerebellar hemispheres (banana sign) (see Chapter 19) (Nicolaides et al. 1986a). Van den Hof et al. (1990) have reported on the diagnosis of OSB in 130 fetuses among 1561 patients at high risk for fetal neural-tube defects who were referred for detailed ultrasound examination. The examinations revealed associated abnormalities of the skull and brain in 129 of the 130 fetuses with OSB. As a result of this evidence of the accuracy of ultrasound in the diagnosis of neural-tube defects, the need for amniocentesis in the evaluation of an elevated MSAFP has been questioned.

At centers adept at diagnosing OSB sonographically, amniocentesis can be reserved for patients with suspicious ultrasound findings or large MSAFP elevations despite a normal scan or when it is impossible to adequately visualize fetal anatomy. At such specialized centers, patients can be counseled that with a normal ultrasound examination, in which good views are obtained of the fetal head and spine, the risk of OSB can be reduced by up to 95%, and therefore patients may elect not to undergo amniocentesis if they so desire

(American College of Obstetricians and Gynecologists, 1996). Patients who are at increased risk for neural-tube defects (i.e., who have elevated MSAFP levels), who have a history of neural-tube defects, or who are taking antifolate medications should be referred to centers with ultrasonographers experienced in diagnostic ultrasound. If ultrasound examination demonstrates a normal spine, cranium, and cerebellum, the chance of an undetected spinal abnormality is low. Therefore, amniocentesis, with a procedure-related risk of up to 1%, is probably unnecessary. Some centers have calculated a revised risk of neural-tube defects on the basis of the MSAFP value and normal results on ultrasound examination at their particular center (Nadel et al. 1990; Richards et al. 1988). For example, in our reference laboratory in a white patient with an a priori risk for OSB of 1 in 1000, an MSAFP of 2.8 multiples of the median (MOM) gives a risk of 1 in 170. When an adequate ultrasound examination is performed by competent ultrasonographers and is interpreted as a normal scan, this risk may be reduced by 95%, giving a reassigned risk of approximately 1 in 3400. In our center, amniocentesis is reserved for cases in which there is incomplete visualization of the fetus (as a result of maternal obesity or fetal position), serum levels of MSAFP greater than 3.5 MOM in the presence of normal sonographic examination, or suspicious ultrasound findings.

The combined use of the maternal serum human chorionic gonadotropin level, unconjugated estriol level, α-fetoprotein (AFP) level, and maternal age can identify 60% of cases of Down syndrome, with a false positive rate of 6.6% (Haddow et al. 1992). Individual estimates of patient risk are used, and amniocentesis is usually offered when the risk is greater than 1 in 270. Addition of a fourth serum marker, Inhibin-A, to this triple-marker screening test may improve the Down syndrome detection rate to 77 to 80%, with a 5 to 7% false-positive rate (Wald et al, 1997). It is now considered the standard of care to offer some form of second trimester multiple marker serum screening for Down syndrome to patients who are less than 35 years of age (American College of Obstetricians and Gynecologists, 1996).

Assessment of the severity of Rh disease and the need for fetal blood transfusion or early delivery has traditionally been based on the results of amniocentesis and the interpretation of the results of spectrophotometric estimation of amniotic fluid bilirubin (Liley 1961). In the assessment of severe Rh sensitization in midtrimester, the only accurate method for predicting the severity of the disease is measurement of the hemoglobin concentration in samples obtained by Nicolaides et al. (1986a; 1986b; 1988). (See section on "Percutaneous Umbilical Blood Sampling.")

Premature delivery is one of the leading causes of perinatal death and long-term handicap. The association between intrauterine infection and premature labor, in the presence and absence of ruptured membranes, has stimulated research into amniocentesis for the diagnosis of subclinical intrauterine infection (Romero et al. 1989). Currently, amniocentesis in the clinical management of preterm labor or preterm rupture of membranes (PROM) is reserved for cases in which there is a suspicion of intrauterine infection.

Measurement of the amniotic fluid lecithin : sphingomyelin ratio (Gluck et al. 1974) and phosphatidylglycerol (Hallman et al. 1976) level is useful for the assessment of fetal lung maturity. However, the need for these tests has declined because of improved neonatal care and the introduction of better methods of ultrasound assessment of gestational age and fetal surveillance. Elective preterm delivery should not be performed without a significant maternal or fetal indication, and therefore assessment of fetal lung maturity adds little to the decision-making process in the vast majority of cases.

Technique

Early attempts at genetic amniocentesis were made transvaginally. Subsequently, the transabdominal approach has been adopted. During the 1960s amniocentesis was performed "blindly." During the 1970s and early 1980s, ultrasonography was used to identify a placenta-free area for entry into a pocket of amniotic fluid. This position was marked on the maternal abdomen, and after a variable length of time, the operator would blindly insert the needle.

In most centers amniocentesis is now performed with continuous ultrasound guidance. An ultrasound scan is first performed to determine the number of fetuses present, to confirm gestational age and fetal viability, and to document normal anatomy. The maternal abdomen is washed with antiseptic solution; it is unnecessary for the technician to scrub and gown. Continuously guided by ultrasound, a 22-gauge needle is introduced into the amniotic cavity (Fig. 2-1). Ultrasound examination may

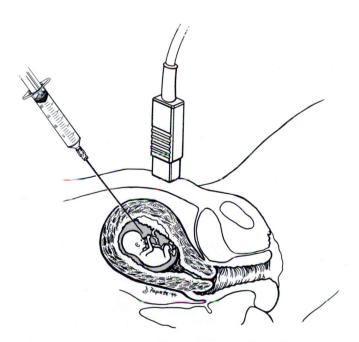

Figure 2-1. Diagrammatic representation of amniocentesis. *(Reprinted, with permission, from D'Alton ME. Prenatal diagnostic procedures. Part 1—Diagnosis and treatment of fetal disease. Semin Perinatol 1994;18: 140–162.)*

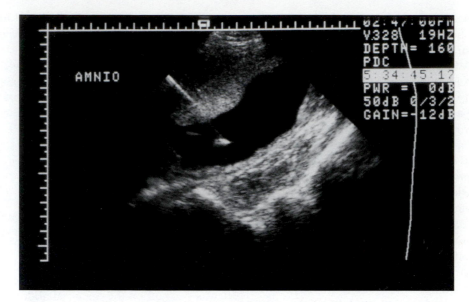

Figure 2-2. Ultrasound image of amniocentesis. See color plate.

be performed with sector or linear-array transducers, and the procedure may be performed either free-hand or with needle guides (Lenke et al. 1985; Jeanty et al. 1983). In our centers, the free-hand technique is preferred because it allows freer manipulation of the needle if the position of the target is abruptly altered by a uterine contraction or fetal movement (Fig. 2-2.) Furthermore, this technique can be easily adapted to all ultrasound-guided diagnostic or therapeutic procedures, such as PUBS and thoracocentesis. Fetal heart rate and activity is documented immediately following the procedure.

Technique in Twins

Amniocentesis in a twin pregnancy involves puncture of the first sac, withdrawal of amniotic fluid, injection of a dye, and then a new needle insertion to puncture the second sac (Elias et al. 1980; Filkins and Russo, 1984). If the fluid aspirated after the second puncture is clear, then the operator knows it does not come from the first sac, which was injected with dye (Fig. 2-3). Indigo carmine is used as an injection dye. Methylene blue should *never* be used because of its association with fetal hemolytic anemia, small intestinal atresia, and fetal demise (Malone and D'Alton, 1999).

A single-puncture method has been described in which the site of needle insertion is determined mainly by the position of the membrane separating the two sacs (Jeanty et al. 1990). After entry into the first sac and aspiration of amniotic fluid, the needle is advanced through the dividing membrane into the second sac. In order to avoid contamination of the second sample with the amniotic fluid from the first sac, the first 1 ml of fluid from the second sample is discarded. We do not

approve of this method, because it could cause iatrogenic rupture of the dividing membrane, creating a monoamniotic sac with an attendant risk of cord entanglement.

Bahado-Singh and colleagues (1992) described a technique of amniocentesis in twins that entails identi-

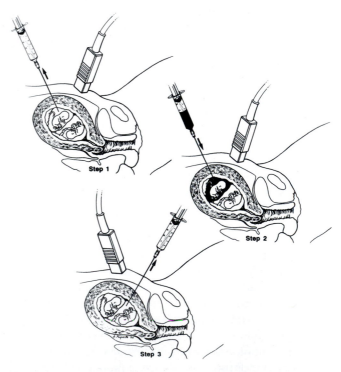

Figure 2-3. Diagrammatic representation of one method of performing amniocentesis in twins. In Step 1, the fluid is aspirated from the first amniotic sac. In Step 2, indigo carmine is injected into the first sac. In Step 3, clear fluid is aspirated from the second sac.

fying the separating membranes with a curvilinear or linear transducer. The first needle and transducer are left in place during the insertion of the second needle. Beekhuis and associates (1992) described another technique that used maternal hemoglobin as a dye marker to differentiate between two sacs. Methylene blue is not recommended as a dye because it has been reported to cause hemolytic anemia or methemoglobinemia (Cowett et al. 1976). An association between fetal intestinal atresia and the use of methylene blue dye for amniocentesis in twins has been reported (Nicolini and Monni 1990; Van der Pol et al. 1992). This association has not been demonstrated with indigo carmine (Cragan et al. 1993).

Fluorescence in Situ Hybridization (FISH)

FISH permits determination of the number and location of specific DNA sequences in human cells, both in interphase nuclei and directly on metaphase chromosomes. The FISH procedure relies on the complementarity between the two strands of the DNA double helix. Probe DNA molecules are nonisotopically labeled by incorporation of a chemically modified nucleotide that is subsequently detected with a fluorescently tagged reporter molecule.

This technology detects aneuploidies caused by monosomies, free trisomies, trisomies associated with robertsonian translocations, triploidy, and other numerical chromosomal abnormalities involving chromosomes 13, 18, 21, X, and Y. The technology was not designed to detect other cytogenetic abnormalities such as mosaicism, translocations, or rare aneuploidies (Ward et al. 1993; Klinger et al. 1992).

Ward et al. (1993) described the first large-scale application of interphase FISH for prenatal diagnosis. FISH was performed on physician request as an adjunct to cytogenetics in 4500 patients. Region-specific DNA probes to chromosomes 13, 18, 21, X, and Y were used to determine ploidy by analysis of signal number in hybridized nuclei. A sample was considered to be euploid when all autosomal probes generated two hybridization signals and when a normal sex chromosome pattern was observed in greater than or equal to 80% of hybridized nuclei. A sample was considered to be aneuploid when greater than or equal to 70% of hybridized nuclei displayed the same abnormal hybridization pattern for a specific probe. Of the attempted analyses, 90% met these criteria and were reported as "informative" to the referring physicians within 48 hours.

The overall detection rate for aneuploidy was 73% (107 of 146). The accuracy rate for informative results for aneuploidies was 93.9% (107 of 114). There were no false positives and seven false negative autosomal aneuploidies. One false positive sex chromosome aneu-

ploidy has been reported (Benn et al. 1992; Ward et al. 1992). The strict reporting criteria used to define and report samples as abnormal led to a lower detection rate of 73% for all aneuploidies. Ward and colleagues are now reevaluating these criteria; for example, if the criteria for reporting a sample as abnormal was changed to include all samples in which greater than 50% of hybridized nuclei were trisomic, the aneuploidy detection rate would improve to 82.9% (107 + 14, of 146). This change in the reporting criteria would have enhanced the detection rate without altering the false positive or false negative rates. In Ward et al.'s study for informative specimens the sensitivity for identification of autosomal trisomy was 92.6%. This was less than anticipated on the basis of initial investigations by Klinger et al. (1992) and Lebo et al. (1992). Undetected contamination of maternal cells, increased background fluorescence as a result of excessive cellular debris, and autofluorescence of the microscope lens contributed to the observed false negative results, thereby decreasing the sensitivity.

The question of which populations should be studied with FISH is debatable. Ward et al. provided the procedure to all patients who requested it. Further study by Strovel et al. (1992) suggested that only cells from patients whose risk of aneuploidy is 1% or greater (on the basis of maternal age, maternal serum findings, or ultrasonographic findings) should be analyzed. Retrospective analyses of 750 consecutive amniotic fluid samples obtained in their laboratory revealed that only 168, or 22%, of these cases had a risk of 1% or greater of being aneuploid. If FISH had only been performed on those 168 cases, 14 aneuploidies would have been detected, whereas only 5 additional abnormalities would have been found in the other 582 cases. Therefore, if the overall goal is to employ interphase FISH as an adjunctive procedure, then a directed analysis optimizing its application by limiting the number of patients studied would yield the highest frequency of abnormalities.

FISH may be useful for rapid confirmation of potential numerical chromosomal aneuploidies when ultrasound examination reveals fetal abnormalities and may be an alternative to PUBS or placental biopsy (D'Alton et al. 1997).

Potential disadvantages of FISH include maternal anxiety after an uninformative result and the negative effect of receiving a disomic FISH result followed by the identification of a chromosome lesion not identified by the initial protocol (Ward et al. 1993). At present there is a lack of laboratories availing themselves of this technology. In order for any technology to gain widespread acceptance, studies must be performed by multiple laboratories to validate its methods and conclusions. Until the method has been used and established in several laboratories, it is not advisable to base pregnancy-management decisions on FISH results alone. FISH clearly cannot yet be used as a totally independent procedure. Aneuploidies will account for only 50 to 70% of all abnormalities detected by standard cytogenetics. It is uncertain what information should be transmitted to the referring physician. The best use of the information is to prioritize existing cases suspected to be abnormal and at most to provide preliminary results. All interphase FISH results must be followed by classical cytogenetic studies. Some authors think that since the information obtained from the interphase FISH studies should not be used for pregnancy management and should only be used in conjunction with classical cytogenetic studies that the patient should not be asked to pay for the test (Schwartz et al. 1993).

Laboratory Considerations

Failure to culture amniocytes occurs in less than 1% of cases. Chromosomal mosaicism occurs in approximately 0.5% of cases. Chromosomal mosaicism is the presence of two or more cell lines with different karyotypes in a single person. This occurs as a result of postzygotic nondisjunction. The observation of multiple cell lines in a prenatal sample does not necessarily mean that the fetus has mosaicism. The most common type of mosaicism detected by amniocentesis is pseudomosaicism (Hsu and Perlis 1984). This phenomenon should be suspected when an abnormality is evident in only one of several cultures of an amniotic fluid specimen. The abnormal cell lines arise during in vitro division; therefore, they are not present in the fetus and are not clinically important. Contamination by maternal cells can be minimized by discarding the first few drops of aspirated amniotic fluid. True fetal mosaicism, diagnosed when the same abnormality is present on more than one cover slip, is rare (0.25%) but clinically important (Hsu and Perlis 1984). The question of whether true mosaicism is present is best resolved by karyotyping fetal lymphocytes obtained on PUBS (Gosden et al. 1988), a method that provides results within 48 hours. Detailed ultrasound examination is also recommended to assess fetal growth and exclude the diagnosis of structural anomalies. If both ultrasound and fetal blood sampling results are normal, the parents can be reassured that the major chromosomal abnormalities have been excluded (Gosden et al. 1988).

More than 100 abnormalities of lipid, mucopolysaccharide, amino acid, and carbohydrate metabolism are amenable to prenatal diagnosis from the study of cultured amniotic fluid cells. However, the substantially larger amount of tissue obtained by chorionic villus sampling (CVS) than by amniocentesis makes CVS the preferred method of diagnosing this group of disorders.

Complications

Fortunately, serious maternal complications such as septic shock are rare in amniocentesis. Amnionitis occurs in 0.1% of cases (Turnbull and Mackenzie 1983).

The development of rhesus isoimmunization (Golbus et al. 1979; Hill et al. 1980) can be avoided by prophylactic administration of anti-D immunoglobulin to Rh-negative women who are about to undergo amniocentesis. Amniotic fluid leak or vaginal blood loss, noted after amniocentesis by 2 to 3% of patients, is usually self limiting, although occasionally leakage of amniotic fluid persists throughout pregnancy (NICHD Amniocentesis Registry 1976; Simpson et al. 1981). Common occurrences are cramping for 1 to 2 hours and lower abdominal discomfort for up to 48 hours after the procedure.

The safety and accuracy of amniocentesis in midtrimester was documented in the mid-1970s by three collaborative studies performed in the United Kingdom, United States, and Canada (Medical Research Council 1977; Working Party on Amniocentesis 1978; NICHD Amniocentesis Registry 1976). However, the only prospective, randomized, controlled trial is a study by Tabor and colleagues (1986), who reported on 4606 low-risk, healthy women. The women, 25 to 34 years old, were randomly allocated to a group that would have amniocentesis or to one that would have ultrasound examination. In this study, the total rate of fetal loss in the patients who underwent amniocentesis was 1.7% and in the control patients 0.7% ($P < 0.01$). The conclusions of this study were initially criticized because an 18-gauge needle (which is associated with higher risks than smaller needles) was used. Tabor et al. (1988) subsequently reported that they had been mistaken in citing the use of an 18-gauge needle and had, in fact, used a 20-gauge needle for most of the procedures. The Danish study also demonstrated that there were significant associations between pregnancy loss and puncture of the placenta, high MSAFP levels, and discolored amniotic fluid (Tabor et al. 1986).

Both the U.K. and Danish studies (Working Party on Amniocentesis 1978; Tabor et al. 1986) found an increase in respiratory distress syndrome and pneumonia in neonates from the amniocentesis groups. Other studies have not found this association. The U.K. study showed an increased incidence of talipes and dislocation of the hip in the amniocentesis group (Working Party on Amniocentesis 1978). More recently, a Danish study on early amniocentesis demonstrated an increased incidence of club foot related to this procedure (Sundberg et al. 1997).

Needle puncture of the fetus, reported in 0.1 to 3.0% of cases (Karp and Hayden 1977; NICHD Amniocentesis Registry 1976), has been suggested as the cause of exsanguination (Young et al. 1977), intestinal atresia

(Therkelsen and Rehder 1981; Swift et al. 1979), ileo-cutaneous fistula (Rickwood 1977), gangrene of a fetal limb (Lamb 1975), uniocular blindness (Merin and Beyth, 1980), porencephalic cysts (Youroukos et al. 1980), patellar-tendon disruption (Epley et al. 1979), skin dimples (Broome et al. 1976), and peripheral-nerve damage (Karp and Hayden 1977). Continuous use of ultrasound to guide the needle minimizes needle puncture of the fetus. Finegan et al. (1990) have reported an increased incidence of middle-ear abnormalities in children whose mothers underwent amniocentesis.

Complications in Multiple Gestation

Results at a single center with 339 mothers with multiple-gestation pregnancies who underwent prenatal diagnosis by amniocentesis revealed a spontaneous abortion rate (up to 28 weeks of gestation) of 3.57%, as compared with an abortion rate of 0.60% in singleton pregnancies (Anderson et al. 1991). It is unclear how much of this increased risk is due to the normal rate of spontaneous abortion in multiple-gestation pregnancies. Unfortunately, there are no reliable data for the spontaneous loss rate in multiple-gestation pregnancies from 16 to 28 weeks of gestation. Coleman et al. (1987) reported a spontaneous abortion rate of 5% in gestations in which twins were detected at 20.5 weeks. Mothers pregnant with twins must also be counseled about the increased risk of having a karyotypically abnormal child. Several reports have noted an increase in chromosomal abnormalities in fetuses in multiple-gestation pregnancies (Lubs and Ruddle 1970; Milunsky 1979). Amniocentesis in twins does raise some very painful questions. Families need first to consider the possibility of a test that will show that one of their twins is normal and the other abnormal.

Early Amniocentesis (EA)

As the technique of mid-trimester amniocentesis gained rapid acceptance, much interest developed in the use of the same diagnostic technique at earlier gestational ages. The term "early amniocentesis" was used to describe the performance of amniocentesis at less than 14 weeks gestation. An assumption was made that since amniocentesis was shown to be a safe and effective procedure in the second trimester of pregnancy, it would be equally safe and effective during the first trimester. However, with the completion of the CEMAT study (Canadian Early and Mid Trimester Amniocentesis Trial) in 1998, it has become clear that early amniocentesis from 11 weeks to 12 weeks 6 days is associated with significant disadvantages (CEMAT Group, 1998).

In the CEMAT study, 4,374 patients were randomized to either early amniocentesis (defined as amniocentesis from 11 weeks to 12 weeks 6 days) or mid-trimester amniocentesis (defined as amniocentesis from 15 weeks to 16 weeks 6 days). It was found that early amniocentesis was significantly more likely to be a technically difficult or unsuccessful procedure when compared with mid-trimester amniocentesis (1.6% versus 0.4%), and it was twice as likely that early amniocentesis would require more than one needle insertion (Johnson et al. 1999). In addition, it was found that early amniocentesis was significantly more likely to result in karyotype culture failure (2.4%) when compared with mid-trimester amniocentesis (0.25%) (Winsor et al. 1999).

The CEMAT investigators also demonstrated significant safety concerns with the early amniocentesis technique. There was a significantly higher rate of total pregnancy losses in the early amniocentesis group (7.6%) versus the mid-trimester group (5.9%) (CEMAT Group, 1998). Also of concern was a significantly higher rate of clubfoot in the early amniocentesis group (1.3%) versus the mid-trimester group (0.1%). Early amniocentesis was also associated with a significantly higher chance of post-procedural amniotic fluid leakage (3.5%) when compared with mid-trimester amniocentesis (1.7%). While it is possible that early amniocentesis between 13 weeks and 14 weeks may be safe, there are no data to counsel patients on the risks of this procedure in this gestational age period. The CEMAT study effectively ends the controversy on the role of early amniocentesis, and suggests that this technique should generally be avoided. If, however, an individual patient desires early amniocentesis, it should only be performed after thorough counseling of the patient about the risks and possible alternatives.

Summary

Indications for amniocentesis have changed considerably over the years and are likely to evolve even further. The most common indication for amniocentesis is to obtain a fetal karyotype in women who will be 35 or more years of age at the time of delivery. The use of amniocentesis in the investigation of elevated MSAFP is declining. Maternal serum triple-panel biochemical screening of chromosomal defects is likely to become a routine antenatal test that may increase the number of second-trimester amniocenteses performed. For the assessment of fetal anemia in severe red-cell isoimmunized pregnancies in the second trimester, amniocentesis is likely to be replaced by PUBS. The use of amniocentesis to test for fetal-lung maturity is likely to continue to decrease as ultrasound dating of pregnancy is now performed in many cases, and premature deliveries are performed only if there are maternal or fetal indications.

► CHORIONIC VILLUS SAMPLING (CVS)

With conventional amniocentesis, results of the karyo-type are received midway through the second trimester. This is a drawback because of the medical risks of performing a dilation-and-evacuation procedure late in the pregnancy. Furthermore, this delay inflicts a severe emotional burden on the patient, especially after experiencing fetal movements. Using chorionic villi as a source for fetal karyotyping during the 10th week of pregnancy was introduced experimentally by Hahnemann and Mohr in 1969, and the use of an endoscopic transvaginal approach was evaluated by Hahnemann in 1974. Clinical use of chorionic villi for fetal sex determination was described in 1975 by a Chinese group performing blind transvaginal aspiration without ultrasound examination (Tietung Hospital 1975). However, CVS became accepted for more widespread use when an ultrasound-guided technique for aspiration was introduced.

Transcervical

Ultrasound examination immediately before the procedure confirms fetal heart activity, appropriate growth, and location of the placenta (Fig. 2-4). The position of the uterus and cervix is determined, and the anticipated catheter path is mentally mapped. If the uterus

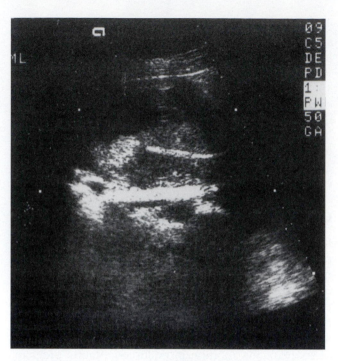

Figure 2-5. Ultrasound image of transcervical chorionic villus sampling demonstrating the catheter in a posterior placenta. *(Reprinted, with permission, from D'Alton ME. Prenatal diagnostic procedures. Part 1—Diagnosis and treatment of fetal disease. Semin Perinatol 1994;18:140–162.)*

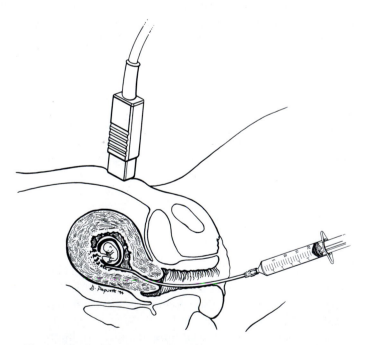

Figure 2-4. Diagrammatic representation of transcervical chorionic villus sampling. *(Reprinted, with permission, from D'Alton ME. Prenatal diagnostic procedures. Part 1—Diagnosis and treatment of fetal disease. Semin Perinatol 1994;18:140–162.)*

is severely anteverted, filling of the bladder frequently straightens its position. If a uterine contraction occurs it could interfere with passage of the catheter, and a decision may be made to delay the procedure until the contraction dissipates. When the uterine condition and location are favorable, the patient is placed in the lithotomy position; and the vulva, vagina, and cervix are aseptically prepared with povidone-iodine. A speculum is inserted, and the anterior lip of the cervix is grasped with a tenaculum to aid in manipulating the uterus. The distal 3 to 5 cm of the catheter is molded into a slightly curved shape and then gently passed through the cervix until a loss of resistance is felt at the endocervix. The operator then waits until the ultrasonographer visualizes the tip of the catheter.

The catheter is inserted parallel to the placenta and passed almost to its distal end (Fig. 2-5). The stylet is then removed and a 20-ml heparinized syringe containing nutrient medium is attached. The syringe is used to apply negative pressure. The catheter and attached syringe are then pulled back slowly, and the syringe is visually inspected for villi, which are easily seen with the naked eye as white branching structures. Once an adequate sample is obtained, the patient is discharged; she is told to contact her physician if she develops heavy bleeding, fever, or unusual vaginal discharge. A follow-up scan and MSAFP assay are performed at 16 weeks of gestation.

Transabdominal

Continuous ultrasound is used to direct a 19- or 20-gauge spinal needle into the long axis of the placenta (Fig. 2-6). After removal of the stylet, villi are aspirated into a 20-ml syringe containing tissue-culture mediums. Unlike transcervical CVS, transabdominal CVS can be performed throughout pregnancy. It therefore constitutes an alternative to amniocentesis or PUBS if karyotype evaluation is needed later in pregnancy. If oligohydramnios is present, transabdominal CVS may be the only approach available to determine fetal karyotype.

Multiple Gestations

Twin and triplet pregnancies have been sampled successfully using CVS, but there are problems inherent with the technique (Brambati et al. 1991b; Pergament et al. 1992). You must be certain that distinct placental sites are identified and sampled individually. When there is any suspicion that two separate samples of placenta are not obtained, a backup amniocentesis should be offered if the fetal genders are concordant (Brambati et al. 1991b).

Another potential difficulty of performing CVS in multiple gestations is the possible cross-contamination of samples. This potential exists when the placentas are

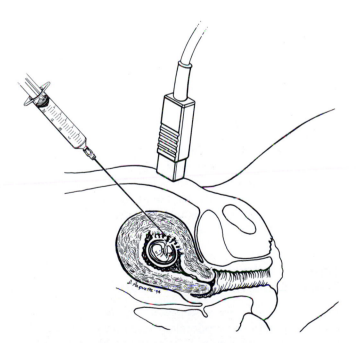

Figure 2-6. Diagrammatic representation of transabdominal chorionic villus sampling. *(Reprinted, with permission, from D'Alton ME. Prenatal diagnostic procedures. Part 1—Diagnosis and treatment of fetal disease. Semin Perinatol 1994;18:140–162.)*

on the same uterine wall (i.e., both anterior or both posterior). In these cases, sampling the lower sac transcervically and the upper sac transabdominally minimizes the chance of contamination. When a biochemical diagnosis is required, the potential for misinterpretation is even greater because a small amount of normal tissue could significantly alter the results. Therefore, unless individual samples can be guaranteed, amniocentesis should be performed.

A detailed drawing of the locations of each placenta and fetus should be made at the time of the procedure. In the case of one abnormal result, this diagram will permit later identification of the affected fetus.

Laboratory Aspects

The average sample from a transcervical aspiration contains 15 to 30 mg of villous material. The villi identified in the syringe are carefully and aseptically transferred for confirmatory inspection and dissection under a microscope. Determining that this is the appropriate tissue is mandatory to minimize maternal decidual contamination. Clean, decidua-free villi are then transferred to Petri dishes for further preparation. Villi are processed for cytogenetic analysis in two ways: Results of direct preparation are available within 3 to 4 days of the procedure; results of tissue culture are usually available within 6 to 8 days. Most laboratories wait to report both results at the same time.

It is recommended that both the direct and culture methods be used with all samples. The direct method gives rapid results on the cytotrophoblast and minimizes maternal decidual contamination. Tissue culture, which is subject to potential contamination from maternal cells, is a better means of identifying and evaluating discrepancies that may exist between the cytotrophoblast and the fetal state (Bianchi et al. 1993).

Any biochemical diagnosis that can be made from amniotic fluid or cultured amniocytes can also be made from chorionic villi (Poenaru 1987). In many cases the results are available more rapidly and efficiently when villi are used, because enzymes are present in sufficient quantity to allow direct analysis rather than requiring the products of tissue culture.

Pregnancy Loss Following CVS

The advantage of earlier diagnosis must be weighed against any increased risk of fetal loss presented by CVS. For statistical purposes, procedure-related spontaneous abortion has generally been defined as spontaneous miscarriage or diagnosed intrauterine fetal death occurring up until 28 completed weeks of gestation. Calculating such procedure-related losses is complicated by background pregnancy loss rates, since 2 to 5% of pregnancies viable at 7 to 12 weeks of gestation are either nonviable when rescanned at 8 to 20 weeks or will

▶ **TABLE 2-3.** TOTAL PREGNANCY LOSS RATES OF CHORIONIC VILLUS SAMPLING (CVS) AND AMNIOCENTESIS (AC) IN THREE COLLABORATIVE TRIALS

Study	Eligible or Attempted (no.)		Total Loss Rate (%)		CVS Excess Loss Rate (%)
	CVS	AC	CVS	AC	
Canadian Collaborative CVS-Amniocentesis Clinical Trial Group (1989)	1191	1200	7.6	7.0	0.6
Rhoads et al. (1989)	2235	651	7.2	5.7	0.8*
MRC Working Party (1991)	1609	1592	13.6	9.0	4.6

*Corrected for difference in maternal age and gestational age.
Reprinted, with permission, from D'Alton ME. Prenatal diagnostic procedures. Part 1—Diagnosis and treatment of fetal disease. Semin Perinatol 1994;18:140–162.

undergo spontaneous miscarriage before 28 weeks of gestation (Gilmore and McNay 1985; Liu et al. 1987; Wilson et al. 1984). The background rate of spontaneous loss increases with maternal age and is therefore highest in the same age range in which women are likely to present for prenatal diagnosis (Gilmore and McNay 1985; Wilson et al. 1984).

Data evaluating the safety of CVS come primarily from three collaborative reports (Table 2-3). In 1989, the Canadian Collaborative CVS/Amniocentesis Clinical Trial Group reported its experience with a prospective randomized trial comparing the safety of CVS to that of amniocentesis. During the study period, patients across Canada were able to undergo CVS only in conjunction with the randomized protocol. The results of the Canadian group confirmed the safety of CVS as a first-trimester diagnostic procedure. There was a 7.6% rate of fetal loss (spontaneous abortions, induced abortions, and late losses) in the CVS group, and a 7.0% rate of loss in the amniocentesis group. An excess rate of loss of 0.6% for CVS over amniocentesis was found, a difference that was not statistically significant. Surprisingly, there was a tendency toward later losses (>28 weeks) in the CVS group. No significant differences were noted between the two groups in the incidence of preterm birth or low birth weight. Maternal complications were equally uncommon in each group.

The U.S. report involved a prospective, though nonrandomized, trial of 2235 women who chose either transcervical CVS or second-trimester amniocentesis (Rhoads et al. 1989). An excess rate of loss of 0.8% in the CVS group over the amniocentesis group was calculated, which was not statistically significant. The rates of loss were lowest in cases in which relatively large amounts of tissue were obtained. Repeated catheter insertions were significantly associated with pregnancy loss. Cases requiring three or more catheter insertions had a 10.8% rate of spontaneous abortion, as compared with a rate of 2.9% in cases that required only one pass.

A prospective, randomized, collaborative comparison of more than 3200 pregnancies, sponsored by the European Medical Research Council, demonstrated that CVS may cause a 4.6% greater rate of pregnancy loss than amniocentesis (95% confidence interval, 1.6 to 7.5%) (MRC Working Party 1991). This difference reflected more spontaneous deaths before 28 weeks of gestation (2.9%), more termination of pregnancy for chromosomal anomalies (1.0%), and more neonatal deaths (0.3%). In this study, villus sampling was performed by both the transcervical and transabdominal routes. The number of repeat procedures was significantly higher in the CVS group as compared with the amniocentesis group.

Exactly what factors contribute to the discrepant results between the European and North American studies remains uncertain. Variability in operator experience might account for part of this discrepancy. The U.S. trial included 7 centers and the Canadian trial 11. In the Medical Research Council Trial there were 31 participating centers contributing various numbers of cases and using different sampling and cytogenetic procedures. There were, on average, 325 cases per center in the U.S. study, 106 in the Canadian study, and only 52 in the European trial. The pregnancy losses in the European series tended to occur before 20 weeks of gestation, as compared with the Canadian study, in which losses occurred significantly later. There is no apparent explanation for these findings.

Transcervical versus Transabdominal Approach

Brambati et al. (1991a) reported the results of a randomized trial of transabdominal versus transcervical CVS by a single operator in 1194 patients. Over 110 cases deviated from the allocated procedure, and more than 80% of the deviations occurred in the transcervical arm of the trial. Moreover, the proportion of cases in which the operator chose to deviate from the allocated procedure increased in each of the 3 years of the study (4.6%, 9.7%, and 15.5%, respectively). More chorionic tissue was obtained by the transcervical method, but the proportion of cases in which less than 10 mg was obtained was similar in both groups. Bleeding was more common following transcervical CVS, whereas cramping was more common with the transabdominal approach. No significant difference was detected in the overall rate of fetal loss (transabdominal approach, 16.5%; transcervical, 15.5%). The transabdominal technique required a significantly smaller proportion of repeat needle insertions (3.3% versus 0.3%), although this did not seem to affect pregnancy outcome. There were also no differences in birth weight, gestational age at delivery, or congenital malformations. The authors commented that a limitation of this study was the operator's eventual preference for the transabdominal approach. They conclude that the two techniques seem equally safe and effective, and the choice to perform one particular technique may depend largely on the operator's preference.

Jackson et al. (1992) conducted a randomized comparison of transcervical and transabdominal CVS at 7 to 12 weeks of gestation. Of 3999 eligible patients, 94% in each arm of the study underwent the allocated procedure. Only one needle insertion was required in 94% of transabdominal CVS cases, and one catheter pass was required in 90% of transcervical CVS procedures. The rate of fetal loss, excluding elective terminations of pregnancy, was 3% in each group.

Smidt-Jensen et al. (1992) published their randomized comparison of routine amniocentesis, transabdominal CVS, and transcervical CVS in 3706 low-risk patients. Patients were randomly assigned to one of the three procedures. The proportion of patients for whom a cytogenetic diagnosis was successfully obtained at the first attempt was 99.7% for amniocentesis, 98.1% for transabdominal CVS, and 96.0% for transcervical CVS ($P < 0.0001$). Total rates of fetal loss were 10.9% for transcervical CVS, 6.3% for transabdominal CVS, and 6.4% for amniocentesis, a statistically significant difference. A large difference was noted between the transabdominal and transcervical CVS groups in the proportion of postprocedural losses of cytogenically normal pregnancies (3.7% for transabdominal and 7.7% for transcervical CVS). The authors conclude that although transabdominal CVS and amniocentesis carry similar risks of fetal loss, transcervical CVS is associated with an overall higher rate of fetal loss, estimated to be in excess of 4.0%.

It is reasonable to speculate that the rate of fetal loss will equilibrate in most centers once equivalent expertise is gained with either approach (Brambati et al. 1987b). It is reasonable to conclude that integration of both transcervical and transabdominal methods of CVS into any program offers the most practical and safe approach to first-trimester diagnosis.

Other Complications

Vaginal bleeding or spotting is relatively uncommon after transabdominal CVS procedures, occurring in 1% or less of cases (Rhoads et al. 1989). Most centers report postprocedure bleeding in 7 to 10% of patients sampled by transcervical CVS (Rhoads et al. 1989). Minimal spotting is more common than bleeding and may occur in almost one third of women sampled by the transcervical route (Rhoads et al. 1989). A subchorionic hematoma may be visualized immediately after sampling in up to 4% of patients sampled transcervically (Brambati et al. 1987b). The hematoma usually disappears before the 16th week of pregnancy and is usually not associated with an adverse outcome.

Since the initial development of transcervical CVS there has been concern that transvaginal passage of an instrument would introduce vaginal flora into the uterus, thereby increasing the risk of infection. Cultures have isolated bacteria in 30% of catheters used for CVS (Brambati and Varotto 1985; Brambati et al. 1987a; Garden et al. 1985; McFadyen et al. 1985; Wass and Bennett 1985). The reported incidence of post-CVS chorioamnionitis, however, is low; it occurs following both transcervical and transabdominal procedures. In the U.S. collaborative trial, infection was suspected as a possible cause of pregnancy loss in only 0.3% of cases (Rhoads et al. 1989). It has been demonstrated that, at least in some cases, infection that occurs after transabdominal CVS is a result of bowel flora introduced by inadvertent puncture by the sampling needle. Early in the development of transcervical CVS, two life-threatening pelvic infections were reported (Barela et al. 1986; Blakemore et al. 1985). A practice of using a new sterile catheter for each insertion has subsequently been universally adopted, and there have been no additional reports of serious infections resulting from the procedure.

Acute rupture of membranes within hours of the procedure can occur but is rare (Rhoads et al. 1989); in 0.3% of cases, rupture has been reported days to weeks after the procedure (Hogge et al. 1986).

An acute rise in MSAFP levels after CVS has been consistently reported, implying a detectable degree of fetomaternal bleeding (Blakemore et al. 1986; Brambati et al. 1986; Shulman et al. 1990). The elevation in MSAFP levels is not related to the technique used to retrieve villi but seems to depend on the quantity of tissue aspirated (Shulman et al. 1990). Levels will return to normal ranges by 16 to 18 weeks of gestation, thus allowing serum screening to proceed according to usual prenatal protocols. All Rh-negative, nonsensitized women who are undergoing CVS should receive $Rh_o(D)$ immune globulin after the procedure. Exacerbation of Rh immunization following CVS has been described. Existing Rh sensitization therefore represents a contraindication to the procedure (Moise and Carpenter 1990).

Risk of Fetal Abnormality

Concern has been raised that CVS might cause severe limb deficiencies. This was first reported by Firth et al. (1991). Their series of 289 CVS pregnancies identified five infants with severe limb abnormalities. Oromandibular-limb hypogenesis syndrome was present in four of the five, and the fifth had a terminal transverse limb-reduction defect. The oromandibular-limb hypogenesis syndrome occurs in 1 of 175,000 live births (Hoyme et al. 1982); therefore, the occurrence of this abnormality in more than 1% of pregnancies in which CVS was performed strongly suggested an association. In Firth's initial report, all the limb abnormalities followed transabdominal sampling performed at a relatively early gestational age: between 55 and 66 days. Burton et al. (1992) also reported transverse limb abnormalities after CVS. Apart from these two reports, most other series have found the incidence of limb-reduction defects to be not significantly different from the expected rates. Using records of the experience of the eight centers participating in the U.S. collaborative evaluation of CVS, Mahoney (1991) reported no cases of oromandibular-limb hypogenesis syndrome and no increased incidence of transverse limb defects. Monni et al. (1991) reviewed their experience of CVS procedures performed before the 66th day of gestation and reported no severe limb defects in the selected population. Two mild finger abnormalities were seen in their series. Defects have also been observed when CVS is performed after 66 days. Reports of limb abnormalities after CVS procedures and population-based studies are summarized in Table 2-4 (see also, Froster and Baird 1992; Froster-Iskenius and Baird 1989).

A variety of mechanisms by which CVS could potentially lead to fetal malformations has been proposed. The occurrence of placental thrombosis with subsequent fetal embolization has been raised as a potential cause. Inadvertent entry into the extraembryonic coelom, resulting in amniotic bands, has also been suggested. This seems unlikely because actual bands have not been observed in any cases. The most plausible proposed mechanism is a form of vascular insult leading to underperfusion of the fetus (Brent 1990). CVS could cause disruption of the vessels supplying the extracorporeal fetal circulation. This disruption would result in the release of vasoactive peptides, producing fetal vasospasm and hypoperfusion of the fetal peripheral circulation. Limb defects have been demonstrated in animal models after exposure to cocaine (Brent 1990; Webster and Brown-Woodman 1990). Theoretically, an overly vigorous technique during the CVS procedure could lead to significant placental damage, with resulting vasospasm and hypovolemia.

Using transcervical embryoscopic visualization of the first-trimester embryo, Quintero et al. (1992) demonstrated the occurrence of fetal facial, head, and thoracic ecchymotic lesions following a traumatic CVS. Although these lesions consistently appeared following significant physical trauma to the placental site, the researchers were not able to produce them by the passage of a standard CVS catheter. Furthermore, these lesions were demonstrated only after the development of a subchorionic hematoma.

A workshop on CVS was convened by the National Institute of Child Health and Human Development (NICHD Workshop 1993) and the American College of Obstetricians and Gynecologists at the National Institutes of Health on April 17, 1992. The most current data suggest that performance of CVS in the usual gestational age time period of 10 to 13 weeks is not associated with an increased risk of limb defects but that performance of the procedure prior to this time may be associated with a risk of severe limb defects as high as 1 to 2% (Jenkins and Wapner, 1999). Some of those attending the workshop concluded that exposure to CVS may have caused limb defects; some did not agree with this conclusion. All who attended agreed that the frequency of oromandibular-limb hypogenesis syndrome seemed to be more common among infants who had been exposed to CVS. This may correlate with, but not be limited to, CVS performed earlier than 7 weeks of gestation. Further studies are needed to determine whether there are factors that correlate with CVS-associated limb defects. These may include gestational age at the time of the procedure, experience of the operator, and the size of the instrument (catheter or needle) used to obtain the sample (NICHD Workshop 1993).

Accuracy of CVS Cytogenetic Results

The overall incidence of chromosomal mosaicism in CVS specimens is estimated to be approximately 1% (Vejerslev and Mikkelsen 1989). Generalized chromosomal mosaicism originates from a mutational event in the first or second postzygotic division, and all tissues of the fetus are affected (Kalousek and Dill 1983). Confined placental mosaicism (CPM), defined as a dichotomy between the chromosomal constitution of placental and fetal tissues, results from mutations occurring in the trophoblast or extraembryonic mesoderm progenitor cells (Kalousek et al. 1991). In most cases of mosaicism diagnosed by CVS, the cytogenetic abnormality is confined to extraembryonic tissue (Breed

▶ **TABLE 2-4.** INCIDENCE OF LIMB-REDUCTION DEFECTS IN GROUPS UNDERGOING CHORIONIC VILLUS SAMPLING AND POPULATION-BASED STUDIES

Chorionic Villus Sampling Series

Study	55 to 66 Days*	Defect	>66 Days*	Defect
Firth et al. (1991)	5/289	1 Transverse limb-reduction defect, 4 combined limb-reduction defects with micrognathia or microglossia	0/250	—
Burton et al.[†] (1992)	—	—	4/394	3 Finger-and-toe abnormalities, 1 finger abnormality
Monni et al. (1991)	0/525	—	2/2227	2 Finger abnormalities
Mahoney[‡] (1991)	1/1025	Longitudinal limb-reduction defect	6/8563	1 Longitudinal limb-reduction defect, 5 transverse limb-reduction defects (2 of the 5 were limited to fingers or toes)
Jackson et al.[‡] (1992)	1/2367	Bilateral aplasia of the thumbs	4/10,496	
Schloo et al. (1992)	1/636	Microglossia and hypodactyly	3/2200	3 Finger abnormalities (2 of the 3 had a family history of limb defects)

Population-based Studies

Study	Defect	Incidence
Froster-Iskenius and Baird (1989)	Combination of limb-reduction defects and micrognathia or microglossia	1/175,000
	Limb-reduction defects	1/1692
	Terminal longitudinal defects	1/2857
	Terminal transverse defects	1/6250
Froster and Baird (1992)	Hand	1/11,035
	Fingers	1/7016
	Foot	1/39,158
	Toes	1/43,354

*The number of days after the beginning of the last menstrual period at the time the procedure was performed.
[†]The number of procedures performed before 67 days was not reported.
[‡]There was some overlap between the series studied by Mahoney and by Jackson et al.
Reprinted, with permission, from D'Alton ME. Prenatal diagnostic procedures. Part 1— Diagnosis and treatment of fetal disease. Semin Perinatol 1994;18:140–162.

et al. 1991; Johnson et al. 1990; Vejerslev and Mikkelsen 1989).

Initially, several studies reported a higher incidence of adverse perinatal outcomes, including increased rates of fetal loss and intrauterine growth restriction (IUGR) in pregnancies complicated by CPM (Johnson et al. 1990; Kalousek et al. 1991). Kalousek et al. (1991) confirmed CPM in only half of placentas studied after birth. IUGR was found only in cases of CPM mosaicism confirmed in term placentas. Wapner et al. (1992) found a significantly higher rate of fetal loss (8.6%) among the 2.5% of patients with CPM, in comparison with patients with a normal karyotype (3.4%). Patients with pseudomosaicism had a rate of pregnancy loss and perinatal outcome similar to that of the normal population. Issues that still need to be investigated are the exact contribution of CPM to IUGR, the significance of the specific chromosome involved in the mosaicism, and the significance of specific tissue sources (i.e., direct cytotrophoblast preparations or mesenchymal tissue cultures) on pregnancy outcome. Counseling before CVS requires a discussion of the frequency and significance of CPM and the potential need for follow-up studies, including ultrasound, amniocentesis, and PUBS (Miny et al. 1991).

Summary

CVS is considered a viable alternative to second-trimester amniocentesis for prenatal diagnosis. Its immediate and long-term safety has been demonstrated. Evaluation of transcervical and transabdominal CVS has demonstrated their comparable safety and efficiency. The techniques are complementary and offer the choice of early prenatal diagnosis to women who have the appropriate indications for the procedure.

► PERCUTANEOUS UMBILICAL BLOOD SAMPLING (PUBS)

In 1983, Daffos et al. described a method of obtaining fetal blood using ultrasonographic guidance. This involved the passage of a 20-gauge spinal needle through the maternal abdomen into the umbilical cord. This technique offered considerable advantage over the fetoscopic methods previously used to obtain fetal blood. The techniques are variously described as percutaneous umbilical blood sampling, fetal blood sampling, cordocentesis, or funipuncture.

Technique

The main differences in the techniques of fetal blood sampling are related to whether the operator uses a needle guide or uses a "free-hand" technique. A variety of needle guides that attach to the transducer can be used. The advantage to this approach is that the needle will be directed precisely to a specific target. The disadvantage is that if the fetus moves or a contraction occurs while the needle is in the uterus, redirection of the tip may be difficult or impossible and will necessitate a repeat procedure. Because of these drawbacks, the authors prefer the free-hand technique to the needle guide. Fetal vessels can be accessed within the cord or the fetus itself. It is easier to enter the cord at the placental insertion site because it is anchored at this location (Figs. 2-7 and 2-8). Color Doppler imaging significantly enhances the ease of visualization of the cord insertion site (Fig. 2-9) and is especially useful when oligohydramnios is present. The hepatic vein is the most accessible vessel for blood sampling within the fetal body.

Once a sample of blood has been aspirated, it is essential to verify that it is fetal in origin. The most definitive way to do this is to compare the mean corpuscular volume (MCV) of the red cells to that of a sample of maternal blood. This is easily performed on small aliquots of blood by a standard channeling instrument. It is preferable to have this instrument in the procedure room. Fetal red cells are considerably larger than those of an adult and therefore afford rapid differentiation. Alternatively, one can inject a small amount of sterile saline, and if the needle is in the umbilical vein, the microbubbles created by the injection will be seen to move toward the fetus. In our centers this method, considered to be somewhat subjective, is not used. Forestier et al. (1988) recommended performing studies on the

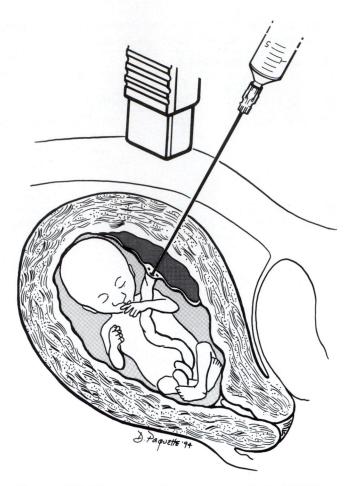

Figure 2-7. Diagrammatic representation of PUBS by ultrasound-guided insertion of the needle into the umbilical vein.

aspirated blood that include a complete blood count with differential analysis and determination of anti-I and anti-i cold agglutinin, β-subunit of hCG, factors IX and VIIIC, and AFP levels. It is not our practice to perform all of these studies. We compare the fetal MCV determination from a Coulter counter in the procedure room with the maternal MCV.

Success Rates and Safety

The rate of fetal loss after PUBS is approximately 2% higher than the background risk for that particular fetus (Daffos et al. 1985; Shulman and Elias 1990). Because many of the fetuses studied have severe congenital malformations, the background loss rate is high in comparison with that of the generally lower-risk population of women who undergo CVS amniocentesis.

The North American PUBS registry, which is maintained at Pennsylvania Hospital in Philadelphia, University of Pennsylvania, collects data from 16 centers in the United States and Canada. As of 1993, information on 7462 diagnostic procedures performed on 6023 patients was available (Ludomirsky 1993). The most common

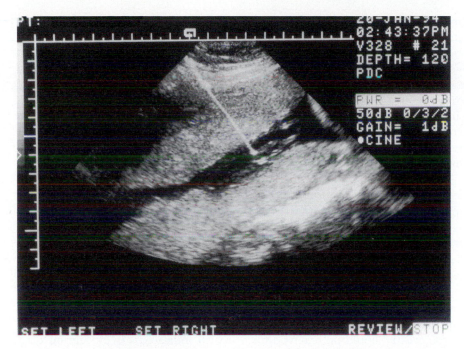

Figure 2-8. Ultrasound image of PUBS demonstrating the needle above the umbilical vein. *(Reprinted, with permission, from D'Alton ME. Prenatal diagnostic procedures. Part 1— Diagnosis and treatment of fetal disease. Semin Perinatol 1994;18:140–162.)*

needle used for procedures is a 22-gauge spinal needle. Fetal loss was defined as intrauterine fetal death within 14 days of the procedure. The rate of fetal loss was calculated to be 1.12% per procedure and 1.33% per patient. There were 84 pregnancies that were considered to be lost as a direct consequence of the fetal

blood sampling. The major causes for fetal loss were chorioamnionitis, rupture of membranes, bleeding from the puncture site, severe bradycardia, and thrombosis. The range of losses for participating centers varied from 1 to 6.7%; this range reflects differing levels of experience of the operators. These figures are subjective, relying

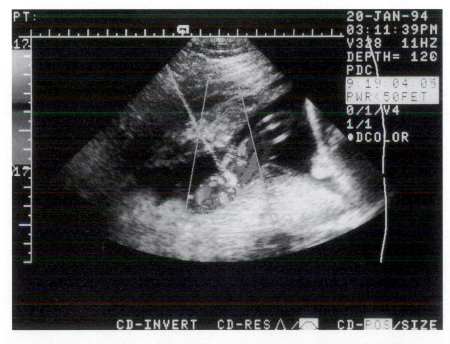

Figure 2-9. Ultrasound image of the same case shown in Figure 2-8, demonstrating the use of color Doppler to enhance visualization of the umbilical cord. See color plate.

on the operator's impression that a pregnancy loss was directly related to the procedure itself and not to the underlying fetal condition that necessitated the procedure. Because many of these fetuses were already compromised at the time of PUBS, it is certainly possible that an in utero death following the procedure might have been entirely unrelated. Nevertheless, this assessment is subjective and could be responsible for an underestimation of the true rates of loss for PUBS. The authors conclude that the intrahepatic vein is an alternative site of sampling or transfusion when access is difficult or failure occurs at the placental cord insertion site. Nicolini et al. (1990b) have described their experience with 214 fetal blood sampling procedures performed from the fetal hepatic vein and report success rates of 91% and 90% for diagnostic and therapeutic procedures, respectively. Rates of fetal loss comparable to those for blood sampling procedures performed at the placental cord insertion site were reported. Because PUBS entails a substantially greater risk of pregnancy loss than does amniocentesis, it should be reserved for situations in which rapid diagnosis is essential or in which diagnostic information cannot be obtained by safer means (D'Alton and DeCherney 1993).

Indications

Approximately two-thirds of the cases of diagnostic fetal blood sampling procedures reported to the PUBS registry were performed either to determine a rapid karyotype or to evaluate hematologic status in pregnancies at risk for red-cell isoimmunization (Ludomirsky 1993). One third of the procedures were performed to rule out fetal infection or to evaluate nonimmune hydrops, fetal acid–base status, twin-to-twin transfusion syndrome, or fetal platelet count.

Chromosome Analysis

The ultrasonographic detection of fetal morphologic malformations is now the most common indication for rapid fetal karyotyping in the United States (Table 2-5). With PUBS, fetal karyotypes are usually available from fetal white cells within 48 to 72 hours. The main advantage cited for PUBS is that it affords rapid availability of results. Its disadvantage is that it entails a greater risk of pregnancy loss than does amniocentesis. We use PUBS only when rapid diagnosis is essential or when diagnostic information cannot be obtained more safely (D'Alton and DeCherney 1993). Amniocentesis for fetal karyotype with the FISH technique for the rapid assay of chromosomes 21, 18, 13, X, and Y is the preferred method in our center (D'Alton and DeCherney 1993). An exception is the case in which the amniotic fluid is stained with blood. FISH studies are then uninformative, and we proceed to PUBS and a placental biopsy if rapid karyotyping is essential. Karyotyping fetal white cells is

▶ **TABLE 2-5.** INDICATIONS FOR PUBS

Most frequent
   Rapid karyotyping
      When ultrasound detects anatomic malformation
      When mosaicism is reported from amniotic fluid or
        CVS specimens
Less frequent
   Fetal red-cell isoimmunization
   Nonimmune hydrops fetalis
   Fetal platelet assessment
   Fetal infection
   Fetal acid–base status
   Diagnosis of twin–twin transfusion
   Hemoglobinopathies
   Coagulation factor deficiencies
   Immunologic deficiencies

Reprinted, with permission, from D'Alton ME. Prenatal diagnostic procedures. Part 1—Diagnosis and treatment of fetal disease. Semin Perinatol 1994;18:140–162.

also indicated for mosaicism detected in material obtained from amniotic fluid or chorionic villi. Although most cases of mosaicism found in chorionic villi can be effectively ruled out by amniocentesis, there have been reports of trisomy 21 mosaicism in which the chorionic villus culture revealed two cell lines, the amniotic fluid culture was entirely normal, yet true mosaicism was demonstrated in fetal blood (Ledbetter et al. 1990).

DNA Analysis

Most inherited hematologic disorders can now be diagnosed by the study of fetal DNA obtained from amniocytes or chorionic villi. Therefore, the antenatal detection of most congenital coagulopathies, hemoglobinopathies, white-cell disorders, and immune disorders does not usually require direct analysis of fetal blood specimens. In some of these cases, family studies are uninformative and PUBS is necessary for diagnosis. This is now the exception rather than the rule.

Fetal Anemia

Assessment of fetal anemia in cases of red-cell isoimmunization requires direct measurement of these parameters in fetal blood. Since Liley's study in 1961, the degree of fetal anemia in Rh-isoimmunized pregnancies has usually been assessed by serial amniocenteses and studies of ΔOD 450 values as a function of gestational age. These values reflect the amount of bilirubin pigment in the amniotic fluid and, as such, are an indirect indicator of the degree of fetal hemolysis. All the data in Liley's original paper, however, were collected at 28 weeks of gestation or later, and extrapolation of the lines dividing the zones in the original graph to earlier gestational ages may not be appropriate (Nicolaides et al. 1986b). Nicolaides found that the ΔOD 450 values accurately reflected the degree of fetal anemia in the third trimester but not in the second trimester when amniotic fluid ΔOD 450 values were compared with fetal hematocrits. Furthermore, there was no pattern to the inaccuracies; in some cases, high ΔOD 450 values inappropriately suggested the need for transfusion, and in other cases, low values were found in fetuses with significant anemia. Therefore, in severely affected cases of Rh isoimmunization, determination of the fetal hemoglobin level is the most accurate way to determine the fetal status and the optimal timing of a transfusion before 28 weeks of gestation.

Fetal blood sampling for determination of fetal anemia in red-cell isoimmunization is the second most common reason for this procedure. It accounts for 23% of all cases reported to the PUBS registry (Ludomirsky 1993). Fetal blood may also be obtained in cases of red-cell isoimmunization to determine the antigen status of the fetus when the father is heterozygous for the discordant antigen. A single invasive procedure can rule out the disease, and no further diagnostic testing will be necessary. Amniocentesis has replaced PUBS as the safest method for fetal RhD type determination, while in the future, a maternal blood sample may replace all invasive tests for fetal RhD type determination (Bennett et al. 1993; Lo et al. 1998).

Fetal Thrombocytopenia

Women with idiopathic thrombocytopenic purpura (ITP) have up to a 15% chance of delivering a neonate with a significantly depressed platelet count. The risk of neonatal bleeding, specifically intracranial hemorrhage, is rare. Nevertheless, some reports advocate delivery by cesarean section if the fetal platelet count is lower than 50,000 per cubic millimeter in order to avoid the trauma that may result from labor. There are no data to show, however, that cesarean section offers an advantage over vaginal delivery. The fetal platelet count can be determined by scalp sampling during labor. This method may not be an accurate reflection of the fetal platelet count and may be falsely low secondary to platelet clumping, or to dilution from amniotic fluid or scalp edema. Furthermore, to allow fetal scalp sampling the patient must be in labor with the cervix dilated, the fetal head must be engaged, and the membranes must be ruptured. In addition, there may not be sufficient time for scalp sampling in women with labor that is progressing rapidly. In cases of fetal thrombocytopenia, the timing of intracranial hemorrhage is unclear. It is possible that it may occur early in labor, before scalp sampling is technically feasible. An alternative approach in women with ITP is to perform PUBS at term, before the onset of labor. A number of studies have determined that PUBS at term reliably predicts the cord platelet count at the time of delivery (Garmel et al. 1994; Moise et al. 1988; Scioscia et al. 1988). It is unclear if cesarean section in the 10 to 15% of patients docu-

mented to have fetal thrombocytopenia will prevent intracranial hemorrhage. We have found documentation of the fetal platelet count before delivery to be helpful in choosing the site of delivery (Garmel et al. 1994). If the fetal platelet count is normal, the patient can deliver at a community hospital. The small percentage of patients carrying severely thrombocytopenic fetuses can deliver at a tertiary-care center, allowing immediate treatment of the newborn. In our series of 41 mothers with ITP there were 6 fetuses with a platelet count of lower than 50,000 per cubic millimeter; all were delivered by cesarean section. In all of these cases, neonatal therapy with steroids and intravenous gamma globulin was required.

Alloimmune thrombocytopenia is the platelet equivalent of Rh disease. In this disorder, the mother makes antibodies to antigens on the fetal platelets, and transplacental passage of these antibodies results in fetal thrombocytopenia. This disorder is associated with a much more marked depression of the fetal platelet count than is found in ITP. Unlike ITP, intracranial hemorrhage may occur in utero long before the onset of labor. Because severe thrombocytopenia and intracranial hemorrhage have been documented in this disorder as early as at 20 weeks of gestation, prolonged antenatal therapy is necessary to protect the fetus against the possibility of spontaneous bleeding. Since platelets have a life span of only 5 to 7 days, repeated in utero transfusions would be required if this were the chosen therapeutic option. Most fetuses with alloimmune thrombocytopenia will respond to intravenous gamma globulin at a dose of 1 g per kilogram administered intravenously once a week to the mother (Bussel et al. 1988; Lynch et al. 1992).

The risk of PUBS is higher in patients with alloimmune thrombocytopenia than in the general population. In these patients, blood sampling should be performed in a facility with access to rapid automated platelet counts at the time of the procedure, and a count should be determined before the sampling needle is withdrawn. A concentrate of washed maternal platelets should be available. If the fetal platelet count is found to be lower than 40,000 to 50,000 per cubic millimeter, a transfusion of maternal platelet concentrate can then be given.

Infectious Disease Diagnosis

Evaluation for fetal infection is the third most common indication for fetal blood sampling in the PUBS registry (8% of all cases). Daffos and colleagues (1988) reported on more than 700 pregnancies exposed to *Toxoplasma gondii* infection and demonstrated that 95% were not infected. Although PUBS has been used for *T. gondii* in the United States, screening for Toxoplasma is not routinely offered to pregnant women; therefore, PUBS is rarely performed for this diagnosis in the United States.

Direct isolation of the organism from fetal blood or amniotic fluid is the most reliable evidence of fetal infection. Technical difficulties and the length of time necessary for culture of the organism often make this approach impractical. Another method is to evaluate the fetal antibody response. Production of specific IgM antibodies is gestational age–dependent and also seems to depend on the organism involved. Almost 100% of fetuses with congenital rubella infection produce specific IgM antibodies after 22 weeks of gestation (Daffos et al. 1984), whereas only 15% of those infected with *T. gondii* tested between 24 and 29 weeks produce specific IgM antibodies against the parasite (Daffos et al. 1988). Therefore, although detection of specific IgM antibodies in fetal blood is reliable evidence of fetal infection, their absence does not rule it out. Nonspecific evidence of infection includes fetal thrombocytopenia, erythroblastosis, leukocytosis, eosinophilia, elevated levels of γ-glutamyltransferase, lactic dehydrogenase, interferon (Raymond et al. 1990; Lebon et al. 1985), and total IgM antibodies.

In recent years polymerase chain reaction (PCR) analysis has been highly reliable in detecting cytomegalovirus in amniotic fluid. Preliminary data suggest that PCR analysis of amniotic fluid is both highly sensitive and specific for the Toxoplasma organism, affording a diagnosis in a few hours (Grover et al. 1990). It is likely that amniocentesis and molecular techniques will replace PUBS for the confirmation of fetal infection.

Fetal Well-Being

Because cord-blood pH at the time of delivery is a well-accepted indicator of neonatal status, it was hoped that fetal blood sampling for blood gases would also accurately predict the fetal condition. Theoretically, PUBS could prove to be useful when more conventional forms of fetal assessment (nonstress testing, biophysical profile) were either equivocal or conflicting. Nicolaides et al. (1989) found significantly more hypoxemia, hypercapnia, hyperlactacidemia, and acidosis when 196 growth-restricted fetuses were compared with 208 who were appropriate in size for gestational age. However, Nicolini and colleagues (1990a) found that acid–base determination did not predict perinatal outcome in a group of growth-restricted fetuses. In their study, 26 growth-restricted fetuses with normal anatomy and karyotypes and absent end-diastolic flow on Doppler examination of the umbilical artery were compared with 20 similar fetuses, with end-diastolic flow evident on Doppler examination. The perinatal mortality was 65.4% in the first group and 0% in the latter. Significant differences in fetal blood values of PO_2, PCO_2, base equivalents, and nucleated red-cell counts were demonstrable between the groups. However, these measurements did not discriminate between surviving fetuses and those who died perinatally. The values in fetuses who survived were similar to those in fetuses who died in the perinatal period. The authors concluded that PUBS has a limited role in monitoring fetal well-being. Appreciable fetal acidosis and hypoxia are found only when the umbilical-artery Doppler waveform and the fetal heart rate pattern are abnormal (Nicolini et al. 1990a; Pardi et al. 1993). Doppler velocimetry of the umbilical artery seems to be a much more powerful predictor than PUBS of the compromised fetus with IUGR. Furthermore, it has been our experience that there is a much higher incidence of nonreassuring fetal testing necessitating emergency cesarean section when PUBS is performed in IUGR fetuses. There is a 15% incidence of fetal bradycardia reported when PUBS is performed in IUGR (Ludomirsky 1993). Because of this, amniocentesis is the preferred technique when determination of fetal karyotype is indicated in the workup of the growth-restricted fetus.

Summary

Access to the fetal circulation has led to important contributions to the understanding of fetal physiology and disease states. PUBS has an overall rate of fetal loss of 2%. There is now a decline in the indications for fetal sampling because of advances in molecular and cytogenetic techniques, which allow for diagnosis from amniotic fluid and chorionic villi. Performance of less invasive procedures that provide the same information is encouraged. PUBS should be reserved for situations in which diagnostic information cannot be obtained by safer methods. However, it is possible that over the next decade we will witness more use of PUBS for intrauterine therapy, such as for stem-cell transplantation.

▶ CONCLUSIONS

Midtrimester amniocentesis created the field of prenatal diagnosis and has become the standard by which all other methods are judged. It remains the procedure of choice when fetal safety is the primary consideration. Earlier prenatal diagnostic methods have increasing appeal for many patients. The most studied of these methods is CVS. Transcervical and transabdominal techniques are equally effective; individual operator experience and placental location are usually the criteria used to choose between the two approaches. Early amniocentesis will be used much less frequently now that compelling evidence regarding its disadvantages has been published. Advances in molecular techniques have led to a declining number of reasons for using PUBS. It is now rarely the procedure chosen for determining fetal karyotype. It is, however, the most direct method of evaluating the severity of Rh sensitization and is the preferred method in severe cases. PUBS is likely to be used more frequently for fetal therapy than for karyotyping over the next decade.

Helping the patient select the most appropriate diagnostic procedure for each indication is a role of crucial importance for the obstetrician and genetic counselor.

REFERENCES

Aburel ME. Le declenchement du travail par injections intra-amniotique de serum sale hypertonique. Gynecol Obstet 1937;36:398.

American College of Obstetricians and Gynecologists. Maternal Serum Screening. American College of Obstetricians and Gynecologists Educational Bulletin #228, The College, Washington, DC, September 1996.

Anderson RL, Goldberg JD, Golbus MS. Prenatal diagnosis in multiple gestation: 20 years' experience with amniocentesis. Prenat Diagn 1991;11:263–270.

Assel BG, Lewis SM, Dickerman LH, et al. Single-operator comparison of early and mid-second trimester amniocentesis. Obstet Gynecol 1992;79:940–944.

Bahado-Singh R, Schmitt R, Hobbins JC. New technique for genetic amniocentesis in twins. Obstet Gynecol 1992;70:304.

Barela AI, Kleinman GE, Golditch IM, et al. Septic shock with renal failure after chorionic villus sampling. Am J Obstet Gynecol 1986;154:1100–1102.

Beekhuis JR, DeBruijn HWA, Van Lith JMN, et al. Second trimester amniocentesis in twins. Br J Obstet Gynaecol 1992;99:126.

Benn P, Ciarleglio L, Lettieri L, et al. A rapid (but wrong) prenatal diagnosis. N Engl J Med 1992;326:1638–1640.

Bennett PR, Le Van Kim C, Colin Y, et al. Prenatal determination of fetal RhD type by DNA amplification. N Engl J Med 1993;329:607–610.

Bevis DCA. Composition of liquor amnii in haemolytic disease of the newborn. Lancet 1950;2:443.

Bianchi DW, Wilkins-Haug LE, Enders AC, et al. Origin of extraembryonic mesoderm in experimental animals: relevance to chorionic mosaicism in humans. Am J Med Genet 1993;46:542–550.

Blakemore KJ, Baumgarten A, Schoenfeld-Dimaio M, et al. Rise in maternal serum alpha-fetoprotein concentration after chorionic villus sampling and the possibility of isoimmunization. Am J Obstet Gynecol 1986;155:988–993.

Blakemore KJ, Mahoney MJ, Hobbins JC. Infection and chorionic villus sampling. Lancet 1985;2:339.

Brambati B, Guercilena S, Bonacchi I, et al. Fetomaternal transfusion after chorionic villus sampling: clinical implications. Hum Reprod 1986;27:37–40.

Brambati B, Matarrelli M, Varotto F. Septic complications after chorionic villus sampling. Lancet 1987a;1:1212.

Brambati B, Oldrini A, Ferrazzi E, et al. Chorionic villus sampling: an analysis of the obstetric experience of 1000 cases. Prenat Diagn 1987b;7:157.

Brambati B, Terzian E, Tognoni G. Randomized clinical trial of transabdominal versus transcervical chorionic villus sampling methods. Prenat Diagn 1991a;11:285–293.

Brambati B, Tului L, Lanzani A, et al. First-trimester genetic diagnosis in multiple pregnancy: principles and potential pitfalls. Prenat Diagn 1991b;11:767–774.

Brambati B, Varotto F. Infection and chorionic villus sampling. Lancet 1985;2:609.

Breed ASPM, Mantingh A, Vosters R, et al. Follow-up and pregnancy outcome after a diagnosis of mosaicism in CVS. Prenat Diagn 1991;11:577–580.

Brent RL. Relationship between uterine vascular clamping, vascular disruption syndrome and cocaine teratology. Teratology 1990;41:757.

Broome DL, Wilson MG, Weiss B, et al. Needle puncture of fetus: a complication of second-trimester amniocentesis. Am J Obstet Gynecol 1976;126:247–252.

Burton BK, Nason LM, DeHenati MJ. False positive acetylcholinesterase with early amniocentesis. Obstet Gynecol 1989;74:607–610.

Burton BK, Schulz CJ, Burd LI. Limb anomalies associated with chorionic villus sampling. Obstet Gynecol 1992;79:726–730.

Bussel J, Berkowitz RL, McFarland JG, et al. Antenatal treatment of neonatal alloimmune thrombocytopenia. N Engl J Med 1988;319:1374.

Byrne D, Azar G, Nicolaides K. Why cell culture is successful after early amniocentesis. Fetal Diagn Ther 1991;6:84–86.

Calhoun BC, Brehm W, Bombard AT. Early genetic amniocentesis and its relationship to respiratory difficulties in paediatric patients: a report of findings in patients and matched controls 3-5 years post-procedure. Prenat Diagn 1994;14:209–212.

Canadian Collaborative CVS/Amniocentesis Clinical Trial Group. Multicentre randomized clinical trial of chorion villus sampling and amniocentesis. Lancet 1989;1:1.

Canadian Early and Mid-Trimester Amniocentesis Trial (CEMAT) Group. Randomized trial to assess safety and fetal outcome of early and mid-trimester amniocentesis. Lancet 1998;351:242–247.

Coleman BG, Grumbach K, Aarger PH, et al. Twin gestations: monitoring of complications and anomalies with US. Radiology 1987;165:449–453.

Cowett R, Hakanson D, Kocon R, et al. Untoward neonatal effect of intraamniotic administration of methylene blue. Obstet Gynecol 1976;48(suppl):745.

Cragan JD, Martin ML, Khoury MJ. Dye use during amniocentesis and birth defects. Lancet 1993;341:1352.

Crandall BF, Hanson FW, Tennant F. Acetylcholinesterase (ACHE) electrophoresis and early amniocentesis (abstract 1010). Am J Hum Genet 1989a;4(suppl):A257.

Crandall BF, Hanson FW, Tennant F, et al. Alpha-fetoprotein levels in amniotic fluid between 11 and 15 weeks. Am J Obstet Gynecol 1989b;160:1204–1206.

Crandall BF, Kulch P, Khalil T. Risk assessment of amniocentesis between 11 and 15 weeks: comparison to later amniocentesis controls. Prenat Diagn 1994;4:913–919.

D'Alton ME. Prenatal diagnostic procedures. Part 1—Diagnosis and treatment of fetal disease. Semin Perinatol 1994;18:140–162.

D'Alton ME, Craigo S, Bianchi D. Prenatal diagnosis procedures. In: Current problems in ob/gyn fertility. Chicago: Mosby, 1994:41–80.

D'Alton ME, DeCherney AH. Prenatal diagnosis. N Engl J Med 1993;328:114–120.

D'Alton ME, Malone FD, Chelmow D, Ward BE, Bianchi DW. Defining the role of fluorescence in situ hybridization on uncultured amniocytes for prenatal diagnosis of aneuploidies. Am J Obstet Gynecol 1997;176(4):769–776.

Daffos F, Capella-Pavlovsky M, Forestier F. Fetal blood sampling during pregnancy with use of a needle guided by ultrasound: a study of 606 consecutive cases. Am J Obstet Gynecol 1985;153:655–660.

Daffos F, Capella-Pavlovsky M, Forestier F. Fetal blood sampling via the umbilical cord using a needle guided by ultrasound. Prenat Diagn 1983;3:271.

Daffos F, Forestier F, Capella-Pavlovsky M, et al. Prenatal management of 746 pregnancies at risk for congenital toxoplasmosis. N Engl J Med 1988;318:271.

Daffos F, Forestier F, Grangeot-Keros L, et al. Prenatal diagnosis of congenital rubella. Lancet 1984;2:1.

Elias S, Gerbie AB, Simpson JL, et al. Genetic amniocentesis in twin gestations. Am J Obstet Gynecol 1980;138:169–174.

Epley SL, Hanson JW, Cruikshank DP. Fetal injury with midtrimester diagnostic amniocentesis. Obstet Gynecol 1979;53:77.

Filkins K, Russo J. Genetic amniocentesis in multiple gestations. Prenat Diagn 1984;4:223.

Finegan JAK, Quarrington BJ, Hughes HE, et al. Child outcome following mid-trimester amniocentesis: development, behaviour, and physical status at age 4 years. Br J Obstet Gynaecol 1990;97:32–40.

Firth HV, Boyd PA, Chamberlain P, et al. Severe limb abnormalities after chorion villus sampling at 56–66 days gestation. Lancet 1991;337:762–763.

Forestier F, Cox WL, Daffos F, et al. The assessment of fetal blood samples. Am J Obstet Gynecol 1988;158:1184.

Froster UG, Baird PA. Limb-reduction defects and chorionic villus sampling. Lancet 1992;339:66.

Froster-Iskenius UG, Baird PA. Limb reduction defects in over one million consecutive livebirths. Teratology 1989;39:127–135.

Fuchs F, Riis P. Antenatal sex determination. Nature 1956;177:330.

Garden AS, Reid G, Benzie RJ. Chorionic villus sampling. Lancet 1985;1:1270.

Garmel S, Craigo S, Morin L, et al. The management of immune thrombocytopenic purpura with percutaneous umbilical blood sampling (abstract). Am J Obstet Gynecol 1994;170:335.

Gilmore DH, McNay MB. Spontaneous fetal loss rate in early pregnancy. Lancet 1985;2:107.

Gluck L, Kulovich MV, Borer RC, et al. The interpretation and significance of the lecithin/sphingomyelin ratio in amniotic fluid. Am J Obstet Gynecol 1974;109:142–155.

Golbus MS, Loughman WD, Epstein CJ. Prenatal genetic diagnosis in 3000 amniocenteses. N Engl J Med 1979;300:157.

Gosden C, Nicolaides KH, Rodeck CH. Fetal blood sampling in investigation of chromosome mosaicism in amniotic fluid cell culture. Lancet 1988;1:613–617.

Grover CM, Thulliez P, Remington JS, et al. Rapid prenatal diagnosis of congenital toxoplasma infection polymerase chain reaction and amniotic fluid. J Clin Microbiol 1990;28:2297.

Hackett GA, Smith JH, Rebello MT, et al. Early amniocentesis at 11–14 weeks gestation for the diagnosis of fetal chromosomal abnormality: a clinical evaluation. Prenatal Diagn 1991;11:311–315.

Haddow JE, Palomaki GE, Knight GJ, et al. Prenatal screening for Down's syndrome with use of maternal serum markers. N Engl J Med 1992;327:588–593.

Hahnemann N. Early prenatal diagnosis; a study of biopsy techniques and cell culturing from extraembryonic membranes. Clin Genet 1974;6:294–306.

Hahnemann N, Mohr J. Antenatal foetal diagnosis in genetic disease. Bull Eur Soc Hum Genet 1969;3:47–54.

Hallman M, Kulovich M, Kirkpatrick E, et al. Phosphatidylinositol and phosphatidylglycerol in amniotic fluid: indices of lung maturity. Am J Obstet Gynecol 1976;125:613–617.

Hanson FW, Tennant FR, Hune S, et al. Early amniocentesis: outcome, risks, and technical problems at ≤12.8 weeks. Am J Obstet Gynecol 1992;166:1707–1711.

Henry GP, Miller WA. Early amniocentesis. J Reprod Med 1992;37:396–402.

Hill LM, Platt LD, Kellogg B. Rh-sensitization after genetic amniocentesis. Obstet Gynecol 1980;56:459.

Hogge WA, Schonberg SA, Golbus MS. Chorionic villus sampling: experience of the first 1000 cases. Am J Obstet Gynecol 1986;154:1249.

Hook EB, Cross PK, Schreinemachers DM. Chromosomal abnormality rates at amniocentesis and in live-born infants. JAMA 1983;249:2034–2038.

Hook EB. Rates of chromosome abnormalities at different maternal ages. Obstet Gynecol 1981;58:282–285.

Hoyme HF, Jones KL, Van Allen MI, et al. Vascular pathogenesis of transverse limb reduction defects. J Pediatr 1982;101:839–843.

Hsu LYF, Perlis T. United States survey on chromosome mosaicism and pseudomosaicism in prenatal diagnosis. Prenat Diagn 1984;4:97.

Jackson LG, Zachary JM, Fowler SE, et al. A randomized comparison of transcervical and transabdominal chorionic villus sampling. N Engl J Med 1992;327:594–598.

Jacobson CB, Barter RH. Intrauterine diagnosis and management of genetic defects. Am J Obstet Gynecol 1967;99:795.

Jeanty P, Rodesch F, Romero R, et al. How to improve your amniocentesis technique. Am J Obstet Gynecol 1983;146:593–596.

Jeanty P, Shah D, Roussis P. Single-needle insertion in twin amniocentesis. J Ultrasound Med 1990;9:11–17.

Jenkins TJ, Wapner RJ. First trimester prenatal diagnosis: chorionic villus sampling. Semin Perinatol 1999;23:403–413.

Johnson A, Wapner RJ, Davis GH, et al. Mosaicism in chorionic villus sampling: an association with poor perinatal outcome. Obstet Gynecol 1990;75:573–577.

Johnson JM, Wilson RD, Singer J, et al. Technical factors in early amniocentesis predict adverse outcome. Results of the Canadian early (EA) versus mid-trimester (MA) amniocentesis trial. Prenat Diagn 1999;19:732–738.

Jorgensen FS, Bang J, Lind AM, et al. Genetic amniocentesis at 7-14 weeks of gestation. Prenat Diagn 1992;12:277–283.

Kalousek D, Dill F. Chromosomal mosaicism confined to the placenta in human conceptions. Science 1983;221:665.

Kalousek DK, Howard-Peebles PN, Olson SB, et al. Confirmation of CVS mosaicism in term placentae and high frequency of intrauterine growth retardation association with confined placental mosaicism. Prenat Diagn 1991;11:743–750.

Karp LE, Hayden PW. Fetal puncture during midtrimester amniocentesis. Obstet Gynecol 1977;49:115.

Klinger K, Landes G, Shook D, et al. Rapid detection of chromosome aneuploidies in uncultured amniocytes by using fluorescence in situ hybridization (FISH). Am J Hum Genet 1992;51:55–65.

Lamb MP. Gangrene of a fetal limb due to amniocentesis. Br J Obstet Gynaecol 1975;82:829.

Lambl D. Ein seltener Fall von Hydramnios. Zentrabl Gynakol 1881;5:329.

Lebo RV, Flandermeyer RR, Diukman R, et al. Prenatal diagnosis with repetitive in situ hybridization probes. Am J Med Genet 1992;43:848–854.

Lebon P, Daffos F, Checoury A, et al. Presence of an acid-labile alpha-interferon in sera from fetuses and children with congenital rubella. J Clin Microbiol 1985;21:775.

Ledbetter DH, Martin AO, Verlinsky Y, et al. Cytogenetic results of chorionic villus sampling: high success rate and diagnostic accuracy in the United States collaborative study. Am J Obstet Gynecol 1990;162:495.

Lenke RR, Cyr DR, Mack LA. Midtrimester genetic amniocentesis with simultaneous ultrasound guidance. J Clin Ultrasound 1985;13:371.

Liley AW. Liquor amnii analysis in the management of the pregnancy complicated by rhesus isoimmunization. Am J Obstet Gynecol 1961;82:1359–1370.

Liu DTV, Jeavons B, Preston C, et al. A prospective study of spontaneous miscarriage in ultrasonically normal pregnancies and relevance to chorion villus sampling. Prenat Diagn 1987;7:223–227.

Lo YM, Hjelm NM, Fidler C, et al. Prenatal diagnosis of fetal RhD status molecular analysis of maternal plasma. N Engl J Med 1998;339:1724–1738.

Lubs HA, Ruddle FH. Chromosomal abnormalities in the human population: estimation of rates based on New Haven newborn study. Science 1970;169:495.

Ludomirsky A. Intrauterine fetal blood sampling—a multicenter registry; evaluation of 7462 procedures between 1987-1991 (abstract). Am J Obstet Gynecol 1993;168:318.

Lynch L, Bussel JB, McFarland JG, et al. Antenatal treatment of alloimmune thrombocytopenia. Obstet Gynecol 1992;80:67.

Mahoney J. Limb abnormalities and chorionic villus sampling. Lancet 1991;337:1422–1443.

Malone FD, D'Alton ME. Multiple gestation: Clinical characteristics and management. In Creasy RK and Resnick R. Maternal-fetal medicine, 4th edition, W.B. Saunders, Philadelphia, 1999; 598–615.

McFadyen IR, Taylor-Robinson D, Furr PM, et al. Infections and chorionic villus sampling. Lancet 1985;2:610.

Medical Research Council. Diagnosis of genetic disease by amniocentesis during the second trimester of pregnancy. Ottawa: Medical Research Council, 1977.

Menees TD, Miller JD, Holly LE. Amniography: preliminary report. Am J Roentgenol Radium Ther 1930;24:363.

Merin MD, Beyth Y. Uniocular congenital blindness as a complication of midtrimester amniocentesis. Am J Ophthalmol 1980;89:299.

Milunsky A. Genetic disorders and the fetus: diagnosis prevention and treatment. New York: Plenum, 1979.

Miny P, Hammer P, Gerlach B, et al. Mosaicism and accuracy of prenatal cytogenetic diagnoses after chorionic villus sampling and placental biopsies. Prenat Diagn 1991;11:581–589.

Moise KJ, Carpenter RJ. Increased severity of fetal hemolytic disease with known Rhesus alloimmunization after first trimester transcervical chorionic villus biopsy. Fetal Diagn Ther 1990;5:76–78.

Moise KJ, Carpenter RJ, Cotton DB, et al. Percutaneous umbilical cord blood sampling in the evaluation of fetal platelet counts in pregnant patients with autoimmune thrombocytopenic purpura. Obstet Gynecol 1988;72:346–350.

Monni G, Ibba RM, Lai R, et al. Limb-reduction defects and chorion villus sampling. Lancet 1991;337:1091.

MRC Working Party on the Evaluation of Chorion Villus Sampling. Medical Research Council European trial of chorionic villus Sampling. Lancet 1991;337:1491.

Nadel AS, Green JK, Holmes LB, et al. Absence of need for amniocentesis in patients with elevated levels of maternal serum alpha-fetoprotein and normal ultrasonographic examinations. N Engl J Med 1990;323:557–561.

Nadler HL. Antenatal detection of hereditary disorders. Pediatrics 1968;42:912.

NICHD Amniocentesis Registry. Midtrimester amniocentesis for prenatal diagnosis: safety and accuracy. JAMA 1976;236:1471.

NICHD Workshop on Chorionic Villus Sampling and Limb and Other Defects, October 20, 1992. Teratology 1993;48:7–13.

Nicolaides KH, Clewell WH, Mibashan RS, et al. Fetal haemoglobin measurement in the assessment of red cell isoimmunization. Lancet 1988;1:1073–75.

Nicolaides KH, Economides DL, Soothill PW. Blood gases, pH, and lactate in appropriate- and small-for-gestational-age fetuses. Am J Obstet Gynecol 1989;161:996.

Nicolaides K, de Lourdes Brizot M, Patel F, et al. Comparison of chorionic villus sampling and early amniocentesis for karyotyping in 1492 singleton pregnancies. Fetal Diagn Ther 1996;1:9–15.

Nicolaides KH, Gabbe SG, Campbell S, et al. Ultrasound screening for spina bifida: cranial and cerebellar signs. Lancet 1986a;2:72–74.

Nicolaides KH, Rodeck CH, Mibashan RS, et al. Have Liley charts outlived their usefulness? Am J Obstet Gynecol 1986b;155:90–94.

Nicolini U, Monni G. Intestinal obstruction in babies exposed in utero to methylene blue. Lancet 1990;336:1258–1259.

Nicolini U, Nicolaides P, Fisk NM, et al. Limited role of fetal blood sampling in prediction of outcome in intrauterine growth retardation. Lancet 1990a;2:768.

Nicolini U, Nicolaides P, Nicholas M, et al. Fetal blood sampling from the intrahepatic vein: analysis of safety and clinical experience with 214 procedures. Obstet Gynecol 1990b;76:47.

Pardi G, Cetin I, Marconi AM, et al. Diagnostic value of blood sampling in fetuses with growth retardation. N Engl J Med 1993;328:692–696.

Penso CA, Sandstrom MM, Garber MF, et al. Early amniocentesis: report of 407 cases with neonatal follow-up. Obstet Gynecol 1990;76:1032–1036.

Pergament E, Schulman JD, Copeland K, et al. The risk and efficacy of chorionic villus sampling in multiple gestations. Prenat Diagn 1992;12:377–384.

Poenaru L. First trimester prenatal diagnosis of metabolic diseases: a survey in countries from the European community. Prenat Diagn 1987;7:333.

Quintero R, Romero R, Mahoney MJ, et al. Fetal haemorrhagic lesions after chorionic villus sampling. Lancet 1992;339:193.

Raymond J, Poissonnier MH, Thulliez PH, et al. Presence of gamma interferon in human acute and congenital toxoplasmosis. J Clin Microbiol 1990;28:1434.

Rhoads GG, Jackson LG, Schlesselman SE, et al. The safety and efficacy of chorionic villus sampling for early prenatal diagnosis of cytogenetic abnormalities. N Engl J Med 1989;320:609–617.

Richards DS, Seeds JW, Katz VL, et al. Elevated maternal serum alpha-fetoprotein with normal ultrasound: is amniocentesis always appropriate? A review of 26,069 screened patients. Obstet Gynecol 1988;71:203–207.

Rickwood AMK. A case of ileal atresia and ileocutaneous fistula caused by amniocentesis. J Pediatr 1977;91:312.

Romero R, Sirtori M, Oyarzun E, et al. Infection and labor. V. Prevalence, microbiology and clinical significance of intraamniotic infection in women with preterm labor and intact membranes. Am J Obstet Gynecol 1989;161:817–824.

Schatz F. Eine besondere Art von ein seitiger Oligohydramnie bei Zwillingen. Arch Gynecol 1992;65:329.

Schloo R, Miny P, Holzgreve W, et al. Distal limb deficiency following chorionic villus sampling? Am J Med Genet 1992;42:404–413.

Schwartz S. Efficacy and applicability of interphase fluorescence in situ hybridization for prenatal diagnosis. Am J Hum Genet 1993;52:851–853.

Scioscia AL, Grannum PAT, Copel JA, et al. The use of percutaneous umbilical blood sampling in immune thrombocytopenic purpura. Am J Obstet Gynecol 1988;159:1066–1068.

Shulman LP, Elias S. Percutaneous umbilical blood sampling, fetal skin sampling, and fetal liver biopsy. Semin Perinatol 1990;14:456–464.

Shulman LP, Meyers CM, Simpson JL, et al. Fetomaternal transfusion depends on amount of chorionic villi aspirated but not on method of chorionic villus sampling. Am J Obstet Gynecol 1990;162:1185–1185.

Simpson JL, Socol ML, Aladjem S, et al. Normal fetal growth despite persistent amniotic fluid leakage after genetic amniocentesis. Prenat Diagn 1981;1:277–279.

Smidt-Jensen S, Permin M, Philip J, et al. Randomised comparison of amniocentesis and transabdominal and transcervical chorionic villus sampling. Lancet 1992;340:1237–1244.

Steele MW, Breg WR, Jr. Chromosome analysis of human amniotic fluid cells. Lancet 1966;1:383.

Strovel JW, Lee KD, Punzalan C, et al. Prenatal diagnosis by direct analysis of uncultured amniotic fluid cells using interphase fluorescence in situ hybridization (FISH). Am J Hum Genet 1992;Suppl S1:A12.

Sundberg K, Bang J, Smidt-Jenson S, et al. Randomised study of risk of fetal loss related to early amniocentesis versus chorionic villus sampling. Lancet 1997;350:697–703.

Swift PGF, Driscoll IB, Vowles KDJ. Neonatal small bowel obstruction associated with amniocentesis. BMJ 1979;1:720.

Tabor A, Philip J, Madsen M, et al. Randomised controlled trial of genetic amniocentesis in 4606 low-risk women. Lancet 1986;1:1287.

Tabor A, Philip J, Bang J, et al. Needle size and risk of miscarriage after amniocentesis. Lancet 1988;1:183–184.

Therkelsen AJ, Rehder, H. Intestinal atresia caused by second trimester amniocentesis: case report. Br J Obstet Gynaecol 1981;88:559–562.

Thompson PJ, Greenough A, Nicolaides KH. Lung function following first-trimester amniocentesis or chorion villus sampling. Fetal Diagn Ther 1991;6:148–152.

Tietung Hospital of Anshan Iron and Steel Co., Anshan, China, Department of Ob/Gyn. Fetal sex prediction by sex chromatin of chorionic villi cells during early pregnancy. Chin Med J 1975;1:117–126.

Turnbull AC, MacKenzie IZ. Second-trimester amniocentesis and termination of pregnancy. Br Med Bull 1983;39:315.

UK Collaborative Study on Alpha-Fetoprotein in Relation to Neural-tube defects. Amniotic fluid alpha-fetoprotein measurements in antenatal diagnosis of anencephaly and open spina bifida in early pregnancy. Lancet 1979;2:652.

Valenti C, Schutta EJ, Kehaty T. Prenatal diagnosis of Down's syndrome. Lancet 1968;2:220.

Van den Hof MC, Nicolaides KH, Campbell J, et al. Evaluation of the lemon and banana signs in 130 fetuses with open spina bifida. Am J Obstet Gynecol 1990;162:322–327.

Van der Pol JG, Volf H, Boer K, et al. Jejunal atresia related to the use of methylene blue in genetic amniocentesis in twins. Br J Obstet Gynaecol 1992;99:141–143.

Vejerslev LO, Mikkelsen M. The European collaborative study on mosaicism in chorionic villus sampling: data from 1986 to 1987. Prenat Diagn 1989;9:575–588.

Walker A. Liquor amnii studies in the prediction of haemolytic disease of the newborn. BMJ 1957;2:376.

Wapner RJ, Simpson JL, Golbus MS, et al. Chorionic mosaicism: association with fetal loss but not with adverse perinatal outcome. Prenat Diagn 1992;12:347–355.

Ward BE, Gersen SL, Carelli MP, et al. Rapid prenatal diagnosis of chromosomal aneuploidies by fluorescence in situ hybridization: clinical experience with 4,500 specimens. Am J Hum Genet 1993;52:854–865.

Ward BE, Gersen SL, Klinger KW. A rapid (but wrong) prenatal diagnosis: integrated genetics replies. N Engl J Med 1992;326:1639.

Wass D, Bennett MJ. Infection and chorionic villus sampling. Lancet 1985;2:338.

Wathen NC, Cass PL, Campbell DJ, et al. Early amniocentesis: alphafetoprotein levels in amniotic fluid, extraembryonic coelomic fluid and maternal serum between 8 and 13 weeks. Br J Obstet Gynaecol 1991;98:866–870.

Webster W, Brown-Woodman T. Cocaine as a cause of congenital malformations of vascular origin: experimental evidence in the rat. Teratology 1990;41:689.

Wilson RD, Kendrick V, Wittman BK, et al. Risk of spontaneous abortion in ultrasonically normal pregnancies. Lancet 1984;2:920.

Working Party on Amniocentesis. An assessment of hazards of amniocentesis. Br J Obstet Gynaecol 1978;85:1.

Winsor EJ, Tomkins DJ, Kalousek D, et al. Cytogenetic aspects of the Canadian early and mid-trimester amniotic fluid trial (CEMAT). Prenat Diagn 1999;19:620-627.

Young PE, Matson MR, Jones OW. Fetal exsanguination and other vascular injuries from mid-trimester genetic amniocentesis. Am J Obstet Gynecol 1977;129:21.

Youroukos S, Papadelis F, Matsaniotis N. Porencephalic cysts after amniocentesis. Arch Dis Child 1980;55:814–815.

CHAPTER 3

Invasive Fetal Therapy and Fetal Surgery

Prenatal diagnosis has become increasingly sophisticated, and technologic advances have enhanced our range of diagnostic capabilities. Invasive therapies have developed as a natural consequence of our expanded understanding of the natural history and pathophysiology of structural anomalies (Adzick et al. 1994b; Garmel et al. 1993). In the 1960s and 1970s, despite rapid progress in prenatal diagnosis, few invasive therapies were considered, much less employed (Adamsons 1966). Once diagnosis was made prenatally, parents had only two alternatives: pregnancy termination, if the diagnosis was made prior to 24 weeks of gestation, or continuing to term (Harrison et al. 1981b). An additional option is altering the site of delivery so that the appropriate pediatric specialists would be available immediately to treat the newborn with a congenital anomaly. As the natural history of many prenatally diagnosed anomalies became better understood, early delivery was recognized as an option to avoid the continuing damage caused by the anomaly in utero (Adzick et al. 1994a, 1994b). Today there are more alternatives. In this chapter we describe the treatment options available, how they were developed, and which therapies may be available in the future.

► FETAL SHUNTING PROCEDURES

A new era in invasive fetal therapy began in the early 1980s, when several independent groups introduced shunting procedures for hydrocephalus and hydronephrosis (Clewell et al. 1982; Frigoletto et al. 1982; Golbus et al. 1982). These first few cases represented an extension of invasive fetal therapy from simple intrauterine blood transfusion for a medical illness to the first attempts at in utero treatment of structural anomalies (Table 3-1).

During this period, hydronephrosis and hydrocephalus were being recognized more frequently with ultrasound examination. The prenatal natural history of these lesions was established by serial sonographic observation of untreated cases (Cendron et al. 1994; Chervenak et al. 1984; Clewell et al. 1985; Crombleholme et al. 1988; Glick et al. 1984a, 1984b; Nakayama et al. 1986). Fetuses with high-grade obstructive uropathy followed to term were often born with advanced hydronephrosis, type IV cystic dysplasia, and pulmonary hypoplasia that were incompatible with life (Cendron et al. 1994; Crombleholme et al. 1988; Potter 1976). In the case of obstructive hydrocephalus, it was known that shunting during the newborn period improved neurologic outcome, and it was reasoned that decompression in utero might avert progressive brain damage (Lawrence et al. 1962; Lorber 1969; Young et al. 1973). At this time, the understanding of the natural history, pathophysiology, and patient selection criteria was rudimentary and incomplete at best. However, work by numerous investigators, in appropriate animal models, helped to define the pathophysiology of these lesions and establish the theoretical basis for intervention (Adzick et al. 1970; Glick et al. 1983, 1984a, 1984b; Harrison et al. 1982d, 1983a; Michejda and Hodgen 1981).

Hydrocephalus

Among the most important things learned about invasive fetal therapy were the necessity of understanding the natural history of the untreated condition and the

▶ **TABLE 3-1.** FETAL MALFORMATIONS TREATABLE BY NEEDLE ASPIRATION AND SHUNTING PROCEDURES

Fetal Malformation	Fetal Presentation	Fetal/Neonatal Consequence
Posterior urethral valves	Hydronephrosis	Renal dysplasia and renal insufficiency
	Oligohydramnios	Pulmonary hypoplasia and respiratory insufficiency
Cystic adenomatoid malformation of the lung	Mediastinal shift Hydrops	Pulmonary hypoplasia
Aqueductal stenosis	Hydrocephalus	Neurologic damage
Fetal hydrothorax	Mediastinal shift, hydrops, polyhydramnios	Pulmonary hypoplasia
Ovarian cyst	Wandering cystic abdominal mass, polyhydramnios	Ovarian torsion

ability to identify which fetuses were the most likely to benefit. Based on the observation that postnatal shunting for hydrocephalus was beneficial, Birnholz et al. used serial percutaneous cephalocentesis to treat hydrocephalus in utero (Birnholz et al. 1981). The results of their efforts were disappointing because the fetus had unrecognized intracranial abnormalities and Becker muscular dystrophy. Shortly thereafter, ventriculoamniotic shunts were developed to provide consistent ventricular decompression (Clewell et al. 1982; Frigoletto et al. 1982). While these procedures enjoyed a brief period of enthusiasm, it soon became clear that results were poor, often related to undetected central nervous system (CNS) and non-CNS anomalies, and that these shunts failed to provide consistent ventricular decompression due to obstruction or migration (Clewell 1991; Manning et al. 1986).

The results of 39 cases reported to the International Fetal Surgery Registry and 5 additional cases from Bologna, Italy, were so disappointing that almost all centers abandoned ventriculoamniotic shunting (Clewell 1991). These cases were reported from a large number of centers for a range of malformations with no consistent selection criteria for intervention (Table 3-2). The

overall mortality in the series was 19%, with half of the deaths thought to be procedure-related. More troubling still was that nearly half the survivors were moderately or severely handicapped and the incidence of handicap appeared to be greater among those who underwent the shunting procedure in utero than among those who were treated conventionally (Clewell 1991; Manning et al. 1986).

The fetus most likely to benefit from ventriculoamniotic shunting is one with isolated, rapidly progressive ventriculomegaly (Chervenak et al. 1985; Clewell 1991; Cochrane et al. 1984; Hudgins et al. 1988; Manning et al. 1986; Pretorius et al. 1985; Rosseau 1991; Serlo et al. 1986). This has been problematic, as the incidence of associated CNS anomalies in reported series has varied from 70 to 84%, with many of these defects not detected prenatally (Chervenak et al. 1985; Cochrane et al. 1984; Hudgins et al. 1988; Pretorius et al. 1985; Rosseau et al. 1991; Serlo et al. 1986) (Table 3-3). Even assuming that our diagnostic capabilities have improved significantly in the past decade, it may be difficult to identify appropriate circumstances for fetal intervention. Previous studies list the incidence of isolated progressive ventriculomegaly from 0 to 56%, with most reports

▶ **TABLE 3-2.** INTERNATIONAL FETAL SURGERY REGISTRY: SHUNTING FOR HYDROCEPHALUS

Postnatal Diagnosis	No. of Cases	% of Cases	No. of Deaths	% Mortality by Diagnosis
Aqueductal stenosis	32	76.9	4	13.3
Associated anomalies	5	12.7	2	40
Holoprosencephaly	1	2.6	1	100
Dandy–Walker malformation	1	2.6	0	0
Porencephalic cyst	1	2.6	0	0
Arnold–Chiari syndrome	1	2.6	0	0
Total	41	100	7	17

Adapted from Manning FA. The fetus with ventriculomegaly: the fetal surgery registry. In: Harrison MR, Golbus MS, Filly RA (eds). The Unborn Patient, 2nd ed. Philadelphia: WB Saunders, 1991:448–452.

► **TABLE 3-3.** OUTCOME OF FETAL VENTRICULOMEGALY

Reference	Associated Anomalies	Therapeutic Abortion (TAB)	Cephalo- centesis	Peri- natal Deaths	Post- natal Deaths	Survivors	NI	Develop- ment Delayed
Chervenack et al. (1985)	53	84%	14	16	14	15	6	8
Cochrane et al. (1984)	41	75%	0	3	24	14	3	11
Pretorius et al. (1985)	40	70%	9	7	18	6	3	3
Serlo et al. (1986)	38	84%	5	—	23	10	6	4
Nyberg et al. (1987)	61		NA	NA	13	10	NA	NA
Hudgins et al. (1988)	47	74%	15	4	9	19	13	6
Drugan et al. (1989)	43	72%	NA			19		
Rosseau et al. (1991)	40	70%	3	NA	9	28	16	12
Total	280		43	5	17	74	31	32

Adapted from Crombleholme TM. Invasive fetal therapy: current notes and future directions. Semin Perinatol 1994;18:385–397.

listing the incidence as only between 4 and 14% (Cochrane et al. 1984; Holzgreve et al. 1993; Hudgins et al. 1988; Rosseau et al. 1991; Serlo et al. 1986). Interestingly, the most recent report to look at prenatally diagnosed ventriculomegaly found no patients with isolated, rapidly progressive ventriculomegaly among 51 fetuses that might otherwise be candidates for decompression (Rosseau et al. 1991).

Before ventriculoamniotic shunting can be reinstated, selection criteria need to be defined. These criteria would include fetuses with isolated, rapidly progressive ventriculomegaly, normal karyotype, accurate exclusion of other CNS and extra-CNS anomalies, and development of a valved shunt less likely than previous versions to clog or become dislodged. As Rosseau et al.'s 1991 study indicated, prenatally diagnosed isolated progressive ventriculomegaly may be quite rare, and given current diagnostic limitations, appropriate selection of fetuses may not be possible. The use of ultrafast fetal MRI has greatly improved the accuracy of prenatal diagnosis of CNS anomalies and may allow more appropriate patient selection (Bilaniuk 1999). However, as noted by Levitsky et al. (1995) the outcome with isolated aqueductal stenosis is extremely poor. Prenatal intervention may be the only treatment option with the potential to improve neurologic outcome.

Hydronephrosis

The first case of a fetus with obstructive uropathy treated in utero by vesicoamniotic shunting was reported by Golbus et al. in 1982. Advances soon followed in diagnosis, technique, shunt design, and patient selection (Crombleholme et al. 1988, 1991, 1994; Harrison et al. 1991; Johnson et al. 1995; Rodeck et al. 1988). The enthusiasm for treating fetal obstructive uropathy has continued unabated during the past decade. In fact, vesicoamniotic shunting, to a certain extent, has become a victim of its own success. The procedure became widely implemented before stringent selection criteria for treat-

ment were developed and the therapeutic efficacy of the procedure was established. The widespread use of vesicoamniotic shunts also had the effects of shifting cases away from the centers where these questions were being studied and limiting attempts to better define the role of vesicoamniotic shunting in the management of fetal obstructive uropathy.

The International Fetal Surgery Registry was established to help answer several important questions, such as: What are the risks of fetal intervention? and Are they outweighed by the benefits of clearly enhanced survival and quality of life (Manning et al. 1987, 1986)? By June 1987, there were reports on 87 patients with hydronephrosis who had been treated in utero. During the subsequent 7 years, only 11 additional patients had been reported, and any additional information obtained from this database is likely to be limited (Manning FA: personal communication). Although the registry did provide useful information about the feasibility and risks of vesicoamniotic shunting, the limitations of this type of registry, with cases submitted from many centers without uniform indications for procedures and limited follow-up, preclude insight into questions of therapeutic efficacy.

The contributors to the International Fetal Surgery Registry were from 20 centers with experience ranging from only 1 to as many as 30 shunts. The overall survival in this cohort was only 40.2% (Manning et al. 1986). The incidence of chromosomal anomalies in treated patients was 8%. A total of 15% underwent termination of pregnancy either because of chromosomal abnormality or sonographic evidence of renal dysplasia. Among the 74 fetuses not aborted, the survival rate was 47.3%. As noted in Table 3-4, there was a spectrum of underlying causes. Survival correlated with underlying cause, with the best survival observed in fetuses with posterior urethral valves (Table 3-4). The worst survival rate was observed with urethral atresia (16.7%) and renal dysplasia (0%). The procedure-related mortality was 4.7%, approximately half that observed

▶ **TABLE 3-4.** FETAL OBSTRUCTIVE UROPATHY: SURVIVAL ACCORDING TO PRIMARY DIAGNOSIS*

Primary Diagnosis	No. of Cases	Percent Surviving
Posterior urethral valves	25	68
Urethral atresia	6	16.7
"Prune belly" syndrome	5	80
Ureteropelvic junction obstruction	2	100
Unknown etiology	36	30.5
Renal dysplasia	6	0
Karyotype abnormality[†]	7	0
	87	40.2

*Primary diagnosis confirmed by either antenatal or neonatal assessment or biopsy.
[†]All seven had elective termination.

Adapted, with permission, from Manning FA. The fetus with obstructive uropathy: the fetal surgery registry. In: Harrison MR, Golbus MS, Filly RA (eds.). The Unborn Patient, 2nd ed. Philadelphia: WB Saunders: 394–398.

for hydrocephalus and approximately the same as that reported for intrauterine transfusion for fetal anemia during the same period (Bowman and Manning 1983; Clewell 1991; Manning et al. 1986).

The limitations of the registry data are evident from the range of underlying diagnoses. The data represent the work of 20 centers, with no consistent approach to diagnosis and no defined patient selection criteria. Also, the patients were treated in the years 1982 to 1985, prior to the establishment of generally accepted criteria for intervention. Not all patients had oligohydramnios, and some were treated despite preserved amniotic fluid volume. The data reported to the International Fetal Surgery Registry did, however, establish the feasibility of treating obstructive uropathy and helped to define the incidence of associated anomalies and the role of intervention in fetal obstructive uropathy. A series of patients treated with a uniform approach is required to develop and refine selection criteria and establish therapeutic efficacy.

The lack of a prospective randomized trial makes the efficacy of prenatal decompression the most difficult question to address in the treatment of fetal obstructive uropathy. The only series that attempted to address this question, albeit in a retrospective analysis, was reported by Crombleholme et al. (1991). In fetuses predicted to have either good or poor prognoses by fetal urine electrolyte and ultrasound criteria, survival was greater among those who underwent decompression in utero, as opposed to those who did not undergo decompression. In the group of fetuses predicted to have a poor prognosis by selection criteria, 10 were treated. Three of these pregnancies were electively terminated, 4 neonates died from pulmonary hypoplasia or renal dysplasia, and 3 survived. All 3 survivors had restoration of normal amniotic fluid (AF) levels and no pul-

monary complications, but in 2 of the 3, renal failure subsequently developed and the patients have undergone renal transplantation. Among the 14 patients with no intervention, there were no survivors (11 terminations and 3 neonatal deaths from pulmonary hypoplasia).

In the group of fetuses predicted by selection criteria to have a good prognosis, there were 9 fetuses who were treated, 1 elective termination (after the development of procedure-related chorioamnionitis), no deaths, and 8 neonatal survivors. Of the 7 patients in the good-prognosis group who were not treated, 5 survived, and 2 died after birth. Renal failure later developed in two of the survivors.

When oligohydramnios develops during the canalicular stage of lung development (16 to 24 weeks of gestation), the fetus usually has pulmonary hypoplasia that precludes survival (Adzick et al. 1970; Nakayama et al. 1986; Harrison et al. 1982b, 1983a, 1987; Hislop et al. 1979). When in utero intervention for obstructive uropathy associated with oligohydramnios restores amniotic fluid volume, neonatal death from pulmonary hypoplasia is clearly averted (Crombleholme et al. 1991; Golbus et al. 1982). In the group of fetuses reported by Crombleholme et al. (1991), there was a preponderance of oligohydramnios in the poor-prognosis group (23 of 24) as compared with the good-prognosis group (7 of 16). Despite this, fetuses from the good-prognosis group seemed to survive as a direct result of fetal treatment. In the good-prognosis group, 6 of the 7 fetuses with oligohydramnios underwent intervention and all 6 survived with normal renal function. However, the 7th patient, with oligohydramnios that was not treated, died at birth from pulmonary hypoplasia. In the entire series, uncorrected oligohydramnios was associated with a 100% neonatal mortality rate. Normal or restored amniotic fluid volume was associated with a 94% survival rate (Crombleholme et al. 1991).

Although in utero decompression seems to prevent neonatal death from pulmonary hypoplasia, the effect on renal function is less clear. The severity of renal dysplasia at birth depends on the timing and severity of obstruction before birth (Crombleholme et al. 1988, 1991; Harrison et al. 1981a, 1981b, 1982b, 1982c, 1987, 1990a; Manning et al. 1986). Experimental work suggests that relief of obstruction during the most active phase of nephrogenesis (20 to 30 weeks of gestation) may obviate further damage and allow normal nephrogenesis to proceed (Adzick et al. 1970; Beck 1971; Glick et al. 1984a, 1984b; Gonzalez et al. 1985; Harrison et al. 1982b, 1987; Peters et al. 1991, Salinas-Madrigal et al. 1988). The development of postnatal renal failure in two infants who were not treated because amniotic fluid volume remained normal raises the question of whether to treat fetuses with obstruction before oligohydramnios develops. Because renal development or maldevelopment is complete at birth, relief of obstruction in infancy or childhood may not prevent the progression to end-stage renal failure (Warshaw et al. 1982). Müller et al. (1993) reported on a group of fetuses with obstructive uropathy, a favorable prognostic profile, and normal amniotic fluid in whom renal insufficiency developed by 1 year of age. The only feature that distinguished this group of fetuses was a urinary level of β_2-microglobulin greater than 2 mg per liter. Elevated fetal urinary levels of β_2-microglobulin may identify fetuses at increased risk for ongoing renal damage from obstruction, even if amniotic fluid is normal. Other investigators have not found β_2-microglobulin levels to be as useful, and levels greater than 10 mg per liter can be a predictor of poor outcome in fetuses over 20 weeks of gestation (Freedman et al. 1997). It remains an open question whether or not in utero decompression could prevent long-term renal insufficiency in these patients.

The maternal morbidity associated with vesicoamniotic shunting has been reported to be minimal, but there has been a high incidence of chorioamnionitis related to the procedure (14%) (Crombleholme et al. 1991; Glick et al. 1985). These cases of chorioamnionitis occurred before the use of prophylactic antibiotics was routine, and during a period when long-term (4 to 16 hours) bladder catheterization rather than aspiration was used for fetal urine sampling. In addition, there have been reports of shunt-induced abdominal-wall defects with herniation of bowel through trochar stab wounds and maternal ascites from leakage of amniotic fluid into the maternal peritoneal cavity (Manning et al. 1986; Robichaux et al. 1991; Ronderos-Dumit et al. 1991).

The utility of vesicoamniotic shunts is limited by the brief duration of decompression, the risk of infection, the risk of catheter obstruction or dislodgment, fetal injury during placement, and potentially inadequate decompression of the fetal urinary tract (Crombleholme et al. 1988, 1991; Estes and Harrison 1993; Glick et al. 1985). These factors make vesicoamniotic shunts inappropriate for long-term decompression of the urinary tract early in gestation and are the impetus for development of open fetal surgical and fetoscopic techniques to treat obstructive uropathy in utero (Crombleholme et al. 1988; Estes and Harrison 1993).

Fetal Hydrothorax

There are two forms of treatment available for fetal hydrothorax (FHT) before 32 weeks of gestation: thoracoamniotic shunting and thoraco-maternal-cutaneous drainage (see Chapter 39). Thoracentesis is a diagnostic maneuver to obtain pleural fluid for differential cell count and culture and to establish whether the effusion is chylous. But even repeated thoracentesis provides inadequate decompression of the fetal chest. There have been several reports of thoracentesis for FHT, performed with either complete resolution or a good outcome de-

spite reaccumulation (Benacerraf et al. 1989; Kurjak et al. 1985; Petres et al. 1982). Others have had disappointing results with repeated thoracentesis for FHT, because of rapid reaccumulation of the effusion and neonatal death from respiratory insufficiency (Longaker et al. 1989; Nicolaides and Azar 1990). Spontaneous resolution of FHT may occur in as many as 10% of cases, and resolution following thoracentesis may or may not be related to the procedure. Thoracentesis alone cannot adequately decompress the fetal chest to allow pulmonary expansion and prevent pulmonary hypoplasia (Laberge et al. 1991).

Thoracoamniotic shunting for FHT, first reported by Rodeck et al. in 1988, provides continuous decompression of the fetal chest, allowing lung expansion. If instituted early enough, this allows compensatory lung growth and prevents neonatal death from pulmonary hypoplasia. Nicolaides and Azar (1990) reported on 48 cases of thoracoamniotic shunting, but there was no attempt to distinguish isolated primary FHT from secondary FHT. Despite intervention, mortality was high. Four of the deaths were due to termination of pregnancy when a chromosomal abnormality was diagnosed. In addition, there were 12 neonatal deaths despite thoracoamniotic shunt placement, but these fetuses seemed to have severe hydrops and secondary FHT. Two fetuses that died in utero also seemed to have had secondary FHT and severe hydrops. If the cases that appear to be secondary FHT are eliminated, the survival of isolated primary FHT treated with thoracoamniotic shunting is 38 of 41 (92%) cases (Moran et al. 1994; Nicolaides and Azar 1990). A similar survival rate with thoracoamniotic shunting was found by Hagay et al. (1993) in their review of fetal pleural effusions. This is a striking improvement when compared with a survival of only 50% in untreated FHT.

The indications for thoracoamniotic shunting are not well defined. Most authors consider the presence of FHT-induced hydrops or polyhydramnios as indications for shunting (Longaker et al. 1989; Nicolaides and Azar 1990; Rodeck et al. 1988). In addition, we recommend thoracoamniotic shunting for primary FHT with evidence of effusion under tension even in the absence of hydrops (Moran et al. 1994). Because spontaneous resolution has been observed even in severe cases of FHT, we reserve thoracoamniotic shunting for cases in which tension hydrothorax recurs after two thoracenteses. The two currently available catheters are the Harrison double-pigtail catheter (VPI Company, Spenser, IN) and the KCH catheter (Rocket USA Inc., Branford, CN) (Fig. 3-1). We have had excellent results with the Rocket catheter, which has the advantage of having the pigtails at 90 degrees to each other so that the outer coil sits flush against the fetal chest.

Another therapeutic option is thoraco-maternal-cutaneous drainage, as reported by Roberts et al. (1986).

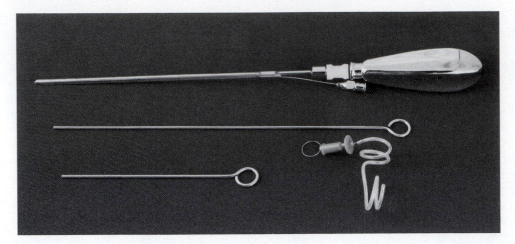

Figure 3-1. The trochar used for KCH catheter insertion, including the obturators and sheath with the KCH catheter for scale. Note the KCH catheter with the pigtail ends at 90 degrees to each other.

Adapting a technique first used for intraperitoneal blood transfusions by Liggins (1986), a catheter is inserted into the fetal pleural cavity. In the single case reported, the chylothorax was successfully decompressed and external drainage was maintained for 7 days, with complete resolution. The catheter was subsequently removed, and the neonatal outcome was good. The advantages of this technique include avoidance of possible repeated shunt insertions, and allowing irrigation of the catheter should it become clogged. Although no adverse effects were reported, there remains a significant risk of infection, dislodgment by the fetus, and cord entanglement.

The limited experience with thoracoamniotic shunting suggests that it is extremely effective in decompressing effusion and improving survival. The risks to mother and fetus of thoracentesis and shunt placement have been minimal and are far outweighed by the potential benefits. Few complications have been reported for either fetal thoracentesis or thoracoamniotic shunts. There has been only one procedure-related fetal death, due to torsion of the umbilical cord thought to be related to thoracentesis (Longaker et al. 1989). One case of migration of the shunt under the fetal skin has been reported, but required no intervention when the infant was born (Rodeck et al. 1988). There have been no maternal complications reported with either thoracentesis or thoracoamniotic shunting. However, it should be recognized that these procedures have the potential for significant complications, including infection, bleeding, premature rupture of membranes, preterm labor, and injury to the fetus (Moran et al. 1994).

Miscellaneous Procedures and Other Indications for Shunts

Small ovarian cysts are common in neonates. They are typically small follicular cysts due to maternal hormonal stimulation and are rarely clinically significant. They usually regress spontaneously (Kirkinen and Jouppila 1985). The prenatal diagnosis of an ovarian cyst should be considered in any female fetus with a cystic pelvic mass (see Chapter 83). Although they can be mistaken for mesenteric cysts, duplications, urachal cysts, or choledochal cysts, ovarian cysts are usually simple pelvic cysts that disappear shortly after delivery. Occasionally, these cysts require surgery for complications due to size, rupture, or torsion (Kirkinen and Jouppila 1985; Kurjak et al. 1984). Once an ovarian cyst becomes symptomatic, salvage of the ovary is unlikely.

Valenti and coworkers were the first to perform cyst decompression in utero, in 1975. A large (7 by 9 cm) ovarian cyst was aspirated to prevent intrapartum cyst rupture. Landrum et al. (1986) reported fetal ovarian cyst aspiration ostensibly to prevent pulmonary hypoplasia. While pulmonary hypoplasia from a pelvic mass is unlikely, aspiration to prevent in utero rupture or torsion and to preserve ovarian tissue is a more appropriate indication for treatment. Holzgreve et al. (1993) have reported their experience with 13 cases of fetal ovarian cysts. This group recommends ovarian cyst decompression to preserve the ovary, especially if the cyst is large, rapidly increasing in size, or observed to be a "wandering mass." Cysts exhibiting these features are more likely to undergo torsion. Cyst tap revealing high levels of prostaglandin F21, progesterone, and testosterone in the fluid confirms the diagnosis. Giorlandino et al. (1990) have reported a case of ovarian cyst treated by cyst aspiration and sclerosis with tetracycline. While this treatment was successful, the use of tetracycline as a sclerosing agent in the fetus is not advised. This group has subsequently reported success in four cases of simple cyst aspiration (Giorlandino et al. 1993). Similarly, D'Addario (1990) aspirated ovarian cysts in two fetuses, but neonatal surgery was still needed. Crombleholme et al. have suggested criteria for intervention in fetal ovarian cysts with diameters of >4 cm, increasing 1 cm per week in size, or as Holzgreve suggested, noted to wander about the abdomen (Crombleholme et al. 1997). Although fetal ovarian cyst decompression seems a relatively benign procedure with the potential for ovarian preservation, the indications for fetal intervention are not uniformly accepted.

In 1987 Nicolaides et al. reported the first case of cystic adenomatoid malformation of the lung (CCAM) treated by shunt insertion in utero. Decompression of a large type I CCAM in a 20-week-old fetus by percutaneous placement of a thoracoamniotic shunt was subsequently reported by Clark in 1988. This procedure resulted in resolution of both mediastinal shift and hydrops and successful delivery at 37 weeks of gestation. Postnatally, the infant underwent uneventful resection of the CCAM. Three subsequent cases of thoracoamniotic shunting in CCAM have been reported by Adzick et al. with a good outcome in two of the three fetuses treated (Adzick 1993; Adzick et al. 1993). These five cases were unusual for CCAM, as they were large cysts resulting in hydrops. More commonly, it is the type III CCAM, or microcystic lesions, that become enlarged, resulting in hydrops and intrauterine fetal death. In these latter cases open fetal surgery and resection are indicated. However, in the rare instances in which there is a single large cyst in CCAM responsible for hydrops, thoracoamniotic shunting appears to be an appropriate treatment option (see Chapter 37).

▶ FETAL CARDIAC PROCEDURES

Fetal Arrhythmias

Fetal arrhythmias are most often ventricular extrasystoles or tachyarrhythmias (see Chapter 54). But bradyarrhythmias account for 9% of cases reported to the Fetal Arrhythmia Registry, half of which occur in structurally normal hearts due to transplacental passage of antibody in mothers with collagen vascular disease (Kleinman and Evans 1988) (see Chapter 44). The other half occur in structurally abnormal hearts, and bradyarrhythmia is almost uniformly fatal in that setting (Kleinman et al. 1982; Stewart et al. 1983). In structurally normal hearts in which complete heart block (CHB) develops in mothers with collagen vascular disease, hydrops will develop in 25%, usually refractory to medical therapy (Altenburger et al. 1977; Carpenter et al. 1986; Machado et al. 1988). If low-output fetal heart failure cannot be reversed by increasing heart rate with β-agonists then fetal cardiac pacing is the only alternative. Carpenter et al. (1986) reported the first fetus treated by implantation of a percutaneous transthoracic pacemaker. Unfortunately, the fetus was severely hydropic and despite successful ventricular capture and

pacing the fetus died within hours. The obvious problems with the percutaneous transthoracic pacemaker are the risks of dislodgment, potential for infection (chorioamnionitis), and the temporary nature of the device in a fetus that will require pacing for the rest of gestation. These limitations prompted a group led by Michael Harrison at UCSF to attempt pacemaker placement by open fetal surgery (Harrison et al. 1993b). Previous work by Crombleholme et al. at this same laboratory had developed the techniques for fetal cardiac pacing and studied the effects of complete heart block in fetal lambs (Crombleholme et al. 1990, 1991). Based on this experimental work, Harrison and coworkers placed a unipolar epicardial pacemaker in a fetus at 22 weeks of gestation with complete heart block and hydrops (Harrison et al. 1993b). Similar to Carpenter et al.'s (1986) experience, although able to achieve ventricular capture and pacing, the heart was irreversibly damaged by 6 weeks of in utero cardiac failure and the procedure was followed by fetal death (Harrison et al. 1993b). It is clear from these two reports that a fetus with CHB and severe hydrops may be unsalvageable. The survival of fetuses with CHB and ventricular escape rates of less than 50 beats per minute is poor (Schmidt et al. 1991). Placement of a pacemaker in the fetus with a ventricular response rate of less than 50 beats per minute before the development of hydrops may allow us to save these otherwise doomed fetuses.

Structural Fetal Heart Disease

Structural cardiac defects, such as pulmonic atresia with an intact ventricular septum (PAIVS) or severe aortic stenosis (AS) (see Chapters 42 and 52), may result in obstruction to blood flow, which in turn alters the development of the heart chambers as well as the pulmonic and systemic vasculature in utero (Vlahakes et al. 1981). The major morbidity from these congenital heart defects often results from the secondary alterations in heart development caused by the primary defect (i.e., hypoplasia of the right ventricle in PAIVS or hypoplastic left heart in AS). In theory, relief of the anatomic obstruction in utero may allow more normal cardiac development, thereby eliminating the need for corrective surgery postnatally.

Aortic stenosis diagnosed prenatally is associated with intrauterine fetal death or neonatal death in fetuses that survive to term. Maxwell et al. (1991) reported a series of 28 fetuses diagnosed prenatally with AS either alone or associated with endocardial fibroblastosis. Only 12 mothers continued the pregnancy to term, and in 2 there was an intrauterine fetal death. None of the 10 neonates survived despite balloon valvuloplasty in 4 of them. Maxwell and coworkers also noted that in 4 fetuses the left ventricle failed to grow, resulting in hypoplastic left heart, which would make the neonate unsuitable for postnatal aortic valve reconstruction. This grim natural history for fetuses with prenatally detected AS prompted Maxwell and colleagues (1991) to attempt the first in utero aortic balloon valvuloplasty. This procedure is performed by direct percutaneous puncture of the left ventricle under ultrasound guidance. A J wire is passed through the stenotic valve, and the balloon catheter is passed over the wire and inflated. All three fetuses treated with this procedure survived to term; two died as neonates and one is doing well at 3 years of age (Maxwell et al. 1991). Two other fetuses were treated unsuccessfully by this technique by another group (Chouri et al. 1994).

Wright et al. (1994) have performed radiofrequency pulmonic valvotomy in a fetus with PAIVS. In the most severe forms of PAIVS, the primary valvular lesion causes secondary alteration in the intracardiac flow pattern, resulting in a hypoplastic right ventricle (Casteneda et al. 1994). In these instances, only palliative pulmonary valvotomy and systemic pulmonary artery shunting can be performed. However, if flow can be reestablished across the pulmonic valve in utero, restoration of intracardiac blood flow may allow subsequent growth of the right ventricle and pulmonary outflow tract. In a 26-week-old fetus with PAIVS, no growth was observed in the right ventricle during 6 weeks of in utero observation. By direct puncture of the right ventricle, a pulmonary valvotomy was performed using a radiofrequency ablation catheter. Although only a minute hole with insignificant flow resulted, this procedure and those reported by Maxwell and Chouri and colleagues have established the feasibility of in utero treatment of structural heart disease. Several centers are actively developing experimental techniques, both by catheter and open fetal surgery to correct structural heart defects in utero (Hanley 1994).

These procedures are certainly not without risk. One of Maxwell's patients died within hours of the procedure and pieces of balloon and guide wire were left within the fetal heart of the other. All three centers have noted pericardial effusions at the conclusion of the procedure, which needed to be evacuated. Despite the risk of these procedures, the dismal outcome for the fetuses with these structural heart defects argues in favor of continued efforts at developing safe and effective invasive fetal therapies.

▶ FETAL SURGERY

Experience has demonstrated the utility of shunting procedures in some fetal conditions, but the limitations of these catheters have also become apparent. In addition to problems with obstruction, dislodgment, and short functional life span, it is evident that for many conditions shunting procedures are not adequate. The experience with open fetal surgery in the 1960s for the treatment of erythroblastosis fetalis was discouraging and was abandoned upon the introduction of percutaneous techniques of fetal transfusion (Asensio et al. 1966; Freda et al. 1964; Liley 1963). In 1982 Harrison et al. introduced open fetal surgery for the treatment of obstructive uropathy (Harrison et al. 1982a). While the procedure (bilateral ureterostomy) was technically successful, the fetus made no urine, oligohydramnios persisted, and the infant died of pulmonary hypoplasia (Table 3-5). Despite this initial unsuccessful result, a new era in fetal therapy was entered. Soon, successful open surgical procedures were reported in the treatment of obstructive uropathy (Crombleholme et al. 1988), congenital diaphragmatic hernia (Harrison et al. 1990c; Harrison and Adzick 1990a, 1993), cystic adenomatoid malformation (Adzick et al. 1993; Harrison et al. 1990b), and sacrococcygeal teratoma (Adzick et al. 1997). An appreciation of the fetal natural history of these conditions and the success of the UCSF group encouraged groups in Philadelphia, Boston, Denver, and Detroit in

---

▶ TABLE 3-5. FETAL MALFORMATIONS TREATABLE BY FETOSCOPIC TECHNIQUES

Fetal Malformation	Fetal Presentation	Fetal/Neonatal Consequences
Posterior urethral valves	Hydronephrosis and oligohydramnios	Renal dysplasia and renal insufficiency Pulmonary hypoplasia
Twin–twin transfusion	Oligohydramnios/polyhydramnios	IUFD, MLE, IUGR
Acephalic-acardiac twin syndrome: Fetoscopic cord ligation Fetoscopic laser ablation Fetoscopic guided cord injection	Polyhydramnios	IUFD, hydrops, cardiac failure Multifocal leukoencephalomalacia
Potential applications Myelomeningocele	Myelomeningocele	Neurologic deficit, hydrocephalus
Amniotic band syndrome	Isolated extremity amniotic bond	Limb amputation
Diaphragmatic hernia	Severe herniation	Pulmonary hypoplosia
Sacrococcygeal teratoma	High output cardiac failure	IUFD; polyhydramnios, preterm labor

IUFD = intrauterine fetal death; MLE = multifocal leukoencephalomalacia; IUGR = intrauterine growth retardation.

the United States as well as in Seoul, Korea; Melbourne, Australia; and Paris, France, to undertake open fetal surgery. Clinical experience is still quite limited, however, with just over 200 cases of open fetal surgery having been performed worldwide.

Embryoscopy and fetoscopy have been used as diagnostic tools since the late 1960s. More recently, they have been used to guide chorionic villus sampling, as well as fetal skin and fetal liver biopsies (see Chapter 2) (Elias 1987; Hahnemann and Mohr 1968; Rodeck et al. 1982). The limitations of the initial fetoscopic procedures were largely related to the primitive optics and instrumentation available at the time. The recent surge in operative laparoscopy has kindled rapid technical advances in optics and instrumentation (Sackier 1992). These advances are illustrated by a report detailing the usefulness of transabdominal fetoscopy in a case of Meckel–Gruber syndrome, in which a diagnosis could not be made by ultrasound examination (Quintero et al. 1993).

The same technologic advances that have made minimally invasive videoendoscopic surgery possible in children and adults offer the potential for minimally invasive fetal surgery (Estes et al. 1992a, 1992b). The small uterine puncture sites required for fetoscopic surgery would, in theory, obviate the morbidity of a large hysterotomy. Specifically, the fetoscopic approach could reduce the risks of preterm labor, hemorrhage, amniotic fluid leak, and uterine rupture and also eliminate the need for cesarean delivery following fetal surgery.

The first experimental work employing the use of fetoscopic surgery was reported by Estes et al. in a model of obstructive uropathy (Estes et al. 1992b). The model was created by ligating the urethra and urachus at 75 days of gestation in fetal lambs. One week later, using the fetoscopic technique, a vesicocutaneous fistula was created by placement of an 8-mm wall stent to effect bladder decompression. This same group has also reported fetoscopic repair of cleft lip in a sheep model in order to take advantage of the unique wound-healing properties of the fetus (Estes et al. 1992a). These initial reports have stimulated similar experimental efforts in other laboratories in developing fetoscopic techniques. Luks et al. (1996) have studied the effects of carbon dioxide (CO_2) insufflation during fetoscopy, documenting significant fetal acidosis as a result. Areas currently under active investigation include studies of the effects of bright light and lasers on the developing fetal eye and optimal techniques of port placement to prevent bleeding and amniotic fluid leak.

Bealer et al. (1995) have reported the use of polymeric foam to "plug the lung until it grows" (PLUG) in a fetal lamb model of congenital diaphragmatic hernia. Although this group performed this by open techniques in fetal lambs, they described how it could easily be performed fetoscopically. Peers et al. (1994) reported their

work with fetal tracheoscopy and described preliminary results with endoluminal tracheal PLUG placement using silicone as a tracheal cast. At the same meeting, Deprest et al. (1994) reported results of first studies of the effects of endoscopic light on the fetal lamb retina.

In addition to adapting fetoscopic techniques to treat conditions currently approached by shunt or open fetal surgery, fetoscopy has the potential to expand the range of fetal intervention (see Table 3-5). Copeland et al. (1993) have developed a fetal sheep model of myelomeningocele that is treated by fetoscopic placement of skin grafts over the neural-tube defect to exclude amniotic fluid and minimize damage to the spinal cord. Crombleholme et al. developed a fetal lamb model of amniotic band syndrome and studied the affected limb's response to fetoscopic release of bands (Crombleholme et al. 1995; Dirkes et al. 1994). Sylvester et al. (1997) have reported the use of fetoscopic tracheoscopy for adenoviral vector delivery in fetal lambs for organ-specific gene therapy. This technique was aimed at developing an in utero gene therapy treatment strategy for surfactant protein B deficiency, for which there is currently no effective therapy short of lung transplantation.

As has been the case during many stages of the development of fetal surgery, because of the pressing need for innovative therapies in fetal disease, clinical application has preceded completion of extensive animal experimentation. Quintero and colleagues (1994) at Hutzel Hospital have used fetoscopic surgical techniques in the treatment of fetuses with obstructive uropathy and the twin-reversed arterial perfusion (TRAP) sequence (see below). Building on previous experience with diagnostic fetoscopy in human fetuses, this group treated a fetus with obstructive uropathy (Quintero et al. 1995). At 26 weeks of gestation, a male fetus with posterior urethral valves underwent fetal cystoscopy and valve ablation using guide wire electrocautery. While this procedure was technically successful, with ablation of valves and restoration of amniotic fluid volume, insufficient attention was given to patient selection. The infant had renal failure at birth, which should have been evident from fetal urine electrolyte analysis prenatally.

Twin-Reversed Arterial Perfusion (TRAP Sequence)

Twin-reversed arterial perfusion (TRAP sequence) occurs only in the setting of a monochorionic pregnancy. It complicates approximately 1% of monochorionic twin gestations, with an incidence of 1 in 35,000 births (James 1977). In the TRAP sequence, the acardiac/acephalic twin receives all of its blood supply from the normal, so-called pump twin. The term *reversed perfusion* is used to describe this scenario as blood enters the acardiac/acephalic twin through its umbilical artery and exits through the umbilical vein. Because the abnormal circulation in TRAP sequence places an increased demand on the heart of the pump twin, cardiac failure is the primary concern in TRAP sequence. If left untreated, the pump twin dies in 50 to 70% of cases. This is especially true when the acardiac/acephalic twin is greater than 50% of the size of the pump twin by estimated weight (Moore et al. 1990).

It is important to exclude chromosomal abnormality prior to offering a fetoscopic procedure in TRAP sequence. The incidence of chromosomal abnormality in the pump twin in TRAP sequence is 9% (Van Allen et al. 1983). Fifty-one percent of these pregnancies are complicated by polyhydramnios and 75% by preterm labor (Healey et al. 1994). The difference in fetal weight between the twins is predictive of outcome. A ratio of the weight of the acardius to that of the pump twin >50% predicts death of the pump twin in 64% of cases (Moore et al. 1990). If this ratio is >75%, the mortality rate for the pump twin is 90%.

Techniques of sectio parva (selective removal of anomalous twin) (Robie et al. 1989) and ultrasound-guided embolization (Porreco et al. 1991) have been used in an attempt to interrupt the vascular connection between the perfused and pump twin. Both of these procedures have associated morbidity and the unreliable outcome led to the development of fetoscopic approaches to the problem. McCurdy et al. was the first to report a case of fetoscopic cord ligation in TRAP sequence performed at 19 weeks of gestation (McCurdy et al. 1993). The pump twin demonstrated significant decompensation despite conservative measures, and difficulty in visualizing umbilical vessels using ultrasound precluded the use of a percutaneous embolization. The patient was offered a fetoscopic approach to this problem, and the acardiac twin's umbilical cord was successfully ligated, but only after the pump twin's cord was ligated and then released when the error was recognized. However, the pump twin had persistent bradycardia and was noted to be dead on ultrasound examination one day after the operation.

Quintero et al. (1994) reported the first successful umbilical-cord ligation for TRAP sequence. The procedure was performed at 19 weeks of gestation using two 12-gauge trocars and a 1.9-mm endoscope. The cord was successfully ligated, and despite some mild uterine irritability postoperatively, the patient did well. Three weeks after the procedure the mother presented with leakage of amniotic fluid that resolved on its own, and the pregnancy continued until 36 weeks of gestation. A healthy boy was delivered after spontaneous labor.

A total of 15 cases of umbilical-cord ligation have now been reported in the literature (Cromblehome et al. 1996; McCurdy et al. 1993; Quintero et al. 1994, 1996;

Willcourt et al. 1995). Ten children survived (67%) without a neurologic deficit. An additional seven cases were treated by umbilical-cord laser coagulation (Arias et al. 1998). The most common complication was the development of premature rupture of membranes (PROM). It is possible that this complication occurred because of the proximity of the placement of the two ports used during the procedure.

In the past 3 years, we have evaluated eight pregnancies complicated by TRAP sequence and fetoscopically treated three. In the first case, the edematous acardius was 200% of the size of the pump twin, with early signs of cardiac decompensation. The size of the acardius precluded an entirely fetoscopic approach, and the cord was ligated with a fetoscopically assisted approach via a 2-cm hysterotomy. The mother delivered a normal infant at 38 weeks of gestation. The second TRAP sequence case was treated by fetoscopic cord ligation at 26 weeks of gestation in an acardius that was 70% of the size of the pump twin. The procedure was technically successful; however, immediately postoperatively preterm labor and cervical changes developed. Preterm labor could not be controlled, and she delivered the acardius and pump twin on postoperative day three. The pump twin subsequently died of respiratory complications related to prematurity. The last case of TRAP sequence was unusual in that the pregnancy was monoamniotic, which occurs in only 25% of cases of TRAP sequence. At presentation at 14 weeks of gestation the size of the acardius was already >70% of the size of the normal pump twin. Because of the ongoing risk of cord entanglement, the cord could not be simply ligated or coagulated, but in addition it had to be cut. Using an entirely percutaneous technique, under combined ultrasonographic and fetoscopic control the cord of the acardius was coagulated using a 3-mm bipolar grasper (Everest Medical Corp., Minneapolis, Minn.) and the cord was cut. The pump twin continues to do well now.

Twin–Twin Transfusion Syndrome

Twin–twin transfusion syndrome (TTTS), or oligohydramnios/polyhydramnios sequence, is a rare syndrome that occurs at an estimated rate of 0.1 to 0.9 in 1000 births. However, this diagnosis can carry an extremely poor prognosis and may be responsible for 15 to 17% of perinatal death in twins. TTTS occurs in the setting of monochorionic twin gestations.

It is estimated that 85% of monochorionic placentas have anomalous vascular connections; however, only 5 to 10% have sufficient imbalance to produce TTTS (Newton 1986). It is also believed that the number of vascular anastomoses as well as the type of anastomoses within a placenta determines if TTTS develops.

The natural history of this disorder has a 60 to 100% mortality for both twins in the most severe cases (Bebbington et al. 1995; Benirschke et al. 1973; Cheschier et al. 1988; Rausen et al. 1965). The most severely affected pregnancies usually present earlier in gestation, with signs of TTTS occurring prior to 20 weeks of gestation. Mothers commonly present during the second trimester of pregnancy with an acute increase in abdominal girth, discomfort, and occasionally respiratory distress or preterm labor. Physical examination reveals tense polyhydramnios. Early presentation prior to 20 weeks of gestation, however, is usually asymtomatic and diagnosis is usually a serendipitous finding on routine ultrasound.

Diagnostic criteria for TTTS include monochorionicity (chorionicity is best determined during the first trimester and is more difficult to determine during the second trimester), a marked discordance in amniotic fluid volume between the twins (thus the term *oligo/poly sequence*), a size discordance with the larger twin in the polyhydramniotic sac, and like-sex twins and a single placental mass (Brennen et al. 1982; Wittman et al. 1981). The most characteristic finding is the presence of a "stuck twin." The larger recipient twin has a large bladder and a polyhydramniotic sac, while the smaller donor twin has a small bladder and is stuck against the uterine wall in an oligohydramniotic sac. The diagnosis of a "stuck twin" can occur from causes other than TTTS, and premature rupture of membranes, placental insufficiency, urinary tract or other structural abnormalities, chromosomal anomalies, and infectious causes should also be ruled out.

Initially, the twins present with a growth discrepancy seen on ultrasound between the larger recipient twin and the growth-restricted donor twin. It is not uncommon for the donor twin to have a velamentous umbilical-cord insertion, which may exacerbate the growth discrepancy. The volume stress on the recipient heart in TTTS often leads to cardiac changes. Cardiomyopathy may develop in the recipient, causing ventricular dysfunction that culminates in fetal hydrops. These cardiac changes include ventricular hypertrophy, tricuspid valvular insufficiency, and in advanced cases, akinetic right ventricle as well as pulmonic valvular insufficiency (Zosmer et al. 1994). Co-twin demise can occur as the fetal hydrops worsens. The surviving co-twin is at risk for severe neurologic injury due to vascular resistance changes with ischemic neurologic events. The surviving co-twin is also at risk for concomitant demise in 4 to 10% of cases (Oglowstein et al. 1993; Fusi et al. 1990).

Several treatment options exist for TTTS, including medical therapy, serial amnioreduction, amniotic septostomy, and fetoscopic approaches. Experience with medical therapy has been anecdotal, with case reports of resolution of TTTS with either digoxin or indomethacin therapy (DeLia et al. 1985a; Roman et al. 1995). These therapies have not been widely accepted or applied to patients diagnosed with TTTS.

Serial amnioreduction is one of the most commonly used and widely accepted therapies for TTTS. Its mechanism of action is unknown but appears to prolong gestation in addition to improving uteroplacental blood flow. Advocates of this therapy believe that amnioreduction increases the survival rate as compared to the natural history of TTTS and with comparable survival to that observed with laser therapy (Elliott et al. 1991). The major criticism of amnioreduction is that it does not prevent the neurologic complications of TTTS.

Amniotic septostomy has been intentionally performed in a small number of cases (Soade et al. 1995). Proponents of amniotic septostomy report equilibrium of amniotic fluid volumes between the two fetuses that lasts for the duration of pregnancy. Although the mechanism of amniotic septostomy is unclear, its success may be related to its effects on fetoplacental hemodynamics. We speculate that amniotic septostomy allows amniotic fluid to cross into the "stuck" twin's sac, resulting in a fluid bolus as the amniotic fluid is imbibed by the fetus. It is likely that cases of amnioreduction that are successful in restoring amniotic fluid volume after just one or two amnioreductions are due to unintentional and unrecognized septostomy. An interesting observation is that TTTS does not seem to occur in monochorionic monoamniotic pregnancies, perhaps for the same reason that amniotic septostomy works. However, as with serial amnioreduction, amniotic septostomy would not be expected to prevent the neurologic sequelae in the event of death of the co-twin. In addition, if too large a septostomy is performed, the twins will be at risk for cord entanglement.

Fetoscopic Laser Ablation

Fetoscopic laser ablation as a treatment for TTTS was initially described by DeLia et al. in 1990. Experimental work in both sheep and rhesus monkey models demonstrated the efficacy of fetoscopic laser ablation using a neodymium: YAG laser prior to its use in the first three cases reported in 1990 (DeLia et al. 1985b, 1989). The three women were treated at 18.5, 22, and 22.5 weeks of gestation after presenting with acute polyhydramnios. Two of the three procedures were uneventful, but one was complicated by a placental vessel perforation. The first two delivered at 27 and 34 weeks due to premature rupture of membranes. In the third patient severe preeclampsia developed at 29 weeks, necessitating delivery. Four of the six infants survived.

A follow-up to these initial cases was published in 1995 (DeLia et al. 1995). DeLia and colleagues reported on 26 patients treated by a fetoscopic approach. Inclusion criteria were ultrasonographic findings consistent with TTTS, posterior placental implantation, gestational age <25 weeks, and clinical hydramnios. The treated patients had a mean gestational age of 20.8 weeks (range, 18 to 24). One patient had surviving triplets, 8 had surviving twins, 9 had a single survivor (2 neonatal and 7 fetal deaths), and 8 had no survivors (all had pregnancy loss within 3 weeks of treatment). The cases with survivors were delivered for obstetric reasons at a mean of 32.2 weeks (range, 26 to 37). Fifty-three percent (28 of 53) of fetuses survived with 96% (27 of 28) demonstrating normal development at a mean of 35.8 months (range, 1 to 68).

A similar experience was reported by Ville et al. (1995). Forty-five women were treated at a median gestational age of 21 weeks (range, 15 to 28). The total number of fetuses surviving to delivery was also 53%. Among the survivors, the median gestational age at delivery was 35 weeks (range, 25 to 40); the median interval between treatment and delivery was 14 weeks (range, 0 to 21). All of the survivors were developing normally at a median age of 12 months (range, 2 to 24).

Some have argued that the vessels on the chorionic plate are only part of the chorioangiopagus and that more vascular connections occur deep within the cotyledon of the placenta. Quintero et al. (1998) have reported a technique of selective photocoagulation for TTTS to address these deep communications. The placental surface is fetoscopically inspected for what have been called nonparticipating vessels (NPVs) and truly participating vessels (TPVs) as well as for the dividing membrane. NPVs are paired vessels with an artery entering a cotyledon and a vein returning to the same umbilical cord. In contrast, a TPV is one that leaves the umbilical cord of the donor headed toward the vascular equator. But TPVs have no vein returning from the cotyledon. The vein draining the cotyledon can be seen on the other side of the vascular equator heading back to the umbilical cord of the recipient fetus. Vessels that are TPVs and cross this membrane are then photocoagulated by an operative endoscope (Quintero et al. 1998). It is unlikely, however, that sufficient pressure could be transmitted across these deep communications within the cotyledons to account for ischemic injury seen in surviving co-twins on fetal death. While these vessels may contribute to TTTS, they are unlikely to be responsible for all of its morbidity.

At the Center for Fetal Diagnosis and Treatment at the Children's Hospital of Philadelphia we have evaluated 19 cases of TTTS and developed an algorithm to assist with the management of the most severely affected TTTS pregnancies presenting prior to 20 weeks of gestation. An extensive workup that includes amniocentesis of both sacs, karyotype analysis, ultrasound examination with amniofusion as needed, echocardio-graphy, and TORCH titers are performed to rule out other anomalies and causes of growth discordance. Once the diagnosis of TTTS is confirmed by exclusion and preserved cardiac function is demonstrated on echocardiography, initial amnioreduction and amniotic septostomy is performed. If cardiac compromise is noted at the time of diagnosis or any time during treatment, fetoscopic cord coagulation is offered. If fluid volume normalizes and the growth discordance stabilizes, the patient is closely followed. If the growth discordance progresses despite restoration of amniotic fluid volume, or if hemodynamic changes develop on Doppler velocimetry, then fetoscopic laser photocoagulation is offered. Comprehensive family counseling is provided prior to offering either fetoscopic cord coagulation or laser ablation based on the specific situation.

As mentioned in the management of anomalous co-twin, several reports in the literature have demonstrated the efficacy of umbilical-cord ligation or coagulation (McCurdy et al. 1993; Quintero et al. 1994). Although this approach has been primarily applied to the management of acardiac/acephalic twin gestations, it is possible to apply either method to the management of TTTS. We have performed a cord coagulation at the Center for Fetal Diagnosis and Treatment for TTTS using a percutaneous fetoscopic approach. An extensive workup revealed a normal karyotype and anatomically normal twins. However, echocardiographic evaluation of the recipient twin revealed an akinetic right ventricle, reversal of flow in the ductus arteriosus, pulmonic valve insufficiency, and reversal of flow in the umbilical-artery Doppler waveforms. This pattern, previously reported in severe TTTS, suggested that this recipient twin was premorbid and that laser coagulation would not be indicated (D'Alton et al. 1995; Audley et al. 1996). While laser photocoagulation would prevent neurologic injury in the stuck twin, it might result in unequal separation of placental mass. This could result in the recipient's dying from cardiac decompensation and the stuck twin from placental insufficiency. Cord coagulation of the premorbid recipient twin offered the advantage of preserving the entire placental mass for the donor twin. Fetoscopic cord coagulation was offered to the patient after five amnioreductions were performed if the stuck twin had not shown improvement and the recipient twin showed clear progression in echocardiographic findings. The case went uneventfully and the patient was discharged home the following day. A healthy infant was delivered at 36 weeks of gestation without signs of neurologic impairment.

Our approach to TTTS differs from that of other groups in that we believe that the treatment should be targeted to the specific conditions of the individual twins. A sequential approach incorporating amnioreduction, amniotic septostomy, fetoscopic laser photocoagulation, and fetoscopic cord coagulation is used as indicated by the amniotic fluid volumes, growth discordance, Doppler velocimetry, and echocardiographic findings.

In monochorionic twin gestations the death of one twin may result in devastating neurologic injury in the surviving twin (Eglowstein et al. 1993; Enbom et al. 1985; Fusi et al. 1990). Crombleholme et al. (1996) reported the first successful application of fetoscopic cord ligation to prevent neurologic injury in a surviving twin. The shared placental circulation of monochorionic twins predisposes a surviving fetus to significant neurologic injury in the event of the death of its twin. The most common neurologic injury is severe multifocal leuko-encephalomalacia, which is secondary to acute ischemia caused by a sudden drop in resistance across the placenta with bleeding into the circulation of the recently deceased twin (D'Alton et al. 1984; Dudley et al. 1986). If the death of a twin could be anticipated, then umbilical cord ligation may prevent neurologic injury to the surviving twin. One twin was structurally normal, but fetal echocardiography performed in the other twin revealed severe congenital heart disease consisting of hypoplastic left heart syndrome associated with severe ventricular dysfunction, marked left ventricular endocardial fibroelastosis, and severe tricuspid regurgitation, as well as pericardial effusion and other early signs of nonimmune hydrops. Together these findings indicated imminent fetal death. The patient underwent an uncomplicated fetoscopic cord ligation. The surviving twin was neurologically normal at birth, 10 weeks after the procedure, and at 1 year of age. Our experience with fetoscopic surgery has shown that pledgeted purse-string sutures are effective in uterine closure and prevention of amniotic fluid leakage. Unlike open fetal surgery, the small puncture sites used in this approach did not preclude normal vaginal delivery. The level I rapid infusion device was particularly helpful in providing a clear aqueous medium at body temperature at a rate controlled so as not to exceed base-line intra-amniotic pressure. The operative technique required only two trocar sites for a fetoscopic port and an operating port. While uterine exposure by laparotomy was necessary, it allowed precise mapping of the amniotic sacs and purse-string closure of the trocar sites. While Quintero et al. (1996) have reported an entirely percutaneous technique, closure of the trocar sites is not possible, and amniotic fluid leak has complicated 30% of their cases.

The indications for fetoscopic cord ligation to prevent neurologic injury in monochorionic twins should be limited to anomalies incompatible with life, in which fetal death is imminent, and a gestational age of less than 28 weeks.

Because fetoscopy can be performed through small (2 to 4 mm) trocar sites instead of a large hysterotomy, it offers several potential advantages over open fetal surgery. The two most important advantages are reduced uterine irritability and the ability to deliver vaginally. These potential advantages have prompted attempts to perform operations by fetoscopic techniques previously performed only by open fetal surgery. Van der Wall et al. (1996) reported fetoscopic tracheal-clip application in a lamb model for the treatment of congenital diaphragmatic hernia. Based on their preliminary experimental work in sheep, this group has attempted fetoscopic clip application in a small series of human fetuses with left-sided diaphragmatic hernia (Van der Wall et al. 1997). These procedures have been extremely long, technically difficult, and complicated by bilateral vocal cord paralysis. There is a great deal of work yet to be done in animal models before application of fetoscopic techniques in more complex fetal anomalies will show the potential benefits of this approach over current open fetal surgical techniques.

► TECHNIQUES IN FETAL SURGERY

The technical aspects of open fetal surgery were developed by Harrison and colleagues in extensive animal experiments using fetal sheep and rhesus monkeys (Harrison et al. 1990). Using these experimental animal models, anesthetic, tocolytic, and surgical techniques were developed and applied clinically. Innovative techniques for opening and closing the gravid uterus were developed that minimize the risks to the mother's health and future reproductive potential (Harrison et al. 1993). This included the development of a uterine stapling device to minimize myometrial bleeding (Adzick et al. 1985; Bond et al. 1989). This group has developed and introduced radiotelemetric fetal monitoring for continuous intraoperative and postoperative fetal electrocardiographic and uterine contraction monitoring (Jennings et al. 1993). The details of techniques used for specific diagnoses requiring fetal surgery are covered under the fetal intervention sections of the chapters on these topics. The approach to entering the gravid uterus, fetal exposure, fetal and maternal monitoring, and anesthetic and tocolytic management are largely the same and are discussed below.

The maternal uterus is exposed through a low transverse abdominal incision. The fascial incision is determined by the position of the placenta. In the case of a posterior placenta a midline fascial incision can be used, as the uterus will not need to be lifted out of the abdomen. In contrast, in an anteriorly placed placenta, the rectus muscles need to be divided in order to allow room to tilt the uterus out of the abdomen, facilitating a posterior hysterotomy. A large abdominal ring retractor (Turner-Warwick, V. Mueller, Berlin, Germany) is used to maintain exposure. Sterile intraoperative ultrasound examination is then used to map the fetal position and the placental location. The edge of the placenta is marked under ultrasound guidance using electrocautery. The position and the orientation of the hysterotomy is planned in order to stay parallel to the closest edge of the placenta and 4 to 5 cm from it.

Two different techniques have been used for performing the hysterotomy. The initial approach used aspiration of approximately 400 ml of amniotic fluid through a trocar passed under ultrasound guidance. The removal of this amniotic fluid relaxes the myometrium and allows the uterine wall to be compressed against the trocar. A 2-cm incision is made through the myometrium and amnion using electrocautery. This hysterotomy incision is then extended using a specially developed absorbable Lactimer stapler (U.S. Surgical Corporation, Norwalk, Conn.) that is fast and hemostatic and seals the membranes to the myometrium (Adzick et al. 1985; Bond et al. 1989). The second technique for performing a hysterotomy uses a trocar attached directly to the uterine stapling device. Two traction sutures are placed to elevate the membrane and myometrial wall from the fetus, and a specially designed trocar attachment that fits on the anvil of the uterine stapling device is inserted directly into the amniotic cavity under ultrasound guidance.

Once the hysterotomy is performed, it is necessary to infuse saline in order to avoid the potential for cord compression. A red rubber catheter attached to a Level I rapid volume infusion device is inserted into the amniotic cavity, which delivers a continuous stream of normal saline at 37°C. The appropriate fetal part is then exposed, leaving the rest of the fetus entirely within the womb. A miniaturized pulse oximeter is wrapped around the fetal palm and protected with a clear plastic adhesive, then shielded from extraneous light with sterile foil wrapping. For certain procedures, a radiotelemeter that is capable of monitoring fetal electrocardiographic changes, temperature, and intra-amniotic pressure can be placed subcutaneously (Jennings et al. 1993).

Once the specific defect has been repaired, the fetal part is then returned to the uterus. Full-thickness number 1 PDS stay sutures are then placed along the length of the hysterotomy. As the staples are made of polyglycolic acid and are absorbable, they are left in place to avoid bleeding from the hysterotomy edges. A watertight two-layer uterine closure is then performed, using a running O PDS. Just prior to completing the first layer, 400 to 500 ml of warm normal saline containing 500 mg of oxacillin is instilled into the amniotic cavity. The stay sutures are then tied and the maternal laparotomy incision is closed in layers. A subcuticular maternal skin closure is used with a transparent adhesive dressing to facilitate postoperative monitoring by a tocodynamometer and ultrasound examination. The hysterotomy used for open fetal surgery remains a weakened area in the myometrium, which is at risk for

rupture during active labor with subsequent pregnancies. The nature of the hysterotomy used in all open fetal surgeries mandates that all future deliveries be by cesarean section.

Tocolysis begins as soon as the uterus is closed with a 6-g load of magnesium sulfate over 1 hour, which then continues at 2 g per hour, or at a higher dose, as clinically indicated by uterine irritability. As the mother emerges from deep anesthesia with isoflurane, there is a tendency for uterine tone to return and for uterine contractions to be observed. To supplement the magnesium sulfate, rectal indomethacin on a schedule of 50 mg every 4 to 6 hours is also used for the first 48 hours. The use of indomethacin requires close fetal monitoring by daily fetal echocardiography for ductal constriction and tricuspid valve regurgitation. Patient-controlled analgesia is also an essential part of the tocolytic management. If the mother is having pain, this will be reflected in increased uterine irritability. We currently use a continuous fentanyl infusion supplemented by bupivacaine for postoperative pain control, delivered through an epidural catheter, with patient-controlled rescue doses. The systemic levels of fentanyl achieved with the use of this epidural technique are sufficient to cross the placenta and provide fetal analgesia.

Far and away the most difficult problem in the management of the maternal–fetal patient following fetal surgery is the control of preterm labor. The large hysterotomy necessary for these procedures uniformly results in preterm labor. This has led to the development of an aggressive tocolytic regimen that often includes combinations of indomethacin, isoflurane anesthesia, magnesium sulfate, terbutaline, calcium-channel blockers, and most recently intravenous nitroglycerin as a nitric oxide donor (Adzick et al. 1994). Despite aggressive tocolytic therapy, the median interval from fetal surgery to delivery is only 5 weeks, with a range of 1 to 15 weeks (Harrison 1993b).

Unlike any other procedure, with the possible exception of organ transplantation from a living, related donor, fetal surgery exposes two patients, the mother as well as the fetus, to the risks of anesthesia, surgery, hysterotomy, and postoperative tocolysis. The most important factor in fetal surgery is the assurance of the mother's safety. Toward this end, extensive maternal monitoring of arterial blood pressure, central venous pressure, and pulse oximetry are necessary. In addition, appropriate fetal monitoring includes telemetric fetal heart monitoring, serial sonography, and surveillance of preterm labor by external tocodynamometer. Optimal monitoring of both patients can best be managed in a setting that combines the capabilities and expertise of both an intensive care unit and a labor floor, in a fetal–maternal intensive care unit (Jennings et al. 1993).

Although the benefits to the fetus with an otherwise lethal congenital malformation are obvious, there

▶ **TABLE 3-6.** FETAL MALFORMATIONS TREATABLE BY OPEN FETAL SURGERY

Fetal Malformation	Fetal Presentation	Fetal/Neonatal Consequences
Posterior urethral valves	Hydronephrosis and oligohydramnios	Renal dysplasia and renal insufficiency Pulmonary hypoplasia and respiratory insufficiency
Cystic adenomatoid malformation of the lung	Chest mass with mediastinal shift and hydrops	Pulmonary hypoplasia and respiratory insufficiency
Congenital diaphragmatic hernia	Herniated viscera in chest	Pulmonary hypoplasia and respiratory insufficiency
Twin–twin transfusion syndrome	Oligohydramnios and polyhydramnios	IUFD, heart failure, MLE
Acephalic-acardiac twin	Intrauterine fetal death	
Sacrococcygeal teratoma	High-output failure hydrops	Intrauterine fetal death, prematurity, hemorrhage
Complete heart block	Hydrops	Intrauterine fetal death
Fetal neck mass	Polyhydramnios	Inability to ventilate due to lack of airway

IUFD = intrauterine fetal death; MLE = multifocal leukoencephalomalacia.

are no direct benefits to the mother, who must assume the risks of fetal surgery and obligatory delivery by cesarean section. There have been no reports of maternal deaths related to open fetal surgery, but the potential for maternal morbidity is formidable. Among the 42 cases reported by Harrison, 5 patients have required perioperative blood transfusions. Amniotic fluid leaks were observed in 5, 2 via the hysterotomy site, requiring reoperation, and 3 via the vagina. Preterm labor was uniformly observed, and the majority of the morbidity occurred as a result of aggressive treatment of preterm labor, including pulmonary edema induced by tocolytic agents (Harrison et al. 1993b). In addition, long-term complications in mothers who undergo fetal surgery include uterine rupture with subsequent pregnancies, as has been seen in two patients. Because the incision used in fetal surgery is not in the lower uterine segment, there is the potential for uterine rupture with labor, so all future deliveries should be by cesarean section. The specific anatomic malformations in which open fetal surgery has already been employed are listed in Table 3-6. Detailed discussion of these conditions are reviewed in the specific chapters that follow.

▶ **CONCLUSIONS**

There have been significant strides made in invasive fetal therapy. In recent years progress seems to be accelerating, providing innovative treatment for fetuses with malformations that would otherwise be fatal. But these pioneering efforts should not be mistaken for establishing invasive fetal therapy as the standard treatment for any condition. Although there is tremendous potential to save fetuses with several highly lethal conditions, much experimental work remains to be done. Assessing the risk:benefit ratio for a mother with a fetus with a life-threatening malformation will evolve as technical advances diminish the potential risks of fetal surgery. Fetal surgery's contribution to advances in perinatal care and tocolytic management have implications far beyond the narrow sphere of fetal therapy. In the last analysis, the collateral advances that occur as a result of invasive fetal therapy may be the most important and lasting contributions of this experimental endeavor. The field of invasive fetal therapy is rapidly evolving and will undoubtedly provide new and exciting therapeutic options for the unborn patient.

REFERENCES

Adamsons K Jr. Fetal surgery. N Engl J Med 1966;275: 204–206.

Adzick NS, Crombleholme TM, Morgan MA, et al. A rapidly growing fetal teratoma. Lancet 1997;349:538.

Adzick NS, Harrison MR, Flake AW, et al. Automatic uterine stapling devices in fetal operation: Experience in a primate model. Surg Forum 1985;36:479–480.

Adzick NS, Harrison MR, Flake AW, et al. Fetal surgery for cystic adenomatoid malformation of the lung. J Pediatr Surg 1993;28:806–812.

Adzick NS, Harrison MR, Hi LM, et al. Pulmonary hypoplasia and renal dysplasia in a fetal urinary tract obstruction model. Surg Forum 1970;38:666–669.

Adzick NS, Harrison MR. Fetal surgical therapy. Lancet 1994a; 343:897–902.

Adzick NS, Harrison MR. The unborn surgical patient. Curr Probl Surg 1994b;31:1–68.

Adzick NS. Fetal thoracic lesions. Semin Pediatr Surg 1993; 2:103–108.

Allan LD, Sharland GS, Tynan M. Natural history of hypoplastic left heart syndrome. Int J Cardiol 1999;25:341–343.

Altenburger KM, Jeljniak M, Roper WL, et al. Congenital complete heart block associated with hydrops fetalis. J Pediatr 1977;91:618–620.

Arias F, Sunderji S, Gimpleson R, et al. Treatment of acardiac twinning. Obstet Gynecol 1998;91:818–821.

Asensio HS, Figueroa-Longo JG, Pelegrina IA. Intrauterine exchange transfusion. Am J Obstet Gynecol 1966;95: 1129–1133.

Bealer J, Sharsgard ED, Hadrick MH, et al. The PLUG (plug the lung until it grows) odyssey: adventures in experimental fetal tracheal occlusion. J Pediatr Surg 1995;30: 361–365.

Bebbington MW, Wilson RD, Machan L, et al. Selective feticide in twin transfusion syndrome using ultrasound-guided insertion of thrombogenic coils. Fetal Diagn Ther 1995;10:32–36.

Beck AD. The effect of intrauterine urinary obstruction upon development of the fetal kidney. J Urol 1971;105: 784–789.

Benacerraf BR, Frigoletto FD, Wilson M, et al. Successful midtrimester thoracocentesis with analysis of lymphocyte population in the pleural fluid. Am J Obstet Gynecol 1989;155:398–399.

Benirschke K, Kim CK. Multiple pregnancy. N Engl J Med 1973;288:1276–1329.

Bilaniuk L. Magnetic resonance imaging of the fetal brain. Semin Roentgenol 1999;34:48–61.

Birnholz JC, Frigoletto FD. Antenatal treatment of hydrocephalus. N Engl J Med 1981;304:1021–1023.

Bond SJ, Harrison MR, Slotnick RN, et al. Cesarean delivery and hysterotomy using an absorbable stapling device. Obstet Gynecol 1989;74:25–28.

Bowman JM, Manning FA. Intrauterine fetal transfusions: Winnipeg, 1982. Obstet Gynecol 1983;61:203–209.

Brennan JN, Diwan RJ, Rosen MG, et al. Fetofetal transfusion syndrome: prenatal ultrasonographic diagnosis. Radiology 1982;143:535–536.

Carpenter RJ, Strasburger JF, Gorson A Jr, et al. Fetal ventricular pacing for hydrops secondary to complete atrioventricular block. J Am Coll Cardiol 1986;8:1434–1436.

Casteneda AR, Jones RA, Mayer JE Jr, Hanley FL. Fetal intervention for congenital heart disease. In: Cardiac surgery of the neonate and infant. Philadelphia: Saunders, 1994:491–496.

Cendron M, D'Alton ME, Crombleholme TM. Prenatal diagnosis and management of fetal hydronephrosis. Semin Perinatol 1994;18(3):163–181.

Chervenak FA, Berkowitz RL, Tortura M, et al. The management of fetal hydrocephalus. Am J Obstet Gynecol 1985; 151:933–937.

Chervenak FA, Duncan C, Ment LR, et al. Outcome of fetal ventriculomegaly. Lancet 1984;2:179–181.

Chescheir NC, Seeds JW. Polyhydramnios and oligohydramnios in twin gestations. Obstet Gynecol 1988;71:882–884.

Chouri R, Bollmann R, Goeldner B. Aortic balloon valvuloplasty in the human fetus: a report of two cases and analysis of the further intrauterine cardiac development. Presented at the 13th International Fetal Medicine and Surgery Society, May 30, 1994, Antwerp, Belgium.

Clark SL, Vitale DJ, Minton SC, et al. Successful fetal therapy for cystic adenomatoid malformation associated with second trimester hydrops. Am J Obstet Gynecol 1987; 157:294–297.

Clewell WH. The fetus with ventriculomegaly: selection and treatment. In: Harrison MR, Golbus MS, Filly RA, eds. The unborn patient: prenatal diagnosis and treatment. 2nd ed. Philadelphia: Saunders, 1991:444–447.

Clewell WH, Meier PR, Manchester DK, et al. Ventriculomegaly: evaluation and management. Semin Perinatol 1985;98–102.

Clewell WH, Johnson ML, Meier RP, et al. A surgical approach to the treatment of fetal hydrocephalus. N Engl J Med 1982;306:1320–1322.

Cochrane DD, Miles ST, Nimrod C, et al. Intrauterine hydrocephalus and ventriculomegaly: associated anomalies and fetal outcome. Can J Neurol Sci 1984;12:51–54.

Copeland ML, Bruner JP, Richards WO, et al. A model for in utero endoscopic treatment of myelomeningocele. Neurosurgery 1993;33:592–545.

Crombleholme TM, Craigo SD, Garmel S, et al. Fetal ovarian cyst decompression to prevent torsion. J Pediatr Surg 1997;32:1447–1449.

Crombleholme TM, Dirkes K, Whitney T, et al. Amniotic band syndrome in fetal lambs: fetoscopic release and morphometric outcome. J Pediatr Surg 1995;30: 979–982.

Crombleholme TM, Harrison MR, Golbus MS, et al. Fetal intervention in obstructive uropathy: prognostic indicators and efficacy of intervention. Am J Obstet Gynecol 1991;162:1239–1244.

Crombleholme TM, Harrison MR, Langer JC, et al. Congenital hydronephrosis: early experience with open fetal surgery. J Pediatr Surg 1988;23:1114–1121.

Crombleholme TM, Harrison MR, Longaker MT, et al. Complete heart block in fetal lambs. I. Technique and acute physiologic response. J Pediatr Surg 1990;25:587–593.

Crombleholme TM, Harrison MR, Longaker MT, et al. Prenatal diagnosis and management of bilateral hydronephrosis. Pediatr Nephrol 1988;2:334–342.

Crombleholme TM, Robertson F, Marx G, Yarnell R, D'Alton ME. Fetoscopic cord ligation to prevent neurologic injury in monozygous twins. Lancet 1996;384:191.

Crombleholme TM, Shiraishi H, Adzick NS, et al. A model of non-immune hydrops in fetal lambs: complete heart block induced hydrops fetalis. Surg Forum 1991;42: 487–489.

Crombleholme TM. Invasive fetal therapy: current status and future directions. Semin Perinatol 1994;18:385–397.

D'Addario V, Volpe G, Kurjak A, et al. Ultrasonic diagnosis and perinatal management of complicated and uncomplicated fetal ovarian cyst: a collaborative study. J Perinat Med 1990;18:375–381.

D'Alton ME, Newton ER, Cetrulo CR. Intrauterine fetal demise in multiple gestation. Acta Genet Med Gemellol 1984;33:43–49.

D'Alton ME, Simpson LL. Syndromes in twins. Semin Perinatol 1995;19:375–386.

DeLia JE, Cruikshank DP, Keye WR. Fetoscopic neodynium:YAG laser occlusion of placental vessels in severe twin–twin transfusion syndrome. Obstet Gynecol 1990;75:1046–1053.

DeLia JE, Cukierski MA, Lundergan DK, et al. Neodynium: YAG laser occlusion of rhesus placental vasculature via fetoscopy. Am J Obstet Gynecol 1989;160:485–489.

DeLia JE, Kuhlmann RS, Harstad TW, et al. Fetoscopic laser ablation of placental vessels in severe previable twin-twin transfusion syndrome. Am J Obstet Gynecol 1995;172: 1202–1211.

DeLia JE, Rogers JG, Dixon JA. Treatment of placental vasculature with a neodymium: YAG laser via fetoscopy. Am J Obstet Gynecol 1985b;151:1126–1127.

DeLia JE, Emery MG, Sheafor SA, et al. Twin transfusion

syndrome: successful in utero treatment with digoxin. Int J Gynecol Obstet 1985a;23:197–201.

Deprest JA, Luks FI, Peers KHE, et al. In utero exposure of the ovine fetal eye to endoscopic light. Presented at the 13th International Fetal Medicine and Surgery Society, June 1, 1994, Antwerp, Belgium.

Dirkes K, Crombleholme TJM, Whitney TW, et al. A model of amniotic band syndrome in fetal lambs. Surg Forum 1994;45:562–564.

Drugan A, Krause B, Canady A, et al. The natural history of prenatally diagnosed cerebral ventriculomegaly. JAMA 1989;261:12–15.

Dudley DK, D'Alton ME. Single fetal death in twin gestation. Semin Perinatol 1986;10:65–72.

Eglowstein M, D'Alton ME. Intrauterine demise in multiple gestation: theory and management. J Matern Fetal Med 1993;2:272–275.

Elias S. Use of fetoscopy for the prenatal diagnosis of hereditary skin disorders. Curr Probl Perinatol 1987;16:1–8.

Elliot JP, Urig MA, Clewell WH. Aggressive therapeutic amniocentesis for treatment of twin-twin transfusion syndrome. Obstet Gynecol 1991;77:537–540.

Enbom JA. Twin pregnancy with intrauterine death of one twin. Am J Obstet Gynecol 1985;152:424–429.

Estes JM, Harrison MR. Fetal obstructive uropathy. Semin Pediatr Surg 1993;2:129–135.

Estes JM, MacGillivray TE, Hedrick MH, et al. Fetoscopic surgery for the treatment of congenital anomalies. J Pediatr Surg 1992a;27:950–954.

Estes JM, Whitley DJ, Lorenz HP, et al. Endoscopic creation and repair of fetal cleft lip. Plast Reconstr Surg 1992b; 90:743–749.

Feingold M, Cetrulo CL, Newton ER, et al. Serial amniocentesis in the treatment of twin–twin transfusion complicated with acute polyhydramnios. Acta Genet Med Gemellol 1986;35:107–113.

Foley M, Clewell W. Management of acardius by umbilical cord ligation in utero. Presented at the 13th Annual International Fetal Medicine and Surgical Society, May 31, 1994, Antwerp, Belgium

Freda VJ, Adamsons K Jr. Exchange transfusion in utero: report of a case. Am J Obstet Gynecol 1964;89:817–821.

Freedman AL, Bukowski TP, Smith CA, et al. Use of urinary beta-2-microglobulin to predict severe renal damage in fetal obstructive uropathy. Fetal Diagn Ther 1997;12(1): 1–6.

Fries MH, Goldberg J, Golbus MS. Treatment of acardiac, acephalic twin gestations by hysterotomy and selective delivery. Obstet Gynecol 1992;79:601–604.

Frigoletto FD Jr, Birnholz JC, Greene MF. Antenatal treatment of hydrocephalus by ventriculoamniotic shunting. JAMA 1982;248:2495–2497.

Fusi L, Gordon H. Multiple pregnancy complicated by single intrauterine death: problems and outcome with conservative management. Br J Obstetr Gynaecol 1990;97: 511–516.

Garmel SH, D'Alton ME. Fetal ultrasonography. West J Med 1993;159:273–285.

Ginsberg NA, Applebaum M, Robin SA, et al. Term birth after midtrimester hysterotomy and selective delivery of an acardiac twin. Am J Obstet Gynecol 1992;167:33–37.

Giorlandino C, Bilanciani E, Bagolan P, et al:. Antenatal ultrasonographic diagnosis and management of fetal ovarian cysts. Int J Gynecol Obstet 1993;44:27–31.

Giorlandino C, Rivosecchi M, Bilanciani P, et al. Successful intrauterine therapy of a large fetal ovarian cyst. Prenat Diagn 1990;10:473–475.

Glick PL, Harrison MR, Adzick NS, et al. Correction of congenital hydronephrosis in utero. IV. In utero decompression prevents renal dysplasia. J Pediatr Surg 1984a;19: 649–655.

Glick PL, Harrison MR, Golbus MS, et al. Management of the fetus with congenital hydronephrosis. II. Prognostic criteria and selection for treatment. J Pediatr Surg 1985; 20:376–381.

Glick PL, Harrison MR, Holks-Miller M, et al. Correction of congenital hydrocephalus in utero. II. Efficacy of in utero shunting. J Pediatr Surg 1984;19:870–881.

Glick PL, Harrison MR, Nakayama DK, et al. Management of ventriculomegaly in the fetus. J Pediatr 1984c;105: 97–105.

Glick PL, Harrison MR, Noall RA, et al. Correction of congenital hydronephrosis in utero. III. Early mid-trimester ureteral obstruction produces renal dysplasia. J Pediatr Surg 1983;98:681–687.

Golbus MS, Harrison MR, Filly RA, et al. In utero treatment of urinary tract obstruction. Am J Obstet Gynecol 1982; 142:383–388.

Gonzalez R, Sheldon CA, Burke B, et al. Renal dysplasia resulting from prenatal urethral obstruction in lambs. J Urol 1985;133:136A.

Hagay Z, Reece A, Roberts A, et al. Isolated fetal pleural effusion: a prenatal management dilemma. Obstet Gynecol 1993;81:147–152.

Hahnemann H, Mohr J. Antenatal fetal diagnosis in the embryo by means of biopsy from the extraembryonic membranes. Bull Eur Soc Hum Genet 1968;2:23–27.

Hanley FL. Fetal cardiac surgery. Adv Cardiac Surg 1994;5: 17–74.

Harrison MR, Adzick NS. Fetal surgical techniques. Semin Pediatr Surg 1993;2:136–142.

Harrison MR, Adzick NS. The fetus as a patient: surgical considerations. Ann Surg 1990a;213:279–291.

Harrison MR, Adzick NS, Flake AW, et al. Correction of congenital diaphragmatic hernia in utero. VI. Hard learned lessons. J Pediatr Surg 1993b;28:1411–1418.

Harrison MR, Adzick NS, Jennings RA, et al. Antenatal intervention for congenital cystic adenomatoid malformation. Lancet 1990b;336:965–967.

Harrison MR, Adzick NS, Langaker MT, et al. Successful repair in utero of a fetal diaphragmatic hernia after removal of herniated viscera from the left thorax. N Engl J Med 1990c;322:1582–1584.

Harrison MR, Filly RA. The fetus with obstructive uropathy: pathophysiology, natural history, selection and treatment. In: Harrison MR, Golbus MS, Filly RA, eds. The unborn patient: prenatal diagnosis and treatment. Philadelphia: Saunders, 1991:328–393.

Harrison MR, Filly RA, Parer JT. Management of the fetus with a urinary tract malformation. JAMA 1981a;246:635–639.

Harrison MR, Golbus MS, Filly RA. Fetal treatment 1982. N Engl J Med 1982b;307:1651–1653.

Harrison MR, Golbus MS, Filly RA. Management of the fetus with a correctable congenital defect. JAMA 1981b;246: 774–777.

Harrison MR, Golbus MD, Filly RA, et al. Fetal hydronephrosis: selection and surgical repair. J Pediatr Surg 1987;22:556–558.

Harrison MR, Golbus MS, Filly RA, et al. Fetal surgery for congenital hydronephrosis. N Engl J Med 1982a;306: 591–593.

Harrison MR, Golbus MS, Filly RA, et al. Management of the fetus with congenital hydronephrosis. J Pediatr Surg 1982c;17:383–388.

Harrison MR, Nakayama DK, Noall RA, et al. Correction of congenital hydronephrosis in utero. II. Decompression reverses effects of obstruction on the fetal lung and urinary tract. J Pediatr Surg 1982d;17:965–974.

Harrison MR, Ross N, Noall R, et al. Correction of congenital hydronephrosis in utero. I. The model: fetal urethral obstruction produces hydronephrosis and pulmonary hypoplasia in fetal lambs. J Pediatr Surg 1983;18:247–256.

Harrison MR. Fetal surgery. West J Med 1993;159:341–349.

Healey MG. Acardia: predictive risk factors for the co-twin's survival. Teratology 1994;50:205–213.

Hislop A, Hey E, Reid L. The lungs in congenital bilateral renal agenesis and dysplasia. Arch Dis Child 1979;54: 32–39.

Holzgreve W, Evans MI. Nonvascular needle and shunt placements for fetal therapy. West J Med 1993;159: 333–340.

Holzgreve W, Feil R, Louwen F, et al. Prenatal diagnosis and management of fetal hydrocephaly and lissencephaly. Child Nerv Syst 1993;9(7):408–412.

Holzgreve W, Tercanli S, Krings W. A simpler technique for umbilical-cord blockade of an acardiac twin. N Engl J Med 1994;330:469–471.

Holzgreve W, Tercanli S. Successful cord blockade by alcoholized suture material through cordocentesis. Presented at the 13th Annual International Fetal Medicine and Surgical Society, May 31, 1994, Antwerp, Belgium.

Hudgins RJ, Edwards MSB, Goldstein R, et al. Natural history of fetal ventriculomegaly. Pediatrics 1988;82:682–698.

Inselman LS, Mellins RB. Growth and development of the lung. J Pediatr 1981;98:1–14.

James WH. A note on the epidemiology of acardiac monsters. Teratology 1977;16:211–216.

Jennings RW, Adzick NS, Longaker MT, et al. Radiotelemetric fetal monitoring during and after open fetal surgery. Surg Gynecol Obstet 1993;176:59–64.

Johnson MP, Corsi P, Bradfield W, et al. Sequential urinalysis improves evaluation of fetal renal function in obstructive uropathy. Am J Obstet Gynecol 1995;173(1):59–65.

Kirkinen A, Jouppila P. Perinatal aspects of pregnancy complicated by fetal ovarian cyst. J Perinat Med 1985;13: 245–251.

Kleinman CS, Donnerstein RL, DeVore GR, et al. Fetal echocardiography for the evaluation of fetal CHF. N Engl J Med 1982;306:568–575.

Kleinman CS, Evans MI. International Fetal Medicine and Surgery Society Fetal Cardiac Registry, 1988.

Kurjak A, Rajhvajn B, Kolger A, et al. Ultrasound diagnosis and fetal malformations of surgical interest. In: Kurjak A,

ed. The fetus as patient. Amsterdam: Excerpta Medica, 1985:243–271.

Kurjak P, Latin V, Mandruzzato P. Ultrasound diagnosis and perinatal management of fetal genito-urinary abnormalities. J Perinat Med 1984;12:291–312.

Laberge JM, Crombleholme TM, Longaker MT. The fetus with pleural effusions. In: Harrison MR, Golbus MS, Filly RA, eds. The unborn patient. 2nd ed. Philadephia: Saunders, 1991:314–319.

Landrum B, Ogburn PL, Feinberg S, et al. Intrauterine aspiration of a large fetal ovarian cyst. Obstet Gynecol 1986; 68:1–14.

Lawrence KM, Coates S. The natural history of hydrocephalus: detailed analysis of 182 unoperated cases. Arch Dis Child 1962;37:345–362.

Levitsky DB, Mack LA, Nyberg DA, et al. Fetal aqueductal stenosis diagnosed sonographically: how grave is the prognosis? AJR Am J Roentgenol 1995;164(3):725–730.

Liggins GC, Kitterman JA. Development of the fetal lung. In Ciba Foundation Symposium 86: The fetus and independent life. London: Pittman, 1981:308–329.

Liggins GC. A self-retaining catheter for fetal peritoneal transfusion. Obstet Gynecol 1986;68:275–277.

Liley AW. Intrauterine transfusion of foetus in haemolytic disease. BMJ 1963;2:1107–1109.

Longaker MT, Laberge TM, Dansereau J, et al. Primary fetal hydrothorax: natural history and management. J Pediatr Surg 1989;24:573–576.

Lorber J. Ventriculo-cardiac shunts in the first week of life: results of a controlled trial in the treatment of hydrocephalus in infants born with spina bifida cystica or cranium bifidum. Dev Med Child Neurol (Suppl) 1969;20: 13–22.

Luks FI, Deprest J, Marcus M, et al. Carbon dioxide pneumo-amnios causes acidosis in fetal lambs. Fetal Diagn Ther 1994;9:105–109.

Machado MVL, Tynan MJ, Curry PVL, et al. Fetal complete heart block. Br Heart J 1988;60:512–515.

Manning FA, Harrison MR, Rodeck C, et al. Catheter shunts for fetal hydronephrosis and hydrocephalus: report of the International Fetal Surgery Registry. N Engl J Med 1986; 315:336–340.

Manning FA: The fetus with ventriculomegaly: the fetal surgery registry. In Harrison, MR, Golbus MS, Filly RA. The Unborn Patient, 2nd ed. Philadelphia: WB Saunders: 448–452.

Maxwell D, Allan L, Tynan MJ. Balloon dilatation of the aortic valve in the fetus: a report of two cases. BMJ 1991;65:256–258.

McCurdy CM, Childers JM, Seeds JW. Ligation of the umbilical cord of an acardiac-acephalus twin with an endoscopic intrauterine technique. Obstet Gynecol 1993;82:708–711.

Michejda M, Hodgen SD. In utero diagnosis and treatment of non-human primate fetal skeletal anomalies. I. Hydrocephalus. JAMA 1981;246:1093–1097.

Moore TR, Gale S, Benirschke K. Perinatal outcome of forty-nine pregnancies complicated by acardiac twinning. Am J Obstet Gynecol 1990;163:907–912.

Moran L, Crombleholme TM, D'Alton ME. Prenatal diagnosis and management of fetal thoracic lesions. Semin Perinatol 1994;18:228–253.

Möller F, Dommergues M, Mandelbrot L, et al. Fetal urinary biochemistry predicts postnatal renal function in children with bilateral obstructive uropathy. Obstet Gynecol 1993;82:813–820.

Nakayama DK, Harrison MR, deLorimier AA, et al. Prognosis of posterior urethral valves presenting at birth. J Pediatr Surg 21:1986;43–45.

Newton ER. Antepartum care in multiple gestation. Semin Perinatol 1986;10:19–29.

Nicolaides KH, Azar GB. Thoraco-amniotic shunting. Fetal Diagn Ther 1990;5:153–164.

Nicolaides KH, Blott AJ, Greenough A. Chronic drainage of fetal pulmonary cysts. Lancet 1987;2:618–619.

Nyberg DA, Mack LA, Hirsh J, et al. Fetal hydrocephalus: sonographic detection and clinical significance of associated anomalies. Radiology 1987;163:187–192.

Peers KHE, Luks FP, Deprest JA, et al. Foregut endoscopy in the fetal lamb and endoscopic placement of tracheal plug. Presented at the 13th International Fetal Medicine and Surgery Society, June 1, 1994, Antwerp, Belgium.

Peters CA, Reid LM, Docimo S, et al. The role of kidney in lung growth and maturation in the setting of obstructive uropathy and oligohydramnios. J Urol 1991;146:597–600.

Petres RE, Redwine FO, Cruikshant DP, et al. Congenital bilateral hydrothorax: antepartum diagnosis and successful intrauterine surgical management. JAMA 1982;248:1360–1362.

Porreco RP, Barton SM, Haverkamp AD. Occlusion of umbilical artery in acardiac, acephalic twin. Lancet 1991;337:326–327.

Potter EL. Kidneys, ureters, urinary bladder, and urethra. In: Potter EL, Craig JM, eds. Pathology of the fetus and neonate. 3rd ed. Chicago: Yearbook, 1976:473–484.

Pretorius DH, Davis K, Manco-Johnson ML, et al. Clinical course of fetal hydrocephalus: 40 cases. Am J Radiol 1985;144:827–832.

Quintero RA, Abuhamad A, Hobbins JC, et al. Transabdominal thin-gauge embryofetoscopy: a technique for early prenatal diagnosis and its use in the diagnosis of a case of Meckel-Gruber syndrome. Am J Obstet Gynecol 1993;168:1552–1557.

Quintero RA, Hume R, Smith C, et al. Percutaneous fetal cystoscopy and endoscopic fulguration of posterior urethral values. Am J Obstet Gynecol 1995;172:206–209.

Quintero RA, Morales WJ, Mendoza G, et al. Selective photocoagulation of placental vessels in twin-twin transfusion syndrome: evaluation of a new technique. Obstet Gynecol Survey 1998;53:S97–S103.

Quintero RA, Reich H, Puder KS, et al. Umbilical-cord ligation of an acardiac twin by fetoscopy at 19 weeks of gestation. N Engl J Med 1994;330:469–471.

Quintero RA, Romero RA, Reich H, et al. In utero percutaneous umbilical cord ligation in the management of complicated monochorionic multiple gestations. Ultrasound Obstet Gynecol 1996;8:16–22.

Rausen AR, Seki M, Strauss L. Twin transfusion syndrome. J Pediatr 1965;66:613–628.

Reid L. The lung: its growth and remodeling in health and disease. Am J Roentgenol 1977;129:777–785.

Roberts AB, Clarkson JM, Pattison NS, et al. Fetal hydrothorax in the second trimester of pregnancy: successful intrauterine treatment at 24 weeks gestation. Fetal Ther 1986;1:203–209.

Roberts RM, Shok DM, Jeanty P, et al. Twin, acardiac ultrasound-guided embolization. Fetus 1991;1:5–10.

Robichaux AG III, Mandell J, Greene MF, et al. Fetal abdominal wall defect: a new complication of vesicoamniotic shunting. Fetal Diagn Ther 1991;6:11–13.

Robie GF, Payne GG Jr, Morgan MA. Selective delivery of an acardiac, acephalic twin. N Engl J Med 1989;320:512–513.

Rodeck CH, et al. Fetal liver biopsy for prenatal diagnosis of ornithine carbamyl transferase deficiency. Lancet 1982;2:297–299.

Rodeck CH, Fish NM, Fraser DI, et al. Long-term in utero drainage of fetal hydrothorax. N Engl J Med 1988;319:1135–1138.

Roman JD, Hare AA. Digoxin and decompression amniocentesis for treatment of feto-fetal transfusion. Br J Obstet Gynecol 1995;102:421–423.

Ronderos-Dumit D, Nicolini U, Vaughan J, et al. Uterine-peritoneal amniotic fluid leakage: an unusual complication of intrauterine shunting. Obstet Gynecol 1991;78:913–915.

Rosseau GL, McCullough DC, Joseph AL. Current prognosis in fetal ventriculomegaly. J Neurosurg 1991;77:551–555.

Saade GR, Olson G, Belfort MA, et al. Amniotomy: a new approach to the 'stuck twin' syndrome. Am J Obstet Gynecol 1995;172:429.

Sackier JM. Laparoscopy in pediatric surgery. J Pediatr Surg 1992;26:1145–1149.

Salinas-Madrigal L, LaReginia M, Vogler G, et al. Induced renal dysplasia in the young opossum. J Pediatr Surg 1988;23:1127–1130.

Schmidt KG, Ulmer HE, Silverman WH, et al. Perinatal outcome of fetal complete heart block: a multicenter experience. J Am Coll Cardial 1991;91:1360–1366.

Schneider KT, Vetter K, Huch R, et al. Acute polyhydramnios complicating twin pregnancies. Acta Genet Med Gemellol 1985;34:179–184.

Serlo W, Kirkinen P, Joupilla P, et al. Prognostic signs in fetal hydrocephalus. Child Nerv Syst 1986;2:93–96.

Simpson PC, Trudinger BJ, Walker A, et al. The intrauterine treatment of fetal cardiac failure in a twin pregnancy with an acardiac, acephalic monster. Am J Obstet Gynecol 1983;147:842–844.

Stewart PA, Tonge HM, Wladimiroff JW, et al. Arrhythmic and structural abnormalities of the heart. Br Health J 1983;50:550–554.

Strong SJ, Corney G. The placenta in twin pregnancy. New York, Pergamon, 1967.

Sylvester K, Yang EY, Cass DL, et al. Fetoscopic gene therapy for congenital lung disease. J Pediatr Surg 1997;32(7):964–969.

Valenti C, Kassner EG, Yermakov V, et al. Antenatal diagnosis of a fetal ovarian cyst. Am J Obstet Gynecol 1975;15:216.

Van Allen MI, Smith DW, Shepard TH. Twin reversed arterial perfusion (TRAP) sequence: a study of 14 twin pregnancies with acardius. Semin Perinatol 1983;7:285–293.

Van der Wall KJ, Bush SW, Meuli M, et al. Fetal endoscopic (Fetendo) tracheal clip. J Pediatr Surg 1996;31:1101–1103.

Van der Wall KJ, Skarsgard CE, Filly RA, et al. Fetendo-clip: a fetal endoscopic tracheal clip procedure in a human fetus. J Pediatr Surg 1997;32:970–972.

Ville Y, Hyett J, Hecher K, et al. Laser treatment of twin–twin transfusion syndrome under sonoendoscopic control. Presented at the 13th International Fetal Medicine and Surgical Society, May 31, 1994, Antwerp, Belgium.

Ville Y, Hyett J, Hecher K, et al. Preliminary experience with endoscopic laser surgery for severe twin-twin transfusion syndrome. N Engl J Med 1995;332:224–227.

Vlahakes GJ, Turley K, Uhlig PN, et al. Experimental model of congenital right ventricular hypertrophy created by pulmonary artery banding in utero. Surg Forum 1981; 32:233–234.

Warshaw BL, Edelbrock HH, Ettinger RB. Progression to end stage renal disease in children with obstructive uropathy. J Pediatr Surg 1982;10:182–188.

Weber AM, Philipson EH. Fetal pleural effusion: A review and meta-analysis for prognostic indicators. Obstet Gynecol 1992;79:281–286.

Weiner CP. Diagnosis and treatment of twin to twin transfusion in the mid-second trimester of pregnancy. Fetal Ther 1987;2:71–74.

Wigglesworth JS, Dejoi R, Guerrini P. Fetal lung hypoplasia: Biochemical and structural variations and their possible significance. Arch Dis Child 56:606–611.

Willcourt RJ, Naughton MJ, Knutzen VK, et al. Laparoscopic ligation of the umbilical cord of an acardiac fetus. J Am Assoc Gynecol Laparosc 1995;2:319–321.

Wittman BK, Baldwin VJ, Nichol F. Antenatal diagnosis of twin transfusion syndrome by ultrasound. Obstet Gynecol 1981;58:123–127.

Wittmann BK, Farquharson PF, Thomas WD, et al. The role of fetocide in the management of severe twin transfusion syndrome. Am J Obstet Gynecol 1986;155:1023–1026.

Wright JGC, Skinner JR, Stumper O, et al. Radiofrequency assisted pulmonary valvotomy in a fetus with pulmonary atresia and intact ventricular system. Presented at the 13th Annual International Fetal Medicine and Surgery Society, May 30, 1994, Antwerp, Belgium.

Young HF, Nielsen FE, Weiss, et al. The relationship of intelligence and cerebral infantile hydrocephalus (IQ potential in hydrocephalic children). Pediatrics 1973;52:38–44.

Zosmer N, Borjoria R, Weiner E, et al. Clinical and echocardiographic features of *in utero* cardiac dysfunction in the recipient twin in twin-to-twin transfusion syndrome. Br Heart J 1994;72:74–79.

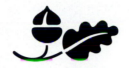

PART II

Management of Fetal Conditions Diagnosed by Sonography

Central Nervous System

CHAPTER 4

Agenesis of the Corpus Callosum

▶ CONDITION

The corpus callosum is a major pathway connecting the two hemispheres of the brain. The development of the corpus callosum begins during the fifth week of fetal life with the formation of the primitive lamina terminalis, which thickens to form the commissural plate. Glial cells coalesce to form a bridgelike structure that serves as a guide for the callosal fibers crossing the longitudinal cerebral fissure to their targets on the contralateral side of the brain (Rakic and Yakovlev 1968). The mature corpus callosum is formed by the seventeenth week of gestation. In agenesis of the corpus callosum (ACC), the commissural fibers do not cross the midline; instead they form thick bundles of fibers, called "Probst bundles," which course in a posterior direction along the medial walls of the lateral ventricles. These bundles indent and separate the anterior horns of the lateral ventricles.

ACC may be an isolated finding; however, it is frequently associated with other malformations and genetic syndromes including chromosomal aberrations and inborn errors of metabolism (Dobyns 1989; Jeret et al. 1987; Parrish et al. 1979). Associated central nervous system (CNS) abnormalities include Chiari malformations, anomalies of neuronal migration including lissencephaly, schizencephaly, pachygyria and polymicrogyria, encephaloceles, Dandy–Walker malformations, holoprosencephaly, and olivopontocerebellar degeneration (Barkovich 1988). Extracranial malformations include abnormalities of the face and of the cardiovascular, genitourinary, gastrointestinal, respiratory, and musculoskeletal systems (Franco et al. 1993; Kozlowski 1993; Parrish et al. 1979).

▶ INCIDENCE

ACC has been estimated to occur in 0.3 to 0.7% of the general population and in 2 to 3% of the developmentally disabled population (Freytag and Lindenberg 1967; Grogono 1968; Jeret et al. 1986). In a large series of patients diagnosed with a metabolic disease by Bamforth et al. (1988), 17% were shown by computed tomography

(CT), ultrasound, or autopsy examination have an abnormality of the corpus callosum.

In a series of 4,122 perinatal or neonatal autopsy specimens, the incidence of CNS malformations was 8.8% and of the 363 CNS malformations diagnosed, agenesis of the corpus callosum accounted for 4.1% (Pinar et al, 1998). These data would suggest that the incidence of agenesis of the corpus callosum is at least 4 per 1,000 births.

► SONOGRAPHIC FINDINGS

Usually only midsagittal and midcoronal scans of the fetal brain allow clear visualization of the corpus callosum. Such views can be obtained with standard transabdominal ultrasound examination of most fetuses in breech position or transverse lie. For fetuses in the vertex position, transvaginal sonography is the preferred technique.

On sagittal scan, the corpus callosum appears as a sonolucent band, demarcated superiorly and inferiorly by two echogenic lines. The superior line arises from the pericallosal cistern; the inferior line derives from the fornix and roof of the cavum septum pellucidum. Color Doppler sonography can demonstrate the pericallosal artery, a branch of the anterior cerebral artery that sweeps in a circular pattern over the corpus callosum. In a coronal scan, the corpus callosum appears to form the roof of the cavum septum pellucidum and frontal horns.

Classic neuroradiologic signs for the diagnosis of ACC on pneumoencephalography were described by Davidoff and Dyke (1934). Their criteria have been applied to the CT diagnosis and also can be applied to sonography (Skidmore et al. 1983). The findings include absence of the corpus callosum and cavum septum pellucidum and a variety of indirect findings, including:

1. Increased separation of the frontal horns and bodies of the lateral ventricles.
2. Relative dilatation of the occipital horns of the lateral ventricles.
3. Concave medial border of the lateral ventricles due to protrusion of the Probst bundles.
4. General dilatation and upward displacement of the third ventricle.
5. Abnormal radial orientation of the medial cerebral gyri. (Bertino et al. 1988; Comstock et al. 1985; Pilu et al. 1993; Sandri et al. 1988, Maheut-Lourmiere and Paillet, 1998).

In a series of 141 cases of fetal cerebral ventriculomegaly, ACC was noted in 16 cases (11%) (Valat et al. 1998). In another series of 82 cases of mild ventriculomegaly, there were 7 cases (9%) of ACC (Vergani et al. 1998). The finding of mild ventriculomegaly

during routine prenatal sonography should, therefore, prompt a targeted search to confirm the presence of the corpus callosum.

It appears that ultrasound diagnosis of ACC is more difficult prenatally than postnatally. The earliest prenatal diagnosis has been made at 19 weeks of gestation (Pilu et al. 1993). Because the corpus callosum is not normally formed until 18 weeks, most reported cases have been diagnosed in the third trimester (Bennett et al. 1996; Bertino et al. 1988). This difficulty in prenatal diagnosis is usually due to the fact that the characteristic ventricular abnormalities can be quite subtle on the axial views of the fetal cranium that are most commonly obtained. It is preferable to use coronal and sagittal views to diagnose the characteristic ventricular abnormalities; however, these views are not as commonly used prenatally.

Routine sonography of the fetal brain is usually performed with axial scans that do not allow visualization of the corpus callosum. However, enlargement of the atria of the lateral ventricles is readily appreciated with these views. In the largest series of prenatally diagnosed ACC, 34 of 35 fetuses had atrial measurements >10 mm (Pilu et al. 1993). Once atrial enlargement has been observed, other ultrasound findings may identify possible ACC. The most consistent and easy-to-identify finding is the teardrop configuration of the lateral ventricles (Fig. 4-1). In the axial plane, enlargement of the atria and occipital horns and separation of the bodies combine to generate a pattern that is readily recognizable. The teardrop configuration of the ventricles has not been documented in conditions other than ACC, and it is believed to be a specific sign for the diagnosis of callosal agenesis (Pilu et al. 1993). In order to document the callosal lesion directly, it is important to obtain midcoronal and midsagittal scans when a dilated atrium or teardrop ventricle is identified.

Prenatal diagnosis of partial ACC has been reported; however, there are very few documented cases (Lockwood et al. 1988; Pilu et al. 1993). The natural history of partial ACC is uncertain, and cerebral findings associated with it are probably more subtle than with the complete form. It is expected that antenatal diagnosis will not be possible in many cases. The cavum septum pellucidum is not identified in cases of complete ACC but may be visualized in cases of partial agenesis. Sonographic evaluation of the structure is potentially helpful in routine screening, alerting the sonologist to perform more coronal and sagittal scans for direct visualization of the corpus callosum. Widening of the interhemispheric fissure and upward displacement of the third ventricle can be documented in approximately half of the prenatal cases. Radial arrangement of the medial cerebral sulci has been seen only in third-trimester studies. This is presumably because the surface of the hemispheres is smooth in the second

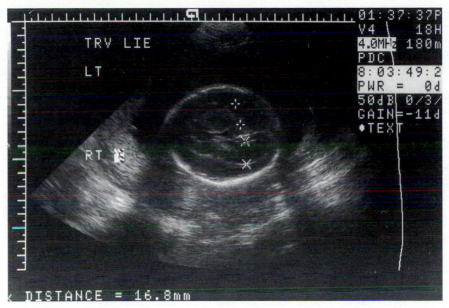

Figure 4-1. Transaxial ultrasound image demonstrating the classic teardrop configuration of the lateral ventricle.

trimester, with secondary sulci appearing only at the onset of the third trimester. In many cases of ACC, prenatal ultrasound may only cause one to suspect the diagnosis, while prenatal magnetic resonance imaging (MRI) may be needed to accurately confirm the diagnosis. In one series of 14 cases of ACC, ultrasonography confirmed the diagnosis in only 4 cases, while MRI confirmed the diagnosis in 13 cases (d'Ercole et al. 1998). In another series of 20 cases of ACC, prenatal MRI made a positive diagnosis in 19 cases (Brisse et al. 1988).

▶ DIFFERENTIAL DIAGNOSIS

Dilatation of the atria and occipital horns is often the most prominent sonographic finding; therefore, anything that causes hydrocephalus is also within the differential diagnosis for ACC (see Chapter 15). In ACC there is usually greater enlargement of the occipital horns, as compared with the remaining ventricular system, than is observed in other forms of hydrocephalus. When a dilated third ventricle is present, differential diagnosis includes other midline cystic spaces such as a cavum septum pellucidum, cavum vergae, interhemispheric arachnoid cyst, and medial porencephalic cyst.

ACC is a feature of Aicardi syndrome, Andermann syndrome, acrocallosal syndrome, Apert syndrome, Shapiro syndrome, oculocerebrocutaneous syndrome, orofaciodigital syndrome, lens dysplasia, and frontal nasal dysplasia (Bamforth et al. 1988). ACC has also been associated with abnormalities of chromosomes 8, 13, and 18 (Jeret et al. 1987). ACC also may be found in association with several inborn errors of metabolism, including nonketotic hyperglycinemia, Zellweger syndrome, adenylosuccinase deficiency, pyruvate dehydrogenase deficiency, neonatal adrenoleukodystrophy, Menkes disease, Leigh syndrome, and glutaric aciduria type II (Blum et al. 1990; Dobyns 1989; Kolodny 1989). Various teratogens have also been implicated as a possible cause of ACC, including alcohol, valproate, cocaine, rubella, and influenza virus (Table 4-1) (Cornover 1990; Dominguez et al. 1991; Friedman 1947; Lindhout 1992).

▶ ANTENATAL NATURAL HISTORY

Little is known about the natural obstetric history of ACC when it occurs as an isolated finding because there have been relatively few accurate prenatal diagnoses, and these are usually made in the third trimester. In one series of 37 pregnancies with prenatally diagnosed ACC, 28 resulted in elective termination of pregnancy, and in the remaining 9 cases liveborn infants were delivered (Hatem-Gantzer et al, 1998). Four of these 9 infants died in the postnatal period. It seems unlikely that the presence of isolated ACC should alter the antenatal course of pregnancy.

▶ MANAGEMENT OF PREGNANCY

Identification of ACC demands a careful search of fetal anatomy for other intracranial and extracranial abnormalities. The association between ACC and chromosomal abnormalities has been addressed by Serur and coworkers (1988), who reviewed 100 cases. Identification of ACC

▶ **TABLE 4-1.** SYNDROMES ASSOCIATED WITH ACC

Autosomal dominant syndromes	Chromosomal syndromes
Fronto nasal dysplasia	Trisomies 13, 18, 8
Autosomal recessive conditions	Teratogens
Apert syndrome	Alcohol, valproate, cocaine
Acrocallosal syndrome	
Andermann syndrome	Infections
Cerebro-oculo facio skeletal syndrome	Rubella
	Influenza
Neu-Laxova syndrome	
Cranio telencephalic dysplasia	Inborn errors of metabolism
Hydrolethalus	Nonketotic hyperglycinemia
	Zellweger syndrome
X-linked dominant syndromes	Neonatal adrenoleukodystrophy
Orofaciodigital syndrome Type I	Menkes syndrome
Aicardi syndrome	Adenylosuccinase deficiency
	Histidinemia
X-linked recessive syndromes	Pyruvate kinase deficiency
Shapiro syndrome	Leigh disease
Len dysplasia	Glutaric aciduria Type II

demands a careful search of fetal anatomy for other intracranial and extracranial abnormalities. MRI may also be of value in confirming the diagnosis and ensuring no other intracranial malformations co-exist (Brisse et al. 1998; d'Ercole et al. 1998). Overall, trisomy 18 was found in 29 cases, full or mosaic trisomy 8 in 21 cases, trisomy 13 in 20, and a variety of other conditions in the remaining cases. It is therefore postulated that chromosomes 8, 13, and 18 have a direct influence on the development of the corpus callosum. In Pilu et al.'s (1993) review of fetal diagnosis of ACC, three fetuses with abnormalities of chromosome 8 had ACC as the only sonographic finding. Therefore, at present, it is our practice to offer amniocentesis for fetal karyotyping independently of the presence of other sonographically detectable abnormalities.

If an isolated ACC is detected and the chromosomes are normal, there is no indication to change the standard of obstetrical care. This diagnosis does not necessitate delivery at a tertiary-care hospital. One should consult with genetics and pediatric neurology specialists. However, the presence of other associated structural abnormalities should prompt referrals to the appropriate pediatric subspecialists, and in this situation the patient should be delivered at a tertiary-care hospital.

Vaginal delivery is recommended unless there is significant hydrocephalus with macrocephaly. Delivery prior to term is not recommended unless an obstetrical indication exists.

▶ TREATMENT OF THE NEWBORN

Detailed examination of the newborn is required. The radiologic procedure of choice postnatally is magnetic resonance imaging (MRI), which allows detection of subtle abnormalities not seen by the other methods, including CT and ultrasound (Barkovich and Norman 1988; Davidson et al. 1985). Additional metabolic investigations may be necessary if inborn errors of metabolism are suspected.

▶ SURGICAL TREATMENT

There are no surgical issues for isolated ACC; however, surgery may be indicated for additional intracranial or extracranial lesions. Some infants may require ventriculoperitoneal shunts for treatment of progressive ventricular dilatation and accelerated head growth (Lacey 1985).

▶ LONG-TERM OUTCOME

Children with ACC and multiple major congenital abnormalities are at high risk for neurodevelopmental retardation, especially if craniofacial defects are present. The presence of either neonatal or infantile seizures is an ominous prognostic sign; most of these children are severely retarded or exhibit delayed development (Lacey 1985). Children with additional intracerebral abnormalities also appear to have a poor prognosis, with most infants experiencing developmental delay. A diagnosis of ACC should alert the physician to the likelihood of severe neurodevelopmental delay and subsequent seizures.

No specific risk figures are available at present to counsel parents regarding neurologic development in children with isolated ACC. Vergani and coworkers

(1988) reported that three infants with prenatal diagnosis of ACC had normal or borderline intelligence quotients at 3-year follow-up examination. In the series by Pilu et al. (1993), a normal developmental quotient was found in 9 of 11 nonfamilial cases with a follow-up ranging between 6 months and 11 years, and borderline development was found in the remaining two. The neurologic development of surviving infants was evaluated with the Brunet–Lezine test and the Stanford–Binet Intelligence Scale. Even in the presence of normal intelligence, ACC may be associated with subtle cognitive defects (Jeeves 1991; Temple et al. 1989, 1990). A possible relationship between ACC and psychotic disorders has also been proposed (Swayze et al. 1990).

In a survey of ACC from the United Kingdom, two thirds of 59 affected patients had epilepsy, half of the adult cases had intellectual impairment, and one-third had a psychotic disorder (Taylor and David, 1998). However, this and other series may be biased by under-ascertainment of asymptomatic cases of ACC. In another series of 10 children who had a diagnosis of ACC made prenatally, all had normal developmental outcome at three years of follow-up, although febrile convulsions were reported to occur more frequently than expected (Moutard et al. 1998).

▶ GENETICS AND RECURRENCE RISK

The recurrence risk of ACC, whether it is isolated or in addition to inborn errors of metabolism or genetic syndromes, depends on the underlying cause. If ACC is associated with aneuploidy the recurrence risk is 1% or the maternal–age related risk for aneuploidy, whichever is greater. If there is an isolated ACC with no known cause, the recurrence risk is probably on the order of 2 to 3% (Young et al. 1985). ACC is a known criterion for the diagnosis of certain syndromes, such as Aicardi, Andermann, and acrocallosal syndromes (Philip et al. 1998). While ACC is generally considered sporadic, familial cases have been reported (Naritomi et al. 1997).

REFERENCES

Bamforth F, Bamforth S, Poskitt K, et al. Abnormalities of corpus callosum in patients with inherited metabolic diseases. Lancet 1988;2:451.

Barkovich AJ, Norman D. Anomalies of the corpus callosum: correlation with further anomalies of the brain. AJR Am J Roentgenol 1988;151:171–179.

Bennett GL, Bromley B, Benacerraf BR. Agenesis of the corpus callosum: prenatal detection usually is not possible before 22 weeks of gestation. Radiology 1996;199:447–450.

Bertino R, Nyberg DA, Cyr DR, et al. Prenatal diagnosis of agenesis of the corpus callosum. J Ultrasound Med 1988;7:251–260.

Blum A, André M, Droullé P, et al. Prenatal echographic diagnosis of corpus callosum agenesis: the Nancy experience 1982–1989. Genet Couns 1990;1:115–126.

Brisse H, Sebag G, Fallet C, Fallet C, et al. Prenatal MRI of corpus callosum agenesis. Study of 20 cases with neuropathological correlations. J Radiol 1998;79:659-666.

Comstock CH, Culp D, Gonzalez J, et al. Agenesis of the corpus callosum in the fetus. J Ultrasound Med 1985;4:613.

Cornover PT, Roessmann U. Malformational complex in an infant with intrauterine influenza viral infection. Arch Pathol Lab Med 1990;114:535–538.

Davidoff LM, Dyke CG. Agenesis of the corpus callosum: its diagnosis by encephalography: report of 3 cases. AJR Am J Roentgenol 1934;32:1–10.

Davidson HD, Abraham R, Steiner RE. Agenesis of the corpus callosum: magnetic resonance imaging. Radiology 1985;155:371–373.

d'Ercole C, Girard N, Carvello L, et al. Prenatal diagnosis of fetal corpus callosum agenesis by ultrasonography and magnetic resonance imaging. Prenat Diagn 1998;18:247–253.

Dobyns WB. Agenesis of the corpus callosum and gyral malformations are frequent manifestations of nonketotic hyperglycinemia. Neurology 1989; 39:817–820.

Dominguez R, Villa Coro AA, Slopis JM, et al. Brain and ocular abnormalities in infants with in utero exposure to cocaine and other street drugs. Am J Dis Child 1991;145:688–95.

Franco I, Kogan S, Fisher J, et al. Genitourinary malformations associated with agenesis of the corpus callosum. J Urol 1993;149:1119–1121.

Freytag E, Lindenberg R. Neuropathologic findings in patients of a hospital for the mentally deficient: a survey of 359 cases. Johns Hopkins Med J 1967;121:379–392.

Friedman M, Cohen P. Agenesis of the corpus callosum as a possible sequel to maternal rubella during pregnancy. Am J Dis Child 1947;7:178–185.

Grogono JL. Children with agenesis of the corpus callosum. Dev Med Child Neurol 1968;10:613–20.

Hatem-Gantzer G, Poulain P, Valleur-Masson D, et al. Agenesis of the corpus callosum. An example of prognosis uncertainty in fetal medicine. J Gynecol Obstet Biol Reprod (Paris) 1998;27:790–797.

Jeeves MA. Stereoperception in callosal agenesis and partial callosotomy. Neuropsychologia 1991;29:19–34.

Jeret JS, Serur D, Wisniewski K, et al. Clinicopathological findings associated with agenesis of the corpus callosum. Brain Dev 1987;9:255–60.

Jeret JS, Serur D, Wisniewski K, et al. Frequency of agenesis of the corpus callosum in the developmentally disabled population as determined by computerized tomography. Pediatr Neurosci 1986;12:101–103.

Kolodny EH. Agenesis of the corpus callosum: a marker for inherited metabolic disease? Neurology 1989;39:847–848.

Kozlowski K, Ouvrier RA. Agenesis of the corpus callosum with mental retardation and osseous lesions. Am J Med Genet 1993;48:6–9.

Lacey DJ. Agenesis of the corpus callosum: clinical features in 40 children. Am J Dis Child 1985;139:953–955.

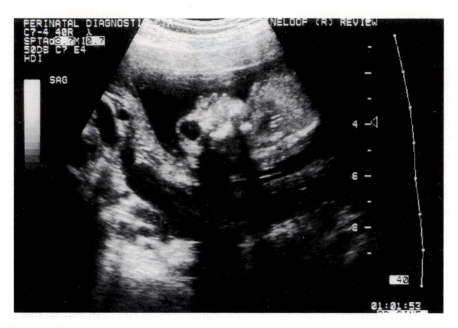

Figure 5-1. Sagittal view of fetal facial profile, demonstrating a lack of cranium above the easily visualized orbit.

is uncommon in isolated anencephaly. Another sonographic finding that may be present is polyhydramnios.

Goldstein and Filly (1988) reviewed the spectrum of prenatal sonographic findings in 20 fetuses with anencephaly. The sonographic diagnosis was based on the absence of brain and calvarium superior to the orbits on coronal views of the fetal head. In 45% of cases, echogenic tissue was seen superior to the orbits. This corresponded to the area cerebrovasculosa and was quite large in four fetuses. In 35% of their cases,

frank polyhydramnios was seen. There were no cases of oligohydramnios. These authors stated that anencephaly can be distinguished from cranial defects associated with the amniotic band syndrome on the basis of symmetry of the cranial defects and the absence of limb, body wall, and spinal anomalies that generally accompany amniotic bands. In this report, prenatal diagnosis was 100% accurate after 14 weeks of gestational age. These authors missed one case initially studied at 12.5 weeks of gestation, but the defect was diagnosed on a

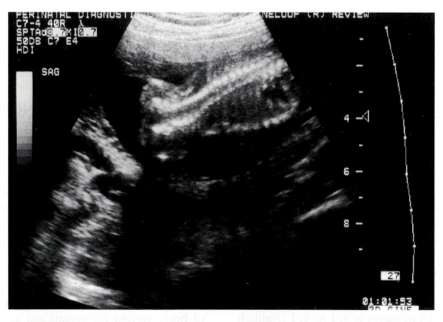

Figure 5-2. Posterior coronal view of an anencephalic fetus demonstrating an abrupt end to the fetal spine. No cranial bones are visualized.

repeat study performed at 26 weeks (Goldstein and Filly 1988).

In postnatal studies, 13 to 33% of anencephalic infants have additional major congenital anomalies. These include congenital heart disease (4 to 15% of cases), hypoplastic lungs (5 to 34%), congenital diaphragmatic hernia (2 to 6%), malrotation of the gut (1 to 9%), renal malformations (25%), including polycystic or dysplastic kidneys (1 to 3%), hypoplasia of the adrenal glands (94%), and omphalocele (16%) (Medical Task Force on Anencephaly 1990; Melnick and Myrianthopoulos 1987). Additional minor anomalies that have been observed in fetuses with anencephaly include a single umbilical artery, a patent ductus arteriosus, and a patent foramen ovale, seen in 2 to 31% of cases.

A unique sonographic finding of academic interest is the presence of dominant right ventricular cardiac output in fetuses with anencephaly. Rizzo and Arduini (1991) studied four fetuses diagnosed with anencephaly during the late second or third trimester, using Doppler echocardiography. As compared with normal fetuses, anencephalic fetuses showed a significant increase in right ventricular cardiac output. These authors concluded that the relationship between brain mass and body weight affects distribution of the cardiac output.

▶ DIFFERENTIAL DIAGNOSIS

The major consideration in the differential diagnosis is to distinguish anencephaly from the presence of amniotic bands. Scalp-covered lesions that include demineralization of the skull can occasionally be confused with anencephaly. It is important to note that the cranial defect associated with anencephaly is always symmetric. With amniotic bands, there should be evidence of other defects, such as limb or digital amputations, asymmetric ventral-wall defects, or spinal defects. Amniotic bands are often associated with oligohydramnios. Other conditions in the differential diagnosis include ruptured encephalocele (see Chapter 11), and iniencephaly (see Chapter 16). The latter condition does not involve the rostral skull or the forebrain. It is very important to distinguish between anencephaly and amniotic bands because of significant differences in their respective recurrence risks. Disorders that are associated with anencephaly are listed in Table 5-1.

▶ ANTENATAL NATURAL HISTORY

There is an increased lethality in utero for fetuses with anencephaly. Approximately 65% abort spontaneously (Medical Task Force on Anencephaly 1990). It is interesting to note that encephaloceles are more typically found in early embryonic abortuses, whereas anen-

▶ **TABLE 5-1.** DISORDERS ASSOCIATED WITH ANENCEPHALY

Folate deficiency
Maternal hyperthermia
Trisomy 13
Trisomy 18
Turner syndrome
Triploidy
Amniotic band syndrome
Limb/body wall defects
Walker-Warburg syndrome

cephaly is a more common finding in later spontaneous abortions (Main and Mennuti 1986).

Van Allen and colleagues (1993) proposed that multisite neural-tube closure provides the best explanation for neural-tube defects in humans. The closure sites are most likely controlled by separate genes expressed during embryogenesis. These authors hypothesized that the majority of neural-tube defects could be explained by a failure of fusion of one of the closures or their contiguous neuropores. Anencephaly results from failure of closure site 2 for meroacranium and closures 2 and 4 for holoacranium. Folate deficiency is thought to affect the closures of sites 2 and 4. This hypothesis has been demonstrated in humans with more than one neural-tube defect (Pantzar et al. 1993).

▶ MANAGEMENT OF PREGNANCY

Maternal serum α-fetoprotein (AFP) levels are elevated in approximately 90% of cases of anencephaly (Medical Task Force on Anencephaly 1990). In cases of significant elevation of maternal serum AFP, the diagnosis of anencephaly is initially confirmed by a level 2 sonographic examination. Prospective parents carrying a fetus with anencephaly should be referred to a tertiary-care center, with ultrasound technicians and physicians who are capable of definitive diagnosis of fetuses with anomalies. If additional fetal structural anomalies are detected, a prenatal karyotype should be offered. In addition, consideration should be given to obtaining a karyotype at birth if the anencephaly is isolated.

Because pregnancy with a fetus with anencephaly carries an increased medical risk for the mother, prospective parents should be offered the opportunity to terminate, if the diagnosis is made before 24 weeks of gestation, as the prognosis for the fetus is uniformly fatal. Because polyhydramnios is often associated with this condition, premature delivery is increased. Labor and delivery are frequently associated with an unstable fetal position, and common maternal complications include dysfunctional labor (poor dilatation or dystocia) and postpartum hemorrhage (Medical Task Force on

Anencephaly 1990). There is an increased incidence of placental abruption with anencephaly (Melnick and Myrianthopoulos 1987).

In a review of over 181 consecutive infants born with anencephaly, Main and Mennuti (1986) found that over half of the cases were stillborn and virtually all others died during the neonatal period. However, over 40% were alive at 24 hours and 5% lived to at least 7 days. Therefore, parents should not be counseled that the infant will die immediately after birth. They should, however, be advised that the prognosis is uniformly fatal for this condition.

▶ FETAL INTERVENTION

There is no fetal intervention for anencephaly.

▶ TREATMENT OF THE NEWBORN

The mean gestational age at delivery for infants with anencephaly is 36.7 ± 5 weeks (Melnick and Myrianthopoulos 1987). The mean birth weight for fetuses with anencephaly, when corrected for the absence of the brain, is within normal limits. The diagnosis of anen-

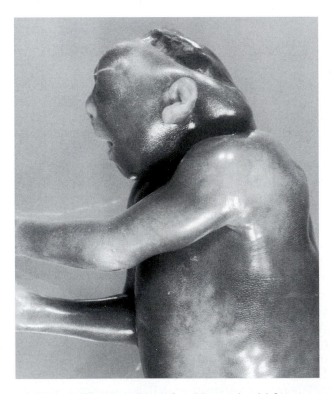

Figure 5-3. Sagittal view of a 20-week-old fetus with anencephaly. Note the total lack of cranial development above the orbits. The area cerebrovasculosa is easily seen. *(Photograph courtesy of Dr. Joseph Semple.)*

cephaly can be confirmed on physical examination when the following criteria are met: A large portion of the skull is absent, the scalp is absent over the skull defect, and a hemorrhagic, fibrotic mass of tissue is exposed to the environment (Fig. 5-3). There are no recognizable cerebral hemispheres present.

Because affected infants lack functioning cerebral cortex, they are permanently unconscious, but brainstem function is present in varying degrees. These patients are not, however, comatose. All infants have spontaneous movements of the extremities and startle myoclonus, although their tone and deep tendon reflexes are increased. Their typical behavior pattern consists of increased extensor tone and spontaneous or stimulus-induced axial myoclonus of the upper and lower extremities (Peabody et al. 1989). They respond to noxious stimuli and exhibit the primitive reflexes associated with feeding and breathing.

Most infants reported have died within the first few days of life, however, survival beyond 1 week of age was between 0 and 9% in three large series. The Medical Task Force on Anencephaly (1990) confirmed that one infant with anencephaly survived for 2 months.

▶ SURGICAL TREATMENT

Surgical treatment is not applicable in anencephaly.

▶ LONG-TERM OUTCOME

The major issue in long-term outcome is the potential use of anencephalic fetuses or infants as organ donors. This is a consideration because nationally, 30 to 50% of children under 2 years of age who are registered for organ transplantation die while waiting for donor organs to become available. Anencephalic infants have been considered as potential organ donors because they have a uniformly fatal prognosis. Difficulties exist, however, because of the traditional means of determining brain death for organ donors. Because anencephalic patients have no functioning cerebral cortex, the usual methods of determining brain death, such as cerebral blood flow testing and electroencephalograms (EEGs), are irrelevant to the diagnosis of anencephaly. For anencephalic patients, the diagnosis of brain death depends on documentation of disappearance of previously existing brain-stem functions, such a positive apnea test or loss of spontaneous movements.

Four different strategies have been suggested for the procurement of organs for transplantation from anencephalic patients:

The first is to place the infant on life support systems at birth and remove the organs as soon as technically possible without regard to the presence or absence of brain-stem function. This strategy has been described by a group in Germany. Holzgreve et al (1987) removed the kidneys from three infants with anencephaly and successfully transplanted them into four recipients. These authors argued that the anencephalic infants were "brain absent." Potential benefit was experienced by the organ recipients, but also by the parents of the anencephalic fetuses, who experienced psychologic benefits and additional moral purpose in carrying the anencephalic pregnancies to term (Holzgreve et al. 1987).

A second strategy is to place the anencephalic infant on life support systems at birth and observe the infant until all brain-stem functions stop. This approach was tested by Peabody et al. (1989), who modified the medical care of 12 live-born infants with anencephaly. For a period of 1 week, they tried to determine whether organ viability could be maintained and whether the criteria of total brain death could be met if these anencephalic infants were placed on life support for 1 week. Only 2 of the 12 infants met these criteria, and no solid organs were procured from these 12 infants. The authors concluded that most organs were suitable for transplantation at birth and that organ function was maintained when intensive care was provided, but only one infant had conclusive evidence of brain-stem death.

A third strategy is to give the infant with anencephaly only comfort care until signs of cardiorespiratory failure develop and then to place the infant on life support awaiting brain death. Peabody et al. (1989) concluded that when intensive care was delayed until brain death was imminent, most organs were damaged to the extent that they were no longer suitable for transplantation.

Most centers currently use a fourth strategy for organ donation from anencephalic infants. They provide standard comfort care until the infant dies. Then cadaver organs are removed, such as the corneas, heart valves, and kidneys.

It is important to note that most of the major organs from anencephalic infants are smaller than average for body size and have somewhat higher rates of malformation, but neither of these findings preclude their use in transplantation (Botkin 1988).

▶ GENETICS AND RECURRENCE RISK

Most cases of anencephaly are compatible with a multifactorial model. An increased incidence of anencephaly and other neural-tube defects occurs in women who have diabetes during pregnancy. Also, women who take valproic acid for a seizure disorder are at increased risk for anencephaly if their medication has been consumed prior to conception or during the first trimester of pregnancy (Main and Mennuti 1986). For the multifactorial model of anencephaly, the recurrence risk is between 2 and 5% (Medical Task Force on Anencephaly 1990).

For fetuses identified with multiple sonographic abnormalities, if a karyotype has not been performed prenatally, it should be obtained at delivery, as some cases of anencephaly are associated with chromosomal abnormalities.

In isolated populations, anencephaly has been described as a single gene disorder. In Iranian Jews, who are highly inbred, anencephaly is inherited as an autosomal recessive condition (Zlotogora 1995).

All women of reproductive age should consume at least 400 mcg of folic acid daily to prevent neural tube defects. For women who have previously had a fetus or infant affected with anencephaly, the Centers for Disease Control and Prevention (CDC) recommends increasing the intake of folic acid to 4000 mcg (4mg) per day beginning at least 1 month prior to conception (Committee on Genetics, 1999). Prenatal diagnosis can be performed in a subsequent pregnancy, either by sonographic examination, or by maternal serum α-fetoprotein analysis.

REFERENCES

Botkin JR. Anencephalic infants as organ donors. Pediatrics 1988;82:250–256.

Committee on Genetics, American Academy of Pediatrics. Folic acid for the prevention of neural tube defects. Pediatrics 1999;104:325–327.

Feuchtbaum LB, Currier RJ, Riggle S, Roberson M, Lorey FW, Cunningham GC. Neural tube defect prevalence in California (1990–1994): eliciting patterns by type of defect and maternal race/ethnicity. Genet Test 1999;3:265–272.

Goldstein RB, Filly RA. Prenatal diagnosis of anencephaly: spectrum of sonographic appearances and distinction from the amniotic band syndrome. AJR Am J Roentgenol 1988;151: 547–550.

Holzgreve W, Beller FK, Buchholz B, Hansman M, Köhler K. Kidney transplantation from anencephalic donors. N Engl J Med 1987;316:1069–1070.

Limb CJ, Holmes LB. Anencephaly: changes in prenatal detection and birth status, 1972 through 1990. Am J Obstet Gynecol 1994;170:1333–1338.

Main DM, Mennuti MT. Neural tube defects: issues in prenatal diagnosis and counseling. Obstet Gynecol 1986;67: 1–16.

Medical Task Force on Anencephaly. The infant with anencephaly. N Engl J Med 1990;332:669–674.

Melnick M, Myrianthopoulos NC. Studies in neural tube defects. II. Pathologic findings in a prospectively collected series of anencephalics. Am J Med Genet 1987;26: 797–810.

Naidich TP, Altman NR, Braffman BH, McLone DG, Zimmerman RA. Cephaloceles and related malformations. AJNR Am J Neuroradiol 1992;13:655–690.

Pantzar J, Ritchie S, Hall JG. Evidence for multi-site closure of the neural tube in humans. Am J Med Genet 1993;47:723–743.

Peabody JL, Emery JR, Ashwal S. Experience with anencephalic infants as prospective organ donors. N Engl J Med 1989;321:344–350.

Rizzo G, Arduini D. Cardiac output in anencephalic fetuses. Gynecol Obstet Invest 1991;32:33–35.

Van Allen MI, Kalousek DK, Chernoff GF, Zlotogora J. Evidence for multi-site closure of the neural tube in humans. Am J Med Genet 1993;47:723–743.

CHAPTER 6

Arachnoid Cyst

▶ CONDITION

Arachnoid cysts represent collections of cerebrospinal fluid enclosed within layers of pia arachnoid. They are lined by arachnoidal cells and collagen. Arachnoid cysts are unilocular, round, oval, or crescentlike in shape. These fluid-filled masses can be distinguished from the fourth ventricle and vallecula. The cerebellar vermis, hemispheres, and brain stem are usually normal in this condition except when the cyst compresses these structures (Altman et al. 1992). Arachnoid cysts are formed by maldevelopment of the leptomeninges. They are located between two layers of the arachnoid membrane. They initially communicate with the subarachnoid space and have the potential to grow due to this continued communication. Fluid accumulates as a result of a ball-valve mechanism (Diakoumakis et al. 1986). Choroid plexus–like tissue can be present within the cyst wall. This ectopic tissue secretes cerebrospinal fluid, resulting in progressive distention of the cyst (Diakoumakis et al. 1986).

Two types of arachnoid cysts exist: the congenital type, which is considered to be the result of maldevelopment of the leptomeninges, and the acquired type, which is the result of hemorrhage, trauma, or infection (Meizner et al. 1988). Two-thirds of prenatally detected cases are supratentorial in location, whereas one-third are located within the posterior fossa (Estroff et al. 1995). In contrast, most postnatally detected cases are located within the posterior fossa (Hogge et al. 1995). Five percent of supratentorial interhemispheric arachnoid cysts are associated with agenesis of the corpus callosum (Lena et al. 1995).

Structural features of the arachnoid cyst wall that distinguish it from the normal arachnoid membrane include:

1. Splitting of the arachnoid membrane at the margin of the cyst

2. A very thick layer of collagen present in the cyst wall

3. Absence of the traversing trabecular processes within the cyst

4. Presence of hyperplastic arachnoid cells located within the cyst wall that presumably participate in collagen synthesis (Rengachary and Watanabe 1981).

Electron micrographic studies of arachnoid cysts reveal a striking and nearly invariable association of the arachnoid cyst with the normal subarachnoid cistern. Some investigators have demonstrated that in their early stages, arachnoid cysts communicate with the subarachnoid space, revealing the exclusively intra-arachnoid nature of the cyst (Rengachary and Watanabe 1981). Other investigators, however, postulate that the retrocerebellar arachnoid cyst may represent a persistent diverticulum of the fourth ventricle that fails to involute, the so-called Blake pouch (Altman et al. 1992). The precise cause for the development of arachnoid cyst is unknown. The factors responsible for the formation of the normal subarachnoid cistern, however, also produce splitting of the arachnoid membrane in that location. This results in a diverticulum or enclosed cystic space. Thus, arachnoid cysts are thought to be a developmental anomaly of the subarachnoid cistern (Rengachary and Watanabe 1981).

▶ INCIDENCE

The incidence of arachnoid cysts is unknown. They are rare in prenatal life. Arachnoid cysts represent 1% of all space-occupying masses in childhood (Estroff et al. 1995) and are an incidental finding in 0.5% of autopsy studies (Rafferty et al. 1998). Arachnoid cysts are more common in males than in females (Kollias et al. 1993;

Lena et al. 1995). The left side of the brain is more commonly affected than the right.

▶ SONOGRAPHIC FINDINGS

Sonographic diagnosis of arachnoid cyst relies on the finding of a sonolucent mass with smooth and thin walls within the brain (Fig. 6-1). This cyst does not communicate with the lateral ventricles, but may be associated with hydrocephalus (Fig. 6-2) due to a mass effect that obstructs the flow of cerebrospinal fluid. In this condition, the cerebellar vermis is normal in size.

In 1986 Diakoumakis et al. described a fetal suprasellar arachnoid cyst that was detected on a routine antenatal sonographic examination performed at 32 weeks of gestation. The patient was followed by repeat sonographic examination, which demonstrated enlargement of the cyst and development of fetal hydrocephalus. These authors also described the characteristic "head of the bunny" appearance on postnatal cranial computed tomographic (CT) examination with a midline cyst and two dilated lateral ventricles (Diakoumakis et al. 1986). In another case report, a fetus was described at 22 weeks of gestation with an isolated extraventricular supratentorial arachnoid cyst (Meizner et al. 1988). No hydrocephalus was present. The axial sonography performed at the level of the cerebral peduncles revealed a rounded, fluid-filled cyst in the right parieto-occipital lobe of the brain. The posteriorly angled coronal scan demonstrated splaying of the right lateral ventricle due to a pressure effect. This fetus was followed with repeated sonographic examinations and the cyst was shown to enlarge progressively over the duration of pregnancy (Meizner et al. 1988).

Most cases of arachnoid cysts are detected at >20 weeks of gestation (Hogge et al. 1995; Rafferty et al. 1998). Only rarely are extracranial abnormalities detected. In one case report, a 1-by-1-cm posterior fossa cyst was detected at 18 weeks of gestation. The pregnancy was aborted because of associated chromosomal abnormalities (Hogge et al. 1995).

Estroff et al. (1995) described two cases of arachnoid cysts that, on the basis of prenatal sonographic findings, were suspected antenatally to be a Dandy–Walker malformation. These authors noted that sonographic distinction between the retrocerebellar arachnoid cysts and the Dandy–Walker cyst may be difficult. Both malformations may be associated with hydrocephalus. In arachnoid cysts, the underlying cerebellar hemispheres and vermis are normal, although they are displaced and compressed anteriorly. Typically, no extracranial abnormalities are present in arachnoid cysts (Estroff et al. 1995).

Rafferty et al. (1998) reported a single case of fetal arachnoid cyst diagnosed at 33 weeks of gestation. Three-dimensional volume scanning was used to confirm that the isolated cystic structure arose from the floor of the middle cerebral fossa.

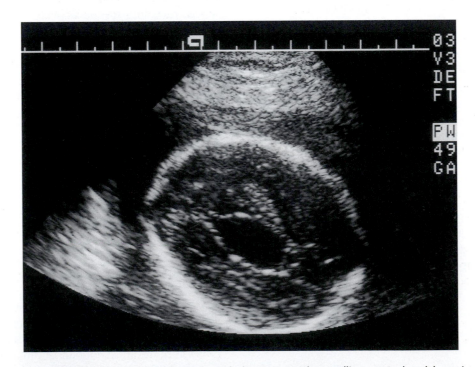

Figure 6-1. Transaxial image of fetal head demonstrating solitary arachnoid cyst.

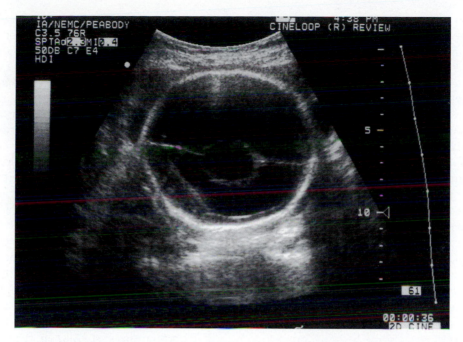

Figure 6-2. Transaxial image of a fetal head demonstrating an arachnoid cyst and associated hydrocephalus.

▶ DIFFERENTIAL DIAGNOSIS

The differential diagnosis for arachnoid cysts is given in Table 6-1. One condition that can be confused with arachnoid cyst is mega cisterna magna. In fetuses with mega cisterna magna, there is no mass effect on the cerebellar hemispheres and no hydrocephalus is present (Estroff et al. 1995). Another consideration in the differential diagnosis is Dandy–Walker malformation (see Chapter 10), which is a well-defined posterior fossa cyst that is separate from the ventricular system (Meizner et al. 1988). Many arachnoid cysts extend anteriorly to the cerebellar hemispheres, which can effectively rule out the Dandy–Walker malformation (Altman et al. 1992). On the other hand, arachnoid cysts in the midline that lie wholly posterior to the cerebellum may be difficult to distinguish from the mega cisterna magna (Altman et al. 1992). It may be quite difficult to distinguish antenatally between Dandy–Walker malformation and arachnoid cysts. This is because the true anatomy of the posterior fossa cannot be seen adequately in utero. The determination of size, shape, and position of the fourth ventricle and cerebellar vermis is critical to accurate antenatal diagnosis (Estroff et al. 1995). The finding of associated agenesis of the corpus callosum may suggest a diagnosis of Dandy–Walker malformation. Postnatally, an invasive procedure, such as instilling radiographic contrast material into the ventricular system (cisternagram) may be necessary to distinguish among Dandy–Walker malformation and its variants (see Chapter 10), mega cisterna magna, or Blake pouch cyst (Estroff et al. 1995). La Torre et al. (1973) recommended angiographic distinction between Dandy–Walker malformation and arachnoid cysts by evaluation of the posterior inferior cerebellar artery and its vermian branch. In arachnoid cysts, all vessels are normal in size and are displaced forward and upward, while in the Dandy–Walker malformation, the posterior inferior cerebellar artery is miniature and the vermian branch of the inferior cerebellar artery and the inferior vermian vein are absent.

An additional consideration in the differential diagnosis of arachnoid cyst is a variant of normal. Knutzon et al. (1991) described a linear hyperechoic structure in the cisterna magna previously thought to be the straight sinus. This structure was identified in 92 to 95 prenatal sonographic examinations. This structure appeared

▶ TABLE 6-1. DIFFERENTIAL DIAGNOSIS OF ARACHNOID CYST

Mega cisterna magna
Dandy–Walker malformation
Normal variant
Alobar holoprosencephaly
Porencephalic cyst
Ependymal cyst
Schizencephaly
Infarct
Tumor

cystlike in 17 of 95 cases studied. On histopathologic correlation in aborted fetuses, this structure was shown to be the subarachnoid septa. It is most likely due to focal concentrations of arachnoid trabeculations in the subarachnoid space (Knutzon et al. 1991). Intrahemispheric arachnoid cysts can be confused with a dorsal cyst present in cases of alobar holoprosencephaly (see Chapter 13) (Lena et al. 1995). Porencephalic cysts are part of the differential diagnosis. They are located within brain matter, communicate with the ventricular system, and do not exert a mass effect. They are often associated with a prenatal or postnatal brain injury (Lena et al. 1995). The final consideration in the differential diagnosis is the presence of ependymal cysts. These occur less frequently than arachnoid cysts and tend to occupy the central white matter of the frontal or temporoparietal lobes (Rengachary and Watanabe 1981). In ependymal cysts, the protein content of the cyst fluid is higher than that of the arachnoid cyst.

▶ ANTENATAL NATURAL HISTORY

Little is known about the antenatal natural history of arachnoid cysts. Some increase in size and others resolve spontaneously. Two cases have been described in the medical literature of arachnoid cysts associated with increased maternal serum α-fetoprotein levels (Hogge et al. 1995; Kwon and Jeanty 1991). It is not known if these are etiologically related or coincidental. From the limited number of prenatal cases reported, it appears that the cyst can grow in size during antenatal life (Diakoumakis et al. 1986; Meizner et al. 1988). In addition, hydrocephalus can develop from obstruction of the foramen of Monro and displacement of the aqueduct posteriorly with blocked basal cisterns.

▶ MANAGEMENT OF PREGNANCY

When an arachnoid cyst is detected within the fetal brain, the patient should be referred to a center capable of complete anatomic sonographic fetal diagnosis. Serial sonographic examination should be performed to monitor potential enlargement of the cyst and subsequent development of ventriculomegaly (Hogge et al. 1995). It is important to seek evidence of associated malformations, as arachnoid cysts may be part of a multiple malformation syndrome. For example, one rare recessively inherited condition consists of absent tibia, polydactyly, cleft palate, and the presence of retrocerebellar cysts (Holmes et al. 1995). Rare cases of arachnoid cyst have been associated with tetralogy of Fallot and neurofibromatosis type 1. Consideration

should be given to performing amniocentesis to obtain a fetal karyotype. In one case, a fetus with a posterior fossa arachnoid cyst was shown to have an abnormal karyotype consisting of 46,X der(X),tX:9(q22;q22). Thus, this fetus had a partial trisomy of the long arm of chromosome 9 with partial monosomy of the long arm of the X chromosome. This was due to a balanced translocation occurring in the mother between chromosomes X and 9 (Hogge et al. 1995).

Prospective parents of a fetus demonstrated to have an arachnoid cyst should be offered the opportunity to consult with a pediatric neurologist, neurosurgeon, and medical geneticist. The presence of an isolated arachnoid cyst is not an indication for cesarean section (Meizner et al. 1988). However, because of the potential for development of ventriculomegaly, the patient should be followed by serial sonograms to determine if the fetal head size is small enough for a vaginal delivery. An additional consideration in the determination of route of delivery is the risk of trauma and hemorrhage within the cyst (Altman et al. 1992).

▶ FETAL INTERVENTION

There is no fetal intervention recommended for arachnoid cyst.

▶ TREATMENT OF THE NEWBORN

Newborns who have been diagnosed with an arachnoid cyst antenatally should undergo a complete physical examination. Arrangements should be made for follow-up with consultants in genetics and neurology. Depending on the location of the cyst, computed tomographic (CT) or magnetic resonance imaging (MRI) scanning is indicated to confirm the presence of the cyst. A careful measurement should be made of the newborn's head circumference, and the presence of asymmetry of the calvarium should be noted. The newborn should be observed for any changes in head circumference, as the potential exists for expansion of the cyst by hemorrhage due to trauma at delivery through the rupture of bridging veins (Altman et al. 1992). Clinical characteristics at birth will depend on the size of the cyst (Kollias et al. 1993). Associated hydrocephalus is present in 30 to 100% of cases (Kollias et al. 1993). In newborns in whom an arachnoid cyst is detected postnatally, the overwhelming presenting symptom is macrocephaly (71.5% of 67 cases reported) (Pascual-Castroviejo et al. 1990). Seizures may occasionally occur in infants with arachnoid cyst. Increased intracranial pressure is rarely a presenting clinical sign.

▶ SURGICAL TREATMENT

The operative procedures for treatment of arachnoid cysts consist of cyst excision, fenestration, or drainage into an adjacent cistern, abdominal cavity, or atrium (Richard et al. 1989). Small asymptomatic cysts do not require any intervention. Surgical excision of the cyst is indicated in the rare cases in which increased intracranial pressure is detected. Craniotomy, however, may result in severe complications. The most common treatment consists of a cystoperitoneal shunt, which results in a high rate of regression of the cyst and rarely produces recurrence or complications. These shunts may need revision due to blockage or growth of the patient (Pascual-Castroviejo et al. 1991). Most neurosurgeons prefer to treat the patient initially with feneshanhim, as the avoidance of a shunt is the primary goal in management (Fewel et al. 1996), More recently, an endoscopic approach to cyst obliteration has been described (Choi et al. 1999).

▶ LONG-TERM OUTCOME

The major complications in the long-term outcome for affected patients include hydrocephalus, seizures, and neurologic abnormalities (Altman et al. 1992; Hogge et al. 1995). Estroff et al. (1995) described the outcome for a fetus diagnosed at 28 weeks of gestation with hydrocephalus and a retrocerebellar cyst. This infant required a complex dual-shunt system, but at 3 months of age the head circumference was following the normal growth curve and the developmental milestones were appropriate for gestational age. These investigators stated that the outcome is often favorable after decompression of the cyst by cystoperitoneal shunt (Estroff et al. 1995).

In a follow-up study of 16 children with symptomatic supratentorial interhemispheric cysts ascertained postnatally, Lena et al. (1995) demonstrated that no cyst became larger but none disappeared completely. These authors had a median follow-up period of 50 months. In 16 children, the preoperative symptoms disappeared completely in 7 and partially in 4. Two of the original patient group were asymptomatic and remained completely normal. Of the 16 children, 12 were entirely neurologically normal, 1 had moderate disability, 2 had severe disability, and 1 died from unrelated pneumonia 3 months after surgery. Seizures developed in 4 of the 16 children (Lena et al. 1995). Richard et al. (1989) followed affected children into adulthood over a 48-year period. These investigators demonstrated a favorable outcome for most patients, with 62 to 93% of all individuals followed over this period having had normal physical and social development and a satisfactory quality of life. The prognosis was also noted to be related to age at operation. Independent of the surgical method used over this 48-year period, the percentage of patients with any disability as compared with all due to arachnoid cyst ranged from approximately 11 to 14%. Patients who died in this study had causes of death unrelated to the arachnoid cyst (Richard et al. 1989).

▶ GENETICS AND RECURRENCE RISK

Most cases of arachnoid cyst appear to be sporadic (Altman et al. 1992). Rare cases of arachnoid cyst are associated with neurofibromatosis type 1 or other multiple congenital anomaly disorders due to single gene mutations (Holmes et al. 1995). For example, an unexpectedly high number of asymptomatic intracranial arachnoid cysts were found in a group of 247 patients with autosomal dominant polycystic kidney disease who underwent high resolution CT scanning or MR imaging (Schievink et al. 1995). If a prenatal karyotype analysis is performed and an unbalanced chromosome abnormality is detected, as in the case reported by Hogge et al. (1995), parental chromosome analysis is strongly suggested.

Occasional families have been described with recurrence of arachnoid cysts. For example, Handa et al. (1981) reported the presence of bilateral arachnoid cysts in the middle cranial fossa in two brothers, aged 10 months and 3 years. Other reports of siblings affected with arachnoid cysts exist in the medical literature (Hendriks et al. 1999; Pomeranz et al. 1991; Tolmie et al. 1997; Wilson et al. 1988). This suggests the possible existence of heritable factors that predispose individuals to the formation of arachnoid cysts.

REFERENCES

Altman NR, Naidich TP, Braffman BH. Posterior fossa malformations. Am J Neuroradiol 1992;13:691–724.

Choi JU, Kim DS, Huh R. Endoscopic approach to arachnoid cyst. Childs Nerv Syst 1999;15:285–291.

Diakoumakis EE, Weinberg B, Mollin J. Prenatal sonographic diagnosis of a suprasellar arachnoid cyst. J Ultrasound Med 1986;5:529–530.

Estroff JA, Parad RB, Barnes PD, Madsen JP, Benacerraf BR. Posterior fossa arachnoid cyst: an in utero mimicker of Dandy–Walker malformation. J Ultrasound Med 1995;14:787–790.

Fewel ME, Levi ML, McComb JG. Surgical treatment of 95 children with 102 intracranial arachnoid cysts. Pediatr Neurosurg 1996;25:165–173.

Handa J, Okamoto K, Sato M. Arachnoid cyst of the middle cranial fossa: report of bilateral cysts in siblings. Surg Neurol 1981;16:127–130.

Hendricks YM, Laan LA, Vielvoye GJ, van Haeringen A. Bilateral sensorineural deafness, partial agensis of the corpus callosum, and arachnoid cysts in two sisters. Am J Med Genet 1999;10:183–186.

Hogge WA, Schnatterly P, Ferguson JE. Early prenatal diagnosis of an infratentorial arachnoid cyst: association with an unbalanced translocation. Prenat Diagn 1995;15:186–188.

Holmes LB, Redline RW, Brown DL, Williams AJ, Collins T. Absence/hypoplasia of tibia, polydactyly, retrocerebellar arachnoid cyst, and other anomalies: an autosomal recessive disorder. J Med Genet 1995;32:896–900.

Knutzon RK, McGahan JP, Salamat MS, Brant WE. Fetal cisterna magna septa: a normal anatomic finding. Radiology 1991;180:799–801.

Kollias SS, Ball WS, Prenger EC. Cystic malformations of the posterior fossa: differential diagnosis clarified through embryologic analysis. Radiographics 1993;13:1211–1231.

Kwon T, Jeanty P. Supratentorial arachnoid cyst. Fetus 1991;1:1.

La Torre E, Fortuna A, Occhipinti E. Angiographic differentiation between Dandy–Walker cyst and arachnoid cyst of the posterior fossa in newborn infants and children. J Neurosurg 1973;38:298–308.

Lena G, van Calenberg F, Genitori L, Choux M. Supratentorial interhemispheric cysts associated with callosal agenesis: surgical treatment and outcome in 16 children. Child Nerv Syst 1995;11:568–573.

Meizner I, Barkai Y, Tadmor R, Katz M. In utero ultrasonic detection of fetal arachnoid cyst. J Clin Ultrasound 1988;16:506–509.

Pascual-Castroviejo I, Roche MC, Bermejo AM, Arcas J, Blazquez MG. Primary intracranial arachnoidal cysts. Child Nerv Syst 1991;7:257–263.

Pomeranz S, Constantini S, Lubetzki-Korn I, Amir N. Familial intracranial arachnoid cyst. Child Nerv Syst 1991;7:100–102.

Rafferty PG, Britton J, Penna L, Ville Y. Prenatal diagnosis of a large fetal arachnoid cyst. Ultrasound Obstet Gynecol 1998;12:358–361.

Rengachary SS, Watanabe I. Ultrastructure and pathogenesis of intracranial arachnoid cysts. J Neuropathol Exp Neurol 1981;40:61–83.

Richard KE, Dahl K, Sanker P. Long-term follow-up of children and juveniles with arachnoid cysts. Child Nerv Syst 1989;5:184–187.

Schievink WI, Huston J 3rd, Torres VE, Marsh WR. Intracranial cysts in autosomal dominant polycystic kidney disease. J Neurosurg 1995;83:1004–1007.

Tolmie JL, Day R, Fredericks B, Galea P, Moffett AW. Dominantly inherited cerebral dysplasia: arachnoid cyst associated with mild mental handicap in a mother and her son. J Med Genet 1997;34:1018–1020.

Wilson W, Deponte KA, McIlhenny J, Dreifuss FE. Arachnoid cysts in a brother and sister. J Med Genet 1988;25:714–715.

CHAPTER 7

Cerebral Calcifications

► CONDITION

Cerebral calcifications are an unusual sonographic finding in the fetus. They are thought to occur late in gestation and result from localized neuronal-cell death. Intracranial calcifications are most commonly associated with the in utero infections due to the TORCH (toxoplasmosis, other agents, rubella, cytomegalovirus, herpesvirus) agents (Ghidini et al. 1989). This chapter covers three types of fetal cerebral calcifications: (1) focal, punctate parenchymal calcifications, (2) periventricular echogenicity, and (3) echogenic blood vessels demonstrated in the thalami and basal ganglia (Estroff et al. 1992).

► INCIDENCE

Fetal intracranial calcifications are rare. Although congenital cytomegalovirus is common (on the order of 0.2 to 2.0% of live births [Hohlfeld et al. 1991]), most cases of congenital cytomegalovirus are not associated with cerebral calcifications. One study found fetal intracranial calcifications in 3 of 18 (17%) of fetuses who were infected congenitally and had prenatal sonographic studies (Drose et al. 1991).

► SONOGRAPHIC FINDINGS

Much of the information regarding the differential diagnosis and outcome for infants with intracranial calcifications derives from the postnatal pediatric radiographic literature. The use of postnatal cranial sonography as an effective means of visualizing intracranial calcifications in newborn infants with congenital infections was first described by Dykes et al. in 1982. She and her colleagues demonstrated the presence of multifocal, high-intensity echoes in infants with infection. What was unusual about this sonographic finding was that there was no acoustical shadowing from these echoes. Subsequently, Teele and colleagues (1988) noted the unique sonographic finding of bright, branching vessels in the thalami and basal ganglia of 12 newborn infants. This finding was strongly associated with the presence of congenital infection. In this group of 12 infants, 5 had congenital cytomegalovirus (CMV), two had congenital rubella, one had congenital syphilis, and 3 had trisomy 13 with no known evidence of infection. These findings later were extended by other investigators, including Ben-Ami and colleagues (1990), who studied 11 infants noted to have bright echogenic stripes in the thalami and basal ganglia. By using duplex sonography, these investigators demonstrated that the stripes derived from the lenticulostriate arteries in the basal ganglia (Fig. 7-1). In their study group, 8 of 11 cases were infected in utero, and 1 additional patient had trisomy 13. In a retrospective review of 2,320 neonatal cranial sonograms, 25 newborns were identified with these linear areas of echogenicity in the basal ganglia (Hughes et al. 1991). Three of the 25 newborns were shown to have abnormal chromosomes (2 had trisomy 21 and 1 had trisomy 13). An additional 4 patients had CMV, and 8 had clinical evidence of either anoxia or other metabolic brain injury. In the remaining 10, there were no signs consistent with infection, but these infants represented a heterogeneous population with associated anomalies (Hughes et al. 1991). These investigators felt that the differential diagnosis of echogenicity of the vessels of the thalami and basal ganglia should be expanded to include a number of associated perinatal conditions.

The first case of intracranial calcifications associated with in utero cytomegalovirus infection was demonstrated in 1989 in a fetus at 21 weeks of gestation (Ghidini et al. 1989). Relatively few cases of fetal intracranial calcifications have been described in the

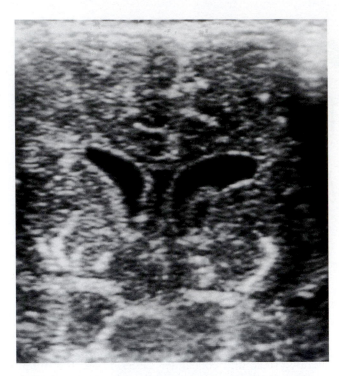

Figure 7-1. Coronal sonogram of a newborn with congenital cytomegalovirus infection, demonstrating branching, echogenic vessels in the basal ganglia. *(Reprinted, with permission, from Ben-Ami T, Yousef-zadeh D, Backus M, Reichman B, Kessler A, Hammer-man-Rozenberg C. Lenticulostriate vasculopathy in infants with infections of the central nervous system: sonographic and Doppler findings. Pediatr Radiol 1990; 20:575–579.)*

literature on prenatal diagnosis. Fakhry and Khoury (1991) reported two cases of fetal intracranial calcifications associated with CMV. In one case, at 32 weeks of gestation, the fetus was also noted to have microcephaly (Fig. 7-2). The other case was studied sequentially. At 17 weeks of gestation, the fetus had a completely normal sonographic examination. At 22 weeks, the fetus was noted to have mild hydrocephalus and subtle hyperechoic foci in the periventricular areas. By 28 weeks of gestation, the ventricular dilation had progressed significantly, and the periventricular hyperechoic foci were more evident. These authors confirmed Dykes et al.'s impressions that acoustic shadowing was not elicited by the periventricular hyperechoic foci. They postulated that this might be due to the small size of the calcifications, which were highly reflective but not absorptive. These authors recommended that in the presence of hydrocephalus, given the prevalence of CMV infection, a careful evaluation of ventricular walls should be undertaken to search for hyperechoic foci. The pattern of bilateral periventricular calcifications may be a specific finding for intrauterine CMV infection (Fig. 7-3) (Tassin et al. 1991). A different fetal manifestation of congenital CMV infection at 20 weeks of gestation was reported by Estroff et al. (1992). The initial transabdominal scan, performed at 20 weeks, demonstrated a hyperechoic rim in the periphery of the fetal cerebral cortex. A follow-up study performed at 31 weeks of gestation, using a transvaginal probe, demonstrated the branching linear areas of echogenicity seen in the fetal

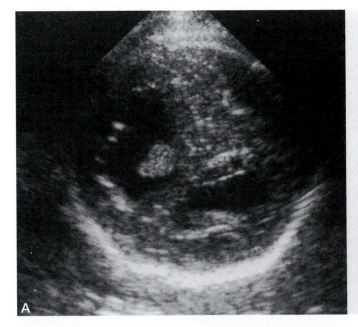
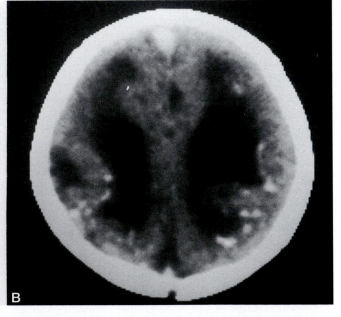

Figure 7-2. (A) Axial scan of a fetal head at 32 weeks of gestation showing periventricular hyperechoic foci with absent acoustic shadowing. The choroid plexi are well seen in the moderately dilated ventricles. (B) CT scan without contrast obtained after birth from the same infant, showing ventriculomegaly and periventricular and parenchymal calcifications. *(Reprinted, with permission, from Fakhry J, Khoury A. Fetal intracranial calcifications: the importance of periventricular hyperechoic foci without shadowing. J Ultrasound Med 1991;10:51–54.)*

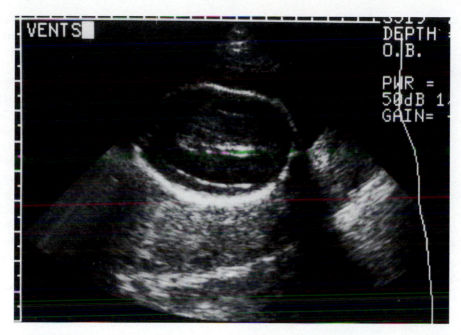

Figure 7-3. Axial scan of a fetal head in a fetus with cytomegalovirus demonstrating ventriculomegaly and bilateral periventricular calcifications. *(Reprinted, with permission, from Drose JA, Dennis MA, Thickman D. Infection in utero: US findings in 19 cases. Radiology 1991;178:369–374.)*

thalami. In addition, punctate hyperechoic foci in the cerebral cortex were seen. This finding is likely to be the fetal equivalent of the lenticulostriate artery echogenicity demonstrated postnatally in several studies (Ben-Ami et al. 1990; Hughes et al. 1991; Teele et al. 1988).

▶ DIFFERENTIAL DIAGNOSIS

The differential diagnosis of fetal intracranial calcifications includes noninfectious and infectious causes. The noninfectious or structural causes include intracranial tumors (Sherer and Onyeije 1998), the bilateral periventricular calcification of subependymal nodules seen in tuberous sclerosis (see Chapter 53), sagittal or transverse sinus thrombosis, Sturge–Weber syndrome, trisomy 13, and intracranial or intraventricular hemorrhage. Why echogenicity of the lenticulostriate arteries in the fetal thalami or basal ganglia are associated with trisomy 13 is currently not known.

The more common cause for fetal intracranial calcification is congenital infection. In many cases, the fetal intracranial calcifications are accompanied by other findings suggestive of infection, including intrauterine growth restriction, placental villitis, hepatosplenomegaly, ascites, hydrops fetalis, ventriculomegaly, or microcephaly (Ghidini et al. 1989). The infections likely to cause intracranial calcifications include CMV (Estroff et al. 1992; Hohlfield et al. 1991), rubella (Yamashita et al. 1991), toxoplasmosis, and herpes simplex., CMV is overwhelmingly the most likely infectious cause for cerebral calcifications (see Figs. 7-1, 7-2, and 7-3) (Fakhry and Khoury 1991).

▶ ANTENATAL NATURAL HISTORY

Toxoplasmosis, CMV, herpes simplex virus type 2, and rubella infections reach the fetal central nervous system via hematogenous dissemination. These viruses are known to have a predilection for rapidly growing subependymal or germinal matrix cells. Once the fetus is infected, these agents cause neuronal- or ganglia-cell necrosis. Necrotic cells may subsequently undergo calcification (Ghidini et al. 1989). Because of this sequence of events, cerebral calcification is rarely documented before the mid- to late second trimester.

In several cases in which a neuropathologic examination was performed on infants who died with the postnatal sonographic finding of echogenic branching thalamic vessels, histopathology demonstrated thickened hypercellular walls with deposits of amorphous basophilic material, suggesting a perinatally acquired vasculitis (Teele et al. 1988). The pathophysiology behind the demonstration of echogenicity was likely due to a vascular injury resulting from a viral infection that affected the fetal central nervous system. Teele and colleagues concluded that postnatal sonography was helpful in detecting early noncalcific inflammation and mineralization in vasculitis due to infection. Fetuses with perinatally acquired infection are at increased risk of spontaneously aborting.

▶ MANAGEMENT OF PREGNANCY

When fetal intracranial calcifications are documented, a careful search must be undertaken for associated structural anomalies, intrauterine growth restriction, and placental problems. The leading candidate in the differential diagnosis is CMV, so further management of pregnancy should include maternal TORCH titers. An amniocentesis is recommended for fetal karyotyping to rule out trisomies 13 and 21, and to obtain amniotic fluid for CMV culture. CMV culture, however, will be positive only 6 weeks after the onset of infection. In one series, two false negative results from amniotic fluid CMV culture were reported (Nicolini et al. 1994). In both cases, the fluid was cultured between 3 and 4 weeks after the infection occurred. After 18 to 20 weeks of gestation, cordocentesis can be performed to measure fetal immunoglobin M (IgM) to CMV and liver-function tests. Two studies have addressed the issue of diagnostic accuracy of various tests to determine fetal infection with CMV (Hohlfeld et al. 1991; Lynch et al. 1991). In the first study, 15 cases of maternal primary CMV were studied. Of these, 8 had documented evidence of fetal infection. All 8 of these cases had a positive CMV culture from amniotic fluid. Six of the 8 affected cases also had positive fetal IgM to CMV. Only 2 of the infected fetuses had abnormal sonograms, and these demonstrated hydrops fetalis and ascites. Of the 7 cases not shown by prenatal diagnostic studies to be infected, the absence of infection was confirmed postnatally. These authors concluded that infection was diagnosed correctly by amniocentesis in all cases but that cordocentesis provided additional clinical information. These data were helpful, because grossly abnormal liver-function tests and complete blood count were associated with a rapidly fatal postnatal outcome (Hohlfeld et al. 1991). In another study, 12 fetuses at risk for CMV were studied. Of these, 6 were diagnosed as infected. The most reliable parameters of fetal infection were isolation of virus from amniotic fluid and elevations of total IgM and γ-glutamine transpeptidase in fetal blood (Lynch et al. 1991).

Polymerase chain reaction (PCR) assays are available for CMV diagnosis, but their sensitivity and specificity for detection of fetal infection have not yet been established (Guerina 1994). Serial sonograms are recommended to monitor fetal growth.

▶ FETAL INTERVENTION

At present there is no effective therapy to treat the fetus in utero (Guerina 1994). The results of treating newborns with ganciclovir have been encouraging, and prompt consideration should be given to fetal treatment with this antiviral agent. Because ganciclovir crosses the placenta by simple diffusion, maternal administration should be possible (Gilstrap et al. 1994).

▶ TREATMENT OF THE NEWBORN

Because of the risk of anemia and cardiovascular complications associated with severe perinatal infection, consideration should be given to delivering potentially infected infants in a tertiary-care center. After delivery, a complete physical examination is indicated, with careful attention to measurements of weight, head circumference, and length. A computed tomographic (CT) scan is useful to confirm the areas of intracranial calcification that were noted on prenatal sonography. However, if bright branching thalamic vessels were demonstrated antenatally, this finding will not be demonstrated on postnatal CT scans (Teele et al. 1988).

If amniocentesis was not performed antenatally, a neonatal urine sample should be obtained for CMV culture. Newborn TORCH titers should be drawn to pair with the maternal samples. If the fetus is infected with CMV, consideration should be given to treatment with ganciclovir over a 6-week course. Ophthalmologic examination may be useful to document the presence of chorioretinitis. Prior to discharge, the newborn infant should undergo hearing tests.

▶ SURGICAL TREATMENT

There is no surgical treatment for cerebral calcifications.

▶ LONG-TERM OUTCOME

The long-term outcome will depend on the cause of the cerebral calcifications. If the underlying diagnosis is trisomy 13, refer to Chapter 132. If the underlying diagnosis is congenital CMV infection, the prognosis is variable. The major complications include hearing loss, microcephaly, developmental delay, seizures, and visual impairment (Ben-Ami et al. 1990; Koga et al. 1990). In a review of 19 cases of prenatally acquired infection due to different agents, Drose et al. (1991) described 6 cases of CMV, 3 of which were detected prenatally by the presence of periventricular calcifications on sonography. An additional 3 were detected postnatally by CT scan or at autopsy. The outcomes for these 6 cases included 2 spontaneous losses at 23 and 24 weeks of gestation, 1 death in the neonatal period, 1 infant who survived with hydrocephalus, 1 infant who survived with hearing loss and abnormal development to 18 months of age, and 1 survivor with only hearing loss (Drose et al. 1991).

The postnatural history of intracranial calcifications in infants with treated congenital toxoplasmosis has been studied by computed tomography (Patel et al. 1996). In infants who were treated with appropriate doses of antibiotics, the majority (75%) of calcifications resolved or diminished.

▶ GENETICS AND RECURRENCE RISK

Fetal intracranial calcifications due to an infectious cause presumably have a low risk of recurrence. Limited case reports exist of recurrence of fetal CMV. If echogenic branching thalamic vessels were demonstrated due to trisomy 21 or 13, the recurrence risk is 1%; there is also an age-related maternal risk if the mother is over age 41 years.

REFERENCES

Ben-Ami T, Yousefzadeh D, Backus M, Reichman B, Kessler A, Hammerman-Rozenberg C. Lenticulostriate vasculopathy in infants with infections of the central nervous system: sonographic and Doppler findings. Pediatr Radiol 1990;20:575–579.

Drose JA, Dennis MA, Thickman D. Infection in utero: US findings in 19 cases. Radiology 1991;178:369–374.

Dykes FD, Ahmann PA, Lazzara A. Cranial ultrasound in the detection of intracranial calcifications. J Pediatr 1982;100: 406–408.

Estroff JA, Parad RB, Teele RL, Benacerraf BR. Echogenic vessels in the fetal thalami and basal ganglia associated with cytomegalovirus infection. J Ultrasound Med 1992; 11:626–688.

Fakhry J, Khoury A. Fetal intracranial calcifications: the importance of periventricular hyperechoic foci without shadowing. J Ultrasound Med 1991;10:51–54.

Ghidini A, Sirtori M, Vergani P, Mariani S, Tucci E, Scola G. Fetal intracranial calcifications. Am J Obstet Gynecol 1989;160:86–87.

Gilstrap LC, Bowdon RE, Roberts SW, Sobhi S. The transfer of the nucleoside analog ganciclovir across the perfused human placenta. Am J Obstet Gynecol 1994;170:967–972.

Guerina NG. Management strategies for infectious diseases in pregnancy. Semin Perinatol 1994;18:305–320.

Hohlfeld P, Vial Y, Maillard-Brignon C, Vaudaux B, Fawer C-L. Cytomegalovirus fetal infection: prenatal diagnosis. Obstet Gynecol 1991;78:615–618.

Hughes P, Weinberger E, Shaw DW. Linear areas of echogenicity in the thalami and basal ganglia of neonates: an expanded association. Radiology 1991;179:103–105.

Koga Y, Mizumoto M, Matsumoto Y et al. Prenatal diagnosis of fetal intracranial calcifications. Am J Obstet Gynecol 1990;163:1543–1544.

Lynch L, Daffos F, Emanuel D et al. Prenatal diagnosis of fetal cytomegalovirus infection. Am J Obstet Gynecol 1991;165:714–718.

Nicolini U, Kustermann A, Tassis B et al. Prenatal diagnosis of human cytomegalovirus infection. Prenat Diagn 1994; 14:903–906.

Patel DV, Holfels EM, Vogel NP et al. Resolution of intracranial calcifications in infants with treated congenital toxoplasmosis. Radiology 1996;199:433–440.

Sherer DM, Onyeije CI. Prenatal ultrasonographic diagnosis of fetal intracranial tumors: a review. Am J Perinatol 1998;15:319–328.

Tassin GB, Maklad NF, Stewart RR, Bell ME. Cytomegalic inclusion disease: intrauterine sonographic diagnosis using findings involving the brain. AJNR Am J Neuroradiol 1991;12:117–122.

Teele R, Hernanz-Schulman M, Sotrel A. Echogenic vasculature in the basal ganglia of neonates: a sonographic sign of vasculopathy. Radiology 1988;169:423–427.

Yamashita Y, Matsuishi T, Murakami Y et al. Neuroimaging findings (ultrasonography, CT, MRI) in 3 infants with congenital rubella syndrome. Pediatr Radiol 1991;21:547–549.

CHAPTER 8
Choroid Plexus Cysts

► **CONDITION**

The choroid plexus is an easily identifiable fetal intracranial structure during the first trimester of pregnancy, and it remains a prominent landmark in the normal fetal brain throughout gestation. Found mainly in the lateral ventricles, the choroid plexus is the major source of cerebrospinal fluid. It begins to develop during the 6th and 7th weeks of gestation (Shuangshoti et al. 1965). Subsequent growth is rapid, and by 9 weeks the choroid plexus fills approximately 75% of the lateral ventricle. The size of the choroid plexus relative to the size of the lateral ventricle decreases progressively as gestation advances, until 20 weeks, when the choroid plexus takes on its adult appearance.

Cysts of the fetal choroid plexus were first described by Chudleigh et al. in 1984. Two years later, Nicolaides et al. (1986) noted an association between the cysts and trisomy 18. Choroid plexus cysts are thought to represent neuroepithelial folds that subsequently fill with cerebrospinal fluid and cellular debris. The cysts are generally less than 1 cm in diameter, may be bilateral or unilateral, and can first be observed as early as 11 weeks gestation (Fig. 8-1) (Guariglia and Rosati 1999). Their appearance correlates with the stage of histogenesis during which the choroidal neuroepithelium becomes

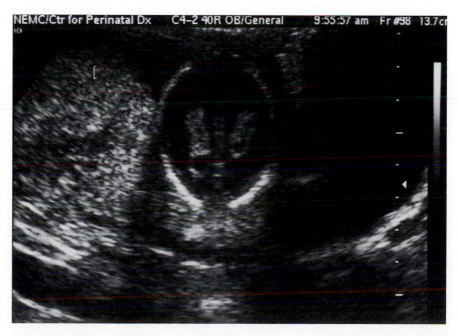

Figure 8-1. Transaxial prenatal sonographic image demonstrating the presence of bilateral choroid plexus cysts.

lobulated and the underlying mesenchymal stroma loosens (Shuangshoti and Metsky 1966). This loose mesenchymal stroma combines with rapid intracellular glycogen deposition and cellular growth to promote formation of the fluid-filled cysts. Between 18 and 25 weeks of gestation, the stroma is replaced by organized fibrous tissue, and the cysts typically regress.

The prenatal identification of choroid plexus cysts has been a cause for concern since a possible association with aneuploidy, particularly trisomy 18, was first reported (Nicolaides et al. 1986). While isolated choroid plexus cysts have been reported in association with trisomy 21 (Twinning et al. 1991; Walkinshaw et al. 1994), this association is generally felt to be coincidental (Gupta et al. 1997). In one series of 143 fetuses with trisomy 21, the frequency of choroid plexus cysts was not significantly different from that in the general population, leading the authors to conclude that the finding of isolated choroid plexus cysts should not be used to increase patients' risk of having a fetus with trisomy 21 (Bromley et al. 1996).

A possible association between isolated choroid plexus cysts and trisomy 18 has however been considerably more controversial. The incidence of choroid plexus cysts in trisomy 18 has been studied at both autopsy and by antenatal sonographic examination. Fitzsimmons et al. (1989) studied seven autopsies of second-trimester fetuses with trisomy 18 and found five fetuses with choroid plexus cysts—an incidence of 71%. A review of the literature by Achiron et al. (1991) revealed that 25 of 38 fetuses (66%) with trisomy 18 had choroid plexus cysts. Two other large series have reported choroid plexus cysts in 29% and 37% of trisomy 18 fetuses (Benacerraf et al. 1990; Nyberg et al. 1993). Combining the series of Achiron, Benacerraf, and Nyberg would suggest an overall incidence of choroid plexus cysts in trisomy 18 of approximately 45%. The risk of trisomy 18 with isolated choroid plexus cysts does not depend on the gestational age at diagnosis, size of cysts, whether they are unilateral or bilateral, or gestational age at resolution of the cysts (Gupta et al. 1995).

However, the vast majority of fetuses with trisomy 18 will have other sonographically identifiable abnormalities, in addition to choroid plexus cysts (see Chapter 133). The question therefore arises as to how great an increase in risk for trisomy 18 exists when no other sonographically identifiable abnormalities are found. The published literature on this subject is very confusing as there is a great degree of variability in populations studied, quality of ultrasound examination, and accuracy of ascertainment of cases. By identifying cases of trisomy 18 from cytogenetic registers and then retrospectively reviewing the ultrasound records of identified cases, the prevalence of isolated choroid plexus cysts during the mid-trimester in trisomy 18 fetuses can

be calculated. Using this approach Gupta et al. (1997) have suggested a prevalence of isolated choroid plexus cysts at mid-trimester in fetuses with trisomy 18 of 4.3%, compared with 0.47% in the general population. This represents a nine-fold increased risk of trisomy 18 following the identification of apparently isolated choroid plexus cysts, although the 95% confidence intervals for this likelihood ratio were wide, ranging from 4 to 19 (Gupta et al. 1997).

The risk of trisomy 18 following the identification of isolated choroid plexus cysts must be interpreted together with the a priori maternal age specific risk. Estimates of maternal age specific risks for trisomy 18 have been published, and are summarized in Table 8-1 (Snijders et al. 1994). By multiplying the maternal age-specific risk for trisomy 18 by the likelihood ratio associated with isolated choroid plexus cysts, specific "posterior" risks can be quoted for individual patients following the identification of an isolated choroid plexus cyst. As shown in Table 8-1, when additional structural abnormalities are discovered together with choroid plexus cysts, the risk of trisomy 18 becomes very high.

Because second trimester multiple marker serum screening programs can also be used to identify pregnancies at increased risk for trisomy 18 (Canick et al. 1990), combining risks from both serum screening programs and sonographic identification of choroid plexus cysts may also be useful. Gratton et al. (1996) have integrated these risks, which are summarized in Table 8-1. As can be seen from this table, the risk for trisomy 18 with isolated choroid plexus cysts and negative multiple-marker serum screening only approaches the loss rate of amniocentesis (1/200) at a maternal age of 38 years or greater. This would suggest that in the presence of an isolated choroid plexus cyst, the maternal age-related risk is the predominant factor that should determine whether or not to undergo amniocentesis (Gratton et al. 1996).

▶ INCIDENCE

Antenatally, choroid plexus cysts have been reported on ultrasound examination with an incidence of 0.18% (Clark et al. 1988) to 3.5% (Chinn et al. 1991) and have an average incidence of approximately 1% at midgestation. The large differences in percentages may be due to whether maternal age was ascertained, the relatively small numbers in each study, the differences in patient population (referral-based versus general screening), sophistication of ultrasound equipment, and underdiagnosis prior to 1986, when the possible correlation with trisomy 18 was first reported (Nicolaides et al. 1986).

Asymptomatic choroid plexus cysts have been reported in approximately 50% of human autopsy studies

► **TABLE 8-1.** CALCULATED RISK OF TRISOMY 18 IN FETUSES WITH ISOLATED CHOROID PLEXUS CYSTS (CPC), AFTER INTEGRATING WITH MULTIPLE-MARKER SERUM SCREENING (MSS) RISK, AND FOLLOWING THE IDENTIFICATION OF ADDITIONAL ABNORMALITIES.

Maternal age (years)	Age-related risk	Isolated CPC	Isolated CPC and normal MSS	CPC with other abnormalities
20	1/4576	1/506	1/1804	1/3
21	1/4514	1/499	1/1779	1/3
22	1/4435	1/491	1/1749	1/3
23	1/4333	1/479	1/1708	1/2
24	1/4204	1/465	1/1658	1/2
25	1/4045	1/447	1/1595	1/2
26	1/3850	1/426	1/1518	1/2
27	1/3619	1/400	1/1427	1/2
28	1/3351	1/371	1/1362	1/2
29	1/3053	1/337	1/1203	1/2
30	1/2724	1/301	1/1074	1/2
31	1/2385	1/264	1/940	>1/2
32	1/2046	1/226	1/806	>1/2
33	1/1721	1/190	1/679	>1/2
34	1/1420	1/157	1/560	>1/2
35	1/1152	1/127	1/454	>1/2
36	1/921	1/102	1/363	>1/2
37	1/727	1/80	1/287	>1/2
38	1/567	1/63	1/223	>1/2
39	1/439	1/49	1/173	>1/2
40	1/338	1/37	1/133	>1/2
41	1/258	1/29	1/102	>1/2
42	1/197	1/22	1/78	>1/2
43	1/149	1/16	1/59	>1/2
44	1/113	1/13	1/45	>1/2
45	1/85	1/9	1/34	>1/2

Modified from, and reprinted with permission from: Gratton et al., Am J Obstet Gynecol 1996;175:1493–1497, and Snijders et al., Prenat Diagn 1994;14:543–552.

(Fakhry et al. 1984; Friday et al. 1985). They are usually less than 1 cm in diameter and have been described with equal frequency in fetuses, neonates, adults, and elderly individuals. Thus, the antenatal finding of a choroid plexus cyst is a relatively common phenomenon. It causes concern because of the association with chromosomal abnormalities (see Chapter 133).

► SONOGRAPHIC FINDINGS

On ultrasound examination, the choroid plexus is highly echogenic because of its juxtaposition with cerebrospinal fluid. Choroid plexus cysts appear as echolucent structures within the plexus and have sharply circumscribed margins. They are easily seen in the standard biparietal diameter view (see Fig. 8-1). The choroid plexus in the hemisphere lying proximal to the ultrasound probe is more difficult to visualize because of reverberation artifact, which degrades the image closest to the transducer. It is therefore important to examine

coronal views of the proximal choroid plexus carefully for the presence of cysts and to use axial and sagittal views as needed. A choroid plexus "pseudocyst" has been described that probably represents the normal corpus striatum (Nelson et al. 1992).

► DIFFERENTIAL DIAGNOSIS

The differential diagnosis of choroid plexus cysts includes other cystic lesions of the central nervous system, such as porencephalic and arachnoidal cysts, as well as congenital neoplasms (see Chapters 6 and 21). Because the cysts are usually small and echolucent, they may be readily distinguished from hemorrhages or choroid plexus papillomas, which are echogenic. The cysts may rarely mimic hydrocephalus, especially when located in the body of the lateral ventricle (Benacerraf 1987).

Hydrocephalus may be differentiated from large choroid plexus cysts by the increased thickness and echogenicity of cyst borders as well as by the eventual sonographic appearance. AJR Am J Roentgenol 1988;151: 179–1181.

DiGiovanni LM, Quinlan MP, Verp MS. Choroid plexus cysts: infant and early childhood developmental outcome. Obstet Gynecol 1997;90:191–194.

Fakhry J, Schecter A, Tenner M, Reale M. Cysts of the choroid plexus in neonates: documentation and review of the literature. J Ultrasound Med 1984;4:561–563.

Fitzsimmons J, Wilson D, Pascoe-Mason J, Shaw C, Cyr D, Mack L. Choroid plexus cysts in fetuses with trisomy 18. Obstet Gynecol 1989;73:257–260.

Friday R, Schwartz D, Tuffli G. Spontaneous intrauterine resolution of intraventricular cystic masses. J Ultrasound Med 1985;4:385.

Gabrielli S, Reece EA, Pilu G, et al. The clinical significance of prenatally diagnosed choroid plexus cysts. Am J Obstet Gynecol 1989;160:1207–1210.

Geary M, Patel S, Lamont R. Isolated choroid plexus cysts and association with fetal aneuploidy in an unselected population. Ultrasound Obstet Gynecol 1997;10:171–173.

Gratton RJ, Hogge WA, Aston CE. Choroid plexus cysts and trisomy 18: risk modification based on maternal age and multiple-marker screening. Am J Obstet Gynecol 1996; 175:1493–1497.

Guariglia L, Rosati P. Prevalence and significance of isolated fetal choroid plexus cysts detected in early pregnancy by transvaginal sonography in women of advanced maternal age. Prenat Diagn 1999;19:128–131.

Gupta JK, Cave M, Lilford RJ, et al. Clinical significance of fetal choroid plexus cysts. Lancet 1995;346:724–729.

Gupta JK, Khan KS, Thornton JG, et al. Management of fetal choroid plexus cysts. Br J Obstet Gynaecol 1997;104: 881–886.

Jones K. Smith's recognizable patterns of human malformation. 4th ed. Philadelphia: Saunders, 1988:16.

Lam A, Villaneuva A. Symptomatic third ventricle choroid plexus cysts. Pediatr Radiol 1992;22:413–416.

Leonardi MR, Wolfe HM, Lanouette JM, et al. The apparently isolated choroid plexus cyst: importance of minor abnormalities in predicting the risk for aneuploidy. Fetal Diagn Ther 1998;13:49–52.

Nadel A, Bromley B, Frigoletto F, et al. Isolated choroid plexus cysts in the second trimester fetus: is amniocentesis really indicated? Radiology 1992;185:545–548.

Nelson NL, Callen PW, Filly RA. The choroid plexus pseudocyst: sonographic identification and characterization. J Ultrasound Med 1992;11:597–601.

Nicolaides KH, Rodeck CH, Gosden CM. Rapid karyotyping for nonlethal fetal malformations. Lancet 1986;1:283–287.

Nyberg D, Kramer D, Resta R, et al. Prenatal sonographic findings of trisomy 18: a review of 48 cases. J Ultrasound 1993;12:103–113.

Ostlere S, Irving H, Lilford R. A prospective study of the incidence and significance of fetal choroid plexus cysts. Prenat Diagn 1989;9:205–211.

Ostlere S, Irving H, Lilford R. Fetal choroid plexus cysts: a report of 100 cases. Radiology 1990;175:753–755.

Perpignano M, Cohen H, Klein V, et al. Fetal choroid plexus cysts: beware the smaller cyst. Radiology 1992; 182:715–717.

Platt LD, Carlson BE, Medearis AL, et al. Fetal choroid plexus cysts in the second trimester of pregnancy: a cause for concern. Am J Obstet Gynecol 1991;164: 1652–1656.

Porto M, Murata Y, Warneke LA, et al. Fetal choroid plexus cysts: an independent risk factor for chromosomal anomalies. J Clin Ultrasound 1993;21:103–108.

Riebel T, Nasir R, Weber K. Choroid plexus cysts: a normal finding on ultrasound. Pediatr Radiol 1992;22:410–412.

Reinsch RC. Choroid plexus cysts—association with trisomy: prospective review of 16,059 patients. Am J Obstet Gynecol 1997;176:1381–1383.

Shuangshoti S, Metsky M. Neuroepithelial cysts of the nervous system. Neurology 1966;887–903.

Shuangshoti S, Roberts M, Metsky M. Neuroepithelial (colloid) cysts: pathogenesis and relation to choroid plexus and ependyma. Arch Pathol 1965;80:214–224.

Snijders R, Shawa L, Nicolaides K. Fetal choroid plexus cysts and trisomy 18: assessment of risk based on ultrasound findings and maternal age. Prenat Diagn 1994;14: 1119–1127.

Sohn C, Gast AS, Krapfl E. Isolated choroid plexus cysts: not an indication for genetic diagnosis? Fetal Diagn Ther 1997;12:255–259.

Sullivan A, Giudice T, Vavelidis F, et al. Choroid plexus cysts: is biochemical testing a valuable adjunct to targeted ultrasonography? Am J Obstet Gynecol 1999;181: 260–265.

Twinning P, Zuccollo J, Clewes J, et al. Fetal choroid plexus cysts: a prospective study and review of the literature. Br J Radiol 1991;64:98–102.

Walkinshaw S, Pilling D, Spriggs A. Isolated choroid plexus cysts—the need for routine offer of karyotyping. Prenat Diagn 1994;14:663–667.

CHAPTER 9

Craniosynostosis

► CONDITION

The term *craniosynostosis* refers to the process of premature bony fusion of the cranial sutures. The term is frequently used interchangeably with the word *craniostenosis,* which technically refers to the aberrant skull shape that results from the process of craniosynostosis (Graham 1981). The weight of the brain doubles during the first year of life, and enlargement of the skull vault is distributed among the main cranial sutures—sagittal, coronal, lambdoid, and metopic. Premature fusion of a suture leads to reduced growth in the direction perpendicular to the fused suture (Thompson et al. 1994). Compensatory growth occurs in the remaining normal sutures. Normally, the cranial sutures are open at birth and become interdigitated by 7.5 months of age. Cranial sutures do not fuse completely until the fourth decade of life (Graham 1981).

It is important to determine whether craniosynostosis is primary or secondary. Primary craniosynostosis is due to an alteration in sutural growth. In primary craniosynostosis, the head of the affected individual is frequently asymmetric. The brain grows at a normal rate but must adjust to confined space. The brain continues to grow in areas where the sutures are open but not in areas where the sutures are closed (Lyon-Jones et al. 1980). Most children affected with primary craniosynostosis are normal neurologically and benefit from surgery. In secondary craniosynostosis, brain growth is impaired and most affected children are neurologically abnormal. In secondary craniosynostosis, a metabolic, storage, hematologic, or structural disorder results in the abnormal brain growth (Table 9-1). In evaluating the fetus with craniosynostosis, it is important to determine whether the craniosynostosis is isolated (simple) or syndromic (complex). To date, over 60 syndromes have been described that include craniosynostosis as an associated feature (Lajeunie et al. 1995).

Isolated craniosynostosis generally presents during the first year of life, and severe neuropsychologic sequelae are unusual (Meilstrup et al. 1995). In most studies, the sagittal suture is the most common site for isolated craniosynostosis (Fig. 9-1). This is called "scaphocephaly," and it results in a head that is elongated from front to back. Physical examination reveals a palpable ridge along the line of the fused suture. The next most commonly affected site is the coronal suture, called "plagiocephaly," and results in asymmetric flattening of the forehead with loss of the supraorbital ridge. This condition is best appreciated when viewed from above the patient. In most reported studies, the least commonly involved suture is the metopic. This is called "trigonocephaly," and produces a keel-shaped forehead and orbital hypotelorism (Thompson et al. 1994). The kleeblattschädel deformity, also described as a cloverleaf skull, has a more symmetric trilobar appearance, which results from premature synostosis of the coronal and lambdoidal sutures (Meilstrup et al. 1995).

► INCIDENCE

The incidence of isolated nonsyndromic craniosynostosis varies between 0.4 and 0.6 per 1000 births (Lajeunie et al. 1995; Shuper et al. 1985; Van Der Ham et al. 1995). Craniosynostosis has been associated with advanced paternal age (Lajeunie et al. 1995), maternal smoking, and higher altitudes (Alderman et al. 1994, 1995). In a study of 154 patients at Johns Hopkins Hospital followed over a 2-year period, Van der Kolk and Beatty (1994) found that 78% of patients had only one suture affected, whereas 16% of patients had multiple sutures involved. Of these 154 patients, 94% had isolated craniosynostosis and 6% had complex or syndromic craniosynostosis. In this study, secondary synostosis occurred in four patients

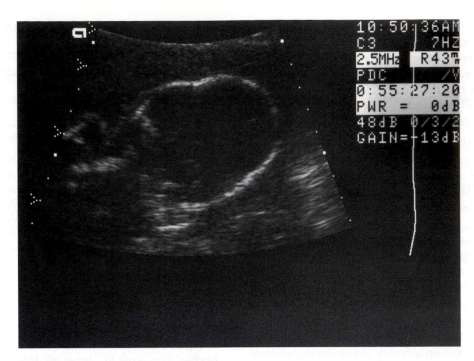

Figure 9-2. Prenatal sonographic image of a fetus at 23 weeks of gestation with Apert syndrome, demonstrating bilateral coronal suture synostosis and a tower-like shape of the skull (turricephaly).

web space (Stankovic et al. 1994). Pfeiffer syndrome has two forms. There is a relatively benign form, known as the type I, which consists of an acrocephalic skull due to bicoronal synostoses. Affected patients have broad thumbs and great toes and soft-tissue syndactyly. Like many of the other syndromes associated with craniosynostosis, affected patients have hypotelorism, maxillary hypoplasia, low-set ears, and normal intelligence (Hill and Grzybeck 1994). Two other subgroups of patients with Pfeiffer syndrome had extreme proctosis and hydrocephalus. These patients have a uniformly poor outcome and are distinguished from each other as the type II form with the cloverleaf skull deformity and the type III form without the cloverleaf skull deformity (Moore et al. 1995). The kleeblattschädel, or cloverleaf, skull deformity is also associated with thanatophoric dysplasia (see Chapter 100). Of all patients with the cloverleaf skull deformity, 20% are due to Pfeiffer syndrome and 40% are due to thanatophoric dysplasia (Hill and Grzybeck 1994). In Carpenter syndrome, affected patients have acrocephaly, soft-tissue syndactyly, preaxial polydactyly, congenital heart disease, and mental retardation. In Baller–Gerold syndrome, affected patients have craniosynostosis and preaxial upper-limb malformations (see Chapter 107) (Boudreaux et al. 1990).

Patients with the Apert syndrome, first described in 1906, have a shortened anterior-posterior diameter of the skull with a high, full forehead, flat occiput, flat facies, shallow orbits, hypotelorism, osseous and cutaneous syndactyly, and associated anomalies (Figs. 9-2 and 9-3). Ten percent of patients have cardiovascular abnormalities, and approximately 10% have genitourinary anomalies, most commonly hydronephrosis and cryptorchidism (Cohen and Kreiborg 1993b). One of the most characteristic findings of patients affected with Apert syndrome includes the complete digital fusion of the soft tissues of the digits 2, 3, and 4, which creates a mid-digital hand mass with a single common nail (see Figures 108-1 through 108-4).

▶ ANTENATAL NATURAL HISTORY

The cranium develops as islands of bone within a fibrous membrane called the "ectomenix." A wedge-shaped proliferation of cells at the periphery is called the "osteogenic front." When osteogenic fronts come in close proximity to each other, a suture develops. The suture allows spatial separation of cranial bones during growth. The suture includes fibrous tissue defined radiographically by lucency and by proliferating osteogenic tissue on the periphery of the bone. The cranial sutures consist of five layers—two cambial and two periosteal layers separated by a middle vascular layer. The suture allows bone growth at sutural margins secondary to distant forces separating sutures (Van der Kolk and Beatty, 1994).

The antenatal natural history for fetuses affected with craniosynostosis depends on whether the condition is isolated or syndromic. In general, fetuses with

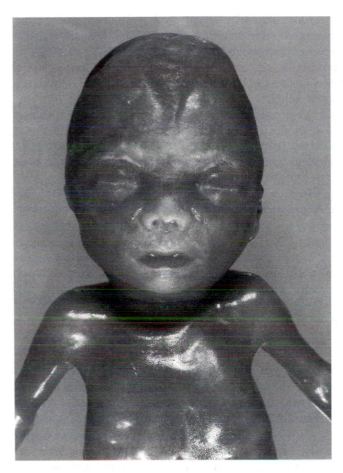

Figure 9-3. Fetus from Figure 9-2 after termination, demonstrating turricephaly and a wide open metopic suture. Prenatal sonograms and post-termination photographs of this fetus' extremities are shown in Figures 108-1 through 108-4.

isolated craniosynostosis grow and develop normally. Fetuses with syndromic craniosynostosis are also generally normal, if not sometimes large for gestational age. There is no indication that any of these syndromes are associated with increased lethality in utero.

▶ MANAGEMENT OF PREGNANCY

One of the most important considerations in the management of pregnancy is to obtain a detailed family history. Both parents should be examined for the presence of facial asymmetry or for partial syndactyly of the fingers or toes. These findings are consistent with the mildest expression of some of the syndromic craniosynostoses. It is also important to remember that parents affected with one of the syndromic craniosynostoses may have had extensive surgical repair and will therefore have a relatively normal appearance.

We recommend referral of the pregnant patient carrying a fetus with presumed craniosynostosis to a tertiary-care center capable of targeted sonographic examination of the fetus. It is particularly important to rule out the presence of associated hand and foot abnormalities as well as the more serious cardiovascular abnormalities that can be present in some of these syndromes. If there is a positive family history of isolated craniosynostosis, no further workup is necessary. If, however, the family history is negative, we recommend prenatal karyotyping to rule out chromosomal abnormalities associated with craniosynostosis. Furthermore, in the setting of a negative family history, if additional sonographic findings suggest a syndromic diagnosis, it is important that the parents meet with a medical geneticist to discuss the implications of the potential diagnoses. Many of the syndromic craniosynostoses are associated with normal intelligence; however, Apert syndrome is associated with a significant chance of developmental delay (see "Long-Term Outcome," which follows).

Magnetic resonance imaging has been used to confirm cranial abnormalities in a case of Apert syndrome (Boog et al. 1999). If the diagnosis is made before 24 weeks of gestation, parents can be given the option of terminating the pregnancy. If the diagnosis is made in the third trimester, however, we recommend that the delivery occur in a tertiary-care center because of the possibility of associated feeding and breathing difficulties in the neonate. In addition, it will be important for a medical geneticist to examine the infant after birth to confirm the presumed clinical diagnosis. Fetuses with skull abnormalities suggesting a head circumference larger than normal may need to be delivered by cesarean section.

▶ FETAL INTERVENTION

There is no intervention for craniosynostosis.

▶ TREATMENT OF THE NEWBORN

Infants with suspected craniosynostosis should have a detailed physical examination at birth. Some of the associated physical findings in the syndromic craniosynostosis are listed in Table 9-3. Anteroposterior and lateral views of the skull should be obtained. On radiography, the prematurely fused suture is either completely absent or represented by a line of increased density. In cases of coronal synostosis, the so-called harlequin appearance of the orbit is due to elevation of the ipsilateral sphenoid wing. Physical examination of the infant should be performed in consultation with a clinical geneticist to seek specific evidence of associated abnormalities. For example, 30% of infants affected with Apert syndrome have submucous cleft palate (Mulliken and Bruneteau 1991).

► **TABLE 9-4.** GENETIC BASIS OF SYNDROMIC CRANIOSYNOSTOSIS

Condition	Chromosome Localization	Gene	Amino Acid Substitution
Craniosynostosis, Boston type	5qter	MSX2 Homeodomain	Pro7His
Greig cephalopolysyndactyly	7p13	GL13	—
Saethre–Chotzen syndrome	7p21.1	*TWIST*	Many
Crouzon syndrome	10q25.3-q26	*FGFR2* Exon 9(B)	Tyr328Cys
			Gly338Arg
			Tyr340His
			Cys342Ser
			Cys342Arg
			Cys342Tyr
			Cys342Trp
			Ala344Ala
			Ala344Gly
			Ser347Cys
			Ser354Cys
		Exon 7(U)	Cys278Phe
			Deletion His, Ile, Glu 287-289
			Gln289Pro
			Trp290Arg
Pfeiffer syndrome	8p11.2-p12	*FGFR1* Exon 5	Pro252Arg
	10q25.3-q26	*FGFR2* Exon 9(B)	Cys342Arg
			Cys342Tyr
			Thr341Pro
			Asp321Ala
			Acceptor splice site
Jackson–Weiss syndrome	10q25.3-q26	*FGFR2* Exon 9(B)	Ala344Gly
			Others?
Apert syndrome	10q25.3-q26	*FGFR2* Exon 7(U)	Ser252Trp
			Pro253Arg
			Others?
Thanatophoric dysplasia, type II	4p16	*FGFR3*	Lys650Glu

the syndrome. In theory, patients with a negative family history do not have an increased incidence of recurrence above background, although gonadal mosaicism is a small possibility. For patients with a negative family history, prenatal sonographic diagnosis in subsequent pregnancies is probably warranted to provide reassurance.

REFERENCES

Alderman BW, Bradley CM, Greene C, Fernbach SK, Baron AE. Increased risk of craniosynostosis with maternal cigarette smoking during pregnancy. Teratology 1994;50: 13–18.

Alderman BW, Zamudio S, Barón AE, et al. Increased risk of craniosynostosis with higher antenatal maternal altitude. Int J Epidemol 1995;24:420–426.

Boog G, LeVaillant C, Winer N, David A, Quere MP, Nomballais MF. Contribution of tridimensional sonography and magnetic resonance imaging to prenatal diagnosis of Apert syndrome at mid-trimester. Fetal Diagn Ther 1999;14:20–23.

Boudreaux JM, Colon MA, Lorusso GD, Parro EA, Pelias MZ. Baller-Gerold syndrome: an 11th case of craniosynostosis and radial aplasia. Am J Med Genet 1990;37:447–450.

Chenowith-Mitchell C, Cohen GR. Prenatal sonographic findings of Apert syndrome. J Clin Ultrasound 1994;22: 510–514.

Cohen MM, Kreiborg S. Growth pattern in the Apert syndrome. Am J Med Genet 1993a;47:617–623.

Cohen MM, Kreiborg S. An updated pediatric perspective on the Apert syndrome. Am J Dis Child 1993b;147: 989–993.

de León GA, de León G, Grover WD, Zaeri N, Alburger PD. Agenesis of the corpus callosum in limbic malformation in Apert syndrome (Type I acrocephalosyndactyly). Arch Neurol 1987;44:979–982.

Fryburg JS, Golden WL. Interstitial deletion of 8q13.3→22.1 associated with craniosynostosis. Am J Med Genet 1993; 45:638–641.

Gorry MC, Preston RA, White GJ, et al. Crouzon syndrome: mutations in two spliceforms of *FGFR2* and a common point mutation shared with Jackson-Weiss syndrome. Hum Mol Genet 1995;4:1387–1390.

Graham JM. Craniostenosis: a new approach to management. Pediatr Ann 1981;10:27–35.

Hill LM, Grzybek PC. Sonographic findings with Pfeiffer syndrome. Prenat Diagn 1994;14:47–49.

Hill LM, Thomas ML, Peterson CS. The ultrasonic detection of Apert syndrome. J Ultrasound Med 1987;6:601–604.

Howard TD, Paznekas WA, Green ED, et al. Mutations in *TWIST,* a basic helix-loop-helix transcription factor, in Saethre-Chotzen syndrome. Nat Genet 1997;15:36–41.

Jabs EW, Li X, Scott AF, et al. Jackson-Weiss and Crouzon syndromes are allelic with mutations in fibroblast growth factor receptor 2. Nat Genet 1994;8:275–279.

Jabs EW, Muller U, Li X, et al. A mutation in the homeo-domain of the human *MSZ2* gene in a family affected with autosomal dominant craniosynostosis. Cell 1993;75:443–450.

Johnson D, Horsley SW, Moloney DM, et al. A comprehensive screen for *TWIST* mutations in patients with craniosynostosis identifies a new microdeletion syndrome of chromosome band 7p21.1. Am J Hum Genet 1998;63:1282–1293.

Kaplan SB, Kemp SS, Oh KS. Radiographic manifestations of congenital anomalies of the skull. Radiol Clin North Am 1916;29:195–218.

Kim R, Uppal V, Wallach R. Apert syndrome and fetal hydrocephaly. Hum Genet 1986;73:93–95.

Lajeunie E, Le Merrer M, Conaiti-Pellie C, Marchac D, Renier D. Genetic study of nonsyndromic coronal craniosynostosis. Am J Med Genet 1995;55:500–504.

Leo MV, Suslak L, Ganesh VL, Adhate A, Apuzzio JJ. Crouzon syndrome: prenatal ultrasound diagnosis by binocular diameters. Obstet Gynecol 1991;78:906–908.

Lewanda AF, Green ED, Weissenbach J, et al. Evidence that the Saethre–Chotzen syndrome locus lies between D7S664 and D7S507, by genetic analysis and detection of a microdeletion in a patient. Am J Hum Genet 1994;55:1195–1201.

Li X, Lewanda AF, Eluma F, et al. Two craniosynostotic syndrome loci, Crouzon and Jackson–Weiss, map to chromosome 10q23-q26. Genomics 1994;22:418–424.

Lyons-Jones K, James HE, Fisher JC. Craniosynostosis and craniofacial anomalies. West J Med 1980;132:500–506.

Meilstrup JW, Botti JJ, MacKay DR, Johnson DL. Prenatal sonographic appearance of asymmetric craniosynostosis: a case report. J Ultrasound Med 1995;14:307–310.

Moloney DM, Slaney SF, Oldridge M, et al. Exclusive paternal origin of new mutations in Apert syndrome. Nat Genet 1996;13:48–53.

Moore MH, Cantrell SB, Trott JA, David DJ. Pfeiffer syndrome: a clinical review. Cleft Palat Craniofac J 1995;32:62–70.

Muenke M, Schell U, Hehr A, et al. A common mutation in the fibroblast growth factor receptor 1 gene in Pfeiffer syndrome. Nat Genet 19948:269–274.

Mulliken JB, Bruneteau RJ. Surgical correction of the craniofacial anomalies in Apert syndrome. Clin Plast Surg 1991;18:277–289.

Munro CS, Wilkie AO. Epidermal mosaicism producing localized acne: somatic mutation in *FGFR2.* Lancet 1998;352:704–705.

Noetzel MJ, Marsh JL, Palkes H, Gado M. Hydrocephalus and mental retardation in craniosynostosis. J Pediatr 1985;107:885–892.

Paznekas WA, Cunningham ML, Howard TD, et al. Genetic heterogeneity of Saethre–Chotzen syndrome, due to *TWIST* and *FGFR* mutations. Am J Hum Genet 1998;62:1370–1380.

Rose CSP, King AAJ, Summers D, et al. Localization of the genetic locus for Saethre–Chotzen syndrome to a 6 cM region of chromosome 7 using four cases with apparently balanced translocations at 7p21.2. Hum Mol Genet 1994;3:1405–1408.

Rutland P, Pulleyn LJ, Reardon W, et al. Identical mutations in the *FGFR2* gene cause both Pfeiffer and Crouzon syndrome phenotypes. Nat Genet 1995;9:173–176.

Schell U, Hehr A, Feldman GJ, et al. Mutations in *FGFR1* and *FGFR2* cause familial and sporadic Pfeiffer syndrome. Hum Mol Genet 1995;4:323–328.

Shuper A, Merlob P, Grunebaum M, Reisner SH. The incidence of isolated craniosynostosis in the newborn infant. Am J Dis Child 1985;139:85–86.

Stankovic B, Krstic V, Stankov B, Jojic L, Magulic M, Artiko G. Jackson–Weiss syndrome registered in four successive generations. Doc Opthalmol 1994;85:281–286.

Thompson D, Jones B, Hayward R, Harkness W. Assessment and treatment of craniosynostosis. Br J Hosp Med 1994;52:17–24.

Van der Ham LI, Cohen-Overbeek TE, Paz Y, Geuze HD, Vermeij-keers C. The ultrasonic detection of an isolated craniosynostosis. Prenat Diagn 1995;15:1189–1192.

van Herwerden L, Rose CSP, Reardon W, et al. Evidence of locus heterogeneity in acrocephalosyndactyly: a refined localization for the Saethre–Chotzen syndrome locus on distal chromosome 7p and exclusion of Jackson–Weiss syndrome from craniosynostosis loci on 7p and 5q. Am J Hum Genet 1994;54:669–674.

Van der Kolk CA, Beatty T. Etiopathogenesis of craniofacial anomalies. Clin Plast Surg 1994;21:481–488.

Whitaker LA, Bartlett SP, Schut L, Bruce D. Craniosynostosis: an analysis of the timing, treatment, and complications in 164 consecutive patients. Plast Reconstr Surg 1987;80:195–206.

CHAPTER 10

Dandy–Walker Malformation and Variants

▶ CONDITION

The Dandy–Walker malformation is a nonspecific congenital brain malformation that results from a number of diverse causes. There are two principal features of the Dandy–Walker malformation: aplasia or hypoplasia of the cerebellar vermis and posterior fossa cysts that represents cystic dilatation of the fourth ventricle (Nyberg et al. 1988).

The first case of Dandy–Walker malformation was reported in 1887 (Murray et al. 1985). In 1914, Blackfan and Dandy described a hindbrain abnormality in a patient with cystic dilatation of the fourth ventricle, hypoplasia of the vermis cerebelli, separation of the cerebellar hemispheres, dilatation of the aqueductus mesencephaly, and absence of the lateral and median apertures of the fourth ventricle (cited in Chang et al. 1984). The term *Dandy–Walker malformation* was first used in 1954, combining case reports of Blackfan and Dandy, and a subsequent report of Taggart and Walker (Chen and Chu 1994).

The Dandy–Walker malformation originates before the sixth or seventh week of embryonic development (Russ et al. 1989). The malformation may occur in single-gene disorders, in chromosomal abnormalities, in environmentally induced malformation syndromes, or in conjunction with other multifactorial anomalies (Cornford and Twining 1992).

The full Dandy–Walker malformation consists of complete vermian agenesis, cystic dilatation of the fourth ventricle, and an enlarged or normal-sized posterior cranial fossa. The condition is commonly associated with obstructive hydrocephalus, which is nearly always present postnatally, but has a variable incidence prenatally.

The full Dandy–Walker malformation should be distinguished from the Dandy–Walker variant and mega cisterna magna (Chen and Chu 1994). The Dandy–Walker variant consists of cerebellar dysgenesis, variable hypoplasia of the cerebellar vermis, without enlargement of the posterior fossa. Ventricular dilatation may or may not be present (Bromley et al. 1994; Estroff et al. 1992). In the Dandy–Walker variant, hypoplasia of the postero-inferior portion of the cerebellar vermis leads to a communication between the fourth ventricle and the cisterna magna (Bromley et al. 1994). In the Dandy–Walker variant, the cerebellar hemispheres are generally small but morphologically within normal limits. In mega cisterna magna, an enlarged cisterna magna is present with an intact cerebellar vermis and fourth ventricle. The cerebellum may be hypoplastic (Estroff et al. 1992). Many authors have tried to distinguish between these three conditions to better delineate the expected prognosis for the affected fetus.

▶ INCIDENCE

The incidence of the full Dandy–Walker malformation is 1 in 25,000 to 35,000 pregnancies (Russ et al. 1989). The Dandy–Walker variant is thought to be more common than the true Dandy–Walker malformation; it accounts for one third of all posterior fossa lesions (Estroff et al. 1992).

In a series of postnatally ascertained Dandy–Walker malformation, it occurred in 12% of cases of congenital hydrocephalus and 2 to 4% of cases of childhood-onset hydrocephalus (Chen and Chu 1994; Murray et al. 1985).

► SONOGRAPHIC FINDINGS

Over the past 10 years, more attention has been paid to the fetal posterior cranial fossa, because of the importance of delineating this area as part of the diagnosis of spina bifida (see Chapter 19). As a result of the increased scrutiny of the posterior fossa, more cases of Dandy–Walker malformation and its variants are being diagnosed antenatally.

A major consideration in the diagnosis of Dandy–Walker malformation is gestational age. Although Dandy–Walker malformation has been diagnosed in the first trimester (Achiron and Achiron 1991; Gembruch et al. 1995), a false positive diagnosis can be made at an early gestational age. Bromley et al. (1994) prospectively evaluated 897 fetuses between 13 and 21 weeks of gestation to determine the normal development of the fetal cerebellum in the second trimester. The pregnant women in the study were all undergoing amniocentesis because of advanced maternal age and were not known to have associated anomalies. Of the fetuses studied, 147 were shown to have an open vermis at the time of initial scanning. Of these 147 fetuses, 56% were open at 14 weeks of gestation, 23% were open at 15 weeks of gestation, and 6% remained open at 17 weeks of gestation. After 17.5 weeks of gestation, all fetuses were noted to have a closed vermis. These authors concluded that prenatal diagnosis of cerebellar malformations, such as the Dandy–Walker variant, should not be made at less than 18 weeks of gestation because development of the cerebellar vermis may be physiologically incomplete. True Dandy–Walker malformations are usually visible earlier in gestation, because the cerebellar hemispheres are hypoplastic and laterally displaced, and in addition, a cyst can be visualized (Fig. 10-1).

The sonographic features of the Dandy–Walker malformation include a central cyst communicating with the fourth ventricle, agenesis or dysgenesis of the cerebellar vermis, and splaying of the cerebellar hemispheres with anterolateral displacement against the tentorium (Russ et al. 1989). Russ et al. (1989) reviewed 15 cases of Dandy–Walker malformation diagnosed between 22 and 36 weeks of gestation. In this study, the anteroposterior diameter of the posterior fossa cyst was between 7 and 45 mm. Most of the cysts were >10 mm. Macrocephaly was seen in 3 of 15 cases (20%). The Dandy–Walker malformation was associated with additional brain anomalies in 68% of cases, including aqueductal stenosis, gyral anomalies, heterotopias, and malformations of the inferior olives. Agenesis of the corpus callosum was seen in 7 to 17% of cases. Importantly, these authors documented that there was a very high incidence of extracranial anomalies. In this study, extracranial anomalies were present in 60% of fetuses studied. The malformations observed involved the cardiac, genitourinary, gastrointestinal, and skeletal systems. Of the 12 fetuses who had karyotyping, one-third were abnormal. Similar findings were noted by Nyberg et al. (1988), who reviewed seven proven cases of Dandy–Walker malformation prenatally diagnosed at a mean of 30 weeks of gestation. These authors stated that the clinical course of children and adults with Dandy–Walker malformation is variable, and this was associated with the presence and severity of central

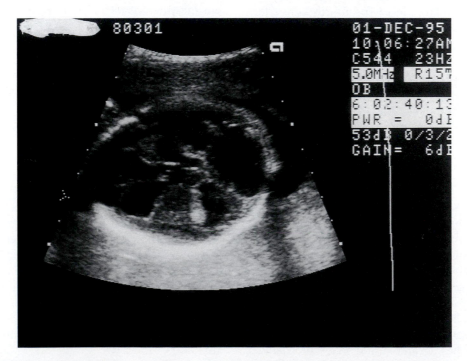

Figure 10-1. Transaxial sonogram of a fetal head demonstrating a posterior fossa cyst. *(Photograph courtesy of Dr. Marjorie C. Treadwell.)*

nervous system (CNS) and extra-CNS malformations. Of the seven patients, five had hydrocephalus. These authors noted an increased incidence of mortality, where five of the seven patients died in the perinatal period. Four of their patients had multiple malformations, and two of these had abnormal karyotypes. These authors concluded that the presence of a Dandy–Walker malformation should prompt a careful search for concurrent abnormalities and consideration of a karyotype. Multiple authors have suggested that the prognosis for Dandy–Walker malformation is influenced by the presence of associated abnormalities. These include the study of Keogan et al. (1994), who reviewed their experience with nine fetuses and tried to distinguish between the presence of the full malformation and isolated vermian hypoplasia. Of the nine fetuses in their report, three had multiple significant CNS and non-CNS abnormalities. Fetuses with an isolated vermian hypoplasia all did well. Similarly, Cowles et al. (1993) described the presence of multiple associated CNS malformations in the Dandy–Walker malformation, including agenesis of the corpus callosum and occasional occipital encephaloceles. In their patient population, they observed extracranial malformations, including cleft lip and cleft palate, cardiac malformations, and urinary tract abnormalities.

The sonographic criteria for the Dandy–Walker variant include partial or complete absence of the cerebellar vermis (Fig. 10-2), a small to normal-sized but near-normal-shaped cerebellar hemisphere, and sonographic continuity between the fourth ventricle and the cisterna magna, which gives the appearance of a cleft (Estroff et al. 1992). In one study, 17 cases of Dandy–

Walker variant were identified. Of these, 15 were identified in the third trimester and 2 in the second. Four of the affected fetuses had ventriculomegaly and 3 had agenesis of the corpus collosum. Almost half of the affected fetuses had other non-CNS abnormalities, including congenital heart disease, gastrointestinal malformations, renal malformations, and intrahepatic calcifications. These authors also found that the presence of the Dandy–Walker variant was associated with a high incidence (29%) of abnormal karyotype (Estroff et al. 1992).

The appearance of the cisterna magna has taken on increasing importance over recent years (Pretorius et al. 1992). The effacement of the cisterna magna gives the "banana sign" of the cerebellum seen in myelomeningocele (see Chapter 19 and Figure 19-2). A small cisterna magna implies an associated neural-tube defect and a Chiari II malformation. In contrast, however, an enlarged cisterna magna can be associated with a Dandy–Walker cyst, cerebellar hypoplasia, and communicating hydrocephalus (Pretorius et al. 1992). Nyberg et al. (1991) studied 33 fetuses with the sonographic appearance of an enlarged cisterna magna. Of these 33 fetuses, 18 (55%) had underlying chromosomal abnormalities. Interestingly, the absence of hydrocephalus and milder enlargement correlated more strongly with the presence of an underlying chromosomal abnormality. The negative correlation between ventriculomegaly and chromosomal abnormality was also seen in another study (Chang et al. 1994). These authors tried to distinguish the prognosis based on the sonographic appearance of the fetal vermis. They reviewed sonographic findings in 65 fetuses with Dandy–Walker

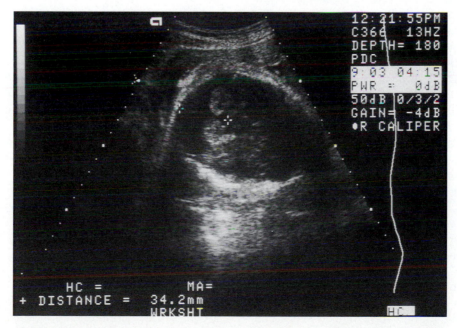

Figure 10-2. Transaxial sonogram demonstrating absence of the cerebellar vermis and splaying of the cerebellar hemispheres.

malformation. Of these, 37 had inferior vermian agenesis, or the milder form of the disorder, and 28 had complete vermian agenesis. Chromosomal abnormalities were seen in 23 of the 51 fetuses who were karyotyped (45%). Chromosomal abnormalities were less prevalent among fetuses with ventriculomegaly. Extracranial abnormalities were seen in 66% of fetuses with inferior vermian agenesis (Chang et al. 1994).

The importance of gestational age at diagnosis was also emphasized by Ulm et al. (1997). These authors compared assocated structural and chromosomal abnormalities in 14 fetuses with Dandy–Walker malformation diagnosed before 21 weeks and 14 fetuses diagnosed after 21 weeks. They concluded that fetuses diagnosed earlier in gestation had a worse prognosis.

▶ DIFFERENTIAL DIAGNOSIS

Major considerations in the differential diagnosis include distinguishing among the Dandy–Walker malformations (true Dandy–Walker cyst versus enlarged cisterna magna versus Dandy–Walker variant), as well as the dorsal cyst seen in holoprosencephaly, and arachnoid cysts (see Chapter 6). The normal depth of the cisterna magna does not exceed 10 mm. Thus, measuring the sagittal dimension of a suspected posterior fossa is useful. The pathognomonic finding in Dandy–Walker malformation is a defect in the vermis through which the cyst communicates with fourth ventricle. The true Dandy–Walker cyst appears as a triangular midline fluid collection with symmetric splaying of the cerebellar hemispheres (see Fig. 10-1) (Russ et al. 1989). Neither arachnoid cysts nor enlarged cisterna magna are associated with vermian defects or other cerebellar or cerebral abnormalities. Retrocerebellar arachnoid cysts compress but do not communicate with the fourth ventricle. In general, arachnoid cysts are asymmetrically positioned in the posterior fossa and tend to be rounded rather than triangular.

The dorsal cyst associated with alobar or semilobar holoprosencephaly can sometimes be confused with the Dandy–Walker malformation. However, in holoprosencephaly, the cyst is supratentorial and communicates directly with the single ventricle seen in this condition. In addition, a hallmark of the diagnosis of holoprosencephaly is the presence of fused or partially fused thalami (see Chapter 13) (Nyberg et al. 1988).

A list of the common conditions associated with Dandy–Walker malformations is given in Table 10-1. Of note are two mendelian (single-gene) disorders that are associated with a very high incidence of Dandy–Walker malformation. In Joubert–Boltshauser syndrome, vermian agenesis is one of the criteria needed for diagnosis. Joubert–Boltshauser syndrome, an autosomal recessive disorder, consists of familial

▶ **TABLE 10-1.** CONDITIONS ASSOCIATED WITH DANDY–WALKER MALFORMATION

Mendelian disorders
  Joubert–Boltshauser syndrome
  Walker–Warburg syndrome
  Coffin–Siris syndrome
  Fraser cryptophthalmos syndrome
  Meckel–Gruber syndrome
  Aicardi syndrome
  Smith–Lemli–Opitz syndrome
Chromosome abnormalities
  Trisomy 9/mosaic trisomy 9
  Triploidy
  45,X
  49,XXX
  6p.24–25 deletion
  Duplication 5p,8p,8q,17q
  Trisomy 13
  Trisomy 18
Teratogens
  Rubella
  Cytomegalovirus
  Toxoplasmosis
  Coumadin
  Alcohol
  Isotretinoin
  Maternal diabetes

Adapted, with permission, from Murray JC, Johnson JA, Bird TD. Dandy–Walker malformation: etiologic heterogeneity and empiric recurrence risks. Clin Genet 1985;28:272–283.

vermian agenesis, episodic hyperpnea, developmental delay, hypotonia, and abnormal eye movements (Keogan et al. 1994). In addition, Dandy–Walker malformation is seen in 53% cases of Walker–Warburg syndrome (Vohra et al. 1993). The Walker–Warburg syndrome consists of lissencephaly with cerebellar malformations, retinal malformations, and congenital muscular dystrophy. The Dandy–Walker malformation is seen in most cases of trisomy 9 or mosaic trisomy 9 (Bureau et al. 1993; McDuffie 1994). An increasing appreciation of the presence of Dandy–Walker malformation is also occurring in Meckel–Gruber syndrome. Dandy–Walker malformation is now being included as one of the CNS malformations needed to make the diagnosis of Meckel–Gruber syndrome (Summers and Donnenfeld 1995).

For an exhaustive list of genetic disorders associated with Dandy–Walker malformation, refer to Chitayat et al. (1994).

▶ ANTENATAL NATURAL HISTORY

The Dandy–Walker malformation is now known to be a complex developmental abnormality of the rhombencephalon. Formerly, it was thought to represent the sequelae of obstruction of the foramina of Lushka and Magendi, which was originally suggested by Dandy and Walker.

The cerebellum develops by cell proliferation from symmetrical centers in the rhomboencephalon. Fusion begins anterosuperiorly at 9 weeks of gestation. This process continues posteroinferiorly, and is completed by 16 to 17 weeks of gestation. This is why defects of only the inferior vermis can occur (Keogan et al. 1994). The defect may represent true rhomboschisis, or it may relate to a transient antenatal rise in ventricular pressure that may prevent normal closure of the vermis.

The natural history for Dandy–Walker malformation in utero is not known. It appears that progressive changes usually occur slowly (Russ et al. 1989). Some degree of enlargement of the posterior fossa cyst and worsening hydrocephalus can be observed in utero, however.

▶ MANAGEMENT OF PREGNANCY

When a suspected diagnosis of fetal Dandy–Walker malformation exists, the prospective parents should be referred to a center capable of a detailed anatomic survey of the fetus. There is a high incidence of associated CNS and extra-CNS malformations in this condition. Importantly, it is the presence of the additional sonographically detected anomalies that appear to adversely affect survival and prognosis for the infant and child with Dandy–Walker malformation. Summarizing many studies, the risk of associated intracranial anomalies appears to be on the order of 25 to 68%, and the risk of additional intracranial anomalies appears to be on the order of 20 to 60% (Chen and Chu 1994). There is an increased incidence of both mental retardation and perinatal mortality for fetuses with this condition. Therefore, if the diagnosis is made earlier than 24 weeks of gestation, the parents should be offered the option of terminating the pregnancy. If the diagnosis is made in the third trimester, conservative management is recommended. In most cases, the cyst, ventricular dilatation, and cisterna magna enlargement occur slowly. Rarely, severe or rapidly increasing ventriculomegaly can necessitate aggressive obstetric intervention (Russ et al. 1989). It is important to recognize that when Dandy–Walker malformation or variant occurs as an isolated finding, the prognosis is variable, and up to 50% of fetuses with this condition have been reported with a normal outcome. When the disorder is associated with an underlying mendelian condition, such as one of those listed in Table 10-1, the prognosis is then based on natural history of that specific disorder.

There are no specific indications for cesarean section in this condition. Similarly, delivery can occur in a community hospital; however, the prospective parents should be advised that the child will need subspecialty evaluation after birth.

▶ FETAL INTERVENTION

There is no fetal intervention for Dandy–Walker malformation.

▶ TREATMENT OF THE NEWBORN

The infant diagnosed prenatally with Dandy–Walker malformation or one of its variants should undergo a complete physical examination at birth. The best imaging study for the posterior fossa is magnetic resonance imaging (MRI). We do not recommend obtaining a postnatal head ultrasound examination through the anterior fontanelle because of the high incidence of false negative diagnoses. Parents should be counseled that hydrocephalus may not be present at birth, but will become apparent in 75% of survivors by 3 months of age (Estroff et al. 1992).

Both prenatal and postnatal consultation should be obtained with pediatric neurology, neurosurgery, and medical genetics specialists. There is a high incidence of associated congenital anomalies, some of which may not be apparent on the antenatal scan. These are summarized in Table 10-2.

▶ TABLE 10-2. ASSOCIATED ABNORMALITIES SEEN IN 148 CASES OF DANDY–WALKER MALFORMATION

	Percent
Cranial	
Agenesis of corpus callosum	14.8
Abnormal gyral pattern	10.8
Occipital encephalocele	7.4
Aqueductal stenosis	3.3
Cardiac	
Ventriculoseptal defects	6.7
Patent ductus arteriosus	3.3
Atrial-septal defects	2.7
Pulmonary stenosis	2.0
Atrioventricular canal defect	2.0
Renal	
Obstructive uropathy	2.0
Polycystic kidneys	2.0
Abnormal uterus	2.0
Cryptorchidism	2.0
Face/hands	
Cleft lip/ cleft palate	6.7
Dysmorphic face	5.4
Facial angioma	5.4
Syndactyly	2.7

Reprinted, with permission, from Cornford E, Twining P. The Dandy–Walker syndrome: the value of antenatal diagnosis. Clin Radiol 1992;45:172–174.

Interestingly, a strong association exists between the presence of large, aggressive facial hemangiomas and the Dandy–Walker malformation or similar posterior fossa abnormalities. In a postnatal study, seven of nine patients with unilateral facial hemangiomas had Dandy–Walker malformation (Reese et al. 1993). This has raised the question of a developmental-field abnormality as the cause of the Dandy–Walker malformation.

▶ SURGICAL TREATMENT

Surgical treatment in the Dandy–Walker malformation consists mainly of placement of a ventriculoperitoneal shunt for cases of symptomatic hydrocephalus (Chen and Chu 1994).

▶ LONG-TERM OUTCOME

Review of the pediatric literature indicates that in general, children diagnosed with the Dandy–Walker malformation have a better prognosis than fetuses diagnosed with the same malformation. In one study, Russ et al. (1989) reviewed the outcome for 15 cases of prenatally diagnosed Dandy–Walker malformation. Excluding the elective terminations, there was an overall mortality of 55% in this group (6 of 11 live-born infants). However, the coexisting structural and chromosomal abnormalities contributed to 83% of the postnatal deaths. In the 6 live-born infants who died, 3 deaths occurred within 5 days of delivery, and 3 between 5 and 24 months of age. Therefore, parents should not be counseled that this condition is associated with immediate postnatal mortality. Review of the pediatric neurosurgical literature indicates a mortality rate of between 12 and 50%. The functional outcome for survivors is variable. An IQ of less than 83 has been documented in 40 to 70% of cases (Russ et al. 1989). Similar results were obtained in a follow-up study by Chang et al. (1994). They reviewed outcome for 65 pregnancies with Dandy–Walker malformation. Of these, 37 (57%) were electively terminated. Five manifested as an in utero fetal demise. Of the 22 live-born neonates, 9 (41%) died. Of these, 7 died within the first 30 days of life and 2 died within the first year of life. Their review of several studies indicate a live-born mortality rate of between 30 and 70% when detected prenatally, but only between 10 and 25% when detected postnatally.

In Estroff's review of patients with the Dandy–Walker variant, a similar percentage (35%) died in utero or during the neonatal period. Of 11 survivors, 1 has trisomy 21 and another is severely handicapped. Nine of the remaining 11 survivors are developing normally. However, 6 of these 9 did not have any associated extracranial abnormalities. Reviewing the long-term prognosis for 8 fetuses with the Dandy–Walker variant who had an isolated anomaly, 6 of 8 (75%) are normal. One died and 1 is deaf and blind (Estroff et al. 1992).

Thus, an appropriate summation of the available follow-up literature seems to indicate that prognosis is significantly better for fetuses with milder anomalies (such as the variant as opposed to the full malformation) and if the Dandy–Walker malformation is isolated. The presence of additional abnormalities contributes significantly to an increased risk of mortality and developmental delay.

▶ GENETICS AND RECURRENCE RISK

The most important consideration in determining the recurrence risk for Dandy–Walker malformation is to determine whether the finding is associated with a mendelian disorder, such as those listed in Table 10-1, or if a chromosomal abnormality is present. If chromosome studies have not been obtained antenatally, they should be obtained during the newborn period.

For isolated Dandy–Walker malformations, familial recurrences are infrequent but do occasionally occur (Obwegeser et al. 1994). Ulm et al. (1999) described a family in which the first child and subsequent dizygotic twins were all affected with isolated Dandy–Walker malformation.

The largest study of the genetics of Dandy–Walker malformation was performed by Murray et al. (1985). These authors describe a retrospective study of 21 autopsy-proven cases of Dandy–Walker malformation. They also reviewed the literature for an additional 92 subjects. These authors noted the increased frequency of association of Dandy–Walker malformation with congenital heart disease, cleft lip and cleft palate, and neural-tube defects. Of the 113 cases studied, 7 had recognizable single-gene disorders, including two cases of Meckel–Gruber syndrome, and one case each of arthrogryposis type 2B, Walker–Warburg syndrome, Ruvalcaba syndrome, Cornelia–De Lange syndrome, and congenital rubella. Excluding the known single-gene diagnoses, of the 106 remaining cases, 22 had other associated major malformations. These authors pooled information available on 44 siblings of the 106 index patients and 54 siblings of 26 patients with Dandy–Walker malformation associated with hydrocephalus. They documented 1 additional case in 98 siblings, thus giving a 1% risk of recurrence.

These authors concluded the Dandy–Walker malformation is a nonspecific CNS abnormality that can occur in single-gene disorders and chromosomal abnormalities. It can be environmentally induced, may exist as an isolated malformation, or may exist in conjunction with other abnormalities. They suggested the following information for genetic counseling: (1) When

Dandy–Walker malformation occurs as part of a mendelian disorder, the recurrence risks are those of the specific disorder. (2) When Dandy–Walker malformation is associated with a chromosomal abnormality, the recurrence risks include those of maternal age for trisomy, and those of the family, depending on whether there is a familial risk for an unbalanced chromosomal abnormality. (3) If the Dandy–Walker malformation is associated with other multifactorial abnormalities, such as cleft lip and palate or congenital heart defects, there is an additional 5% recurrence risk for those abnormalities. (4) If the Dandy–Walker malformation was isolated, there is an empiric recurrence risk of between 1 and 5% (Murray et al. 1985).

If the presence of an unbalanced karyotype has been documented in the fetus or newborn, parental chromosomes should be studied prior to judging recurrence risks. Prenatal diagnosis is available in subsequent pregnancies through the use of targeted ultrasound examination, ideally performed in the second trimester.

REFERENCES

Achiron R, Achiron A. Transvaginal ultrasonic assessment of the early fetal brain. Ultrasound Obstet Gynecol 1991;1: 336–344.

Bromley B, Nadel AS, Pauker S, Estroff JA, Benacerraf BR. Closure of the cerebellar vermis: evaluation with second trimester US. Radiology 1994;193:761–763.

Bureau Y-A, Fraser W, Fouquett B. Prenatal diagnosis of trisomy 9 mosaic presenting as a case of Dandy–Walker malformation. Prenat Diagn 1993;1379–1385.

Chang MC, Russell SA, Callen PW, Filly RA, Goldstein R. Sonographic detection of inferior vermian agenesis in Dandy–Walker malformations: prognostic implications. Radiology 1994;193:765–770.

Chen F-P, Chu K-K. Prenatal diagnosis of Dandy–Walker malformation: report of a case. J Formos Med Assoc 1994;93:967–970.

Chitayat D, Moore L, Del Bigio MR, et al. Familial Dandy–Walker malformation associated with macrocephaly, facial anomalies, developmental delay, and brain stem dysgenesis: prenatal diagnosis and postnatal outcome in brothers. A new syndrome? Am J Med Genet 1994;52:406–415.

Cornford E, Twining P. The Dandy–Walker syndrome: the value of antenatal diagnosis. Clin Radiol 1992;45:172–174.

Cowles T, Furman P, Wilkins I. Prenatal diagnosis of Dandy–Walker malformation in a family displaying X-linked inheritance. Prenat Diagn 1993;13:87–91.

Estroff JA, Scott MR, Benacerraf BR. Dandy–Walker variant: prenatal sonographic features and clinical outcome. Radiology 1992;185:755–758.

Gembruch U, Baschat AA, Reushe E, Wallner SJ, Greiwe M. First trimester diagnosis of holoprosencephaly with a Dandy–Walker malformation by transvaginal ultrasonography. J Ultrasound Med 1995;14:619–622.

Keogan MT, De Atkine AB, Hertzberg BS. Cerebellar vermian defects: antenatal sonographic appearance and clinical significance. J Ultrasound Med 1994;13:607–611.

McDuffie RS. Complete trisomy 9: case report with ultrasound findings. Am J Perinat 1994;11(2):80–84.

Murray JC, Johnson JA, Bird TD. Dandy–Walker malformation: etiologic heterogeneity and empiric recurrence risks. Clin Genet 1985;28:272–283.

Nyberg DA, Cyr DR, Mack LA, Fitzsimmons J, Hickok D, Mahony BS. The Dandy-Walker malformation: prenatal sonographic diagnosis and its clinical significance. J Ultrasound Med 1988;7:65–71.

Nyberg DA, Mahony BS, Hegge FN, Hickok D, Luthy D, Kapur R. Enlarged cisterna magna and the Dandy–Walker malformation: factors associated with chromosome abnormalities. Obstet Gynecol 1991;77:436.

Obwegeser R, Deutinger J, Brenaschek G. Recurrent Dandy-Walker malformation. Arch Gynecol Obstet 1994; 255:161–163.

Pretorius DH, Kallman CE, Grafe MR, Budorick NE, Stamm ER. Linear echoes in the fetal cisterna magna. J Ultrasound Med 1992;11:125–128.

Reese V, Frieden IJ, Paller AS, et al. Association of facial hemangiomas with Dandy–Walker and other posterior fossa malformations. J Pediatr 1993;122:379–384.

Russ PD, Pretorius DH, Johnson MJ. Dandy–Walker syndrome: a review of fifteen cases evaluated by prenatal sonography. Am J Obstet Gynecol 1989;161:401–406.

Summers MC, Donnenfeld AE. Dandy–Walker malformation in the Meckel syndrome. Am J Med Genet 1995;55:57–61.

Ulm B, Ulm MR, Dentinger J, Bernaschek G. Dandy–Walker malformation diagnosed before 21 weeks of gestation: associated malformations and chromosomal abnormalities. Ultrasound Obstet Gynecol 1997;10:167–170.

Ulm B, Ulm MR, Deutinger J, Bernaschek G. Isolated Dandy–Walker malformation: prenatal diagnosis in two consecutive pregnancies. Am J Perinatol 1999;16:61–63.

Vohra N, Ghidini A, Alvarez M, Lockwood C. Walker–Warburg syndrome: prenatal ultrasound findings. Prenat Diagn 1993;13:575–579.

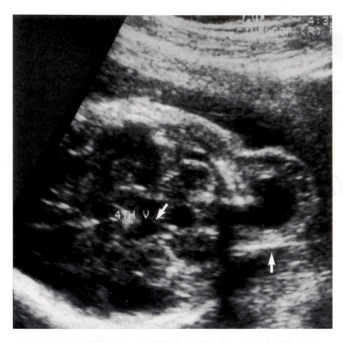

Figure 11-1. Transaxial sonogram demonstrating an occipital encephalocele with the appearance of a cyst within a cyst. The arrow indicates the location of the encephalocele. 4th v = the fourth ventricle.

To diagnose an encephalocele sonographically, the following criteria should be met:

1. The mass should be seen attached to the fetal head or move with the fetal head.
2. A bony defect should be revealed.
3. Intracranial anatomic abnormalities should be detected, such as hydrocephalus.
4. The spine should be scanned to diagnose associated spina bifida.
5. The fetal kidneys should be examined, because of a high incidence of association with renal cystic disease.

In 7 to 15% of cases, neural-tube defects are shown to be present in association with the encephalocele (Fleming et al. 1991). In addition, microcephaly is seen in 20% of cases. Other associated central nervous system (CNS) anomalies that occur with encephalocele include absence of the corpus callosum, orofacial clefting, craniosynostosis, Dandy–Walker malformation, Arnold–Chiari malformation, ectrodactyly, hemifacial microsomia, Klippel–Feil anomaly, iniencephaly, and myelomeningocele (Cohen and Lemire 1982).

In one study, Budorick et al. (1985) reviewed 26 cases of prenatally diagnosed encephalocele. Seventy-one percent of these cases were in the occipital location. Sixty-five percent of cases had associated major congenital anomalies. CNS features that were observed and helped with the diagnosis of encephalocele included:

1. A visible skull defect (seen in 96% of cases).
2. Ventriculomegaly (23% of cases).
3. Microcephaly (seen in 50% of cases).
4. A beaked tectal plate (38% of cases).
5. A flattened basio-occiput (38% of cases).

These authors demonstrated that if more than 50% of the intracranial contents were exteriorized, postnatal survival was poor.

In another study, Goldstein et al. (1991) reviewed the prenatal sonograms of encephaloceles in 15 fetuses. Of these, 13 were in the occipital location, 1 in the ethmoidal, and 1 in the frontoparietal. These authors could not accurately distinguish between meningocele and meningoencephalocele. They also noted an inward depression of the frontal bones (the lemon sign) in 33% of fetuses with encephalocele. The long-term outcome for these fetuses was uniformly poor. Only 3 of 14 fetuses with adequate follow-up were born alive (21%). Of the 9 patients who had prenatal chromosome studies performed, 4 (44%) were abnormal. Abnormalities included trisomy 13, trisomy 18, mosaic trisomy 20, and an unbalanced chromosome translocation. The outcome for the remaining 11 patients included 5 therapeutic terminations of pregnancy, 2 stillbirths, and 4 neonatal deaths. Similarly, Wininger and Donnenfeld (1984) reviewed 15 cases of prenatally diagnosed encephalocele. These authors also demonstrated a high incidence of associated major anomalies (60% of cases). The indications for prenatal sonography in this study were fairly nonspecific and included seven routine scans performed for gestational age dating, three performed prior to amniocentesis for advanced maternal age, three for a positive family history of an unrelated genetic disorder, and two for elevated maternal serum α-fetoprotein. The mean gestational age at detection of these cases was 12 to 14 weeks. These authors identified three multifactorial disorders, two cases of chromosomal abnormalities, and two autosomal recessive syndromes. The outcome for the fetuses in their study was poor. One fetus miscarried at 23 weeks of gestation. There were six terminations of pregnancy. Of the eight live-born infants, only five survived beyond the neonatal period, and all of the three for whom follow-up information was available had developmental delay.

▶ DIFFERENTIAL DIAGNOSIS

Important considerations in the sonographic differential diagnosis of encephalocele include location of the extracranial mass (midline or lateral), consistency of the mass (cystic or solid), and whether or not the anomaly is associated with an underlying cranial bony defect (Sherer et al. 1993). Encephaloceles are typically midline, cystic structures that overlie or project through a defect in the

▶ **TABLE 11-1.** DIFFERENTIAL DIAGNOSIS BETWEEN CYSTIC HYGROMA AND ENCEPHALOCELE

Sonographic Finding	Cystic Hygroma	Encephalocele
Bone defect in skull	Never	Always
Septae	Present and bilateral; often extend to neck	If present, only in midline; continuous with fetal brain
Contents of sac	Fluid only	Variable
Associated microcephaly	Rare	Common
Location	Posterolateral aspect of neck	Occipital, 70%; frontal, parietal, or nasofrontal, 30%

Modified, with permission, from Pearce JM, Griffin D, Campbell S. The differential prenatal diagnosis of cystic hygromata and encephalocele by ultrasound examination. J Clin Ultrasound 1985;13:317–320.

calvarium. The diagnosis is helped by the identification of herniated brain tissue and associated hydrocephalus.

A major consideration in the differential diagnosis is cystic hygroma (Table 11-1). An occipital meningocele that contains only cerebrospinal fluid can be confused with a cystic hygroma. With cystic hygromas, however, the margins of the mass blend into the skin line. Cystic hygromas frequently contain septations. There are fewer CNS anomalies associated with cystic hygromas. In addition, other findings of hydrops, such as pleural effusions and ascites, can be found with cystic hygroma (Goldstein et al. 1991; Pearce et al. 1985). Encephaloceles can also be confused with teratomas, which are solid or heterogeneous but have no demonstrable brain tissue. Hemangioma is an additional soft-tissue mass that can be confused with encephalocele; they are heterogeneously echogenic, with no identifiable skull defects. They form an obtuse angle with the adjacent skull, as opposed to cephaloceles, which typically form an acute angle with the adjacent skull (Bronshtein et al. 1992; Winter et al. 1991). Sherer et al. (1993)

described the case of a 27-week-old fetus with a right retroauricular mass thought to overlay a bony defect of the skull. This was initially diagnosed as an encephalocele, but it was later shown to be a subcutaneous hemangioma. The prognosis is significantly better for a hemangioma (Bronshtein et al. 1992). Other considerations in the differential diagnosis include scalp edema (Winter et al. 1991) and branchial cleft cysts.

Once the encephalocele has been verified, a careful search must be made for associated anomalies. Encephaloceles are frequently associated with other anomalies, and the demonstration of other anomalies may help to make a syndromic diagnosis. A significant cause of encephaloceles is amniotic band or amniotic rupture (see Chapter 101). Encephaloceles due to amniotic bands tend to have irregular surfaces, and asymmetric placement. Amniotic bands or aberrant tissue bands become entangled in oral and nasal orifices or become attached directly to the face or cranium.

A listing of the major syndromes of which encephalocele is a component is given in Table 11-2. The most

▶ **TABLE 11-2.** SYNDROMES IN WHICH ENCEPHALOCELE IS A MAJOR COMPONENT

Condition	Pattern of Inheritance	Associated Findings
Chemke syndrome	Autosomal Recessive	Hydrocephalus, cerebellar dysgenesis, retinal dysplasia, corneal opacities, cataracts
Cryptophthalmos syndrome (Fraser)	Autosomal Recessive	Skin of forehead covers one or both eyes; total/partial syndactyly of fingers or toes
Dyssegmental dwarfism	Autosomal Recessive	Short tubular bones, bowing of extremities, vertebral anomalies, small thorax, cleft palate, micrognathia
Frontonasal dysplasia	Sporadic	Ocular hypertelorism, median cleft lip
Knobloch syndrome	Autosomal Recessive	Retinal detachment, myopia, normal intelligence
Meckel–Gruber syndrome	Autosomal Recessive	Polydactyly, polycystic kidneys, oligohydramnios, other CNS abnormalities
Amniotic band (rupture)	Sporadic	Limb amputations, facial clefts, thoracoabdominal wall defects, skull malformations
Roberts syndrome	Autosomal Recessive	Short or absent limbs, facial cleft, hypertelorism, heart and kidney defects

Modified, with permission, from Cohen MM, Lemire RJ. Syndromes with cephaloceles. Teratology 1982;25:161–172; Chervenak FA, Isaacson G, Mahoney MJ, Berkowitz RL, Tortora M, Hobbins JC. Diagnosis and management of fetal cephalocele. Obstet Gynecol 1984;64:86–90.

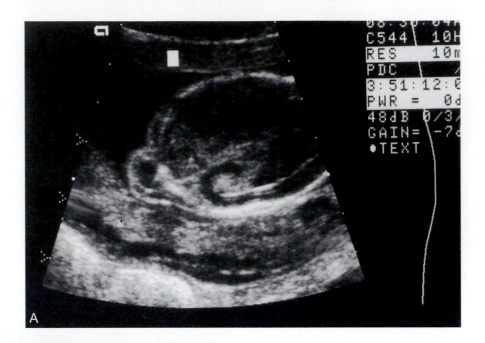

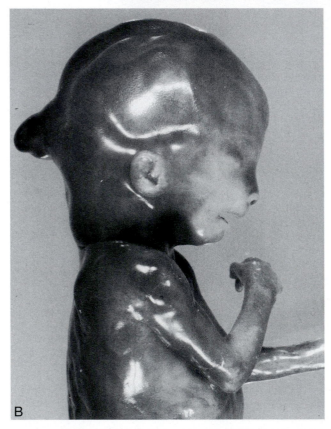

Figure 11-2. (A) Transaxial sonogram of a fetal head demonstrating a small occipital encelphalocele. This fetus has Meckel–Gruber syndrome. (B) Corresponding autopsy photograph of the same fetus with an intact encephalocele. The fetus also has micrognathia. *(Photograph courtesy of Dr. Joseph Semple.)*

common of these is Meckel–Gruber syndrome, an autosomal recessive condition that is characterized by the presence of an occipital encephalocele, polydactyly, polycystic kidneys, and multiple associated anomalies (Figs. 11-2A and 11-2B). Up to 5% of neural-tube defects occur as part of Meckel–Gruber syndrome (Chervenak et al. 1984).

Meckel–Gruber syndrome should be suspected in fetuses with encephalocele and oligohydramnios. In one study, four of five patients with oligohydramnios and encephalocele had Meckel–Gruber syndrome (Budorick et al. 1995). Encephalocele is found in association with several different chromosome abnormalities.

► ANTENATAL NATURAL HISTORY

The failure of the rostral end of the neural tube to close results in an encephalocele. During the fourth week of fetal life, fusion begins in the region of the fourth somite and extends both rostrally and caudally. Encephaloceles are due either to primary overgrowth of neural tissue in the line of closure or failure of induction by adjacent mesodermal tissues that may interrupt the process of closure. The majority of encephaloceles occur in the midline; however, they may also result from disruption of fetal-skull formation, such as in the amnion rupture sequence (Chervenak et al. 1984). Encephaloceles occur between 25 and 50 days of gestation for anterior defects and up to 60 days for posterior defects (Brown and Sheridan-Pereira 1992).

The presence of encephalocele is associated with an increased incidence of death in utero. An encephalocele is the predominant neural-axis anomaly found in fetuses spontaneously aborted at less than 20 weeks of gestational age (Goldstein et al. 1991).

An interesting case reported by Bronshtein and Zimmer (1991) documented by sonography the formation of a cephalocele in two stages. Initially, an occipital meningocele was detected by transvaginal study at 13 weeks of gestation. By 14 weeks, brain tissue was visualized, and the diagnosis was changed to a meningoencephalocele. At 15 to 16 weeks of gestation, the lesion disappeared, but was detected again at 19 weeks of gestation. On repeated sonographic examinations, this case illustrated that the primary process was the formation of the meningocele, but that once an opening became present, brain tissue protruded into it at a later stage.

► MANAGEMENT OF PREGNANCY

Fetuses in which encephalocele is suspected should be referred to a center capable of thorough anatomic study of the fetus. Detailed sonography should be performed to verify the presence of the encephalocele and to search for associated anomalies. Because of the high incidence of associated anomalies and chromosomal abnormalities, a prenatal karyotype should be offered. Most encephaloceles will be diagnosed as an incidental finding. Most encephaloceles are covered by skin, so typically there is no increase in the maternal serum α-fetoprotein level.

Once the encephalocele is diagnosed, further obstetrical management is affected by the size of the defect, the gestational age at diagnosis, and the presence or absence of associated anomalies. A thorough discussion should be held with the prospective parents that describes the expected prognosis for the infant. Prognosis depends on

1. The presence and amount of brain in the herniated sac. (This is the most important consideration.)
2. The presence or absence of hydrocephalus.
3. The presence or absence of microcephaly.
4. The presence or absence of other anomalies that suggest a syndromic diagnosis. (Fleming et al. 1991).

Magnetic resonance imaging may help to better delineate fetal CNS anatomy (Fig. 11-3). Encephaloceles in the sincipital or frontal location have a better prognosis. This is probably because the defects are in general smaller, resulting in less herniation of the brain. Also, apparently the loss of the frontal cortex produces fewer neurologic defects (Chervenak et al. 1984). If the encephalocele is diagnosed at less than 24 weeks of gestation, termination of the pregnancy can be offered to the parents. If the parents want to continue the pregnancy, they should meet with a neurosurgeon, neonatologist, and medical geneticist.

The route of delivery is determined by sonographic findings in the fetus. If a large amount of brain tissue is observed in the sac, or if associated anomalies are present, minimizing maternal risk should be the primary consideration, and cesarean section is probably not advisable. Cesarean section can be considered when

1. The encephalocele is large enough to cause cephalopelvic disproportion.
2. Other obstetric considerations are present, such as a previous low vertical cesarean section.
3. A coincident viable twin is present.
4. If the parents are aware of the risk of significant developmental defects in the infant and accept the risk involved (Chatterjee et al. 1985; Chervenak et al. 1984).

We recommend that the baby be delivered at a tertiary-care center to facilitate coordination of services for the newborn.

► FETAL INTERVENTION

There is no fetal intervention indicated for encephalocele.

► TREATMENT OF THE NEWBORN

Treatment of the newborn with encephalocele depends to a large extent on the size and location of the lesion and whether or not associated anomalies are present. For large occipital encephaloceles, the long-term outcome is

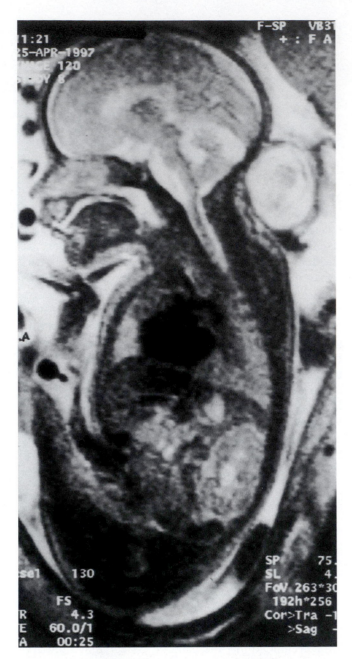

Figure 11-3. Sagittal half-Fourier single-shot turbo spin-echo sequence (HASTE) magnetic resonance image of the fetus with a posterior encephalocele shown in Figure 11-1. A small amount of brain tissue is seen within the sac. The remainder of the fetal brain appears normal except for the posterior aspect of the occipital lobe. *(Image courtesy of Dr. Deborah Levine.)*

nearly uniformly poor. Even if parents have decided not to terminate the pregnancy, they may decide that no aggressive intervention should be taken. On the other hand, certain parents may desire that everything be done for their newborn. In any event, cephaloceles typically have an intact skin cover. The intracranial volume is reduced by herniation, and children with large

encephaloceles generally have microcephaly at birth. A complete physical examination is indicated to rule out an associated syndrome (see Table 11-2). Consultation with a medical genetics specialist should be obtained. If the parents want surgery to be performed, a neurosurgical consultation should be obtained. In general, surgical treatment is performed as soon as possible, although few data exist that correlate timing of surgery with ultimate developmental outcome.

▶ SURGICAL TREATMENT

The surgical challenges in cases of encephalocele include closing the anatomical defect in the cranial vault and achieving as near normal functional outcome as possible with minimal psychomotor defects (Habal 1993). Surgical repair in encephalocele consists of opening and exploring the sac, excising malformed brain tissue, and closing the basal dural defect. Surgical repair is generally timed for 0 to 4 months of age (Date et al. 1993). In cases of giant occipital encephaloceles with microcephaly secondary to massive brain herniation, the use of a fine mesh has been described to provide a rigid extracranial compartment for the encephalocele. Daily digital compression is performed and the mesh is gradually imbricated into the calvarium (Gallo 1992).

Surgical considerations for sincipital encephaloceles are different because of the associated craniofacial deformities. In general, surgical treatment for frontal or sincipital encephaloceles include removal of the encephalocele, closure of the dura intracranially, followed by transcranial bone grafting, and correction of orbital hypertelorism or dystopia (David and Proudman 1989). Hockley et al. (1990) described treatment of the patient with an anterior encephalocele. They listed the following indications for urgent surgery: absence of skin cover, hemorrhage, airway obstruction, or impairment of vision. For most cases of frontal encephalocele, surgery was elective, and the indications included protection of the brain; facilitation of nursing; prevention of infection; improvement of the airway, speech, and vision; or treatment of associated anomalies, such as hydrocephalus and hypertelorism.

▶ LONG-TERM OUTCOME

The most important consideration in the long-term follow-up of a patient with encephalocele appears to be whether or not brain tissue is present in the extracranial sac. There is no question that the prognosis is much better for a fetus with a meningocele as opposed to a meningoencephalocele. In one report of 24 patients with surgically repaired encephalocele, follow-up information was available on 22 patients who survived.

In this study, 1 patient died from pneumonia at 8 months of age and another at 4 years. Of the 22 surviving patients, 14 had meningoceles. All of these surviving children were normal. Of the eight survivors with meningoencephalocele two were normal, four were ambulatory and had mild to moderate retardation, and two were bedridden with marked retardation. These authors concluded that presence of gross brain tissue in the sac was the most important prognostic factor (Date et al. 1993).

Similar results were seen by Simpson et al. (1984), who studied the outcome for 74 patients with cephaloceles. Of these infants, 17 had meningoceles; all did well, even if associated hydrocephalus developed. Of the 57 infants with meningoencephalocele, almost all did poorly despite surgical expansion of the cranial cavity or decompression of enlarged ventricles.

Docherty et al. (1991) described the outcome for 52 patients with occipital cephaloceles between 1971 and 1990. This study was biased, in that no information was given regarding whether the lesion was a meningocele or a meningoencephalocele. Hydrocephalus developed in 57% of patients, and over half of these required shunting. Twenty-three percent of patients died within the first year. Of the 23 survivors or their caretakers who returned a questionnaire, 14 were normal and 9 were significantly handicapped, but this study was limited in that the underlying pathology of the lesion was not described in the article. Based on the available literature, it seems reasonable to conclude that outcome for fetuses with meningocele is reasonably good, whereas outcome for fetuses with demonstrable brain tissue in the mass is uniformly poor.

▶ GENETICS AND RECURRENCE RISK

An important consideration in the genetics of encephalocele is to determine whether the lesion is isolated. Isolated encephaloceles have not been shown to be familial. There is no evidence in the literature of an increased incidence of affected siblings. This is different from other neural-tube defects, in which the genetics appear to be multifactorial. On the other hand, many encephaloceles are associated with specific syndromes, and many of these are inherited as autosomal recessive conditions (see Table 11-2). It is therefore extremely important to determine whether the encephalocele has associated anomalies, making it consistent with a syndromic diagnosis.

An attempt should be made to study chromosomes either prenatally or postnatally. Previously reported chromosomal abnormalities that have been demonstrated in fetuses with encephaloceles include trisomies 13 and 18 and mosaic trisomy 20, as well as unbalanced translocations and inversions.

Although isolated encephalocele is not considered to have an increased risk of recurrence, parents can be offered prenatal sonography in a subsequent pregnancy. Encephaloceles have been diagnosed as early as 12 weeks of gestation by transvaginal sonography (Cullen et al. 1990; Fleming et al. 1991).

REFERENCES

Adetiloye VA, Dare FO, Oyelami OA. A ten year review of encephalocele in a teaching hospital. Int J Gynecol Obstet 199341:241–249.

Bronshtein M, Bar-Hava I, Blumenfeld Z. Early second-trimester sonographic appearance of occipital haemangioma simulating encephalocele. Prenat Diagn 1992;12:695–698.

Bronshtein M, Zimmer EZ. Transvaginal sonographic follow-up on the formation of fetal cephalocele at 13–19 weeks' gestation. Obstet Gynecol 1991;78:528–530.

Brown MS, Sheridan-Pereira M. Outlook for the child with a cephalocele. Pediatrics 1992;90:914–919.

Budorick NE, Pretorius DH, McGahan JP, Grafe MR, James HE, Slivka J. Cephalocele detection in utero: sonogaphic and clinical features. Ultrasound Obstet Gynecol 1995;5:77–85.

Chatterjee MS, Bondoc B, Adhate A. Prenatal diagnosis of occipital encephalocele. Am J Obstet Gynecol 1985;153:646–647.

Chervenak FA, Isaacson G, Mahoney MJ, Berkowitz RL, Tortora M, Hobbins JC. Diagnosis and management of fetal cephalocele. Obstet Gynecol 1984;64:86–90.

Cohen MM, Lemire RJ. Syndromes with cephaloceles. Teratology 1982;25:161–172.

Cullen MT, Athanassiadis AP, Romero R. Prenatal diagnosis of anterior parietal encephalocele with transvaginal sonography. Obstet Gynecol 1990;75:489–491.

Date I, Yagyu Y, Asari S, Ohmoto T. Long-term outcome in surgically treated encephalocele. Surg Neurol 1993;40:125–130.

David DJ, Proudman TW. Cephaloceles: classification, pathology, and management. World J Surg 1989;13:349–357.

Docherty JG, Daly JC, Carachi R. Encephaloceles: a review 1971–1990. Eur J Pediatr Surg 1991;1(Suppl):11–13.

Fleming AD, Vintzileos AM, Scorza WE. Prenatal diagnosis of occipital encephalocele with transvaginal sonography. J Ultrasound Med 1991;10:285–286.

Gallo AE. Repair of giant occipital encephaloceles with microcephaly secondary to massive brain herniation. Child Nerv Syst 1992;8:229–230.

Goldstein RB, LaPidus AS, Filly RA. Fetal cephaloceles: diagnosis with US. Radiology 1991;180:803–808.

Graham D, Johnson RB, Winn K, Sanders RC. The role of sonography in the prenatal diagnosis and management of encephalocele. J Ultrasound Med 1982;1:111–115.

Habal MB. Craniofacial correction of the occipital encephalocele. J Craniofac Surg 1993;4:215–222.

Hockley AD, Goldin JH, Wake MJC. Management of anterior encephalocele. Child Nerv Syst 1990;6:444–446.

Kalien B, Robert E, Harris J. Associated malformations in infants and fetuses with upper or lower neural tube defects. Teratology 1998;57:56–63.

Pearce JM, Griffin D, Campbell S. The differential prenatal diagnosis of cystic hygromata and encephalocele by ultrasound examination. J Clin Ultrasound 1985;13:317–320.

Richards CG. Frontoethmoidal meningoencephalocele: a common and severe congenital abnormality in South East Asia. Arch Dis Child 1992;67:717–719.

Sherer DM, Perillo AM, Abramowicz JS. Fetal hemangioma overlying the temporal occipital suture, initially diagnosed by ultrasonography as an encephlocele. J Ultrasound Med 1993;12:691–693.

Simpson DA, David DJ, White J. Cephaloceles: treatment, outcome, and antenatal diagnosis. Neurosurgery 1984;15:14–21.

Wininger SJ, Donnenfeld AE. Syndromes identified in fetuses with prenatally diagnosed cephaloceles. Prenat Diagn 1994;14:839–843.

Winter TC, Mack LA, Cyr DR. Prenatal sonographic diagnosis of scalp edema/cephalohematoma mimicking an encephalocele. AJR Am J Roentgenol 1993;161:1247–1248.

Wiswell TE, Tuttle DJ, Northam RS, Simonds GR. Major congenital neurologic malformations. Am J Dis Child 1990;144:61–67.

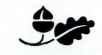

CHAPTER 12

Exencephaly

▶ CONDITION

Exencephaly is a rare fetal anomaly that is incompatible with extrauterine life. In exencephaly, the bones of the cranial vault are absent, but the facial structures and bones of the base of the skull are preserved (Casellas et al. 1993). Exencephaly is considered to be a precursor to anencephaly, but it differs from anencephaly because residual brain tissue is present and floating free in the amniotic fluid.

Exencephaly is frequently noted in animal teratogen studies. Human exencephaly appears to be confined to early gestation. Only rare reports exist of a third-trimester diagnosis of an exencephalic fetus (Wilkins-Haug and Freedman 1991). However, anencephaly is more common in humans than in animals. The greater prevalence of anencephaly in humans is attributed to a longer gestational period, which presents the opportunity for destruction of the free-floating brain matter.

Exencephaly is due to the failure of the neural tube to close during the fourth week of embryonic development, but reopening or degeneration of a previously closed neural tube is also possible. The underlying defect is thought to be due to a failure in mesenchymal migration (Stagiannis et al. 1995). In pathologic studies, the exencephalic brain is noted to be covered by a highly vascular epithelial layer. In exencephaly, two relatively equivalent cerebral hemispheric remnants are present within a reddish mass of disorganized tissues, remnants of deep cerebral neural elements, blood vessels, fibrous tissues, and fluid-filled spaces (Hendricks et al. 1988). This brain remnant has been termed the "anencephalic area cerebrovasculosa." In exencephalic brain tissue, the gyri and sulci are shallow, flattened, and disorganized. All surfaces of the brain are highly vascular. The remaining central nervous system tissue is dysplastic, with little or no neuronal differentiation,

and very little normal cortex is present (Hendricks et al. 1988).

▶ INCIDENCE

Papp et al. (1986) reviewed cases of neural-tube defect detected by maternal serum α-fetoprotein (AFP) screening. In 36,075 screened pregnancies, 10 cases of exencephaly were detected. This equals an incidence of 3 cases per 10,000 screened pregnancies. The same population had 14 cases of anencephaly per 10,000 screened pregnancies. In this report from Hungary, the mean age of the mothers of fetuses with exencephaly was 22 years. Of the 10 affected pregnancies detected, 9 were singletons and 1 was a twin gestation. In 8 of the 9 cases described, the maternal serum AFP levels were greater than 2.5 multiples of the median.

In experimental animals, there is an increased incidence of exencephaly in fetuses of female mice injected with clomiphene citrate prior to ovulation (Dziadek 1993). In addition, hyperglycemia in mice induces exencephaly (Sadler 1980). The phenomenon in mice is similar to the inhibition of neural-tube closure seen in infants of mothers with diabetes.

▶ SONOGRAPHIC FINDINGS

Exencephaly can be detected early and late in gestation. In the normal fetus, at approximately 11 weeks of gestation, echogenic images can be seen that correspond to calcification of the cranial bones. If calcification is absent at this point in gestation, exencephaly should be considered. Later in gestation, the most common finding in exencephalic fetuses is the presence of a large quantity of disorganized brain tissue that is not

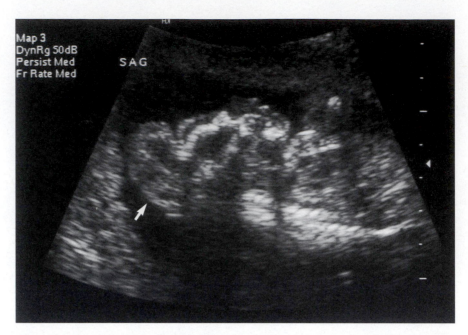

Figure 12-1. Sagittal view of a fetus demonstrating a large quantity of disorganized brain tissue not covered by skull bones (arrow).

covered by the bones of the skull, with concomitant preservation of facial structures and bones at the base of the skull (Fig. 12-1).

The first prenatal sonographic diagnosis of exencephaly at 39 weeks of gestation was described by Cox et al. in 1985. Subsequently, multiple case reports have contributed to the information available regarding sonographic diagnosis. In one report, in a routine sonographic examination performed at 29 weeks of gestation, the flat bones of the skull were noted to be absent with only a small part of the occipital bone present (meroacrania). Disorganized brain tissue was noted to be floating free in the amniotic cavity. In addition, no evidence was seen of cerebral ventricles, and the gyri were noted be extremely disorganized (Casellas et al. 1993).

Exencephaly is often associated with other malformations. Hendricks et al. (1988) described four cases of exencephaly. Two of these were associated with amniotic bands and multiple asymmetric additional anomalies. Two of the patients in this report had associated omphalocele. All of these cases were diagnosed in the second or third trimester. First-trimester diagnosis of exencephaly is also possible (Bognoni et al. 1999; Nishi and Nakano 1994). In one report (Kennedy et al. 1990), a vaginal sonogram performed at 10.5 weeks of gestation revealed the absence of the normal calvarium, choroid, and echolucent areas seen in the brain at that point in gestation. In the affected fetus, the brain appeared echodense, with pulsatile prominence in the area of the forebrain. Because of the concern regarding lack of cranial calcification, repeat sonography was performed at 14 weeks of gestation. At this later time,

the cranium was noted to be absent above the occipital bones, a widened cervical spine was present, and fragments of neural tissue were seen attached but floating in the amniotic fluid in the process of degeneration (Kennedy et al. 1990). Several reports describe prenatal diagnosis of pentalogy of Cantrell with exencephaly (Bognoni et al. 1999).

▶ DIFFERENTIAL DIAGNOSIS

The differential diagnosis for exencephaly includes massive meningoencephalocele, amniotic bands or amniotic rupture, limb–body-wall complex, and skeletal dysplasias. It is important to distinguish exencephaly from massive meningoencephalocele because the latter condition is not lethal. In massive meningoencephalocele, the cranial vault is always detected, and part of the brain is intracranial (Abu Musa et al. 1990). In meningoencephalocele, the exposed brain tissue appears more normal than in exencephaly, in which marked dysplasia and disorganized development of rudimentary brain tissue exists.

In the amniotic band syndrome, rupture of the amnion leads to subsequent entanglement of fetal parts by fibrous mesodermic bands. This condition is suggested by the presence of asymmetric lesions in the brain, with associated defects of the spine, abdominal wall, and limbs (Abu Musa et al. 1990; Casellas et al. 1993; Hendricks et al. 1988). In limb–body-wall complex, exencephaly or encephalocele are associated with facial clefts, limb defects, and scoliosis. This condition is diagnosed by disruption of the body wall in association with multiple severe abnormalities. Pentalogy of Cantrell (see Chapter 64) consists of a supraumbilical-wall defect, defect of the lower sternum, deficiency of the anterior diaphragm, defect of the diaphragmatic pericardium, and the presence of intracardiac defects. In several reports, approximately 10% of patients with pentalogy of Cantrell have associated central nervous system malformations, including exencephaly (Denath et al. 1994; Hori et al. 1984)(see Chapter 64).

A final consideration in the differential diagnosis is the presence of a skeletal dysplasia. This can be suggested by lack of mineralization of skull bones, such as is seen in hypophosphatasia (see Chapter 96) and osteogenesis imperfecta type II (see Chapter 98). In the skeletal dysplasias, however, the intracranial anatomy is normal. Typical of the skeletal dysplasias are the abnormalities of the long bones, which include shortening or bowing.

▶ ANTENATAL NATURAL HISTORY

Exencephaly is considered to be a precursor to anencephaly. In animals with short gestational periods, exencephaly is frequently observed. However, if the gestation is prolonged artificially, the exposed cerebral structures experience obstruction, resulting in anencephaly (Casellas et al. 1993). Wood and Smith (1984) developed an experimental model for anencephaly by administering vitamin A to pregnant rats. The fetuses were noted to have exencephaly that spontaneously disintegrated and eventually became anencephaly. It is thought that the chemical and physical trauma to which the cerebral tissue (unprotected by its sheltering bone cover) is exposed determines its eventual destruction. In humans, destruction of exposed developing brain structures may be complete by 8 to 10 weeks of gestation (Abu Musa et al. 1990).

It has now been demonstrated in humans that a similar progression from exencephaly to anencephaly exists. Wilkins-Haug and Freedman (1991) described a case in which progression to anencephaly was demonstrated by multiple sonograms in a continuing pregnancy. In their case, a 16-week-old fetus was diagnosed with exencephaly. In the cranial area, a well-circumscribed tissue mass was demonstrated without sonographic evidence of cranial calcification. At 18 weeks of gestation, these findings were unchanged, and the parents elected to continue the pregnancy. Repeat sonography was performed at 24 weeks of gestation, when polyhydramnios was demonstrated, and the brain tissue appearance had changed significantly. The disorganized tissue mass was no longer well circumscribed. It was convoluted and floating free in the amniotic fluid cephalad to the frontal bones. At 29 weeks of gestation,

the volume of the free-floating brain tissue had significantly decreased. Only a thin layer of tissue remained above the frontal bones. A female infant was delivered by spontaneous vaginal delivery at 30 weeks of gestation with Apgar scores of 1 and 0. The physical appearance of this infant was consistent with classic anencephaly. Physical examination of the cranial area revealed a minimal amount of erythematous, spongy tissue, without cranial or skin covering. This case demonstrates the destruction and disorganization of the developing brain that eventually results in the development of the anencephalic area cerebrovasculosa. A similar phenomenon has been described in another case report, in which selective feticide was performed in a twin pregnancy at 18 weeks of gestation. One twin was normal and the other affected with exencephaly (Papp et al. 1986). This case was followed by repeated sonograms for the healthy twin, and the exposed cerebral mass in the affected twin also regressed over time.

▶ MANAGEMENT OF PREGNANCY

Fetuses with exencephaly may be detected by abnormal maternal serum screening results. Maternal serum AFP, maternal serum human chorionic gonadotropin (hCG), and urinary β-core hCG levels are all elevated in this condition (Hayashi et al. 1994). Fetuses in which exencephaly is suspected should be referred to a center capable of detailed anatomic sonographic screening to confirm the diagnosis. Pregnancies in which amniocenteses have been performed also reveal extremely high levels of amniotic-fluid AFP (Papp et al. 1986). In addition, large numbers of actively phagocytic macrophages can be demonstrated in the amniotic fluid of fetuses with exencephaly (Papp et al. 1986). It is thought that the degeneration of the exposed neural tissue is potentiated by the macrophages, although it is not known whether these macrophages are fetal or maternal in origin.

Typically, exencephaly is not associated with chromosomal abnormalities, although one case reported deletion of the long arm of chromosome 13 (Lam et al. 1998). However, because of the severity of the defect, a chromosome analysis should be performed to permit accurate genetic counseling. Exencephaly is not compatible with postnatal life. Therefore, the parents should be given the option of termination of pregnancy if this condition is diagnosed before 24 weeks of gestation. There is no indication for cesarean delivery.

▶ FETAL INTERVENTION

There is no fetal intervention for exencephaly.

▶ TREATMENT OF THE NEWBORN

Exencephaly is a lethal condition. There is no indication for resuscitation of the newborn.

▶ SURGICAL TREATMENT

There is no surgical treatment for exencephaly.

▶ LONG-TERM OUTCOME

Exencephaly is uniformly fatal.

▶ GENETICS AND RECURRENCE RISK

Exencephaly may be one part of a multiple congenital anomaly syndrome that is inherited as a single-gene disorder. For example, exencephaly is part of the Roberts syndrome, which is inherited as an autosomal recessive condition and consists of limb-reduction anomalies, unilateral anophthalmia, and premature centromeric splitting on karyotype (Verloes et al. 1989). Exencephaly has also been reported to be associated with an autosomal dominant brachydactyly pedigree (Stagiannis et al. 1995). Exencephaly can also be an extreme manifestation of the Adams–Oliver syndrome, which is inherited as an autosomal dominant gene. This condition consists of congenital scalp defects and distal limb anomalies. Every attempt should be made to determine whether the exencephaly is isolated or part of a multiple malformation syndrome. If the fetus is terminated, an autopsy should be performed and chromosome analysis should be performed at the time of termination.

Exencephaly has been described in a product of a consanguineous (brother/sister) mating in which both parents had Waardenburg syndrome. This mating raised the question of homozygosity for a mutation in the PAX3 gene. The PAX3 gene is analogous to the mouse splotch gene. In splotch homozygotes, exencephaly develops in half of litters. This human mating possibly demonstrates the role of PAX3 in neurulation, neural-crest-cell migration, and development of limb muscles in the human as well as the mouse (Aymé and Philip 1995).

The recurrence risk for exencephaly depends on its underlying etiology. Cases that are associated with amnion rupture do not have an increased risk of recurrence. If a single-gene disorder is present, the recurrence risk will depend on whether it is autosomal recessive, autosomal dominant, or X-linked. Exencephaly is considered to be within the spectrum of neural-tube defects, which have an increased risk of recurrence on the order to 2 to 5%. Preconceptual folic acid and sonographic examination are recommended in subsequent pregnancies.

REFERENCES

Abu Musa A, Hata T, Senoh D, et al. Antenatal sonographic diagnosis of exencephaly. Gynecol Obstet Invest 1990; 29:75–77.

Aymé S, Philip N. Possible homozygous Waardenburg syndrome in a fetus with exencephaly. Am J Med Genet 1995;59:263–265.

Bognoni V, Quartuccio A, Quartuccio A. First-trimester sonographic diagnosis of Cantrell's pentalogy with exencephaly. J Clin Ultrasound 1999;27:276–278.

Casellas M, Ferrer M, Rovira M, Pla F, Martinez A, Cabero L. Prenatal diagnosis of exencephaly. Prenat Diagn 1993;13: 417–422.

Cox GG, Rosenthal SJ, Holsapple JW. Exencephaly: sonographic findings and radiologic pathologic correlation. Radiology 1985;155:755–756.

Denath FM, Romano W, Solez M, Donnelly D. Ultrasonographic findings of exencephaly in pentalogy of Cantrell: case report and review of the literature. J Clin Ultrasound 1994;22:351–354.

Dziadek M. Preovulatory administration of clomiphene citrate to mice causes fetal growth restriction and neural tube defects (exencephaly) by an indirect maternal effect. Teratology 1993;47:263–273.

Hayashi M, Itoh H, Sodemoto T, Shinagawa T. Prenatal diagnosis of exencephaly associated with high levels of maternal serum human chorionic gonadotropin and urinary β-core fragment of hCG/creatinine ratio. Prenat Diagn 1994;14:1173–1177.

Hendricks SK, Cyr DR, Nyberg DA, Raabe R, Mack LA. Exencephaly—clinical and ultrasonic correlation to anencephaly. Obstet Gynecol 1988;72:898–901.

Hori A, Roessmann U, Eubel R, Ulbrich R, Dietrich-Schott B. Exencephaly in Cantrell-Haller-Ravitsch syndrome. Acta Neuropathol 1984;65:158–162.

Kennedy KA, Flick KJ, Thurmond AS. First trimester diagnosis of exencephaly. Am J Obstet Gynecol 1990;162: 461–463.

Lam YH, Tang MH, Ng LK. 13q⁻ in a fetus with ultrasonographic diagnosis of exencephaly in the first trimester. Prenat Diagn 1998;18:634–635.

Nishi T, Nakano R. First-trimester diagnosis of exencephaly by transvaginal ultrasonography. J Ultrasound Med 1994; 13:149–151.

Papp Z, Csecsei K, Toth Z, Polgar K, Szeifert GT. Exencephaly in human fetuses. Clin Genet 1986;30:440–444.

Sadler TW. Effects of maternal diabetes on early embryogenesis. II. Hyperglycemia-induced exencephaly. Teratology 1980;21:349–356.

Stagiannis KD, Sepulveda W, Fusi L, Garrett C, Fisk NM. Exencephaly in autosomal dominant brachydactyly syndrome. Prenat Diagn 1995;15:70–73.

Verloes A, Herens C, Van Maldergem L, Retz MC, Dodinval P. Roberts-SC phocomelia syndrome with exencephaly. Ann Génét 1989;32:169–170.

Wilkins-Haug L, Freedman W. Progression of exencephaly to anencephaly in the human fetus—an ultrasound perspective. Prenat Diagn 1991;11:227–233.

Wood LR, Smith MT. Generation of anencephaly: 1) aberrant neurulation; and 2) conversion of exencephaly to anencephaly. J Neuropathol Exp Neurol 1984;43:620–633.

CHAPTER 13

Holoprosencephaly

► CONDITION

The term holoprosencephaly describes a spectrum of cerebral and facial malformations that result from absent or incomplete division of the embryonic forebrain, the prosencephalon. The abnormality occurs during the third week of gestation (Müller and O'Rahilly 1989). Two separate sets of terms are used to describe the facial and brain anomalies. DeMyer (1964) proposed a subclassification of holoprosencephaly based on the extent of sagittal division of the cerebral cortex, thalamus, and hypothalamus. In the most severe form, alobar holoprosencephaly, midline structures are absent and there is no division of the hemispheres. A single common ventricle is present and the thalami are fused. In semilobar holoprosencephaly, incomplete division of the forebrain results in partial separation of the hemispheres. In lobar holoprosencephaly, there is normal cortical division and two thalami, but abnormalities exist in the corpus callosum, septum pellucidum, or olfactory tract or bulbs. The facial abnormalities accompanying holoprosencephaly range from subtle to grotesque (Fig. 13-1). In general, the more severe facial malformations are associated with alobar holoprosencephaly, but exceptions do occur (Table 13-1). The most severe facial malformation is cyclopia, a single or fused double eye and absent nasal structures (Figs. 13-1A and 13-1B). A proboscis, a cylindrical protuberance, may also be present (Fig. 13-1C). In ethmocephaly, the eyes are separate but closely placed (hypotelorism); a proboscis is present (Fig. 13-1D). Ethmocephaly is the rarest of the facial malformations seen in holoprosencephaly.

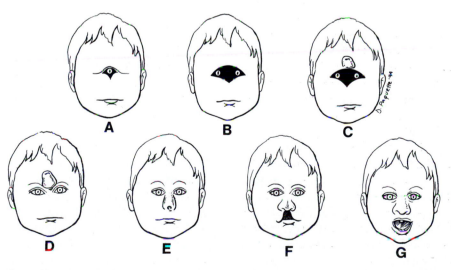

Figure 13-1. The spectrum of facial malformations that can accompany holoprosencephaly. See text for details.

▶ **TABLE 13-1.** RELATIONSHIP BETWEEN BRAIN AND FACIAL ABNORMALITIES SEEN IN HOLOPROSENCEPHALY (HP)

Brain	Face	Clinical Findings
Alobar HP	Cyclopia	Median single or fused eyes; may have no eye; proboscis present or absent
Alobar HP	Ethmocephaly	Rarest facial type; severe ocular hypotelorism with proboscis
Generally alobar HP	Cebocephaly	Ocular hypotelorism and blind-ended, single nostril nose
Generally alobar HP	Median cleft lip	Ocular hypotelorism, flat nose, median cleft lip
Semilobar or lobar HP	Mild dysmorphism	Spectrum of milder abnormalities, or normal, including ocular hypotelorism, flattened midface and nose, unilateral or bilateral cleft lip, iris coloboma, single central incisor

Source: Zeman W, Palmer CG. The face predicts the brain: the diagnostic significance of median facial anomalies for holoprosencephaly (arhinencephaly). Pediatrics 1964;34:256–263; Cohen MM Jr, Jirasek JE, Guzman RT, Gorlin RJ, Peterson MQ. Holoprosencephaly and facial dysmorphia: nosology, etiology and pathogenesis. Birth Defects 1971;7:125–135; Cohen MM. Perspectives on holoprosencephaly. Part I. Epidemiology, genetics, and syndromology. Teratology 1989a;40:211–235.

In cebocephaly, ocular hypotelorism is present along with a nasal structure that has a single nostril (Fig. 13-1E). In the milder forms of holoprosencephaly, ocular hypotelorism, flat nose, and a median cleft lip occur (Fig. 13-1F). Arrhinencephaly refers to the absence of the olfactory tracts and bulbs. Subtle, often missed forms of holoprosencephaly include mild hypotelorism, eye abnormalities (iris or retinal colobomas), mild midface hypoplasia, bifid uvula, and single central maxillary incisor tooth (Fig. 13-1G).

▶ **INCIDENCE**

The true incidence of holoprosencephaly is unknown, as presumably there is a high incidence of death in early embryonic life. In a study of 36,380 spontaneous abortions, Matsunaga and Shiota (1977) noted 150 embryos with holoprosencephaly. This equals a prevalence of 40 per 10,000. Using data from a population-based birth defects registry from California, Croen et al. (1996) identified 121 cases among a cohort of 1,035,386 live births and fetal deaths. This equaled a prevalence of 1.2 per 10,000 births. Of all cases, 41% (50 of 121) had a chromosomal abnormality, most commonly, trisomy 13. Among cases with normal chromosomes, increased risks were observed among Hispanic women. There is an excess of female conceptuses in alobar (3:1), as opposed to lobar (1:1) holoprosencephaly (Cohen 1989a). Prevalence is also increased in twins (Suslak et al. 1987). The only confirmed human teratogen is maternal diabetes, which increases the risk of holoprosencephaly 200-fold as compared with controls (Barr et al. 1983).

Other postulated teratogens include ethanol (Jellinger et al. 1981; Ronen and Andrews 1991), salicylate (Benawra et al. 1980), and cytomegalovirus (Byrne et al. 1987). Holoprosencephaly accounts for 16% of cases of fetal "hydrocephalus" diagnosed in utero (Nyberg et al. 1987).

▶ **SONOGRAPHIC FINDINGS**

In most fetuses, a midline echo is normally generated by the reflection of sound waves from acoustic interfaces at the interhemispheric fissure. This echo is absent in alobar holoprosencephaly (Fig. 13-2) (Pilu et al. 1987). In addition, in the standard transverse view of the fetal head obtained during measurement of the biparietal diameter (BPD), ventriculomegaly may be noted. The extent of thalamic fusion is best evaluated on a coronal scan (Figs. 13-3A and 13-3B). When a large cystic abnormality of the fetal head is detected, evaluation of the midline structures of the fetal face is recommended. Greene and colleagues (1987) have described the use of two sonographic criteria for the diagnosis of holoprosencephaly: intracranial abnormalities and structural abnormalities of the face. In any case of suspected holoprosencephaly, the bony orbits should be visualized (Fig. 13-4). Normal standards exist for the distance between orbits; this is important in the diagnosis of ocular hypotelorism (Mayden et al. 1982). Facial views will also demonstrate the presence of a proboscis (see Fig. 13-4). First-trimester holoprosencephaly has been diagnosed by transvaginal sonography (Bronshtein et al. 1991; Hamada et al. 1992;

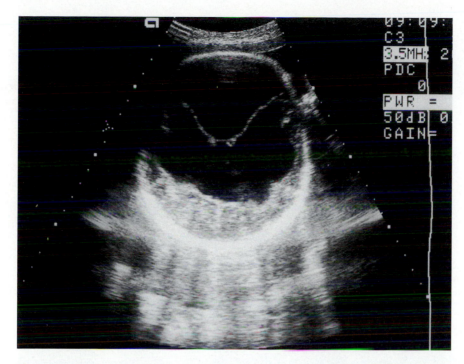

Figure 13-2. Coronal sonographic image demonstrating alobar holoprosencephaly. Note the complete absence of an interhemispheric fissure and the large cystic abnormality.

Stagiannis et al. 1995; Tongsong et al. 1999). Several studies have shown that extracranial abnormalities occur in approximately 50% of cases (Berry et al. 1990; McGahan et al. 1990). The most common anomalies are meningomyelocele, renal dysplasia, cardiac defects, and polydactyly.

▶ DIFFERENTIAL DIAGNOSIS

The main considerations in the differential diagnosis of holoprosencephaly include hydrocephalus, midline cerebral defects, such as septo-optic dysplasia, hydranencephaly, and porencephalic cysts. Holoprosencephaly may be distinguished from fetal hydrocephalus by demonstration of the absence of the midline echo and fusion of the thalami. Hydrocephalus due to aqueductal stenosis or an Arnold–Chiari malformation displays an intact falx cerebri, distinct and separate ventricles, and splayed thalami (Nyberg et al. 1987). In hydranencephaly, a thinned cerebral cortex may be noted. Finally, although both hydranencephaly and porencephalic cyst can demonstrate an absent or deviated falx, with these diagnoses, the thalami should be distinct (Nyberg et al. 1987). Holoprosencephaly can occur as an isolated finding or in combination with other anomalies in a single gene disorder, such as Smith–Lemli–Opitz syndrome (Peebles 1998).

▶ ANTENATAL NATURAL HISTORY

Holoprosencephaly is highly lethal during fetal life. It has been estimated that only 3% of holoprosencephalic conceptuses survive long enough to be considered a live birth (Cohen 1989b). In a retrospective study, 40% of cases were associated with vaginal bleeding and were considered threatened miscarriages (Berry et al. 1990). The perinatal mortality rate is on the order of 89% (McGahan et al. 1990). It is important to recognize, however, that some neonates do survive and leave the hospital with this condition.

▶ MANAGEMENT OF PREGNANCY

Holoprosencephaly is a profound fetal brain anomaly that cannot be altered or treated. Considerations for the subsequent management of the pregnancy include elective termination of pregnancy if the diagnosis is made earlier than 24 weeks, determining the cause of the holoprosencephaly, and planning the route of delivery. Because approximately 30 to 50% of fetuses with holoprosencephaly have chromosomal abnormalities, prenatal karyotype is recommended. A chromosomal abnormality is more likely to be present if extrafacial abnormalities are detected on sonography (Berry et al.

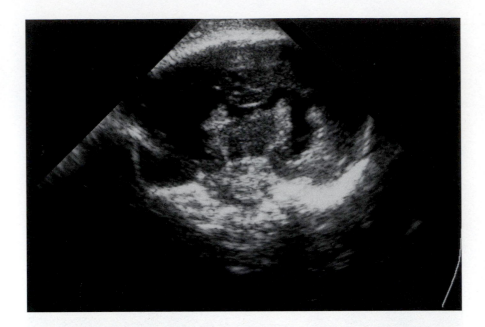

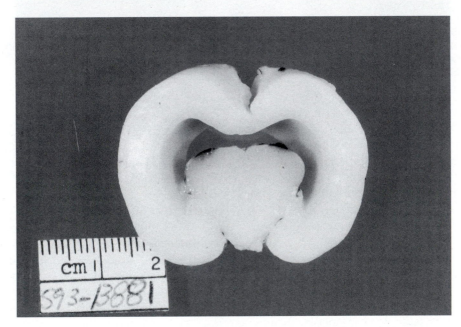

Figure 13-3. Top: Coronal sonographic image demonstrating thalamic fusion. Bottom: Corresponding pathologic specimen from a fetal brain, demonstrating a single ventricle and thalamic fusion. *(Photograph courtesy of Dr. Joseph Semple.)*

1990). The most common chromosomal abnormality is trisomy 13; a wide variety of other chromosomal abnormalities have also been described (Fig. 13-5) (Aronson et al. 1987; Estabrooks et al. 1990; Gillerot et al. 1987; Hamada et al. 1991; Hatziioannou et al. 1991; Helmuth et al. 1989; Isada et al. 1980; Kuchle et al. 1991; Lurie et al. 1990; Münke 1989, 1988; Petit et al. 1991; Urioste et al. 1988; Van Allen et al. 1993).

Since familial recurrences of holoprosencephaly have been reported, a family history should be obtained to elicit information on family members with mental retardation, microcephaly, cleft lip and/or cleft palate, eye abnormalities, flattening of the midface, or the presence of a single central incisor (Fig. 13-6) (Berry et al. 1984; Hattori et al. 1987). The mother should be asked whether she has a history of diabetes mellitus or was exposed to ethanol or salicylates. TORCH (toxoplasmosis, other agents, rubella, cytomegalovirus, herpes simplex) titers should be considered, given the reports that associate holoprosencephaly with cytomegalovirus.

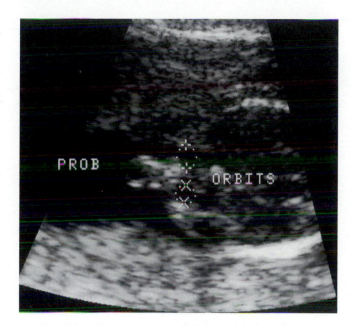

Figure 13-4. Sonographic image demonstrating hypotelorism and the presence of a proboscis.

Although sonography should adequately identify the presence of holoprosencephaly, magnetic resonance imaging (MRI) has been reported as an alternative to improve antenatal definition of the central nervous system (CNS) anatomy (Horvath et al. 1989; Toma et al. 1990).

Cesarean delivery should be considered only for maternal indications. Occasionally, macrocephaly due to ventriculomegaly may prevent vaginal delivery. In cases of alobar holoprosencephaly, cephalocentesis may facilitate a nonoperative delivery.

▶ **FETAL INTERVENTION**

There is no fetal intervention for this condition.

▶ **TREATMENT OF THE NEWBORN**

Infants with cyclopia, ethmocephaly, and cebocephaly do not survive the perinatal period. Given the expectations for severe mental retardation in infants who survive with alobar holoprosencephaly, aggressive resuscitation, including mechanical ventilation, is contraindicated. In the delivery room, the infant should be warmed and dried. A thorough physical examination is recommended to document the presence of associated anomalies. If a karyotype was not obtained prenatally, it should be at birth. Some infants will breathe and maintain their own temperature. Potential problems for

HOLOPROSENCEPHALY

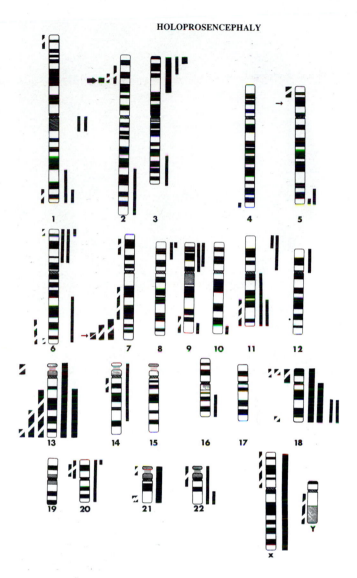

TRIPLOIDY

Figure 13-5. Genetic map demonstrating cytogenetic location of chromosomal abnormalities documented in patients with holoprosencephaly. The broken bars to the left of each chromosome identify the location of genes proposed to be involved in holoprosencephaly. *(Reprinted from Münke M. Clinical, cytogenetic, and molecular approaches to the genetic heterogeneity of holoprosencephaly. Am J Med Genet 1989;34:237–245. Copyright © 1989 John Wiley & Sons, Inc. Reprinted, by permission, of John Wiley & Sons, Inc.)*

the newborn include seizures, apnea, and feeding difficulties. If the parents are willing to take the infant home, they can be taught to feed the infant by gavage. Postnatal sonography of the neonatal head may help to further define anatomy and prognosis.

When prolonged survival is not expected, but the parents want to take the infant home, the following arrangements should be made prior to discharge: primary pediatric follow-up, autopsy, and organ donation (in accordance with parental wishes). In our experience, term infants with major anomalies such as holoprosencephaly are still considered candidates for donation of corneas and heart valves. The autopsy is critical for determining whether the holoprosencephaly was an isolated finding or part of a syndrome.

▶ LONG-TERM OUTCOME

Occasionally, patients with the milder forms of holoprosencephaly do survive and thrive (Fig. 13-7). At several months of age, a computed tomographic (CT) scan is recommended to redefine the extent of CNS malformation. An endocrine evaluation is also indicated to assess the hypothalamic/pituitary/thyroid/adrenal axis. Elias et al. (1992) have proposed a treatment plan for patients with the mildest forms of holoprosencephaly—those with normal brains but midline craniofacial defects centered around abnormalities of the ethmoid bone. They recommend a multidisciplinary evaluation that consists of physical examination, family history, psychometric testing, and CT scan. If mental development is normal, the patient is then considered a candidate for craniofacial reconstruction.

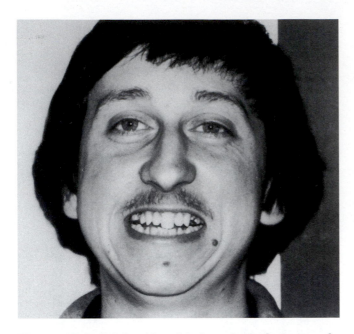

Figure 13-6. Adult with mild phenotypic features of holoprosencephaly, including a central incisor tooth and hypotelorism. These features may not be noticed in apparently normal individuals, yet they place the parent at high risk for offspring with more severe forms of holoprosencephaly. *(Reprinted from Johnson VP. Holoprosencephaly: a developmental field defect. Am J Med Genet 1989;34:258–264. Copyright © 1989 John Wiley & Sons, Inc. Reprinted, by permission, of John Wiley & Sons, Inc.)*

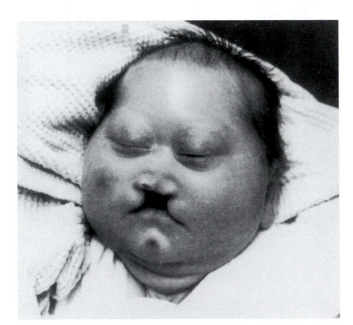 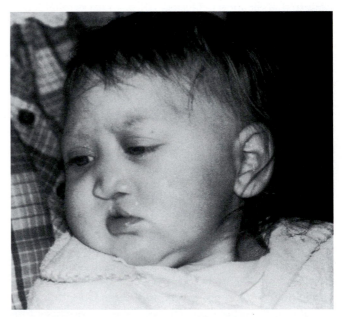

Figure 13-7. Postnatal photographs of surviving infants with milder forms of holoprosencephaly. (Left) Infant with severe hypotelorism, upslanting palpebral fissures, severe midface and nasal hypoplasia, and median cleft lip and palate. (Right) More mildly affected infant with midface hypoplasia, and a median cleft lip and palate that have been repaired. She is the daughter of the man shown in Figure 13-6. *(Reprinted from Johnson VP. Holoprosencephaly: a developmental field defect. Am J Med Genet 1989;34:258–264. Copyright © 1989 John Wiley & Sons, Inc. Reprinted, by permission, of John Wiley & Sons, Inc.)*

▶ **TABLE 13-2.** HOLOPROSENCEPHALY (HPE) GENES

Gene	Map Location	Linked Loci
HPE 1	21q 22.3	Down syndrome critical region
HPE 2/SIX 3	2p 21	Human homeobox
HPE 3/SHH	7q 36	Engrailed-2
		Limb deformity
HPE 4	18p 11.3	Bipolar affective disorder
		Multiple cutaneous leiomyomata
HPE 5/ZIC 2	13q32	Drosophila forkhead homologue
		Caudal-type homeobox transcription factor

Adapted, with permission, from Dean M. Polarity, proliferation and hedgehog pathway. Nat Genet 1996;14: 245–247.

▶ GENETICS AND RECURRENCE RISK

Holoprosencephaly due to sporadic, nonchromosomal, nonsyndromic reasons carries an empiric recurrence risk of 6% (Roach et al. 1975). In a 20-year review of cases from Western Scotland, Whiteford and Tolmie (1996) suggested that holoprosencephaly does not necessarily breed true, and that affected families had a 12% recurrence risk for serious neurologic disability. If a chromosomal abnormality is detected, the recurrence risk may be approximately 1% (in the case of trisomy 13 or 18) or higher (if a balanced translocation was found in a parent). In women with diabetes mellitus, the recurrence risk is 1% (Barr et al. 1983). A careful search must be made for relatives with the subtle findings of holoprosencephaly. The autosomal dominant form is notable for variation in the phenotype (see Figs. 13-6, 13-7A, and 13-7B). Penetrance of the gene is on the order of 30% (Collins et al. 1993). In addition, DeMyer et al. (1963) described an autosomal recessive pattern of inheritance for holoprosencephaly.

Much progress has occurred recently in the molecular understanding of the development of holoprosencephaly (Münke et al. 1989). At least five different genes have been identified that are involved in the development of holoprosencephaly (Table 13-2) (Dean 1996). The human sonic hedgehog gene (SHH) has been shown to be the same as the holoprosencephaly 3 (HPE 3) gene located on chromosome 7q 36 (Belloni et al. 1996; Roessler et al. 1996). SHH is a segment polarity gene that plays a role in development of the notochord, somites, and limbs (Dean 1996). In humans, loss of one SHH allele is sufficient to cause holoprosencephaly (Roessler et al. 1996, 1997).

Results of a complete DNA analysis of the SHH gene in 344 unrelated cases of holoprosencephaly has identified 23 different mutations (Nanni et al. 1999). These include nonsense and missense mutations, deletions, and an insertion. No genotype-phenotype correlation is apparent based upon this mutational analysis. Furthermore, Smith–Lemli–Opitz syndrome, a recessively inherited disorder of cholesterol biosynthesis, is associated with holoprosencephaly. Low cholesterol levels lead to abnormal or incomplete modification of the SHH protein. Other genes involved in the etiology of holoprosencephaly include SIX3, the HPE2 locus on human chromosome 2p21. This homeobox gene contains information that is essential for the development of the anterior neural plate and eye in humans (Wallis et al. 1999). ZIC2, a human homologue of the Drosophila odd-paired gene, maps to chromosome 13q32. Heterozygous mutations in ZIC2 are associated with holoprosencephaly (Brown et al. 1998).

Many additional genes important in forebrain development are currently being cloned and studied in vertebrate model organisms (Wallis and Muenke 1999). It is believed that as many as 12 genetic loci are associated with the development of holoprosencephaly (Wallis et al. 1999). This is clearly an evolving area. Table 13-3 summarizes our recommendations for post-delivery assessment of a fetus or infant with holoprosencephaly. Given the rapid progress in human genetic and developmental research, we recommend obtaining a skin biopsy or placental material to establish a fibroblast cell line for future DNA studies. Finally, in all cases of holoprosencephaly, it is essential to hold a follow-up meeting with the parents after delivery or termination to review all pathologic studies and to summarize the understanding of the cause, genetics, and recurrence risk.

▶ **TABLE 13-3.** POST-DELIVERY ASSESSMENT OF A FETUS/INFANT WITH HOLOPROSENCEPHALY

Rule out chromosomal abnormality with high resolution banding
Obtain a detailed family history
Examine the proband's family to rule out subtle abnormalities
Obtain an autopsy
Bank DNA for future genetic studies
Hold follow-up meeting to summarize results of above studies

REFERENCES

Aronson DC, Jansweijer MC, Hoovers JM, Barth PG. A male infant with holoprosencephaly, associated with ring chromosome 21. Clin Genet 1987;31:48–52.

Barr M Jr, Hanson JW, Currey K, et al. Holoprosencephaly in infants of diabetic mothers. J Pediatr 1983;102:565–568.

Belloni E, Muenke M, Roessler E, et al. Identification of Sonic hedgehog as a candidate gene responsible for holoprosencephaly. Nat Genet 1996;14:353–356.

Benawra R, Mangurten HH, Duffell DR. Cyclopia and other anomalies following maternal ingestion of salicylates. J Pediatr 1980;96:1069.

Berry SA, Pierpont ME, Gorlin RJ. Single central incisor in familial holoprosencephaly. J Pediatr 1984;104:877–879.

Berry SM, Gosden C, Snijders RJ, Nicolaides KH. Fetal holoprosencephaly: associated malformation and chromosomal defects. Fetal Diagn Ther 1990;5:92–99.

Bronshtein M, Wiener Z. Early transvaginal sonographic diagnosis of alobar holoprosencephaly. Prenat Diagn 1991;11:459–462.

Brown SA, Warburton D, Brown LY, et al. Holoprosencephaly due to mutations in ZIC2, a homologue of Drosophila odd-paired. Nat Genet 1998;20:180–183.

Byrne PK, Siliver MM, Gilbert JM, Cadera W, Tanswell AK. Cyclopia and congenital cytomegalovirus infection. Am J Med Genet 1987;28:61–65.

Cohen MM. Perspectives on holoprosencephaly. Part I. Epidemiology, genetics, and syndromology. Teratology 1989a;40:211–235.

Cohen MM. Perspectives on holoprosencephaly. Part III. Spectra, distinctions, continuities, and discontinuities. Am J Med Genet 1989b;34:271–288.

Cohen MM Jr, Jirasek JE, Guzman RT, Gorlin RJ, Peterson MQ. Holoprosencephaly and facial dysmorphia: nosology, etiology and pathogenesis. Birth Defects 1971;7:125–135.

Collins AL, Lunt PW, Garrett C, Dennis NR. Holoprosencephaly: a family showing dominant inheritance and variable expression. J Med Genet 1993;30:36–40.

Croen LA, Shaw GM, Lammer EJ. Holoprosencephaly: epidemiologic and clinical characteristics of a California population. Am J Med Genet 1996;64:465–472.

Dean M. Polarity, proliferation and hedgehog pathway. Nat Genet 1996;14:245–247.

DeMyer WE, Zeman W, Palmer CG. Familial alobar holoprosencephaly (arhinencephaly) with median cleft lip and palate: report of patient with 46 chromosomes. Neurology 1963;13:913–991.

DeMyer W, Zeman W, Palmer CG. The face predicts the brain: diagnostic significance of median facial anomalies for holoprosencephaly (arhinencephaly). Pediatrics 1964; 34:256–263.

Elias DL, Kawamoto HK, Wilson LF. Holoprosencephaly and midline facial anomalies: redefining classification and management. Plast Reconstr Surg 1992;90:951–958.

Estabrooks LL, Rao KW, Donahue RP, Aylsworth AS. Holoprosencephaly in an infant with a minute deletion of chromosome 21(q22.3). Am J Med Genet 1990;36:306–309.

Gillerot Y, Hustin J, Koulischer L, Viteux V. Prenatal diagnosis of a dup(3p) with holoprosencephaly. Am J Med Genet 1987;26:225–227.

Greene MF, Benacerraf BR, Frigoletto FD. Reliable criteria for the prenatal sonographic diagnosis of alobar holoprosencephaly. Am J Obstet Gynecol 1987;156:687–689.

Hamada H, Arinami T, Koresawa M, Kubo T, Hamaguchi H, Iwasaki H. A case of trisomy 21 with holoprosencephaly: the fifth case. Jinrui Idengaku Zasshi 1991;36:159–163.

Hamada H, Oki A, Tsunoda H, Kubo T. Prenatal diagnosis of holoprosencephaly by transvaginal ultrasonography in the first trimester. Asia Oceania J Obstet Gynaecol 1992; 18:125–129.

Hattori H, Okuno T, Momoi R, Kataoka K, Mikawa H, Shiota K. Single central maxillary incisor and holoprosencephaly. Am J Med Genet 1987;28:483–487.

Hatziioannou AG, Krauss CM, Lewis MB, Halazonetis TD. Familial holoprosencephaly associated with a translocation breakpoint at chromosomal position 7q36. Am J Med Genet 1991;40:201–205.

Helmuth RA, Weaver DD, Wills ER. Holoprosencephaly, ear abnormalities, congenital heart defect, and microphallus in a patient with 11q- mosaicism. Am J Med Genet 1989; 32:178–181.

Horvath L, Seeds JW. Temporary arrest of fetal movement with pancuronium bromide to enable antenatal magnetic resonance imaging of holoprosencephaly. Am J Perinatol 1989;6:418–420.

Isada NB, Bolan JC, Larsen JW, Kent SG. Trisomy 22 with holoprosencephaly: a clinicopathologic study. Teratology 1990;42:333–336.

Jellinger K, Gross H, Kaltenback E. Holoprosencephaly and agenesis of the corpus callosum: frequency of associated malformations. Acta Neuropathol (Berl) 1981;55:1–10.

Johnson VP. Holoprosencephaly: a developmental field defect. Am J Med Genet 1989;34:258–264.

Kuchle M, Kraus J, Rummelt C, Naumann GO. Synophthalmia and holoprosencephaly in chromosome 18p deletion defect. Arch Ophthalmol 1991;109:136–137.

Lurie IW, Ilyina HG, Podleschuk LV, Gorelik LB, Zaletajev DV. Chromosome 7 abnormalities in parents of children with holoprosencephaly and hydronephrosis. Am J Med Genet 1990;35:286–288.

Matsunaga E, Shiota K. Holoprosencephaly in human embryos: epidemiologic studies of 150 cases. Teratology 1977;16:261–272.

Mayden KC, Tortora M, Berkowitz RL, Bracken M, Hobbins JC. Orbital diameters: a new parameter for prenatal diagnosis and dating. Am J Obstet Gynecol 1982;144:289–297.

McGahan JP, Nyberg DA, Mack LA. Sonography of facial features of alobar and semilobar holoprosencephaly. AJR Am J Roentgenol 1990;154:143–148.

Müller F, O'Rahilly R. Mediobasal prosencephalic defects, including holoprosencephaly and cyclopia, in relation to the development of the human forebrain. Am J Anat 1989;185:391–414.

Münke M. Clinical, cytogenetic, and molecular approaches to the genetic heterogeneity of holoprosencephaly. Am J Med Genet 1989;34:237–245.

Münke M, Emanuel BS, Zackai EH. Holoprosencephaly: association with interstitial deletion of 2p and review of the cytogenetic literature. Am J Med Genet 1988;30:929–938.

Nanni L, Ming JE, Bocian M, et al. The mutational spectrum of the sonic hedgehog gene in holoprosencephaly: SHH mutations cause a significant proportion of autosomal dominant holoprosencephaly. Hum Mol Genet 1998: 2479–2488.

Nyberg DA, Mack LA, Bronstein A, Hirsch J, Pagon RA. Holoprosencephaly: prenatal sonographic diagnosis. AJR Am J Roentgenol 1987;149:1051–1058.

Peebles DM, Holoprosencephaly. Prenat Diagn 1998;18: 477–480.

Petit P, Moerman P, Fryns JP. Lobar holoprosencephaly and Xq22 deletion. Genet Couns 1991;2:119–121.

Pilu G, Romero R, Rizzo N, Jeanty P, Bovicelli L, Hobbins JC. Criteria for the prenatal diagnosis of holoprosencephaly. Am J Perinatol 1987;4:41–49.

Roach EW, DeMyer K, Palmer M, Connelly A, Merrit A. Holoprosencephaly: birth data, genetic and demographic analysis of 30 families. Birth Defects 1975;11:294–313.

Roessler E, Belloni E, Gaudenz K, et al. Mutations in the human Sonic Hedgehog gene cause holoprosencephaly. Nature Genet 1996;14:357–360.

Roessler E, Ward DE, Gaudenz K, et al. Cytogenetic rearrangements involving the loss of the Sonic Hedgehog gene at 7q36 cause holoprosencephaly. Hum Genet 1997; 100:172–181.

Ronen GM, Andrews WL. Holoprosencephaly as a possible embryonic alcohol effect. Am J Med Genet 1991;40: 151–154.

Stagiannis KD, Sepulveda W, Bower S. Early prenatal diagnosis of holoprosencephaly: the value of transvaginal ultrasonography. Eur J Obstet Gynecol Reprod 1995;61: 175–176.

Suslak L, Mimms GM, Desposito F. Monozygosity and holoprosencephaly: cleavage disorders of the "midline field." Am J Med Genet 1987;28:99–102.

Toma P, Costa A, Magnano GM, Cariati M, Lituania M. Holoprosencephaly: prenatal diagnosis by sonography and magnetic resonance imaging. Prenat Diagn 1990;10: 429–436.

Tongsong T, Wanapirak, C, Chanprapaph P, Siriangkul S. First trimester sonographic diagnosis of holoprosencephaly. Int J Gynaecol Obstet 1999;66:165–169.

Urioste M, Valcarcel E, Gomez MA, et al. Holoprosencephaly and trisomy 21 in a child born to a nondiabetic mother. Am J Med Genet 1988;30:925–928.

Van Allen MI, Ritchie S, Toi A, Fong K, Winsor E. Trisomy 4 in a fetus with cyclopia and other anomalies. Am J Med Genet 1993;46:193–197.

Wallis DE, Muenke M. Molecular mechanisms of holoprosencephaly. Mol Genet Metab 1999;68:126–138.

Wallis DE, Roessler E, Hehr U, et al. Mutations in the homeodomain of the human SIX3 gene cause holoprosencephaly. Nat Genet 1999;22:196–198.

Whiteford ML, Tolmie JL. Holoprosencephaly in the west of Scotland 1975–1994. J Med Genet 1996;33:578–584.

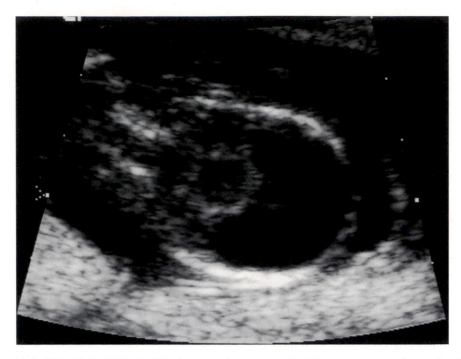

Figure 14-1. Prenatal sonographic image demonstrating the absence of cerebral cortex and presence of a large fluid-filled mass.

(Romero et al. 1988). The falx is usually present but may be partially or completely absent. Macrocephaly is usually present and is attributed to continuing production of cerebrospinal fluid by the choroid plexus (Greene et al. 1985; Raybaud 1983). Polyhydramnios can be a common associated finding (Fleischer and Brown 1977).

The sonographic appearance of hydranencephaly may sometimes be difficult, because visualization of a completely anechoic cystic mass is dependent on the timing of sonography in relation to the vascular insult. The diagnosis of hydranencephaly may not be clear when the infarction and hemorrhage form an evolving process. Recent hemorrhage appears echogenic, and as a clot lyses it assumes the characteristic anechoic appearance of hydranencephaly (Edmondson et al. 1992; Greene et al. 1985). Serial sonography may therefore be necessary to confirm the diagnosis, as hydranencephaly is an evolving process.

▶ DIFFERENTIAL DIAGNOSIS

The most common differential diagnoses that should be considered include extreme hydrocephalus, porencephaly, and lobar holoprosencephaly. When hydrocephalus is extreme the cerebral cortex may be very thin and closely applied to the cranium, thereby making it difficult to differentiate from cases of hydranencephaly with preserved falx. The presence of even minimal cerebral cortex indicates extreme hydrocephalus

rather than hydranencephaly. In addition, hydranencephaly usually demonstrates a pronounced bulging of the brain stem into the cystic cavity, while in extreme hydrocephalus the presence of residual cortical matter prevents this characteristic appearance (Romero et al. 1988). Magnetic resonance imaging (MRI) has been reported as a complementary technique for the definitive intrauterine diagnosis of hydranencephaly (Vila-Coro and Dominguez 1989).

Porencephaly may be differentiated from hydranencephaly by the asymmetric appearance of porencephalic cysts, although complete differentiation of the two conditions can be difficult because they may represent a continuum (Sanders et al. 1996). Features that help differentiate lobar holoprosencephaly from hydranencephaly include absence of the falx and midline structures, absence of the third ventricle, fusion of the thalami, and preservation of some cortical tissue in holoprosencephaly. Furthermore, facial anomalies and additional central nervous system anomalies are usually present with alobar holoprosencephaly. A list of the conditions that have been associated with hydranencephaly is given in Table 14-1.

▶ ANTENATAL NATURAL HISTORY

Little is known about the antenatal natural history of hydranencephaly. In one reported case, the initial sonographic evaluation was normal at 18 weeks gestation. Follow-up ultrasound examination at 25 weeks revealed

► **TABLE 14-1.** REPORTED ASSOCIATIONS WITH HYDRANENCEPHALY

Infections
  Cytomegalovirus (Kubo et al. 1994)
  Herpes simplex (Christie et al. 1986; Hutto et al. 1987)
  Rubella (Deshmukh et al. 1993)
  Toxoplasmosis (Altshuler 1973; Plantaz et al. 1987)
Chromosomal Abnormalities
  Trisomy 13 (Dixon 1988)
Neoplasms
  Congenital rhabdoid tumor of the brain (Velasco et al. 1993)
Bleeding disorders
  Factor XIII deficiency (Takada et al. 1989)
Syndromes associated with hydranencephaly
  Agnathia malformation complex (Persutte et al. 1990)
  Hypoplastic thumbs (Norman and Donnai 1992)
  Renal dysplasia (Bendon et al. 1987; Gschwendtner et al. 1997)
  Polyvalvular heart defect (Bendon et al. 1987)
  Lethal multiple pterygium syndrome (Mbakop et al. 1986)

sonographic evidence of hydranencephaly (Sanders 1996). Other case reports document the intrauterine diagnosis of massive intracranial hemorrhage at 27 and 30 weeks of gestation, with subsequent development of hydranencephaly over a period of weeks (Edmondson et al. 1992; Greene et al. 1985). These findings confirm the theory that hydranencephaly represents an evolving intrauterine process that may be secondary to a profound vascular insult.

► **MANAGEMENT OF PREGNANCY**

An accurate prenatal diagnosis is necessary for appropriate management decisions. It is particularly important to make the distinction between hydranencephaly and extreme hydrocephalus. If there is any doubt left after sonographic examination, MRI of the fetus should be performed, especially if consideration is given to therapeutic action such as cephalocentesis or termination (Vila-Coro and Dominguez 1989). Serology and/or cultures for toxoplasmosis, cytomegalovirus, rubella, and herpes should also be performed. If there is any sonographic suspicion of other abnormalities, fetal karyotyping should be offered.

Termination of pregnancy as late as the third trimester may be justified in light of a reliable prenatal diagnosis of hydranencephaly. The criteria for third-trimester termination include the availability of reliable diagnostic tests that can accurately predict a condition that is either incompatible with postnatal life or characterized by the absence of cognitive function (Chervenak et al. 1984).

Vaginal delivery is preferred. Inasmuch as macrocephaly is commonly associated with hydranencephaly, cephalocentesis may be necessary to allow successful vaginal delivery (Greene et al. 1985). Serial ultrasound examinations should be performed during the pregnancy to evaluate for the development of macrocephaly. Cephalocentesis is performed by inserting an 18- or 20-gauge spinal needle into the fetal head under ultrasound guidance and aspirating cerebrospinal fluid. The fluid removed is usually dark brown (Greene et al. 1985). If the fluid obtained is not dark brown, it should prompt analysis for protein concentration because in hydranencephaly a highly proteinaceous fluid is suggestive of an intracranial neoplasm (Velasco et al. 1993).

If there is any doubt about the diagnosis, delivery is optimally performed in a setting where qualified subspecialists are available for resuscitation and syndrome diagnosis. If there is no doubt regarding the diagnosis, there is no advantage to delivery in a tertiary-care setting. Fetal monitoring is not indicated. If fetal monitoring is performed and the results are not reassuring, cesarean delivery is not recommended.

► **FETAL INTERVENTION**

No fetal interventions have been described following the prenatal diagnosis of hydranencephaly.

► **TREATMENT OF THE NEWBORN**

The neonate with hydranencephaly usually presents with macrocephaly and frequent seizures, although the diagnosis may be delayed for several months because of relatively appropriate early behavior. In one series of 22 patients, the average age at diagnosis was 12 weeks, with a range of 1 day to 10.5 months (Herman et al. 1988). Common presenting symptoms include increasing head size, psychomotor retardation, and increasing spasticity. Most patients have ophthalmic abnormalities involving optic-nerve abnormalities, strabismus, and inferior displacement of the globe (the "setting sun" sign). Transillumination of the skull was the traditional method of postnatal diagnosis of hydranencephaly. However, transillumination of the skull may also be seen with extreme hydrocephalus. Computed tomographic (CT) scanning is helpful in distinguishing hydranencephaly from extreme hydrocephalus and may demonstrate maximal preservation of the frontal cortex and a normal cerebral vascular architecture in hydrocephalus (Herman et al. 1988). MRI is the most definitive imaging technique for the diagnosis of hydranencephaly (Hanigan and Aldrich 1988).

Electrophysiologic studies, specifically electroencephalography (EEG) and visual evoked responses, may also be helpful in distinguishing extreme hydrocephalus from hydranencephaly (Iinuma et al. 1989). The EEG in hydranencephaly is typically flat, and visual evoked potentials show no response. By contrast, in neonates with extreme hydrocephalus there is some EEG activity and normal visual evoked potentials (Herman et al. 1988; Iinuma et al. 1989). Auditory evoked potentials in hydranencephaly show an absent middle latency response, while somatic evoked potentials show an absent cortical response (Hanigan and Aldrich 1988). If prenatal testing was not performed for cytomegalovirus, toxoplasmosis, rubella, and herpes infections, then appropriate serologic and microbiologic studies should be done during the newborn period.

▶ SURGICAL TREATMENT

Unlike extreme hydrocephalus, in hydranencephaly shunting procedures are not indicated. Sutton and associates (1980) followed neonates with hydranencephaly with serial CT, EEG, and developmental evaluations for 4 to 23 months. No improvement was demonstrated in these five infants by radiologic or neurologic criteria despite aggressive surgical treatment and shunt placement. In contrast, five infants with extreme hydrocephalus treated during the same period improved dramatically after shunt placement (Sutton et al. 1980). In cases of unilateral hydranencephaly, shunting to prevent increasing compromise of the uninvolved side is indicated and has demonstrated favorable results (van Doornik and Hennekam 1992). No other surgical interventions are recommended for hydranencephaly.

▶ LONG-TERM OUTCOME

The outcome for children with complete hydranencephaly is universally poor. There is no specific treatment, and active medical intervention is not indicated. Almost half of infants with hydranencephaly die within 1 month, and fewer than 15% survive 1 year (Dixon 1985). In a series of 22 patients, only 3 were alive at ages 9, 12, and 17 years, and all 3 required constant custodial care (Herman et al. 1988).

In contrast, the prognosis for unilateral hydranencephaly is more favorable. Of the six patients described in the literature, four demonstrated only mild developmental delay (van Doornik and Hennekam 1992). No data were provided for one patient. Another patient had multiple congenital defects combined with hemihydranencephaly and severe retardation (van Doornik and Hennekam 1992).

▶ GENETICS AND RECURRENCE RISK

Hydranencephaly is usually the result of a destructive process in a previously normally formed brain rather than a primary malformation. There has been a reported association with trisomy 13 (Dixon 1988). Therefore, for most cases there will be no recurrence risk. Familial cases are extremely rare, and such families should be offered prenatal diagnosis with ultrasound examination in a subsequent pregnancy.

REFERENCES

Altshuler G. Toxoplasmosis as a cause of hydranencephaly. Am J Dis Child 1973;125:251–252.

Bendon RW, Siddiqi T, de Courten-Myers G, et al. Recurrent developmental anomalies. 1. Syndrome of hydranencephaly with renal aplastic dysplasia; 2. Polyvalvular developmental heart defect. Am J Med Genet Suppl 1987;3:357–365.

Chervenak F, Farley MA, Walters L, et al. When is termination of pregnancy during the third trimester morally justifiable? N Engl J Med 1984;310:501–504.

Christie JD, Rakusan TA, Martinez MA, et al. Hydranencephaly caused by congenital infection with herpes simplex virus. Pediatr Infect Dis 1986;5:473–478.

Deshmukh CT, Nadkarni UB, Nair K, et al. Hydranencephaly/multicystic encephalomalacia: association with congenital rubella infection. Indian Pediatr 1993;30:253–257.

Dixon A: Hydranencephaly. Radiography 1988;54:12–13.

Edmondson SR, Hallak M, Carpenter, et al. Evolution of hydranencephaly following intracranial hemorrhage. Obstet Gynecol 1992;75:870–871.

Fleischer A, Brown M. Hydramnios associated with fetal hydranencephaly. J Clin Ultrasound 1977;5:41–43.

Greene MF, Benacerraf B, Crawford JM. Hydranencephaly: US appearance during in utero evolution. Radiology 1985;156:779–780.

Gschwendtner A, Mairinger T, Soelder E, et al. Hydranencephaly with renal dysgenesis: a coincidental finding? Case report with review of the literature. Gynecol Obstet Invest 1997;44:206–210.

Hamby WB, Krauss RF, Beswick WF. Hydranencephaly: clinical diagnosis. Pediatrics 1950;6:371–383.

Hanigan WC, Aldrich WM. MRI and evoked potentials in a child with hydranencephaly. Pediatr Neurol 1988;4:185–187.

Herman DC, Bartley GB, Bullock JD. Ophthalmic findings of hydranencephaly. J Pediatr Ophthalmol Strabismus 1988;25:106–111.

Hutto C, Arvin A, Jacobs R, et al. Intrauterine herpes simplex infections. J Pediatr 1987;110:97–101.

Iinuma K, Handa I, Kojima A, et al. Hydranencephaly and maximal hydrocephalus: usefulness of electrophysiological studies for their differentiation. J Child Neurol 1989;4:114–117.

Kubo S, Kishino T, Satake N, et al. A neonatal case of hydranencephaly caused by atheromatous plaque obstruction of aortic arch: possible association with a congenital cytomegalovirus infection? J Perinatol 1994;14:483–486.

Lin YS, Chang FM, Liu CH. Antenatal detection of hydranencephaly at 12 weeks menstrual age. J Clin Ultrasound 1992;20:62–64.

Mbakop A, Cox JN, Stormann C, et al. Lethal multiple pterygium syndrome: report of a new case with hydranencephaly. Am J Med Genet 1986;25:575–579.

Moser RP, Seljeskog EL. Unilateral hydranencephaly: case report. Neurosurgery 1981;9:703–705.

Muir CS. Hydranencephaly and allied disorders. Arch Dis Child 1959;34:231–246.

Myers RE. Brain pathology following fetal vascular occlusion: an experimental study. Invest Ophthalmol 1969;8:41–50.

Najafzadeh TM, Reinisch L, Dumars KW. Etiologic heterogeneity in hydranencephaly. Birth Defects: Original Article Series 1982;18:229–235.

Norman AM, Donnai D. Hypoplastic thumbs and hydranencephaly: a new syndrome? Clin Dysmorphol 1992;1:121–123.

Ohtsuka H. A rare patient with a false median cleft lip associated with multiple congenital anomalies. Ann Plast Surg 1986;17:155–160.

Persutte WH, Yeasting RA, Kurczynski TW, et al. Agnathia malformation complex associated with a cystic distention of the oral cavity and hydranencephaly. J Craniofac Genet Dev Biol 1990;10:391–397.

Plantaz D, Joannard A, Pasquier B, et al. Hydranencéphalie et toxoplasmose congénitale: a propos de quatre observations. Pédiatrie 1987;42:161–165.

Raybaud C. Destructive lesions of the brain. Neuroradiology 1983;25:265–291.

Regec SP, Bernstine RL. Hydranencephaly in a twin gestation. Obstet Gynecol 197954:369–371.

Romero R, Pilu G, Jeanty P, et al. Hydranencephaly. In: Romero R, Pilu G, Jeanty P, Ghidini A, Hobbins JC, eds. Prenatal diagnosis of congenital anomalies. East Norwalk, CT: Appleton and Lange 1988:52–54.

Sanders RC, Blackmon LR, Hogge WA, et al. Hydranencephaly. In: Sanders RC, Blackmon LR, Hogge WA, Wulfsberg EZ, eds. Structural fetal abnormalities: the total picture. St. Louis: Mosby 1996:37–38.

Sutton LN, Bruce DA, Schut L. Hydranencephaly versus maximal hydrocephalus: an important clinical distinction. Neurosurgery 1980;6:34–38.

Suzuki M, Seki H, Yoshimoto T. Unilateral hydrocephalus combined with occlusion of the ipsilateral internal carotid artery. Surg Neurol 1985;24:27–30.

Takada K, Shiota M, Ando M, et al. Porencephaly and hydranencephaly: a neuropathological study of four autopsy cases. Brain Dev 1989;11:51–56.

van Doornik MC, Hennekam RC. Hemi-hydranencephaly with favourable outcome. Dev Med Child Neurol 1992;34:454–458.

Velasco ME, Brown JA, Kini J, et al. Primary congenital rhabdoid tumor of the brain with neoplastic hydranencephaly. Child Nerv Syst 1993;9:185–190.

Vila-Coro AA, Dominguez R. Intrauterine diagnosis of hydranencephaly by magnetic resonance. Magn Reson Imaging 1989;7:105–107.

Warkany I. Congenital malformations: notes and comments. Chicago: Year Book 1971:231–233.

CHAPTER 15

Hydrocephalus

► CONDITION

Hydrocephalus is a pathologic increase in intracranial cerebrospinal fluid (CSF) volume, whether intraparenchymal or extraparenchymal, independent of hydrostatic or barometric pressure (Raimondi 1994). This may result from either fluid production that exceeds absorption or primary atrophy of the cerebral parenchyma. Most cases are due to mechanical obstruction to the flow of CSF at some level (DeLange 1977). The site of obstruction may be inside the ventricular system (noncommunicating or internal hydrocephalus) or outside the ventricles (communicating or external hydrocephalus) (Pilu 1986). Aqueductal stenosis comprises one-third of the cases of hydrocephalus in postnatal series; it is less common in prenatal studies. The aqueduct of Sylvius is the narrowest portion of the spaces through which the CSF flows (Raimondi 1994). *Ventriculomegaly* is a descriptive term of a pathologic process that has many causes. It may occur due to obstruction of CSF flow, or as a consequence of maldevelopment of the ventricle in anomalies such as agenesis of the corpus callosum (colpocephaly) or as an ex vacuo (destructive) phenomenon secondary to cerebral atrophy (Cardoza et al. 1988a). Ventriculomegaly is an indicator of underlying central nervous system (CNS) anomalies. It may also be the first sign of associated extra-CNS anomalies.

The existence of hydrocephalus has been known since ancient times. Hippocrates knew that accumulation of water within the head caused it to enlarge, but the physiology of hydrocephalus was not understood at that time. It was not until the 16th century that Vesalius demonstrated that the water was accumulating within the ventricles (Hirsch 1994). The hereditary nature of hydrocephalus was first appreciated by Bickers and Adams in 1949. In hereditary stenosis of the aqueduct

of Sylvius, an X-linked condition, the range of severity of hydrocephalus is wide; it ranges from minimal involvement to gross hydrocephalus that results in prenatal or perinatal death (Willems et al. 1990).

► INCIDENCE

The incidence of isolated fetal ventriculomegaly is 0.64 per 1000 pregnancies. (Wilson et al. 1989). Wiswell et al. (1990) performed a retrospective analysis of all live-born and stillborn infants in U.S. Army hospitals between 1971 and 1987. All fetuses and infants were included if they achieved more than 20 weeks of gestation. Of 763,364 pregnancies studied, 370 had hydrocephalus. This equaled an incidence of 0.48 per 1000 total births, or one per 2063 total births. Of the infants with hydrocephalus, 37% had additional anomalies unrelated to the primary defect. No significant racial differences were seen, but an increased incidence of affected males was noted (64% male, 36% were female). A predominance of males is consistently observed in all studies of hydrocephalus due to the inherited X-linked forms of the abnormality.

► SONOGRAPHIC FINDINGS

The diagnostic impression of hydrocephalus is usually qualitative due to the fact that the sonographic appearance of enlarged ventricles is striking (Fig. 15-1). It is important to note that the fetal biparietal diameter may not be increased when the ventricles are definitely dilated. The lateral ventricles can be visualized as early as 12 weeks of gestation. Early in the second trimester, the choroid plexus is very echogenic and large relative to the volume of the cerebral hemispheres. The choroid

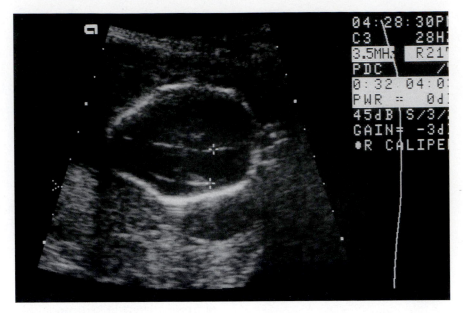

Figure 15-1. Axial sonographic image of a fetal head with hydrocephalus.

plexus normally fills the entire lateral ventricle posterior to the foramen of Monro. This tends to obscure the lateral ventricular wall to which it is closely applied (Fadel 1989). This, together with the hypoechoic brain mantle, may falsely be interpreted as dilated ventricles filled with CSF. In second-trimester fetuses with hydrocephalus, the first recognizable abnormality is generally the relative shrinkage of the normally prominent choroid plexus (Fadel 1989).

Several different methods have been proposed by different authors to quantitatively evaluate increased CSF. These methods include measurement of the ratio of the lateral ventricular width (LVW) to the hemispheric width (HW) or measurement of the ventricular atria. The LVW:HW ratio is not sensitive in early pregnancy. The first measurement of lateral ventricular dilation is the displacement of the medial wall of the lateral ventricle toward the midline. This does not change the LVW:HW ratio (Fadel 1989). Furthermore, the echo-genic outer lines originally thought to represent the lateral walls of the lateral ventricle in an axial scan of the fetal head have been shown by Hertzberg et al. (1987) to originate from deep cerebral veins. These reflections from small venous structures and deep fetal white matter may be displaced in the presence of hydrocephalus. In 1988, Cardoza et al. demonstrated that the position of the fetal choroid plexus was dependent on gravity. These authors suggested using the choroid angle (the angle between the long axis of the choroid plexus and the linear midline echo on a transverse axial sonogram through the body of the lateral ventricle), which was shown to vary directly with ventricular size. In normal-sized ventricles, the mean angle was 14 degrees, with a range between 6 and 22 degrees. In

fetuses with ventriculomegaly the angles varied between 29 and 90 degrees, and a normal distribution was not observed (Cardoza et al. 1988a). The choroid angle was shown to increase with the severity of hydrocephalus.

Subsequently, the same group of investigators measured the ventricular atria in 100 healthy fetuses between 14 and 38 weeks of gestation (Cardoza et al. 1988b). They compared these measurements with 38 fetuses in whom ventriculomegaly had already been diagnosed. Axial sonograms of the fetal brain taken through the atrium of the lateral ventricle demonstrated that the normal atrial diameter remained relatively constant throughout gestation despite growth of the surrounding brain. The mean diameter of the atrium was 7.6 ± 0.6 mm. These authors suggested that atrial diameters >10 mm, which were greater than 4 SD above the mean, suggested the presence of ventriculomegaly. This measurement was quickly performed and was reproducible. There were no statistically significant differences observed in the mean atrial diameter among fetuses of different gestational ages. Close interobserver and intraobserver reproducibility was demonstrated in this study (Cardoza et al. 1988b). The ease of measurement and ease of remembering the normal and abnormal values have popularized this approach to the diagnosis of ventriculomegaly.

If an atrial diameter of >10 mm is considered abnormal, borderline ventriculomegaly has been defined as an atrial measurement of between 10 and 12 mm or 10 and 15 mm. The presence of borderline ventriculomegaly has been associated with an increased risk of central nervous system (CNS) and non-CNS abnormalities, and suggests the need for a fetal anatomic examination. Several studies have substantiated this recommendation. Mahony et al. (1988) performed a prospective study of 20 fetuses with mild isolated ventriculomegaly. These authors defined borderline ventriculomegaly as a 3- to 8-mm separation existing between the choroid plexus in the atrium of the lateral cerebral ventricle and the adjacent ventricular wall on an axial scan. Of the 20 fetuses identified, 8 had a normal outcome (40%). The remaining 12 fetuses had additional sonographic abnormalities. Of these 12, 4 had an uncertain prognosis and 8 died.

Goldstein et al. (1990) used the transverse diameter of a ventricular atrium of 10 mm or more and reviewed the medical records of 55 fetuses retrospectively identified with mild ventriculomegaly. Of these 55 fetuses, 13 had isolated ventriculomegaly and 42 had associated abnormalities. There was a significant difference in mortality between the fetuses who had the isolated finding and those fetuses with associated abnormalities. Of 15 living children who could be identified, 9 (60%) were normal at 6 to 30 months of postnatal age, 3 (20%) were abnormal, and 3 (20%) were lost to follow-up. These authors concluded that isolated mild ventriculomegaly was associated with a better prognosis than more substantial ventriculomegaly.

In a third study, Achiron et al. (1993) identified eight cases of mild isolated ventriculomegaly among 5400 routine antenatal sonographic studies performed between 16 and 22 weeks of gestation Of the eight, three were normal postnatally, five were abnormal and two of these five had serious chromosomal abnormalities. These authors reviewed the medical literature and found 109 cases described with mild ventriculomegaly. Of these, 92 were isolated and 11 had an abnormal karyotype. The incidence of abnormal chromosomes was 12%, so these authors recommended that karyotyping be performed in all cases of mild ventriculomegaly.

Similarly, Bromley et al. (1991) performed a retrospective study on the clinical course and outcome for 44 fetuses identified with mild ventriculomegaly between 1987 and 1990. These authors also used a definition of an axial scan measurement of the fetal brain between 10 and 12 mm. In their patient population, 17 of the 44 (39%) had other sonographic abnormalities, 6 of them in the CNS. These authors also had a 12% incidence of abnormal karyotypes, including 3 cases of trisomy 21, 1 case of trisomy 18, and 1 case of deletion of the short arm of chromosome 7. There were 5 elective terminations of pregnancy and 3 neonatal deaths. Of 36 liveborn neonates, 26 were developmentally and clinically normal at 3 to 18 months of postnatal age. Ten of the 36 were developmentally impaired, including 5 cases of apparently isolated ventriculomegaly. These authors concluded, however, that these fetuses with mild ventriculomegaly have a decreased incidence of associated abnormalities and a better outcome than fetuses with more severe dilatation.

Unilateral hydrocephalus is extremely uncommon. This condition carries a better prognosis than bilateral hydrocephalus. Of eight reported cases identified in utero, five were due to congenital absence or stenosis of the foramen of Monro, one was due to transient obstruction of CSF flow by a hematoma, one was due to holoprosencephaly, and one was due to unknown causes (Patten et al. 1991). Chari et al. (1993) described a fetus diagnosed at 34 weeks of gestation with a dilated right ventricle due to a frontoethmoidal encephalocele. These authors speculated that the right foramen of Monro was atretic and that pressure from the progressive ventriculomegaly led to the development of the encephalocele. All reports thus far seem to indicate that unilateral hydrocephalus is not associated with the presence of extracranial anomalies. Furthermore, all patients have required postnatal placement of a ventriculoperitoneal shunt (Anderson et al. 1993; Chari et al. 1993; Paten et al. 1991). In a study of 27 fetuses with isolated, borderline ventriculomegaly, 25 had a normal neurological outcome, 1 had petit mal seizures, and one was electively terminated (Lipitz et al. 1998).

▶ DIFFERENTIAL DIAGNOSIS

In the differential diagnosis of hydrocephalus, it is important to rule out associated intrauterine infection, such as cytomegalovirus, toxoplasmosis, syphilis, intracranial hemorrhage, or a central nervous system tumor. Furthermore, myelomeningocele can be the underlying reason for the hydrocephalus (see Chapter 19).

In hydranencephaly, only remnants of the cortex remain. Fluid-filled sacs that are lined by leptomeninges replace the rest of the brain. In porencephaly the parenchyma of the brain contains one or more fluid-filled cavities (see Chapter 21). The Dandy–Walker malformation includes ventricular dilation (see Chapter 10). Demonstration of the absence of falx cerebri and fusion of the thalami can distinguish holoprosencephaly from other causes of hydrocephalus (see Chapter 13). Consideration should also be given to the possibility of underlying single gene disorder.

One of the major concerns with the antenatal sonographic finding of hydrocephalus is the fact that ventriculomegaly is frequently associated with additional anomalies within and outside of the fetal brain. Associated intracranial anomalies (such as agenesis of the corpus callosum or the Dandy–Walker malformation) are present in at least one-third of cases. Extracranial abnormalities have been demonstrated in two-thirds of cases (Fadel 1989). Nyberg et al. (1987) reviewed 61 cases of fetal hydrocephalus. In this report, 51 of 61 (84%) of fetuses had associated malformations. Thirty-five of 39 CNS abnormalities were correctly identified. Thirty-four fetuses had anomalies outside the brain, and

27 of these were multiple. Only 7 of their patients had isolated hydrocephalus. In this series, fetal mortality was directly related to the presence of abnormalities outside the CNS. Of concern was the fact that false negative diagnoses were common, and included esophageal atresia, spinal abnormalities, lung hypoplasia, and cardiac defects. In this series, 41 of 61 fetuses ultimately died from associated conditions such as asphyxiating thoracic dystrophy (Jeune syndrome) (Singh et al. 1988) (see Chapter 90), Apert syndrome, in which hydrocephalus is considered a major associated malformation (Hyon et al. 1986), and the Walker–Warburg syndrome. This latter recessively inherited condition includes hydrocephalus, multiple CNS malformations, microophthalmia, severe mental retardation, congenital myopathy, and a limited life span (Crowe et al. 1986). Finally, inborn errors of metabolism, such as fumarase deficiency, can cause polyhydramnios and hydrocephalus in utero (Remes et al. 1992). In this condition, enlargement of the cerebral ventricles is due to cerebral atrophy and polyhydramnios is due to intrauterine hypotonia, causing poor swallowing.

▶ ANTENATAL NATURAL HISTORY

CSF is formed within the ventricular system—50% from the choroid plexus and 50% from the cerebral capillaries. The circulation of CSF is unidirectional (Vintzileos et al. 1983). It flows from the lateral ventricles through the foramen of Monro into the third ventricle. It then flows from the third ventricle to the aqueduct of Sylvius through the fourth ventricle into the spinal subarachnoid space (foramen of Magendie) or to the basal cisterns (foramen of Luschka) over the cerebral hemispheres. CSF is reabsorbed by arachnoid villi in venous sinuses. The flow of CSF is partially derived by arterial pulsations of the choroid plexus (Vintzileos et al. 1983). In the newborn, the normal flow rate of CSF is 0.35 ml per minute.

Oi et al. (1990) reviewed their experience with 24 cases of fetal hydrocephalus. Four fetuses underwent transabdominal or transvaginal cephalocentesis prenatally and intracranial pressures were measured. The results suggested that the fetal brain is subjected to extremely high intracranial pressures, resulting from a mixture of hydrocephalic pressure and intermittent uterine constriction. A similar experience has been observed in animals in the rhesus monkey model. The intracranial pressure in normal monkey fetuses was 55 to 66 mm of water, and in hydrocephalic fetuses the pressures were 100 to 250 mm of water. Experimental in utero shunt procedures in primate models were encouraging, with improvement in CT findings after surgery. The human model is different because a variety of CNS anomalies are associated with human hydrocephalus.

In a similar study, Simpson et al. (1988) presented a series of patients with fetal CNS defects who had cephalocentesis performed at the time of termination of pregnancy. The intracranial CSF pressures and volumes were quite variable. There was no correlation between the type of lesion and intracranial pressure observed.

▶ MANAGEMENT OF PREGNANCY

The finding of prenatal ventriculomegaly mandates referral to a center capable of targeted sonographic examination of the fetus due to the high incidence of CNS and extra-CNS anomalies. Prospective parents should be counseled regarding the diversity of conditions that can be labeled as hydrocephalus and associated with hydrocephalus (Pober et al. 1986). They should be counseled that ventriculomegaly is progressive in 2.5 to 4.5% of cases and that the incidence of associated abnormalities varies from 54 to 84% (Rosseau et al. 1992). Consideration should be given to obtaining a fetal karyotype, due to the 12 to 25% incidence of abnormalities. Consideration should also be given to performance of an infectious workup for the presence of cytomegalovirus and toxoplasmosis. Serial sonograms should be performed to determine whether the hydrocephalus is stable, progressive, or resolving. The major factor that influences prognosis is the presence of associated abnormalities (Pober et al. 1986). For this reason, we recommend obtaining a fetal magnetic resonance image (MRI). Termination of pregnancy can be offered if the diagnosis is made before 24 weeks of gestation. In general, decisions about management options depend on the gestational age at the time of diagnosis and the presence and nature of associated abnormalities.

Chervenak and McCullough (1987) discussed an ethical analysis of the management of pregnancy complicated by fetal hydrocephalus and macrocephaly, balancing the needs of the mother and the child. In general, a cesarean delivery after demonstrating pulmonary maturity is recommended to permit prompt postnatal neurosurgical therapy. If severe abnormalities incompatible with extrauterine life are present, such as thanatophoric dysplasia, cephalocentesis (removal of CSF from the ventricular system) to reduce head size to permit vaginal delivery can be considered.

▶ FETAL INTERVENTION

In utero treatment has been attempted for hydrocephalus to try to prevent progressive damage to the fetal brain caused by the chronically increased CSF pressure. In utero treatment was first attempted by Clewell et al. (1982), who used an indwelling shunt to drain fetal CSF, and Birnholz and Frigoletto (1981), who reported the use of serial sonographically guided percutaneous cephalocenteses. Specific criteria for intrauterine therapy were set down by the International Fetal Medicine and Surgery Society. These included ventriculomegaly, gestational age of less than 30 weeks, sonographic evidence of continued ventricular enlargement, singleton pregnancy, the pregnant patient's understanding of the experimental treatment, and the pregnant patient's commitment to long-term follow-up (Oi et al. 1989). A registry was formed in 1982 under the auspices of the International Fetal Medicine and Surgery Society (Drugen et al. 1989; Manning et al. 1986). This group analyzed the results of 39 antenatal procedures performed in the United States and 5 in Italy. Between 1982 and 1985 these 44 cases were selected for in utero treatment based on the guidelines set up by the society. Of the 44 cases, 36 (82%) fetuses survived and 8 (19%) died in utero or during the perinatal period. Four of these deaths were related to the in utero procedure. Twenty-two of 36 survivors were left with varying neurologic and physical handicaps. Forty-eight percent of the infants were severely handicapped (Manning et al. 1986). Because of the high rate of procedure-related death and lack of significant improvement in outcome, the in utero treatment has been abandoned for the present.

Hudgins et al. (1988) retrospectively reviewed the outcomes of 47 fetuses evaluated during a 4-year period in the fetal treatment program at the University of California at San Francisco. Twenty-five of these 47 fetuses with ventriculomegaly had severe associated abnormalities and were either electively terminated or died during the perinatal period. Of the remaining 22, 19 had stable ventriculomegaly, 2 had progressive ventriculomegaly, and 1 resolved in utero. Of the 19 postnatal long-term survivors, 13 (68%) were normal and 6 (32%) had moderate to severe developmental delay. Associated abnormalities were detected in 74% of fetuses, and there was a 20% false negative rate of detection of associated abnormalities. These authors concluded that they were unable to define a group of patients that would benefit from in utero shunting. In their series, only a 14% incidence of isolated, progressive ventriculomegaly was noted.

Fetuses with isolated, progressive ventriculomegaly are the most likely to benefit from in utero treatment. However, these fetuses represent such a small minority of the total population of fetuses with fetal ventriculomegaly that in utero treatment is currently not recommended.

Fetal intervention for hydrocephalus occurring secondary to myelomeningocele is discussed in Chapter 19.

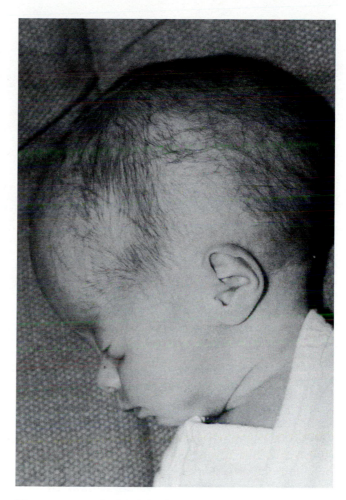

Figure 15-2. Postnatal photograph of a newborn infant diagnosed prenatally with hydrocephalus. Note enlarged head and prominent venous pattern on scalp.

(Fig. 15-2). Consultation with a medical geneticist and a neurosurgeon is recommended. Postnatal diagnostic imaging of the central nervous system may include computed tomographic (CT) scan and magnetic resonance imaging (MRI). If a chromosome analysis was not performed prenatally, it should be performed during the newborn period. The major goals of treatment of the newborn are to determine an underlying cause for the hydrocephalus and to stabilize the infant for the placement of a ventriculoperitoneal shunt.

If the infant has been found to have multiple associated abnormalities incompatible with survival, a detailed autopsy is recommended if death occurs during the neonatal period.

▶ TREATMENT OF THE NEWBORN

Infants who are delivered with a prenatal diagnosis of ventriculomegaly need a detailed physical examination

▶ SURGICAL TREATMENT

The major treatment of hydrocephalus is the placement of a ventriculoperitoneal shunt. Surgical therapy was not successful until the work of Dandy and Blackfan, who in 1914 accurately described the circulation of CSF. This stimulated development of surgical treatment in the first half of the 20th century (Hirsch 1994). The introduction of the Holter valve in 1956 significantly decreased the postoperative mortality seen with the placement of the ventriculoperitoneal shunt. Mortality related to this surgery is minimal. The major morbidities are associated with blockage of the shunt and infection.

▶ LONG-TERM OUTCOME

The most important factor in the long-term outcome is the presence of associated abnormalities. In one study Rosseau et al. (1992) reviewed follow-up data on 40 patients identified prenatally with hydrocephalus in a community-acquired series. Of these 40 patients, 3 were electively terminated and 37 delivered. Of the 37, 26 (70%) underwent the placement of a ventriculoperitoneal shunt. Ten of these 26 (38%) had satisfactory cognitive ability. Of the 11 patients who were not treated, reasons for nontreatment included misdiagnosis, resolution of hydrocephalus, or parental refusal. Multiple studies seem to indicate that approximately 40 to 50% of survivors have a normal IQ. The IQs are not proportional to brain expansion after the placement of the shunt. Ventricular dilatation is not responsible for the long-term outcome (Hirsch 1994). Similarly, the site of obstruction does not affect long-term intelligence. Approximately 10% of survivors have a seizure disorder (Hirsch 1994). In a study of intelligence outcome in 44 children with shunted hydrocephalus, the site of obstruction, the number of shunt revisions, the number of postsurgical complications such as infection or hematoma, or the presence of seizures did not correlate with abnormalities in neuropsychologic functioning. Verbal intelligence was shown to be affected by the presence of motor deficits and the need for antiepileptic therapy. Nonverbal intelligence was affected by the presence of a brain malformation or the age at the time of shunt placement. In this study, if a shunt was placed later in life it indicated that the aqueductal stenosis developed slowly (Riva et al. 1994).

▶ GENETICS AND RECURRENCE RISK

The major considerations in the genetics of hydrocephalus are related to the underlying cause. In a review of the causes of hydrocephalus in live-born infants, Burton (1979) performed a retrospective analysis of 205 patients. In this patient population, 83% had isolated hydrocephalus. Forty-three percent of cases were due to aqueductal obstruction, 38% were due to communicating hydrocephalus, 13% were due to Dandy–

Walker malformation, and 6% were due to other anatomic lesions. In the majority of cases of the postnatally identified hydrocephalus, a specific nongenetic cause was not documented. Review of 353 siblings of the 205 patients demonstrated that 1.4% had hydrocephalus. Importantly, specific subgroups were identified to be at high risk. These included males with aqueductal stenosis. Classic X-linked recessive hydrocephalus, known as Bickers–Adams disease, or hereditary stenosis of the aqueduct of Sylvius (HSAS) has been mapped to chromosome Xq28 by linkage analysis (Willems et al. 1990). This disease may be genetically heterogeneous. Another gene has been mapped to Xq27.3 (Strain et al. 1994). In a fetus identified with hydrocephalus, a complete family history is essential. It is important to note that males affected with X-linked HSAS may be normocephalic and nondysmorphic, but they will have mental retardation (Kelley et al. 1988). Families with a recessively inherited form of hydrocephalus have been identified, but in general consanguinity has also been identified (Zlotogora et al. 1994). A family with dominantly inherited disease has been described in which the mother and her three daughters have a syndrome consisting of delayed psychomotor development, psychosis, hydrocephalus with white-matter alterations, arachnoid cysts, brachydactyly, and Sprengel anomaly (Ferlini et al. 1995). This condition has been described as an X-linked dominant trait.

A family history should alert the health care provider to the potential presence of an X-linked disorder in the family. For families with a negative family history, the recurrence rate of hydrocephalus is 4%. This figure was ascertained from a prospective study performed of 251 pregnancies with couples with at least one previous child with hydrocephalus (Váradi et al. 1988). Of 261 pregnancies, 4 aborted spontaneously before 22 weeks of gestation. In 15 pregnancies, fetal CNS malformations were identified, including 12 cases of hydrocephalus and 3 cases of isolated neural-tube defects. In 261 pregnancies, the recurrence of hydrocephalus was 4.6%. In couples who had had only one previous child with hydrocephalus there was a recurrence of 9 in 224 total pregnancies (4.0%).

In recent years, much progress has ensued regarding the molecular understanding of a variety of conditions inherited as X-linked recessive disorders and include hydrocephalus as one manifestation. It is thought that X-linked hydrocephalus comprises approximately 5% of all cases of hydrocephalus (Schrander-Stumpel and Fryns, 1998). These conditions include HSAS (hydrocephalus due to aqueductal stenosis, mental retardation, clasped thumbs, and spastic paraparesis). Related conditions include MASA (mental retardation, aphasia, shuffling gate, and adducted thumbs) and spastic paraplegia type I (SPG1). MASA syndrome and SPG1 present with milder symptoms and a longer life expectancy than HSAS. These three conditions are all now known to be caused by heterogeneous mutations in the gene encoding the neural-cell adhesion molecule L1. L1 is involved in intracellular recognition and neuronal migration in the CNS (Jouet et al. 1995). A wide variation is observed in patients belonging to the same family, as well as in patients from different families. HSAS is known to account for 7% of cases of hydrocephalus in males (Strain et al. 1994).

The L1 cell-adhesion molecule is a multidomain cell-surface glycoprotein expressed on the axons of post-mitotic neurones. L1 is involved in neuronal migration and neurite extension. It may also have a role in myelinization of neurons in the peripheral nervous system. Jouet et al. (1995) reviewed the 23 mutations described thus far in the L1 gene. Twelve were missense mutations, 3 were deletions, 1 was a duplication, and 2 were nonsense changes. L1 is a member of the immunoglobulin superfamily. Three mutations have been identified that affect different fibronectin domains. These are critical for L1 function in brain development. These authors recommended that X-linked hydrocephalus and the MASA sydrome should be considered as variable manifestations of the same disorder and consideration should be given to renaming these conditions as L1 syndrome. Thus, heterogeneous mutations in the L1 gene form a clinical spectrum of disorders that can be recognized both prenatally and postnatally (Takechi et al. 1996). Families who have a history that suggests the presence of an X-linked disorder should have DNA collected on a research basis to try to prospectively identify L1 gene mutations.

Families in whom no genetic etiology can be identified can be offered prenatal sonographic studies in a subsequent pregnancy due to the recurrence risk of 4%.

REFERENCES

Achiron R, Schimmel M, Achiron A, and Mashiach S. Fetal mild idiopathic lateral ventriculomegaly: is there a correlation with fetal trisomy? Ultrasound Obstet Gynecol 1993:89–92.

Anderson N, Malpas T, Davison M. Prenatal diagnosis of unilateral hydrocephalus. Pediatr Radiol 1993;23:69–70.

Bickers DS, Adams RD. Hereditary stenosis of the aqueduct of Sylvius as a cause of congenital hydrocephalus. Brain 1949;72:246–262.

Birnholz JC, Frigoletto FD. Antenatal treatment of hydrocephalus. N Engl J Med 1981;304:1021–1023.

Bromley B, Frigoletto FD, Benacerraf BR. Mild fetal lateral cerebral ventriculomegaly: clinical course and outcome. Am J Obstet Gynecol 1991;164:863–867.

Burton B. Recurrence risks for congenital hydrocephalus. Clin Genet 1979;16:47–53.

Cardoza JD, Filly RA, Podrasky AE. The dangling choroid plexus: a sonographic observation of value in excluding ventriculomegaly. AJR Am J Roentgenol 1988a;151:767–770.

Cardoza JD, Goldstein RB, Filly RA. Exclusion of fetal ventriculomegaly with a single measurement: the width of the lateral ventricular atrium. Pediatr Radiol 1988b;169:711–714.

Chari R, Bhargava R, Hammond I, Ventureyra ECG, Lalonde AB. Pitfall to avoid: antenatal unilateral hydrocephalus. Can Assoc Radiol J 1993;44:57–59.

Chervenak FA, McCullough LB. Ethical challenges in perinatal medicine: the intrapartum management of pregnancy complicated by fetal hydrocephalus with macrocephaly. Semin Perinatol 1987;11:232–239.

Clewell WH, Johnson ML, Meier PR, et al. A surgical approach to the treatment of fetal hydrocephalus. N Engl J Med 1982;306:1320–1325.

Crowe C, Jassani M, Dickerman L. The prenatal diagnosis of the Walker–Warburg syndrome. Prenat Diagn 1986;6:177–185.

DeLange SA. Progressive hydrocephalus. In: Vinken PJ, Bruyn GW, eds. Handbook of clinical neurology. Amsterdam: Elsevier, 1977:526–563.

Drugan A, Krause B, Canady A, Zador IE, Sacks AJ, Evans MI. The natural history of prenatally diagnosed cerebral ventriculomegaly. JAMA 1989;261:1785–1788.

Fadel HE. Antenatal diagnosis of fetal intracranial anomalies. J Child Neurol 1989;4:S107–S112.

Ferlini A, Ragno M, Gobbi P, et al. Hydrocephalus, skeletal anomalies, and mental disturbances in a mother and three daughters: a new syndrome. Am J Med Genet 1995;59:506–511.

Goldstein RB, LaPidus AS, Filly RA, Cardoza J. Mild lateral cerebral ventricular dilatation in utero: clinical significance and prognosis. Radiology 1990;176:237–240.

Hertzberg BS, Bowie JD, Burger PC, Marshburn PB, Djang WT. The three lines: origin of sonographic landmarks in the fetal head. AJR Am J Roentgenol 1987;149:1009–1012.

Hirsch JF. Consensus: long-term outcome in hydrocephalus. Child Nerv Syst 1994;10:64–69.

Hudgins RJ, Edwards MSB, Goldstein R, et al. Natural history of fetal ventriculomegaly. Pediatrics 1988;82:692–697.

Hyon K, Uppal V, Wallach R. Apert syndrome and fetal hydrocephaly: clinical case reports. Hum Genet 1986;73:93–95.

Jouet M, Moncla A, Paterson J, et al. New domains of neural cell-adhesion molecule LI implicated in X-linked hydrocephalus and MASA syndrome. Am J Hum Genet 1995;56:1303–1314.

Kelley RI, Mennuti MT, Hickey WF, Zackai EH. X-linked recessive aqueductal stenosis without macrocephaly. Clin Genet 1988;33:390–394.

Lipitz S, Yagel S, Malinger G, Meizner I, Zalel Y, Achiron R. Outcome of fetuses with isolated borderline unilateral ventriculomegaly diagnosed at mid-gestation. Ultrasound Obstet Gynecol 1998;12:23–26.

Mahony BS, Nyberg DA, Hirsch JH, Petty CN, Hendricks SK, Mack LA. Mild idiopathic lateral cerebral ventricular dilatation in utero: sonographic evaluation. Radiology 1988;169:715–721.

Manning FA, Harrison MR, Rodeck C, et al. Catheter shunts for fetal hydronephrosis and hydrocephalus: report of the

International Fetal Surgery registry. N Engl J Med 1986; 315:336–340.

Nyberg DA, Mack LA, Hirsch J, Pagon RO, Shepard TH. Fetal hydrocephalus: sonographic detection and clinical significance of associated anomalies. Radiology 1987;163: 187–191.

Oi S, Matsumoto S, Katayama K., Mochizuki M. Pathophysiology and postnatal outcome of fetal hydrocephalus. Child Nerv Syst 1990;6:338–345.

Patten RM, Mack LA, Finberg HJ. Unilateral hydrocephalus: prenatal sonographic diagnosis. AJR Am J Roentgenol 1991;156:359–363.

Pober BR, Greene MF, Holmes LB. Complexities of intraventricular abnormalities. J Pediatr 1986;108:545–551.

Raimondi AJ. A unifying theory for the definition and classification of hydrocephalus. Child Nerv Syst 1994;10:2–12.

Remes AM, Rantala H, Hiltunen JK, Leisti J, Ruokonen A. Fumarase deficiency: two siblings with enlarged cerebral ventricles and polyhydramnios in utero. Pediatrics 1992; 89:730–734.

Riva D, Milani N, Giorgi C, Pantaleoni C, Zorzi C, Devoti M. Intelligence outcome in children with shunted hydrocephalus of different etiology. Child Nerv Syst 1994;10: 70–73.

Rosseau GL, McCullough DC, Joseph AL. Current prognosis in fetal ventriculomegaly. J Neurosurg 1992;77:551–555.

Schrander-Stumpel C, Fryns JP. Congenital hydrocephalus: nosology and guidelines for clinical approach and genetic counseling. Eur J Pediatr 1998;157:355–362.

Simpson GF, Edwards MSB, Callen P, Filly RF, Anderson RL, Golbus MS. Pressure, biochemical, and culture characteristics of CSF associated with the in utero drainage of various fetal CNS defects. Am J Med Genet 1988;29:343–351.

Singh M, Ray D, Paul VK, Kumar A. Hydrocephalus in asphyxiating thoracic dystrophy. Am J Med Genet 1988; 29:391–395.

Strain L, Gosden CM, Brock DJH, Bonthron DT. Genetic heterogeneity in X-linked hydrocephalus: linkage to markers within Xq27.3. Am J Hum Genet 1994;54: 236–243.

Takechi T, Tohyama J, Kurashige T, et al. A deletion of five nucleotides in the L1CAM gene in a Japanese family with X-linked hydrocephalus. Hum Genet 1996;97:353–356.

Váradi V, Zoltan T, Torok O, Zoltan P. Heterogeneity and recurrence risk for congenital hydrocephalus. Am J Med Genet 1988;29:305–310.

Vintzileos AM, Ingardia CJ, Nochimson DJ. Congenital hydrocephalus: a review and protocol for perinatal management. Obstet Gynecol 1983;62:539–549.

Willems PJ, Dijkstra I, Van Der Auwera BJ, et al. Assignment of X-linked hydrocephalus to Xq28 by linkage analysis. Genomics 1990;8:367–370.

Wilson RD, Hitchman D, Wittman BK. Clinical follow-up of prenatally diagnosed isolated ventriculomegaly, microcephaly and encephalocele. Fetal Ther 1989;4:49–57.

Wiswell T, Tuttle DJ, Northam RS, Simonds GR. Major congenital neurologic malformations. Am J Dis Child 1990; 144:61–67.

Zlotogora J, Sagi M, Cohen T. Familial hydrocephalus of prenatal onset. Am J Med Genet 1994;49:202–204.

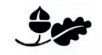

CHAPTER 16

Iniencephaly

► CONDITION

The term *iniencephaly,* first used by St. Hilaire in 1836, derives from the Greek word *inion,* meaning the nape of the neck. It is a rare, lethal malformation. The diagnosis of iniencephaly is based on three features: deficiency of the occipital bone, cervicothoracic spinal retroflexion, and rachischisis. The majority of affected patients also have visceral malformations (Scherrer et al. 1992).

Lewis (1897) classified iniencephalus into two types: iniencephalus apertus, in which there is involvement of the brain with an encephalocele present, and iniencephalus clausus, in which no malformation of the occipital bone or brain is present.

A more complete clinical description of iniencephaly was given by Hrgovic et al. (1989) in which they described iniencephaly as a defect of the occipital bone with the presence of an accompanying enlarged foramen magnum. Partial or total absence of the thoracic and cervical vertebrae exists. The vertebrae present are irregularly fused and demonstrate an incomplete closure of the vertebral arch and/or body. A significant shortening of the fetal spine exists as a result of extreme lordosis and hyperextension (or retroflexion) of a malformed spinal column on the neck. The fetal face is upturned and the skin in the mandibular area joins the breast due to complete absence of the neck (Hrgovic et al. 1989).

► INCIDENCE

The incidence of iniencephaly is between 1 in 1000 to less than 1 in 100,000 (Gartman et al. 1991). The vast majority of cases result in fetal death or stillbirth, which makes it difficult to estimate the true incidence accurately. In one report, the incidence of iniencephaly was 1 in 896 in Edinburgh, Scotland (Paterson 1944). The condition affects predominantly females, who account for 90% of cases (Rodriguez et al. 1991). The cause of iniencephaly is unknown. It has been noted, however, that in geographical areas where there is an increased incidence of anencephaly there is also an increased incidence of iniencephaly (Katz et al. 1989). In 1991, Rodriguez et al. reported a cluster of five cases of iniencephaly over a 4-month period in Miami. The mothers were all of Hispanic ethnic background, but had no other common causal factors (Rodriguez et al. 1991). Other factors reported in the literature to be associated with iniencephaly include parental consanguinity, maternal syphilis, and maternal ingestion of tetracycline or sedatives (Scherrer et al. 1992).

► SONOGRAPHIC FINDINGS

The sonographic diagnosis of iniencephaly is based on two diagnostic clues: extreme dorsal flexion of the head and an abnormally short and deformed spine. This allows the fetal thorax and head to be seen in the same scanning plane. The other diagnostic clue is the presence of an abnormal fetal spine (Meizner et al. 1992). Polyhydramnios is frequently present because of the fetus's inability to swallow.

Multiple associated malformations are generally present in cases of fetal iniencephaly. In one report, David and Nixon (1976) examined 50 pathologic specimens from fetuses with iniencephaly. There were significant associated malformations in 84% of these cases. The most frequent malformations were hydronephrosis, cardiovascular malformations, single umbilical artery, and diaphragmatic hernia. Also noted were the presence of cyclopia, facial clefts, omphalocele, and club foot (David and Nixon 1976). Iniencephaly is associated with a variety of central nervous system abnormalities, including encephalocele, hydrocephalus, hydromyelia, anencephaly, microcephaly, polymicrogyria, agenesis of the cerebellar vermis, and the presence of a cerebellar cyst (Scherrer et al. 1992). In a review of 19 cases at one institution, Dogan et al. (1996) noted associated encephalocele in 5 of the 19 cases, and anencephaly in 15 of the 19 cases.

Prenatal diagnosis of iniencephaly was initially detected on radiography of the maternal abdomen that was performed because the uterine size was larger than indicated for the gestational date. In this report, the presence of a single fetus with a large head and hyperextension were shown on radiography (Kapoor and Saha 1987). The first prenatal sonographic diagnosis of iniencephaly was performed in the same year, when a fetus at 22 weeks of gestation was noted to have hyperextension of the neck and a large neural-tube defect involving the thoracolumbar spine (Foderaro et al. 1987). Shoham et al. (1988) described a fetus at 19 weeks of gestation in which iniencephaly was detected because of an increased maternal serum α-fetoprotein (AFP) level. On sonography, the fetus was noted to be in the breech position. The head was described as an echogenic mass with the absence of clearly identifiable parietal bones. The fetal head was noted to be in continuity with the shoulders. Overt rachischisis of the cervical and thoracic vertebral column were seen on sagittal section. In the coronal view, increased separation of the vertebral lamina in the affected area were noted. A soft-tissue mass, thought to be a myelomeningocele, extended posteriorly from the distorted spine. In addition, there was marked hyperextension of the head with crowding of the ribs, and no fetal neck was identified. These authors suggested the following sonographic criteria for the diagnosis of iniencephaly:

1. Absence of normal parietal bones.
2. Absence of normal brain tissue.
3. Overriding of the head on the shoulders without identification of a normal neck structure.
4. Rachischisis.
5. Myelomeningocele (Shoham et al. 1988).

In another case report, a fetus with iniencephaly apertus was diagnosed at 21 weeks of gestation based on extreme dorsiflexion of the head accompanied by an abnormally short and deformed spine. Severe polyhydramnios was present. These authors stated that it was difficult to scan the fetus in the longitudinal axis because of marked retroflexion of the head accompanied by extreme cervicothoracic lordosis. The spinal vertebrae were malformed and the vertebral column was twisted into a U-shape. The marked, fixed retroflexion of the fetal head was so prominent that the fetal head and both thighs could be observed in a transverse scan (Meizner et al. 1992).

Iniencephaly has also been diagnosed as early as 13 weeks of gestation by transvaginal sonography. Sherer et al. (1993) diagnosed the presence of a persistently hyperextended fetal head with the occipital area in close association with the fetal back. In longitudinal and transverse transvaginal scanning, spinal dysraphism was also shown. The calvarium was noted to be absent but brain tissue was present in this 13-week-old affected fetus.

▶ DIFFERENTIAL DIAGNOSIS

The differential diagnosis of iniencephaly includes anencephaly (see Chapter 5). Fetuses with anencephaly share many uncommon malformations with iniencephaly, including congenital diaphragmatic hernia. In anencephalic fetuses, although the calvarium is absent, the head is not as retroflexed as it is in iniencephaly and usually a normal neck structure is demonstrated. Another consideration in the differential diagnosis is cervical myelomeningocele.

The Klippel–Feil malformation complex is sometimes considered the mildest form of iniencephaly. Klippel–Feil malformation consists of shortness of the neck with fusion of the cervical vertebrae. The condition is compatible with life. The distinction between iniencephaly and Klippel–Feil malformation complex has been debated in the literature, but they probably represent opposite aspects of a continuum of the same developmental abnormality. This is illustrated by a case report in which a 17-year-old boy diagnosed with severe Klippel–Feil anomaly had a three-dimensional computed tomographic (CT) scan performed. This study confirmed complete fusion of the bodies of the cervical and upper thoracic spine into a solid, curved vertebral block. In addition, an enlarged foramen magnum opened into wide posterior defects in neural arches of C1 through C3. The posterior elements of the lower cervical and upper thoracic spines were completely fused. The presence of the enlarged foramen magnum indicated that the true diagnosis in this patient was mild iniencephaly. In both Klippel–Feil anomaly and iniencephaly, fibrous bands connect the occiput to the posterior aspect of the cervical spine. In iniencephaly, however, an enlarged foramen magnum communicates directly with the spinal canal through neural-arch defects, such as those that were present in this patient (Munden et al. 1993). Three-dimensional CT scans are recommended for patients with severe Klippel–Feil anomaly to identify the presence of iniencephaly, which would change the surgical plans if surgical release of the retroflexed head is anticipated. Distinction between iniencephaly and Klippel–Feil anomaly is important because the prognosis for iniencephaly is generally lethal, but the prognosis for Klippel–Feil anomaly is not.

▶ ANTENATAL NATURAL HISTORY

In iniencephaly, developmental disturbances of the neural tube and spine arise very early in embryogenesis, generally between day 26 and 30 after conception. The lesions in iniencephaly have been experimentally reproduced with administration of vinblastine, streptonigrin, and triparanol (Scherrer et al. 1992). Two hypotheses for the pathogenesis of iniencephaly have been advanced: dilation and rupture of a previously closed neural tube and failure of the neural tube to close during embryogenesis (Scherrer et al. 1992). Other authors describe a developmental arrest of the normal physiologic retroflexion of the embryo that takes place at 3 weeks of gestation. In the normal embryo, forward bending subsequently occurs at 4 weeks of gestation. This does not occur in fetuses with iniencephaly (Rodriguez et al. 1991). The persistent cervical retroflexion leads to failure of the neural groove to close in the area of the cervical spine. The abnormal fetal growth occurring at such an early stage in gestation is thought to be the reason for the multiple associated malformations, due to subsequent hindering and cramping of structures related to the retroflexed fetal neck (David and Nixon 1976).

▶ MANAGEMENT OF PREGNANCY

Pregnancies in which there is a fetus with iniencephaly can be associated with increased maternal serum AFP levels, due to the open neural-tube defect (Shoham et al. 1988). Pregnant women carrying fetuses in which iniencephaly is suspected should be referred to a center capable of fetal anatomic diagnosis. A complete ultrasound examination should be performed to look for associated malformations and to document the extent of the neural-tube defect. An amniocentesis should be performed to obtain a fetal karyotype, an amniotic fluid AFP level, and an acetylcholinesterase level. The amniotic fluid AFP and acetylcholinesterase levels will help to determine if the neural-tube defect is covered by skin. Some authors have indicated that survival outside the womb is possible if the neural-tube defect is covered by skin, no encephalocele is present, and no other malformations are detected in the fetus (Katz et al. 1989).

With rare exceptions, the diagnosis of iniencephaly is not compatible with life outside the womb. If the diagnosis is made earlier than 24 weeks of gestation, the prospective parents should be counseled regarding the option of termination of pregnancy. If the diagnosis is made later than 24 weeks of gestation, or if the parents opt to continue the pregnancy to term, the presence of the hyperextended fetal head might cause dystocia. Consideration should be given to the performance of a cesarean section for safe delivery of the fetus with iniencephaly (Kapoor and Saha 1987).

▶ FETAL INTERVENTION

There is no fetal intervention for iniencephaly.

▶ TREATMENT OF THE NEWBORN

There is no indication for aggressive resuscitation of infants with iniencephaly. For the few long-term survivors reported in the literature, heroic measures were not performed (Katz et al. 1989). A physical examination, however, is indicated to confirm the suspected prenatal diagnosis. In addition, postmortem radiographs can be obtained. These may demonstrate cervicothoracic spinal retroflexion with severe shortening of the spine, ill-defined vertebral bodies, and overcrowding of the ribs that extend upward to the base of the skull (Scherrer et al. 1992).

An autopsy should be performed. This will demonstrate the absence of the neck and the presence of the head positioned directly on top of a markedly shortened trunk. The vertebral column is generally extremely shortened and retroflexed. There may also be fusion of the vertebral bodies and aplasia of ossification centers in the cervicothoracic spine (Scherrer et al. 1992). Multiple associated malformations are generally present (David and Nixon 1976).

▶ SURGICAL TREATMENT

Two reports discuss the same patient who survived to at least 21 months of age (Gartman et al. 1991; Katz et al. 1989) (Fig. 16-1). This was a male infant who was the product of a twin gestation. Prenatal sonographic diagnosis was made at 17 weeks of gestation, but due to expected lethality for the fetus with iniencephaly and the concern that selective termination would harm the other normal twin, the pregnancy was followed conservatively to delivery. The twins were delivered at 36 weeks of gestation by cesarean section following spontaneous rupture of membranes. It was previously decided that no heroic measures would be performed on the infant with iniencephaly. Despite this, he survived and was initially fed by orogastric tube and required oxygen supplementation by hood for 3 days. He was discharged to home at 5 days of age. Initially, feeding was difficult and slow, but he gained weight at a normal rate. At 6 weeks of postnatal age, he had persistent vomiting due to pyloric stenosis and had an uncomplicated pyloromyotomy performed. At 12 weeks of postnatal life, magnetic resonance imaging (MRI) was

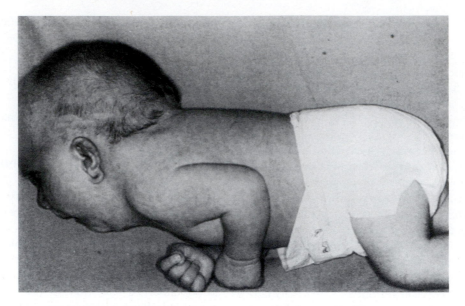

Figure 16-1. Postnatal photograph of a 6-week-old infant with iniencephaly. *(Reprinted, with permission, from Katz VL, Aylsworth AS, Albright SG. Iniencephaly is not uniformly fatal. Prenat Diagn 1989;9:595–599.)*

performed on the head and spine, which demonstrated agenesis of the corpus callosum. At that point, the decision was made to repair the flexion deformity, which was done at 14 weeks of age (Gartman et al. 1991).

During the operation, the subcutaneous fat in the neck was noted to contain many thick fibrous bands, which contributed to the retroflexion deformity. These bands were sectioned. The surgeons noted enlargement of the foramen magnum and an atrophied cerebellar vermis. The infant's head was flexed to a nearly neutral position under direct visualization of the cerebellum and brain stem. A pericranial graft was harvested from the occipital bones. Postoperatively, the patient was maintained in a soft cervical collar. At 7 months of age, MRI demonstrated relief of the brain-stem compression and partial correction of the flexion deformity. The child did well postoperatively, but at 1 year of age hydrocephalus developed, requiring placement of a ventriculoperitoneal shunt.

▶ LONG-TERM OUTCOME

Developmental outcome for the toddler reported by Gartman et al. (1991) and Katz et al. (1989) was at the 9- to 11-month level at 21 months of chronologic age. These authors indicated that formal developmental testing was hampered because restricted cervical flexion limited inferior vision. In addition, gross motor development was delayed due to a decreased range of motion of the shoulders. In infancy, for example, the child could stand but not push up. These authors felt that the developmental outcome was better than that indi-

cated by formal testing, because verbal and social milestones were age-appropriate (Gartman et al. 1991; Katz et al. 1989).

Other long-term survivors with iniencephaly have been reported only rarely.

▶ GENETICS AND RECURRENCE RISK

Little is known about the genetics of iniencephaly because of the rarity of the condition. Based on the similarities between iniencephaly and anencephaly, iniencephaly is considered to be a multifactorial disorder with a presumed 5% recurrence risk (Shoham et al. 1988). In most cases of isolated iniencephaly, the chromosomes have been normal. Prenatal sonographic examination is indicated for future pregnancies.

REFERENCES

David TJ, Nixon A. Congenital malformations associated with anencephaly and iniencephaly. J Med Genet 1976; 13:263–265.

Dogan MM, Ekic E, Yapa EG, Soysal ME, Soysal SK, Gokmen O. Iniencephaly: Sonographic-pathologic correlation of 19 cases. J Perinat Med 1996;24:501–511.

Foderaro AE, Abu-Yousef MM, Benda JA, Williamson RA, Smith WL. Antenatal ultrasound diagnosis of iniencephaly. J Clin Ultrasound 1987;15:550–554.

Gartman JJ, Melin TE, Lawrence WT, Powers SK. Deformity correction and long-term survival in an infant with iniencephaly. J Neurosurg 1991;75:126–130.

Hrgovic Z, Pantiz HG, Kurjak A, Jurkovic D. Contribution to the recognition of iniencephaly on the basis of a new case. J Perinat Med 1989;17:375–379.

Kapoor R, Saha MM. Prenatal diagnosis of iniencephaly—report of 2 cases. Australas Radiol 1987;31:400–403.

Katz VL, Aylsworth AS, Albright SG. Iniencephaly is not uniformly fatal. Prenat Diagn 1989;9:595–599.

Lewis HF. Iniencephalus. Am J Obstet Gynecol 1897;35:11–53.

Meizner I, Levi A, Katz M, Maor E. Iniencephaly: a case report. J Reprod Med 1992;37:885–888.

Munden MM, Macpherson RI, Cure J. Iniencephaly: 3D-computed tomography imaging. Pediatr Radiol 1993;23:572.

Paterson SJ. Iniencephalus. J Obstet Gynaecol Brit Emp 1944;51:330–335.

Rodriguez MM, Reik RA, Carreno TD, Fojaco RM. Cluster of iniencephaly in Miami. Pediatr Pathol 1991;11:211–221.

Saint-Hilaire IG. Histoire des anomalies de l' organisation. Paris: Baillière, 1836:308.

Scherrer CC, Hammer F, Schinzel A, Briner J. Brain stem and cervical cord dysraphic lesions in iniencephaly. Pediatr Pathol 1992;12:469–476.

Sherer DM, Hearn-Stebbins B, Harvey W, Metlay LA, Abramowicz JS. Endovaginal sonographic diagnosis of iniencephaly apertus and craniorachischisis at 13 weeks, menstrual age. J Clin Ultrasound 1993;21:124–127.

Shoham Z, Caspi B, Chemke J, Dgani R, Lancet M. Iniencephaly: prenatal ultrasonographic diagnosis—a case report. J Perinat Med 1988;16:139–143.

CHAPTER 17

Intracranial Hemorrhage

▶ CONDITION

Fetal intracranial hemorrhage refers to bleeding that occurs antenatally from a blood vessel into the ventricles, subdural space, or parenchyma of the brain. Whereas neonatal hemorrhage is a relatively common occurrence, affecting 40 to 60% of infants delivered before 32 weeks of gestation, fetal intracranial hemorrhage is quite rare. Factors that may place the fetus at risk for intracranial hemorrhage include alterations in maternal blood pressure, a maternal seizure disorder, placental abruption, or alloimmune platelet disorders (Kuhn et al. 1992).

Three types of intracranial hemorrhages can occur: periventricular or intraventricular, intraparenchymal, and subdural. Periventricular or intraventricular hemorrhages are the most common, emanating from small vessels within the subependymal germinal matrix before 33 weeks of gestation (McGahan et al. 1984). The pathogenesis of intraventricular hemorrhage (IVH) is related to fragility of the capillary bed of germinal matrix, a disproportionate amount of total cerebral blood flow to the periventricular area, and the lack of auto-regulation of cerebral blood flow in the fetus or premature infant.

Sonographic diagnosis of fetal intracranial hemorrhage was first reported in 1982 in a woman with recurrent episodes of pancreatitis and a fetal death at 29 weeks of gestation (Kim and Elyaderani 1982). Subsequently, the majority of reported antenatally detected cases of intracranial hemorrhage have occurred during the third trimester (Catanzarite et al. 1995).

Parenchymal hemorrhages may be identified as distinct echogenic areas within the cerebral tissue, with or without displacement of the underlying ventricular or outer surfaces of the brain. As these hemorrhages evolve, they become hypoechoic and flattened as the hematoma liquefies. Residual changes may include development of a porencephalic cyst or ventricular enlargement. Clots in the ventricular system are seen as bright echogenic areas that are similar to choroid plexus. A subdural hematoma generally presents as fetal macrocephaly, with separation of the skull from the cerebral cortex. Hyperechoic and hypoechoic areas are identified, filling the space between the brain gyri and the skull. The presence of cerebral edema may cause acoustic enhancement of brain gyri. Catanzarite et al. (1995) have reported on the diagnosis of fetal subdural hemorrhage. They recommended imaging the fetal head in the axial or coronal plane at one level of the sylvian fissure. Normally the separation between the cortex and the inner table of the skull is less than 4 mm. Subdural bleeding can be seen as a collection of echodense material outlining the cortex and separating the sylvian fissure from the inner table of the skull. An additional report on fetal subdural hematoma came from Rottmensch et al. (1991), who identified enhanced echogenicity of the sulci as an indication of brain edema. These authors stated that brain function cannot be predicted sonographically except in the most severe cases.

In a retrospective survey of pregnant women in whom diagnosis of fetal intracranial hemorrhage was made, Achiron et al. (1993) identified five fetuses between 26 and 36 weeks of gestation at the time of diagnosis. They used both transabdominal and transvaginal sonography. In the patients studied by transabdominal sonography, hyperechoic lesions were shown in the brain parenchyma and lateral ventricles in three of five fetuses. Transvaginal sonography permitted enhanced visualization of ventriculomegaly in one fetus and periventricular leukomalacia in the second fetus. Of the five fetuses studied, three were appropriate for gestational age and two were growth-restricted. The two growth-restricted fetuses had abnormal nonstress tests and abnormal flow velocity wave forms, and these infants died after birth. Of the three survivors described in this report, two had normal long-term development and hydrocephalus developed in one. This latter infant suffered from neurodevelopmental retardation and eventually died at age 7 months (Achiron et al. 1993).

In the largest review to date, Vergani et al. (1996) described their experience with six cases diagnosed at the University of Milan and 35 cases identified from the English literature. Of the 41 cases of fetal intracranial hemorrhage reviewed, 20 had isolated IVH, 13 had parenchymal hemorrhage, and eight had subdural or subarachnoid hemorrhage. These investigators devised a prognostic scoring system for IVH. A favorable outcome was seen in 50% (6 of 12) fetuses observed with grade 2 IVH, but none of the fetuses with the equivalent of a grade 3 IVH (blood filling the ventricles) had a favorable outcome.

▶ INCIDENCE

In one study performed at a single institution, the University of Milan, six cases of antenatal intracranial hemorrhage was detected in 6651 fetuses studied. This equals an incidence of 0.9 per 1000 fetuses (Vergani et al. 1996). An unusually high incidence of prenatal subdural intracranial hemorrhage has been documented in Pacific Islanders who emigrate to New Zealand (Becroft et al. 1989). The cause for this high incidence is unknown, but it suspected to be due to traditional forms of abdominal massage used to change fetal position in utero.

In one study, Sims et al. (1985) reviewed the clinical features and neuropathology of intracranial hemorrhage in 433 consecutive stillbirth autopsies. The authors identified 25 cases of periventricular or intraventricular hemorrhage or gliosis. Of the 25 cases, 10 had IVH alone, 5 had IVH plus an additional intraparenchymal hemorrhage, 5 had parenchymal hemorrhage only, and 5 had gliosis, indicating a remote neurologic injury. Other studies have shown that IVH is present in 6% of stillbirths at autopsy (Minkoff et al. 1985).

Immune thrombocytopenic purpura is the most common autoimmune disorder affecting pregnant women, with an incidence of 1 in 1000 to 1 in 10,000 pregnancies. Fewer than 1% of these women will have babies in whom an intracranial hemorrhage develops.

Alloimmune thrombocytopenia develops as a result of maternal sensitization to fetal platelet antigens. This occurs in 1 in 2000 to 1 in 5000 pregnancies. Of these cases, approximately 10 to 30% are at risk for intracranial hemorrhage (Bussel et al. 1988; Johnson et al. 1997).

▶ SONOGRAPHIC FINDINGS

Intracranial hemorrhage is identified as an echogenic area within the ventricles or brain parenchyma. Blood clots are usually echogenic (Fig. 17-1) and evolve to characteristic echolucent cystic areas. The sonographic

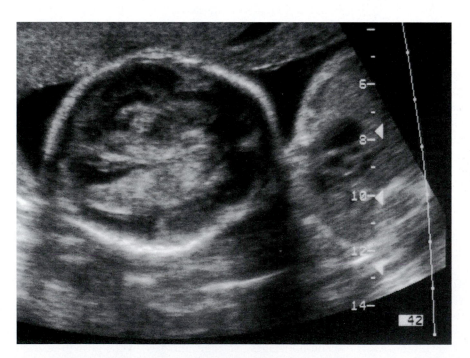

Figure 17-1. Antenatal sonographic image of a twin fetus with a large intracranial hemorrhage. Note the presence of multiple echogenic areas consistent with blood clots.

criteria for an intracranial hemorrhage include the presence of an echogenic mass, unilateral or bilateral ventriculomegaly with the presence of intraventricular echogenic foci, germinal matrix, echogenicity, or the presence of periventricular hypoechoic lesions (cysts).

▶ DIFFERENTIAL DIAGNOSIS

The major considerations in the differential diagnosis include identifying other potential causes of intraparenchymal or intraventricular masses, as well as identifying potential causes for hemorrhage. It is important to rule out the presence of a prominent choroid plexus. This may present as a densely echogenic mass within the ventricles. The choroid plexus can occupy a large proportion of ventricular space, but this is a normal finding with an expected normal prognosis (Kim and Elyaderani 1982). Other causes of an echogenic midbrain mass include intracranial neoplasm or infection.

Considerations in the differential diagnosis of the cause of hemorrhage include coagulopathies such as factor V and X deficiency as well as fetal thrombocytopenia due to maternal immune thrombocytopenia or maternal platelet antigen incompatibility.

▶ ANTENATAL NATURAL HISTORY

Two main factors are implicated in the pathogenesis of neonatal intracranial hemorrhage, and the same factors are relevant for fetal intracranial hemorrhage: sudden changes in cerebral blood pressure, which cause subependymal hemorrhage in the fragile premature capillary bed of germinal matrix, and perinatal asphyxia, with its attendant hypoxia that tends to induce fluctuations in cerebral blood pressure, resulting in intracranial hemorrhage (Volpe 1981). The pathogenesis of spontaneous intrauterine subdural hematoma remains less clear. It has been postulated that subdural hematoma may be due to the presence of intermittent aqueductal obstruction, which results in intermittent decompression. This can result in tearing of bridging veins and the development of subdural hematoma (Atluru and Kumar 1987).

The natural history of intracranial hemorrhage can evolve from bleeding to clot formation to obstruction of spinal fluid drainage, which results in hydrocephalus, or the clot can destroy brain parenchyma and develop into a porencephalic cyst (Fig. 17-2).

Porencephaly is defined as a fluid-filled cavity present within the cerebral hemispheres, which may or may not communicate with the spaces that contain cerebrospinal fluid (Eller and Kuller 1995). A porencephalic cyst results from destruction of cerebral tissues secondary to trauma, infection, or hemorrhage. Type 1 porencephaly is a condition that is acquired during the

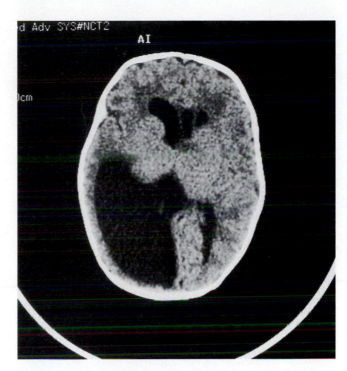

Figure 17-2. Postnatal CT scan taken in an infant noted antenatally to have an intracranial hemorrhage. The scan shows the evolution of the hemorrhage into a massive porencephalic cyst.

third trimester, due to a destructive process. The area of destroyed cerebral parenchyma is replaced with cerebrospinal fluid. The germinal matrix is especially vulnerable to hypoxia and ischemia between 24 to 32 weeks of gestation due to the sparse supportive stroma, delicate vasculature, and increased metabolic activity of this area (Eller and Kuller 1995).

Another complication in the evolution of fetal intracranial hemorrhage is hydranencephaly. Hydranencephaly is a congenital anomaly of the central nervous system marked by absence of cerebral tissue. Hydranencephaly (see Chapter 14) can evolve following a subacute intraparenchymal hemorrhage. Edmondson et al. (1992) described a circumscribed hyperechoic mass that progressively became more sonolucent with increased fluid accumulation and resulted in loss of identifiable cerebral cortex over the left parietal and occipital lobes. Macrocephaly developed. The infant eventually died on day 4 of life. At autopsy, an organizing hematoma and extensive resorption of the underlying cortex was seen, leaving a fluid-filled cavity with a meningeal covering.

▶ MANAGEMENT OF PREGNANCY

The major consideration in the management of pregnancy is to determine the cause of the intracranial hemorrhage. The pregnant patient should be questioned regarding her medical history or the possibility of drug exposure. Maternal conditions associated with fetal intracranial hemorrhage include pancreatitis, preeclampsia, seizures, immune and alloimmune thrombocytopenia, and other disorders of coagulation. Fetal conditions that have been reported to be associated with intracranial hemorrhage include factors V and X deficiency (summarized in Catanzarite et al. 1995). Alterations in maternal blood pressure, such as hypotension or hypertension associated with preeclampsia, can result in fetal intracranial hemorrhage.

An extensive history regarding the possibility of drug exposure should be obtained. For example, maternal exposure to warfarin has been associated with fetal subdural hemorrhage and evolution to hydrocephalus (Robinson et al. 1980; Ville et al. 1993). The pregnant patient who requires anticoagulation should be changed to heparin during pregnancy. In the normal second-trimester fetus, vitamin K_2 is 20% of adult levels and vitamin K_1 is undetectable. Even in subtherapeutic doses, warfarin further reduces the bioavailability of vitamin K to the fetus (Ville et al. 1993). Also, maternal cholestasis and ingestion of cholestyramine can lead to vitamin K deficiency (Sadler et al. 1995). Furthermore, ingestion of aspirin has also been shown to result in fetal hemorrhage (Karlowicz and White 1993). Salicylate competes with vitamin K at prosthetic group sites on enzymes that synthesize coagulant proteins. Cocaine has also been postulated to be important as a cause of fetal intrauterine hemorrhage because cocaine use leads to destructive lesions of the fetal brain, particularly cerebral infarction (Volpe 1992). In another study, however, although maternal cocaine exposure was shown to lead to placental abruption, investigators did not find an association between prenatal cocaine use and fetal or neonatal intracranial hemorrhage (Dusick et al. 1993). Fetal trauma, such as in the traditional Polynesian maternal massage, can result in fetal subdural hemorrhage (Gunn et al. 1988).

The presence of a maternal seizure disorder can predispose to fetal intracranial hemorrhage. Neonates exposed to anticonvulsants in utero can have coagulation defects. Fetal anoxia that occurs during a maternal seizure may lead to redistribution of blood flow to the brain and to arterial hypertension (Minkoff et al. 1985). These authors recommended that the fetus of a patient with a seizure disorder who has seizures during pregnancy should be evaluated after the seizure for the presence of intracranial hemorrhage. They emphasized the importance of strict maternal seizure control.

The fetus identified antenatally with an intracranial hemorrhage may have abnormal fetal heart rate patterns (Catanzarite et al. 1995), a nonreactive nonstress test, fetal tachycardia, or a positive oxytocin challenge test related to fetal anemia. No relationship, however, has been demonstrated between the umbilical and cerebral artery pulsatility index and severe intracranial hemorrhage (Scherjon et al. 1993).

Repeated sonography is indicated to monitor the evolution of the bleeding, to monitor for the development of hydrocephalus, and to check for the presence of hydrops fetalis secondary to fetal anemia. Depending on the cause of the hemorrhage, the fetus may require transfusion with red cells, platelets, and intravenous γ-globulin (in the case of alloimmune thrombocytopenia). Some investigators have suggested daily nonstress tests and contraction stress tests, daily biophysical profiles, and weekly sonography until there is evidence of fetal lung maturity (Pretorius et al. 1986)

Aggressive antenatal management may be indicated for fetuses with alloimmune thrombocytopenia (AIT). Bussel et al. (1988) described antenatal treatment of AIT in seven pregnant women with previously affected infants. These authors gave intravenous γ-globulin with or without dexamethasone, and none of the treated fetuses had intracranial hemorrhage. This therapy either reduces maternal antibody production or transport across the placenta or delays the destruction of antibody-coated platelets in the fetal reticuloendothelial system. A follow-up study by this same group concluded that dexamethasone produced no added therapeutic effect; however, intravenous γ-globulin was appropriate for thrombocytopenic fetuses before the use of weekly in utero platelet transfusions (Bussel et al. 1996).

The serologic diagnosis of AIT can be made by satisfying three requirements: demonstration of a platelet antigen incompatibility between the parents, demonstration of a platelet antibody in maternal serum that binds paternal but not maternal platelets, and identification of an antibody as specific for platelet antigen incompatibility. When a prior sibling has had an antenatal intracranial hemorrhage due to AIT, the clinical manifestations are the same or worse in subsequent fetuses who carry the same antigen (Bussel et al. 1997). To prevent antenatal intracranial hemorrhage, treatment must be initiated as early as possible in the subsequent pregnancy.

We recommend that the fetus with an intracranial hemorrhage be delivered at a tertiary-care center capable of resuscitation of the newborn infant. Cesarean delivery should be considered for fetuses known to have AIT (Burrows et al. 1988).

Aggressive management may or may not be indicated in the case of fetal subdural hematoma. In one report, a fetus with subdural hematoma was detected in utero at 32 weeks of gestation by the presence of multiple blood clots in the subdural space with secondary compression of brain tissue. Cordocentesis detected anemia in the fetus, who was treated aggressively with transfusion of packed red cells and platelets. Following transfusion, the nonstress test and biophysical profile improved, but delivery was delayed to reduce anticipated complications of prematurity. Nine days later, a second episode of intracerebral bleeding occurred, prompting delivery by emergency cesarean section. Despite the aggressive treatment, the infant died at 6 hours of age (Rottmensch et al 1991).

▶ FETAL INTERVENTION

No specific intervention is indicated for the fetus other than transfusion of intravenous γ-globulin and/or platelets.

▶ TREATMENT OF THE NEWBORN

Specific attention should be paid to evidence of increased intracranial pressure, by measurement of the head circumference and palpation of the sutures and fontanelles. The infant should also be specifically examined for the presence of petechiae or ecchymoses as evidence of coagulopathy. A blood count is indicated to determine whether the infant is anemic. Depending on the cause of the hemorrhage, postnatal transfusion with intravenous γ-globulin, packed red blood cells, or platelets lacking an incompatible antigen or steroid therapy in the case of AIT, may be indicated. A diagnostic workup for viral sepsis should also be considered.

Postnatally, cranial anatomy should be assessed by computed tomography (CT) scan or magnetic resonance imaging (MRI). Specific consideration should be given to monitoring for the presence of posthemorrhagic hydrocephalus. Hydrocephalus develops as a consequence of acute obstruction to cerebrospinal fluid flow by a blood clot. If posthemorrhagic hydrocephalus is present, consultation with a neurosurgeon is appropriate.

▶ SURGICAL TREATMENT

If posthemorrhagic hydrocephalus is present, the infant may need the placement of a ventriculoperitoneal shunt to drain cerebrospinal fluid.

▶ LONG-TERM OUTCOME

In their review of 41 antenatally detected cases of intracranial hemorrhage, Vergani et al. (1996) documented that a poor outcome was present in 68% of fetuses. The outcome was directly related to the location and extent of the hemorrhage. A poor outcome was present in 7 of 8 (88%) fetuses with subdural or subarachnoid hemorrhage. Similarly, a poor outcome was present for 12 of 13 (92%) of fetuses with parenchymal hemorrhage. A more favorable prognosis was present for fetuses with IVH, in which 9 of 20 cases (45%) had a poor outcome,

but these were all observed in grade 2 and 3 hemorrhages. Therefore, the presence of a grade 1 IVH observed antenatally is generally associated with a favorable prognosis.

All fetuses with intracranial hemorrhage are at an increased risk for the postnatal development of seizures and cerebral palsy (Scher et al. 1991). Similarly, the potential exists for the prenatal or postnatal developmental of hydrocephalus and neurodevelopmental delay.

The clinical course for fetuses diagnosed with AIT is more variable. The outcome ranges from benign resolution within 2 to 3 weeks after birth to an occasional fatal hemorrhage (Kuhn et al. 1992).

▶ GENETICS AND RECURRENCE RISK

The genetic causes of intracranial hemorrhage include the platelet disorders and the coagulopathies. Every attempt should be made to diagnose the underlying basis of the hemorrhage, as a number of the coagulopathies that involve protein or factor deficiencies are inherited in an autosomal dominant manner and are expected to have a 50% risk of recurrence.

Ninety-eight percent of the population of fetuses with alloimmune thrombocytopenia are phospholipase A_1 (PLA1)-positive. The transmission of the gene for this platelet antigen is autosomal dominant (Morales and Stroup 1985). Two percent of the population lacks this platelet antigen. Mothers who lack the platelet antigen can be sensitized from fetal platelets carrying this antigen that cross into their circulation. Immunoglobulin G from the sensitized mother then crosses the placenta and causes destruction of the fetal platelets. The affected infant is generally diagnosed only after an initial hemorrhagic episode. The chance of recurrence depends on whether the father of the baby is homozygous, meaning that both of his chromosomes carry the gene for the platelet antigen. If the father is a homozygote, there is a 100% chance of having a subsequently affected child. However, if the father is heterozygous there is only a 50% chance that a subsequent child will inherit the chromosome carrying the gene for PLA1 (Kuhn et al. 1992). A review of the medical literature shows an overall 75% chance of having a subsequently affected child, but it is important to remember that the risk is either 50% or 100% for an individual couple.

For many of the inherited coagulopathies or platelet disorders, parental diagnosis is available on a DNA basis from chorionic villi or amniotic fluid cells, or by obtaining fetal blood at cordocentesis. Because of the relatively high recurrence risk for these conditions, careful sonographic monitoring in a subsequent pregnancy is indicated to monitor for the potential for fetal intracranial hemorrhage.

▶ COND

Macrocepha
greater than
terms *macro*
used interch
cates an inc
drocephalus
ated with su
lesions, an u
ber and Pri
ally weigh le
sidered abr
normal brai
cases of ma
a normal lai

The mo
nign familial
of cases. It is
inant patterr
a male:fema
ley 1981). Is
idence of fa
1972; Pettit
sociated wit
18.1, such
Beckwith–W
and achondr
son 1969).

Several
with macroc
tiple hemar
1960). Consi
the nomencl
cephaly–han
nayan–Riley
Macrocephal

REFERE

Achiron R, F
  hemorrha;
  graphic di
Atluru VL, K
  hematoma
  Pediatr Ne
Becroft DMC
  Pacific Isl;
  NZ Med J
Burrows RF,
  thrombocy
  hemorrha;
Bussel, JB, I
  ment of a
  gamma-gl
  low-dose
  Obstet Gy
Bussel JB, B
  U. Antena
  cytopenia
Bussel JB, Z
  alloimmur
  22–26.
Catanzarite '
  natal sonc
  case with
  of the lite
Dusick AM,
  tracranial
  cocaine e:
  weight inl
Edmondson
  tion of hy
  rhage. Ot
Eller KM, Ki
  ogy, diagi
  50:684–68
Gunn TR, M
  secondary
  Obstet Gy
Johnson JA,
  Prenatal c
  immune t
  45–52.
Karlowicz M
  a term ne
  acid inges

CHAPTER 19

Myelomeningocele

► CONDITION

Neural-tube defects are the second most prevalent neonatal anomaly in the United States, ranking behind only cardiac malformations. Worldwide, 400,000 infants are born each year with a neural-tube defect (Rieder 1994). Myelomeningocele is an open spinal-cord defect that protrudes dorsally, is not covered by skin, and is usually associated with spinal-nerve paralysis. Technically, *spina bifida* refers to a cleft or opening in the vertebral body; this term is also used to collectively describe a group of disorders that involve the spinal cord. Lumbosacral lipomas are subcutaneous masses of fat in the lumbosacral region (Shurtleff and Lemire 1995). Myelomeningoceles are malformations that result from failure of the neural tube to fuse during early embryogenesis, at approximately 26 days postovulation, when the caudal neuropore is closing. Skin-covered defects, such as lipomyelomeningocele, result from abnormalities in secondary neurulation and retrogressive differentiation occurring between days 28 and 56 postovulation (Shurtleff and Lemire 1995).

The first medical report of a myelomeningocele was made by a Dutch physician, Nicholas Tulp, who practiced between 1593 and 1674. He described a series of six cases of patients with spina bifida (Tulp, 1716).

"Open" neural-tube defects are myelomeningoceles that are not covered by skin. Leakage of α-fetoprotein (AFP) from the cerebrospinal fluid (CSF) into the amniotic fluid results in an increased transport of AFP into the maternal circulation. Screening by maternal serum AFP analysis has resulted in an increased ability to detect these lesions prenatally.

Herniation of the spinal cord probably reduces intraspinal pressure. This allows the hindbrain to become downwardly displaced, resulting in the Chiari type II malformation, which is seen almost exclusively in patients affected with myelodysplasia. It is characterized by caudal movement of the cerebellar vermis, brain stem, and fourth ventricle. The Chiari type II malformation is responsible for many of the deaths during the first two years of life seen in patients affected with myelodysplasia. Chiari, a professor of pathology in Prague, wrote two papers in 1891 and 1896 that described four types of pathologic changes occurring in 40 affected patients (Rauzzino and Oakes, 1995). These changes concerned the abnormal position of the cerebellum in relation to the foramen magnum. Arnold, in contrast, published a single case report in 1894 that described a single patient with myelodysplasia and other congenital anomalies (Rauzzino and Oakes 1995).

► INCIDENCE

The incidence and live-birth prevalence of myelomeningocele are correlated strongly with ethnic and geographic factors. The highest frequencies of neural-tube defects are found in Great Britain, Ireland, Pakistan, Northern India, Egypt, and Arab countries. The lowest incidences are found in Finland, Japan, and Israel. Even in the United States, a geographic distribution of these defects occurs, with the frequency being the highest in the East and the South, and the lowest in the West (Harmon et al. 1995). There is an increased incidence of neural-tube defects in Hispanics, especially if the mother was born in Mexico (Shaw et al. 1994).

The live-birth prevalence of infants with myelomeningocele has changed dramatically since the advent of widespread maternal serum screening for AFP. Before 1980, the live-birth prevalence of infants with neural-tube defects was between 1.5 and 4.5 per 1000 live births. After 1980, this decreased to 0.74 to 2.5 per 1000 live births (Shurtleff and Lemire 1995). In the

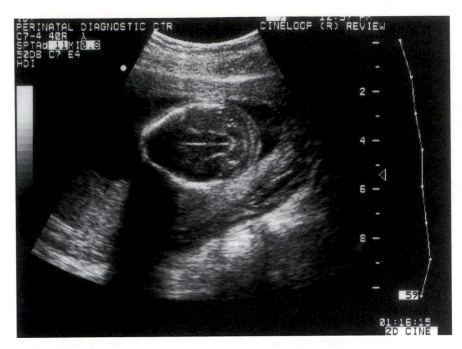

Figure 19-2. Suboccipital bregmatic view of a fetal head demonstrating the "banana sign," which derives from anterior curving of the cerebellar hemispheres with simultaneous obliteration of the cisterna magna.

normal parallel configuration of the vertebral arches (Fig. 19-3). In the transverse plane, ossification centers in the neural arch either diverge or take on a **U**-shaped configuration (Fig. 19-4). The presence of scoliosis or kyphosis is associated with neural-tube defects.

Other sonographic findings that may suggest a myelomeningocele include a cystic meningeal sac, which may have a shimmering effect with fetal motion

(Fig. 19-5) (Budorick et al. 1995). The sonographer should also examine the fetus's lower extremities for the possibility of clubbed feet.

The incidence of associated anomalies in meningomyelocele is lower in reports derived from living children versus those in autopsy series. In one series of 181 patients with myelodysplasia, 5 had renal malformations and 3 had congenital heart disease (Kreder et al. 1992).

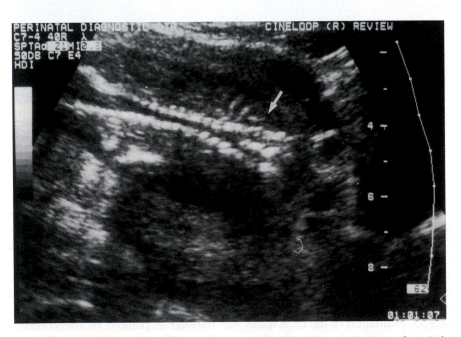

Figure 19-3. Sonographic view of fetal spine demonstrating widening of vertebral arches in a case of meningomyelocele. *(Photograph courtesy of Dr. Michael Paidas.)*

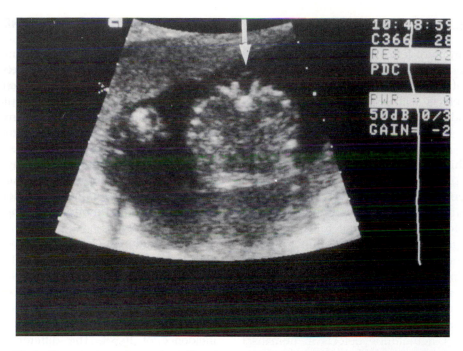

Figure 19-4. Transverse view of ossification centers in the neural arch with a U-shaped configuration.

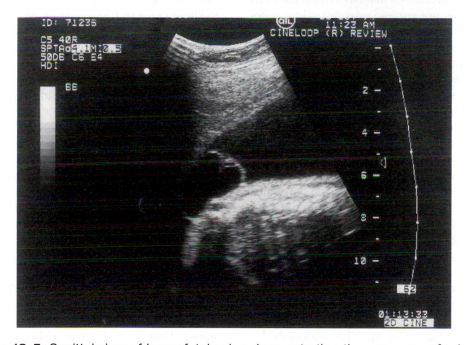

Figure 19-5. Sagittal view of lower fetal spine demonstrating the presence of a large sac. *(Photograph courtesy of Dr. Marjorie Treadwell.)*

▶ DIFFERENTIAL DIAGNOSIS

The differential diagnosis for myelomeningocele includes isolated hemivertebrae (see Chapter 95). The lemon sign, as stated earlier, has also been seen in encephalocele (see Chapter 11), thanatophoric dysplasia (see Chapter 100), cystic hygroma (see Chapter 32), and craniosynostosis (see Chapter 9 and Fig. 19-1 B). The demonstration of a mass near the fetal sacrum must also call to mind the possible diagnosis of sacrococcygeal teratoma (see Chapter 116). Sacrococcygeal teratomas are large cystic or solid masses arising from the coccyx. These masses may be associated with fetal hydrops or polyhydramnios. If the fetal sacral bones cannot be visualized, considerations in the differential diagnosis also include the caudal regression syndrome and sirenomelia (see Chapter 87).

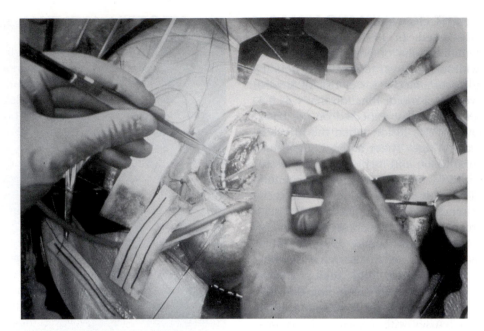

Figure 19-7. Intraoperative view of fetal surgical procedure to repair the meningo-myelocele seen on the MRI in Figure 19-6. The cyst has been excised and skin flaps have been mobilized and a valved shunt is being inserted just prior to completing the skin closure.

Postnatal MRI revealed that the Arnold–Chiari type II malformation was no longer present and there was no hydrocephalus. Developmental milestones at 6 months of age were within normal limits. These authors concluded that in utero repair of neural-tube defects may prevent the secondary complications of an Arnold–Chiari malformation, including the need for postnatal shunt procedures (Adzick et al. 1998). Other authors have described the successful repair of myelomeningocele in utero (Bruner et al. 1999; Dias et al. 1999; Tulipan and Bruner 1998). MRI scans of four infants who had undergone intrauterine myelomeningocele repair were compared to a retrospective group of controls. In the infants who were treated antenatally, there was no evidence of hindbrain herniation while other stigmata of the Chiari II malformation persisted (Tulipan et al. 1998). These authors hypothesized that intrauterine repair may decrease the morbidity associated with the Chiari II malformation, including brainstem dysfunction, hydrocephalus, and syringomyelia. Preliminary reports are now appearing in literature using an endoscopic approach to cover the neural tube defect in utero (Bruner et al. 1999).

▶ TREATMENT OF THE NEWBORN

The newborn infant with myelomeningocele should be handled in as sterile a manner as possible. The lesion should be immediately covered with warm physiologic Ringer's lactate or normal saline. A firm, protective ring of sterile dressings should be placed around the sac, and the sac should be covered with a nonadhesive dressing (Hahn 1995; Shurtleff and Lemire 1995). If the infant needs to be intubated, this should be performed in the prone or in the lateral recumbent position. At all times, normothermia must be maintained.

An initial physical examination should be performed by the neonatologist and the pediatric neurologist or neurosurgeon to assess the functional level and the extent of the neurologic deficit. The sensory level can be determined by stimulating dermatomes with pinpricks. The spinal column should be examined for evidence of early scoliosis or kyphosis. Consideration should be given to performing a cranial computed tomographic (CT) and/or MRI scan so that the neurosurgeon can plan the surgical approach. The parents should be informed that if hydrocephalus is not present antenatally, it may develop after repair of the neural-tube defect. Generally, if a shunt is necessary, it is placed before subsequent urologic or orthopedic repair.

The Arnold–Chiari type II malformation is present in 95% of patients with myelomeningocele. In 6% of affected patients, central ventilatory dysfunction may be present, as demonstrated by central apnea, stridor, respiratory distress, or aspiration. Bulbar involvement may result in vocal-cord paralysis or dysphagia. Unfortunately, approximately half of all newborns with meningomyelocele have pneumographic abnormalities or abnormal responses to increasing CO_2 content in inspired air (Petersen et al. 1995). Therefore, standard tests of respiratory function are not useful to predict which infants will become symptomatic because of an Arnold–Chiari malformation.

▶ SURGICAL TREATMENT

The earliest recorded surgical treatment of a child with spina bifida was performed in 1910 (Hahn 1995). With the development of antibiotics, there was increased interest in treating this condition. It is currently recommended that surgical closure should occur within the first 24 to 48 hours of life to decrease morbidity and mortality.

Exposure of neural tissue to trauma during birth potentially causes a shock-like state to the neural placode. The goals of operative repair include preserving all viable neural tissue, reconstituting a normal anatomic environment, and minimizing the chance of infection or preventing ascending infection of the neural axis (Hahn 1995). During repair, the neurosurgeon must:

1. Identify the neural placode, intermediate epithelial layer, and the pia, arachnoid, and dura.
2. Preserve neural tissues.
3. Reconstitute a normal neural environment with reconstitution of the pia—arachnoidal, dural, fascial, and skin layers.
4. Complete skin closure.
5. Prevent leakage of cerebrospinal fluid (Pang 1995).

The operative mortality for myelomeningocele repair is near 0%. Currently there is expected to be a 95% or higher survival rate for the first 2 years of life (Hahn 1995).

Hydrocephalus develops in 80% of cases of myelomeningocele. This is often not apparent until the neural-tube defect is repaired. It is not uncommon to require a shunt placement within a few days after neural-tube defect repair.

▶ LONG-TERM OUTCOME

The long-term considerations for the infant and child with myelomeningocele include neuromuscular and urologic function, as well prevention of orthopedic abnormalities. To stand erect, motor function is needed to at least the third lumbar level. To walk, the child must exhibit motor function from the fourth to the fifth lumbar level. To function sexually as an adult, the individual must have motor function to at least the second to fourth sacral level.

The degree of handicap and survival rate depends on the level of spinal segments, the severity of the lesion, the treatment program, and the associated anomalies (Budorick et al. 1995). The lower the spinal level,

the better the prognosis. Prediction of long-term IQ is impossible. Approximately one-fourth of patients have an IQ below 50, one-fourth of patients have an IQ above 100, and 50% of patients have a learning disability (Budorick et al. 1995).

The Arnold–Chiari malformation is the most common cause of death. Hindbrain dysfunction causes death within the first year of life in 10 to 15% of patients (Rauzzino and Oakes 1995). Symptomatic patients present with apnea, aspiration, swallowing difficulties, and opisthotonos. Considerations for surgical decompression of the hindbrain include:

1. Inspiratory stridor at rest.
2. Aspiration pneumonia due to palatal dysfunction or gastroesophageal reflux.
3. The presence of central apnea with or without cyanosis, especially during sleep.
4. Opisthotonos.
5. Functionally significant or progressive spasticity of the upper extremities or truncal or appendicular ataxia (Rauzzino and Oakes 1995).

In recent years, there has been an increased appreciation of the long-term consequences of renal failure in adulthood (Zawin and Lebowitz 1992). Therefore, urologic management is more aggressive and directed toward maintaining normal renal function (Stone 1995). After the neural-tube defect has been closed and a shunt has been placed, urodynamic studies are recommended. If the patient has high pressures due to bladder–sphincter dyssynergia, a voiding cystourethrogram (VCUG) can be performed to rule out vesicoureteric reflux. For many cases, anticholinergics or smooth muscle relaxants are recommended to alter the overreactivity of the abnormal detrusor. This treatment is meant to increase the capacity of the bladder. Prophylactic antibiotics are used to prevent urinary tract infection. Children are taught how to perform clean, intermittent bladder catheterization. This technique safely and effectively empties the bladder, preventing both upper-tract deterioration and overflow incontinence (Zawin and Lebowitz 1992). If frequent urinary tract infection is a problem, a vesicostomy can be performed, creating a fistula between the bladder and the abdominal wall. Eighty percent of children with neural-tube defects achieve continence by intermittent catheterization and the use of anticholinergic medications.

Surgical treatment is complicated by a widespread latex allergy seen in affected children.

The presence of myelodysplasia can lead to musculoskeletal deformities. The goals of the orthopedic surgeon are to maintain mobile and pain-free joints, as well as to prevent decubitus ulcers in insensate limbs (Karol 1995). The spine is at risk for the subsequent development of kyphosis and scoliosis. Significant spine deformities that require surgery develop in 10% of

▶ **TABLE 20-1.** CLASSIFICATION OF MICROCEPHALY BY ETIOLOGY

Microcephaly with Associated Malformations		Microcephaly without Associated Malformations
Genetic		Genetic
Chromosomal abnormalities		Primary microcephaly
Trisomy 21		Alpers syndrome
Trisomy 13		Paine syndrome
Trisomy 18		Inborn errors of metabolism
Trisomy 22		Disorders of folic acid metabolism
4p−		Hyperlysinemia
5p−		Methylmalonic acidemia
18p−		Phenylketonuria
18q−		
Single gene defects	Mode of inheritance	
Angelman syndrome	Deletion 15q	
Bloom syndrome	Autosomal recessive	
Borjeson-Forssman-Lehmann syndrome	Sex-linked recessive	
Cockayne syndrome	Autosomal recessive	
Coffin-Siris syndrome	Autosomal recessive	
DeLange syndrome	Autosomal dominant ?	
DeSanctis-Cacchione syndrome	Autosomal recessive	
Dubowitz syndrome	Autosomal recessive	
Fanconi pancytopenia	Autosomal recessive	
Focal dermal hypoplasia	X-linked dominant	
Incontinentia pigmenti	X-linked dominant	
Johanson-Blizzard syndrome	Autosomal recessive	
Langer-Giedion syndrome	Deletion 8q	
Lissencephaly syndrome	Autosomal recessive	
Meckel-Gruber syndrome	Autosomal recessive	
Menkes syndrome	Sex-linked recessive	
Roberts syndrome	Autosomal recessive	
Rubinstein-Taybi syndrome	Autosomal dominant/ new mutation	
Seckel bird-headed dwarfism	Autosomal recessive	
Smith-Lemli-Opitz syndrome	Autosomal recessive	
Williams syndrome	Elastin mutation	
Environmental		Environmental
Prenatal exposure to infections		Prenatal exposure to radiation
Rubella syndrome		Fetal malnutrition
Cytomegalovirus disease		Perinatal trauma or hypoxia
Herpes virus		Postnatal infections
Toxoplasmosis		
Varicella zoster		
Prenatal exposure to drugs or chemicals		
Fetal alcohol syndrome		
Fetal hydantoin syndrome		
Vitamin A or vitamin A analogues		
Aminopterin syndrome		
Cocaine exposure		
Methylmercury exposure		
Solvent exposure: toluene, gasoline		
Carbon monoxide poisoning		
Irradiation		
Maternal phenylketonuria		

Adapted from: Ross JJ, Frias JL: Microcephaly. In "Handbook of Clinical Neurology." Amsterdam: Elsevier Holland Biomedical Press, Vol 30, pp 507–524 1977. 1993.

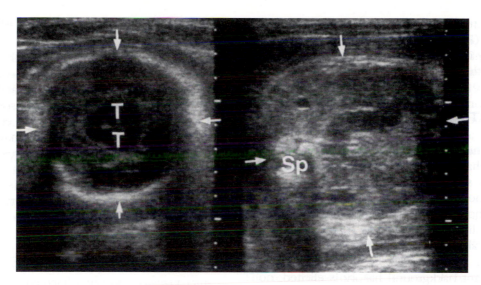

Figure 20-1. Prenatal sonographic image of the head of a 35-week-old fetus (on left), which is considerably smaller than its abdomen (shown on the right). T = thalami, Sp = spine. *(Reprinted, with permission, from Romero R, Pilu G, Jeanty P, et al. Microcephaly. In: Romero R, Pilu G, Jeanty P, Ghidini A, Hobbins JC, eds. Prenatal diagnosis of congenital anomalies. Norwalk, CT: Appleton and Lange, 1988:54–59.)*

fetal head and abdominal circumferences is invariably present (Fig. 20-1). The use of head circumference rather than biparietal diameter (BPD) is more appropriate in the diagnosis of microcephaly. The BPD can be inaccurate in breech presentations and conditions that cause intrauterine molding, such as oligohydramnios and multiple gestation. By contrast, the fetal head circumference should not be affected by molding. One series found that a BPD smaller than 3 SD below the mean was associated with a normal outcome in 44% of cases (Chervenak et al. 1984). This high incidence of falsely abnormal results was probably due to the inclusion of fetuses with simple intrauterine molding. In a later series of 24 fetuses with BPD values of more than 3 SD below the mean, only 4 proved to have microcephalyc after birth, and 3 of these 4 fetuses had additional major malformations (Chervenak et al. 1987).

Microcephaly may also be diagnosed based on an abnormal ratio of head circumference to femur length or of head circumference to abdominal circumference. Normograms for these ratios have been published (Romero et al. 1988). A diagnosis of microcephaly should be made with caution when using such normograms, because some causes of microcephaly may be associated with intrauterine growth restriction or abnormal long bone growth.

When microcephaly is present, the most affected part of the fetal brain is the forebrain. This has prompted investigators to evaluate the role of frontal-lobe measurements in the diagnosis of microcephaly. Ultrasonographic measurements of the frontal lobe and thalamic-frontal-lobe distance were below 2 SD in three cases of microcephaly diagnosed in utero and confirmed af-

ter birth (Goldstein et al. 1988). In two of the three cases, other conventional diagnostic measurements (BPD, occipitofrontal diameter, and head circumference) were also reduced. In one case in which the conventional parameters were equivocal, the authors found that additional measurements of the frontal lobe were diagnostic of microcephaly. Neonatal evaluation confirmed the diagnosis. The authors advocate adding the frontal-lobe and the thalamic-frontal-lobe measurements to other conventional measurements to enhance the prenatal detection of microcephaly (see Fig. 20-1).

In a report on the prospective prenatal diagnosis of microcephaly in 21 pregnancies occurring in 15 families with a previously affected child with microcephaly, serial measurements of the fetal head, abdomen, and femur were made by ultrasound examination at intervals of approximately four weeks (Tolmie et al. 1987). Four fetuses with microcephaly were detected in the third trimester. One affected fetus was missed because no scans were performed after 24 weeks of gestation. The main reason for late diagnosis of affected fetuses was that the head growth did not slow appreciably until the third trimester (Tolmie ct al. 1987). Therefore, a diagnosis of microcephaly cannot be excluded by ultrasonography performed during the second trimester of pregnancy.

A detailed fetal sonographic evaluation for associated anomalies should be performed in all cases. In the absence of associated abnormalities the diagnosis of microcephaly is made on the basis of the head circumference alone.

More recently, power Doppler ultrasonography has been used during the second trimester to diag-

population-based study from British Columbia that attempted total ascertainment, a 6% recurrence risk for microcephaly with mental retardation was noted (Herbst and Baird 1982). It was not clear from this study whether microcephaly was defined as a head circumference of less than 2 or less than 3 SD below the mean. In a further series, a recurrence risk of 19% was reported from 29 cases of microcephaly in a referral genetic service for the west of Scotland (Tolmie et al. 1987).

A possible explanation for the higher risk of recurrence found in selected population studies (Bartley and Hall 1978; Bundey and Carter 1974; Tolmie et al. 1987) in comparison to other studies (Herbst and Baird 1982) may be ascertainment bias. Nevertheless, these studies provide a useful source of information for prenatal diagnosis and counseling of parents with a diagnosis of fetal microcephaly.

REFERENCES

Alzial C, Dufier JL, Aicardi J, et al. Ocular abnormalities of true microcephaly. Ophthalmologica 1980;180:333–339.

Avery GB, Meneses L, Lodge A. The critical significance of measurement microcephaly. Am J Dis Child 1972;123:214–217.

Bartley JA, Hall BD. Mental retardation and multiple congenital anomalies of unknown etiology: frequency of occurrence in similarly affected sibs of the proband. Birth Defects 1978;14:127–137.

Book JA, Schut JW, Reed SC. A clinical and genetical study of microcephaly. Am J Ment Defic 1953;57:637–660.

Brandon MWG, Kirman BH, Williams CE. Microcephaly. J Ment Sci 1959;105:721–747.

Bundey S, Carter CO. Recurrence risks in severe undiagnosed mental deficiency. J Ment Defic Res 1974;18:115–134.

Bundey S, Griffiths MI. Recurrence risks in families of children with symmetrical spasticity. Dev Med Child Neurol 1977;19:179–191.

Chervenak FA, Jeanty P, Cantraine F, et al. The diagnosis of fetal microcephaly. Am J Obstet Gynecol 1984;149:512–517.

Chervenak FA, Rosenberg J, Brightman RC, et al. A prospective study of the accuracy of ultrasound in predicting fetal microcephaly. Obstet Gynecol 1987;69:908–910.

Cowie VA. Microcephaly: a review of genetic implications in its causation. J Ment Defic Res 1987;31:229–233.

Davies H, Kirman BH. Microcephaly. Arch Dis Child 1962;37:623.

Dolk H. The predictive value of microcephaly during the first year of life for mental retardation at seven years. Dev Med Child Neurol 1991;33:.974–983.

Goldstein I, Reece EA, Pilu G, et al. Sonographic assessment of the fetal frontal lobe: a potential tool for prenatal diagnosis of microcephaly. Am J Obstet Gynecol 1988;158:1057–1062.

Herbst DS, Baird PA. Sib risks for non-specific mental retardation in British Columbia. Am J Med Genet 1982:13:197–208.

Hughes HE, Miskin M. Congenital microcephaly due to vascular disruption: in utero documentation. Pediatrics 1986;78:85–87.

Hunter AGW. Brain. In: Stevenson RE, Hall JG, Goodman RM, eds. Human malformations and related anomalies. Vol. 2. New York: Oxford University Press, 1993:1–19.

Martin HP. Microcephaly and mental retardation. Am J Dis Child 1970;119:128–131.

Myrianthopoulos NC, Chung CS. Congenital malformations in singletons: epidemiological survey: report from the Collaborative Perinatal Project. Birth Defects 1974;10:1–58.

Nelson KB, Deutschberger J. Head size at one year as a predictor of four year IQ. Dev Med Child Neurol 1970;12:487–495.

Opitz JM, Kaveggia EG, Durkin-Stamm MV, et al. Diagnostic/genetic studies in severe mental retardation. Birth Defects 1978;14:1–38.

Penrose LS. The biology of mental defect. 4th ed. London: Sidgwick and Jackson, 1972:170–174.

Persutte WH, Kurczynski TW, Chaudhuri K, et al. Prenatal diagnosis of autosomal dominant microcephaly and postnatal evaluation with magnetic resonance imaging. Prenat Diagn 1990;10:631–642.

Pilu G, Falco P, Milano V, et al. Prenatal diagnosis of microcephaly assisted by vaginal sonography and power Doppler. Ultrasound Obstet Gynecol 1998;11:357–360.

Romero R, Pilu G, Jeanty P, et al. Microcephaly. In: Romero R, Pilu G, Jeanty P, Ghidini A, Hobbins JC, eds. Prenatal diagnosis of congenital anomalies. Norwalk, CT: Appleton and Lange, 1988:54–59.

Ross JJ, Frias JL. Microcephaly. In: Vipken PJ and Bruyn, AW, ed. Handbook of clinical neurology. Vol. 30. Amsterdam: Elsevier, 1977:507–524.

Sells CJ. Microcephaly in a normal school population. Pediatrics 1977;59:262–265.

Sherer DM, Abramowicz JS, Jaffe R, et al. Twin-twin transfusion with abrupt onset of microcephaly in the surviving recipient following spontaneous death of the donor twin. Am J Obstet Gynecol 1993;169:85–88.

Siber M. X-linked recessive microencephaly, microphthalmia with corneal opacities, spastic quadriplegia, hypospadias and cryptorchidism. Clin Genet 1984;26:453–456.

Tenconi R, Clementi M, Audino G. Autosomal dominant microcephaly. J Pediatr 1983;102:644.

Tolmie JL, McNay M, Stephenson JBP. Microcephaly: genetic counseling and antenatal diagnosis after the birth of an affected child. Am J Med Genet 1987;27:583–594.

Van Den Bosch J. Microcephaly in the Netherlands: a clinical and genetical study. Ann Hum Genet 1959;23:91–116.

Volpe JJ. Neurology of the newborn. Philadelphia: Saunders, 1987:36.

Warkany J, Lemire RJ, Cohen MM. Mental retardation and congenital abnormalities of the nervous system. Chicago: Year Book, 1981:13–40.

Webster MH, Smith CS. Congenital anomalies and maternal herpes zoster. BMJ 1977;2:1193.

CHAPTER 21

Porencephaly

▶ CONDITION

The term *porencephaly* is often used interchangeably with *porencephalic cyst, schizencephaly, cystic brain degeneration,* and *congenital brain clefts*. Porencephaly was first described in 1859 as a cavity or cleft of the cerebral cortex (Heschl 1859). These lesions may or may not communicate with the ventricular and subarachnoid systems. Two major subgroups are described: developmental porencephaly, which includes schizencephaly and simple porencephaly and congenital encephaloclastic porencephaly (Hall 1993).

Developmental porencephaly represents primary failure of neuronal development and migration. Synonyms include *true porencephaly, schizencephaly,* and *congenital porencephaly*. Congenital midline porencephaly is a more recently described malformation, consisting of the triad of a midline parietal scalp anomaly (such as alopecia or cephalocele), hydrocephalus, and a midline intracranial cyst (Vintzileos et al. 1987; Yokota and Matsukado 1979). While this malformation most likely represents a form of porencephaly, some authors consider it a variant of holoprosencephaly (Vintzileos et al. 1987).

In contrast, congenital encephaloclastic porencephaly results from cortical destruction due to an external insult in an otherwise normal brain. Synonyms include *pseudoporencephaly, false porencephaly,* and *cystic brain degeneration*. This destruction results in an intracerebral cystic cavity containing cerebrospinal fluid, and such a cyst may be single or multiple (Fig. 2-1) (Hall 1993). Congenital encephaloclastic porencephaly may have many different causes; of these, fetal vascular occlusion is considered the most common (Dekaban 1965; Nixon et al. 1974). The cause of fetal vascular occlusion is usually unknown but has been reported in the surviving fetus of a monochorionic twin pregnancy with a single intrauterine death (Jung et al. 1984), and

also following in utero exposure to cocaine (Dominguez et al. 1991). Other causes of porencephaly include inflammatory diseases, such as coxsackievirus or cytomegalovirus infection (Chalhub et al. 1977; Tominaga et al. 1963); trauma resulting from ventricular puncture

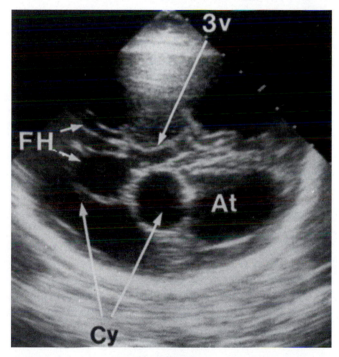

Figure 21-1. Prenatal sonographic image demonstrating the presence of multiple cystic lesions (Cy) within the cerebral parenchyma in a fetus with infectious pseudoporencephaly. An asymmetric enlargement of the lateral ventricles is also seen. At = atria of lateral ventricles; FH = frontal horns of lateral ventricle; 3v = third ventricle. *(Reprinted, with permission, from Romero R, Pilu G, Jeanty P, et al. Porencephaly. In: Romero R, Pilu G, Jeanty P, Ghidini A, Hobbins JC, eds. Prenatal diagnosis of congenital anomalies. Norwalk, CT: Appleton & Lange, 1988:50–52.)*

(Lorber and Grainger 1963), amniocentesis (Eller and Kuller 1994), or chorionic villus sampling (Sharma and Phadke, 1991); and vascular insults from hemorrhage or embolism (Cantue and LeMay 1967). Familial porencephaly consistent with both autosomal dominant and recessive patterns of inheritance has also been reported (Berg et al. 1983; Haverkamp et al. 1995; Sensi et al. 1990).

▶ INCIDENCE

Porencephaly is an extremely rare condition whose incidence is unknown.

▶ SONOGRAPHIC FINDINGS

Porencephaly has been successfully diagnosed prenatally using both sonography and magnetic resonance imaging (Komarniski et al. 1990; Levine et al. 1997; Lithuania et al. 1989; Meizner and Elchalal, 1996; Pilu et al. 1997). The sonographic appearance is that of a fluid-filled space in the normal brain parenchyma. The cyst is more commonly unilateral but may be bilateral (Fig. 21-2). When cysts are multiple they are frequently symmetric in appearance (Klingensmith and Cioffi-Ragan 1986). Loss of cerebral tissue is often easily visible on coronal scans. Color Doppler sonography may be helpful in delineating a particular vascular abnormality associated with the cystic lesion (Suchet 1994). Communication with the lateral ventricles or subarachnoid space is often visible. The ipsilateral ventricle is usually enlarged to compensate for the smaller brain mass. The diagnosis of porencephaly should be considered whenever marked asymmetric ventriculomegaly is found (Chervenak et al. 1983; Toma et al. 1990).

▶ DIFFERENTIAL DIAGNOSIS

The differential diagnosis includes other cystic brain lesions such as arachnoid cyst (see Chapter 6) and, more rarely, cystic tumors (Sauerbrei and Cooperberg 1983). In one case of asymmetric hydrocephalus the diagnosis of porencephaly was suspected but could not be confirmed with an ultrasound examination. Magnetic resonance imaging correctly identified the porencephalic cavity communicating with the lateral ventricle (Toma et al. 1990). If severe hydrocephalus is also present it must be distinguished from hydranencephaly. Hydranencephaly is considered to be an extreme form of encephaloclastic porencephaly.

▶ ANTENATAL HISTORY

In keeping with the vascular cause of many cases of porencephaly, in utero deterioration of porencephalic

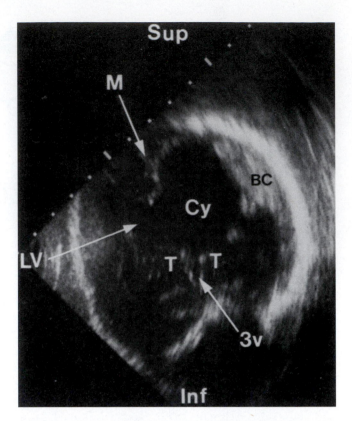

Figure 21-2. Cranial coronal scan of a 30-week-old fetus with severe porencephaly. A large cystic cavity (Cy) occupies most of one hemisphere, and it communicates with the contralateral lateral ventricle (LV). BC = blood clot; Inf = inferior, Sup = superior, T = thalami, M = midline. *(Reprinted, with permission, from Romero R, Pilu G, Jeanty P, et al. Porencephaly. In: Romero R, Pilu G, Jeanty P, Ghidini A, Hobbins JC, eds. Prenatal diagnosis of congenital anomalies. Norwalk, CT: Appleton & Lange, 1988:50–52.)*

cystic masses has been documented (Klingensmith and Cioffi-Ragan 1986). In this case, significant deterioration of cystic areas was noted between ultrasound examinations performed at 31 and at 36 weeks of gestation. In addition, the cystic deterioration corresponded to the distribution of the middle cerebral arteries (Klingensmith and Cioffi-Ragan 1986). Other than this case report, little information is available to guide counseling of the patient with fetal porencephaly.

▶ MANAGEMENT OF PREGNANCY

Serologic testing for cytomegalovirus, coxsackievirus, and toxoplasma should be considered. Because there are no reported associations with chromosomal disorders, amniocentesis for karyotyping is not indicated. The parents should be counseled that the prognosis depends on the location and size of the lesion. However, in almost all cases of true porencephaly, the neonatal outcome will be poor, with severe intellectual and neurologic sequelae (Romero et al. 1988). Neurologic sequelae can include spastic tetraplegia, blindness, and severe speech impediment. Prenatal magnetic resonance imaging may be helpful in differentiating fetal intracranial cystic lesions (Levine et al. 1997). Prenatal consultation with a pediatric neurologist and a neonatalogist is recommended to discuss neonatal management. Termination of pregnancy should be offered, if diagnosed before 24 weeks of gestation. Delivery should occur in a tertiary-care center. Vaginal delivery should be allowed in almost all cases because of the invariably poor neonatal outcome. In cases of associated macrocephaly initial cephalocentesis to allow vaginal delivery should be considered (Romero et al. 1998).

▶ FETAL INTERVENTION

No fetal intervention has been described for this condition, and none is likely, as porencephaly appears as a result of the absence of cerebral tissue.

▶ TREATMENT OF THE NEWBORN

The infant should be evaluated promptly after birth by a pediatric neurologist. Imaging of the neonatal brain, using sonography and magnetic resonance imaging should be performed to aid in defining the extent of neurologic deficit. The initial signs and symptoms of porencephaly depend on the location of the defect and include seizures, varying degrees of developmental delay, visual and sensory deficits, and hydrocephalus. Porencephaly should be considered in any child with unexplained hemiparesis. The degree of impairment is variable, with some patients initially showing only mild to borderline impairment, while other infants are profoundly impaired (Tardieu et al. 1981; Nixon et al. 1974). No specific treatment is indicated, although appropriate medical therapy to control seizures is often needed.

▶ SURGICAL TREATMENT

In some cases of porencephaly with associated hydrocephalus, there may be a role for surgical intervention to prevent further hydrocephalus-associated injury. This may be especially helpful in cases of a unilateral intracerebral cyst, resulting in a midline shift toward the contralateral side. Progression of impairment may therefore occur, unless a shunt is placed to collapse the cyst (Hall 1993). In one series of nine children with progressive porencephaly, improvement was demonstrated following surgical placement of a ventriculoperitoneal shunt (Tardieu et al. 1981). The authors suggested shunts for any patient with progressive clinical signs of neurologic deterioration. They recommended shunts in patients under 2 years of age in whom a large cyst is demonstrated, with hydrocephalus, macrocephaly, and developmental delay (Tardieu et al. 1981).

▶ LONG-TERM OUTCOME

The long-term outcome for infants with porencephaly depends on the extent of the cystic destruction of cerebral tissue. Minimal data are available for accurate counseling. In most cases there is severe cerebral destruction, and the long-term outcome for such infants is extremely poor. A severe variety of postnatal encephaloclastic porencephaly has been described in 15 neonates with a birth weight of 600 to 1270 g and a gestational age at delivery of 24 to 32 weeks (Cross et al. 1992). Cerebral ultrasound examinations were characterized by irregular cystic lesions involving the periphery of the brain. Fourteen of the 15 infants died in the first 6 weeks of life, and 8 had clinical evidence of neurologic abnormality resulting in seizures. The only survivor had severe neurologic deficit at 12 months of age (Cross et al. 1992).

▶ GENETICS AND RECURRENCE RISK

In the majority of cases the underlying cause for porencephaly will not be identified. Prevention of encephaloclastic porencephaly may be possible in cases of monochorionic twins with the impending death of one fetus. In such cases, consideration of elective preterm delivery, or fetoscopic cord ligation of the abnormal twin, may prevent porencephaly, which is usually caused by profound hypotension at the time of death of the twin (see Chapter 120).

In general, the recurrence risk for porencephaly is extremely low. However, familial cases of porencephaly have been described, and may be associated with a 25% to 50% chance of recurrence (Berg et al. 1983; Haverkamp et al. 1995; Sensi et al. 1990). The majority of familial cases of porencephaly have shown a dominant inheritance, and the affected parent may only be mildly affected. It is therefore important to maintain a high index of suspicion when deciding whether to investigate possible milder forms of porencephaly in family members.

REFERENCES

Berg RA, Aleck KA, Kaplan AM. Familial porencephaly. Arch Neurol 1983;40:567–569.

Cantu RC, LeMay M. Porencephaly caused by intracerebral hemorrhage. Radiology 1967;88:526–530.

Chalhub EG, Devivo DC, Siegel BA, et al. Coxsackie A9 focal encephalitis associated with acute infantile hemiplegia and porencephaly. Neurology 1977;27:574–579.

Chervenak FA, Berkowitz FL, Romero R, et al. The diagnosis of fetal hydrocephalus. Am J Obstet Gynecol 1983;147:703–716.

Cross JH, Harrison CJ, Preston PR, et al. Postnatal encephaloclastic porencephaly—a new lesion? Arch Dis Child 1992;67:307–311.

Dekaban A. Large defects in cerebral hemispheres associated with cortical dysgenesis. J Neuropathol Exp Neurol 1965;24:512–530.

Dominguez R, Vila-Coro AA, Slopis JM, et al. Brain and ocular abnormalities in infants with in utero exposure to cocaine and other street drugs. Am J Dis Child 1991;145:688–695.

Eller KM, Kuller JA. Porencephaly secondary to fetal trauma during amniocentesis. Am J Hum Genet 1994;55:2210.

Hall JG. In: Stevenson RE, Hall JG, Goodman RM, eds. Human malformations and related anomalies. Volume 2. New York: Oxford University Press, 1993:78–82.

Haverkamp F, Zerres K, Ostertum B, et al. Familial schizencephaly: further delineation of a rare disorder. J Med Genet 1995;32:242–244.

Heschl R. Gehirndefekt und Hydrocelphalus. Prager Vierteljahrsch Prakt Heilkunde 1859;61:59.

Jung JH, Graham JM, Schultz N, et al. Congenital hydranencephaly/porencephaly due to vascular disruption in monozygotic twins. Pediatrics 1984;73:467–469.

Klingensmith WC, Cioffi-Ragan DT. Schizencephaly: diagnosis and progression in utero. Radiology 1986;159:617–618.

Komarniski CA, Cyr DR, Mack LA, et al. Prenatal diagnosis of schizencephaly. J Ultrasound Med 1990;9:305–307.

Levine D, Barnes PD, Madsen JR, et al. Fetal central nervous system anomalies: MR imaging augments sonographic diagnosis. Radiology 1997;204:635–636.

Lithuania M, Passamonti U, Cordone MS, et al. Schizencephaly: prenatal diagnosis by computed sonography and magnetic resonance imaging. Prenat Diagn 1989;9:649–655.

Lorber J, Grainger RG. Cerebral cavities following ventricular punctures in infants. Clin Radiol 1963;14:98.

Meizner I, Elchalal U. Prenatal sonographic diagnosis of anterior fossa porencephaly. J Clin Ultrasound 1996;24:96–99.

Nixon GW, Johns RE Jr, Myers GG. Congenital porencephaly. Pediatrics 1974;54:43–50.

Pilu G, Falco P, Perolo A, et al. Differential diagnosis and outcome of fetal intracranial hypoechoic lesions: report of 21 cases. Ultrasound Obstet Gynecol 1997;9:229–236.

Romero R, Pilu G, Jeanty P, et al. Porencephaly. In: Romero R, Pilu G, Jeanty P, Ghidini A, Hobbins JC (eds). Prenatal diagnosis of congenital anomalies. Norwalk, CT: Appleton & Lange, 1988:50–52.

Sauerbrei EE, Cooperberg PL. Cystic tumors of the fetal and neonatal cerebrum: ultrasound and computed tomographic evaluation. Radiology 1983;147:689–692.

Sensi A, Cerruti S, Calzolari E, et al. Familial porencephaly. Clin Genet 1990;38:396–397.

Sharma AK, Phadke S. Porencephaly: a possible complication of chorion villus sampling? Ind Pediatr 1991;28:1061–1063.

Suchet IB. Schizencephaly: antenatal and postnatal assessment with colour-flow Doppler imaging. Can Assoc Radiol J 1994;45:193–200.

Tardieu M, Evrard P, Lyon G. Progressive expanding congenital porencephalies: a treatable cause of progressive encephalopathy. Pediatrics 1981;68:198–202.

Toma P, Lucigrai G, Ravegnani M, et al. Hydrocephalus and porencephaly: prenatal diagnosis by ultrasonography and MR imaging. J Comput Assist Tomogr 1990;14:843–845.

Tominaga I, Kaihou M, Kimura T, et al. Cytomegalovirus fetal infection: porencephaly with polymicrogyria in a 15-year-old boy. Rev Neurol 1996;152:479–482.

Vintzileos AM, Hovick TJ, Escoto DT, et al. Congenital midline porencephaly: prenatal sonographic findings and review of the literature. Am J Perinatol 1987;4:125–128.

Yokota A, Matsukado Y. Congenital midline porencephaly: a new brain malformation associated with scalp anomaly. Child Brain 1979;5:380–397.

CHAPTER 22

Vein of Galen Aneurysm

► CONDITION

Vein of Galen aneurysm is also referred to as a varix of the vein of Galen or vein of Galen malformation. This anomaly is a complex arteriovenous malformation affecting the vein of Galen and the cerebral arteries. The vein of Galen is a single, midline structure formed by the convergence of the two internal cerebral veins and the basal veins of Rosenthal posterior to the splenium of the corpus callosum; the vein courses posteriorly to empty into the straight sinus. During embryologic development, cerebral arteries and veins cross in close proximity to each other; fistulous connections may exist because only a few cell layers separate these vessels (Padget 1956). These fistulas persist because of an arteriovenous pressure gradient. The size and number of arteriovenous fistulous connections determine the eventual size of a vein of Galen aneurysm.

Aneurysm of the vein of Galen was first described in 1937 by Jaeger and colleagues. The first precise anatomical definitions of these vascular malformations was described in 1960 (Litvak et al. 1960). Malformations of the vein of Galen most probably arise early in embryogenesis in the 20- to 40-mm fetus, when arteries and veins are still simple endothelial tubes (Padget 1956). Following an anatomic analysis of 23 cases of vein of Galen aneurysm, it was concluded that the venous sac most probably represents persistence of the embryonic median prosencephalic vein of Markowski, not the vein of Galen per se (Raybaud et al. 1989). Even though there is plausible evidence that the aneurysmal sac is the persistent embryonic median prosencephalic vein of Markowski rather than the true vein of Galen, this author concluded that it was reasonable to retain the generally accepted nomenclature of *vein of Galen aneurysm,* but to restrict its use to cases in which the arteriovenous fistulas are within the wall of the venous

sac. Vein of Galen aneurysms may be defined as direct arteriovenous fistulas situated between choroidal and/or quadrigeminal arteries and an overlying single median venous sac.

The size of the aneurysm of the vein of Galen determines its clinical presentation. When the aneurysm is large, as much as 50 to 60% of the cardiac output may be shunted through the lesion (Cumming 1980). This arteriovenous shunt may result in high-output congestive heart failure, and these patients tend to present with hydrops in utero, or with cardiac failure in early neonatal life.

Other cases of vein of Galen aneurysm are not associated with cardiac failure and may not present until the first year of life. Hydrocephalus may also occur in association with a large vein of Galen aneurysm, although the cause is uncertain. Possible mechanisms for the development of hydrocephalus include compression of the sylvian aqueduct by the aneurysmal mass and defective cerebrospinal fluid resorption resulting from intracranial venous hypertension (Diebler et al. 1981; Gold et al. 1964).

Cerebral damage including cerebral infarction, periventricular leukomalacia, and hemorrhagic infarction may also occur in association with aneurysm of the vein of Galen (Norman and Becker 1974). Suggested mechanisms by which such cerebral parenchymal injury may occur include:

1. A steal-induced ischemic phenomenon from overlying abnormal vessels.
2. Cerebral ischemia due to compromised perfusion from congestive heart failure.
3. Hemorrhagic infarction from thrombosis of the dilated vein of Galen.
4. Atrophy resulting from compression of adjacent structures by the aneurysm.

therapy with embolization techniques (Friedman et al. 1993). Approximately 50% of neonates suffering from severe progressive cardiac failure can be expected to survive following such embolization techniques (Mickle and Quisling 1994).

► LONG-TERM OUTCOME

Little information is available on the long-term follow-up of prenatally diagnosed cases of vein of Galen aneurysm. In one series of 18 patients diagnosed prenatally, 13 infants survived the immediate neonatal period and 12 underwent embolization of the aneurysm (Rodesch et al. 1994). Total occlusion of the aneurysm was obtained in 8 cases. Sixty-seven percent of the newborns were neurologically normal when assessed with Denver Development Tests (Rodesch et al. 1994).

In another series of 22 patients with vein of Galen aneurysm treated with embolization techniques, there was a 50% mortality rate and a 37% incidence of severe mental retardation in survivors of procedures performed soon after the introduction of the technique (Friedman et al. 1993). For procedures performed after modification of the original technique, there was no mortality, and 6 of the 11 patients were functionally normal at 30 months of follow-up. Two patients had severe neurologic deficiency, and some developmental delay was observed in one other patient. The improvement in outcome results were attributed to earlier diagnosis, improvement in the microcatheters used for embolization, avoidance of overly aggressive neurosurgical procedures, and general improvements in neonatal care (Friedman et al. 1993). In addition, when vein of Galen aneurysm first presents in the older child, results of therapy are more favorable, with mortality rates as low as 20% (Hoffman et al. 1982).

Infants who require shunting for hydrocephalus with vein of Galen aneurysm appear to have a less favorable neurologic outcome (Zerah et al. 1992). For these infants, a significant difference in the clinical outcome was noted between the groups with shunting and those with no shunting (Zerah et al. 1992). Of the patients without shunts, 67% were free of any neurologic deficit or mental retardation, and fewer than 5% had significant mental retardation. In contrast, only 33% of the patients with a shunt had a favorable outcome, and significant mental retardation developed in more than 15% (Zerah et al. 1992). The authors' conclusion was that treatment of hydrocephalus in vein of Galen aneurysm can be achieved through obliteration of the malformation and that shunting should not be the preferred treatment for hydrocephalus in this condition.

The prognosis for patients with thrombosed vein of Galen aneurysm seems to be more favorable. The impact of treatment on outcome for thrombosed vein of Galen aneurysms is controversial. Some authors believe a clotted vein of Galen aneurysm may constitute a risk to the motor and mental development of the patient, whereas others feel that the thrombosed vein may shrink or fibrose without intervention and therefore may not be clinically significant (Six et al. 1980). In one case report of thrombosed vein of Galen aneurysm, spontaneous resolution of hydrocephalus occurred, and shunting was unnecessary (Six et al. 1980). In two other cases radiologic evidence of progressive shrinking of the clotted aneurysm to a residual inert calcification was demonstrated, without the need for therapeutic intervention (Beltramello et al. 1991).

► GENETICS AND RECURRENCE RISK

There have been no reported cases of recurrent vein of Galen aneurysm. The inheritance pattern appears to be sporadic.

REFERENCES

Amacher AL, Shillito J. The syndromes and surgical treatment of aneurysm of the great vein of Galen. J Neurosurg 1973;39:89–98.

Baenziger O, Martin E, Willi U, et al. Prenatal brain atrophy due to a giant vein of Galen malformation. Neuroradiology 1993;35:105–106.

Ballester MJ, Raga F, Serra-Serra V, et al. Early prenatal diagnosis of an ominous aneurysm of the vein of Galen by color Doppler ultrasound. Acta Obstet Gynecol Scand 1994;73:592–595.

Beltramello A, Perini S, Mazza C. Spontaneously healed vein of Galen aneurysms. Child Nerv Syst 1991;7:129–134.

Boldry E, Miller ER. Arteriovenous fistula (aneurysm) of the great cerebral vein (of Galen) and circle of Willis: report on two cases treated by ligation. Arch Neurol Psychiatry 1949;62:77–83.

Ciricillo SF, Edwards MSB, Schmidt KG, et al. Interventional neuroradiological management of vein of Galen malformations in the neonate. Neurosurgery 1990;27:22–28.

Comstock CH, Kirk JS. Arteriovenous malformations: locations and evolution in the fetal brain. J Ultrasound Med 1991;10:361–365.

Cumming GR. Circulation in neonates with intracranial arteriovenous fistula and cardiac failure. Am J Cardiol 1980;45:1019–1024.

Diebler C, Dulac O, Renier D, et al. Aneurysms of the vein of Galen in infants aged 2 to 15 months: diagnosis and natural evolution. Neuroradiology 1981;21:185–197.

Doren M, Tercanli S, Holzgreve W. Prenatal sonographic diagnosis of a vein of Galen aneurysm: relevance of associated malformations for timing and mode of delivery. Ultrasound Obstet Gynecol 1995;6:287–289.

Friedman DM, Verma R, Madrid M, et al. Recent improvement in outcome using transcatheter embolization techniques for neonatal aneurysmal malformations of the vein of Galen. Pediatrics 1993;91:583–586.

Gold AP, Ransohoff J, Carter S. Vein of Galen malformation. Acta Neurol Scand 1964;40:5–31.

Hirsch JH, Cyr D, Eberhardt H, et al. Ultrasonographic diagnosis of an aneurysm of the vein of Galen in utero by duplex scanning. J Ultrasound Med 1983;2:231–233.

Hoffman HJ, Chuang S, Hendrick EB, et al. Aneurysms of the vein of Galen: experience at the Hospital for Sick Children, Toronto. J Neurosurg 1982;57:316–322.

Horowitz MB, Jungreis CA, Quisling RG, et al. Vein of Galen aneurysms: a review and current perspective. Am J Neuroradiol 1994;15:1486–1496.

Jaeger J, Forbes RP, Dandy WE. Bilateral congenital cerebral arteriovenous communications aneurysm. Trans Am Neurol Assoc 1937;63:173–176.

Jeanty P, Kepple D, Roussis P, et al. In utero detection of cardiac failure from an aneurysm of the vein of Galen. Am J Obstet Gynecol 1990;163:50–51.

Johnston IH, Whittle IR, Besser M, et al. Vein of Galen malformation: diagnosis and management. Neurosurgery 1987;20:747–758.

Koh AS, Grundy HO. Fetal heart rate tracing with congenital aneurysm of the great vein of Galen. Am J Perinatol 1988;5:98–100.

Lasjaunias P, Garcia-Monaco R, Rodesch G, et al. Vein of Galen malformation: endovascular management of 43 cases. Child Nerv Syst 1991;7:360–367.

Litvak J, Yahr MD, Ransohoff J. Aneurysms of the great vein of Galen and midline cerebral anteriovenous anomalies. J Neurosurg 1960;17:945–954.

Martínez-Lage JF, Garcia Santos JM, Poza M, et al. Prenatal magnetic resonance imaging detection of a vein of Galen aneurysm. Child Nerv Syst 1993;9:377–378.

Matjasko J, Robinson W, Eudaily D. Successful surgical and anesthetic management of vein of Galen aneurysm in a neonate in congestive heart failure. Neurosurgery 1988; 22:908–910.

McLeod ME, Creighton RE, Humphreys RP. Anaesthetic management of arteriovenous malformations of the vein of Galen. Can Anaesth Soc J 1982;29:307–312.

Mickle JP, Quisling RG. The transtorcular embolization of vein of Galen aneurysms. J Neurosurg 1986;64:731–735.

Mickle JP, Quisling RG. Vein of Galen fistulas. Neurosurg Clin North Am 1994;5:529–540.

Mickle JP, Quisling R, Ryan P. Transtorcular approach to vein of Galen aneurysms. Pediatr Neurosurg 1994;20: 163–168.

Norman MG, Becker LE. Cerebral damage in neonates resulting from arteriovenous malformation of the vein of Galen. J Neurol Neurosurg Psychiatry 1974;37:252–258.

O'Donnabhain D, Duff DF. Aneurysms of the vein of Galen. Arch Dis Child 1989;64:1612–1617.

Osherwitz D, Davidoff LM. Midline calcified intracranial aneurysms between occipital lobes. J Neurosurg 1947;4:539–541.

Padget DH. The cranial venous system in man in reference to development, adult configuration and relation to the arteries. Am J Anat 1956;98:307–355.

Raybaud CA, Strother CM, Hald JK. Aneurysms of the vein of Galen: embryonic considerations and anatomical features relating to the pathogenesis of the malformation. Neuroradiology 1989;31:109–128.

Reiter AA, Huhta JC, Carpenter RJ, et al. Prenatal diagnosis of arteriovenous malformation of the vein of Galen. J Clin Ultrasound 1986;14:623–628.

Rodesch G, Hui F, Alvarez H, et al. Prognosis of antenatally diagnosed vein of Galen aneurysmal malformations. Child Nerv Syst 1994;10:79–83.

Sepulveda W, Platt CC, Fisk NM. Prenatal diagnosis of cerebral arteriovenous malformation using color Doppler ultrasonography: case report and review of the literature. Ultrasound Obstet Gynecol 1995;6:282–286.

Six EG, Cowley AR, Kelly DL, et al. Thrombosed aneurysm of the vein of Galen. Neurosurgery 1980;7:274–278.

Stockberger S, Smith R, Don S. Color Doppler sonography as a primary diagnostic tool in the diagnosis of vein of Galen aneurysm in a critically ill neonate. Neuroradiology 1993;35:616–618.

Suma V, Marini A, Saia OS, et al. Vein of Galen aneurysm. Fetus 1981;1:1–6.

Warkany J. Cerebrovascular malformations. Congenital Malform 1971;1:249.

Watson DG, Smith RR, Brann AW. Arteriovenous malformation of the vein of Galen: treatment in a neonate. Am J Dis Child 1976;130:520–525.

Yamashita Y, Abe T, Ohara N, et al. Successful treatment of neonatal aneurysmal dilatation of the vein of Galen: the role of prenatal diagnosis and trans-arterial embolization. Neuroradiology 1992;34:457–459.

Yasargil MG, Antic J, Laciga R, et al. Arteriovenous malformations of vein of Galen: microsurgical treatment. Surg Neurol 1976;6:195–200.

Zerah M, Garcia-Monaco R, Rodesch G, et al. Hydrodynamics in vein of Galen malformations. Child Nerv Syst 1992;8:111–117.

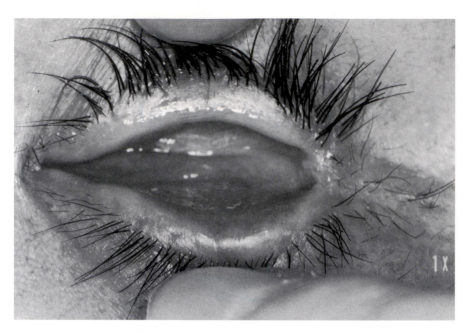

Figure 23-1. Absence of the globe with a normal appearance to the eyelids and eyelashes in anophthalmos. *(Reprinted, with permission, from Matsui H, Hayasaka S, Setogawa T. Congenital cataract in the right eye and primary clinical anophthalmos of the left eye in a patient with cerebellar hypoplasia. Ann Ophthalmol 1993;25:315–318.)*

degenerative anophthalmos, the optic tract and vesicles are initially normally developed, but subsequently undergo degeneration and disappear. Most cases of degenerative anophthalmos result in severe microphthalmos. Because the lens depends on the optic vesicle for its differentiation, in primary and secondary anophthalmos the lens is absent. In cases of anophthalmos, the nonneuroectodermal structures are usually normally formed. The orbits, eyelids, cilia, lacrimal apparatus, conjunctiva, and extraocular muscles are usually normal (Fig. 23-1) (Brunquell et al. 1984). In cryptophthalmos, the eyelid fails to develop. Cryptophthalmos is also known as "hidden eyes"; in these patients the palpebral fissures are absent. In these cases, fusion generally occurs between the skin and the anterior aspect of the eye; therefore, useful vision does not develop in these patients.

▶ INCIDENCE

Anophthalmos is extremely rare. A prospective study performed in the United States involving 50,000 pregnancies documented the combined incidence of anophthalmos and microphthalmos to be 0.22 per 1000 live births (Gilbert 1993; Warburg 1993). The incidence of isolated anophthalmos is rarer, reported to be 0.4 per 10,000 live births. The overall prevalence of anophthalmia and microphthalmia in Britain is 1.0 per 10,000 births (Dolk et al. 1998). Clinical anophthalmos is frequently associated with central nervous system anomalies, cytomegalovirus infection, chromosomal abnormalities, and mental retardation (Matsui et al. 1993). Anophthalmos also has been associated with attempted mechanical termination of the pregnancy, and severe maternal vitamin A deficiency (O'Keefe et al. 1987), as well as multiple viral infections, including rubella, influenza, varicella, and parvovirus B19 (Gilbert 1993). Medications taken by the pregnant woman that are suspected to cause anophthalmos include lysergide, ethambutol, thalidomide, and vitamin A. Recently, the pesticide benomyl has been investigated as the potential cause of a cluster of cases of anophthalmos occurring in Europe (Gilbert 1993).

In a British study of individuals with severe anophthalmia or microphthalmia, 51% of cases were bilateral, 72% were associated with other eye malformations, and 65% were associated with malformations outside the eye (Busby et al. 1998).

▶ SONOGRAPHIC FINDINGS

In the sonographic diagnosis of anophthalmos, consideration should be given to measurement of the orbit as well as the globe. In 1982, Mayden et al. published nomograms for fetal inner and outer orbital diameters measured in the occipital transverse and posterior positions of 180 normal pregnancies. They documented that the outer orbital diameter was closely related to biparietal diameter, and can be used as a substitute for gestational age when the position of the fetal head precludes measurement. They subsequently studied 463 fetuses at risk for congenital anomalies and diagnosed three with abnormal orbital diameters that were below the fifth percentile. They made an antenatal sonographic diagnosis of hypotelorism, which was confirmed in one of the three products of conception. In a second fetus, severe microcephaly and cebocephaly were confirmed after birth (Mayden et al. 1982). In the same year, de Elejalde and de Elejalde (1982) reported the presence of the fetal globe at 48 days of gestation. They recommended analyzing the fetal eyes in the transverse and coronal planes. In the transverse plane, the long axis of the transducer was positioned perpendicular to the fetal sagittal plane and moved from the top of the skull across the fetal face to analyze the malar and ethmoidal nasal walls or the orbits. By studying the posterior aspect of the eye, they could study the opening of the optic nerve and artery, and by moving anteriorly, they could study the eyelids. Immediately posterior to the eyelids, they could study the anterior and posterior chambers of the eye by looking for fluid content. In the coronal plane, the irides, sclerae, and lens were studied. The eyelids were noted to be closed before week 25 of gestation but opened after 26 weeks. The border of the closed eyelids can be recognized as a thick sonolucent line. In the coronal plane, the iris can be located and observed for horizontal movement, which is easier to document after 17 weeks of gestation (de Elejalde and de Elejalde 1982). The sagittal plane was not recommended except during very early pregnancy. This group recommended measurement of the interethmoidal and intermalar distances, as they are roughly comparable to inner and outer canthal distances, permitting diagnosis of hypotelorism or hypertelorism. This report confirmed the presence of the fetal iris in a family at risk for aniridia.

The sonographic diagnosis of anophthalmia can be challenging. Abnormalities in the fetal orbits are more easily recognized than abnormalities in the fetal globe. A specific finding appears to be flattened or concave eyelids when the fetal globes are missing (Fig. 23-2). Nomograms for fetal eye measurements from 12 weeks of gestation onwards have been published (Achiron et al. 1995).

▶ DIFFERENTIAL DIAGNOSIS

The major consideration in the differential diagnosis of anophthalmos is to determine whether the anophthalmos is isolated or part of a syndrome. Table 23-1 lists some of the disorders in the differential diagnosis of anophthalmos. Many of these have a chromosomal abnormality as the underlying basis for the anophthalmos. When the anophthalmos is apparently isolated, it is important to determine whether other family members are also affected. Single-gene disorders that include anophthalmos as part of their findings include Fraser (cryptophthalmos-syndactyly) syndrome (Feldman et al. 1985; Pankau et al. 1994; Ramsing et al. 1990; Schauer et al. 1990), Goltz syndrome (Gottlieb et al. 1973; Marcus et al. 1990), Goldenhar syndrome, Waardenburg syndrome, type II (Richieri-Costa et al. 1983), and Lenz syndrome, which can be associated with unilateral anophthalmos.

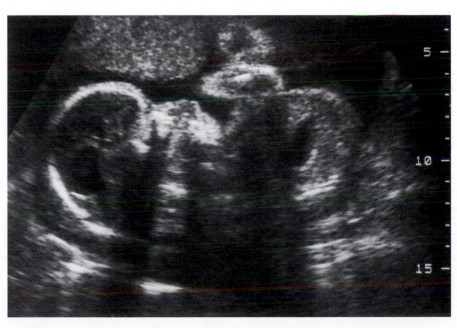

Figure 23-2. Antenatal sonogram, performed at 27 weeks of gestation, demonstrating anophthalmia and severe midface hypoplasia in a fetus with trisomy 13.

▶ **TABLE 23-1.** CONDITIONS ASSOCIATED WITH ANOPHTHALMOS

Condition	Additional Findings
Trisomy 13	Multiple congenital anomalies
Fraser syndrome	Renal agenesis, cryptophthalmos, laryngeal atresia, cutaneous syndactyly, ambiguous genitalia
Goltz syndrome	Linear depressed skin lesions with herniation of fetal nodules; bone, tooth, and nail abnormalities
Waardenberg syndrome, type II	Hand malformations, club foot, missing digits

▶ ANTENATAL NATURAL HISTORY

The overall fetal prognosis will be highly dependent on the underlying cause of the anophthalmos. If the condition is isolated, the fetus will be blind if the anophthalmos is bilateral, but otherwise should be expected to do well. If the fetus has an underlying chromosomal abnormality, however, the prognosis for survival will be much worse. Prognosis also will be related to the presence of additional malformations.

Although chorioretinitis is thought to be the most common ocular manifestation of rubella, anophthalmos has also been reported with in utero cytomegalovirus infection (Frenkel et al. 1980; McCarthy et al. 1980). Anophthalmos is also associated with midline defects of the brain and face, including cleft lip and cleft palate, hypothalamic disorders, panhypopituitarism, diabetes insipidus, and seizure disorders (Bierich et al. 1991; Leichtman et al. 1994).

Conditions that affect the development of the forebrain, such as maternal diabetes, ingestion of ethanol, or the presence of holoprosencephaly, place the fetus at risk for the development of anophthalmos as well as microphthalmos.

▶ MANAGEMENT OF PREGNANCY

Anophthalmos is commonly seen as part of a multiple malformation syndrome. It is therefore important to refer a patient in whom fetal anophthalmos is suspected to a center experienced in the antenatal detection of congenital malformations. Because of the rarity of anophthalmos and its association with severe abnormalities and blindness, we recommend obtaining a fetal karyotype to rule out chromosomal abnormalities as the underlying cause of the anophthalmos. It is important to ascertain the mother's medication history, maternal diabetes (as indicated in the results of glucose-tolerance testing), and a history of ethanol ingestion as potential causes for the anophthalmos. We also recommend obtaining TORCH (toxoplasmosis, other agents, rubella, cytomegalovirus, herpesvirus) titers to diagnose in utero cytomegalovirus, rubella, or toxoplasmosis infection. It is also important to obtain a maternal history of varicella infection.

▶ FETAL INTERVENTION

At present there is no fetal intervention indicated for anophthalmos.

▶ TREATMENT OF THE NEWBORN

The newborn with unilateral or bilateral anophthalmos should have a complete physical examination to rule out associated congenital anomalies. A computed tomographic (CT) scan or magnetic resonance imaging (MRI) should be performed to differentiate between true anophthalmos and clinical anophthalmos (Fig. 23-3). If fetal karyotyping has not been performed, it should be performed during the newborn period. In addition, urine should be collected for cytomegalovirus culture. TORCH titers should be obtained from the infant and mother (if not obtained prenatally). A pediatric ophthalmologic consultation should be obtained to discuss plans for prosthetic fitting and plastic surgery.

▶ SURGICAL TREATMENT

The development of the orbital region is correlated with the outgrowth of the eyeball; therefore, in the setting of anophthalmos, there is underdevelopment of the orbit as well as hypoplasia of the affected side of the face with underdevelopment of the malar bone, zygomatic arch, and frontal bone. The resulting facial asymmetry is apparent at birth. Most surgeons recommend progressive dilation of the orbit as soon as possible after birth. The long-term goal is to create a suitable pocket for a cosmetically acceptable prosthesis (Marchac et al. 1977). The presence of the prosthesis will stimulate further growth of the bony orbit. However, surgical treatment is frequently necessary to achieve sufficient posterior stability of the prosthesis.

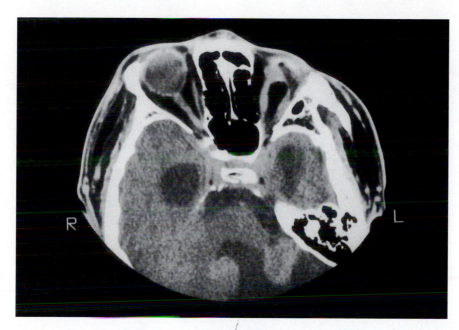

Figure 23-3. Postnatal CT scan showing on the patient's left side, a small nodular mass with well-developed extraocular muscles in a case of primary anophthalmos. A normal eye is present on the right. *(Reprinted, with permission, from Matsui H, Hayasaka S, Setogawa T. Congenital cataract in the right eye and primary clinical anophthalmos of the left eye in a patient with cerebellar hypoplasia. Ann Ophthalmol 1993;25:315–318.)*

A new procedure has been described that uses a lens-shaped hydrogel device that expands the eyelids and mucosal socket to allow insertion of the eye prosthesis (Wiese et al. 1999).

▶ LONG-TERM OUTCOME

In a review of 15 patients with clinical anophthalmos, those who had prosthetic therapy initiated in the first year of life had acceptable cosmetic results. Of this group, 2 patients had bilateral anophthalmos, 10 had systemic abnormalities, 5 had mental retardation (all of these patients had midline facial clefts), and 6 had abnormalities of the remaining eye, including coloboma of the iris, microphthalmia, epibulbar dermoid, and nystagmus (O'Keefe et al. 1987). A more recent technique of three-dimensional orbital bone expansion has achieved the best results (O'Keefe et al. 1987; Marchac et al. 1977) (Fig. 23-4).

▶ GENETICS AND RECURRENCE RISK

Most cases of bilateral anophthalmos are sporadic. Clinical anophthalmos has been reported to be inherited in families as an autosomal dominant trait (Sensi et al. 1987), an X-linked condition (Brunquell et al. 1984), and an autosomal recessive disorder (Kohn et al. 1988).

Kohn reported a three-generation pedigree with 19 affected individuals who all had bilateral anophthalmos and normal intelligence. This family was highly inbred. Sensi et al. (1987) described a family in which only the extreme anophthalmic form occurred, transmitted as an autosomal dominant with incomplete penetrance. This family had six affected members. All of them had normal intelligence, and karyotypes were normal. Richieri-Costa et al. (1983) have described a different autosomal recessive syndrome in consanguineous Brazilian parents whose children had anophthalmos and distal extremity abnormalities.

Other rare conditions, inherited as autosomal recessive mutations, include the anophthalmia-esophageal genital syndrome (Shah et al. 1997), anophthalmia-Waardenburg syndrome (Suyugul et al. 1996), and "anophthalmia-plus" syndrome (Fryns et al. 1995). A variety of chromosomal abnormalities have been reported in association with anophthalmos, including trisomy 13, a 7;15 translocation (Wajntal et al. 1978), a 14q22-23 deletion (Bennett et al. 1991), and an unbalanced subtelomeric translocation involving the long arms of chromosomes 2 and 7 (Brackley et al. 1999). The patient with the 14q deletion had an absent pituitary gland, hypoplastic adrenal glands, absent left horn of the uterus, and clinodactyly in addition to the bilateral anophthalmos. Other conditions associated with anophthalmos and chromosomal abnormalities include a case of Klinefelter syndrome (Welter et al. 1974) and mosaicism for polyploidy (Masket et al. 1970).

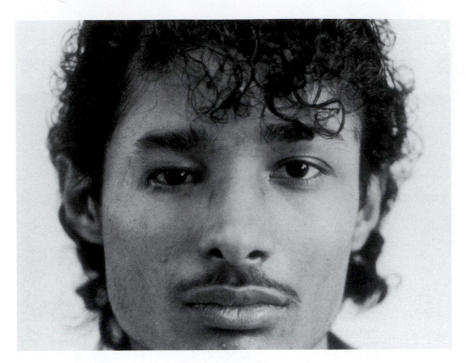

Figure 23-4. Patient with unilateral anophthalmos, treated with early prosthetic therapy but no surgical eyelid revisions, demonstrating an acceptable cosmetic result. *(Reprinted, with permission, from O'Keefe M, Webb M, Pashby RC, et al. Clinical anophthalmos. Br J Ophthalmol 1987;71:635–638.)*

Any patient with anophthalmos should be referred to a medical genetics unit for complete pedigree interpretation and counseling regarding recurrence risk. Specific genetic counseling will depend on the underlying cause of the anophthalmos. If an unbalanced chromosomal abnormality is detected, parental blood samples should be obtained to study their karyotypes. Any infant with anophthalmos should be examined by a clinical geneticist to seek additional dysmorphic features that will permit diagnosis of a genetic syndrome.

REFERENCES

Achiron R, Gottlieb Z, Yarm Y, Gabbey M, Gavvay U, Lipitz S, Mashiach S. The development of the fetal eye: in utero ultrasonographic measurements of the vitreous and lens. Prenat Diagn 1995;15:155—160.

Bennett CP, Betts DR, Seller MJ. Deletion 14q (q22q23) associated with anophthalmia, absent pituitary, and other abnormalities. J Med Genet 1991;28:280–281.

Bierich JR, Christie M, Heinrich JJ, Martinez, AS. New observations on midline defects: coincidence of anophthalmos, microphthalmos and cryptophthalmos with hypothalamic disorders. Eur J Pediatr 1991;150:246–249.

Brackley KJ, Kilby MD, Morton J, Whittle MJ, Knight SJ, Flint J. A case of recurrent congenital fetal anomalies associated with a familial subtelomeric translocation. Prenat Diagn 1999;19:570–574.

Brunquell PJ, Papale JH, Horton JC, Williams RS, Zgrabik MJ, Albert DM, Headley-White ET. Sex-linked hereditary bilateral anophthalmos: pathologic and radiologic correlation. Arch Ophthalmol 1984;102:108–113.

Busby A, Dolk H, Collin R, Jones RB, Winter R. Compiling a national register of babies born with anophthalmia/microphthalmia in England 1988–1994, Arch Dis Child Fetal Neonatal Ed 1998;79:F168–173.

de Elejalde MM, de Elejalde BR. Ultrasonographic visualization of the fetal eye. J Craniofac Genet Dev Biol 1985;5:319–326.

Dolk H, Busby A, Armstrong BG, Walls PH. Geographical variation in anophthalmia and microphthalmia in England, 1988–1994. BMJ 1998;317:905–909.

Feldman E, Shalev E, Weiner E, Cohen H, Zuckerman H. Microphthalmia-prenatal ultrasonic diagnosis: a case report. Prenat Diagn 1985;5:205–207.

Frenkel LD, Keys MP, Hefferen SJ, Rola-Pleszczynski M, Bellanti JA. Unusual eye abnormalities associated with congenital cytomegalovirus infection. Pediatrics 1980;66:763–766.

Fryns JP, Legius E, Moerman P, Var den Berghe K, Van den Berghe H. Apparently new "anophthalmia-plus" syndrome in sibs. Am J Med Genet 1995;58:113–114.

Gilbert R. "Cluster" of anophthalmia in Britain. BMJ 1993;307:340–341.

Gottlieb SK, Fisher BK, Violin GA. Focal dermal hypoplasia. A nine-year follow up study. Arch Dermatol 1973;108:551–553.

Kohn G, el Shawwa R, Rayyes E. Isolated "clinical anophthalmia" in an extensively affected Arab kindred. Clin Genet 1988;33:321–324.

Leichtman LG, Wood B, Rohn R. Anophthalmia, cleft lip/palate, facial anomalies, and CNS anomalies and hypothalamic disorder in a newborn: a midline developmental field defect. Am J Med Genet 1994;50:39–41.

Marchac D, Cophignon J, Achard E, Dufourmental C. Orbital expansion for anophthalmia and micro-orbitism. Plast Reconstr Surg 1977;59:486–491.

Marcus DM, Shore JW, Albert DM. Anophthalmia in the focal dermal hypoplasia syndrome. Arch Ophthalmol 1990;108:96–100.

Masket S, Galioto FM, Jr., Best M. Anophthalmia, multiple abnormalities, and unusual karyotype. Am J Ophthalmol 1970;70:381–383.

Matsui H, Hayasaka S, Setogawa T. Congenital cataract in the right eye and primary clinical anophthalmos of the left eye in a patient with cerebellar hypoplasia. Ann Ophthalmol 1993;25:315–318.

Mayden KL, Tortora M, Berkowitz RL, et al. Orbital diameters: A new parameter for prenatal diagnosis and dating. Am J Obstet Gynecol 1982;144:289–297.

McCarthy RW, Frenkel LD, Kollarits CR, Keys MP. Clinical anophthalmia associated with congenital cytomegalovirus infection. Am J Ophthalmol 1980;90:558–561.

Moore KL. The developing human. Philadelphia: Saunders, 1974:345–352.

O'Keefe M, Webb M, Pashby RC, et al. Clinical anophthalmos. Br J Ophthalmol 1987;71:635–638.

Pankau R, Partsch CJ, Janig U, Meinecke R. Fraser syndrome: A case with bilateral anophthalmia but presence of normal eyelids. Genet Couns 1994;5:191–194.

Ramsing M, Rehder H, Holzgreve W, Meinecke P, Lenz W. Fraser syndrome in the fetus and newborn. Clin Genet 1990;37:84–96.

Richieri-Costa A, Gollop TR, Otto PG. Autosomal recessive anophthalmia with multiple congenital abnormalities—type Waardenberg. Am J Med Genet 1983;14:607–615.

Sassani JW, Yanoff M. Anophthalmos in an infant with multiple congenital anomalies. Am J Ophthalmol 1977;83: 43–48.

Schauer GM, Dunn LK, Godmilow L, Eagle RC, Jr., Knisley AS. Prenatal diagnosis of Fraser syndrome at 18.5 weeks gestation with autopsy findings at 19 weeks. Am J Med Genet 1990;37:583–591.

Sensi A, Incorvaia C, Sebastiani A, Calzolari E. Clinical anophthalmos in a family. Clin Genet 1987;32:156–159.

Shah D, Jones R, Porter H, Turnpenny P. Bilateral microphthalmia, esophageal atresia, and cryptorchidism: the anophthalmia-esophageal-genital syndrome. Am J Med Genet 1997;70:171–173.

Suyugul Z, Seven M, Hacihanefioglu S, Kartal A, Suyugul N, Cenani A. Anophthalmia-Waardenburg syndrome: a report of three cases. Am J Med Genet 1996;62:391–397.

Wajntal A, Olazabal LC, Billerbeck AEC, Malta RFS, Alves MR, Diament AJ. Clinical anophthalmia and translocation 7/15. Rev Bras Genet 1978;1:67–75.

Warburg M. Classification of microphthalmos and coloboma. J Med Genet 1993;30:664–669.

Welter DA, Lewis LW, Jr., Scharff L, III, Smith WS. Klinefelter's syndrome with anophthalmos. Am J Ophthalmol 1974;77:895–898.

Wiese KG, Vogel M, Guthoff R, Gundlach KK. Treatment of congenital anophthalmos with self-inflating polymer expanders: a new method. J Craniomaxillofac Surg 1989; 27:72–76.

CHAPTER 24
Cleft Lip and Cleft Palate

▶ CONDITION

Cleft lip and cleft palate are relatively common facial malformations that occur early in gestation. Although they are distinct anomalies, they frequently occur together (Seeds and Cefalo 1983). In all cases of orofacial clefting, 60 to 75% involve cleft lip, with or without cleft palate, and 25 to 40% are isolated cleft palate (Fig. 24-1). Most cases (80%) are unilateral, occurring twice as commonly on the left side as on the right (Bronshtein et al. 1991; Gorlin et al. 1971; Seeds and Cefalo 1983). Isolated cleft palate is more frequently associated with other anomalies (Jones MC 1988).

Orofacial clefts derive from abnormalities in the migration and proliferation of facial mesenchyme, a neural-crest–cell derivative. Coalescence of facial mesenchyme results in the formation of the primary palate, which creates the initial separation between oral and nasal cavities, eventually creating part of the upper lip and anterior maxilla (Ross and Johnston 1972). Cleft lip with or without cleft palate results from failure of the nasal and maxillary facial processes to fuse. Fusion of these processes may be affected by the amount of mesenchyme present, its rate of migration, and the distance over which this migration occurs (Lynch and Kimberling 1981). Syndromes that involve relatively broad

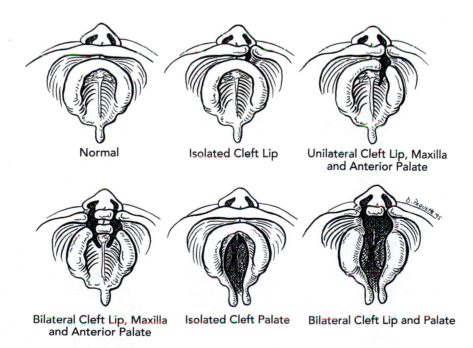

Normal

Isolated Cleft Lip

Unilateral Cleft Lip, Maxilla and Anterior Palate

Bilateral Cleft Lip, Maxilla and Anterior Palate

Isolated Cleft Palate

Bilateral Cleft Lip and Palate

Figure 24-1. Schematic representation of the different types of malformations found in cases of orofacial clefting. The perspective is from the inside of the mouth looking upward toward the nose.

facies, such as Crouzon or Waardenburg syndrome, are associated with an increased incidence of facial clefts.

Isolated cleft palate has a different pathophysiology than either cleft lip or cleft lip associated with cleft palate. It results from interference in any of the following processes that occur during normal closure of the palate:

1. The palatal shelves move from bilateral vertical positions lateral to each side of the tongue to horizontal positions overlying the tongue.
2. The tongue exerts resistance to the movement of the palatal shelves.
3. The tongue moves downward to below the palatal shelves.
4. The horizontal palatal shelves become flattened and extend their leading edges toward the midline.
5. The shelves meet in the midline and fuse. Their respective epithelia then dissolve at the point of contact.

(Lynch and Kimberling 1981). From the foregoing description, it is apparent that the tongue plays a role in the etiology of cleft palate. Any factor that interferes with downward displacement of the tongue, tongue movement, or tongue pressure may interfere with palatal fusion. Neurologic and myopathic conditions, such as Stickler syndrome, can be associated with cleft palate.

▶ INCIDENCE

The overall incidence of facial clefts in white populations is 1 in 1000 live-born infants (Bronshtein et al. 1991, 1994; Fogh-Andersen 1942; Lynch and Kimberling 1981; Stoll et al. 1991), although marked variation occurs in different racial and ethnic groups. Black infants have a lower incidence (1 in 2273 births), whereas that among Japanese and Native Americans is higher (1 in 584 and 1 in 276, respectively) (Lynch and Kimberling 1981; Tretsven 1963). Cleft lip and cleft palate occur twice as often in males as in females (Bronshtein et al. 1991). In some studies, orofacial clefting has been shown to occur more commonly in fetuses whose mothers are of advanced age (Shaw et al. 1991; Womersley and Stone 1987); in a large population-based registry, however, no association between maternal age and cleft disorders was seen (Baird et al. 1994). Although there are case reports of associations of facial clefts with prenatal exposure to anticonvulsants, agricultural pesticides, retinoid medications, nitrate compounds, organic solvents, alcohol, and a vitamin-deficient diet (Shaw et al. 1991), no chemical or biologic agent has been shown to consistently and reliably cause facial clefts in humans. The most controversial association—maternal cigarette smoking—has generated data that argue both for (Khoury et al. 1987) and against (Werler et al. 1990) the association. Periconceptual multivitamin use may reduce the incidence of cleft palate (Werler et al. 1999).

▶ SONOGRAPHIC FINDINGS

The fetal face assumes its normal contour by 14 weeks of gestation. The earliest prenatal sonographic diagnosis of fetal cleft was described at 11 weeks by embryoscopy (Dommergues et al. 1995). Seeds and Cefalo (1983) were the first investigators to advocate a combination of frontal and coronal scanning of the midface. In 1984, Benacerraf et al. recommended routinely examining the face as part of a complete antenatal sonographic examination. They described a coronal view through fetal facial structures that encompassed both orbits, the maxilla, and the anterior portion of the mandible in one vertical plane. Sherer and colleagues (1991) described an oblique coronal facial view that was achieved by aiming the transducer beneath the fetal chin using the nares as a landmark. They sought echogenic evidence of an intact fissure created by the closed lips (Fig. 24-2). The two advantages of this approach are that rarely was this view unobtainable due to position of the fetus and that the appearance of the philtrum was clearly defined. Using a combination of transverse, coronal, and profile views, Turner and Twining (1993) were able to define fetal facial structures in 95 to 97% of fetuses at 16 to 20 weeks of gestation.

Despite these studies, sonographic diagnosis of small or incomplete facial clefts remains challenging. The detection rate varies from 21 to 91% (Bronshtein et al. 1994). In general, cleft lip is easier to demonstrate than cleft palate. Bronshtein et al. (1991) advocated the use of the sagittal paramedian view to detect pseudoprognathism, a protrusion of the mandible relative to the maxilla. In bilateral cleft lip and palate, a paranasal echogenic mass may be present due to premaxillary protrusion of the prolabial structure that exists in this condition (Nyberg et al. 1992, 1993). Sherer and colleagues (1993) have advocated for the use of color Doppler imaging to demonstrate abnormal amniotic fluid flow across the fetal pharyngeal bone defect.

Bronshtein et al. (1994) described the use of transvaginal sonography to detect facial clefts in the early second trimester. In 14,988 examinations performed, 11 cases of orofacial clefts were detected. Of these, 10 were cases of cleft lip and cleft palate and 1 was isolated cleft lip. All diagnoses were confirmed after termination of the pregnancy or at birth.

Despite these encouraging results, most cases of cleft lip and palate are not diagnosed antenatally. The American Institute of Ultrasound in Medicine (AIUM) and American College of Obstetrics and Gynecology

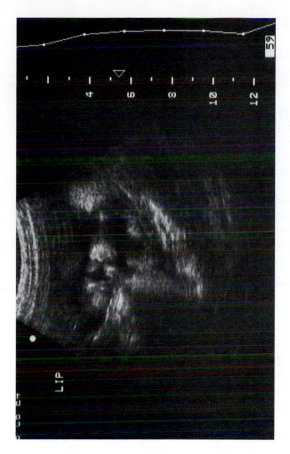

Figure 24-2. Sagittal view of a fetal face demonstrating a large midline cleft lip.

(ACOG) guidelines do not recommend routine views of the fetal face. The best data regarding the sensitivity of sonographic screening for detection of cleft lip and palate is from the RADIUS trial (Crane et al. 1994), a multicenter study of pregnant women at low risk for adverse outcome in pregnancy, designed to test the hypothesis that routine ultrasonography performed on two occasions during pregnancy would reduce perinatal mortality and morbidity (Ewigman et al. 1993). The secondary outcomes of anomaly detection were reported separately. In the screened population of 7685 patients, there were 10 cases of cleft lip and palate. Three were prenatally diagnosed, a detection rate of 30%. In the control population of 7596 patients there were 7 cases of cleft lip and palate. One was diagnosed prenatally, for a detection rate of 14%. One of the criticisms of the RADIUS trial was that the rate of anomaly detection did not reflect the diagnostic capability of ultrasound screening at the time the study was performed. In the setting of a positive family history or a patient at increased risk for cleft lip and/or cleft palate, we recommend that a prenatal ultrasound examination be performed in a center experienced in the diagnosis of congenital anomalies.

One study examined the use of three-dimensional sonographic visualization fetal tooth buds as a means of improving antenatal characterization of fetal facial clefts (Ulm et al. 1999). In all 17 fetuses studied, it was possible to classify the clefts as either cleft lip alone or unilateral or bilateral cleft lip and palate.

▶ DIFFERENTIAL DIAGNOSIS

The most important consideration in the differential diagnosis of cleft lip is to distinguish between the normal vertical midline appearance of the philtrum and a pathologic median cleft lip. Although most cleft lips are left-sided and unilateral, a median cleft lip can be associated with syndromes such as orofacialdigital, type I, or frontonasal dysplasia. Consideration should also be given to detection of premaxillary agenesis, which is almost always associated with alobar holoprosencephaly (see Chapter 13).

When a paranasal echogenic mass is detected in cases of bilateral cleft lip and palate, the differential diagnosis includes hemangioma, anterior meningocele, teratoma, and enlarged tongue and proboscis (Nyberg et al. 1992). Of these conditions, only premaxillary protrusion associated with cleft lip and palate contains bone within the mass, resulting from anterior migration of maxillary and alveolar bones (Nyberg et al. 1992).

Once a cleft is identified, a diligent search should be made to detect associated anomalies. The finding of additional anomalies will significantly affect the differential diagnosis. Over 250 syndromes are associated with facial clefts (Shprintzen et al. 1985). Common syndromes include Goldenhar (facioauriculovertebral dysplasia), Treacher–Collins (mandibulofacial dysostosis), Pierre–Robin, Stickler, DiGeorge, and Shprintzen (velocardiofacial) (Table 24-1). Additional anomalies seen in cases of Pierre–Robin sequence include micrognathia and polyhydramnios (Hsich et al. 1999).

▶ ANTENATAL NATURAL HISTORY

Cleft lip and palate are seen more frequently in first-trimester abortuses than in newborns. In one study of 3216 pregnancy losses, Kraus et al. (1963) demonstrated that 11.5% of fetuses spontaneously aborted at 8 weeks of gestation, 1.8% of abortuses at 6 to 19 weeks of gestation, and 0.16% of live-born infants had orofacial clefts. Thus, fetuses with cleft lip and palate are at increased risk for intrauterine demise. The risk for fetal loss is related to the presence of associated anomalies, which were found in 61.7% of cases studied (Kraus et al. 1963).

In general, the detection of a facial cleft in a fetus is more likely to be associated with other malformations than the detection of a cleft at birth. In one study,

▶ **TABLE 24-1.** COMMON SYNDROMES ASSOCIATED WITH FACIAL CLEFTS

Syndrome	Associated Findings
Goldenhar (facioauriculovertebral dysplasia)	Asymmetric facial hypoplasia, microtia, preauricular skin tags, hemivertebrae, cardiac defects
Pierre–Robin sequence	Micrognathia, U-shaped cleft of soft palate
Shprintzen (velocardiofacial syndrome)	Cardiac defects, hypotonia, growth restriction, chromosome 22q microdeletion; autosomal dominant
Stickler (hereditary arthro-ophthalmopathy)	Flat facies, micrognathia, hypotonia, myopia, scoliosis; autosomal dominant
Treacher–Collins (mandibulofacial dysostosis)	Malar and mandibular hypoplasia, downslanting palpebral fissures, ear malformations, absent lower eyelashes; autosomal dominant
Trisomy 13	Polydactyly, congenital heart disease, central nervous system abnormalities
Trisomy 18	Intrauterine growth restriction, congenital heart disease
Van der Woude (lip pit–cleft lip syndrome)	Lower lip pits, missing teeth; autosomal dominant

Saltzman et al. (1986) described 12 cases of orofacial clefts diagnosed prenatally. Other malformations were detected in 10 (83%) of these fetuses. The chromosomes of 7 of these fetuses were studied prenatally or postnatally; 4 were abnormal due to trisomy 13 or 18. In a slightly larger study, Turner and Twining (1993) demonstrated additional anomalies in 88% of fetuses with facial clefts. Notable in this study were the large number of fetuses (9) with clefts and skeletal dysplasia. Benacerraf and Mulliken (1993) described a group of 32 fetuses at 16 to 40 weeks of gestation and over a 3.5-year period ascertained that 17 (53%) had associated anomalies. Five cases of trisomy 13 and 1 case of trisomy 18 were reported, giving a 35% rate of chromosomal aneuploidy in the setting of cleft with multiple anomalies. The associated malformations involved the central nervous system (11 cases), heart (9), kidneys (9), skeleton (10), and abdomen (2). Among the 15 fetuses without associated anomalies, 4 were terminated electively, 1 spontaneously aborted, 1 died from pulmonic stenosis and vertebral anomalies, and 9 survived and underwent successful postnatal surgical correction. Interestingly, this study included 3 cases of unilateral incomplete cleft lip that were undetected at 20 weeks of gestation but were diagnosed at 27 weeks. The overall false negative rate of detection of cleft lip and palate were not addressed in this report.

In postnatal studies, approximately 25% of infants with clefts have associated malformations (Kraus et al. 1963). Isolated cleft lip has the lowest frequency (range, 7 to 45% of cases). The highest incidence of multiple and complex anomalies occurs with isolated cleft palate (range, 13 to 72% of cases) (Ademiluyi et al. 1989; Gorlin et al. 1971; Jones MC 1988; Shprintzen et al. 1985). Shprintzen and colleagues (1985) described an extensive study of 1000 patients attending a craniofacial clinic, all of whom were seen by a clinical geneticist for a thorough dysmorphology examination. Associated anomalies were documented in 63.4% of patients. Craniofacial anomalies were most frequently represented, but short stature, microcephaly, and mental retardation (in 28% of cases) were also common findings.

▶ **MANAGEMENT OF PREGNANCY**

The suspected diagnosis of orofacial cleft necessitates a thorough search for associated anomalies, ideally at a sonographic facility with experience in prenatal diagnosis of anatomic defects. If a facial cleft and an additional anomaly are demonstrated, a prenatal karyotype should be obtained. Orofacial clefting is seen in 75% of cases of trisomy 13, 15% of cases of trisomy 18, 1.5% of cases of trisomy 21, and as stated earlier, approximately 0.1 to 0.15% of chromosomally normal fetuses (Warkany 1971). If a karyotype is performed, additional consideration should be given to fluorescence *in situ* hybridization (FISH) studies to rule out a microdeletion of chromosome 22 that is associated with DiGeorge and Shprintzen syndromes. For the apparently isolated cleft palate or cleft lip–cleft palate complex, we recommend offering the parents the opportunity to obtain the fetal karyotype because of the high incidence of associated anomalies noted in postnatal studies. Because the infant will require multiple operations postnatally, the presence of an abnormal karyotype may influence the parents' decisions regarding continuation of the pregnancy. It is highly likely that maternal ultrasound examination will diagnose trisomies 18 and 13, but it is not as reliable for the diagnosis of trisomy 21.

For the fetus with an apparently isolated cleft lip located lateral to the midline, the recommendations are less clear. There is no evidence in the medical literature of a case of unilateral isolated cleft lip diagnosed antenatally associated with an abnormal karyotype. On the other hand, even cleft lip has a significant rate of associated anomalies in postnatal studies. Thus, while the yield of cytogenetic abnormal results is likely to be extremely low, we recommend discussing with prospective parents the risk of the amniocentesis procedure versus the perceived benefits of knowing that the fetal chromosomes are normal.

Other than sonographic examination and karyotype, management of the pregnancy should continue in a routine manner. Fetuses with isolated cleft lip and palate can be delivered in a community hospital. Fetuses with multiple anomalies should be delivered in a setting where qualified subspecialists are available for newborn resuscitation, syndromic diagnosis, and therapy. We recommend that the prospective parents meet with a pediatric craniofacial surgeon soon after the antenatal diagnosis of facial cleft to discuss the steps involved in surgical treatment. Parents can then have the opportunity to observe the physical appearance of children with repaired facial clefts (Fig. 24-3).

▶ FETAL INTERVENTION

Because the fetal skin has unique scarless wound-healing properties, in utero repair of fetal facial clefts

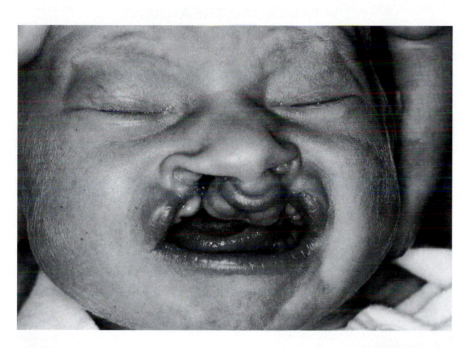

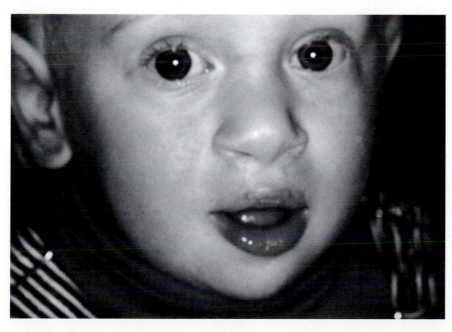

Figure 24-3. Top: Postnatal photograph of an infant who was diagnosed at 20 weeks of gestation with a bilateral cleft lip and palate. Bottom: Follow-up photograph of the same patient at 1 year of age following complete surgical repair. *(Photographs courtesy of Dr. Michael Lewis.)*

has been proposed (Dado et al. 1990; Longaker et al. 1991; Strauss and Davis 1990). It is well recognized that the characteristic facies following repair of cleft lip and cleft palate, with midface retrusion and maxillary deficiency, are often the result of surgical scar formation that inhibits facial and maxillary growth. Because studies of mice and sheep have demonstrated that scarless cleft lip repair is possible antenatally, some have postulated that in the presence of normal functional maturity in the growing fetus, human facial appearance would be enhanced by the absence of scar and unimpaired facial growth. However, the current state of fetal surgery precludes intervention for purely cosmetic defects, although this remains an intriguing theoretical possibility. Reports in the literature on plastic surgery have enthusiastically embraced the potential esthetic advantages of in utero repair, but lack any mention of the risks of fetal surgery to the affected fetus and the mother (Hallock et al. 1985).

However, a precedent for in utero repair of nonlethal fetal malformations has been established with myelomenigocele (see Chapter 19). Recently, the successful in utero repair of a congenital cleft palate model has been described in the goat (Weinzweig et al. 1999).

▶ TREATMENT OF THE NEWBORN

Studies have shown that infants with clefting disorders have lower mean birth and placental weights than normal infants (Lilius and Nordstrom 1992). The immediate concerns in treatment of the newborn infant with a cleft involve clearing of the airway and the ability to feed. Many hospitals have specialized feeding teams or individuals available with expertise in feeding infants with orofacial clefts. It is wise to involve these specialists early to help select a nipple and advise parents on feeding techniques. Breast-feeding is possible but considerably more difficult than for the infant without a cleft palate. Infants with isolated cleft lip feed most easily and grow the most quickly. The mean weekly weight gain for all infants with clefts is 145 g, which is lower than the rate in normal infants (Jones W 1988). This may be due to the nipple rubbing against the delicate nasal mucosa, which causes ulceration.

The infant with a cleft requires a thorough physical examination to look for associated anomalies that may have been missed on sonographic examination. If additional anomalies are detected, the infant should be referred to a clinical geneticist. One author recommends consideration of an ophthalmologic evaluation during the first year of life in all infants with cleft palate because of the relatively high frequency of Stickler syndrome (Jones M 1988). Severe myopia, glaucoma, and retinal detachment can develop in individuals affected with

Stickler syndrome, but the disorder may be extremely difficult to diagnose during infancy. Chromosome analysis, including a FISH test to rule out microdeletion of chromosome 22, should be considered in all infants with cleft palate.

Subsequent treatment of the infant should occur in the setting of a cleft palate multidisciplinary team approach (NIH Consensus Panel 1993). Hearing should be assessed as soon as possible. A plan should be made in conjunction with the primary pediatrician to ensure weekly assessment of nutritional intake and weight gain during the first month of life.

▶ SURGICAL TREATMENT

The exact time of the first surgical repair depends on the anatomy of the malformation. For a unilateral complete cleft, a preliminary lip–nasal adhesion is often performed within the first month of life, followed by the more definitive repair at 4 to 6 months of age. For a unilateral or bilateral incomplete cleft, nose and lip correction can be performed any time within the first 6 months of life. For a bilateral complete cleft lip and palate, presurgical maxillary orthodontics may be indicated prior to surgical closure of the lip within the first few weeks (see Fig. 24-3A). Bilateral cleft lip and nose correction and closure of the alveolar cleft are performed at 4 to 6 months (see Fig. 24-3B) (NIH Consensus Panel 1993). For lip repairs, the infant stays in the hospital for 1 day; for palate repairs, 2 days. In otherwise healthy infants, there is virtually no mortality associated with these procedures (Dado et al. 1990).

Surgical closure of the hard and soft palate is usually complete by 1 year of age. The goal of palate surgery is to restore normal function. Generally, speech results are excellent in 75 to 85% of children, with no need for further surgical procedures. In the small percentage of children in whom velopharyngeal insufficiency persists, secondary surgical procedures can be performed at 3 to 7 years of age, bringing the percentage of children with normal speech to 90 to 95%.

▶ LONG-TERM OUTCOME

The salient long-term issues for a child with cleft lip and palate include midface hypoplasia, appearance (and related psychologic problems), dental abnormalities, speech disorders, and reduced body growth (Felix-Schollaart et al. 1992). Cleft palate has also been shown to be associated with olfactory deficits, more often in boys than in girls (Richman et al. 1988). Children with cleft lip and palate are prone to multiple progressive problems as they grow. As many as 25 to 35% have speech abnormalities requiring secondary palate surgery and speech therapy. All children with cleft palate require speech evaluation, and some will need therapy. Speech and language evaluations are recommended at least annually until 4 years of age (NIH Consensus Panel 1993). Common dental anomalies include missing, extra, or malpositioned teeth. In addition, there are secondary defects that result from the surgical corrective procedures. In patients with unilateral cleft lip and palate, a secondary nasal deformity from a depressed alar base and tip and deviation of the septum can exist. Bilateral cleft lip–cleft palate deformity predisposes to bilateral widening of the alar base and a short columella. Scarring from surgical repair results in midface growth deficiency, with maxillary retrusion and relative mandibular prognathism (Hallock 1985).

Infants with cleft lip and palate have hearing abnormalities that begin surprisingly early in postnatal life. They require frequent and ongoing audiologic surveillance (NIH Consensus Panel 1993). In one study of 23 infants less than 1 year of age, only 2 had normal hearing at age 6 months (Hélias et al. 1988). Of the 19 infants affected by hearing abnormalities, evidence of conduction deafness was documented by abnormal brain-stem auditory evoked responses. Fifteen infants had chronic otitis media with effusion, presumably due to the fact that the eustachian tube is smaller in patients with cleft palate. Obstruction of the eustachian tube is related to the inability of the tensor veli palatine muscle to dilate the eustachian tube actively during swallowing (Hélias et al. 1988). Early myringotomy with placement of bilateral tympanotomy tubes improved hearing acuity and consonant articulation in patients with cleft palate (Grant et al. 1988; Hubbard et al. 1985).

In infants with cleft lip and cleft palate, decidual tooth formation and eruption is normal, but permanent dentition may be delayed (Poyry and Ranta 1986; Poyry et al. 1989). Almost all children with cleft palate defects will require fixed orthodontic appliances (braces) on their permanent teeth. During the period of mixed dentition, removable or fixed appliances may be necessary for expansion and alignment of the incisors (Asher-McDade and Shaw 1990).

Regular psychologic screening, preferably by an expert in craniofacial disorders, is also recommended to assess the child's cognitive development, behavior, and self-image (NIH Consensus Panel 1993).

▶ GENETICS AND RECURRENCE RISK

Cleft lip and cleft palate are considered to be polygenic, multifactorial traits (Kousseff et al. 1992). Approximately 3% of cases are due to a single-gene defect (Lynch and Kimberling 1981). Over 250 syndromes are associated with clefting. It is therefore important to rule out a syndromic diagnosis before discussing the risk of recurrence. Several families have been described with X-linked and autosomal dominant patterns of inheritance (Rollnick and Kaye 1986). A complete family history should indicate other cases occurring within the same pedigree.

When counseling families regarding recurrence risk, it is important to examine parents for the so-called microforms of cleft palate, including a bifid uvula, submucous cleft of the soft palate, and linear lip indentations. This latter finding is characteristic of Van der Woude syndrome, a dominantly inherited disorder in which there is a high penetrance of cleft lip and palate but no extrafacial associated anomalies. The incidence of Van der Woude syndrome is 1 in 33,600 live births (Sander et al. 1995). The finding of lip pits in a parent and an affected infant with a cleft disorder strongly suggests Van der Woude syndrome and a 50% risk of recurrence. The gene for Van der Woude syndrome has been localized on the basis of linkage studies and microdeletion to chromosome 1q32-41 (Sander et al. 1995; Schutte et al. 1999). Embryoscopy has been used to diagnose cleft lip as early as 11 weeks of gestation in a fetus at risk for Van der Woude syndrome (Dommergues et al. 1995).

If the parents have a negative physical examination and family history, the empiric risk for a second affected child is 4% (Lynch and Kimberling 1981; Tenconi et al. 1988). Table 24-2 summarizes empiric recurrence risks for several clinical scenarios.

To date, no specific gene for isolated cleft lip or palate has been demonstrated, although linkage analyses in several families have suggested a possible role for the proto-oncogene *bcl* 3 (Stein et al. 1995), and studies in mice and humans have suggested that transforming growth factor-alpha is a candidate gene (Machida et al. 1999; Miettinen et al. 1999).

A study of 21 families in northern Italy with at least 2 affected individuals showed linkage to the marker D6S89 on chromosome 6p23 (Carinci et al. 1995). Another proposed locus for a candidate gene for isolated cleft palate is chromosome 2q32 (Brewer et al. 1999).

It is not currently known why extra copies of genes on chromosomes 13 and 18 result in facial clefts. The submicroscopic deletions of chromosome 22 seen in DiGeorge and Shprintzen syndrome are associated with cleft palate. Many other chromosomal rearrangements and deletions are associated with clefting. It is not known whether this is due to a gene dosage effect or an overall interference with early development. An approach to identification of candidate genes causing cleft palate was summarized by Wilson (1992).

▶ **TABLE 24-2.** EMPIRICAL RECURRENCE RISK FIGURES FOR OROFACIAL CLEFTS

			Cleft Lip and Palate (%)	Cleft Palate Alone (%)
Normal parents	Number of affected children	Number of normal children		
	1	0	4.0	3.5
	1	1	4.0	3.0
	2	0	14.0	13.0
One parent affected	Number of affected children	Number of normal children		
	0	0	4.0	3.5
	1	0	12.0	10.0
	1	1	10.0	9.0
	2	0	25.0	24.0
Both parents affected	Number of affected children	Number of normal children		
	0	0	35.0	25.0
	1	0	45.0	40.0
	1	1	40.0	35.0
	2	0	50.0	45.0

Modified, with permission, from Cohen MM Jr. Craniofacial disorders. In: Emery AE, Rimoin DL, eds. Principles and practice of medical genetics. New York: Churchill Livingstone, 1983:593–595.

REFERENCES

Ademiluyi S, Oyeneyin J, Sowemimo G. Associated congenital abnormalities in Nigerian children with cleft lip and palate. West Afr J Med 1989;8:135–138.

Asher-McDade C, Shaw MC. Current cleft lip and palate management in the United Kingdom. Br J Plast Surg 1990;43:318–321.

Baird PA, Sadovnick AD, Yee IML. Maternal age and oral cleft malformations: data from a population-based series of 576,815 consecutive livebirths. Teratology 1994;49:448–451.

Benacerraf BR, Frigoletto FD Jr, Bieber FR. The fetal face: ultrasound examination. Radiology 1984;153:495–497.

Benacerraf BR, Mulliken JB. Fetal cleft lip and palate: sonographic diagnosis and postnatal outcome. Plast Reconstr Surg 1993;92:1045–1051.

Brewer CM, Leek JP, Green AJ, et al. A locus for isolated cleft palate located on human chromosome 2q23. Am J Hum Genet 1999;65:387–396.

Bronshtein M, Blumenfeld I, Kohn J, Blumenfeld Z. Detection of cleft lip by early second trimester transvaginal sonography. Obstet Gynecol 1994;84:73–76.

Bronshtein M, Mashiah N, Blumenfeld I, Blumenfeld Z. Pseudoprognathism—an auxiliary ultrasonographic sign for transvaginal ultrasonographic diagnosis of cleft lip and palate in the early second trimester. Am J Obstet Gynecol 1991;165:1314–1316.

Carinci F, Pezzetti F, Scapoli L, et al. Nonsyndromic cleft lip and palate: evidence of linkage to a microsatellite marker on 6p23. Am J Hum Genet 1995;56:337–339.

Cohen MM Jr. Craniofacial disorders. In: Emery AE, Rimoin DL, eds. Principles and practice of medical genetics. New York: Churchill and Livingstone, 1983:593–595.

Crane JP, LeFevre ML, Winborn RC, et al. A randomized trial of prenatal ultrasonographic screening: impact on the detection, management, and outcome of anomalous fetuses. Am J Obstet Gynecol 1994;171:392–399.

Dado DV, Kernahan DA, Gianopoulos JG. Intrauterine repair of cleft lip: what's involved? Plast Reconstr Surg 1990;85:461–465.

Dommergues M, LeMerrer M, Couly G, DeLeZoide AL, Dumez Y. Prenatal diagnosis of cleft lip at 11 menstrual weeks using embryoscopy in the Van der Woude syndrome. Prenat Diagn 1995;15:378–381.

Ewigman BG, Crane JP, Frigoletto FD, LeFevre ML, Bain RP, McNellis D. Effect of prenatal ultrasound screening on perinatal outcome. N Engl J Med 1993;329:821–827.

Felix-Schollaart B, Hoeksma JB, Prahl-Andersen B. Growth comparison between children with cleft lip and/or palate and controls. Cleft Palate Craniofac J 1992;29:475–480.

Fogh-Andersen P. Inheritance of harelip and cleft palate. Copenhagen: Nyt Nordisk Forlag. Arnold Busck, 1942.

Gorlin RJ, Cervenka J, Pruzansky S. Facial clefting and its syndromes. Birth Defects Original Article Series 1971;7:3–49.

Grant HR, Quiney RE, Mercer DM, Lodge S. Cleft palate and glue ear. Arch Dis Child 1988;63:176–179.

Hallock GG. In utero cleft lip repair in A/J mice. Plast Reconstr Surg 1985;75:785–789.

Hélias J, Chobaut J, Mourot M, Lafon JC. Early detection of hearing loss in children with cleft palates by brain-stem auditory response. Arch Otolaryngol Head Neck Surg 1988;114:154–156.

Hsieh YY, Chang CC, Tsai TD, Yang TC, Lee CC, Tsai CH. The prenatal diagnosis of Pierre–Robin sequence. Prenat Diagn 1999;19:567–569.

Hubbard T, Paradise J, McWilliams B, Elster B, Taylor F. Consequences of unremitting middle-ear disease in early life. N Engl J Med 1985;312:1529–1534.

Jones MC. Etiology of facial clefts: prospective evaluation of 428 patients. Cleft Palate J 1988;25:16–20.

Jones W. Weight gain and feeding in the neonate with cleft: a three-center study. Cleft Palate J 1988;25:379–384.

Khoury MJ, Weinstein A, Panny S, et al. Maternal cigarette smoking and oral clefts: a population-based study. Am J Public Health 1987;77:623–625.

Kousseff B, Papenhausen P, Neu R, Essign YP, Saraceno C. Cleft palate and complex chromosome rearrangements. Clin Genet 1992;42:135–142.

Kraus BS, Kitamura H, Ooe T. Malformations associated with cleft lip and palate in human embryo and fetuses. Am J Obstet Gynecol 1963;321–328.

Lilius GP, Nordstrom REA. Birth weight and placental weight in cleft probands. Scand J Plast Reconstr Hand Surg 1992;26:51–54.

Longaker MT, Whitby DJ, Adzick NS, et al. Fetal surgery for cleft lip: a plea for caution. Plast Reconstr Surg 1991;88: 1087–1092.

Lynch HT, Kimberling WJ. Genetic counseling in cleft lip and cleft palate. Plast Reconstr Surg 1981;68:800–815.

Machida J, Yoshiura KI, Funkhauser CD, Natsume N, Kawai T, Murray JC. Transforming growth factor-alpha (*TGFA*): genomic structure boundary sequences, and mutation analysis in nonsyndromic cleft lip/palate and cleft palate only. Genomics 1999;61:237–242.

Miettinen PJ, Chin JR, Shumb L, et al. Epidermal growth factor receptor function is necessary for normal craniofacial development and palate closure. Nat Genet 1999;22: 69–73.

NIH Consensus Panel. Parameters for the evaluation and treatment of patients with cleft lip/palate or other craniofacial anomalies. Cleft Palate Craniofacial J 1993; 30(Suppl).

Nyberg DA, Hegge FG, Kramer D, Mahony BS, Kropp RH. Premaxillary protrusion: a sonographic clue to bilateral cleft lip and palate. J Ultrasound Med 1993;12:331–335.

Nyberg DA, Mahony BS, Kramer D. Paranasal echogenic mass: sonographic sign of bilateral complete cleft lip and palate before 20 menstrual weeks. Radiology 1992;184: 757–759.

Poyry M, Nystrom M, Ranta R. Tooth development in children with cleft lip and palate: a longitudinal study from birth to adolescence. Eur J Orthodont 1989;11:125–130.

Poyry M, Ranta R. Formation of anterior maxillary teeth in 0–3 year old children with cleft lip and palate and prenatal risk factors for delayed development. J Craniofac Genet Dev Biol 1986;6:15–26.

Richman RA, Sheehe PR, McCanty T, et al. Olfactory deficits in boys with cleft palate. Pediatrics 1988;82:840–844.

Rollnick BR, Kaye CI. Mendelian inheritance of isolated nonsyndromic cleft palate. Am J Med Genet 1986;24: 465–473.

Ross RB, Johnston MC. Cleft lip and palate. Baltimore: Williams & Wilkins, 1972.

Saltzman DH, Benacerraf BR, Frigoletto FD. Diagnosis and management of fetal facial clefts. Am J Obstet Gynecol 1986;155:377–379.

Sander A, Murray JC, Scherpbier-Heddema T, et al. Microsatellite-based fine mapping of the Van der Woude syndrome locus to an interval of 4.1 cM between D1S245 and D1S414. Am J Hum Genet 1995;56:310–318.

Schutte BC, Basart AM, Watanabe Y, et al. Microdeletions at chromosome bands 1q32-q41 as a cause of Van der Woude syndrome. Am J Med Genet 1999;84:145–150.

Seeds JW, Cefalo RC. Technique of early sonographic diagnosis of bilateral cleft lip and palate. Obstet Gynecol 1983;62:2S.

Shaw G, Croen L, Curry C. Isolated oral cleft malformations: associations with maternal and infant characteristics in a California population. Teratology 1991;43:225–228.

Sherer DM, Abramowicz JS, Jaffe R, Woods JR Jr. Cleft palate: confirmation of prenatal diagnosis by colour Doppler ultrasound. Prenat Diagn 1993;13:953–956.

Sherer DM, Hearn B, Abramowicz J. Echogenic oral labial fissure: an aid to rule out fetal cleft lip. J Ultrasound Med 1991;10:239.

Shprintzen RJ, Siegel-Sadewitz VL, Amato J, Goldberg RB. Anomalies associated with cleft lip, cleft palate, or both. Am J Med Genet 1985;20:585–595.

Stein J, Mulliken JB, Stal S, et al. Non-syndromic cleft lip with or without cleft palate: evidence of linkage to BCL3 in 17 multigenerational families. Am J Hum Genet 1995; 57:257–272.

Stoll C, Alembik Y, Dott B, Roth MP. Epidemiological and genetic study in 207 cases of oral clefts in Alsace, northeastern France. J Med Genet 1991;28:325–329.

Strauss RP, Davis JU. Prenatal detection and fetal surgery of cleft and craniofacial abnormalities in humans: social and ethical issues. Cleft Palate Craniofac J 1990;27:176–182.

Tenconi R, Clementi M, Turolla L. Theoretical recurrence risks for cleft lip derived from a population of consecutive newborns. J Med Genet 1988;25:243–246.

Tretsven VE. Incidence of cleft lip and palate in Montana Indians. J Speech Hear Disord 1963;28:52–57.

Turner G, Twining P. The facial profile in the diagnosis of fetal abnormalities. Clin Radiol 1993;47:389–395.

Ulm MR, Kratochwil A, Ulm B, Lee A, Bettelheim D, Bernaschek G. Three-dimensional ultrasonographic imaging of fetal tooth buds for characterization of facial clefts. Early Hum Dev 1999;55:67–75.

Warkany J. Congenital malformations. Chicago: Year Book, 1971.

Weinzweig J, Panter KE, Pantaloni M, et al. The fetal cleft palate: II. Scarless healing after in utero repair of congenital model. Plast Reconstr Surg 1999;104:1356–1364.

Werler MM, Hayes C, Louik C, Shapiro S, Mitchell AA. Multivitamin supplementation and risk of birth defects. Am J Epidemiol 1999;150:675–682.

Werler MM, Lammer EJ, Rosenberg L, Mitchell AA. Maternal cigarette smoking during pregnancy in relation to oral clefts. Am J Epidemiol 1990;132:926–932.

Wilson GN. Human congenital anomalies: application of new genetic tools and concepts. Semin Perinatol 1992; 16:385–400.

Womersley J, Stone DH. Epidemiology of facial clefts. Arch Dis Child 1987;62:717–720.

CHAPTER 25
Hemifacial Microsomia

▶ CONDITION

Hemifacial microsomia is a predominantly unilateral malformation of craniofacial structures that originally develop from the first and second branchial arches. The characteristic findings of hemifacial microsomia include hypoplasia of the malar, maxillary, and/or mandibular regions of the face with associated abnormalities of the ears and vertebrae (Burck 1983). The term *hemifacial microsomia* was first used by Gorlin and Pindborg (1964), who described a condition consisting of unilateral microtia, macrostomia, and failure of formation of the mandibular ramus and condyle. Since then, hemifacial microsomia has been considered one phenotypic manifestation of a group of disorders that affect the face, ears, eyes, vertebrae, heart, and kidneys. This spectrum of disorders has been called "oculoauriculovertebral dysplasia," although this is technically incorrect because the term *dysplasia* refers to abnormalities of cellular differentiation. An association between hemifacial microsomia, auricular malformations, and specific malformations of the eye known as epibulbar dermoids was first recognized by Goldenhar in 1952 (Heffez and Doku 1984). Although the name *Goldenhar syndrome* is widely used, the use of the word *syndrome* is also incorrect because there is no known unique cause for this phenotype. At present, hemifacial microsomia is considered to be part of a complex developmental field defect known as the oculoauriculo-vertebral (OAV) anomaly. There is no agreement on the minimal diagnostic criteria and the phenotypic spectrum for this condition (Rollnick 1988). It is not known whether OAV anomaly represents one entity with variability in the phenotype or whether there are several different entities with similar phenotypes. Causal heterogeneity for this group of conditions has been described (Rollnick 1988). However, any fetus identified with asymmetry of the facial structures or hemifacial microsomia should be considered to be at risk for associated eye, ear, vertebral, cardiac, and renal malformations.

▶ INCIDENCE

The incidence of hemifacial microsomia varies considerably according to the minimal diagnostic criteria used to define the condition. When the most mildly affected individuals are included, the incidence is on the order of 1 in 3000 to 1 in 5000 live births (Benacerraf and Frigoletto 1988). When only the most severely affected patients are included, the incidence was on the order of 1 in 45,000 live births in one study performed in northern Ireland (Morrison et al. 1992). Approximately two-thirds of cases of hemifacial microsomia are unilateral (Singer et al. 1994). When unilateral, the right side is more commonly involved. When the condition is bilateral, one side is more severely affected than the other (Heffez and Doku 1984). In one report of 294 patients affected with the oculo-auriculovertebral anomaly, a male:female ratio of 2:1 was observed (Rollnick et al. 1987). In the same study, 78% of affected individuals were white. In this study, 154 patients (52%) had no other congenital anomaly in addition to the anomalies required for diagnosis, which consisted of microtia, mandibular hypoplasia, anomalies of the cervical spine, and/or anomalies of the eye, including epibulbar dermoids or lipodermoids. Of the remaining patients, 51 (18%) had one additional anomaly and 89 (30%) had two or more additional anomalies (Rollnick et al. 1987).

▶ SONOGRAPHIC FINDINGS

Relatively few reports of hemifacial microsomia have been described in the literature on prenatal sonography.

In 1986, Tamas et al. described a fetus with polyhydramnios, unilateral anophthalmia, and a malformed, low-set ipsilateral ear. This was followed by a report in 1988 from Benacerraf and Frigoletto, who described a fetus at 29 weeks of gestation with moderate polyhydramnios, an abnormal fetal facial profile with micrognathia, a right-kidney hydronephrosis and hydroureter, an enlarged echogenic left lung, a ventriculoseptal cardiac defect, and a two-vessel umbilical cord. Prenatally, a cystic adenomatoid malformation of the lung was suspected, but this was refuted postnatally when it was found that the right lung was absent and the left lung was hyperexpanded. The infant died during the newborn period. Physical examination at birth revealed a right-sided mandibular hypoplasia, an abnormal right ear, and vertebral anomalies that were not appreciated antenatally. Goldenhar syndrome was diagnosed postnatally (Benacerraf and Frigoletto 1988).

Potential sonographic findings in cases of hemifacial microsomia or OAV anomaly might include polyhydramnios due to impaired fetal swallowing. This is likely to be the result of either unilateral mandibular hypoplasia or micrognathia due to hypoplasia of the condyle and ramus, which has been documented in 60% of infants affected with these conditions (Heffez and Doku 1984). Some infants with OAV anomaly are intrauterine-growth-restricted (Kobrynski et al. 1993). In one fetus with Goldenhar syndrome, a lipoma of the corpus callosum, which presented as a hyperechoic midline structure, was described (Jeanty et al. 1991). In

another case, the prenatal sonographic diagnosis of OAV anomaly at 15 weeks' gestation was suggested by the presence of a maxillary cleft in association with unilateral microphthamia (DeCatte et al. 1996).

In any fetus in whom facial asymmetry is suspected, an attempt should be made to sonographically examine the fetal ears, because microtia or other ear abnormalities are frequently seen in association with the mandibular hypoplasia (Fig. 25-1). The spine should be observed closely, as there is an increased incidence of spinal malformations, most commonly, hemivertebrae. The prevalence of associated congenital heart disease in infants with OAV anomaly has been reported to range from 5 to 58% (Kumar et al. 1993). Two-thirds of these cases are either tetralogy of Fallot or a ventriculoseptal defect. In one study 19% (6 of 32) of patients with OAV anomaly had congenital heart disease. The cardiac lesions in this study were varied and more complex than previously reported, including double-outlet ventricle, pulmonary atresia with ventriculoseptal defect, and total anomalous pulmonary venous return. Five of the 6 cases were conotruncal malformations. Pulmonary and renal anomalies were noted to be more common in the patients with congenital heart disease. Morrison et al. (1992) also reported that 8 of their 25 patients with OAV anomaly had congenital heart disease. In fetuses with hemifacial microsomia, the presence of congenital heart disease is an important prognostic factor because of the very high neonatal mortality rate when congenital heart disease exists. In Morrison's study (1992), 6 of 8 infants

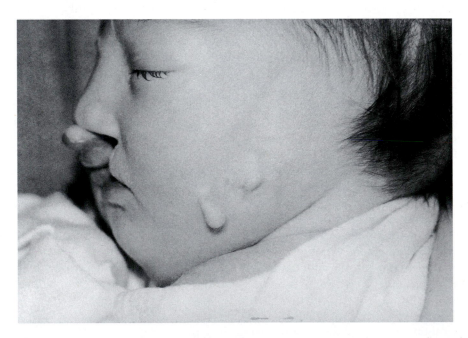

Figure 25-1. Postnatal photograph of a newborn who was noted antenatally to have hemifacial microsomia and a bilateral cleft lip and palate. Note the lack of ear development but the presence of two small ear tags.

died before 2 years of age, and in Kumar's (1993) study, 4 of 6 infants died during the newborn period.

A high incidence of urinary tract abnormalities has also been demonstrated in infants with OAV anomaly. Of 20 infants with OAV anomaly, 14 were demonstrated to have a variety of renal and urinary anomalies, including ectopic or fused kidneys, renal agenesis, vesicoureteral reflux, ureteropelvic obstruction, ureteral duplication, and multicystic kidneys (Ritchey et al. 1994). Therefore, any fetus identified with hemifacial microsomia should undergo a detailed sonographic study with particular attention paid to the ears, heart, vertebrae, and kidneys.

► DIFFERENTIAL DIAGNOSIS

The differential diagnosis includes conditions that are considered to be part of the phenotypic spectrum of hemifacial microsomia and OAV anomaly, as well as other syndromes that include hemifacial microsomia as one component. The differential diagnosis of hemifacial microsomia variants includes microtia, hemifacial microsomia, Goldenhar syndrome, OAV dysplasia, and otomandibular dysostosis. The minimal criteria for these conditions are given in Table 25-1. Other conditions associated with the hemifacial microsomia phenotype include branchio-oto-renal syndrome, a dominantly inherited disorder that consists of hemifacial microsomia, preauricular and branchial sinuses and kidney anomalies; Townes–Brock syndrome, another dominantly inherited disorder that consists of hemifacial microsomia and anal and digital anomalies; and hemifacial microsomia/radial limb defects, which includes the additional finding of triphalangeal thumbs. There have been other case reports of hemifacial microsomia in association with other, more severe anomalies (Dodinval 1979; Rollnick 1988).

► ANTENATAL NATURAL HISTORY

Little is known about the antenatal natural history for fetuses with hemifacial microsomia. More information is available regarding its pathogenesis. Experiments performed in animals have suggested that abnormalities of blood flow to the first and second branchial arches may produce malformations similar to those found in hemifacial microsomia and its variants (Poswillo 1974). Poswillo showed that the presence of an expanding hematoma in the region of the ear and jaw produced a branchial-arch abnormality that destroyed the differentiating tissues in that region. Additional studies using triazene in the pregnant rat or thalidomide in the pregnant monkey produced hemorrhage and formation of hematoma in the anatomic distribution of the stapedial

▶ **TABLE 25-1.** MINIMAL CRITERIA FOR DIAGNOSIS OF HEMIFACIAL MICROSOMIA VARIANTS

Diagnosis	Minimal Criteria
Microtia	Isolated microtia
Hemifacial microsomia	Unilateral microtia
	Small and/or malformed mandible
	Anomalies of cervical spine
Goldenhar syndrome	Unilateral microtia
	Small and/or malformed mandible
	Epibulbar dermoids and/or lipodermoids
Oculo-auriculo-vertebral dysplasia	Unilateral microtia
	Small and/or malformed mandible
	Epibulbar dermoids and/or lipodermoids
	Anomalies of the cervical spine

Reprinted, with permission, from Rollnick BR, Kaye CI. Hemifacial microsomia and variants: pedigree data. Am J Med Genet 1983;15:233–253.

artery. A clinical correlation in humans has been documented by Robinson et al. (1987), who described three unrelated children with unilateral craniofacial defects. Abnormal cartoid-artery blood flow studies were documented in two of the three patients described. This group hypothesized that the craniofacial defects were the result of an in utero vascular accident, most likely due to interruption of blood flow to structures supplied by the stapedial artery. Interestingly, these patients also had unilateral cerebral atrophy. In one patient, a decreased right carotid pulse was documented. This patient also had colonic stenosis, which has also been postulated to be the result of an in utero vascular compromise.

The vascular theory for the pathogenesis of hemifacial microsomia and OAV anomaly could explain abnormalities of the facial features, but it does not explain some of the associated findings, including epibulbar dermoids and other eye malformations and congenital heart disease. These associated abnormalities could be explained by an abnormality in the interaction of neural-crest–cell derivatives with branchial-arch mesenchyme. This could be the result of exposure to a teratogen such as retinoic acid (Lammer et al. 1985). Abnormalities of cranial neural-crest–cell derivatives would also affect conotruncal development of the heart and the anterior chamber of the eye. Also known to cause anomalies of the first and second branchial arches in humans and animals are primidone, thalidomide, and maternal diabetes (Rollnick 1988). Another theory regarding the cause of hemifacial microsomia is that this condition is the result of a local deficit of oxygen or a brief, total hypoxic insult to the embryo, resulting in decreased oxygen for tissue formation.

▶ MANAGEMENT OF PREGNANCY

When a fetus is identified with hemifacial microsomia, a detailed sonographic survey should be performed to examine the fetus for the aforementioned associated anomalies, including microtia, micrognathia, vertebral malformations (most commonly hemivertebrae), congenital heart disease (especially conotruncal defects), and renal abnormalities. An attempt should be made to examine the parents for subtle manifestations of OAV anomaly, such as preauricular tags or fistulae, small or abnormally shaped ears, narrow external auditory canals, or micrognathia. Isolated microtia is considered to be a minimal expression of OAV anomaly (Llano-Rivas et al. 1999). The parents should be asked if there is any history of hearing deficit in the family. If hemifacial microsomia is demonstrated in the fetus, consideration should be given to obtaining a fetal karyotype. Many chromosomal abnormalities have been described in association with facial asymmetry and the OAV anomaly (Table 25-2) (Rollnick 1988). In addition, a case of complete trisomy 22 has been described using fluorescence in situ hybridization studies (Kobrynski et al. 1993). Knowledge of the fetal karyotype will certainly help in establishing a prognosis for the infant and in guiding further treatment. There is no indication for cesarean delivery other than for standard obstetric reasons. We recommend that these infants be delivered in a tertiary-care center if polyhydramnios is present, suggesting micrognathia, and if there is the potential for airway compromise at birth. Most infants with OAV anomaly can be delivered in a community hospital, but should receive multispecialty evaluation, including a clinical genetics examination shortly after birth.

▶ FETAL INTERVENTION

There are no fetal interventions indicated for hemifacial microsomia.

▶ TREATMENT OF THE NEWBORN

The overall goal in the treatment of the newborn with hemifacial microsomia is to determine whether the anatomic defects are localized to the head or whether there are associated anomalies that will influence long-term health. The most important aspect of newborn treatment is a detailed physical examination, with specific attention to the ears, documenting the presence of auricular or preauricular appendages, blind-ending preauricular fistula, abnormalities in ear size or shape, presence of epibulbar dermoids or lipomas, colobomas (notching) of the upper eyelid, hemivertebrae, con-

▶ **TABLE 25-2.** CHROMOSOME ABNORMALITIES ASSOCIATED WITH OAV ANOMALY

Chromosome 5p deletion
Monosomy 6q
Mosaic trisomy 7
Duplication of 7q and 8q
Mosaic trisomy 9
Chromosome 18q deletion
Trisomy 18
Recombinant chromosome 18
Ring chromosome 21
Deletion chromosome 22q 13.31
47,XXY
49,XXXXY

Reprinted, with permission, from Rollnick BR. Oculoauriculovertebral anomaly: variability and causal heterogeneity. Am J Med Genet Suppl 1988;4:41–53.

genital heart disease, and renal anomalies (Thomas 1980). If the vertebrae were not adequately visualized antenatally, we recommend obtaining a postnatal radiograph of the vertebrae to look for malformations of the spine. In addition, we recommend obtaining a postnatal echocardiogram, because of the relatively high incidence of congenital heart lesions. It is especially important to document cardiac anatomy, because of the relatively high postnatal mortality for infants identified with hemifacial microsomia and congenital heart disease (Morrison et al. 1992; Kumar et al. 1993). In addition, because of the high incidence of genitourinary malformations in infants with the OAV anomaly, we recommend that a screening ultrasound examination be performed in the neonatal period to identify significant urologic abnormalities before functional consequences ensue (Ritchey et al. 1994).

▶ SURGICAL TREATMENT

The goals of surgical treatment include improving facial symmetry, stimulating further facial growth, correcting maxillary deficiency, providing a growth center in the temporomandibular joint, improving chewing, allowing for early soft-tissue expansion, and minimizing psychologic trauma associated with an asymmetric facial appearance (Heffez and Doku 1984). The surgical treatment depends on the severity of the mandibular hypoplasia. Mandibular hypoplasia has been classified according to its severity. Grade 1 is a small but normal temporomandibular joint and ramus; Grade 2 is an abnormal but functional temporomandibular joint and ramus; and Grade 3 is an absent temporo-mandibular joint and ramus. With increasing severity of the bony abnormalities, there is more severe hypoplasia of the associated facial and lingual muscles, which exaggerates the asymmetry of the facial appearance. In addition, there is generally a correlation between severity of the microtia and the mandibular anomalies. The mandibular deformity is surgically corrected in two or more stages. The first operation generally is performed when the child is between 5 and 12 years of age and can cooperate with the required postoperative orthodontic therapy. For severely affected patients who have an absent mandibular ramus, an augmentation procedure is performed using costochondral bone grafts (Heffez and Doku 1984). A second operation is generally required during the teenage years, after the majority of facial growth has occurred.

▶ LONG-TERM OUTCOME

For patients with hemifacial microsomia or the OAV anomaly, the long-term health outcome is good. Over 90% of these patients have normal intelligence. Except for those who have severe conotruncal cardiac defects, the general health and life expectancy of these patients are excellent.

▶ GENETICS AND RECURRENCE RISK

The cause of hemifacial microsomia and OAV anomaly is heterogeneous. The majority of patients with hemifacial microsomia occur sporadically within a family. A scarcity of reports of concordance of the defects in monozygotic or dizygotic twins supports this interpretation of the genetics (Boles et al. 1987; Burck 1983; Setzer et al. 1981). However, there have been multiple reports of autosomal dominant inheritance with variable expression of the phenotype (Burck 1983; Singer et al. 1994). There also have been multiple case reports of this finding with two affected siblings and unaffected parents, suggesting autosomal recessive inheritance (Rollnick 1988). As previously discussed, many chromosomal abnormalities have been associated with hemifacial microsomia. Therefore, if a chromosome study was not obtained prenatally, it should be obtained during the newborn period. Rollnick and Kaye (1983) described 97 individuals affected with hemifacial microsomia. Of these, 44 (45%) had relatives with either ear anomalies, mandibular hypoplasia, or early-onset hearing loss. The most frequent malformations included preauricular skin tags. In this study, 8% of first-degree relatives had at least a minor manifestation of hemifacial microsomia.

When counseling the family for recurrence of hemifacial microsomia, the physician must examine the parents and siblings and obtain a complete family history. If the family history is negative and the parental physical examination is negative for the milder forms of hemifacial microsomia, the recurrence risk is 2 to 3% (Burck 1983; Rollnick and Kaye 1983).

REFERENCES

Benacerraf BR, Frigoletto FD. Prenatal ultrasonographic recognition of Goldenhar's syndrome. Am J Obstet Gynecol 1988;159:950–952.

Boles DJ, Bodurtha J, Nance WE. Goldenhar complex in discordant monozygotic twins: a case report and review of the literature. Am J Med Genet 1987;28:103–109.

Burck U. Genetic aspects of hemifacial microsomia. Hum Genet 1983;64:291–296.

DeCatte L, Laubach M, Legein J, Gossens A. Early prenatal diagnosis of oculoauriculovertebral dysplasia or the Goldenhar Syndrome. Ultrasound Obstet Gynecol 1996;8:422–424.

Dodinval P. Facial asymmetries: problems in genetic counseling. J Genet Hum 1979;27:189–203.

Gorlin RJ, Pindborg JJ. Syndromes of the head and neck. New York: McGrawHill, 1964:261–425.

Heffez L, Doku HC. The Goldenhar syndrome: diagnosis and early surgical management. Oral Surg Oral Med Oral Pathol 1984;58:2–9.

Jeanty P, Zaleski W, Fleischer AC. Prenatal sonographic diagnosis of lipoma of the corpus callosum in a fetus with Goldenhar syndrome. Am J Perinatol 1991;8:89–90.

Kobrynski L, Chitayat D, Zahed L, et al. Trisomy 22 and facioauriculovertebral (Goldenhar) sequence. Am J Med Genet 1993;46:68–71.

Kumar A, Friedman JM, Taylor GP, et al. Pattern of cardiac malformation in oculoauriculovertebral spectrum. Am J Med Genet 1993;46:423–426.

Lammer EJ, Chen DT, Hoar RM, et al. Retinoic acid embryopathy. N Engl J Med 1985;313:837–841.

Llano-Rivas I, Gonzalez-Angel A, del Castillo V, Reyes R, Carnevale A. Microtia: a clinical and genetic study at the National Institue of Pediatrics in Mexico City. Arch Med Res 1999;30:120–124.

Morrison PJ, Mulholland HC, Craig BG, et al. Cardovascular abnormalities in the oculo-auriculo-vertebral spectrum (Goldenhar syndrome). Am J Med Genet 1992;44:425–428.

Poswillo D. Otomandibular deformity: Pathogenesis as a guide to reconstruction. J Maxillofac Surg 1974;2:64–73.

Ritchey ML, Norbeck J, Huang C, et al. Urologic manifestations of Goldenhar syndrome. Urology 1994;43:88–91.

Robinson LK, Hoyme HE, Edwards DK, Jones KL. Vascular pathogenesis of unilateral craniofacial defects. J Pediatr 1987;111:236–239.

Rollnick BR. Oculoauriculovertebral anomaly: variability and causal heterogeneity. Am J Med Genet Suppl 1988;4:41–53.

Rollnick BR, Kaye CI. Hemifacial microsomia and variants: pedigree data. Am J Med Genet 1983;15:233–253.

Rollnick BR, Kaye CI, Nagatoshi K, et al. Oculoauriculovertebral dysplasia and variants: phenotypic characteristics of 294 patients. Am J Med Genet 1987;26:361–375.

Schrander-Stumpel CT, de Die-Smulders CE, Hennekam RC, et al. Oculoauriculovertebral spectrum and cerebral anomalies. J Med Genet 1992;29:326–331.

Setzer ES, Ruiz-Castaneda N, Severn C, et al. Etiologic heterogeneity in the oculoauriculovertebral syndrome. J Pediatr 1981;98:88–90.

Singer SL, Haan E, Slee J, et al. Familial hemifacial microsomia due to autosomal dominant inheritance: case reports. Aust Dent J 1994;39:287–291.

Tamas DE, Mahony BS, Bowie JD, et al. Prenatal sonographic diagnosis of hemifacial microsomia (Goldenhar-Gorlin syndrome). J Ultrasound Med 1986;5:461–463.

Thomas P. Goldenhar syndrome and hemifacial microsomia: observations on three patients. Eur J Pediatr 1980;133: 287–292.

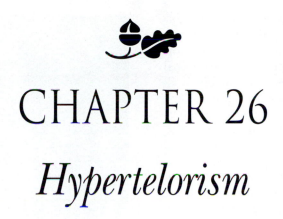

CHAPTER 26

Hypertelorism

▶ CONDITION

Hypertelorism is a condition in which a larger-than-average distance exists between the orbits. The distances between the medial canthi and pupils are also increased (Kirkham et al. 1975). The term was first used by Greig in 1924, who described hypertelorism as a "great breadth between the eyes." Ocular hypertelorism is defined as an increased distance between the medial orbital walls. This can be demonstrated either radiographically or clinically by an increased interpupillary distance. If the interpupillary distance is greater than 2 SD above the mean for the patient's age, hypertelorism is said to exist (Brodsky et al. 1990). More recently, it has been recommended that the diagnosis of hypertelorism be made radiographically by interorbital measurements. The difficulty with using intercanthal distance to define hypertelorism is that soft-tissue changes of the face can increase the intercanthal distance without affecting the interorbital distance (Trout et al. 1994). Telecanthus is an increased distance between the median canthi. This can either be primary, defined as an increase in soft tissue with normal interpupillary and interbony distance, or secondary, which is really orbital hypertelorism, with an increased interbony or interpupillary distance (Murphy and Laskin 1990). The major concern regarding the fetal finding of hypertelorism is its association with median facial and brain defects, such as encephalocele, facial cleft, and craniosynostosis.

▶ INCIDENCE

Hypertelorism is rare. Its exact incidence is unknown. Hypertelorism may occur as an isolated fetal defect or in association with other anomalies.

▶ SONOGRAPHIC FINDINGS

Imaging of the fetal orbits and measurements of the interorbital distance are not routinely performed in most centers that offer targeted fetal sonographic studies. Measurement of the fetal interorbital distance is not included in either the American Institute of Ultrasound in Medicine (AIUM) or American College of Obstetrics and Gynecology (ACOG) guidelines for obstetrical sonography (American College of Obstetrics and Gynecology 1993). Fetal orbital measurements should be performed in any pregnant woman known to have had a previously affected child with a condition associated with hypertelorism, such as Opitz syndrome. Detection of fetal hypertelorism in any structural survey should alert the sonographer to the possibility of other anomalies. The finding should be taken seriously.

In 1985, de Elejalde and de Elejalde studied 1108 pregnant women and measured the interorbital distances in their fetuses between 7 and 38 weeks of gestation. They constructed a chart that derived normal growth percentiles for the intermalar and interethmoidal distances for fetuses between 10 and 40 weeks of gestation. The intermalar and interethmoidal distances were comparable to the postnatal measurements of inner and outer canthal distances. In 1982, Mayden and colleagues described fetal inner and outer orbital diameter measurements in 180 normal pregnancies. The outer orbital diameter was demonstrated to be closely related to the biparietal diameter. Fetal orbits were identified in three different head positions, including occipitotransverse, occipitoposterior, and occipitoanterior. Twelve years after this report, the validity of this nomogram was tested in a high-risk antenatal population by another group of investigators, who obtained inner and outer orbital measurements from 422 fetuses between 12 and 37 weeks of gestation (Trout et al. 1994). This group identified three cases of hypertelorism, with inner orbital measurements above the 95th percentile for gestational age and outer orbital distances within the normal limits but near the 95th percentile for gestational age. In the three cases of hypertelorism identified, all fetuses had serious associated abnormalities, including cleft palate, diaphragmatic hernia, imperforate anus, porencephaly, encephalocele, and truncus arteriosus. The three fetuses with hypertelorism were all diagnosed between 20 and 33 weeks of gestation. These investigators recommended routine measurement of the interorbital distance at the level of the thalamus at the same time that the conventional biparietal diameter measurement was taken. They measured outer orbital diameter from outer to outer bony margins of the orbit, whereas the inner orbital diameter was measured from inner to inner bony margin of the orbits. The bony orbits were seen reliably from 12 weeks of gestation onward. These investigators stressed that it was the inner orbital diameter measurement that was most clearly associated with postnatal hypertelorism. The three affected fetuses described in this study had inner orbital diameter measurements that were more than 2 SD from the mean for gestational age, whereas the outer orbital diameter measurements were borderline high.

In another report of 1600 fetuses screened by transvaginal sonography at 12 to 18 weeks of gestation, 8 ocular abnormalities were found, but no cases of hypertelorism were described (Bronshtein et al. 1991). To date, there have been no reports of fetal hypertelorism in the first trimester.

In one case report, a fetus at 20 weeks of gestation was diagnosed with Opitz syndrome (Hogdall et al. 1989). This syndrome consists primarily of hypertelorism and hypospadias. This fetus was described as an "at-risk" member of a large kindred affected with Opitz syndrome, which is inherited as an autosomal dominant condition. At 18 weeks of gestation, a prenatal sonogram was within normal limits. At that time, the outer orbital measurement was 30 mm (the normal mean for gestational age is 29 mm; range, 24 to 33 mm). The inner orbital measurement was 15 mm (mean for gestational age, 11 mm; range, 8 to 15 mm). At 20 weeks, the study was repeated and a small phallus with hypospadias was noted. In addition, the outer orbital measurement was 36 mm (mean for gestational age, 33 mm; range, 28 to 37 mm) (Fig. 26-1). The inner orbital measurement was 17 mm (mean for gestational age, 13 mm; range, 10 to 16 mm). Because of the provisional diagnosis of an affected fetus with Opitz syndrome, the pregnancy was terminated. Perinatal autopsy studies revealed widely separated eyes and an enlarged fourth ventricle, as well as hypospadias, and imperforate anus. Thus, the fetus was confirmed as affected. This study also reinforced the findings of Trout et al. (1994), who determined that the inner orbital measurement is the more sensitive indicator of the affected fetus with hypertelorism.

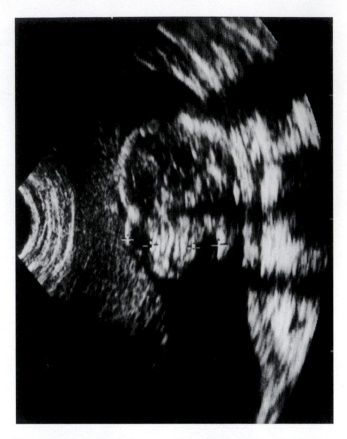

Figure 26-1. Prenatal sonographic image of a fetus at 20 weeks of gestation with Opitz BBB syndrome. Lateral view of orbits demonstrating increased distance between inner aspects of the globes. *(Reprinted, with permission, from Hogdall C, Siegel-Bartelt J, Toi A, Ritchie S. Prenatal diagnosis of Opitz (BBB) syndrome in the second trimester by ultrasound detection of hypospadias and hypertelorism. Prenat Diagn 1989;9:783–793. Copyright 1989 John Wiley & Sons, Inc. Reprinted, by permission, of John Wiley & Sons, Ltd.)*

▶ DIFFERENTIAL DIAGNOSIS

Hypertelorism is strongly associated with other abnormalities, especially of the frontal part of the brain. A number of conditions are associated with hypertelorism, and these are summarized in Table 26-1. Most significantly, these consist of chromosomal abnormalities, single-gene disorders, developmental abnormalities of the skull or brain, and rare syndromes of unknown cause.

▶ ANTENATAL NATURAL HISTORY

The antenatal natural history depends on the underlying condition responsible for the hypertelorism. For example, there is a higher-than-normal rate of miscarriage in fetuses affected with Opitz syndrome (Patton et al. 1986). The natural history for isolated fetal hypertelorism is unknown.

▶ **TABLE 26-1.** CONDITIONS ASSOCIATED WITH HYPERTELORISM

Chromosomal abnormalities
  Trisomy 9p (Centerwall and Beatty-DeSana 1975)
  45,X (Chrousos et al. 1984)
  Interstitial deletion of chromosome 1 (Sarda et al. 1992)
  Interstitial deletion of chromosome 13 (Dean et al. 1991)
  Interstitial deletion of chromosome 17 (Park et al. 1992)
  Chromosome 22q11.2 deletion (Fryburg et al. 1996)
Single gene disorders
Facial–genital disorders
  G syndrome (Opitz–Frias syndrome)
  BBB syndrome (Opitz syndrome)
  Aarskog syndrome
Other single-gene disorders
  Apert syndrome
  Coffin–Lowry syndrome
  Crouzon syndrome
  Frontonasal dysplasia
  LEOPARD syndrome
  Neurofibromatosis
  Noonan syndrome
Developmental abnormalities
  Anterior cephalocele
  Median cleft face
  Frontal, ethmoidal, sphenoidal meningoencephalocele
  Craniosynostosis
  Megalencephaly
Rare syndromes
  Sclerocornea, hypertelorism, syndactyly, ambiguous
    genitalia (Martinez-Frias et al. 1994)
  Diaphragmatic hernia, exomphalos, absent corpus
    callosum, hypertelorism, myopia, deafness (Donnai
    and Barrow 1993)
  Hypertelorism, hypospadias, tetralogy of Fallot (Farag
    and Teebi 1990)
  Hypertelorism, downslanting palpebral fissures, malar
    hypoplasia, low-set ears, joint and scrotal abnormali-
    ties (Seaver and Cassidy 1991)

Hypertelorism has been shown to be the result of first-trimester fetal trauma. In one report, two fetuses were described who were exposed to dilation and curettage during the first trimester of pregnancy (Holmes 1995). The cause of hypertelorism was hypothesized to be the result of exposure to marked and acute mechanical forces on the fetal circulatory system. This resulted in shear stress with release of vasoactive modulators and potentially resulted in the multiple congenital abnormalities described in these two fetuses.

▶ **MANAGEMENT OF PREGNANCY**

When fetal orbital hypertelorism is documented, a detailed anatomic survey should be performed to look for associated malformations, especially in the central nervous system. Strongly associated findings include anterior cephalocele; clefts of the face, lip, palate, and nose; megalencephaly; and craniosynostosis. Because multiple chromosomal abnormalities have been documented in association with fetal hypertelorism, a karyotype should be obtained. Recently, an association between Opitz syndrome and microdeletion of chromosome 22q11.2 has been demonstrated (Fryburg et al. 1996; Lacassie and Arriaza 1996). Both parents should have their inner and outer canthal distances measured and compared with normal standards for adults (Fig. 26-2). If the hypertelorism is apparently isolated, there is no indication for a change in the standard management of pregnancy. If, however, the orbital hypertelorism is found to be associated with a severe brain defect, the parents should be counseled regarding the grim prognosis for this condition. Termination of pregnancy can be discussed if the abnormality is found before 24 weeks of gestation.

Families at risk for many of the single-gene disorders listed in Table 26-1 should have fetal orbital

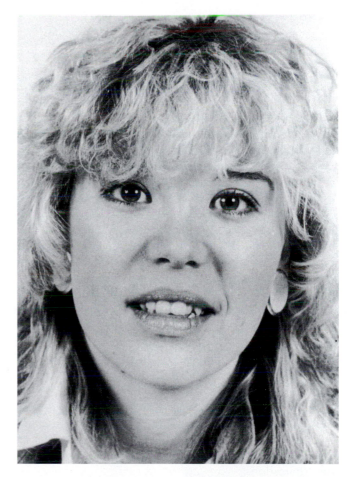

Figure 26-2. The mother of the fetus in Figure 26-1 also had hypertelorism. *(Reprinted, with permission, from Hogdall C, Siegel-Bartelt J, Toi A, Ritchie S. Prenatal diagnosis of Optiz (BBB) syndrome in the second trimester by ultrasound detection of hypospadias and hypertelorism. Prenat Diagn 1989;9:783–793. Copyright 1989 John Wiley & Sons, Inc. Reprinted, by permission, of John Wiley & Sons, Ltd.)*

measurements taken during serial sonographic studies. In one study, hypertelorism was considered to herald a severe expression of brain involvement in neurofibromatosis. In this report, 11 patients with neurofibromatosis were described who had hypertelorism. All the patients had severe central nervous system abnormalities. In an additional 23 patients with neurofibromatosis but no hypertelorism, no central nervous system abnormalities were demonstrated, despite extensive skin involvement with neurofibromas (Westerhof et al. 1984). Although this finding has not been validated prenatally, it would be of interest to routinely measure orbital distances in fetuses at risk for neurofibromatosis, and to correlate those distances with neurologic abnormalities observed postnatally.

▶ FETAL INTERVENTION

There are no fetal interventions recommended for hypertelorism.

▶ TREATMENT OF THE NEWBORN

The infant with isolated hypertelorism should have a detailed physical examination, including postnatal measurements of the inner and outer canthal distances. If a fetal chromosomal analysis was not obtained antenatally, it should be obtained in the immediate postnatal period. In addition, consultation with a medical geneticist is recommended. Consideration should be given to postnatal assessment of the affected infant's intracranial anatomy by computed tomographic (CT) scan. In the absence of documentation of cerebral abnormalities, or in the setting of a family with isolated hypertelorism as a physical trait, the infant affected with isolated hypertelorism should require only routine newborn care.

Infants with hypertelorism and hypospadias should be considered to be at risk for the Opitz-G syndrome (Fig. 26-3) (Cappa et al. 1987). Affected infants have a 30% chance of having laryngotracheal or esophageal clefts. These infants are at high risk for stridor, wheezing, and choking upon feeding. Infants who are clinically diagnosed with this condition should have a barium swallow examination and endoscopy to rule out the presence of these clefts. Many affected infants require tracheostomy, feeding gastrostomy, or a Nissen fundoplication.

▶ SURGICAL TREATMENT

Surgical treatment is not indicated during the newborn period or during very early childhood. Surgical treat-

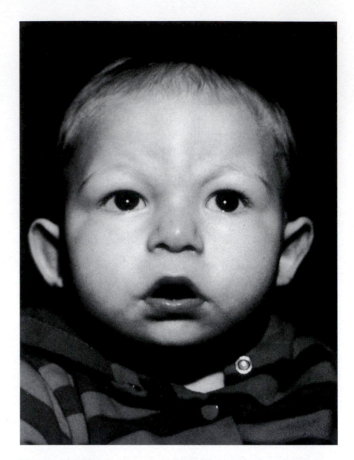

Figure 26-3. A 14-month-old boy with hypertelorism and hypospadias, who was given a clinical diagnosis of Opitz G/BBB syndrome. He had a chromosome deletion of 22q11.2. *(Reprinted, with permission, from Fryburg JS, Lin KY, Golden WL. Chromosome 22q11.2 deletion in a boy with Opitz (G/BBB) syndrome. Am J Med Genet 1996;62:274–275. Copyright ©1996 John Wiley & Sons, Inc. Reprinted, by permission, of Wiley-Liss, Inc., a subsidiary of John Wiley & Sons, Inc.)*

ment should be contemplated only after evaluation by a craniofacial team. The surgical treatment for hypertelorism was first described by Tessier (1974). This treatment involves mobilization of the orbits and their contents to the midline to achieve normal separation between the orbits (Ortiz-Monasterio et al. 1990). In Tessier's description of the surgical technique for hypertelorism, it was demonstrated that

1. Extensive areas of the craniofacial skeleton could be completely devascularized and repositioned and still survive.
2. The orbits could be circumferentially mobilized and repositioned without affecting the patient's vision.
3. Intracranial and extracranial surgery could be combined to treat serious deformities of physical appearance (Tessier 1974; Whitaker and Vander Kolk 1988).

Plastic surgery for hypertelorism is generally not performed before 24 months of age because of the small size of the facial structures and the position of the tooth buds in the maxilla (Whitaker and Vander Kolk 1988). In one report, however, McCarthy et al. (1990) described surgical treatment of hypertelorism as safe, desirable, and effective even in a child under 5 years of age.

▶ LONG-TERM OUTCOME

The long-term outcome for a child with isolated hypertelorism is good. If the hypertelorism is associated with severe cerebral abnormalities, the prognosis will depend on the extent of the severity of the associated anomalies. Many of the single-gene disorders that have been described in association with hypertelorism (Table 26-1) do involve mental retardation or mild developmental disabilities. The reader is referred to Chapter 9 for further information on disorders such as Apert and Crouzon syndromes, which include hypertelorism and craniosynostosis as physical findings.

▶ GENETICS AND RECURRENCE RISK

The genetics of hypertelorism will depend on the underlying cause for this finding. If a chromosomal abnormality such as an interstitial deletion or partial trisomy is detected, parental chromosomes must be studied. Further genetic counseling will depend on whether the parents are shown to be carriers of a balanced translocation. Ten percent of cases of Turner syndrome (45,X) have hypertelorism (Chrousos et al. 1984). The recurrence risk for Turner syndrome is not considered to be increased above background, and it is independent of maternal age. In one case report, a deletion of chromosome 22q11.2 was found in a male with Opitz G/BBB syndrome (Fryburg et al. 1996).

Every attempt should be made to make a definitive diagnosis in the infant with hypertelorism. This will permit accurate estimates of recurrence risk and counseling, as many of the conditions associated with hypertelorism described in Table 26-1 are inherited as autosomal dominant traits. If one of the parents is diagnosed retrospectively as having a single-gene disorder, such as Opitz syndrome, the parents can be counseled about the 50% recurrence risk in future children.

No specific gene has been identified for hypertelorism. Prenatal diagnosis in subsequent pregnancies can be made by sonographic measurement of the fetal orbits.

REFERENCES

American College of Obstetrics and Gynecology. Ultrasonography in pregnancy. ACOG Tech Bull 1993; December:187.

Brodsky MC, Keppen LD, Rice CD, Ranells JD. Ocular and systemic findings in the Aarskog (facial-digital-genital) syndrome. Am J Ophthalmol 1990;109:450–456.

Bronshtein M, Zimmer E, Gershoni-Baruch R, Yoffe N, Meyer H, Blumenfeld Z. First and second trimester diagnosis of fetal ocular defects and associated anomalies: report of eight cases. Obstet Gynecol 1991;77:443–449.

Cappa M, Borrelli P, Marini R, Neri G. The Opitz syndrome: a new designation for the clinically indistinguishable BBB and G syndromes. Am J Med Genet 1987;28:303–309.

Centerwall WR, Beatty-DeSana JW. The trisomy 9p syndrome. Pediatrics 1975;56:748–755.

Chrousos GA, Ross JL, Chrousos G, et al. Ocular findings in Turner sydrome: a prospective study. Ophthalmology 1984;91:926–928.

Dean JC, Simpson S, Couzin DA, Stephen GS. Interstitial deletion of chromosome 13: prognosis and adult phenotype. J Med Genet 1991;28:533–535.

de Elejalde MM, de Elejalde BR. Ultrasonographic visualization of the fetal eye. J Craniofac Genet Dev Biol 1985; 5:319–326.

Donnai D, Barrow M. Diaphragmatic hernia, exomphalos, absent corpus callosum, hypertelorism, myopia, and sensorineural deafness: a newly recognized autosomal recessive disorder? Am J Med Genet 1993;47:679–682.

Farag TI, Teebi AS. Autosomal recessive inheritance of a syndrome of hypertelorism, hypospadias, and tetralogy of Fallot? Am J Med Genet 1990;35:516–518.

Fryburg JS, Lin KY, Golden WL. Chromosome 22q11.2 deletion in a boy with Opitz (G/BBB) syndrome. Am J Med Genet 1996;62:274–275.

Greig DM. Hypertelorism: A hitherto undifferentiated congenital cranio-facial deformity. Edin Med J 1924;31:560.

Hogdall C, Siegel-Bartelt J, Toi A, Ritchie S. Prenatal diagnosis of Opitz (BBB) syndrome in the second trimester by ultrasound detection of hypospadias and hypertelorism. Prenat Diagn 1989;9:783–793.

Holmes LB. Possible fetal effects of cervical dilation and uterine curettage during the first trimester of pregnancy. J Pediatr 1995;126:131–134.

Kirkham TH, Milot J, Berman P. Ophthalmic manifestations of Aarskog (facial-digital-genital) syndrome. Am J Ophthalmol 1975;79:441–445.

Lacassie Y, Arriaza MI. Opitz G/BBB syndrome and the 22q11.2 deletion. Am J Med Genet 1996;62:318.

Martinez-Frias ML, Bermejo E, Sanchez-Otero T, Urioste M, Morena V, Cruz E. Sclerocornea, hypertelorism, syndactyly, and ambiguous genitalia. Am J Med Genet 1994; 49:195–197.

Mayden KL, Tortora M, Berkowitz RL, Bracken M, Hobbins JC. Orbital diameters: a new parameter for prenatal diagnosis and dating. Am J Obstet Gynecol 1982;144:289–297.

McCarthy JG, La Trenta GS, Breitbart AS, Zide BM, Cutting CB. Hypertelorism correction in the young child. Plast Reconstr Surg 1990;86:214–225.

Murphy WK, Laskin DM. Intercanthal and interpupillary distance in the black population. Oral Surg Oral Med Oral Pathol 1990;69:676–680.

Ortiz-Monasterio F, Medina O, Musolas A. Geometrical planning for the correction of orbital hypertelorism. Plast Reconstr Surg 1990;86:650–657.

Park JP, Moeschler JB, Berg SZ, Bauer RM, Wurster-Hill DH. A unique de novo interstitial deletion del (17) (q21.3q23) in a phenotypically abnormal infant. Clin Genet 1992;41:54–56.

Patton MA, Baraitser M, Nickolaides K, Rodeck CH, Gamsu H. Prenatal treatment of fetal hydrops associated with the hypertelorism-dysphagia syndrome. Prenat Diagn 1986; 6:109–115.

Sarda P, Lefort G, Taviaux S, Humeau C, Rieu D. Interstitial deletion of chromosome 1 del (1) (q32 q42): case report and review of the literature. Clin Genet 1992;441:25–27.

Seaver LH, Cassidy SB. New syndrome: mother and son with hypertelorism, downslanting palpebral fissures, malar hypoplasia, and apparently low-set ears associated with joint and scrotal anomalies. Am J Med Genet 1991;41: 405–409.

Tessier P. Experiences in the treatment of orbital hypertelorism. Plast Reconstr Surg 1974;53:1–19.

Trout T, Budorick NE, Pretorius DH, McGahan JP. Significance of orbital measurements in the fetus. J Ultrasound Med 1994;13:937–943.

Westerhof W, Delleman JW, Wolters E, Dijkstra P. Neurofibromatosis and hypertelorism. Arch Dermatol 1984;120: 1579–1581.

Whitaker LA, Vander Kolk C. Orbital reconstruction in hypertelorism. Otolaryngol Clin North Am 1988;21: 199–214.

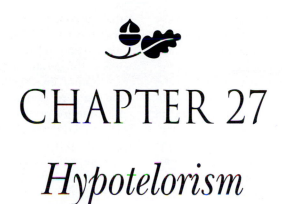

CHAPTER 27

Hypotelorism

► CONDITION

The term *hypotelorism* was used as early as 1960 to indicate a decrease in interorbital distance (Judisch et al. 1984). *Ocular hypotelorism* is defined as a decreased distance between the eyes or pupils, whereas *orbital hypotelorism* is defined as a shortened distance between the medial aspects of the orbital walls (Converse et al. 1975; Judisch et al. 1984). The major concern regarding the finding of fetal hypotelorism is its association with midline craniofacial defects and major cerebral anomalies.

Orbital hypotelorism results from developmental abnormalities of the telencephalon, which is a derivative of the forebrain. It is strongly associated with holoprosencephaly (see Chapter 13) (Achiron et al. 1995; Converse et al. 1975). Frequently, hypotelorism is more obvious radiographically or sonographically than clinically. In one study, the normal range of interorbital distances was documented in anteroposterior facial radiographs obtained in 250 normal children. The mean values ranged from 15 mm in infancy to 23 mm at 12 years of age. The interorbital distance was found to be narrower for girls than for boys. The interorbital distance normally remains small until 18 months of age, when distance gradually increases in both sexes. Interorbital growth levels off in females at age 13 years, but in males this distance continues to increase until 21 years of age (Converse et al. 1975). Interorbital distances are closely related to ethnic background. Individuals who trace their ancestry to Eskimos or Mongolians may have hypotelorism as a normal genetic variation (Awan 1977).

► INCIDENCE

Hypotelorism is uncommon. Most references list the incidence of hypotelorism as unknown, but one reference documented hypotelorism in 1 in 1220 deliveries in Taiwan (a frequency of 0.08% live births) (Kuo et al. 1990).

► SONOGRAPHIC FINDINGS

Imaging of the fetal orbits and measurements of the interorbital distance are not routine in most centers that provide antenatal sonography. Measurement of the interorbital distance is not included in the American Institute of Ultrasound in Medicine (AIUM) or American College of Obstetrics and Gynecology (ACOG) guidelines for obstetrical sonography (American College of Obstetrics and Gynecology 1993). Fetal orbital measurements should be taken in any pregnant woman with a previously affected child, or in the setting of a central nervous system malformation such as hydrocephalus or holoprosencephaly or a facial cleft. When orbital hypotelorism is discovered, the finding should be taken seriously, because of its strong association with cerebral abnormalities (Trout et al. 1994). In 1982, Jeanty and colleagues determined the ocular diameter, interocular distances, and binocular distances in a group of fetuses. They proposed the use of inner and outer canthal distances as an indication of fetal growth. In another study of 1108 pregnant women, the interorbital distances were analyzed in fetuses between 7 and 38 weeks of gestation. A chart consisting of normal growth percentiles for the intermalar and interethmoidal distances was created for fetuses between 10 and 40 weeks of gestation (de Elejalde and de Elejalde 1985). These investigators thought that the intermalar and interethmoidal distances were comparable to postnatal measurements of inner and outer canthal distances. In 1982, Mayden and colleagues constructed a nomogram from measurements of fetal inner and outer orbital diameters obtained in 180 normal pregnancies. These investigators demonstrated that the outer orbital diameter was closely related to the biparietal diameter. After constructing this nomogram, they studied an additional 463 fetuses considered to be at high risk for anomalies. They diagnosed three cases of hypotelorism because fetal orbital measurements were below the 95th percentile confidence limits. In two of these three fetuses, hypotelorism was confirmed postnatally, and the other was lost to follow-up. This nomogram was also used to examine six fetuses at risk for ocular abnormalities due to prior affected children in the family. In all six cases, normal antenatal measurements were predicted and correlated with normal neonatal interocular distances (Mayden et al. 1982). Twelve years after this report, the validity of this nomogram was tested in a high-risk antenatal population. The new investigators obtained inner and outer canthal measurements of 422 fetuses studied prospectively over a period of 12 months. These fetuses were between 12 and 37 weeks of gestation (Trout et al. 1994). This group identified six cases of hypotelorism and two cases of cyclopia. For all of these affected fetuses, both the inner and outer canthal measurements fell clearly below 2 SD of the mean. Most cases had measurements that were 3 or 4 SD below the mean and were very clearly abnormal. In all the cases of hypotelorism, there were associated intracranial or extracranial abnormalities, including holoprosencephaly, encephalocele, cleft palate, cardiac anomalies, imperforate anus, congenital diaphragmatic hernia, and digital anomalies. These investigators recommended measurement of the interorbital distance at the level of the thalamus at the same time that the biparietal diameter was measured (Fig. 27-1). They stated that bony orbits were seen reliably in transabdominal scans from 12 weeks of gestation and later.

Other investigators recommend a coronal view of the fetus to demonstrate both orbits, the maxilla, and the anterior portion of the mandible in a vertical plane. They recommend moving the transducer posteriorly to image both bony orbits (Meizner et al. 1987). In one case report, a fetus at 38 weeks of gestation was demonstrated to have hypotelorism in association with microphthalmia, microcephaly, and alobar holoprosencephaly (Kuo et al. 1990). These investigators stressed the importance of using measurements based on normal standards for the patient's specific ethnic group, which in this case was Chinese.

More recently, transvaginal sonography has been used to detect fetal ocular abnormalities. In one report of 1600 cases screened at 12 to 18 weeks of gestation, 8 cases of ocular abnormalities were seen. There were associated defects of the central nervous system in 5 of the 8. These authors recommended that the optimal section in a transvaginal scan consists of a transverse image of the fetal skull at the orbital plane. They also recommended an oblique tangential section from the nasal bridge, which can also detect hypoechogenic circles lateral to the nose in the anterior part of the orbits representing the fetal lens. Using this approach, Bronshtein and colleagues (1991) were able to detect the fetal eyes within the orbits in 40% of cases at 11 weeks of gestation and 100% of cases at 12 weeks of gestation.

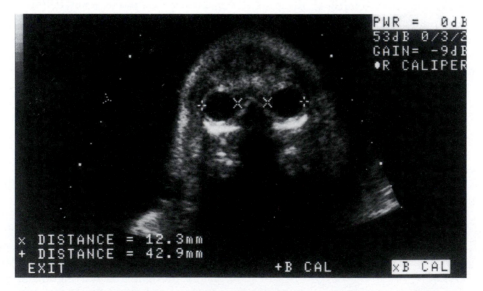

Figure 23-1. Antenatal sonogram demonstrating the presence of hypotelorism. The Xs mark the inner orbital measurement (12.3 mm) and the +s mark the outer orbital measurement (42.9 mm). Both of these measurements are abnormal for gestational age. *(Photograph courtesy of Dr. Marjorie C. Treadwell.)*

▶ DIFFERENTIAL DIAGNOSIS

Fetal hypotelorism is strongly associated with abnormalities of the brain, specifically telencephalon derivatives, including the spectrum of malformations seen in holoprosencephaly (see Chapter 13) (Wong et al. 1999). The associated conditions include arrhinencephalia, cebocephaly, ethmocephaly, otocephaly, and cyclopia (Lin et al. 1998). Many chromosomal abnormalities are associated with orbital hypotelorism. The most common is trisomy 13, but trisomy 20p, partial trisomy 15p, trisomy 21, and chromosome 5p deletion have also been seen. In one study, three of six fetuses with orbital hypotelorism had chromosomal abnormalities including trisomy 13, ring 21, and chromosome 7 short arm deletion (Trout et al. 1994). Hypotelorism is also associated with abnormalities of head shape, including microcephaly and trigonocephaly. Syndromes associated with hypotelorism include Meckel–Gruber, Williams, Coffin–Siris, Langer–Giedion, oculodentodigital dysplasia, nasal maxillary dysostosis (Binder syndrome), and craniosynostosis-medial aplasia (Jeanty et al. 1982; Judisch et al. 1984).

▶ ANTENATAL NATURAL HISTORY

The antenatal natural history depends on the underlying condition responsible for the hypotelorism. The natural history for isolated fetal hypotelorism is unknown.

▶ MANAGEMENT OF PREGNANCY

When orbital hypotelorism is documented, a detailed anatomic survey should be performed to look for associated malformations, particularly in the central nervous system. Holoprosencephaly should be ruled out. In addition, because of the multiple chromosomal abnormalities seen in association with hypotelorism, a fetal karyotype should be obtained. Both parents should have their inner and outer canthal distances measured and compared with normal standards for adults. If the hypotelorism is apparently isolated, there is no indication for a change in the standard management of pregnancy. If the orbital hypotelorism is found to be associated with holoprosencephaly, the parents should be counseled regarding the grim prognosis for this condition. Termination of pregnancy should be discussed if the abnormality is found before 24 weeks of gestation.

▶ FETAL INTERVENTION

There are no fetal interventions for hypotelorism.

▶ TREATMENT OF THE NEWBORN

The infant with isolated hypotelorism should have a detailed physical examination, including postnatal measurements of the inner and outer canthal distances. If a chromosomal analysis was not obtained antenatally, it should be obtained during the postnatal period. In addition, consultation with a medical geneticist is recommended. Consideration should be given to postnatal assessment of the infant's intracranial anatomy by computed tomographic (CT) scan. In the absence of documentation of cerebral abnormalities, the infant with isolated hypotelorism should require only routine newborn care.

▶ SURGICAL TREATMENT

Surgical treatment is not indicated during the newborn period or during early childhood. For the patient who has isolated severe orbital hypotelorism resulting from a syndrome, plastic surgery is possible later in life. In one report, severe orbital hypotelorism was successfully corrected surgically in a 14-year-old girl with nasomaxillary dysostosis (Binder syndrome) (Converse et al. 1975).

▶ LONG-TERM OUTCOME

The long-term outcome for a child with isolated hypotelorism is expected to be good. If the hypotelorism is associated with severe cerebral abnormalities, prognosis will depend on the severity of the associated anomalies. The reader is referred to Chapter 13 for further information on this condition.

▶ GENETICS AND RECURRENCE RISK

The genetics of hypotelorism will depend on the underlying cause for this finding. If a chromosomal deletion or partial trisomy is detected, parental chromosomes should be studied. Further genetic counseling will depend on whether the parents are shown to be carriers of a balanced translocation. If the underlying diagnosis is trisomy 13, the parents should be counseled that there is a recurrence risk of 1% in addition to the maternal-age–related risks. Hypotelorism has been reported as an isolated trait inherited as an autosomal dominant in a three-generation pedigree (Judisch et al. 1984). In this family, intelligence was completely normal. If parental measurements are consistent with a familial trait of hypotelorism, the parents can be counseled about the 50% recurrence risk.

At present, no specific gene has been identified for hypotelorism.

REFERENCES

Achiron R, Gottlieb Z, Yaron Y, Gabbay M, Lipitz S, Mashiach S. The development of the fetal eye: in utero ultrasonographic measurements of the vitreous and lens. Prenat Diagn 1995;15:155–160.

American College of Obstetrics and Gynecology. Ultrasonography in pregnancy. ACOG Tech Bull 1993;December:187.

Awan KJ. Hypotelorism and optic disc anomalies: an ignored ocular syndrome. Ann Ophthalmol 1977;9:771–777.

Bronshtein M, Zimmer E, Gershoni-Baruch R, Yoffe N, Meyer H, Blumenfeld Z. First and second trimester diagnosis of fetal ocular defects and associated anomalies: report of eight cases. Obstet Gynecol 1991;77:443–449.

Converse JM, McCarthy JG, Wood–Smith D. Orbital hypotelorism: pathogenesis, associated facio-cerebral anomalies, surgical correction. Plast Reconstr Surg 1975;56: 389–394.

de Elejalde MM, de Elejalde BR. Ultrasonographic visualization of the fetal eye. J Craniofac Genet Dev Biol 1985;5: 319–326.

Jeanty P, Dramaix-Wilmet M, Van Gansbeke O, Van Regemorter V, Rodesch R. Fetal ocular biometry by ultrasound. Radiology 1982;143:513–516.

Judisch GF, Kraft SP, Bartley JA, Jacoby CG. Orbital hypotelorism: an isolated autosomal dominant trait. Arch Ophthalmol 1984;102:995–997.

Kuo H-C, Chang F-M, Wu C-H, Yao B-L, Liu C-H. Antenatal ultrasonographic diagnosis of hypertelorism. J Formos Med Assoc 1990;89:803–805.

Lin HH, Liang RI, Chang FM, Chang CH, Yu CH, Yang HB. Prenatal diagnosis of otocephaly using two-dimensional and three-dimensional ultrasonography. Ultrasound Obstet Gynecol 1998;11:361–363.

Mayden KL, Tortora M, Berkowitz RL, Bracken M, Hobbins JC. Orbital diameters: a new parameter for prenatal diagnosis and dating. Am J Obstet Gynecol 1982;144:289–297.

Meizner I, Katz M, Bar-Ziv J, Insler V. Prenatal sonographic detection of fetal facial malformations. Isr J Med Sci 1987; 23:881–885.

Trout T, Budorick NE, Pretorius DH, McGahan JP. Significance of orbital measurements in the fetus. J Ultrasound Med 1994;13:937–943.

Wong HS, Lam YH, Tang MH, Cheung LW, Ng LK, Yan KW. First-trimester ultrasound diagnosis of holoprosencephaly: three case reports. Ultrasound Obstet Gynecol 1999; 13:356–359.

CHAPTER 28

Macroglossia

► CONDITION

Macroglossia is defined in children as a resting tongue that protrudes beyond the teeth or the alveolar ridge (Weiss and White 1990; Weissman et al. 1995). The antenatal diagnosis of macroglossia is subjective because no standard measurements of tongue size exist for the fetus or neonate. In the neonate, the tongue grows faster than the other oral structures. Growth of the tongue is also not limited by the presence of teeth. Some normal neonates at rest may exhibit apparent enlargement of the tongue and protrusion through the lips. For the majority of these newborns, however, the tongue recedes into place with normal anatomic growth of the mouth (Myer et al. 1986). The first scientific report of macroglossia occurred in 1854, when Virchow and Uber described a lingual lymphatic malformation that arose from dilation of lymphatic spaces in the tongue (Vogel et al. 1986).

Vogel and colleagues (1986) have defined two types of macroglossia: "true" and "relative." *True macroglossia* means that histologic abnormalities of the tongue are present that correlate with the clinical findings of tongue enlargement. Examples of such findings include vascular malformations, muscular hypoplasia, tumor infiltrate, or the presence of abnormal elements within the tongue, including edema, inflammation, or storage material. *Relative macroglossia* means that there is apparent tongue enlargement, but no histologic changes within the tongue are demonstrated. An example of relative macroglossia is trisomy 21, in which the tongue is normal but appears large due to mandibular or maxillary underdevelopment or generalized oropharyngeal hypotonia. In Beckwith–Wiedemann syndrome, the histology of the tongue is normal, and the macroglossia is due to hyperplasia of the muscle fibers. In lymphangioma, histologic analysis reveals numerous endothelial-lined cystic spaces that contain lymphatic fluid, erythrocytes, and lymphocytes in a thin stroma of connective tissue. The striated muscle in the tongue subsequently atrophies where compression has occurred from dilated lymphatics (Rice and Carson 1985).

► INCIDENCE

Macroglossia is a rare fetal finding (Weismann et al. 1995). To our knowledge, there are no published reports of the true incidence of macroglossia presenting in utero. An estimate of the incidence of macroglossia may be calculated indirectly from the incidences of three common conditions that are associated with macroglossia—Beckwith–Wiedemann syndrome, congenital hypothyroidism, and trisomy 21. The incidence of Beckwith–Wiedemann syndrome is one in 13,500 births (Patterson et al. 1988). Approximately 82 to 99% of infants with Beckwith–Wiedemann syndrome have macroglossia (Elliott and Maher 1994; McManamny and Barnett 1985). Taking the more conservative estimate of macroglossia in Beckwith–Wiedemann syndrome (82%), this would give an approximate incidence of 1 in 16,000 live births with macroglossia due to Beckwith–Wiedemann syndrome. Overall, trisomy 21 occurs in 1 in 1000 live births. Approximately 8.9% of fetuses with trisomy 21 have macroglossia (Weismann et al. 1995). This would give a live-birth incidence of macroglossia due to trisomy 21 of 1 in 11,000 live births. Congenital hypothyroidism occurs in 1 in 5000 live births (Kourides et al. 1984). Approximately 20% of newborns with hypothyroidism have macroglossia (Grant et al. 1992). This would equal a live-birth incidence of 1 in 25,000 live births with hypothyroidism and macroglossia. Summation of these studies gives a range of 1 in 11,000 to 1 in 25,000 live births presenting with macroglossia as a symptom.

▶ SONOGRAPHIC FINDINGS

The tongue can be successfully imaged by an inferior coronal view of the fetal face. The tongue can also be visualized by the sagittal profile face view, if the tongue is extending from the mouth (Fig. 28-1A) (Weismann et al. 1995). Fetuses with macroglossia have a large protruding tongue (Fig. 28-2A). Although nomograms have been published for both first and second trimester fetal tongue size (Achiron et al. 1997; Bronshtein et al. 1998), the diagnosis is usually subjective. Additional sonographic findings include polyhydramnios due to impairment in fetal swallowing. Considerations in the further assessment of fetuses with macroglossia include a detailed search for associated anomalies. Specifically, it is important to rule out fetal goiter (Kourides et al.

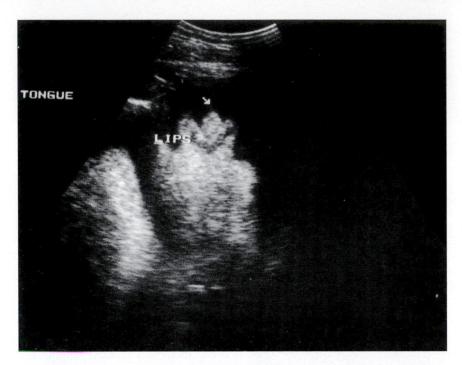

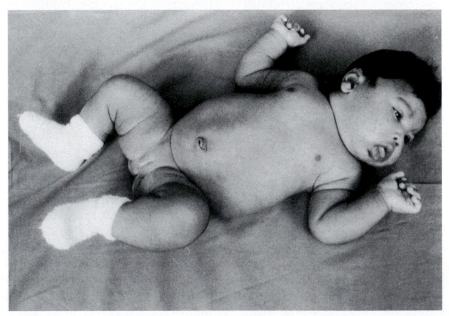

Figure 28-1. Top: Prenatal sagittal scan performed at 34 weeks of gestation, demonstrating a large tongue that protrudes beyond the fetal lips. Bottom: Postnatal photograph of same individual at 2 months of age. The macrosomia, macroglossia, and lax abdominal musculature were consistent with a diagnosis of Beckwith–Wiedemann syndrome. *(Reprinted, with permission, from Viljoen DL, Jaquire Z, Woods DL. Prenatal diagnosis in autosomal dominant Beckwith-Wiedemann syndrome. Prenat Diagn 1991;11:167–175. Copyright 1991 John Wiley & Sons Ltd. Reprinted, by permission, of John Wiley & Sons Ltd.)*

1984). A large-for-gestational-age fetus with polyhydramnios might also suggest maternal diabetes. A macrosomic fetus with macroglossia and other findings, such as omphalocele, increased abdominal circumference, adrenal gland cyst, nephromegaly, and cardiovascular abnormalities, is likely to have Beckwith–Wiedemann syndrome. Table 28-1 summarizes the prenatal ultrasonographic findings in six cases of Beckwith–Wiedemann syndrome. Macrosomia due to Beckwith–Wiedemann syndrome is a constant finding and can be diagnosed between 16 and 22 weeks of gestation (Viljoen et al. 1991). Prenatal diagnosis of Beckwith–Wiedemann syndrome

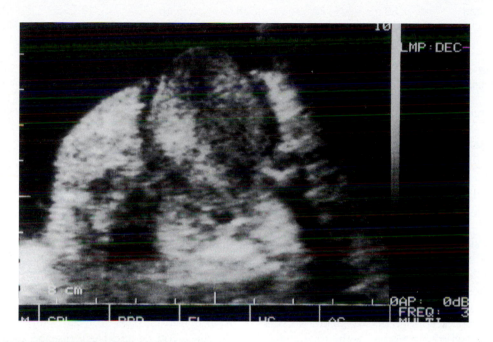

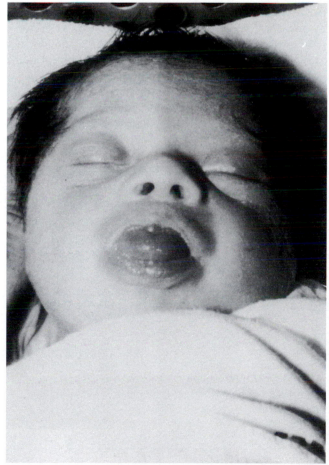

Figure 28-2. Top: Axial scan through the floor of the fetal mouth, performed at 22 weeks of gestation, demonstrating a large tongue that extends outside of the mouth. This was the only abnormal finding. Bottom: Postnatal photograph of same infant during the neonatal period, showing an enlarged tongue. The karyotype revealed trisomy 21. *(Reprinted, with permission, from Weissman A, Mashiach S, Achiron R. Macroglossia: prenatal ultrasonographic diagnosis and proposed management. Prenat Diagn 1995;15:66–69. Copyright 1995 John Wiley & Sons Ltd. Reprinted, by permission, of John Wiley & Sons Ltd.)*

▶ **TABLE 28-1.** ULTRASONOGRAPHIC AND CLINICAL FINDINGS IN SIX FETUSES WITH BECKWITH–WIEDEMANN SYNDROME

Clinical Characteristics	Case 1	Case 2	Case 3	Case 4	Case 5	Case 6	Total
Family history of BWS	Sporadic	Affected Sibling	Affected Sibling	Affected Sibling	Affected Sibling	Mother has BWS	5/6
Ultrasound feature (wga*)							
Diagnosis suspected	20	20	18	16	18	22	—
Hydramnios	+(20)	—	+	+	+	Mild (22)	5/6
Macroglossia	—	—	—	—	—	+(34)	1/6
Macrosomia	+(20)	+	+	+	+(18)	+(34)	6/6
Renal hyperplasia	+(20)	—	—	—	—	+(22)	2/6
Adrenal hyperplasia	—	—	+	—	—	—	1/6
Omphalocele	+	+	+	+	+(18–19)	—	5/6
Abdominal circumference	—	—	—	—	+(19)	+(22)	2/6
Hepatomegaly	—	—	—	—	—	+(29)	1/6
Termination of pregnancy	—	—	+(19)	—	+(21)	—	2/6
Birth weight (g)	4285	4600	—	5100	—	5300	

*wga = Gestational age in weeks.

(from Viljoen et al. 1991)

has been reported at 19 weeks of gestation (Winter et al. 1986), 28 weeks of gestation (Wieacker et al. 1989), and 30 weeks of gestation (Cobellis et al. 1988). Prenatal sonographic diagnosis is not always conclusive for this condition. Even in the setting of a positive family history and multiple prenatal sonograms, the diagnosis was missed in a fetus who presented with severe hydronephrosis, cardiomegaly, and hepatomegaly in utero (Nowotny et al. 1994). An additional important consideration in fetal sonographic assessment of macroglossia is the possibility of lingual lymphatic malformations, often seen in association with other lymphatic malformations, such as cystic hygroma. Prenatal sonographic assessment should also specifically exclude abnormalities associated with trisomy 21, such as shortening of the long bones, an increased nuchal fold, cardiovascular defects, widening of the space between the first and second toes, and renal pyelectasis.

▶ DIFFERENTIAL DIAGNOSIS

The differential diagnosis of conditions associated with macroglossia is given in Table 28-2. The most important considerations in the differential diagnosis include Beckwith–Wiedemann syndrome (exomphalos-macroglossia-gigantism, or EMG, syndrome) (Fig. 28-1B), trisomy 21 (Fig. 28-2B), congenital hypothyroidism, lingual lymphatic malformations, tumor/epignathus, and hemangiomas/vascular malformations. Prior to the recognition of Beckwith–Wiedemann syndrome in 1963, lymphangioma was the most common cause of macroglossia presenting during the newborn period. Sixty percent of lymphangiomas that involve the tongue present at birth (Rice and Carson 1985). Lingual lymphatic

malformations are the most common vascular abnormalities of the tongue and are frequently localized to the anterior two-thirds of the tongue. Inborn errors of metabolism that can be associated with macroglossia include Hunter, Hurler, Maroteaux–Lamy, and Sanfilippo syndromes, as well as Pompe (glycogen storage disease, type II) and I-cell disease, and GM_1 gangliosidosis. Of these, the disorders that can present during the newborn period are Hurler, I-cell, GM_1 gangliosidosis, and possibly Pompe. Patients with I-cell disease are typically growth-restricted and have abnormal neurologic signs. Farber's lipogranulomatosis, in its most severe form, can present during the neonatal period. These infants will have the classic triad of subcutaneous nodules, hoarseness, and joint involvement.

▶ ANTENATAL NATURAL HISTORY

The antenatal natural history of macroglossia is unremarkable. As an isolated finding, there is no evidence

▶ **TABLE 28-2.** DIFFERENTIAL DIAGNOSIS OF CONDITIONS ASSOCIATED WITH MACROGLOSSIA

Beckwith–Wiedemann syndrome
Trisomy 21
Congenital hypothyroidism
Lymphangioma
Hemangioma
Inborn error of metabolism
Isolated autosomal dominant trait
Lingual thyroid
Neurofibroma
Epignathus

for in utero lethality due to the presence of macroglossia. However, macroglossia due to trisomy 21 does have an increased risk for pregnancy loss. As stated earlier, there can be polyhydramnios associated with macroglossia due to impairment of swallowing.

▶ MANAGEMENT OF PREGNANCY

When macroglossia is documented in utero, detailed level II sonography is indicated to look for associated anomalies. It is important to rule out the anomalies associated with Beckwith–Wiedemann syndrome, such as omphalocele, macrosomia, and nephromegaly. It is also important to rule out trisomy 21. Nicolaides et al. (1992, 1993) described a series of 13 fetuses with macroglossia. In 10, a chromosomal abnormality was found, and 9 of the 10 had trisomy 21. None of these patients had isolated macroglossia; additional anomalies were always documented. However, Weismann et al. (1995), have described a case of isolated macroglossia due to trisomy 21 (see Fig. 28-2). Given the fact that macroglossia is a relatively rare finding, we recommend obtaining a chromosomal analysis on the fetus with macroglossia. This is important for two reasons: one is to rule out trisomy 21 as the cause of the macroglossia. The other consideration is that in some cases of Beckwith–Wiedemann syndrome, there are abnormalities seen in chromosome 11p15.

If hypothyroidism is suspected in the fetus, particularly in the presence of a goiter, it has been recommended to obtain amniotic fluid thyroid-stimulating hormone (TSH) levels to confirm the diagnosis. According to Kourides et al. (1984), the normal TSH levels in amniotic fluid at 26 and 38 weeks of gestation are 0.44 ± 0.21 μU per milliliter and 0.27 ± 0.15 μU per milliliter, respectively. The fetus reported by Kourides et al. had markedly elevated TSH values of 2.4 and 2.9 μU per milliliter at 26 and 38 weeks. These authors advocate the early diagnosis of hypothyroidism to permit treatment of the infant on day 1 of life. Although newborn screening for hypothyroidism is routine in most states, the diagnosis is not usually communicated to the pediatrician until 2 to 3 weeks after birth. Thus, the infant does not generally receive treatment until approximately 3 to 4 weeks of age. If hypothyroidism is prenatally diagnosed, treatment can begin immediately after birth and reduce symptoms. If the macroglossia is due to Beckwith–Wiedemann syndrome, the fetus may be large for gestational age, and cesarean delivery may be necessary because of dystocia.

▶ FETAL INTERVENTION

There are no fetal interventions indicated for macroglossia.

▶ TREATMENT OF THE NEWBORN

The immediate considerations in treatment of the newborn with macroglossia include preventing airway obstruction, monitoring for difficulties in feeding and swallowing, and monitoring for hypoglycemia if a clinical diagnosis of Beckwith–Wiedemann syndrome is suspected. Physical examination should confirm the macroglossia. During the newborn period this will be notable for the tongue protruding through the lips. Palpation of the tongue is generally unremarkable and unrevealing. The diagnosis of Beckwith–Wiedemann syndrome is important to make because of the increased rate of infant mortality associated with this condition. Babies with Beckwith–Wiedemann syndrome are at risk for severe neonatal hypoglycemia, seizures, and congestive heart failure (Viljoen et al. 1991).

In infants with trisomy 21, the tongue is not actually enlarged. In a radiographic study of the tongue of several patients with Down syndrome, Ardran et al. (1972) demonstrated that the problem in Down syndrome was due to large lingual tonsils, which narrowed the airway. They hypothesized that the gaping mouth of the patient with Down syndrome related to the need to provide an airway. The major problems in Down syndrome relate to oropharyngeal hypotonia and midface underdevelopment. The tongue protrusion present during the first year of life in infants with trisomy 21 tends to disappear with improved muscular tone as the patients grow older. Limbrock et al. (1991) advocate the use of a palatal plate to stimulate oral muscular tone to improve spontaneous tongue positioning, drooling, and the open-mouthed posture seen in infants and children with trisomy 21.

If no prenatal studies have been obtained, the physical examination is the most important component of the assessment of the newborn with macroglossia. If physical findings suggest Down syndrome, a chromosomal study should be performed. If physical findings suggest Beckwith–Wiedemann syndrome, a chromosomal study should also be performed to look for abnormalities of 11p15 (Slavotinek et al. 1997). Special efforts should be made to verify the results of newborn screening thyroid-function tests. In the absence of any other diagnosis, consideration should be given to the diagnosis of inborn errors of metabolism. Urine for mucopolysaccharides, oligosaccharides, and sialyloligosaccharides will identify most metabolic diseases. Pompe (glycogen storage disease, type III) would not be identified by the urine tests, but the clinical findings of cardiomyopathy and significant hypotonia should suggest the diagnosis. Similarly, the clinical findings present in Farber lipogranulomatosis should help in diagnosis, although the assay for acid ceramidase in leukocytes, fibroblasts, and amniocytes will be definitive.

▶ SURGICAL TREATMENT

Many infants with macroglossia will have spontaneous resolution of the problem due to normal growth of the oropharynx, mandible, and maxilla. The major treatment for this condition is a partial glossectomy early in life to restore adequate breathing and swallowing, and to leave a tongue capable of normal speech, taste sensation, and further orofacial development (Rice and Carson 1985). Most surgeons recommend operative intervention by 6 months of age to prevent dental abnormalities such as prognathism and malocclusion. McManamny and Barnett (1985), who are strong advocates for partial glossectomy, state that macroglossia is unsightly, predisposes to drooling, and gives a false impression of mental retardation. Macroglossia affects dentition and prevents orthodontic treatment until the tongue is reduced. Macroglossia also affects the pronunciation of consonants, thereby impairing clarity of speech.

The goals of surgery include preservation of normal taste sensation, restoration of normal size and shape of the tongue for proper articulation after incision, and correction of a dental-arch deformity and malocclusion of the teeth by later orthodontics (Gupta 1971). Surgical methods include an anterior V-shaped wedge resection, a bilateral marginal resection, a U-shaped resection with the open end facing posteriorly, and a combined transoral–transcervical approach for an extremely large lesion (Myer et al. 1986). Partial glossectomy is curative, and postoperatively there is no recurrence. In occasional cases in which the initial resection is inadequate, a second procedure is performed to remove more of the tongue. For most patients, however, the treatment is completely curative and these lesions heal well. Even in cases of Beckwith–Wiedemann syndrome, there is no evidence that the muscular hyperplasia causes the tongue to increase in size after surgery.

▶ LONG-TERM OUTCOME

Patients with macroglossia need to be followed for evidence of chronic alveolar hypoventilation, which has been documented in patients with Beckwith–Wiedemann syndrome and has been noted to cause a secondary reversible pulmonary hypertension syndrome (Smith et al. 1982). If there is a suggestion of airway obstruction, patients should be monitored closely for evidence of hypoventilation with intermittent blood-gas evaluation. In rare cases, tracheostomy has been recommended. Symptomatic macroglossia can lead to noisy breathing, difficulty with chewing and swallowing, drooling, slurred speech, an open bite deformity, a dry cracked tongue, and ulceration and secondary infection of the tongue (Vogel et al. 1986). In patients who are diagnosed

with Beckwith–Wiedemann syndrome, close follow-up for development of embryonal tumors is warranted (Schneid et al. 1997). These include frequent postnatal sonographic studies to assess for Wilms tumor, hepatoblastoma, and nephroblastoma (McManamny and Barnett 1985).

In a long-term follow-up of 13 children with Beckwith–Wiedemann syndrome ascertained by congenital macroglossia, Hunter and Allanson (1994) described normalization of the craniofacial appearance by adolescence, leaving little clue as to the original diagnosis. None of the patients described in this series were retarded.

▶ GENETICS AND RECURRENCE RISK

Isolated macroglossia has been described as a familial trait inherited as an autosomal dominant in two unrelated families (Reynoso et al. 1986). Recurrence risks for trisomy 21 are described more fully in Chapter 134. Beckwith–Wiedemann syndrome is a genetically heterogeneous condition. Most cases are chromosomally normal. The gene has been localized to chromosome 11p15 by linkage analysis in the 15% of families that appear to have a familial transmission of this condition (Slavotinek et al. 1997). Chromosomal analysis is recommended in cases of Beckwith–Wiedemann syndrome to rule out duplications or abnormalities of chromosome 11p15. Although most cases of Beckwith–Wiedemann syndrome are sporadic, recessive and multifactorial inheritance have also been suggested (Viljoen et al. 1991). Overexpression of insulin-like growth factor 2 (IGF2), the gene involved in Beckwith–Wiedemann syndrome, is maternally imprinted and functions as a growth factor and tumor suppressor (Weksberg et al. 1993). In 28% of parents who carry informative DNA polymorphisms, uniparental disomy has been demonstrated (Slatter et al. 1994). In all the cases studied by Slatter and colleagues, there was paternal uniparental disomy present as a mosaic cell line. Therefore, there is good evidence in sporadic cases that uniparental disomy of chromosome 11 occurs as a postzygotic event. In families in which this is demonstrated, there should theoretically be no recurrence risk. In parents who have an affected infant with Beckwith–Wiedemann syndrome, a family history should be obtained to rule out dominant patterns of inheritance.

Recently, germline mutations in the cyclin dependent kinase inhibitor gene *CDKN1C* (p57KIP2) have been reported in some patients with Beckwith–Wiedemann syndrome. A higher frequency of omphalocele has been shown in the cases associated with *CDKN1C* mutations (Lam et al. 1999).

Macroglossia due to inborn errors of metabolism is inherited in a pattern consistent with a single gene defect. Recurrence risk is related to the underlying disorder, whether it is an autosomal recessive or X-linked condition.

REFERENCES

Achiron R, Ben Arie A, Gabbay U, Mashiach S, Rotstein Z, Lipitz S. Development of the fetal tongue between 14 and 26 weeks of gestation: in utero ultrasonographic measurements. Ultrasound Obstet Gynecol 1997;9:39–41.

Ardran GM, Harker P, Kemp FH. Tongue size in Down's syndrome. J Ment Defic Res 1972;16:160–166.

Bronshtein M, Zimmer EZ, Tzidony D, Hajos J, Jaeger M, Blazer S. Transvaginal sonographic measurement of fetal lingual width in early pregnancy. Prenat Diagn 1998; 18:577–580.

Cobellis C, Iannoto P, Stabile M, et al. Prenatal ultrasound diagnosis of macroglossia in the Beckwith–Wiedemann syndrome. Prenat Diagn 1988;8:79–81.

Elliott M, Maher ER. Beckwith–Wiedemann sydrome. J Med Genet 1994;31:560–564.

Grant DB, Smith I, Fuggle PW, Tokar S, Chapple J. Congenital hypothyroidism detected by neonatal screening: relationship between biochemical severity and early clinical features. Arch Dis Child 1992;67:87–90.

Gupta OP. Congenital macroglossia. Arch Otolaryngol 1971; 93:378–383.

Hunter AGW, Allanson JE. Follow-up study of patients with Beckwith–Wiedemann syndrome with emphasis on the change in facial appearance over time. Am J Med Genet 1994;51:102–107.

Kourides IA, Berkowitz RL, Pang S, Van Natta FC, Barone CM, Ginsberg-Fellner F. Antepartum diagnosis of goitrous hypothyroidism by fetal ultrasonography and amniotic fluid thyrotropin concentration. J Clin Endocrinol Metab 1984;59:1016–1018.

Lam WW, Hatada I, Ohishi S, et al. Analysis of germline CDKN1C (P57K1P2) mutations in familial and sporadic Beckwith–Wiedemann syndrome (BWS) provides a novel genotype-phenotype correlation. J Med Genet 1999;36: 518–523.

Limbrock GJ, Fischer-Brandies H, Avalle C. Castillo-Morales' orofacial therapy: treatment of 67 children with Down syndrome. Dev Med Child Neurol 1991;33:296–303.

McManamny DS, Barnett JS. Macroglossia as a presentation of the Beckwith–Wiedemann syndrome. Plast Reconstr Surg 1985;75:170–176.

Myer CM III, Hotaling AJ, Reilly JS. The diagnosis and treatment of macroglossia in children. Ear Nose Throat J 1986;65:444–448.

Nicolaides KH, Salvesen DR, Snijders RJ, Gosden CM. Fetal facial defects: associated malformations and chromosomal abnormalities. Fetal Diagn Ther 1993;8:1–9.

Nicolaides KH, Snijiders RJ, Gosden CM, Berry C, Campbell S. Ultrasonographically detectable markers of fetal chromosomal abnormalities. Lancet 1992;340:704–707.

Nowotny T, Bollmann R, Pfeifer L, Windt E. Beckwith–Wiedemann syndrome: difficulties with prenatal diagnosis. Fetal Diagn Ther 1994;9:256–260.

Patterson GT, Ramasastry SS, Davis JU. Macroglossia and ankyloglossia in Beckwith–Wiedemann syndrome. Oral Surg Oral Med Oral Pathol 1988;65:29–31.

Reynoso MC, Hernandez A, Soto F, Garcia-Cruz O, Martinez y Martinez R, Cantu JM. Autosomal dominant macroglossia in two unrelated families. Hum Genet 1986;74: 200–202.

Rice JP, Carson SH. A case report of lingual lymphangioma presenting as recurrent massive tongue enlargement. Clin Pediatr 1985;24:47–50.

Schneid H, Vazquez MP, Vacher C, Gourmelen M, Cabrol S, Le Bonc Y. The Beckwith–Wiedmann syndrome phenotype and the risk of cancer. Med Pediatr Oncol 1997;28: 411–415.

Slatter RE, Elliott M, Welham K, et al. Mosaic uniparental disomy in Beckwith–Wiedemann syndrome. J Med Genet 1994;31:749–753.

Slavotinek A, Gaunt L, Donnai D. Paternally inherited duplications of 11p15.5 and Beckwith–Wiedemann syndrome. J Med Genet 1997;34:819–826.

Smith DF, Mihm FG, Flynn M. Chronic alveolar hypoventilation secondary to macroglossia in the Beckwith–Wiedemann syndrome. Pediatrics 1982;70:695–697.

Viljoen DL, Jaquire Z, Woods DL. Prenatal diagnosis in autosomal dominant Beckwith–Wiedemann syndrome. Prenat Diagn 1991;11:167–175.

Vogel JE, Mulliken JB, Kaban LB. Macroglossia: a review of the condition and a new classification. Plast Reconst Surg 1986;78:715–723.

Weiss LS, White JA. Macroglossia: a review. J LA State Med Soc 1990;142:13–16.

Weissman A, Mashiach S, Achiron R. Macroglossia: prenatal ultrasonographic diagnosis and proposed management. Prenat Diagn 1995;15:66–69.

Weksberg R, Shen DR, Fei YL, Song QL, Squire J. Disruption of insulin-like growth factor 2 imprinting in Beckwith–Wiedemann syndrome. Nat Genet 1993;5:143–150.

Wieacker P, Wilhelm C, Greiner P, Schillinger H. Prenatal diagnosis of Wiedemann–Beckwith syndrome. J Perinatol Med 1989;17:351–355.

Winter SC, Curry CJR, Smith C, Kassel S, Miller L, Andrea J. Prenatal diagnosis of the Beckwith–Wiedemann syndrome. Am J Med Genet 1986;24:137–141.

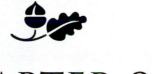

CHAPTER 29

Micrognathia

► CONDITION

Micrognathia is a facial malformation characterized by mandibular hypoplasia and a small, receding chin that fails to maintain the tongue in a forward position. Micrognathia has been described in at least 77 syndromes (Sherer et al. 1995).

Early in embryonic development, the mandible grows slowly. Between 4 and 8 weeks of gestation, the developing tongue remains in the nasal cavity, between the palatine shelves, and a physiologic micrognathia is present. Around the eighth week of gestation, the mandible grows rapidly, and the tongue is normally pulled downward and forward. This allows the palatine shelves to come together to form the secondary palate. At this point in gestation, the mandible extends beyond the maxilla, but continued growth of the maxilla once again produces a relative micrognathia in the fourth and fifth months of gestation. The mandible continues to grow during the third trimester. If the compensatory growth of the mandible is incomplete at birth, a relative micrognathia can exist (Hawkins and Simpson 1974).

Micrognathia may result from environmental or genetic factors. For example, sharp flexion of the fetal neck in utero results in continuous pressure of the chin against the sternum, which impedes mandibular growth (Hawkins and Simpson 1974). Micrognathia is also one component of many chromosomal and genetic syndromes (see below).

Micrognathia is commonly thought of as one component of the Pierre Robin syndrome. This clinical triad consists of micrognathia, upper-airway obstruction, and a U-shaped cleft palate. The name derives from a 1923 report by Pierre Robin, a French stomatologist, who described the association between newborn micrognathia and upper-airway obstruction caused by glossoptosis

(posterior displacement of the tongue). The symptoms associated with this "syndrome" are primarily due to an underlying mandibular abnormality. During fetal life, when the mandible is hypoplastic, the tongue cannot descend normally into the oral cavity at 7 to 11 weeks of gestation. If the tongue does not descend, it will remain pressed against the base of the cranium. This will then interfere with fusion of the medially growing palatal shelf and ultimately result in a cleft palate (Shprintzen 1988).

Normal mandibular growth may depend on the presence of mandibular movement during intrauterine development. In one study, Sherer and colleagues (1995) examined the correlation between lack of mandibular movement, manifested by the absence of fetal swallowing, and the development of subsequent micrognathia. Over a 4-year period, these investigators studied 28 fetuses with polyhydramnios, defined as an amniotic fluid volume of >20 cm^3. The study group consisted of 14 fetuses studied sonographically with absent mandibular movement and a nonvisualized stomach. These findings were interpreted as being consistent with absent fetal swallowing. The control group consisted of 14 fetuses with polyhydramnios but who had sonographic evidence of swallowing. In the study group, 2 fetuses were stillborn. Of the 12 live-born infants, 11 died in the neonatal period between 1 hour and 7 days of life. All the fetuses in the study group had micrognathia confirmed at birth, whereas none of the fetuses in the control group had micrognathia. These authors concluded that lack of fetal swallowing movements were likely to be important in the development of micrognathia. In this study, four major groups of underlying anomalies were identified in cases of absent fetal swallowing:

1. Complete absence of any fetal movements (fetal hypokinesia/akinesia sequence).

2. Major central nervous system abnormalities with neurologic impairment of the swallowing mechanism.
3. Abnormal karyotype.
4. Isolated absent swallowing due to Moebius sequence (sixth and seventh cranial nerve palsy). (Sherer et al. 1995).

The most severe form of micrognathia is agnathia—total or virtual absence of the mandible. This extremely rare and lethal anomaly is the result of a developmental field defect thought to be secondary to an insult to developing neural-crest–cell derivatives (Persutte et al. 1990). Prenatal sonographic diagnosis has been reported for this condition (Persutte et al. 1990).

▶ INCIDENCE

The incidence of mild-to-moderate micrognathia in the general population is unknown. In one study, 56 cases of micrognathia were identified in 2086 high-risk fetuses studied in a tertiary sonographic unit over 8 years (Nicolaides et al. 1993). The incidence of micrognathia in this series of high-risk referrals was 2.6%.

▶ SONOGRAPHIC FINDINGS

The first prenatal diagnosis of micrognathia was made in a patient deemed to be at risk for Robin malformation because the parents already had an affected child. At 23 weeks of gestation, the facial structures were studied and considered to be within normal limits. The same patient returned at 35 weeks of gestation, when polyhydramnios and a striking micrognathia were demonstrated. This report indicated that significant fetal mandibular growth occurs during the third trimester (Pilu et al. 1986). In a later study of 2086 high-risk fetuses, severe micrognathia was diagnosed by the presence of a prominent upper lip and a small chin in 56 cases (Nicolaides et al. 1993). Significantly, all cases with micrognathia in this study had additional malformations or evidence of intrauterine growth restriction. More recently, a review of 20 prenatally diagnosed cases of Pierre Robin sequence noted a high incidence of associated polyhydramnios (60% of cases) and cleft palate (45% of cases) (Hsich et al. 1999).

All reports of sonographic studies performed on fetuses with micrognathia stress the extremely high incidence of associated anomalies and the grim prognosis for this finding. Bromley and Benacerraf (1994) described their experience with 20 fetuses diagnosed with micrognathia between 15 weeks of gestation and full term. Thirteen of these fetuses had polyhydramnios (a 70% incidence). These authors hypothesized that the

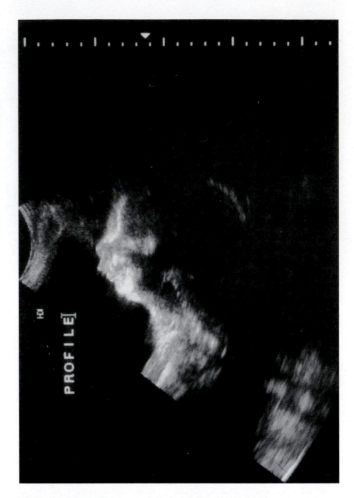

Figure 29-1. Severe fetal micrognathia demonstrated in sagittal view obtained at 29 weeks of gestation.

polyhydramnios was due to difficulty in fetal swallowing. These authors recommended a full sonographic evaluation of the fetal face, which optimally includes a midsagittal profile, coronal sections of the lower face, and axial evaluation of the orbital area. In this report, micrognathia was subjectively defined as an unusually small mandible with a receding chin demonstrated on the midsagittal view of the fetal face (Fig. 29-1). The fetal mandible was not measured.

To date, four reports have attempted to establish sonographic nomograms of fetal mandibular length in relationship to gestational age (Otto and Platt 1991; Paladini et al. 1999). To provide objective evidence of micrognathia, Chitty et al. (1993) created a growth chart for mandibular length in 184 normal fetuses between 12 and 27 weeks of gestation. The fetal mandible was measured from the proximal end of the ramus at its insertion site into the temporomandibular joint to its distal end where it meets the cartilaginous symphysis mentis. The measurement was made in a plane that visualized one ramus of the jaw. The ultrasound beam

▶ **TABLE 29-1.** MEAN FETAL MANDIBULAR MEASUREMENT

Gestation (wk)	25th Percentile (mm)	50th Percentile (mm)	97.5th Percentile (mm)
12	6.3	8.0	9.7
13	8.2	10.2	12.3
14	10.0	12.4	14.7
15	11.7	14.4	17.2
16	13.4	16.4	19.5
17	15.0	18.4	21.8
18	16.5	20.2	24.0
19	18.0	22.1	26.2
20	19.4	23.9	28.3
21	20.8	25.6	30.4
22	22.2	27.3	32.4
23	23.5	28.9	34.4
24	24.8	30.6	36.4
25	26.0	32.2	38.3
26	27.3	33.7	40.2
27	28.4	35.2	42.1
28	29.6	36.7	43.9

Reprinted from Chitty LS, Campbell S, Altman DG. Measurement of the fetal mandible—feasibility and construction of a centile chart. Prenat Diagn 1993;13:749–756. Copyright 1993 John Wiley & Sons. Reprinted by permission of John Wiley & Sons, Ltd.

was placed at a right angle to the plane of the mandible. A single measurement was recorded. Normal values obtained in this study are given in Table 29-1. At more than 28 weeks of gestation, it became difficult to identify and define fetal facial landmarks. This was due to change in fetal positioning and adjacent bony structure shadowing. These authors as well as others stated that accurate and reliable measurements of the mandible were not possible in the third trimester. In another study, fetal mandibular measurements were obtained in a scan plane parallel to the mandible that included the fetal hypopharynx. In this report of 204 women with uncomplicated pregnancies and reliable gestational dating, the anterior, posterior, and transverse fetal jaw measurements were shown to increase with gestational age (Watson and Katz 1993).

Paladini et al. (1999) developed the jaw index (anteroposterior mandibular diameter/BPD × 100) to objectively diagnose micrognathia. In a population of 198 fetuses with malformations, they compared the jaw index to subjective assessment of micrognathia. The jaw index had a 100% sensitivity and a 98.1% specificity in diagnosing micrognathia at a cutoff level of less than 23.

Fetal micrognathia is highly associated with the presence of additional structural abnormalities, including intrauterine growth restriction, skeletal dysplasias, congenital heart disease, and polyhydramnios. In one study of 3200 scans performed at a single center in the United Kingdom, facial anomalies were detected in 24 fetuses; 9 of these had micrognathia. All of the fetuses with micrognathia had associated abnormalities, most commonly, trisomy 18 and skeletal dysplasias (Turner and Twining 1993).

▶ **DIFFERENTIAL DIAGNOSIS**

Micrognathia is diagnosed either subjectively or objectively, by comparing individual fetal jaw measurements with the nomograms for fetal mandible measurements as a function of gestational age. The differential diagnosis must include conditions that are known to be associated with micrognathia. These are summarized in Table 29-2, and include chromosomal abnormalities, neuromuscular abnormalities, single-gene (mendelian) disorders, other syndromes, and teratogen exposure. Stickler syndrome, an autosomal dominant disorder consisting of micrognathia, myopia, epiphyseal dysplasia, juvenile arthropathy, cleft palate, mild sensorineural hearing loss, and airway obstruction, is frequently missed during the newborn period. In a retrospective review of patients with micrognathia and symptoms consistent with the Robin malformation, Shprintzen (1988) found a very high incidence of Stickler syndrome. Most of these cases were diagnosed later in childhood. Treacher Collins syndrome, a dominantly inherited disorder consisting of micrognathia, small ears, downslanting palpebral fissures, malar hypoplasia, lower eyelid coloboma, and abnormal hair growth, has been diagnosed prenatally by noting the presence of a hypoplastic mandible, absent ears, and severe polyhydramnios (Cohen et al. 1995; Crane and Beaver 1986; Meizner et al. 1991). Similarly, Nager syndrome (acrofacial

difficulties in breathing and feeding simultaneously. Most patients can maintain an adequate airway as long as they are awake and actively moving their tongue. When they fall asleep, however, the tongue musculature relaxes and the airway can become obstructed. Relief of obstruction can be achieved by pulling the tongue forward or by placing the patient in the prone position (Hawkins and Simpson 1974). Any infant with micrognathia should be admitted to a special-care nursery and observed by pulse oximetry. The propensity for respiratory obstruction thus can be monitored while the infant is under supervision in the prone position.

These infants also have difficulty with oral feedings. Feedings should be offered with a soft nipple in an almost upright position. In some centers, these infants are offered a nasopharyngeal positive-pressure tube with nasogastric feedings to promote weight gain and maintain patency of the airway. If the infant appears to be stable and pulse oximetry is normal, conservative (nonoperative) treatment is best.

▶ SURGICAL TREATMENT

There are multiple options for surgical treatment, including glossopexy (anchoring of the tongue to the mandible and lower lip) and tracheostomy. Most infants are given an initial trial of conservative management, but if multiple pneumonias develop, consideration should be given to performing tracheostomy to maintain the airway. Monroe and Ogo (1972) described their experience with 65 infants with micrognathia. Of these, 9 had a tracheostomy tube placed for an average of 19.2 months. Two of these 9 infants died. There was a very high incidence of associated abnormalities. They described the case histories of an additional 7 patients who did not have a tracheostomy tube placed. These authors concluded that 5 of the deaths could have been prevented by performing tracheostomy. If the infant is failing to thrive because of difficulties with swallowing, gastrostomy-tube placement may be considered to allow improved nutrition.

▶ LONG-TERM OUTCOME

Monroe and Ogo (1972) reviewed records of 65 patients with micrognathia treated at the Children's Memorial Hospital in Chicago between the years 1950 and 1969. Eight deaths occurred in this group of patients. All were due to aspiration with or without pneumonia. Of the 65 patients, 51 (78%) failed to thrive. In addition, there was a high incidence of associated anomalies (56% of patients). These included congenital heart disease (14 patients), ear abnormalities (7), club foot (4), congenital hip dislocation (3), and syndactyly (3). Of the long-term

survivors in the Bromley and Benacerraf (1994) study, 1 had Treacher Collins syndrome, 1 had Pierre Robin malformation, 1 had intrauterine growth restriction but is now normal, and one had multiple congenital anomalies but survived postsurgical repair.

The long-term outcome for many infants with micrognathia will depend on the extent and severity of the associated malformations. For the infant with isolated micrognathia, the potential for mandibular growth means that symptoms will potentially disappear over the first few years of life. If any concerns exist over the long term regarding physical appearance, orthodontic therapy and jaw advancement can be offered during adolescence (Kennett and Curran 1973).

▶ GENETICS AND RECURRENCE RISK

The recurrence risk for the syndromes listed in Table 29-2 with a known pattern of inheritance will be 25 or 50%, depending on whether the syndrome is autosomal recessive or dominant, respectively. The recurrence risk for a fetal chromosomal abnormality will be 1%, or the age-related maternal risk, whichever is higher.

A few reports suggest that a single gene exists that predisposes to micrognathia or related orofacial defects. In one report, 10 of 65 patients with micrognathia had at least one family member with cleft palate (Monroe and Oto 1972). In another case report of a consanguineous Middle Eastern family (in which the parents were first cousins), three children with polyhydramnios and micrognathia were noted. This family apparently had an autosomal recessive gene that predisposed them to lethal micrognathia. All three fetuses affected by this condition died during the newborn period because of hyaline membrane disease and asphyxia. Amniography performed during pregnancy in affected infants showed that no contrast material was swallowed into the fetal intestinal tract (Berant et al. 1978).

REFERENCES

Benson CB, Pober BR, Hirsh MP, Doubilet PM. Sonography of Nager acrofacial dysostosis syndrome in utero. J Ultrasound Med 1988;7:163–167.

Berant M, Grauer M, Grunstein S. Hydramnios with familial micrognathia. J Pediatr 1978;92:157–158.

Bromley B, Benacerraf BR. Fetal micrognathia: associated anomalies and outcome. J Ultrasound Med 1994;13:529–533.

Chitty LS, Campbell S, Altman DG. Measurement of the fetal mandible—feasibility and construction of a centile chart. Prenat Diagn 1993;13:749–756.

Cohen J, Ghezzi F, Goncalves L, Fuentes JD, Paulyson KJ, Sherer DM. Prenatal sonographic diagnosis of Treacher

Collins syndrome: a case and review of the literature. Am J Perinatol 1995;12:416–419.

Crane JP, Beaver HA. Midtrimester sonographic diagnosis of mandibulofacial dysostosis. Am J Med Genet 1986;25: 251–255.

Hawkins DB, Simpson JV. Micrognathia and glossoptosis in the newborn: surgical tacking of the tongue in small jaw syndromes. Clin Pediatr 1974;13:1066–1073.

Hsich YY, Chang CC, Tsai HD, Yang TC, Lee CC, Tsai CH. The prenatal diagnosis of Pierre Robin sequence. Prenat Diagn 1999;19:567–569.

Kennett S, Curran JB. Mandibular micrognathia: etiology and surgical management. J Oral Surg 1973;31:8–17.

Meizner I, Carmi R, Katz M. Prenatal ultrasonic diagnosis of mandibulofacial dysostosis (Treacher Collins syndrome). J Clin Ultrasound 1991;19:124–127.

Monroe CW, Ogo K. Treatment of micrognathia in the neonatal period: report of 65 cases. Plast Reconstr Surg 1972;50:317–325.

Nicolaides KH, Salvesen DR, Snijders RJM, Gosden CM. Fetal facial defects: associated malformations and chromosomal abnormalities. Fetal Diagn Ther 1993;8:1–9.

Otto C, Platt LD. The fetal mandible measurement: An objective determination of fetal jaw size. Ultrasound Obstet Gynecol 1991;1:12–17.

Paladini D, Morra T, Teodoro A, Lamberti A, Tremolaterra A, Martinelli P. Objective diagnosis of micrognathia in the fetus: the jaw index. Obstet Gynecol 1999;93:382–386.

Persutte WH, Lenke RR, DeRosa RT. Prenatal ultrasonographic appearance of the agnathia malformation complex. J Ultrasound Med 1990;9:725–728.

Pilu G, Romero R, Reece EA, Jeanty P, Hobbins JC. The prenatal diagnosis of Robin anomalad. Am J Obstet Gynecol 1986;154:630–632.

Sherer DM, Metlay LA, Woods JR, Jr. Lack of mandibular movement manifested by absent fetal swallowing: a possible factor in the pathogenesis of micrognathia. Am J Perinatol 1995;12:30–33.

Shprintzen RJ. Pierre Robin, micrognathia, and airway obstruction: the dependency of treatment on accurate diagnosis. Int Anesthesiol Clin 1988;26:64–71.

Turner GM, Twining P. The facial profile in the diagnosis of fetal abnormalities. Clin Radiol 1993;47:389–395.

Watson WJ, Katz VL. Sonographic measurement of the fetal mandible: standards of normal pregnancy. Am J Perinatol 1993;10:226–228.

CHAPTER 30

Microphthalmos

► CONDITION

Microphthalmos is one stage in a spectrum of developmental abnormalities that affect the eye. The most extreme form of microphthalmos is anophthalmos (see Chapter 23). Other conditions included in the spectrum of microphthalmos are listed in Table 30-1. Simple microphthalmos (nanophthalmos) has been defined as an eye with a normal anterior segment length and a posterior segment length greater than 2 SD below the mean (Weiss et al. 1989a). When intraocular malformations are also present, the anomaly is referred to as complex microphthalmos (Weiss et al. 1989b). Although microphthalmos can present as an isolated finding, it is more commonly appreciated as part of a syndrome involving multiple malformations (Bronshtein et al. 1991). Microphthalmos is strongly associated with abnormalities of the central nervous system.

Warburg (1993) proposed a phenotypic classification of microphthalmos that consists of three groups: genetic (monogenic and chromosomal), prenatally acquired (teratologic agents and intrauterine deformations), and associations. Genetic disorders commonly result in malformations of the eye, whereas prenatally acquired insults result in disruption or deformation of an initially normal eye.

Microphthalmos is a deformity that results from arrest of ocular growth and development. The eye is considered microphthalmic at birth if its greatest diameter is smaller than 15 mm. The normal newborn eye has a diameter of 16 to 19 mm (Price et al. 1986).

The eye derives from three embryologic germ layers. Neuroectoderm gives rise to the optic vesicle; neural-crest cells are responsible for migration to the anterior chamber of the developing eye. Ectoderm is responsible for the formation of the lens placode. Neuroectodermal and mesodermal cells participate in the closure of the optic fissure. The variety of cells and tissue types involved explains variability of phenotypic abnormalities of the eye (Warburg 1993). The embryonic optic fissure is formed from invagination along the inferior aspect of the optic cup and optic stalk at the 5-to-8-mm stage of gestation. This fissure allows the ingress of the hyaloid artery and egress of retinal axons through the optic nerve. In the normal eye, the embryonic optic fissure closes at 33 to 44 days after conception. If the fissure fails to fuse, a defect in the neuroectodermal and uveal tissues will be produced, forming a coloboma. The coloboma is a layer of sclera lined by maldeveloped neuroectoderm (Leatherbarrow et al. 1990). Colobomas of the uvea are frequently associated with microphthalmos and microcornea. Congenital cystic eye is a malformation that results from failure of

► TABLE 30-1. SPECTRUM OF CONDITIONS INCLUDED IN MICROPHTHALMOS

Total microphthalmos
  Congenital cystic eye
  Apparent anophthalmos
  Simple microphthalmos
  Microphthalmos with intraocular malformations
    (complex microphthalmos)
    Congenital cataract
    Anterior chamber malformation
    Colobomata
      Uveal
      Optic-nerve
      Cystic
    Multiple ocular malformations
  Partial microphthalmos
    Anterior segment
    Posterior segment

Source: Warburg M. Classification of microphthalmos and coloboma. J Med Genet 1993;30:664–669.

invagination of the optic vesicle. Cysts frequently develop from proliferation of neuroectodermal tissue at the edge of the persistently open embryonic fissure. The optic cup originates from localized evagination of forebrain. The optic cup is the supporting framework for further optic development. Thus, conditions that result in abnormalities of the forebrain also potentially affect the optic cup (Weiss et al. 1989a).

► INCIDENCE

The incidence of microphthalmos is 0.12 to 0.22 per 1000 live births (Price et al. 1986; Warburg 1993). In a study of 1600 prenatal sonograms obtained in pregnancies at high risk for fetal anomalies, Bronshtein et al. (1991) detected 2 cases of microphthalmos. A study of over 15,000 blind schoolchildren in Japan noted an association between advanced maternal age and/or increased birth order with microphthalmos. This study presumably excluded the severe trisomies by ascertaining a school-based population (Nakajima et al. 1979). More recently, a national birth registry in the United Kingdom noted a prevalence of either anophthalmia or microphthalmia of 1.0 per 10,000 births (Busby et al. 1998). Thirty-four percent of affected infants had mild microphthalmia. Of the severely affected infants, 51% of cases were bilateral, other non-eye malformations were present in 65% of cases, and 72% had other eye malformations.

► SONOGRAPHIC FINDINGS

The ability to measure the human fetal eye and orbits antenatally was first documented in 1982, when in two separate reports, sonographic measurements of fetal ocular diameters, interocular distance, and binocular distance were published (Jeanty et al. 1982; Mayden et al. 1982). Using transvaginal sonography, Bronshtein et al. (1991) detected fetal eyes within their orbits in 40% of screened fetuses at 11 weeks of gestation and 100% of fetuses at 12 weeks of gestation. They also noted the presence of a hypoechogenic ring that represented the fetal lens in 75% of fetuses at 12 weeks and 100% of fetuses at 14 weeks of gestation (Fig. 30-1). Fetal eyelid motion was detectable by the beginning of the second trimester. This group recommended that the optimal section for the examination of the fetal eye is a transverse plane taken at the level of the skull at the orbits. An oblique tangential section taken from the fetal nasal bridge may detect hypoechogenic circles lateral to the nose consistent with the developing lens (Bronshtein et al. 1991).

Nomograms have been established for measurements of the fetal eye taken from 12 to 37 weeks of

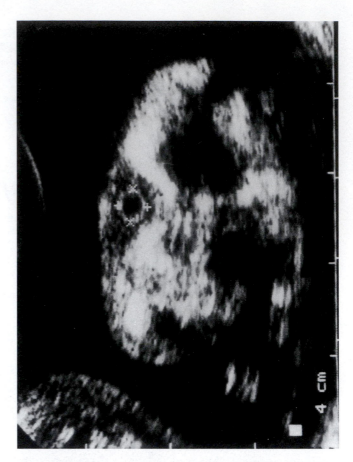

Figure 30-1. Transvaginal lateral coronal sonogram performed at 14 weeks of gestation demonstrating caliper measurements of the fetal lens. *(Reprinted, with permission, from Achiron R, Gottlieb Z, Yaron Y, Gabbay M, Lipitz S, Mashiach S. The development of the fetal eye: in utero ultrasonographic measurements of the vitreous and lens. Prenat Diagn 1995;15:155–160.)*

gestation using a combination of transvaginal and transabdominal high-resolution ultrasound techniques (Achiron et al. 1995). In this study, the fetal eye was evaluated by a coronal–facial view with the ultrasound probe positioned lateral to the fetal orbit. This group measured the transverse and supero-inferior diameters of the vitreous, and the outer-edge-to-outer-edge measurement of the lens as a function of gestational age. Only one observer made the measurements, but three separate measurements were obtained on each fetal eye. An intraobserver variation of $3.1 \pm 1.5\%$ existed. This group studied 12 fetuses at risk for eye abnormalities and found 3 with vitreous and lens measurements above or below the 95% confidence intervals for gestational age (Achiron et al. 1995). An additional study documented the normal growth percentiles for intermalar and interethmoidal distances from 10 to 40 weeks of gestation (de Elejalde and de Elejalde 1985).

Although investigators have advocated routine study of the fetal face with prenatal sonography (Benacerraf

▶ **TABLE 30-2.** ETIOLOGIC CLASSIFICATION OF MICROPHTHALMOS

Genetic		Prenatally Acquired		Unknown	
Malformations and syndromes		*Disruptions*		*Deformations*	*Associations*
Single-Gene Disorder	Chromosomal Abnormality	Drugs/Irradiation	Maternal Disease		
Autosomal dominant	Trisomy 13	Ionizing radiation	Diabetes	Encephalocele	CHARGE
Autosomal recessive	Trisomy 18	(4–11 weeks)	Cytomegalovirus	Tumors	VATER
X-linked	18p−	Ethanol	Rubella		
	13q−	Thalidomide	Toxoplasmosis		
	4p−	Isotretinoic acid			
	Triploidy				
	Other Deletions/ Duplications				

Modified, with permission, from Warburg M. Classification of microphthalmos and coloboma. J Med Genet 1993;30:664–669.

et al. 1984), the American Institute of Ultrasound and Medicine (AIUM), American College of Radiology (ACR), and American College of Obstetrics and Gynecology (ACOG) do not include this view with their recommendations for a fetal scan performed for anatomic survey in the second or third trimester of pregnancy. Microphthalmos, even in the setting of a fetal face examination, may be difficult to detect antenatally. Bronshtein et al. (1991) reported two false negative results for fetuses at prior genetic risk for microphthalmos.

▶ DIFFERENTIAL DIAGNOSIS

The major consideration in the differential diagnosis is to determine whether the microphthalmos is isolated or part of a syndrome or association. Table 30-2 lists the etiologic classification of microphthalmos. If the condition is isolated, it is important to determine whether other family members are also affected. Many chromosomal abnormalities include microphthalmos as part of a multiple congenital anomaly syndrome; trisomy 13 is one of the more common ones (Allen et al. 1977). Microphthalmos can be the consequence of exposure to certain drugs, ionizing radiation, or infectious agents. Microphthalmos can also be the result of single-gene multiple-congenital-abnormality syndromes (Table 30-3), including Walker-Warburg syndrome (Crowe et al. 1986; Dobyns et al. 1990), Fraser syndrome (Schauer et al. 1990), Meckel–Gruber syndrome (Bateman 1983), cerebro-oculo-facio-skeletal syndrome (Bateman 1983), Lenz syndrome (Traboulsi et al. 1988), focal dermal hypoplasia (Goltz syndrome) (Gottlieb et al. 1973), Norrie disease, Hallermann–Strieff syndrome, oculodentodigital syndrome, frontonasal dysplasia, and microphthalmia with linear skin defects. Any fetus diagnosed with

▶ **TABLE 30-3.** SYNDROMES ASSOCIATED WITH MICROPHTHALMOS

Syndrome	Associated Findings	Inheritance
Walker–Warburg	Pachygyria, cerebellar hypoplasia, encephalocele, Dandy–Walker cyst, hydrocephalus, cataract	Autosomal recessive
Fraser	Mental retardation, syndactyly, genital abnormalities	Autosomal recessive
Meckel–Gruber	Microcephaly, encephalocele, polydactyly, cystic renal dysplasia, cleft lip and palate	Autosomal recessive
Cerebro-oculo-facio-skeletal	Microcephaly, cataracts, micrognathia, flexion contractures	Autosomal recessive
Lenz	Microcephaly; mental retardation; digital, skeletal, dental abnormalities	X-linked
Focal dermal hypoplasia (Goltz)	Microcephaly, syndactyly, skin lesions, dental anomalies	X-linked (lethal in males)
Norrie	Cataracts, deafness, mental retardation	X-linked
Hallermann–Streiff	Brachycephaly, micrognathia, cataracts, thin small nose, skin atrophy, hypotrichosis	Autosomal recessive
Oculodentodigital	Small nares, enamel hypoplasia, syndactyly, sparse hair	Autosomal dominant
Frontonasal dyplasia (median cleft face)	Hypertelorism, defect in midline frontal bone, cleft lip, notched nose	Unknown

microphthalmia should have specific studies performed to rule out holoprosencephaly (see Chapter 13; Artman and Boyden 1990). Microphthalmos also can result from masses, such as encephalocele and tumors pressing on the developing eye. Finally, microphthalmos is seen in associations of congenital anomalies, such as CHARGE and VATER.

▶ ANTENATAL NATURAL HISTORY

The overall fetal prognosis will depend to a large extent on the underlying cause of the microphthalmos. Fetuses who have isolated microphthalmos do well during gestation. Fetuses who have an underlying chromosomal abnormality will have a much worse prognosis. In a Japanese study, Amemiya and Nishimura (1977) studied 60 intact human fetal specimens that were selected on the basis of the presence of nonocular abnormalities. This study showed a very high association of eye abnormalities with other malformations. Overall, 18 (30%) of the fetuses had eye malformations and 12 (16.7%) had an asymmetric insertion of the recti muscles that would predispose the infant to severe strabismus later in life. The incidence of ocular malformation in fetuses with heart abnormalities was 40%, and central nervous system abnormalities was 37.5%. Abnormalities in the endocrine organs had a 31.6% chance of having associated ocular malformations. This study suggested that when severe malformations of other organs were detected early in fetal life, a specific study of the fetal eye was also indicated.

Microphthalmia is one of the most common consequences of ionizing radiation delivered to the pregnant woman. In a review of 26 cases of pregnant women who received large doses of radiation during pregnancy, Dekaban (1968) demonstrated that the fetus was especially vulnerable to development of severe microphthalmos between 4 and 11 weeks of gestation. Radiation after 12 weeks resulted in microcephaly, servere brain abnormalities, and growth restriction, but after 12 weeks the eyes were relatively protected. Any condition that affects development of the forebrain, such as maternal diabetes or maternal ingestion of ethanol, will also put the fetus at risk for development of microphthalmos.

▶ MANAGEMENT OF PREGNANCY

Microphthalmos is more commonly seen as part of a multiple malformation syndrome than as an isolated finding. In one study, six of eight cases of ocular malformations were associated with intracranial defects or other organ malformations (Bronshtein et al. 1991). Agenesis of the corpus callosum is associated with ocular abnormalities in 25% of cases (Waring et al. 1976). It is therefore important to refer a patient in whom fetal microphthalmos is suspected to a center experienced in the detection of congenital malformations. In addition, a referral center is more likely to be familiar with the normal measurements of the fetal eye (Achiron et al. 1995). It is important to obtain a history from the mother regarding medication exposures, ethanol ingestion, and the results of glucose-tolerance testing to rule out maternal diabetes as an cause for microphthalmos. Isotretinoic acid, a commonly prescribed acne medication, can cause microphthalmos, so consideration should be given to the possibility of exposure to this medication in teenage patients or in older patients with severe cystic acne.

In the setting of isolated microphthalmos, it is important to examine both parents and to ask specifically about the history of visual difficulties and/or consanguinity. Because of the rarity of microphthalmos and its association with severe abnormalities, we recommend obtaining a fetal karyotype to rule out the large number of chromosomal abnormalities that can result in microphthalmos. We also recommend obtaining TORCH (toxoplasmosis, other agents, rubella, cytomegalovirus, herpesvirus) titers because cytomegalovirus, rubella, and toxoplasmosis can all result in microphthalmos.

▶ FETAL INTERVENTION

There are no fetal interventions indicated for microphthalmos.

▶ TREATMENT OF THE NEWBORN

Microphthalmos can be a subtle finding that can be missed during the newborn period. Asymmetry of the globes or an abnormal red reflex should prompt a pediatric ophthalmologic consultation. A newborn who has microphthalmos and a corneal diameter of 5 mm or less has a very poor prognosis for useful vision (Elder 1994). The globe serves as a scaffold for further development of eyelids. Infants who have had severe microphthalmos in utero will have foreshortening of the palpebral fissure and flattening of the eyelids. The abnormal appearance becomes more apparent as facial growth occurs over the first year of life. Price et al. (1986) recommend fitting infants who have unilateral microphthalmos with cosmetic scleral shells. This permits the development of a symmetric ocular appearance without any need for surgery. They recommend initial fitting of the prosthesis at 2 months of age, with refittings twice or more yearly during the first 2 years of life. The adult eye size is normally reached at age 13 years, so fittings are required only throughout the childhood years.

▶ SURGICAL TREATMENT

When microphthalmos is present with a cyst, the cyst may be aspirated repeatedly or surgically excised. Enucleation should be performed only if the cyst aspiration is unsuccessful. Once the eye is enucleated, later orbital and eyelid reconstruction will become necessary (Waring et al. 1976). A lensectomy can be performed for congenital cataract. Corneal transplantation has successfully restored vision in some infants with microphthalmos (Feldman et al. 1987).

▶ LONG-TERM OUTCOME

Elder et al. (1994) described 27 patients with bilateral microphthalmos, who had visual acuity of less than 6/60. All patients had nystagmus. Of the 27, 12 had congenital cataracts as their primary cause of blindness. An additional 6 had chorioretinal colobomas; 2 had degenerative myopia. There was no light perception in 8 of the 27. This study was performed in a very poor Middle Eastern area, where patients had no access to surgical treatment. Most patients with microphthalmos have high hyperopia and require lens correction. During adulthood, microphthalmic eyes are at high risk for glaucoma, retinal detachment, and spontaneous uveal effusion (Weiss et al. 1989). A retrospective follow-up study of 30 children with microphthalmos revealed that 7 had mental retardation, but a surprisingly high number of the others were described as extremely good students (Whiteman and Crawford 1980). Long-term follow-up by a pediatric ophthalmologist is recommended.

▶ GENETICS AND RECURRENCE RISK

Isolated microphthalmos usually occurs sporadically, although there have been reports of autosomal dominant inheritance (Vingolo et al. 1994) and autosomal recessive inheritance in a large inbred Arab kindred (Kohn et al. 1988), a Swiss Anabaptist kindred (Cross and Yoder 1976) and an Iranian Jewish inbred community (Zlotogora et al. 1994). Additionally, X-linked forms have been reported (Warburg 1981). Shulman et al. described a family initially thought to have microphthalmos presenting as an autosomal recessive condition, but later found to be autosomal dominant with incomplete penetrance (Shulman et al. 1993).

Multiple chromosomal abnormalities have been associated with microphthalmia. These include triploidy; trisomies 13 and 18; deletion of the short arm of chromosome X (Xp22.2 to ter) (Ogata et al. 1998; Temple et al. 1990); deletion of 4p−, 4q−, 13q−, 13 ring, 18q−, and 18 ring; and duplications of 4q+, 7p+, 9+, 10q+, 13q+, 22q+, and partial trisomy 22. In addition, microphthalmos has been found in at least 10 patients with trisomy 4p (Lurie and Samochvalov 1994). Common chromosomal abnormalities to be suspected in the setting of microphthalmos with coloboma are trisomy 13, 13q−, triploidy, and trisomy 4p. More than 100 genetic conditions have been described for microphthalmos with coloboma. Of these, at least 50 are syndromes inherited as autosomal dominants, 67 are syndromes described as autosomal recessives, and 16 conditions are described with X-linked inheritance (Warburg 1993).

Any patient found to have microphthalmos should be referred to a medical genetics unit for complete pedigree interpretation and counseling regarding recurrence risk. Specific genetic counseling will depend on the underlying cause of the microphthalmos. If unbalanced chromosomal abnormalities are detected, parental blood samples should be obtained to study the parental karyotypes. Infants with microphthalmos should be examined by a clinical geneticist to seek additional dysmorphic features to permit diagnosis of a genetic syndrome.

The mouse microphthalmia (mi) gene encodes a protein whose mutations result in early-onset deafness, reduced eye size, and loss of pigmentation in the eye, inner ear, and skin. A human homolog of this gene exists and maps to human chromosome 3p12-14 (Tachibana et al. 1994). This gene is responsible for Waardenburg syndrome, type 2, a dominantly inherited disorder with sensorineural hearing loss and heterochromic irides but no microphthalmia (Hughes et al. 1994). The gene for microphthalmia with linear skin defects has been cloned and mapped to chromosome Xp22 (Ogata et al. 1998; Wapenaar et al. 1993).

REFERENCES

Achiron R, Gottlieb Z, Yaron Y, Gabbay M, Lipitz S, Mashiach S. The development of the fetal eye: in utero ultrasonographic measurements of the vitreous and lens. Prenat Diagn 1995;15:155–160.

Allen JC, Venecia G, Opitz JM. Eye findings in the 13 trisomy syndrome. Eur J Pediatr 1977;124:179–183.

Amemiya T, Nishimura H. Ocular malformations in human fetuses with external malformations. J Pediatr Ophthalmol 1977;14:165–170.

Artman HG, Boyden E. Microphthalmia with single central incisor and hypopituitarism. Am J Med Genet 1990;27:192–193.

Bateman JB. Genetics in pediatric ophthalmology. Pediatr Clin North Am 1983;30:1015–1031.

Benacerraf BR, Frigoletto FD Jr, Bieber FR. The fetal face: ultrasound examination. Radiology 1984;153:495–497.

Bronshtein M, Zimmer E, Gershoni-Baruch R, Yoffe N, Meyer N, Blumenfeld Z. First and second trimester diagnosis of fetal ocular defects and associated anomalies: report of eight cases. Obstet Gynecol 1991;77:443.

Bushby A, Dolk H, Collin R, Jones RB, Winter R. Compiling a national register of babies born with anophthalmia/

cord is clamped and the infant is handed over to the neonatologists. It is crucial that the timing of the delivery of the baby, after obtaining an airway, is carefully orchestrated with the anesthesiologist, because uterine relaxation is essential for an EXIT procedure. After delivery of the baby and placenta, massive uterine bleeding may occur unless uterine tone is rapidly reestablished. This is best accomplished by turning off the halogenated anesthetic agent to allow uterine tone to return to normal, as well as beginning an oxytocin infusion. After the infant and placenta are delivered, vigorous massage of the uterus stimulates contraction and minimizes blood loss (Langer et al. 1992; Mychatisha et al. 1997; Skarsgard et al. 1996; Sylvester et al. 1998).

Crombleholme et al. (2000) reported the first successful salvage and long term survival of a fetus with CHAOS due to complete tracheal atresia. The fetus was originally diagnosed with bilateral cystic adenomatoid malformation of the lung and nonimmune hydrops at 19 weeks of gestation. Although intrauterine fetal death was anticipated, 12 weeks after diagnosis the fetus was doing well, albeit with massive ascites and severe polyhydramnios. The EXIT procedure performed at 31 weeks of gestation demonstrated complete tracheal occlusion due to subglottic atresia (see Fig. 31-5). A tracheostomy was performed and the newborn did well, requiring ventilatory support due to diaphragmatic dysfunction but was weaned to room air in 24 hours.

▶ FETAL INTERVENTION

Adzick and colleagues (Adzick NS: personal communication, 1997) have reproduced the pathophysiology of CHAOS in a fetal lamb model (Crombleholme et al. 2000). Tracheal ligation at 80 days of gestation produces extremely large hyperplastic fetal lungs, with secondary nonimmune hydrops and polyhydramnios. The fetal lambs die in utero if left untreated. Performing a tracheostomy in utero reverses these changes and allows the lambs to be delivered at term. There has never been a case of CHAOS treated in utero, although techniques that might be used to treat this lethal condition are currently available. Because of the possibility of a simple laryngeal web or cyst, in utero bronchoscopy should be performed first. If a more significant airway obstruction exists, a tracheostomy can then be performed. Although there are many unanswered questions about the long-term effects of in utero tracheostomy on lung development, it is clear that CHAOS, when associated with hydrops carries a high risk of intrauterine fetal death. In addition, in a fetal lamb model of this condition, tracheostomy reversed the pathophysiology. However, the case reported by Crombleholme et al. suggests that in some cases hydrops can be tolerated for prolonged periods. If close monitoring is available, intervention may be deferred until 32 weeks of gestation, when an EXIT procedure can be considered with acceptable risks of prematurity.

▶ TREATMENT OF THE NEWBORN

In cases of CHAOS in which an EXIT procedure is performed, the infant should have an airway in place before being handed over to the neonatologist. It is important to examine the infant for possible associated anomalies. Blood for karyotype analysis should be sent if a karyotype was not obtained during the pregnancy. Depending on physical findings, plain radiography to exclude vertebral anomalies, sonography to exclude genitourinary anomalies, and echocardiography should all be considered. The possibility of a communication existing between trachea and esophagus must be excluded in all patients with CHAOS. The pathophysiology of CHAOS results in a capillary leak syndrome after delivery by EXIT procedure. The neonate reported by Crombleholme et al. required careful fluid management because of capillary leak, and the massive ascites was initially refractory to diuretic therapy. Because of chronic tracheal obstruction, this newborn had diffuse tracheobronchial malacia, which required 6-to-7-cm. H_2O positive end-expiratory pressure (PEEP) to maintain his airway. In addition, diaphragmatic dysfunction, secondary to distention in utero, was severe at birth. Phrenic-nerve stimulation confirmed that the neuromuscular unit was intact. There was progressive improvement during the first 5 months of life. The infant was weaned from mechanical ventilatory support by 9 months of age and underwent tracheal reconstruction at 14 months of age.

▶ SURGICAL TREATMENT

The most important aspect of the care of the newborn diagnosed with CHAOS is securing and maintaining the airway. Once potential associated anomalies have been excluded, and the infant's cardiorespiratory status is stable, an elective approach to evaluating the newborn's airway can be taken. In the absence of tracheoesophageal fistula, the surgical management of CHAOS is elective. The initial evaluation should be directed toward diagnosing the level of obstruction to allow planning of definitive surgical repair. It is important that prospective parents understand that, depending on the nature of the malformation, perfect laryngeal reconstruction and adequate speech may not be possible. The ideal timing of reconstruction in these extremely rare cases has not been established. However, bronchoscopy performed during the newborn period will exclude simple causes of laryngeal obstruction, such as laryngeal cyst or web. The majority of webs are located at the level of the glottis or are immediately subglottic and are readily diagnosed by laryngoscopy or bronchoscopy. These webs can occasionally be lysed endoscopically with a knife or laser. Although lasers can be used, the small airway of the newborn may make it difficult to avoid thermal damage to surrounding tissues. An infant urethral resectoscope with a narrow cutting loop can be used with brief bursts of cutting current. There are only anecdotal reports of successful reconstruction and long-term outcome in this condition (Richards et al. 1992; Smith et al. 1965).

▶ LONG-TERM OUTCOME

Because of the nature of the malformation in CHAOS, very little information exists regarding the long-term outcome for affected children. In cases of simple laryngeal cyst or web, normal laryngeal function can be anticipated. The outcome in cases of more significant laryngeal malformation is less certain. Most infants with this problem have not survived.

▶ GENETICS AND RECURRENCE RISK

Most cases of CHAOS occur as sporadic, isolated malformations without known risk of recurrence. In cases of CHAOS associated with Fraser syndrome, there is a 25% chance of recurrence, as this syndrome is believed to be inherited as an autosomal recessive disorder (Fraser et al. 1962). There has been one report of Fraser syndrome with inversion of p11;q21 in chromosome 9. While pericentric inversions in chromosome 9 are frequent and considered normal variants (Kaiser et al. 1994), it has been suggested that this inversion may result in disruption of the autosomal recessive gene responsible for Fraser syndrome.

REFERENCES

Arizawa M, Imai S, Suchara N, et al. Prenatal diagnosis of pulmonary atresia. Cesta Obst Gynaec 1989;41: 907–910.

Baarsma R, Bekedam DJ, Visser GH. Qualitatively abnormal fetal breathing movements associated with tracheal atresia. Early Hum Dev 1993;32:63–69.

Canty TG, Hendren WH. Upper airway obstruction from frequent cysts of the hypopharynx. J Pediatr Surg 1975; 10:807–812.

Cohen SR. Congenital atresia of the larynx with endolaryngeal surgical correction: a case report. Laryngoscope 1971;81:1607–1615.

Crombleholme TM, Albonese C. The fetus with airway obstruction in the unborn patient. In Harrison MR, Evans

MI, Adzick NS, Holzgreve W, eds. 3rd ed, (in press) Philadelphia, PA: WB Saunders 2000.

Crombleholme TM, Sylvester K, Flake AW, et al. Salvage of a fetus with congenital high airway obstruction syndrome (Chaos), Fet Diagnos Ther (in press).

Delechotte P, Lemery D, Vanlieferinghen P. Association atresie laryngee et agenesie renale bilaterale: hyperplasie versus hypoplasie pulmonaire. Presented at Quaterereinae journee de la Societe Francaise de Foetopathologie, Paris-Bichat, France, 1988.

Didier F, Droulle P, Marchal C. A propos du depistage antenatal dis atresies tracheale at laryngee. Arch Fr Pediatr 1990;47:396–397.

Fang SH, Ocejo R, Sin M, et al. Congenital laryngeal atresia. Arch Dis Child 1989;143:625–627.

Feldman E, Shalev E, Weiner E, et al. Microphthalmic-prenatal ultrasound diagnosis: a case report. Prenat Diagn 1995;5:205–207.

Fox H, Cocker J. Laryngeal atresia. Arch Dis Child 1964;39: 641–645.

Fraser GR. Our genetic "load": a review of some aspects of genetic variation. Ann Hum Genet 1962;25:387–415.

Hedrick MH, Martinez-Ferro, Filly RA, et al. Congenital high airway obstruction syndrome (CHAOS): a potential for perinatal intervention. J Pediatr Surg 1994;29:271–274.

Kaiser P. Pericentric inversions—problems and significance for clinical genetics. Hum Genet 1984;65:1–47.

Langer JC, Tabb T, Thompson P, et al. Management of prenatally diagnosed tracheal obstruction: accent to the airway in utero prior to delivery. Fetal Diagn Ther 1992;7: 12–16.

Liechty KW, Crombleholme TM, Flake AW, et al. Intrapartum airway management for giant fetal neck masses: the exit procedure (ex utero intrapartum treatment). Am J Obstet Gynecol 1997;177:870–874.

Mychatisha G, Bealer J, Graf J, et al. Operating a placental support: the ex utero interpartum treatment (EXIT) procedure. J Pediatr Surg 1997;32:227–230.

Richards DS, Yancey MK, Duff P, et al. The perinatal management of severe laryngeal stenosis. Obstet Gynecol 1992;80:537–540.

Schauer GM, Dunn LK, Godmilow L, et al. Prenatal diagnosis of Fraser syndrome at 18.5 weeks' gestation, with autopsy findings at 19 weeks'. Am J Med Genet 1990; 37:583–591.

Scurry JP, Adamson TM, Cussen LJ. Fetal lung growth in laryngeal atresia and tracheal agenesis. Aust Paediatr J 1989;25:47–51.

Skarsgard ED, Chitkara U, Krane EJ, et al. The OOPS procedure (operation on placental support): in utero airway management of the fetus with prenatally diagnosed tracheal obstruction. J Pediatr Surg 1996;31:826–828.

Silver MM, Thurston WA, Patrick JE. Perinatal pulmonary hypoplasia due to laryngeal atresia. Hum Pathol 1988;19: 110–113.

Smith II, Bain AD. Congenital atresia of the larynx: a report of nine cases. Ann Otol Rhinol Laryngol 1965;74:338–349.

Sylvester KG, Rosanen Y, Kitano Y, et al. Tracheal occlusion reverses the high impedance to flow in the fetal pulmonary circulation and normalizes its physiologic response to oxygenation at term. J Pediatr Surg 1998;33:1071–1075.

The mortality rate for cystic hygromas diagnosed prior to 30 weeks of gestation, with posterior location, is extremely high because of the high incidence of nonimmune hydrops and associated chromosomal defects. In the report by Langer et al. of 27 cases diagnosed prior to 30 weeks of gestation, all but 2 fetuses died. Of the 25 that did not survive, nonimmune hydrops developed in 21, 4 spontaneously aborted, and 21 were electively terminated. The only 2 survivors had spontaneous regression and were subsequently diagnosed with Noonan syndrome at birth (Langer et al. 1990). Cystic hygroma associated with nonimmune hydrops is almost uniformly fatal. There are chromosomal abnormalities in approximately 80% of these cases. Fetuses with normal chromosomes have a higher incidence of consanguinity (Langer et al. 1990). These cases of cystic hygroma are also more likely to be associated with familial conditions, such as Noonan syndrome (Zarabi et al. 1983), multiple pterygium syndrome (Chen et al. 1982), polysplenia syndrome, Roberts syndrome (Graham et al. 1983), or an isolated recessive trait (Cowchock et al. 1982). In a review of 100 fetuses with nuchal thickening or cystic hygroma detected sonographically at 10 to 15 weeks of gestation, Nadel et al. (1993) found that a good prognosis could be expected if the karyotype was normal, there were no separations in the mass, and there were no associated hydrops.

In marked contrast to cystic hygromas with associated karyotypic abnormalities, there is a small group of fetuses with an isolated cystic hygroma without chromosomal abnormality, structural anomaly, or familial condition and in which hydrops does not develop; they have an excellent prognosis. The major concern in fetuses with large cystic cervical masses later in gestation is airway compromise at birth. The fetuses often require delivery by EXIT procedure (see below).

▶ MANAGEMENT OF PREGNANCY

The management of a pregnancy complicated by a fetus with cystic hygroma depends on the presence or absence of nonimmune hydrops, chromosomal abnormalities, or other associated anomalies. Once a cystic hygroma has been detected, a detailed sonographic examination should be performed to search for fetal skin edema, ascites, and pleural or pericardial effusions. In addition, other structural anomalies should be excluded, especially genitourinary and cardiac defects. Genetic amniocentesis is recommended in all cases of cystic hygroma because of the high incidence of associated chromosomal abnormalities. In the presence of nonimmune hydrops the prognosis is grim, and appropriate counseling is indicated. In the presence of severe associated anomalies or a chromosomal abnormality prior to 24 weeks of gestation, elective termination may be offered.

Echocardiography should be offered in cases in which no chromosomal abnormalities are detected to exclude cardiac defects. An isolated cystic hygroma diagnosed in the third trimester has a much more favorable prognosis, and attention should be focused on site and mode of delivery. Because of risks of airway compromise, delivery in a tertiary-care center with neonatologists and pediatric surgeons standing by is recommended. Because of the risks of airway compromise, consideration should be given to the EXIT procedure (Liechty et al. 1997). While a cervical mass of any size can cause airway compromise, masses sufficiently large enough to cause polyhydramnios can obstruct the pharynx or larynx, making intubation exceedingly difficult. Pregnancies with a cystic hygroma should be followed closely for the development of polyhydramnios and secondary uterine irritability. Polyhydramnios in fetuses with large cystic hygromas may be so severe as to require amnioreduction to treat maternal respiratory difficulties and preterm labor.

▶ FETAL INTERVENTION

A few cases of lymphangioma have undergone in utero drainage by ultrasound-guided cyst aspiration. Chen et al. (1996) reported two fetuses that underwent multiple cyst aspirations. In each case karyotype analysis was normal and there were no associated structural anomalies. The rationale for this approach is to prevent polyhydramnios, irreversible facial deformity, and progression to hydrops fetalis. It is unclear, however, that these multiple cyst aspirations had any effect on outcome. While cyst aspiration as an adjunct to securing an airway at birth may be indicated, there are few data to support in utero decompression to prevent progression to nonimmune hydrops or facial deformity. The lack of benefit and risk of repeated aspirations make this fetal intervention difficult to justify. Kaufman et al. (1996) did report successful percutaneous decompression of a large axillary lymphangioma that would have caused skeletal dystocia. Ultrasound-guided aspiration was followed by normal spontaneous vaginal delivery. Figure 32-3 demonstrates an axillary lymphangioma detected antenatally and aspirated prior to birth to allow vaginal delivery.

A group in Sapporo, Japan, has attempted intrauterine sclerotherapy using OK-432 at 27 and 28 weeks of gestation (Wattori et al. 1996). OK-432 is a lyophilized mixture of a low-virulence strain of *Streptococcus pyogenes* of human origin incubated with penicillin G. The fetuses had involution of the cystic hygroma, and at birth only a slight skinfold was noted. There are few data on the use of this agent postnatally and none are available on its potential effects in the developing fetus. Currently, the only fetal procedure indicated for large

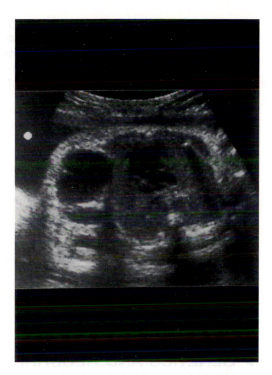 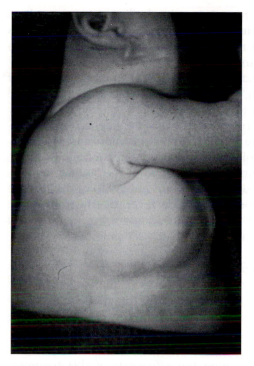

Figure 32-3. (A) Prenatal sonographic image of an axillary lymphangioma that was aspirated prior to vaginal delivery. (B) Postnatal photograph of same child prior to surgical removal of the lymphangioma.

cystic hygromas is EXIT (ex utero intrapartum treatment), which involves placement of an endotracheal tube before the fetus is separated from the placenta (Liechty et al. 1997).

▶ TREATMENT OF THE NEWBORN

Treatment of the fetus with a large cystic hygroma includes an EXIT procedure to secure the airway (Liechty et al. 1997). The EXIT procedure allows up to 1 hour with excellent uteroplacental gas exchange for laryngoscopy, bronchoscopy and, if necessary, tracheostomy with or without partial resection of the mass (Liechty et al. 1997). If the fetus is premature and at increased risk for respiratory distress syndrome, surfactant replacement therapy can be administered while on placental support. In addition, in a three-vessel cord, an umbilical artery catheter, and even an umbilical venous catheter can be placed while on placental support to facilitate newborn resuscitation.

▶ SURGICAL TREATMENT

Once an airway has been established, the care of the newborn should focus on any underlying lung disease and exclusion of any associated anomalies and chromosomal abnormalities, if this has not already been done. Once the newborn is able to be transported to a tertiary-care facility, a computed tomographic (CT) scan and MRI scan with magnetic resonance angiography should be obtained of the infant's head and neck to confirm the diagnosis of lymphangioma and to determine the extent of the hygroma. Of particular concern is to define whether there is extension into the mediastinum or the floor of the mouth and tongue.

The infant with a large cystic hygroma has an intrinsically unstable airway, and resection should proceed as soon as the diagnostic evaluation is completed. Cystic hygromas of a modest size can be dealt with on a more elective basis if they do not pose a risk for airway compromise. The nature of the lymphangioma often precludes a complete resection. The surgical approach is focused on resection of as much of the mass as possible without sacrificing vital structures. Some surgeons have recommended a conservative approach in asymptomatic lymphangiomas because of occasional spontaneous regression. More commonly, these lesions grow proportionately with the growth of the infant. There may also be acute increases in the size of the cyst due to hemorrhage or infection. Because of difficulty in achieving a complete resection, alternative treatments have been tried with variable results.

Cystic aspiration is of little benefit except in the rare instance of a large dominant cyst as a means of emergency decompression. However, the cysts rapidly reaccumulate. Sclerosing agents have been used as an

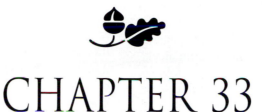

CHAPTER 33

Goiter

► CONDITION

Fetal goiter, or thyromegaly, is a diffuse enlargement of the fetal thyroid gland. Goiter in the fetus can occur as part of a hypothyroid, hyperthyroid, or euthyroid state. Hypothyroid fetal goiters are more common than those associated with either the hyperthyroid or euthyroid states.

Goiter associated with fetal hypothyroidism can be caused by transplacental passage of antithyroid medications being used by a mother with hyperthyroidism, iodine deficiency, iodine intoxication, transplacental passage of antithyroid antibodies, congenital metabolic disorders of thyroid hormone synthesis, or hypothalamic-pituitary hypothroidism (Bruner and Dellinger 1997; Noia et al. 1992; Romero et al. 1988; Soliman et al. 1994; Van Loon et al. 1995; Vicens-Calvet et al. 1998; Weiner et al. 1980). Most cases of hypothyroid goiter will not become apparent until the neonatal period. When goiter associated with hypothyroidism is recognized in utero it is most likely to be secondary to transplacental passage of drugs or congenital dyshormonogenesis because of an inherited enzymatic deficiency (Romero et al. 1988). Congenital hypothyroidism is a serious condition, which if not treated within the first 3 months of life is likely to result in irreversible mental retardation. Although newborn screening programs for congenital hypothroidism have been extremely successful in reducing the incidence of mental retardation associated with this condition, it is possible that the presence of a hypothyroid state in utero may result in some degree of hearing, speech, and other intellectual impairment, despite early neonatal therapy (Rovet et al. 1987). This emphasizes the importance of thorough evaluation and treatment of fetal goiter whenever it is suspected prenatally.

Goiter associated with fetal hyperthyroidism is almost always caused by transplacental passage of a thyroid-stimulating IgG antibody from the mother (Belfar et al. 1991; Hadi and Strickland 1995; Heckel et al. 1997; Hatjis 1993; Wenstrom et al. 1990). Such antibodies are present in at least 95% of women with Graves disease. Thyroid-stimulating antibody levels in Graves disease may not reflect maternal thyroid status, as they are detectable in women who are clinically hyperthyroid, euthyroid, or hypothyroid. Therefore, whenever a patient with a history of Graves disease becomes pregnant, the fetus is at risk for hyperthyroid goiter, irrespective of the mother's clinical thyroid state. The fetal thyroid gland becomes fully responsive to thyroid-stimulating substances, such as maternal IgG, only in the second trimester, so the detection of a fetal goiter before 20 to 24 weeks of gestation is unlikely.

► INCIDENCE

Fetal goiter is extremely rare, with no published series sufficient to allow an estimation of its incidence. Hypothyroid goiter is more common than hyperthyroid goiter. Congenital hypothyroidism has an incidence of 1 in 4000 live births. Only a small fraction of these will be complicated by fetal goiter, because in the vast majority of cases goiter becomes clinically apparent only during neonatal life (Fisher et al. 1979). Inborn errors of thyroid hormone biosynthesis that result in congenital dyshormonogenesis and cause hypothyroid fetal goiter are rare, being present in 1 in 30,000 live births. Graves disease is seen in about 1% of pregnant women, and hyperthyroidism or hypothyroidism will develop in 2 to 12% of these fetuses or neonates (Hatjis 1993). However, only a small fraction of this number of at-risk fetuses will be diagnosed prenatally with a fetal goiter.

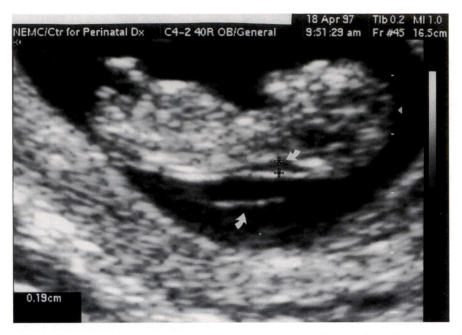

Figure 34-1. Sonographic image of a fetus at 12 weeks of gestation demonstrating the requirements for an adequate nuchal translucency measurement. The fetus is in the midsagittal plane and occupies 75% of the image. The measurement is taken when the fetus has moved away from the amnion (lower arrow), and the calipers are placed on the inner borders of the nuchal fold (upper arrow).

conditions during the first trimester, in general, simple nuchal edema is smaller and is never septated. However, simple nuchal edema may extend over the entire crown-to-rump length, with many similarities to cystic hygroma.

In addition to being associated with aneuploidy, increased nuchal translucency is also strongly associated with structural fetal malformations, in particular cardiac malformations. In a series of 29,154 pregnancies screened using nuchal translucency measurement, 28 of the 50 cases (56%) of major fetal cardiac defects were in the group with increased nuchal translucency (Hyett et al. 1999).

▶ ANTENATAL NATURAL HISTORY

Because increased nuchal translucency is a marker for aneuploidy, there is a high degree of intrauterine lethality associated with this finding. It has been estimated that over 40% of fetuses with Down syndrome die between 12 weeks of gestation and term (Snijders et al. 1995). However, fetuses identified with Down syndrome based on increased nuchal translucency do not appear to be at higher risk of intrauterine death than those identified using more traditional means. In a series of six cases of Down syndrome identified by increased nuchal translucency and managed expectantly, the nuchal edema resolved in five, and all six fetuses survived to term (Pandya et al. 1995b).

▶ MANAGEMENT OF PREGNANCY

The association between nuchal-fold thickening and increased incidence of aneuploidies was first noted in high-risk populations, such as women of advanced maternal age or those with a previous pregnancy complicated by an aneuploid fetus. In 22 studies of nuchal translucency measurement in populations at high risk for aneuploidy, 30% of fetuses were found to have chromosomal abnormalities, with almost half of these abnormalities being Down syndrome (Stewart and Malone 1999). The precise magnitude of the association between increased nuchal translucency and aneuploidy in high-risk populations is unclear because different studies used different gestational-age ranges and different measurements to define increased thickness. While a wide variety of values were used to define an abnormal nuchal-translucency measurement, most studies used a cutoff value of 3 mm. In addition, many of these studies included both fetuses with simple nuchal edema and those with cystic hygroma, which may explain the high incidence of Turner syndrome. Before deciding on a role for nuchal translucency screening in the general population, however, studies evaluating its efficacy in such populations were needed.

At least eight studies have been published evaluating the role of nuchal translucency screening in the general population. These studies are summarized in Table 34-1. There is a great degree of variation between the studies in the detection rate for Down syndrome—

▶ **TABLE 34-1.** STUDIES OF NUCHAL TRANSLUCENCY SCREENING IN GENERAL PATIENT POPULATIONS

Study	Abnormal Nuchal Translucency	Number of Fetuses	Positive Predictive Value*	Down Syndrome Detection Rate
Bewley et al. (1995)	≥3.0 mm	1,368	3% (2/70)	33% (1/3)
Kornman et al. (1996)	≥3.0 mm	923	6% (2/36)	29% (2/7)
Taipale et al. (1997)	≥3.0 mm	10,010	24% (18/76)	54% (7/13)
Hafner et al. (1998)	≥2.5 mm	4,233	15% (11/74)	43% (3/7)
Orlandi et al. (1997)	Delta value[†]	744	19% (8/43)	57% (4/7)
Pajkrt et al. (1998)	≥3.0 mm	1,473	24% (8/33)	67% (6/9)
Theodoropoulos et al. (1998)	>95th%[‡]	3,550	22% (20/101)	91% (10/11)
Snijders et al. (1998)	>95th%[‡]	96,127	10% (463/4672)	72% (234/326)
Total	Varied	118,428	10% (532/5105)	70% (267/383)

*For an abnormal fetal karyotype, given an increased nuchal translucency.
[†]Nuchal translucency defined as abnormal based on a value added to the expected measurement (delta value).
[‡]Nuchal translucency defined as abnormal if greater than the 95th percentile value based on fetal crown-to-rump length.

ranging from 29% to 91% (Stewart and Malone 1999). The largest study enrolled 96,127 patients and suggested a detection rate for Down syndrome of 72% (Snijders et al. 1998). However, a critical reappraisal of this study suggested a true detection rate for Down syndrome of 60% for nuchal translucency screening (Haddow 1998).

Currently, it is recommended that screening for Down syndrome using increased nuchal translucency should be considered an investigational tool, and that interventions such as chorionic villus sampling and amniocentesis should not be performed in clinical practice for this reason (Stewart and Malone 1999). At present it is not possible to quote a specific risk for aneuploidy based on nuchal translucency measurements and maternal age. In the absence of these data, counseling should involve informing patients of an unquantified increase in the risk of aneuploidy whenever a nuchal translucency measurement of >3 mm is found. However, patients with increased nuchal translucency could be referred for appropriate counseling and intervention to a center participating in one of the trials of nuchal translucency screening. If the research trials underway in the United States and the United Kingdom confirm previous reports on the role of nuchal translucency screening, there may then be a place for offering invasive testing to such patients during the first trimester (Stewart and Malone 1999).

When increased nuchal translucency is noted on ultrasonography, a careful search for other abnormalities or markers for aneuploidy is recommended. There is increasing evidence that nuchal translucency is associated with congenital heart disease (Hyett et al. 1996). In such cases, increased nuchal translucency may be a result of the abnormal cardiac development. It has even been hypothesized that the increased fluid collection may be an early sign of congestive heart failure. A careful follow-up ultrasound evaluation is recommended at 18 to 20 weeks to assess the fetal anatomy and to confirm the absence of fetal hydrops.

▶ **FETAL INTERVENTION**

No fetal intervention has been described for increased nuchal translucency.

▶ **TREATMENT OF THE NEWBORN**

In euploid fetuses there appears to be no additional risk from increased nuchal translucency, and no specific neonatal interventions appear necessary. However, because of an association between increased nuchal translucency and congenital diaphragmatic hernia (Sebire et al. 1997), coarctation of the aorta (Hyett et al. 1995), cardiac malformations (Hyett et al. 1996), and congenital arthrogryposis (Hyett et al. 1997), a careful physical examination is recommended to exclude any additional congenital malformations. In newborn infants with Down syndrome, excess tissue at the back of the neck may be a residual effect of the nuchal edema (Fig. 34-2).

▶ **SURGICAL TREATMENT**

There is no surgical treatment for increased nuchal translucency.

▶ **LONG-TERM OUTCOME**

There are no data on long-term outcome of euploid fetuses that had increased nuchal translucency during the first trimester. Long-term outcome depends also on the presence of any associated malformations, such as aneuploidy, cardiac malformations, or congenital diaphragmatic hernia.

Thoracic

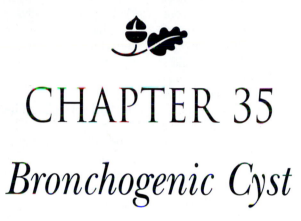

CHAPTER 35

Bronchogenic Cyst

▶ CONDITION

Bronchogenic cysts are embryonic abnormalities that fall within the group of bronchopulmonary foregut malformations (Gerle et al. 1968). Bronchogenic cysts are most often unilocular thin-walled cysts that are found in proximity to the membranous portion of the posterior trachea. However, bronchogenic cysts may also be found intraparenchymally, intrapericardially, mediastinally, infradiaphragmatically in the retroperitoneum, and in subcutaneous tissues of the cervical region (Bailey et al. 1990; Boue et al. 1994; Foerster et al. 1991; Hayashi et al. 1992; Khalil et al. 1995; Liam et al. 1994; Lippmann et al. 1992; Pierson et al. 1995; Resl et al. 1996; Ribet et al. 1995; Shimizu et al. 1990; Suen et al. 1993; Swanson et al. 1991;Wilkinson et al. 1992). The bronchogenic cysts may or may not have communication with the tracheobronchial tree (Pierson et al. 1995). Similarly, as with other foregut malformations, bronchogenic cysts may communicate with the gastrointestinal tract, usually the esophagus or stomach (Braffman et al. 1988; Gerle et al. 1968; Yang et al. 1994). It may be difficult to distinguish these cysts, which may be intimately associated

with the esophagus, from enteric duplication cysts. However, while bronchogenic cysts may have scattered smooth muscle present, they lack two well-developed muscular layers and nervous plexuses. In addition, bronchogenic cysts often have cartilaginous rests, mucous glands, and ciliated respiratory epithelium within them.

Bronchogenic cysts have been diagnosed prenatally in 10 fetuses (Albright et al. 1988; Mayden et al. 1984; Meizner et al. 1994; Rahmani et al. 1995; Vergnes et al. 1989). In each case the lesion was asymptomatic. However, because of the potential postnatal complications associated with bronchogenic cysts, the prenatal findings should never be ignored. The propensity of these lesions to cause symptoms relates to their position and size. Symptoms are most commonly related to intrinsic compression of the tracheobronchial tree, pulmonary artery, or esophagus (Coran et al. 1994; Dale et al. 1994; Worsnop et al. 1993). These cysts can compress the bronchi, thereby obstructing the distal airway. Under these circumstances, the prenatal sonographic abnormality detected may be the increased echogenicity of the lung distal to the obstructed bronchus (Young et al. 1989). This pattern may mimic the prenatal presentation of congenital lobar emphysema (Ahel et al. 1994; Barker 1996). Even when asymptomatic prenatally, these lesions require close management postnatally as they may cause stridor, bronchial obstruction, and possibly, respiratory distress or infection (Dale et al. 1994; Suen et al. 1993). All bronchogenic cysts require surgical resection because of the uncertainty of diagnosis and the potential for infection, hemoptysis, enlargement and obstruction, and malignant transformation.

▶ INCIDENCE

The true incidence of bronchogenic cyst is difficult to determine because of the asymptomatic nature of most bronchogenic cysts. In a report from Kousseff et al. from the University of South Florida (1997), the incidence of bronchopulmonary foregut malformations between 1984 to 1994 was only 2 cases among 24,000 families evaluated. Based on a review of noncardiac fetal intrathoracic lesions by Meizner et al. from a single center (1994), three cases of bronchogenic cysts were diagnosed prenatally. During the same period, this center had 46,281 births, yielding an estimated incidence of 1 in 15,427 live births.

▶ SONOGRAPHIC FINDINGS

Bronchogenic cysts are most often thin-walled unilocular cysts seen posterior to the trachea in the subcari-

nal region (Figs. 35-1 and 35-2). Bronchogenic cysts can be multilocular and can be seen at any point from the cervical subcutaneous position to any level of the mediastinum (Bagwell et al. 1988; Boue et al. 1994; Khalil et al. 1995; Lippmann et al. 1992). Bronchogenic cysts can be seen in unusual locations, mistaken for intrapericardial lesions, and may even be seen in the mouth or as an intradural lesion (Roos-Hesselink et al. 1996, Shimizu et al. 1990, Wilkinson et al. 1992).

Bronchogenic cysts may also be seen in proximity to the diaphragm, both intrathoracically and intra-abdominally. These lesions can be seen in the retroperitoneum, making it difficult to establish a definite cause.

Because these cysts are often intimately associated with the bronchi, they can cause extrinsic compression. Young et al. (1989) reported one case that was sonographically evident only by the obstruction of a bronchus, resulting in increased echogenicity of the lung distal to the cyst.

▶ DIFFERENTIAL DIAGNOSIS

The differential diagnosis of bronchogenic cysts depends on their location. Most bronchogenic cysts that have been recognized prenatally were mediastinal in location. In the anterior mediastinum, the differential diagnosis includes lymphangioma, pericardial cyst, diaphragmatic hernia, and thymic cyst. In the posterior mediastinum, the differential diagnosis should include enteric duplication cyst, anterior meningomyelocele, cystic neurogenic tumor,

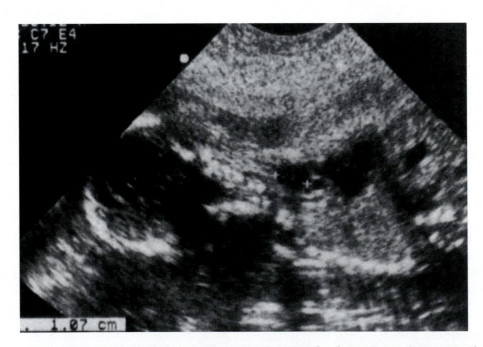

Figure 35-1. Transverse prenatal sonographic image of a fetal chest demonstrating a 1.0-cm unilocular cyst. *(Reprinted, with permission, from Rahmani MR, Filler RM, Shuckett B. Bronchogenic cyst occurring in the antenatal period. J Ultrasound Med 1995;14:971–973.)*

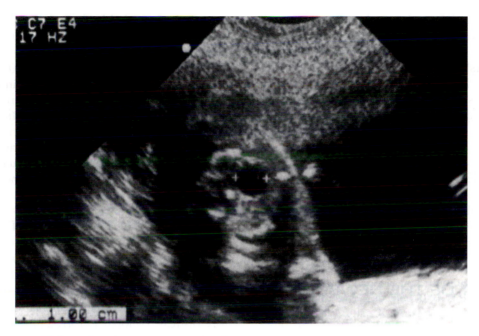

Figure 35-2. Longitudimal sonographic image of the same fetus shown in Figure 35-1. *(Reprinted, with permission, from Rahmani MR, Filler RM, Shuckett B. Bronchogenic cyst occurring in the antenatal period. J Ultrasound Med 1995;14:971–973.)*

and diaphragmatic hernia. Intraparenchymal cyst can be difficult to distinguish from cystic adenomatoid malformation of the lung. Infradiaphragmatic cysts, most commonly in the retroperitoneum, may be mistaken for adrenal cysts (Foerster et al. 1991; Swanson et al. 1991) or for enteric duplication cysts, or mesenteric cysts. These rare bronchogenic cysts are often misdiagnosed until resection and histologic diagnosis are performed.

▶ ANTENATAL NATURAL HISTORY

Our understanding of the antenatal natural history of bronchogenic cyst is quite limited, as only 10 cases have been diagnosed prenatally (Albright et al. 1988; Mayden et al. 1984; Meizner et al. 1994; Rahmani et al. 1985; Romero et al. 1980; Vergnes 1989). In each case, the bronchogenic cyst was asymptomatic and there were no adverse prenatal events. These cysts were isolated and unilocular, except in one case in which there were two, one in each lung (Romero et al. 1980). None of the prenatally diagnosed bronchogenic cysts have been associated with nonimmune hydrops, polyhydramnios, preterm labor, or intrauterine fetal death. Despite the apparently benign appearing prenatal history, it is important to recognize the limited number of cases on which these observations are based, and the potential complications that may been seen postnatally.

▶ MANAGEMENT OF PREGNANCY

In cases of suspected fetal bronchogenic cyst, the pregnant patient should undergo detailed sonographic evaluation to exclude other anomalies and consider alternative diagnoses such as cystic adenomatoid malformation, thymic cyst, diaphragmatic hernia, or enteric duplication cyst. Intrathoracic cysts should be examined for impingement on adjacent structures, including the tracheobronchial tree, pulmonary artery, and pericardium (Younis et al 1991; Yerman et al 1990). In the case of impingement on the tracheobronchial tree, subtle differences in the echotexture of the lung distal to the point of airway obstruction should be seen (Young et al. 1989). The position of the mediastinum and the presence or absence of polyhydramnios should also be noted. Bronchogenic cysts are part of a spectrum of bronchopulmonary foregut malformations that can be associated with each other (Black et al. 1988; Grewa et al. 1994). Other bronchopulmonary foregut malformations include esophageal duplication cysts, esophageal diverticulum, tracheoesophageal fistula, neurenteric cysts, and bronchopulmonary sequestrations (Demos et al. 1975; Gerle et al. 1968; O'Connell et al. 1979; Black et al. 1988). Vertebral anomalies have also been reported in association with bronchogenic cysts (Fallon et al. 1954). In cases of suspected pericardial bronchogenic cysts, an echocardiogram should be obtained. In infradiaphragmatic bronchogenic cysts, care should be taken to define the location and distinguish it from adrenal cysts,

Panicek DM, Heitzman ER, Randall PA. The continuum of pulmonary developmental anomalies. Radiographics 1987; 7:747–772.

Rodgers BM, Harmon PK, Johnson AM. Bronchopulmonary foregut malformations: the spectrum of anomalies. Ann Surg 1986;203:517–524.

Romero R, Chevernak FA, Kotzen J, et al. Antenatal sonographic findings of extralobar sequestration. J Ultrasound Med 1982;1:131–132.

Sade RM, Clause M, Ellis FH. The spectrum of pulmonary sequestration. Ann Thorac Surg 1974;18:644–658.

Sauerbrei E. Lung sequestration: duplex doppler diagnosis at 12 weeks' gestation. J Ultrasound Med 1992;10:101–105.

Savic B, Birtel FJ, Thalen W, et al. Lung sequestration: report of seven cases and review of 540 published cases. Thorax 1979;34:96.

Siffling PA, Forrest TS, Hill WC. Prenatal sonographic diagnosis of bronchopulmonary foregut malformation. J Ultrasound Med 1989;8:277–280.

Slotnick RN, McGahan J, Milio L, et al. Antenatal diagnosis and treatment of fetal bronchopulmonary sequestration. Fetal Diagn 1990;5:33–39.

Stern E, Brill PW, Winchester P. Imaging of prenatally detected intraabdominal extralobar pulmonary sequestration. Clin Imag 1990;14:152–156.

Thilenius OG, Ruschhaupt DG, Replogh RL, et al. Spectrum of pulmonary sequestration: association with anomalous pulmonary venous drainage in infants. Pediatr Cardiol 1983;4:97–100.

Thomas CS, Leopold GR, Hilton S, et al. Fetal hydrops associated with extralobar pulmonary sequestration. J Ultrasound Med 1987;5:668–671.

van Nayenberg H, Ein fall vox intrathorokaler nebenlunge. Zentralbl Allg Pathol 1914;25:673–680.

Vode A, Kramer L. Extralobar pulmonary sequestration presenting as intractable pleural effusion. Pediatr Radiol 1989;19:333–334.

Warner CL, Britt RL, Riley HD Jr. Bronchopulmonary sequestration in infancy or childhood. J Pediatr 1958;53:521–528.

Weinbaum PJ, Bars-Koefoed R, Green KW et al. Antenatal sonographic findings in a case of intraabdominal pulmonary sequestration. Obstet Gynecol 1989;73:860.

Weiner C, Yarner M, Pringle K, et al. Antenatal diagnosis and palliative treatment of nonimmune hydrops fetalis secondary to pulmonary extralobar sequestration. Obstet Gynecol 1986;68:275–280.

White JJ, Donahoo JS, Ostrow PT et al. Cardiovascular and respiratory manifestations of pulmonary sequestration in childhood. Ann Thorac Surg 1974;18:286–292.

Williams AD, Enumah FI. Extralobar pulmonary sequestration. Thorax 1968;23:200–205.

CHAPTER 37

Cystic Adenomatoid Malformation

► CONDITION

Congenital cystic adenomatoid malformation of the lung (CCAM) is a rare lesion characterized by a multicystic mass of pulmonary tissue with a proliferation of bronchial structures (Miller et al. 1980; Stocker et al. 1977). One theory holds that CCAM represents a failure of maturation of bronchiolar structures and occurs at approximately the fifth or sixth week of gestation during the pseudoglandular stage of lung development (Miller et al. 1980; Shanji et al. 1988; Stocker et al. 1977). Others have considered CCAM to represent a focal pulmonary dysplasia, since skeletal muscle has been identified within the cyst walls (Leninger and Haight 1973).

CCAM is slightly more common in males and may affect any lobe of the lung (Hernanz-Schulman 1993). The lesion is unilobar in 80 to 95% of cases and bilateral in fewer than 2% (Stocker et al. 1977). Unlike bronchopulmonary sequestration (BPS), CCAMs have a communication with the tracheobronchial tree, albeit via a

minute tortuous passage. In contrast to BPS, CCAMs derive their arterial blood supply and venous drainage from normal pulmonary circulation, but anomalous arterial and venous drainage of CCAM has been also reported (Rashad et al. 1988) as well as so called "hybrid" lesions which have a systemic blood supply (Cass et al. 1997).

Stocker et al. have subdivided CCAM into three types based on their pathologic characteristics (Fig. 37-1) (Stocker et al. 1977). Type I lesions account for 50% of postnatal cases of CCAM, and consist of single or multiple cysts lined by ciliated pseudostratified epithelium. These cysts are usually quite large (on the order of 3 to 10 cm) and few in number (1 to 4). Type I lesions are usually associated with a favorable outcome. Type II lesions account for 40% of postnatal cases of CCAM and consist of more numerous cysts of smaller diameter (usually less than 1 cm) lined by ciliated, cuboidal, or columnar epithelium. Respiratory bronchioles and distended alveoli may be present between these cysts. There is a high frequency of associated congenital

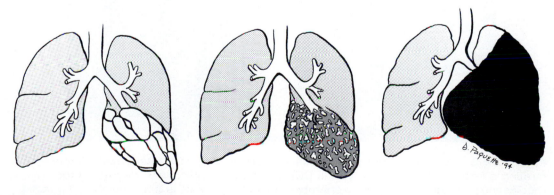

Figure 37-1. Depiction of Stocker's classification of type I, II, and III CCAM.

anomalies with type II lesions. The prognosis in the type II lesions often depends on the severity of associated anomalies. The most commonly associated anomalies include genitourinary, such as renal agenesis or dysgenesis; cardiac, including truncus arteriosus and tetralogy of Fallot; jejunal atresia; diaphragmatic hernia; hydrocephalus; and skeletal anomalies (Stocker et al. 1977). The high incidence of associated anomalies has led to speculation that this type of CCAM may occur as a result of events occurring prior to 31 days of gestation (Walker and Cudmore 1990). The type III lesions account for only 10% of cases and are usually large homogeneous microcystic masses that cause mediastinal shift. These lesions have bronchiole-like structures lined by ciliated cuboidal epithelium, separated by masses of alveolar-sized structures lined by nonciliated cuboidal epithelium. The mixture of epithelial and mesenchymal structures in type III lesions has led to speculation that its development is related to events occurring prior to 28 days of gestation, after the formation of the lung buds (Walker and Cudmore 1990). The prognosis in type III CCAMs is usually poor, presenting with nonimmune hydrops in utero and cardiorespiratory compromise in the newborn (Adzick et al. 1985B; Harrison et al. 1990A).

▶ INCIDENCE

CCAM is a relatively rare lesion, with only 421 cases in infants and children reported at the time of this writing, in the world literature since its original description in 1949. In more recent years, with the widespread use of obstetrical ultrasound, there has been a rapid increase in the number of cases detected prenatally. Since the initial report of a prenatal sonographic diagnosis of CCAM, there have been over 300 antenatally detected cases reported (Adzick et al. 1998; Nicolaides et al. 1987).

▶ SONOGRAPHIC FINDINGS

CCAMs are diagnosed prenatally by the demonstration of a lung tumor that may be solid or cystic in the absence of vascular flow detected by Doppler studies (Fig. 37-2) (Bezzuti and Isler 1983; Cone and Adam 1984; Dann et al. 1981; Deacon et al. 1990; Diwan et al. 1983; Johnson et al. 1984; Marcus et al. 1986; Mendoza et al. 1986). Types I and II CCAM appear as cystic or echolucent pulmonary masses. It is important to note that on ultrasound examination, diaphragmatic hernias, cystic hygromas, and other cystic lesions, such as bronchogenic or enteric cysts, and pericardial cysts, can be mistaken for type I or type II CCAM (Boulot et al. 1991). A type III CCAM typically appears as a large hyperechogenic mass, often associated with mediastinal shift and hydrops (Adzick et al. 1985B).

The sonographic appearance of CCAMs can range from solid echodense mass filling the chest to a dominant cyst with a similar effect on the mediastinum. The vast majority of CCAMs derive their blood supply from

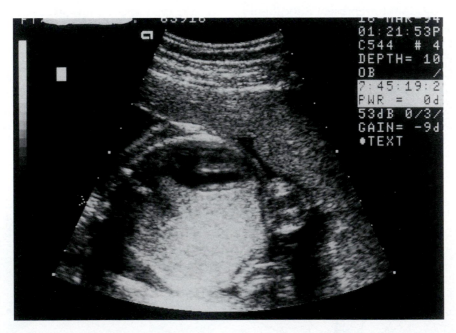

Figure 37-2. Prenatal sonographic cross-sectional image of a fetal chest, demonstrating a large homogeneous type III CCAM filling the right chest, displacing the mediastinum to the left. The four-chamber view of the heart is seen displaced against the left chest wall *(Courtesy of Dr. Marjorie Treadwell).*

the pulmonary circulation and drain via the pulmonary veins. However, color doppler should be used to search for the presence of a systemic feeding vessel. This may be observed in most bronchopulmonary sequestrations (the main differential diagnosis in CCAMs) and in hybrid lesions (Cass et al. 1997). The systemic feeding vessel in hybrid CCAM lesions usually comes directly off the descending aorta; however, transdiaphragmatic systemic feeding vessels have been observed in CCAMs.

▶ DIFFERENTIAL DIAGNOSIS

The differential diagnosis of fetal thoracic masses includes congenital diaphragmatic hernia (CDH) (see Chapter 38), bronchogenic or enteric cysts, BPS (see Chapter 36), mediastinal cystic hygroma (see Chapter 32), bronchial atresia or stenosis, neuroblastoma, and brain heterotopia (Chinn et al. 1983; Gonzalez-Cuezzi et al. 1980; Hobbins et al. 1979; Romero et al. 1982). The sonographic appearance of CCAM will influence the differential diagnosis. Type I CCAMs are more likely to be confused with a CDH. Observing peristalsis in the loops of herniated intestine or emptying of the stomach herniated through the diaphragm may help to differentiate the two (May et al. 1993). In rare cases, amniography and computed tomographic (CT) scanning have been employed to distinguish CDH from

other thoracic lesions (Adzick 1993). More recently, fetal magnetic resonance imaging (MRI) has proved extremely helpful in evaluating fetal chest masses and distinguishing them from diaphragmatic hernia (Fig. 37-3) (Hubbard and Crombleholme 1998). It is also worth noting that there have been cases of CCAM occurring with CDH (Stocker et al. 1977). The microcystic type III CCAMs are highly echogenic. This is helpful in distinguishing CCAM from solid tumors such as neuroblastoma. Bronchogenic cysts are unilocular and are usually adjacent to major bronchi, which may be confused with a type I CCAM. However, the main differential diagnosis in CCAM is usually BPS. Unlike most CCAMs, BPS derives its blood supply from the systemic circulation (Carter 1959). This systemic blood supply to BPS can often be demonstrated with the use of color flow Doppler studies (Fig. 37-4) (Hernanz-Schulman et al. 1991; Morin et al. 1994). There has been an anecdotal report of CCAM associated with anomalous blood supply (Rashad et al. 1988). With the exception of this case, the demonstration of systemic blood supply to a thoracic mass has been thought to be pathognomonic of BPS. More recently, Cass et al. (1997) described six cases of cystic adenomatoid malformation that had systemic blood supply. These lesions were called "hybrid" lesions as they had features of both CCAMs and BPSs and their natural history was also a mixture of the two lesions.

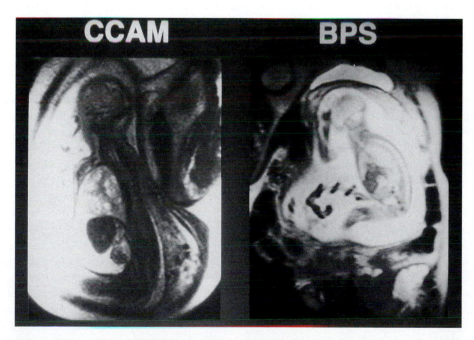

Figure 37-3. Fetal MRI in CCAM and BPS. The left panel is a sagittal section of a fetus with complex multicystic cystic adenomatoid malformation with associated hydrops and ascites. The right panel is a sagittal section of a fetus with a bright-intensity homogeneous wedge-shaped mass due to bronchopulmonary sequestration.

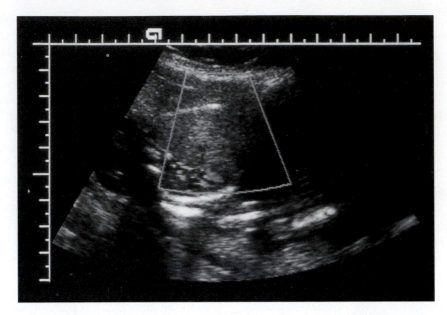

Figure 37-4. Color Doppler sonogram demonstrating systemic feeding vessel arising from the aorta supplying an echogenic lung mass, in this case a bronchopulmonary sequestration. See color plate.

▶ ANTENATAL NATURAL HISTORY

The postnatal natural history of CCAM can be quite variable (Adzick 1993, 1998; Atkinson et al. 1972; Cloutier et al. 1993; Heij et al. 1990; Kuller et al. 1992; Neilson et al. 1991; Nishiboyoshi et al. 1982; Pulpeiro et al. 1987; Stocker et al. 1977). The lesion can be completely asymptomatic and come to medical attention only when chest radiography is performed for other reasons, such as a history of mild respiratory complaints with recurrent infections in infancy or childhood (Stocker et al. 1977). However, fewer than 10% of CCAMs present after the first year of life. Eighty percent of postnatal patients will present at birth with severe cardiorespiratory compromise due to severe pulmonary hypoplasia (Atkinson et al. 1972; Cloutier et al. 1993; Heij et al. 1990; Hernanz-Schulman et al. 1991; Kuller et al. 1992; Neilson et al. 1991; Nishiboyoshi et al. 1981; Pulpeiro et al. 1987; Stocker et al. 1977). Even before the advent of obstetrical sonography, it was recognized that up to 14% of cases of CCAM result in stillbirths (Stocker et al. 1977). This observation hinted at the different prenatal natural history of CCAM.

The outcome of fetuses diagnosed prenatally with CCAM has only recently been reported, and our understanding of the natural history of CCAM is still evolving. We know that the worst outcome is observed in fetuses in which hydrops develops (Adzick 1993; Adzick et al. 1985B, 1998; Harrison et al. 1990A). Hydrops is usually seen in very large type III lesions, which cause mediastinal shift and vena caval obstruction (Fig. 37-5). Hydrops may also be exacerbated by the loss of pro-

tein from the CCAM into the amniotic fluid, thus reducing the fetal colloid oncotic pressure from hypoproteinemia (Hernanz-Schulman et al. 1991). Rarely has a fetus with CCAM survived after the onset of hydrops, and these only when fetal surgery has been performed (Adzick et al. 1998).

Adzick et al. have proposed a modification of Stocker's classification of CCAMs, based on anatomy and sonographic appearance to assist in predicting outcome in cases detected in utero (Adzick et al. 1985B). In this classification, macrocystic CCAMs have single or multiple cysts >5 mm in diameter. Microcystic CCAMs are more solid and bulky, with cysts that are <5 mm in diameter. This distinction can easily be made sonographically in the fetus. Macrocystic lesions appear sonographically as fluid-filled cysts, while microcystic lesions appear solid due to fine interfaces with the ultrasound beam creating an almost homogeneous appearance (Adzick et al. 1985B). This is a useful sonographic distinction, because microcystic lesions are almost invariably fatal. The high mortality rate of microcystic lesions is due to the large size these lesions attain and secondary sequelae, including mediastinal shift, pulmonary hypoplasia, polyhydramnios, and nonimmune hydrops (Adzick et al. 1985B, 1993, 1998; Harrison et al. 1990A). Despite the type of lesions, however, the overall prognosis depends primarily on the size of the lesion. Polyhydramnios is seen in up to 70% of CCAMs diagnosed antenatally (Adzick et al. 1998). The pathogenesis of polyhydramnios is not completely understood but is thought to relate to esophageal obstruction from mediastinal shift and interference with

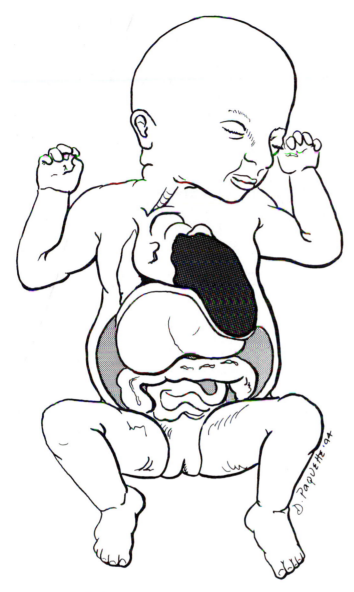

Figure 37-5. Schematic illustration of the pathophysiology of large CCAMs. The rapid growth of the chest mass compresses the lungs, depresses the diaphragm, shifts the mediastinum, compromising venous return to the heart. Ascites, placentomegaly, and anasarca of nonimmune hydrops develop.

fetal swallowing of amniotic fluid (Miller et al. 1980; Murayama et al. 1987). This is supported by the absence of fluid in the stomachs of many of these fetuses.

The diagnosis of CCAM may also have implications for the health of the mother. Adzick et al. (1993) reported a mother with a fetus with CCAM that developed the "mirror syndrome," a hyperdynamic preeclamptic state that may be life-threatening. The "mirror syndrome" has been seen in molar pregnancies, sacrococcygeal teratoma, and in fetal conditions that result in poor placental perfusion, which leads to endothelial cell injury (Roberts et al. 1989; Creasy 1979). The only

treatment for this syndrome is immediate delivery of the baby.

The antenatal diagnosis of a large CCAM might at first appear to be an ominous finding; however, several reports have described disappearing fetal lung masses (Adzick and Harrison 1993; Adzick et al. 1993; Budorick et al. 1992; Fine et al. 1988; MacGillivray et al. 1993; Saltzman et al. 1988). MacGillivray et al. (1993) have reported six cases of large CCAM with associated mediastinal shift that progressively decreased in size over the course of gestation. These lesions were all of the microcystic, or type III, variety but none was associated with nonimmune hydrops. The percentage of cases that will undergo spontaneous regression is not known for certain, but the experience at two tertiary-care centers was between 6 and 11% of evaluated cases (Adzick et al. 1998; MacGillivray et al. 1993). The reason for regression of fetal CCAM is not understood. Decompression of the fluid from the CCAM into the tracheobronchial tree or outgrowing its blood supply have been suggested as possible mechanisms (Adzick et al. 1993). There has been no biochemical or sonographic marker that allows us to distinguish between a CCAM that will regress and one that will progress to hydrops.

Recently, Crombleholme et al (1999) reported the use of CCAM volume and the CCAM volume ratio as a predictor of the development of hydrops. The CCAM volume is calculated using the formula for the volume of an ellipse ($h \times w \times l \times 0.52$) in cm^3 with the measurement of the greatest length in the saggital section and the width and height taken at 90 degrees to the saggital measurement. The CCAM volume ratio (CVR) is obtained by dividing the CCAM volume by the head circumference (in cm) to correct for any differences in gestational age. Based on 20 fetuses with CCAMs, the CCAM volume and the CVR were found to be significantly higher in fetuses with hydrops. In addition, when the mean of the group that did not develop hydrops plus two standard deviations were added a cutoff value of 1.2 was obtained. No fetuses with CVR less than 1.2 ever developed hydrops. The numbers from this study were too small to predict which CCAMs would progress to hydrops as several were already hydropic at presentation. The CVR is a useful criterion to select fetuses at greatest risk for the development of hydrops and those at low risk for development of hydrops.

The single largest experience with prenatally diagnosed CCAMs has been reported by Adzick et al. (1998). This series reflected the combined experience of The Center for Fetal Diagnosis and Treatment at the Children's Hospital of Philadelphia, and The Fetal Treatment Center at The University of California, San Francisco, comprising a 12–year retrospective study at the two centers and 175 fetal lung lesions. There were 134 fetuses with CCAMs in this group. Of these, 14 pregnancies

lung growth was observed in five of the eight cases in which complete tracheal occlusion was achieved. In three cases in which complete occlusion was not achieved, either because the polymeric foam or the aneurysm clip could not completely occlude the trachea, no acceleration of lung growth was observed. In the remaining five patients, despite biologic response to tracheal occlusion, none survived because of non-pulmonary complications, including small-bowel obstruction, intracranial hemorrhage, cerebral atrophy, and intrauterine fetal death (Harrison et al. 1997).

Despite excellent biologic response with complete tracheal occlusion, there was only one survivor in this initial series. The group at The Children's Hospital of Philadelphia had similar problems when the procedure was performed at 28 weeks of gestation (Fig. 38-5). Survival increased to 40% in fetuses with a predicted mortality rate in excess of 90% when fetal tracheal clip application was performed at 26 weeks of gestation (Flake et al. 2000). The UCSF group recently reported their experience with fetoscopic tracheal clip application (Mychaliska et al. 1998). There were 4 survivors among the 10 patients in which it was attempted. In 4 patients the fetoscopic procedure had to be converted to an open procedure and none survived. There were 2 other deaths, 1 due to multiple pterygium syndrome (Mychaliska et al. 1998). Of note, 2 of the 4 survivors have bilateral vocal-cord paralysis secondary to recurrent laryngeal-nerve injury requiring permanent tracheostomy. Although the fetoscopic clip procedure has

been advocated by the UCSF group to reduce preterm labor and lengthen postoperative gestation, the data thus far have not supported this contention. In addition, the selection criteria for fetoscopic clip procedure has been an LHR <1.4 (Mychaliska et al. 1998). However, this group's own data on LHR suggests 100% survival with conventional postnatal therapy with an LHR >1.35 (Metkus et al. 1996). We currently recommend the fetal tracheal-clip procedure only for isolated diaphragmatic hernia with herniation of the liver and an LHR <1.0. In other words, with a predicted survival on only 10% with conventional postnatal therapy in order to limit the maternal risks of fetal surgery to only the most severe cases of CDH.

Accurate preoperative assessment of the extent of herniation of the left lobe of the liver is an essential prerequisite before considering fetal surgery (Harrison et al. 1993a). Careful evaluation of the umbilical vein by color flow Doppler studies can diagnose herniated left lobe of the liver (Boostaylor et al. 1995). When the umbilical vein is deviated far to the left, the liver is usually herniated. If there is no kinking of the sinus venosus, the left lobe of the liver is not herniated or is amenable to reduction. Other signs of herniated left lobe of the liver include a posteriorly displaced stomach or a soft-tissue density between the lateral border of the heart and the herniated stomach (Harrison et al. 1993). Hubbard et al. (1997) have reported the use of fetal magnetic resonance imaging (MRI) to assess herniation of the left lobe of the liver. The exquisite

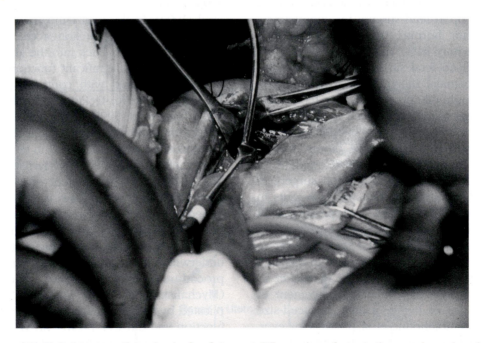

Figure 38-5. Intraoperative view of a fetus at 26 weeks of gestation undergoing fetal tracheal clip application. The fetal arms are retracted down through the hysterotomy and the head is extended within the uterus. The fetal neck is opened above the sternal notch to expose the fetal trachea.

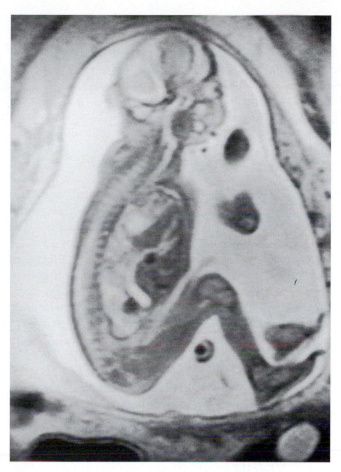

Figure 38-6. Fetal MRI performed in a fetus at 24 weeks of gestation, demonstrating marked herniation of the left lobe of the liver. The bright signal in the left portal vein can be seen tacking up into the left chest.

anatomic detail obtained with HASTE and echoplanar MRI have made this the test of choice to assess herniation of the left lobe of the liver (Fig. 38-6) (Hubbard et al. 1997).

▶ TREATMENT OF THE NEWBORN

All fetuses with CDH are at high risk for severe pulmonary hypoplasia and are optimally managed by delivery in a perinatal center with neonatal and pediatric surgical experts immediately available, preferably in a center capable of performing ECMO (Crombleholme 1996; Harrison et al. 1990). The resuscitation of a newborn includes immediate endotracheal intubation, neuromuscular blockade, and positive-pressure ventilation. Strategies to minimize barotrauma should be employed, whether by conventional ventilation via "gentilation" or by high-frequency oscillatory ventilation (Hi Fi). The infant should have a sump-style nasogastric tube inserted in the delivery room to perform con-

tinuous suction to avoid dilation of the intrathoracic bowel from the infant swallowing air. In the delivery room the infant should have umbilical arterial and umbilical venous catheters placed to monitor arterial blood gases and provide venous access. Preductal and postductal transcutaneous oxygen saturation monitors can help to continuously monitor right-to-left shunting across the ductus arteriosus.

Judicious volume resuscitation is important; however, many infants with diaphragmatic hernia require fluid boluses and vasopressor support with dopamine and occasionally dobutamine.

There has been interest in minimizing the damage to the hypoplastic lung by the use of gentilation (Wung et al. 1995). This strategy limits inspiratory pressures to 30 cm of water and permits hypercapnea to pCO_2 levels of 58. This strategy has been successfully employed in a select group of fetuses with mild to moderately severe diaphragmatic hernia. In the most severely affected infants, the limits of this ventilatory strategy are soon exceeded, and support with ECMO must be initiated.

The use of inhaled nitric oxide in congenital diaphragmatic hernia has met with mixed results. Inhaled nitric oxide has not clearly been shown to benefit newborns with diaphragmatic hernia. However, inhaled nitric oxide has been beneficial in preventing the need for ECMO during the postoperative period (Dillon et al. 1995; Frostell et al. 1993).

▶ SURGICAL TREATMENT

It was once believed that immediate operation to decompress the chest was necessary. However, in recent years, it has been recognized that this is not the case. The more important variable is the degree of underlying pulmonary hypoplasia. Emergency surgical repair may, in fact, be detrimental to the infant's tenuous pulmonary status after birth and relative pulmonary artery hypertension (Hazebrock et al. 1989; Langer et al. 1989). It is better to delay repair until the infant has stabilized. This may take hours or days. If the infant deteriorates during this so-called honeymoon period, ECMO can be initiated. The infant can undergo repair of CDH while on ECMO and be weaned from the circuit postoperatively (Connors et al. 1990).

Repair of CDH is usually performed via a left-upper-quadrant transverse or subcostal incision, which allows exposure of the defect and reduction of the herniated viscera. The diaphragm can occasionally be primarily repaired but in severe cases the defect is large or there may be complete diaphragmatic aplasia, both of which require a prosthetic patch. A chest tube is usually inserted after repair of CDH, as well as a subdiaphragmatic closed suction drain. The chest tube is placed only to water seal, and no suction is applied.

▶ LONG-TERM OUTCOME

The long-term outcome of infants with CDH who survive the neonatal period depends on the severity of pulmonary hypoplasia, and the degree of bronchopulmonary dysplasia resulting from long-term ventilatory support (Bales et al. 1979). In addition, extrapulmonary complications are now being noted more commonly in survivors of CDH (Glass et al. 1989; Lund et al. 1994). There is a high incidence of neurologic problems in children with CDH, independent of exposure to ECMO. Other complications such as reactive airway disease, sensorineural hearing loss due to prolonged need for antibiotics and/or furosemide (Lasix), seizures, and developmental delay may be seen in up to 20 to 30% of patients (Lund et al. 1994). Long-term follow-up evaluation and early intervention are indicated in this group of high-risk patients.

Failure to thrive has been noted in many survivors of diaphragmatic hernia (Atkinson et al. 1992; Cunniff et al. 1990a; D'Agostino et al. 1995; Van Meers et al. 1993). Many infants with diaphragmatic hernia have feeding difficulties that may require gavage feedings and may contribute to failure to thrive. The causes of failure to thrive may be multifactorial but Nobuhora et al. (1996) noted that 30% remained below the fifth percentile despite optimization of caloric intake; 68% of the patients in this group were ECMO survivors. Van Meers et al. (1993) also noted a high percentage (50%) of CDH survivors supported with ECMO who had failure to thrive.

Gastroesophageal reflux may affect as many as 50 to 62% of diaphragmatic hernia survivors (Kieffer et al. 1995; Koot et al. 1993). While some have reported good response to medical therapy (Stolar et al. 1990), the need for antireflux surgery varied from 9.6 to 14.8% (Kieffer et al. 1995; Koot et al. 1995; Nagaya et al. 1994).

Musculoskeletal deformities, such as pectus excavatum and scoliosis, may also develop in survivors of diaphragmatic hernia. The cause of these deformities may be the asymmetric lung size, the diaphragmatic repair, or the increased work of breathing some patients may have. In the series reported by Nobuhora et al. (1996) the incidence of pectus excavatum was 21% and scoliosis was 10.5%.

▶ GENETICS AND RECURRENCE RISK

Although the vast majority of cases of CDH are sporadic, there have been anecdotal reports of familial CDH that is inherited as an autosomal dominant (Crane et al. 1979; Gibbs et al. 1997; Norio et al. 1984; Pollock et al. 1979; Wolfe et al. 1990). The pattern of inheritance in sporadic CDH is poorly understood, but the recurrence risk for siblings has been estimated to be as high as 2%

(Brachen et al. 1983; Norio et al. 1984; Pollock et al. 1979). CDH occurs more commonly in females than in males, with a ratio 3:2 (Butler and Claireaux 1962; Crane et al. 1979; Fitzgerald et al. 1979). Although no specific features of CDH identify a familial predisposition, there is a higher incidence of bilateral hernias and a lower incidence of associated life-threatening malformations in familial rather than sporadic cases (Puri et al. 1984). CDH occurs as part of Fryns syndrome (Bamforth et al. 1989; Cunniff et al. 1990a; Moerman et al. 1988), an autosomal recessive condition that is usually lethal. It comprises CDH with cleft palate, hypoplastic nails and terminal phalanges, cystic kidneys, genital and central nervous system anomalies, and dysmorphic facies. Fryns syndrome is a single-gene defect inherited in an autosomal recessive manner and carries a 25% chance of recurrence. Twenty-five cases have been reported to date. The thoracoabdominal syndrome (TAS) is composed of CDH and ventral hernias, hypoplastic lung, and cardiac anomalies. Its inheritance in one family suggests X-linked dominant inheritance (Carmi et al. 1990). David and Illingsworth's (1976) study of 143 patients in England showed that 50% had other malformations. Cunniff et al. (1990a), studied 102 children. Of these 39% had a major nonpulmonary malformation, especially cardiac defects (18%). Karyotype was abnormal in 5% (trisomy 18, Turner syndrome, 10:X translocation). CDH associated with mosaic tetrasomy 12p (46, XY/47, XY, +i12p, see Chapter 130) has been reported (Bressen et al. 1991). Rarely, CDH can be found in association with VATER or Poland anomalies. Associated anomalies include lung hypoplasia, malrotation of the intestine, and patent ductus arteriosus. Cardiovascular anomalies have been reported in up to 23% of cases. These include ventricular septal defect, vascular ring, and coarctation of the aorta. There is also a higher incidence of neural-tube defects, genitourinary anomalies, esophageal atresia, omphalocele, and cleft palate.

In cases of perinatal loss, every attempt should be made to have autopsy studies performed to document the presence of additional anomalies not detected on sonographic examination. A follow-up meeting with a clinical geneticist is useful to summarize autopsy results and discuss possible genetic diagnoses. In conditions such as Fryns syndrome, single-gene defects are present that are inherited in an autosomal recessive manner and carry a 25% chance of recurrence. Familial diaphragmatic hernia, which is inherited as an autosomal dominant condition with a 50% chance of recurrence, should have prenatal screening by early prenatal sonography in subsequent pregnancies.

REFERENCES

Adzick NS. On the horizon: neonatal lung transplantation. Arch Dis Child 1992;67:455–457.

Adzick NS, Harrison MR. Fetal surgical therapy. Lancet 1994;343:897–902.

Adzick NS, Harrison MR, Glick PL, et al. Diaphragmatic hernia in the fetus: prenatal diagnosis and outcome in 94 cases. J Pediatr Surg 1985a;20:357–362.

Adzick NS, Outwater KM, Harrison MR, et al. Correction of congenital diaphragmatic hernia in utero IV: an early gestational fetal lamb model for pulmonary vascular morphometric analysis. J Pediatr Surg 1985b;20:673–680.

Adzick NS, Vacanti JP, Lillehei CW, et al. Fetal diaphragmatic hernia: ultrasound diagnosis and clinical outcome in 38 cases from a single medical center. J Pediatr Surg 1981; 24:654–660.

Alcorn D, Adamson T, Lambert T: Morphologic effects of chronic tracheal ligation and drainage in the fetal lamb lung. J Anat 1976;22:649–657.

Areechon W, Reid L. Hypoplasia of the lung associated with congenital diaphragmatic hernia. BMJ 1963;1:230–233.

Bales ET, Anderson G. Diaphragmatic hernia in the newborn: mortality, complications and long-term follow-up observations. In: Kiesewetter WB, ed. Long term follow-up in congenital anomalies. Proceedings from the Pediatric Surgical Symposium. Pittsburgh, 1979;10–20.

Bamforth J, et al. Congenital diaphragmatic hernia, coarse facies, and acral hypoplasia: Fryns Syndrome. Am J Med Genet 1989;32:93–99.

Bealer JF, Skorsgard ED, Hedrick NH, et al. The "plug" odyssey: adventures in experimental fetal tracheal oclusion. J Pediatr Surg 1995;30:361–367.

Beierle EA, Langhorn MR, Cassin S. In utero lung growth in fetal sheep with diaphragmatic hernia and tracheal stenosis. J Pediatr Surg 1996;31:141–146.

Boostaylor BS, Filly RA, Harrison MR, Adzick NS. Prenatal sonographic predictors of liver herniation in congenital diaphragmatic hernia. J Ultrasound Med 1995;14: 515–520.

Boyden EA. Development and growth of the airways. In: Hodson WA, ed. Development of the lung. New York: Marcel Dekker 1977:37–86.

Brachen MB, Berg A. Bendictin (Debendax) and congenital diaphragmatic hernia. Lancet 1983;1:586–587.

Butler N, Claireaux AE. Congenital diaphragmatic hernia as a cause of perinatal mortality. Lancet 1962;1:659–661.

Carmel JA, Friedman F, Adams FH, et al. Fetal tracheal ligation and lung development. Am J Dis Child 1965;109: 452–457.

Carmi R et al. Fryns syndrome: an autosomal recessive disorder associated with craniofacial anomalies, diaphagmatic hernia. Am J Med Genet 1990;36:109–114.

Companale RD, Rowland RH. Hypoplasia of the lung associated with congenital diaphragmatic hernia. Ann Surg 1955;142:17–28.

Connors RH, Tracy T, Bailey PV, et al. Congenital diaphragmatic hernia repair on ECMO. J Pediatr Surg 1990;25: 1043–1047.

Crane JP. Familial congenital diaphragmatic hernia: prenatal diagnostic approach and analysis of twelve families. Clin Genet 1979;16:244–248

Crombleholme TM, Adzick NS, Hardy K, et al. Pulmonary lobar lung transplantation in neonatal swine: a model for the treatment of congenital diaphragmatic hernia. J Pediatr Surg 1990;25:11–18.

Cunniff C, Jones KL, Jones MC. Patterns of malformation in children with congenital diaphragmatic defects. J Pediatr 1990a;116:258–261.

Cunniff C, et al. Fryns syndrome: an autosomal recessive disorder associated with cariofacial anomalies, diaphagmatic hernia, and distal digital hypoplosia. Pediatrics 1990b;85:499–504.

David TJ, Illingworth CA. Diaphragmatic hernia in the southwest of England. J Med Genet 1976;13:253–256.

DeFiore JW, Fauza DO, Slavin R, et al. Experimental tracheal ligation reverses the structural and physiologic effects of pulmonary hypoplasia in congenital diaphragmatic hernia. J Pediatr Surg 1994;29:248–252.

Dillon PW, Filley RE, Hudome SM, et al. Nitric oxide reversal of recurrent pulmonary hypertension and respiratory failure in an infant with CDH after successful ECMO therapy. J Pediatr Surg 1995;30:743–744.

Evans JNG, MacLachlan RF. Choanal atresia. J Laryngol 1971;85:903–905.

Fitzgerald RJ. Congenital diaphragmatic hernia as a cause of perinatal mortality. J Med Sci 1979;146:280–284.

Flake AW, Crombleholme TM, Johnson MD, et al. Treatment of severe congenital diaphragmatic hernia by fetal tracheal occlusion: chemical experience with fifteen cases. Am J Obstet Gynecol (in press).

Frostell CG, Lannquist PA, Sonesson SE, et al. Near fatal pulmonary hypertension after surgical repair of congenital diaphragmatic hernia: successful use of inhaled nitric oxide. Anaesthesia 1993;48:679–683.

Geggel RL, Reid LM. The structural basis of PPHN. Clin Perinatol 1984;2:525–585.

Geggel RL, Murphy JD, Langleben D, et al. Congenital diaphragmatic hernia: Arterial structural changes and persistent pulmonary hypertension after surgical repair. J Pediatr 1985;107:757–764.

Gibbs DL, Rice HE, Farrell JA, et al. Familial diaphragmatic agenesis: an autosomal-recessive syndrome with a poor prognosis. J Pediatr Surg 1997;32:366–368.

Greenwood RD, Rosenthal A, Nodes A. Cardiovascular abnormalities associated with congenital diaphragmatic hernia. Pediatrics 1976;57:92–96.

Harrison MR, Adzick NS, Bullard K, et al. Correction of congenital diaphragmatic hernia in utero VII: a prospective trial. J pediatr Surg 1997;31:1637–1642.

Harrison MR, Adzick NS, Estes JM, et al. A prospective study of the outcome of fetuses with diaphragmatic hernia. JAMA 1994;271:382–384.

Harrison MR, Adzick NS, Flake AW. Congenital diaphragmatic hernia: an unsolved problem. Semin Pediatr Surg 1993a;2:109–112.

Harrison MR, Adzick NS, Flake AW, et al. Correction of congenital diaphragmatic hernia. VI. Hard earned lessons. J Pediatr Surg 1993b;28:1411–1418.

Harrison MR, Adzick NS, Flake AW, et al. Correction of congenital diaphragmatic hernia in utero VIII: response of the hypoplastic lung to tracheal occlusion in fetuses with diaphragmatic hernia. J Pediatr Surg 1996;31: 1339–1348.

Harrison MR, Adzick NS, Longaker MT, et al. Successful repair in utero of a fetal diaphragmatic hernia after removal of herniated viscera from the left thorax. N Engl J Med 1990a;322:1582–1584.

Holzgreve W, Holzgreve B, Curry CJR: Non-immune hydrops fetalis: diagnosis and management. Semin Perinatol 1985;19:52–67.

Hook A, Schneider I, Jorde A, et al. Diagnotic and theropie eines falles von Kangenitalem hydrothorax infolge extraloborere lungen-separation. Kinderarztl Prox 1987;55:81–84.

Hunter WS, Becroft DM. Congenital pulmonary lymphangiectasias associated with pleural effusions. Arch Dis Child 1984;59:278–281.

Hutchison AA, Drew JH, Yu VYH, et al. Nonimmunologic hydrops fetalis: a review of 61 cases. Obstet Gynecol 1982;59:347–353.

Im SS, Rizos N, Joutsi P, et al. Nonimmunologic hydrops fetalis. Am J Obstet Gynecol 1984;148:566–571.

Inselman LS, Mellins RB. Growth and development of the lung. J Pediatr 1981;98:1–15.

Jaffe R, DiSegni E, Altaras M, et al. Chylothorax spontanie neonatal: diagnostic antenatal. Arch Fr Pediatr 1986;43:752–755.

Jauppela P, Kirkinen P, Huna R, et al. Prenatal diagnosis of pleural effusions by ultrasound. J Clin Ultrasound 1983;11:516–519.

Keeling JW, Gough DJ, Iliff PJ. The pathology of non-rhesus hydrops. Diagn Histopathol 1983;6:89–111.

Kerr-Wilson RHJ, Duncan A, Hume R. Prenatal pleural effusion associated with congenital pulmonary lymphangiectasia. Prenat Diagn 1985;5:73.

Kitohara M. A case report of congenital lymphedema with chylothorax. Nippon Kyobu Shikkan Gakkai Zasshi 1985;23:106–108.

Kristofferson SE, Ipsen L. Ultrasound real time diagnosis of hydrothorax before delivery in an infant with extralobar lung sequestration. Acta Obstet Gynecol Scand 1984;63:723–726.

Kurjak A, Rajhvajn B, Kolger A, et al. Ultrasound diagnosis and fetal malformations of surgical interest. In: Kurjak A, ed. The fetus as a patient. Amsterdam: Excerpta Medica, 1985:243–271.

Laberge JM, Crombleholme TM, Langaker MT. The fetus with pleural effusions. In: Harrison MR, Golbus MS, Filly RA, eds. The unborn patient. 2nd ed. Philadelphia: Saunders 1991;314–319.

Landy HJ, Daly V, Heyl PS, et al. Fetal thoracentesis with unsuccessful outcome. J Clin Ultrasound 1990;18:50–53.

Lange IR, Harman CR, Ash KM, et al. Twin with hydramnios: treating premature labor at source. Am J Obstet Gynecol 1989;160:152–157.

Lazarus KH, McCurdy FA. Multiple congenital anomalies in a patient with Diamond-Blackfan syndrome. Clin Pediatr 1984;23:520–523.

Levin DL. Morphologic analysis of the pulmonary vascular bed in congenital left-sided diaphragmatic hernia. J Pediatr 1978;92:80–85.

Lewis WH. The development of the muscular system. In: Keibel F, Mall FP, eds. Manual of human embryology. Philadelphia: Lippincott, 1910:454–522.

Lien JM, Colmargen GH, Gehret JF, et al. Spontaneous resolution of fetal pleural effusion diagnosed during the second trimester. J Clin Ultrasound 1990;18:54–56.

Liggins GC. A self retaining catheter for fetal peritoneal transfusion. Obstet Gynecol 1986;68:275–277.

Longaker MT, Laberge JM, Dansereau J, et al. Primary fetal hydrothorax: natural history and management. J Pediatr Surg 1989;24:573–576.

Manning D, O'Brien NG. Congenital pleural effusion with multiple associated anomalies. Ir Med J 1983;76:497–499.

Milsom JW, Kron IL, Rheuban KS, et al. Chylothorax: an assessment of current surgical management. J Thorac Cardiovasc Surg 1985;89:221–227.

Morin L, Crombleholme TM, D'Alton ME: Prenatal diagnosis and management of fetal thoracic lesions. Semin Perinatol 1994;18:228–253.

Murayoma K, Jimbo T, Matsumoto Y, et al. Fetal pulmonary hypoplasia with hydrothorax. Am J Obstet Gynecol 1987;157:119–120.

Murphy MC, Newman BM, Rodgers BM: Pleuroperitoneal shunts in the management of persistent chylothorax. Ann Thorac Surg 1989;48:195.

Nicolaides KH, Azar GB: Thoraco-amniotic shunting. Fetal Diagn Ther 1990;5:153–164.

Nicolaides KH, Rodeck CH, Lange I, et al. Fetoscopy in the assessment of unexplained fetal hydrops. Br J Obstet Gynaecol 1985;92:671–679.

Parker M, James D. Spontaneous variation in fetal pleural effusions: case report. Br J Obstet Gynaecol 1991;98:403–405.

Pearl KN, Wilson RG: Management problem of child with congenital marble skin and chylothorax requiring repeated drainage. Lancet 1981;2:90–91.

Peleg D, Golichowski KM, Rogan WD. Fetal hydrothorax and bilateral pulmonary hypoplasia: ultrasonic diagnosis. Acta Obstet Gynecol Scand 1985;64:451–453.

Petres RE, Redwine FO, Cruikshank DP. Congenital bilateral chylothorax: antepartum diagnosis and successful inrauterine surgical management. JAMA 1982;248:1360–1362.

Pijpess L, Reuss A, Stewart PA, et al. Noninvasive management of isolated bilateral fetal hydrothorax. Am J Obstet Gynecol 1989;161:330–332.

Puntis WL, Roberts KD, Handy D. How should chylothorax be managed? Arch Dis Child 1987;62:593–596.

Reece EA, Lockwood CJ, Rizzo N et al. Intrinsic intrathoracic malformations of the fetus: sonographic detection and clinical presentation. Obstet Gynecol 1987;70:627–632.

Reynolds M. Disorders of the thoracic cavity and pleura and infections of the lung, pleura, and mediastinum. In: O'Neill JA, Rowe MI, Grosfeld JA, Fonkalsund EW, Coran AG, eds. Pediatric Surgery. 5th ed. St. Louis: Mosby-Year Book, 1998:899–919.

Rigsby R, Crombleholme TM, Green K, D'Alton M. Algorithm for the management of fetal hydrothorax. Fetal Diag Ther (in press).

Roberts AB, Clarkson JM, Pattison NS, et al. Fetal hydrothorax in the second trimester of pregnancy: successful intrauterine treatment at 24 weeks gestation. Fetal Ther 1986;1:203–209.

Rodeck CH, Fisk NM, Fraser DI, Nicolini U. Long-term in utero drainage of fetal hydrothorax. N Engl J Med 1988;319:1135–1138.

Roth A. Lymphangiectasies dissemunies cutonies congenitalis pleurales et intestinales. Arch Anat Cytol Pathol 1984;32:349–353.

Smelzer DM, Stickler GM, Fleming RE. Primary lymphatic dysplasia in children: chylothorax, chylous ascites, and generalized lymphatic dysplasia. Eur J Pediatr 1986;145: 386–391.

Smith DW. Recognizable patterns of human malformation: genetic, embryologic and clinical aspects. 3rd ed. Philadelphia: Saunders, 1982.

Stenzl W. Treatment of postsurgical chylorthorax with fibrin glue. Thorac Cardiovasc Surg 1983;31:35.

Van Gerde J, Campbell AN, Symth JA, et al. Spontaneous chylothorax in newborns. Am J Dis Child 1984;138: 961–967.

Weber AM, Philipson EH. Fetal pleural effusion: a review and meta-analysis for prognostic indicators. Obstet Gynecol 1992;79:281–286.

Weiner C, Yarner M, Pringle K, et al. Antenatal diagnosis and palliative treatment of nonimmune hydrops fetalis secondary to extralobar sequestration. Obstet Gynecol 1986;68:275–280.

Wilson RH, Duncan A, Hume R, et al. Prenatal pleural effusion associated with congenital pulmonary lymphangectasia. Prenat Diagn 1985;5:73–76.

Yaghoobian J, Comrie M. Transitory bilateral isolated fetal pleural effusions. J Ultrasound Med 1988;7:231–232.

CHAPTER 40

Pulmonary Agenesis

► CONDITION

Pulmonary agenesis is a rare developmental condition in which there is complete absence or severe hypoplasia of one or both lungs (Booth et al. 1967; Borja et al. 1970; Boxer et al. 1978; Costas et al. 1977; McCormick et al. 1979; Mygind et al. 1980; Oyamada et al. 1953; Shenoy et al. 1979; Yaghmai 1970). Although quite rare, it was initially recognized by dePozzi in 1673 (Skandalakis et al. 1994). Munchmeyer was the first to diagnose unilateral agenesis of the lung clinically in 1885 (Ferguson et al. 1944). There have since been over 200 cases of unilateral agenesis of the lung reported. However, only 14 cases have been reported of bilateral agenesis of the lung (Allen and Affelbach 1925; Claireaux et al. 1957; Devi et al. 1966; Diaz et al. 1989; Engellenner et al. 1989; Faro et al. 1979; Ostor et al. 1978; Tuynman et al. 1952). In some cases, bilateral pulmonary agenesis was an isolated finding. In other cases pulmonary agenesis was found in association with other anomalies in the gastrointestinal, genitourinary, and ocular systems (Claireaux et al. 1957; Devi et al. 1966; Ostor et al. 1978; Tuynman et al. 1952).

A number of theories have been advanced to explain the pathogenesis of lung aplasia. Lung aplasia has been observed in experimental animals fed a diet deficient in vitamin A (Warkany et al. 1948). Some authors have suggested that there may be a vascular cause of pulmonary agenesis, similar to that invoked for intestinal atresia (Louw 1959). Other authors have suggested a genetic cause for the pulmonary agenesis. Booth and McKenzie and their colleagues linked unilateral pulmonary agenesis to ipsilateral facial and jaw abnormalities, an association noted more recently by Kenawi et al. (Booth et al. 1967; Kenawi et al. 1976; McKenzie and Craig 1955). The gene involved may have a variable expressivity and penetrance. However, the ac-

tual cause of this type of pulmonary agenesis remains obscure.

Schneider (1909) proposed a classification for the degree of underdevelopment of the lung that has been adopted by many authors. In Class I there is agenesis of the lung or total absence of the bronchus and lung. In Class II there is aplasia in which there is a rudimentary bronchus without lung tissue. In Class III hypoplasia there is bronchial hypoplasia and a variably reduced amount of lung tissue present. Bilateral agenesis of the lung is incompatible with life and, fortunately, is exceedingly rare (Engellenner et al. 1989). Unilateral agenesis occurs about 25 times more commonly, and it may be compatible with a normal life (Booth et al. 1967; Maltz et al. 1968). This classification scheme is most appropriately referred to as agenesis and hypoplasia, with Class I and II representing cases of agenesis, and Class III representing cases of hypoplasia.

Unilateral pulmonary agenesis is associated with a broad range of anomalies of other organ systems. The most common cardiac defect associated with unilateral agenesis is patent ductus arteriosus. Although noted to be present fairly frequently, because this is a common neonatal finding, it may or may not relate directly to the nature of the underlying cause of the pulmonary agenesis. Another common finding is anomalous pulmonary venous drainage, either to the azygos vein or to a persistent left superior vena cava. Other cardiovascular anomalies that have been reported include left pulmonary artery posterior to the left bronchus, aorta anterior to the trachea and compressing it with the left pulmonary artery posterior to the trachea, an anomalous pulmonary venous drainage of the left lung to the right atrium, and four pulmonary veins on the right side. In addition, atrial and ventricular septal defects have been reported in association with pulmonary agenesis.

Although tracheoesophageal anomalies may accompany unilateral pulmonary agenesis, only 13 cases have been recorded thus far, one of which was tracheoesophageal fistula (Kitagawa et al. 1995; Steadland et al. 1995). Other gastrointestinal anomalies associated with pulmonary agenesis include duodenal atresia, annular pancreas, malrotation, Meckel diverticulum, and imperforate anus. Barium contrast studies may demonstrate deviation of the esophagus to the agenetic side, particularly when the right lung is absent. Occasionally the diaphragm may be deficient on either the ipsilateral or contralateral side, allowing eventration of the abdominal viscera. However, this diaphragmatic anomaly is more commonly seen accompanying pulmonary hypoplasia than agenesis.

The most common spinal abnormality seen in association with pulmonary agenesis is hemivertebrae (see Chapter 95). This can be seen in both agenesis of the lung and hypoplasia of the lung. The resulting scoliosis may be quite severe and produce an additional handicap in the child already suffering from recurrent respiratory infection. Such scoliosis may also be due to a rudimentary rim of lung tissue on the affected side. An abnormality of the spine or ribs in the cervical or thoracic regions may be attended by a more prominent scapula on the affected side.

In at least six cases, there have been associated facial or jaw abnormalities ipsilateral to the side of the pulmonary agenesis or hypoplasia (Cunningham et al. 1997; David et al. 1996). These abnormalities have included hemifacial microsomia, deformed left external ear, seventh nerve paralysis, small deformed right ear without a patent external auditory canal, facial asymmetry, torticollis, and unilateral mandibulofacial dysostosis (see Chapter 25).

Ipsilateral limb abnormalities have also been observed in many of these cases. These usually involve the upper extremity on the ipsilateral side (Cunningham et al. 1997). While abnormalities of both the ulna and the radius and malformation of the carpus result in a smaller, less powerful hand and arm, the most characteristic abnormalities have been noted in the ipsilateral thumb. These included triphalangia; angulated thumb, in which the middle phalanx is hypoplastic; a preaxial polydactyly; and an abnormal thumb with a short first metacarpal. Some of these digital radial dysplasias fit the pattern of the Holt–Oram syndrome (Holt and Oram 1960) and the ventriculoradial dysplasia syndrome (Harris et al. 1966).

▶ INCIDENCE

The incidence of agenesis, either unilateral or bilateral, is uncertain. Based on a report of four cases among 114,569 hospital admissions Borja et al. (1970) suggested a prevalence of 0.0034%. During a 6-year period, four other patients were noted with unilateral agenesis among 41,403 admissions to the King Feisel Specialist Hospital and Research Center, which would represent a prevalence of 0.0097% or about 1 in 10,000 admissions, or 0.67% of the 596 patients who underwent cardiac catherization at that center (Mardini et al. 1985). Agenesis of the right lung and left lung are about equally common. Females are affected slightly more commonly than males, and the condition may be inherited (Mardini et al. 1985; Schechter et al. 1968).

There is no estimate of the prenatal incidence of pulmonary aplasia; however, Schechter et al. (1968) have estimated an incidence of 1 in 15,000 based on autopsies. Both lungs are affected with equal frequency, although patients with left lung aplasia have a much better prognosis.

▶ SONOGRAPHIC FINDINGS

The diagnosis of pulmonary agenesis is often made only at the time of autopsy. However, in recent years cases of unilateral pulmonary agenesis have been recognized prenatally (Becker et al. 1993; Bromley and Benacerraf 1997; Engellenner et al. 1989; Yancey and Richards 1993). Sonographically, the mediastinum is shifted toward the affected side and the diaphragm on the ipsilateral side is elevated. Care should be taken to distinguish pulmonary hypoplasia caused by compression from a diaphragmatic hernia or cystic adenomatoid malformation from unilateral agenesis. The sonographic features of unilateral pulmonary agenesis include medial mediastinal shift to the agenetic side and enlarged echogenic lung herniating into the contralateral chest anterior and/or posterior to the mediastinum. There may be associated scoliosis with a curve toward the agenetic side with or without hemivertebrae. Because of the frequency of associated anomalies in pulmonary agenesis affecting other organ systems, a careful sonographic examination should be performed, including scanning of the vertebrae, heart, and limbs and the genitourinary and central nervous systems. There is an association with ipsilateral radial ray defects and hemifacial microsomia. The presence of bilateral facial or radial ray anomalies may be seen in bilateral pulmonary agenesis (Cunningham et al. 1997). Renal abnormalities including dysplasia and horseshoe kidney have been reported with unilateral pulmonary agenesis, as has encephalocele (Becker et al. 1993; Cunningham et al. 1997). Both polyhydramnios and oligohydramnios have been reported in pulmonary agenesis (Engellenner et al. 1989). In the single case of nonimmune hydrops reported in a fetus with unilateral pulmonary agenesis, it was thought to be due to partial closure of the ductus arteriosus in an otherwise structurally normal heart (Engellenner et al. 1989).

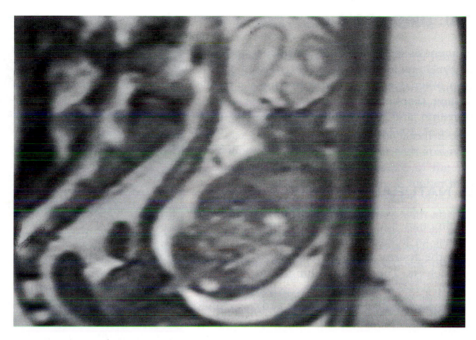

Figure 40-1. Fetal MRI of a fetus with right pulmonary agenesis. This coronal section demonstrates the enlarged left lung herniating over into the right chest with shift of the heart and mediastinum to the agenetic side.

While opacification of the ipsilateral hemithorax with displacement of the mediastinum occurs in the direction of the agenetic lung, Roque et al. (1997) reported a postnatal patient in which this was not the case. In that patient the mediastinum was not displaced, but the liver and the intact diaphragm were displaced cephalad. Fetal magnetic resonance imaging (MRI) has been helpful in distinguishing unilateral pulmonary agenesis from other causes of mediastinal shift. MRI clearly demonstrates the compensatorily enlarged unilateral lung shifting over into the contralateral hemithorax with shift of the heart and mediastinal structures to the agenetic side (Figs. 40-1 and 40-2).

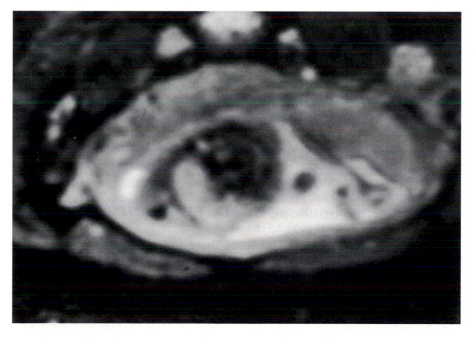

Figure 40-2. Fetal MRI in transverse section in a fetus with right pulmonary agenesis demonstrating enlarged unilateral lung with shift of mediastinum.

made. In general, there is no need to transfer care to a tertiary-care center. However, the patient should be aware that if esophageal atresia is confirmed postnatally the newborn will require immediate transport to a tertiary-care center with pediatric surgeons capable of reconstructing the anomaly. The presence of esophageal atresia has no implications for the mode of delivery. Cesarean section should be reserved for obstetric indications and there is no need to alter the timing of delivery.

▶ FETAL INTERVENTION

There are no fetal interventions for esophageal atresia and tracheoesophageal fistula.

▶ TREATMENT OF THE NEWBORN

When esophageal atresia is strongly suspected, consideration should be given to delivery in a tertiary-care center. A Replogle sump tube should be positioned in the proximal esophageal pouch and placed to low, continuous suction to prevent aspiration of secretions. Chest radiography showing the sump tube coiled in the proximal pouch is consistent with a diagnosis of esophageal atresia. However, rarely a Replogle tube will coil in the pharynx of a normal infant. In isolated esophageal atresia, plain radiography reveals a gasless abdomen. If a tracheoesophageal fistula is present, bowel gas will be seen on plain radiography. The infant should be maintained in an upright position and given antibiotics, and H_2 blockers intravenously. Because of the reported 7% incidence of proximal esophageal pouch–tracheal fistulas (Fig. 41D) and the possibility of coiling of a sump tube in the pharynx, despite a normal esophagus, some groups perform contrast studies or bronchoscopy/esophagoscopy at the time of repair.

▶ SURGICAL TREATMENT

After considering gestational age, birth weight, pulmonary function, and the presence of other associated anomalies, a decision is made whether to perform a reconstructive procedure or a staged repair with initial closure of the tracheoesophageal fistula and placement of a gastrostomy tube for enteral feedings. In the extremely premature infant, or a newborn of any gestational age with tracheoesophageal fistula complicated by pneumonia, a feeding gastrostomy can be performed, with or without closure of the tracheoesophageal fistula, and definitive repair can be deferred until the infant's clinical status improves.

In cases of isolated esophageal atresia, the gap between proximal and distal pouches is usually prohibitively long (Fig. 41-1A). In these cases, a gastrostomy tube is placed to allow enteral feeding. Bolus feedings are employed to encourage gastroesophageal reflux to facilitate growth and dilation of the distal pouch. The growth of the proximal and distal pouches will be maximal between 10 and 12 weeks of postnatal age (Puri et al. 1981). In the meantime, nasopharyngeal suction is maintained to clear saliva, and H_2 blockers are administered to prevent severe esophagitis. Serial contrast studies are performed every few weeks to assess growth of the pouches so that reconstruction may be undertaken as soon as possible. One risk of this approach is aspiration pneumonia. If the infant's respiratory status has been compromised because of aspiration of secretions, this form of therapy must be abandoned. A cervical esophagostomy is then performed to drain salivary secretions. This results in foreshortening of the proximal esophageal pouch and necessitates an esophageal replacement procedure using either colon interposition or a gastric tube. These procedures are usually not performed until approximately 1 year of age.

The prolonged hospitalization, expense, risk of salivary aspiration, and, most importantly, lost opportunity to reconstruct the infant's native esophagus have led some surgeons to attempt a primary repair during the newborn period. Spitz et al. (1987) have reported some success with the gastric pullup of so-called long-gap esophageal atresia. The advantages of this approach include brief hospitalization, lower cost, and early return to normal feeding. The use of this procedure in the United States is not widespread because of the ongoing risk of aspiration from pooling of secretions in the intrathoracic gastric reservoir and compromise of respiratory function secondary to mass effect of the gastric pullup in the posterior mediastinum.

A basic tenet of all reconstructive esophageal surgery is the preservation of the native esophagus whenever possible. True to this tenet, Kimura et al. (1984) have proposed an ingenious operation for long-gap esophageal atresia. The infant's proximal esophagus is mobilized through an incision into the right neck and a spiral myotomy is performed to lengthen the esophagus. The esophagus telescopes like a "barber shop pole" and the muscular layers are reapproximated. This gives sufficient length to create an esophagostomy at the level of the nipples. A gastrostomy tube is placed for enteral feeding, but sham feedings can be commenced to preserve the coordination of normal swallowing. In addition, an esophagostomy positioned on the chest instead of at the clavicle allows placement of an ostomy appliance for ease of care. Normal neck movement then stretches the proximal esophagus. In a series of two or three procedures, the stoma is advanced

1.5 to 2.5 cm to lengthen the proximal esophagus. When sufficient length has been obtained, the esophagus can be reconstructed through a right thoracotomy. The advantages of this approach include discharge from hospital within the first 10 days of life, maintenance of normal swallowing coordination by sham feedings, cost reduction, and, most importantly, a reconstruction that preserves the infant's native esophagus. There is limited experience with this approach and no data on long-term outcome are yet available.

▶ LONG-TERM OUTCOME

In cases of esophageal atresia, the motor function of the distal esophageal pouch never becomes normal because of its interruption during embryologic life. Manometric studies of the distal esophageal pouch have demonstrated that it lacks normal peristalsis and the stripping activity usually observed after reflux of acid into the distal esophagus. In addition to motor disturbances, the sensory innervation of the distal esophagus does not appear to be as robust as that of the normal esophagus. Also, due to foreshortening of the intraabdominal esophagus, the lower esophageal sphincter appears to be less competent than in normal infants. All these factors predispose to gastroesophageal reflux and the potential for severe esophagitis. A more significant consequence is the development of strictures at the anastomosis, which occurs as a result of acid injury in this area. To prevent these complications, all infants with tracheoesophageal fistula should be on H_2-blocker therapy to prevent injury from gastroesophageal reflux. In instances in which recurrent anastomotic stricturing occurs despite repeated dilations and adequate medical therapy, antireflux procedures such as Nissen fundoplication are often indicated.

As experience has grown with repair of esophageal atresia and tracheoesophageal fistula, it has become more widely recognized that these are children at risk for the subsequent development of Barrett's mucosa from prolonged and severe gastroesophageal reflux. Barrett's mucosa is the result of metaplastic changes in the mucosa of the distal esophagus. This is a premalignant condition and requires close endoscopic surveillance with biopsies to detect dysplastic changes that precede the development of esophageal carcinoma. Esophageal carcinoma has developed after repair of tracheoesophageal fistula in patients as young as 21 years of age (Adzick et al. 1989). It is presumed that these malignancies arose within areas of Barrett's mucosa, which were caused by severe untreated gastroesophageal reflux. While both Barrett's mucosa and esophageal carcinoma are rare in children with repair of esophageal atresia and tracheoesophageal fistula, the incidence is uncertain. It is recommended that all children with this anomaly undergo endoscopic surveillance periodically to ensure that clinically silent gastroesophageal reflux has not resulted in severe esophagitis predisposing to the development of Barrett's mucosa.

Because of the abnormal motility in the reconstructed esophagus of the child with esophageal atresia with tracheoesophageal fistula, the motility in this organ is never quite normal. These children are prone to the impaction of food boluses at the anastomosis. This may occur even in the absence of a true anastomotic stricture. The reason for this is the disordered motility in the distal esophageal pouch, which does not move the food bolus normally into the stomach. All parents should be advised that once their infant begins eating solid food the pieces should be small and that they should learn to chew their food very well. This problem with impaction of food in the esophagus usually becomes less frequent as the child grows and the caliber of the esophagus increases.

▶ GENETICS AND RECURRENCE RISK

Although these anomalies are thought to be sporadic and there is no strong evidence that the anomalies are transmitted in a mendelian pattern, there are clinical data to suggest that there may be some genetic background for the transmission of the abnormality. A number of patients who survive repair of esophageal atresia have produced offspring with the same anomaly (Pletcher et al. 1991; Van Staey et al. 1984). Siblings with esophageal atresia have been reported, including one family with three affected children (Pletcher et al. 1991; Van Staey et al. 1984). Esophageal atresia and tracheoesophageal atresia are more common in twins (Ohkama 1978). One series of 102 patients reported an incidence of 6% of both twins affected with esophageal atresia (David et al. 1975). The literature suggests that parents of a single affected child should be given an empiric recurrence risk between 0.5 and 2%, rising to more than 20% if a second sibling is affected (Pletcher et al. 1991).

REFERENCES

Adzick NS, Fisher JH, Winter HS, et al. Esophageal adenocarcinoma 20 years after esophageal atresia repair. J Pediatr Surg 1989;24:741–744.

Bovicelli L, Rizzo N, Orsini LF, et al. Prenatal diagnosis and management of fetal gastrointestinal abnormalities. Semin Perinatol 1983;7:109–117.

Bowie JD, Clair MR. Fetal swallowing and regurgitation: observation of normal and abnormal activity. Radiology 1982;144:877–878.

Crombleholme TM, D'Alton ME, Cendron M, et al. Prenatal diagnosis and the pediatric surgeon: the impact of prenatal consultation on perinatal management. J Pediatr Surg 1996;31:156–162.

David TJ, O'Callaghan SE. Oesophageal atresia in the Southwest of England. J Med Genet 1975;12:1–11.

Estroff JA, Parad RB, Share JC, et al. Second trimester prenatal findings in duodenal and esophageal atresia without tracheoesophageal fistula. J Ultrasound Med 1994;13:375–379.

Eyeheremendy E, Pfister M. Antenatal real-time diagnosis of esophageal atresia. J Clin Ultrasound 1983;11:395–399.

Farrant P. The antenatal diagnosis of esophageal atresia by ultrasound. Br J Radiol 1980;53:1202–1203.

Greenwood RD, Rosenthal A. Cardiovascular malformations associated with tracheoesophageal fistula and esophageal atresia. Pediatrics 1976;57:87–91.

Gross R. The surgery of infancy and childhood. Philadelphia: Saunders, 1977.

Holder TM, Cloud DT, Lewis JE, et al. Esophageal atresia and tracheoesophageal fistula: a survey of its members by the Surgical Section of the American Academy of Pediatrics. Pediatrics 1964;34:542–549.

Kimura K, Soper RT. Multistaged extrathoracic esophageal elongation for long gaps esophageal atresia. J Pediatr Surg 1984;29:566–568.

Landing BH. Syndromes of congenital heart disease with tracheobronchial anomalies. AJR Am J Roentgenol 1975;123:679–686.

Louhimo I, Lindahl H. Esophageal atresia: primary results of 500 consecutively treated patients. J Pediatr Surg 1983;18:217–229.

Manning PB, Morgan RA, Coran AG, et al. Fifty years' experience with esophageal atresia and tracheoesophageal fistula. Ann Surg 1986;204:446–451.

Moore KL, Pessaud TUN. The developing human: clinically oriented embryology. 5th ed. Philadelphia: Saunders, 1993;251:70–72.

Ohkama R. Congenital esophageal atresia with tracheoesophageal fistula in identical twins. J Pediatr Surg 1978;13:361–262.

Pletcher BA, Friedes JS, Breg WR, et al. Familial occurrence of esophageal atresia with and without tracheoesophageal fistula: report of two unusual kindreds. Am J Med Genet 1991;39:380–384.

Pretorius DH, Drose JA, Dennis MA, et al. Tracheoesophageal fistula in utero. J Ultrasound Med 1987;6:509–513.

Puri P, Blake N, O'Donnell B, et al. Delayed primary anastomosis following spontaneous growth of esophageal segments in esophageal atresia. J Pediatr Surg 1981;16:180–183.

Robertson FM, Crombleholme TM, Paidas M, et al. Prenatal diagnosis and management of gastrointestinal anomalies. Semin Perinatol 1994;18:182–195.

Skandalakis JE, Gray SW, et al. Esophagus. In: Skandalakis JE, Gray SW (eds). Embryology for surgeons. Baltimore, MD: Williams and Wilkins, 1994:65–112.

Smith EI: The early development of the trachea and esophagus in relation to atresia of the esophagus and tracheoesophageal fistula. Contrib Embryol 1957;245:43–57.

Spitz L, Keily E, Spornan T. Gastric transposition for esophageal replacement in children. Ann Surg 1987;206:69–77.

Spitz L, Keily E, Biereton RJ, et al. Management of esophageal atresia. World J Surg 1993;17:296–300.

Stringer MD, McKenna KM, Goldstein RB, et al. Prenatal diagnosis of esophageal atresia. J Pediatric Surg 1995;30:1258–1263.

Van Staey M, De Bie S, Matten MT, et al. Familial congenital esophageal atresia: personal case report and review of the literature. Hum Genet 1984;66:260–266.

Zemlyn S. Prenatal detection of esophageal atresia. J Clin Ultrasound 1981;9:453–454.

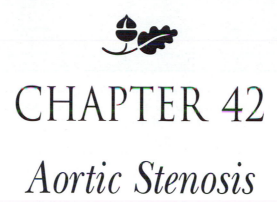

CHAPTER 42

Aortic Stenosis

▶ CONDITION

Aortic stenosis is the congenital obstruction of the left ventricular outflow tract of the heart. Stenosis can occur at, above, or below the aortic valve (Becker and Anderson 1981). Subvalvular aortic stenosis can be either fixed or dynamic. Fixed aortic stenosis is due to the presence of a discrete membranous diaphragm or a diffuse fibromuscular ring below the valve. Dynamic subvalvular aortic stenosis demonstrates a constantly changing pressure gradient across the valve and is most commonly due to muscular thickening of the septum. This form of subvalvular aortic stenosis is often called "asymmetric septal hypertrophy" (ASH), "idiopathic hypertrophic subaortic stenosis" (IHSS), or "hypertrophic obstructive cardiomyopathy" (HOCM). A transient form of dynamic subvalvular aortic stenosis has also been described, secondary to fetal hyperglycemia (Gutgesell et al. 1976).

Valvular aortic stenosis occurs secondary to abnormalities of the cusps of the aortic valve. Congenital unicuspid or bicuspid aortic valves may be stenotic at birth or they may become stenotic later in adult life. Other causes of valvular aortic stenosis include dysplastic or thickened cusps and fusion of the commissures that separate the cusps.

Supravalvular aortic stenosis can occur secondary to a localized narrowing of the ascending aorta, the presence of a membrane just superior to the origin of the coronary arteries, or a diffuse narrowing of the aortic arch and great arteries (Fig. 42-1). Because the obstruction occurs above the origin of the coronary arteries at the sinuses of Valsalva, the coronary arteries are also exposed to the elevated left ventricular pressures.

With all types of congenital aortic stenosis, if the stenosis becomes severe, secondary endocardial fibroelastosis can occur, leading to thickening of the endocardium and subsequent mitral insufficiency or cardiomyopathy. Aortic stenosis diagnosed early in gestation may evolve over time into hypoplastic left heart syndrome (Sharland et al. 1991).

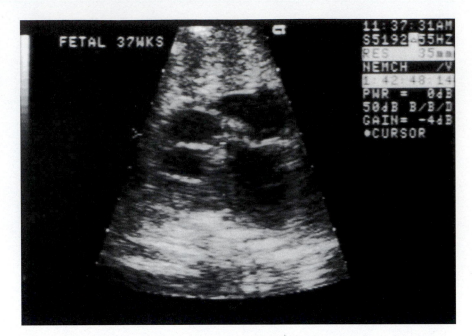

Figure 42-1. Antenatal sonographic image of a fetus at 37 weeks of gestation, demonstrating thickened aortic valve and narrowed left ventricular outflow tract.

▶ INCIDENCE

The overall incidence of congenital heart disease is 4 in 1000 to 10 in 1000 live births (Hoffman 1990). Aortic stenosis accounts for 3 to 6% of all congenital cardiovascular malformations, although it makes up 1 to 3% of all cardiac lesions in newborns presenting with significant cardiac defects (Kitchener et al. 1993; Rowe et al. 1981). It occurs up to four times more commonly in males than in females, although this sex predominance may be less marked in newborn populations. Overall, aortic stenosis has an incidence of 3.5 in 10,000 live births, while congenital bicuspid aortic valve may be as common as 1 in 100 live births.

▶ SONOGRAPHIC FINDINGS

Prenatal diagnosis of aortic stenosis is unreliable. Because supravalvular and subvalvular forms of aortic stenosis are usually not clinically apparent during the newborn period, prenatal diagnosis of these conditions is rarely successful. Prenatal sonographic features suspicious for aortic stenosis include enlargement or hypoplasia of the left ventricle. However, it is important to realize that left ventricular size can also be normal despite the presence of significant aortic stenosis. The right ventricle is also usually dilated with critical aortic stenosis, as blood flow is redistributed to the right ventricle and through the ductus arteriosus. In addition, critical aortic stenosis is usually associated with poststenotic aortic root dilation.

Incomplete opening of the aortic valve and increased aortic turbulence on Doppler echocardiography are both sonographic signs consistent with aortic stenosis during the newborn period, but prenatal visualization of these signs is extremely difficult because of the small size of the fetal aortic root. Prenatal diagnosis of a significant pressure drop (more than 50 mm Hg) across the valve is also suggestive of aortic stenosis (Jouk and Rambaud 1991)(Fig. 42-2). Prenatal visualization of abnormal thickening of the interventricular septum in aortic stenosis has been documented (Stewart et al. 1986). In severe cases of congenital aortic stenosis, antenatal Doppler studies may demonstrate significant mitral regurgitation. Aortic stenosis may also be the underlying cause of some cases of hydrops fetalis or intrauterine growth restriction, and therefore aortic stenosis should always be considered during the sonographic assessment of these conditions.

▶ DIFFERENTIAL DIAGNOSIS

The main alternatives that must be considered in the prenatal diagnosis of aortic stenosis include primary cardiomyopathy (see Chapter 45) and hypoplastic left heart (see Chapter 51) (Huhta et al. 1987). In addition, coarctation of the aorta must be considered, but the prenatal diagnosis of this condition is also very limited (see Chapter 46). Unlike aortic stenosis, primary cardiomyopathy is usually associated with a normal aortic valve and no evidence of poststenotic dilation. Such

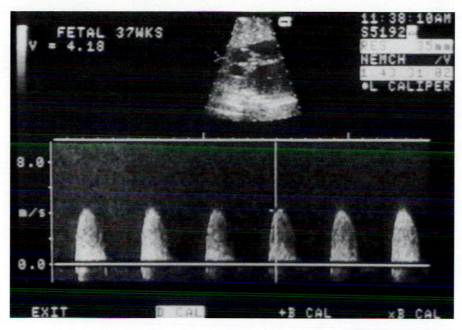

Figure 42-2. Doppler studies of same stenotic valve shown in Figure 42-1. A 65 mm Hg gradient was present across this valve.

primary cardiomyopathies may be secondary to endocardial fibroelastosis, viral or bacterial myocarditis, or some glycogen storage diseases.

Hypoplastic left heart syndrome is usually associated with both mitral- and aortic-valve atresia. In addition, the hypoplastic left ventricle may be globular in shape, rather than ellipsoid, which can be demonstrated on a four-chamber cardiac view by the left ventricle failing to reach the apex of the heart. In some cases differentiation of aortic stenosis from hypoplastic left heart syndrome can be difficult because the enlarged right ventricle seen with aortic stenosis may make the left ventricle appear small or even hypoplastic. Other features that aid in differentiating aortic stenosis from hypoplastic left heart syndrome include failure of growth in left ventricular, aortic, or mitral dimensions on serial examinations, as well as severe restriction of interatrial shunting in cases of hypoplastic left heart syndrome (McCaffrey and Sherman 1997).

▶ **ANTENATAL NATURAL HISTORY**

The antenatal natural history of congenital aortic stenosis can be quite varied, with almost all cases of sub-valvular and supravalvular aortic stenosis resulting in no fetal compromise, while critical valvular aortic stenosis can lead to intrauterine growth restriction, hydrops fetalis, and severe hemodynamic compromise during the early newborn period. The presence of hydrops

with a structural cardiac malformation is usually considered an ominous finding.

Left ventricular pressure overload may lead to ventricular enlargement, relative coronary hypoperfusion, subendocardial ischemia, and consequently, significant impairment of cardiac function. This can result in severe metabolic acidosis, leading to death in a significant number of cases, either before or soon after birth (Sharland et al. 1991). Sustained elevated left ventricular pressure secondary to outflow-tract obstruction can also lead to the intrauterine development of endocardial fibroelastosis and subsequent cardiomyopathy, which also increases the mortality rate for congenital aortic stenosis. In cases of aortic stenosis diagnosed prenatally, left ventricular volume and aortic-root dimensions tend to fall off from the normal percentiles as gestation progresses, and this information may be useful in predicting the appropriate form of repair during the newborn period (Simpson and Sharland 1997).

In one series of 30 cases of prenatally diagnosed left ventricular dysfunction, an initial appearance of aortic stenosis evolved over time into complete hypoplastic left heart syndrome in five cases (Sharland et al. 1991). There may be a spectrum of diseases in the fetus, involving primary left ventricular endocardial fibroelastosis, critical aortic stenosis, and hypoplastic left heart syndrome. Therefore, if screening takes place early enough, an initial clinical presentation of aortic stenosis may evolve over time into hypoplastic left heart syndrome (Sharland et al. 1991).

▶ MANAGEMENT OF PREGNANCY

Following the prenatal diagnosis of aortic stenosis, careful assessment of the remainder of the fetal anatomy is mandatory to rule out associated cardiac and noncardiac abnormalities. A referral for prenatal consultation with a pediatric cardiologist and neonatologist is recommended. Fetal echocardiography should be performed by an appropriately trained specialist if it has not already been done, as associated defects that may also be present include coarctation of the aorta, ventricular septal defect, and endocardial fibroelastosis. Karyotyping is also recommended because of the association between aortic stenosis and chromosomal abnormalities such as Turner syndrome. The fetus should be monitored with serial ultrasound examinations to detect early signs of congestive heart failure or hydrops fetalis. If hydrops develops, the prognosis is usually poor, although there are insufficient data at present to recommend changes in obstetric management. While it may be reasonable to offer early delivery in the setting of aortic stenosis with hydrops, it is as yet unclear if such an intervention will change the already poor fetal prognosis.

In the absence of hydrops, continued sonographic surveillance is recommended, followed by delivery for standard obstetric reasons in a tertiary-care facility, with the immediate availability of a pediatric cardiologist and cardiothoracic surgeon. Although some pediatric specialists have recommended elective cesarean delivery in the presence of critical aortic stenosis (Robertson et al. 1989), at present there are insufficient data to support routine cesarean delivery in this setting.

▶ FETAL INTERVENTION

Because of the high neonatal mortality rate associated with critical aortic stenosis, invasive attempts have been made in utero to correct the underlying valve abnormality. In one case report, a 16-gauge needle was placed transabdominally at 27 weeks of gestation and then inserted through the apex of the fetal heart, followed by a balloon catheter, which was threaded through the left ventricle into the ascending aorta (Lopes et al. 1996). Inflation of the balloon reportedly improved flow through the aortic valve, resulting in sonographic resolution of hydrops. The fetus was delivered by cesarean section but died from recurrent ventricular fibrillation soon after birth. In one other case report, in utero balloon dilation for aortic stenosis was technically successful in one of two fetuses, but did not affect fetal outcome (Maxwell et al. 1991). One survivor has been described following in utero balloon dilation of a stenotic aortic valve (Allan et al. 1995). The criteria to select appropriate fetal candidates for in utero intervention are not yet clear, although the presence of endocardial fibroelastosis may contraindicate intervention. Fetal intervention by means of in utero balloon dilation should therefore be considered experimental at this time.

In addition to balloon dilation, the only other form of in utero intervention described for aortic stenosis is digoxin therapy for the mother, which was reported in two cases of hydrops fetalis secondary to severe aortic stenosis, followed by postnatal balloon valvuloplasty (Bitar et al. 1997).

▶ TREATMENT OF THE NEWBORN

The initial treatment of newborns with congenital aortic stenosis involves diagnosing the severity of the condition followed by medical stabilization. Postnatal echocardiography should be performed promptly to confirm the diagnosis, establish its severity, and rule out other associated cardiac malformations. Echocardiography with Doppler studies should be sufficient to obtain this information without having to perform to cardiac catheterization (Fig. 42-3) (Huhta et al. 1987).

Medical management of aortic stenosis centers around stabilizing the infant while awaiting surgical intervention. Supplemental oxygen therapy, with or without mechanical ventilation, correction of metabolic acidosis, maintenance of normal hematocrit, inotropic support with digoxin, and cautious use of diuretics to alleviate pulmonary edema are all recommended (Kiel 1990). Prostaglandin E_1 infusion is recommended to maintain patency of the ductus arteriosus and improve tissue perfusion (Leoni et al. 1984). Balloon valvuloplasty via the umbilical artery may be useful as either a palliative procedure until definitive surgical repair takes place or as the primary repair procedure (Kiel 1990).

Definitive therapeutic options for the repair of critical aortic stenosis include biventricular repair, univentricular repair, or cardiac transplantation. Biventricular repair involves aortic valvulotomy (either open surgical or percutaneous balloon approaches). Univentricular repair is by means of a Norwood-type surgical procedure (anastomosis of the main pulmonary artery to the aorta followed later by creation of an atriopulmonary connection). Often within hours or days of birth the physician must decide which of these therapeutic options to follow. The presence of multiple small left heart structures may suggest improved survival following a Norwood-type repair rather than a valvulotomy (Rhodes et al. 1991). Aortic valvulotomy may yield better results when the aortic root measures 5 mm or greater (Turley et al. 1990).

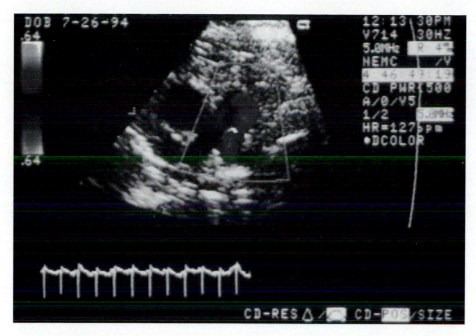

Figure 42-3. Color Doppler studies in a newborn with aortic stenosis, pulmonic atresia, and intact ventricular septum. See color plate.

▶ SURGICAL TREATMENT

Aortic valvulotomy is indicated when congestive heart failure is present or when the valve area is less than 0.5 cm^2 per square meter. Valvulotomy can be successfully performed via a closed, percutaneous approach, using a no. 5 Cook balloon catheter, which avoids the need for open surgery and cardiopulmonary bypass (Lababidi et al. 1984). Alternatively, an open surgical approach can be performed with the aid of hypothermia and cardiopulmonary bypass, in which commissural incisions are made in the stenotic valve, relieving stenosis but avoiding aortic incompetence. The disadvantage of this surgical approach is the need for cardiopulmonary bypass, which can significantly add to the morbidity for an already critically ill infant (Beeman and Hammon 1990). An alternative surgical approach involves closed valvulotomy through a median sternotomy with insertion of a valvulotome through a left ventricular stab wound. The Norwood-type surgical repair is described in more detail in the chapter on hypoplastic left ventricle (see Chapter 51). More detailed description of surgical techniques for repair of congenital aortic stenosis is beyond the scope of this textbook but is readily available in the literature (Gaynor and Elliott 1993).

Operative mortality for aortic stenosis typically occurs within 48 hours of surgery. The operative mortality rate for corrective surgery has been given as 1.9% for valvular stenosis, 6% for fixed subvalvular stenosis, and 5.5% for dynamic subvalvular stenosis (Jones et al.

1982). An overall operative mortality of 9% to 18% has been quoted for valvulotomy in cases of severe neonatal aortic stenosis (Gildein et al. 1996; Messina et al. 1984).

▶ LONG-TERM OUTCOME

Without treatment, almost all clinically significant cases of congenital aortic stenosis result in death. Even when aortic stenosis is mild at presentation, it may become progressive, eventually requiring surgery (Kitchener et al. 1993). Later complications after repair include aortic incompetence or regurgitation and bacterial endocarditis. The long-term mortality rate from aortic stenosis is 23% during the first year of life and falls to 1.2% during the first two decades, 3% in the third, 3.5% in the fourth, 6% in the fifth, and 8.5% in the sixth decade of life (Campbell 1968). In a more recent series, survival was 90% at age 10 years and 73% at age 25 years (Elkins et al. 1997). Twenty-five-year survival for aortic stenosis is 76% (Morris and Menashe 1991).

Approximately 50 to 70% of neonates who had surgical correction of aortic stenosis had satisfactory results when evaluated 5 to 14 years postoperatively (Jones et al. 1982). Almost one third of patients will require repeat aortic valve repair within 15 to 20 years of the original operation (Beeman and Hammon 1990; Gaynor et al. 1995). In another series, there was a 28% reoperation rate after a median duration of 8.7 years (Kitchener et al. 1993). A further 5% of patients may require a third operation later in childhood for aortic-valve stenosis (Wheller et al. 1988). Sudden deaths comprise more than one-third of all late cardiac deaths for aortic stenosis (Morris and Menashe 1991)

▶ GENETICS AND RECURRENCE RISK

Between 5 and 8% of all cases of congenital heart disease also involve a chromosomal abnormality, usually trisomy 21, and therefore the recurrence risk is that of the chromosomal defect itself (Hoffman 1990). Only a minority of cases of congenital heart disease (approximately 3%) are inherited in a classical mendelian pattern. The dynamic form of subvalvular aortic stenosis (IHSS or HOCM) is most often inherited in an autosomal dominant pattern. Subvalvular aortic stenosis may also occur as part of Turner and Noonan syndromes. Noonan syndrome is inherited as an autosomal dominant gene, and Turner syndrome is most commonly sporadic. Isolated supravalvular aortic stenosis may be inherited in an autosomal dominant pattern. Supravalvular aortic stenosis may also occur as part of the Williams syndrome, together with developmental delay and an unusual facies. Williams syndrome is due to the deletion of one copy of the elastin gene and may be diagnosed using a fluorescence in situ hybridization probe that maps to the elastin gene on chromosome 7.

Without a history suggestive of a mendelian or chromosomal disorder, the recurrence risk for a couple with one previously affected child with aortic stenosis is 2%. If there have been two affected children, the risk is 6%. Interestingly, the chance of having an affected infant if the mother has aortic stenosis is 13 to 18%, but if the father is affected, it is only 3% (Nora and Nora 1988).

REFERENCES

Allan LD, Maxwell DJ, Carminati M, et al. Survival after fetal aortic balloon valvoplasty. Ultrasound Obstet Gynecol 1995;5:90–91.

Becker AE, Anderson RH. Pathology of congenital heart disease. London: Butterworths, 1981.

Beeman SK, Hammon JW: Neonatal left ventricular outflow tract surgery. In: Long WA, ed. Fetal and neonatal cardiology. Philadelphia: Saunders, 1990:760–769.

Bitar FF, Byrum CJ, Kveselis DA, et al. In utero management of hydrops fetalis caused by critical aortic stenosis. Am J Perinatol 1997;14:389–391.

Campbell M. The natural history of congenital aortic stenosis. Br Heart J 1968;30:514–526.

Elkins RC, Knott-Craig CJ, McCue C, Lane MM. Congenital aortic valve disease: improved survival and quality of life. Ann Surg 1997;225:503–511.

Gaynor JW, Bull C, Sullivan ID, et al. Late outcome of survivors of intervention for neonatal aortic valve stenosis. Ann Thorac Surg 1995;60:122–126.

Gaynor JW, Elliott MJ: Congenital left ventricular outflow tract obstruction. J Heart Valve Dis 1993;2:80–93.

Gildein HP, Kleinert S, Weintraub RG, Wilkinson JL, Karl TR, Mee RBB. Surgical commissurotomy of the aortic valve: outcome of open valvotomy in neonates with critical aortic stenosis. Am Heart J 1996;131:754–759.

Gutgesell HP, Mullins CE, Gilette PC, et al. Transient hypertrophic subaortic stenosis in infants of diabetic mothers. J Pediatr 1976;89:120.

Hoffman JIE. Congenital heart disease: Incidence and inheritance. Pediatr Clin North Am 1990;37:25–43.

Huhta JC, Carpenter RJ, Moise KJ, et al. Prenatal diagnosis and postnatal management of critical aortic stenosis. Circulation 1987;75:573–576.

Jones M, Barnhart GR, Morrow AG. Late results after operations for left ventricular outflow tract obstruction. Am J Cardiol 1982;50:569–579.

Jouk PS, Rambaud P. Prediction of outcome by prenatal Doppler analysis in a patient with aortic stenosis. Br Heart J 1991;65:53–54.

Kiel EA. Aortic valve obstruction. In: Long WA, ed. Fetal and neonatal cardiology. Philadelphia: Saunders, 1990: 465–476.

Kitchener DJ, Jackson M, Walsh K, Peart I, Arnold R. Incidence and prognosis of congenital aortic stenosis in Liverpool (1960–1990). Br Heart J 1993;69:71–79.

Lababidi Z, Wu JR, Walls JT. Percutaneous balloon aortic valvuloplasty. Am J Cardiol 1984;53:194–197.

Leoni F, Huhta JC, Stark J, et al. Effect of prostaglandin on early surgical mortality in obstructive lesions of the systemic circulation. Br Heart J 1984;52:654–659.

Lopes LM, Cha SC, Kajita LJ, et al. Balloon dilatation of the aortic valve in the fetus. Fetal Diagn Ther 1996;11:296–300.

McCaffrey FM, Sherman FS. Prenatal diagnosis of severe aortic stenosis. Pediatr Cardiol 1997;18:276–281.

Maxwell D, Allan L, Tynan MJ. Balloon dilatation of the aortic valve in the fetus: a report of two cases. Br Heart J 1991;65:256–258.

Messina LM, Turley K, Stanger P, et al. Successful aortic valvulotomy for severe congenital valvular aortic stenosis in the newborn infant. J Thorac Cardiovasc Surg 1984;88: 92–96.

Morris CD, Menashe VD. 25-year mortality after surgical repair of congenital heart defect in childhood. JAMA 1991;266:3447–3452.

Nora JJ, Nora AH. Update on counseling the family with a first-degree relative with a congenital heart defect. Am J Med Genet 1988;29:137–142.

Rhodes LA, Colan SD, Perry SB, et al. Predictors of survival in neonates with critical aortic stenosis. Circulation 1991;84:2325–2335.

Robertson MA, Byrne PJ, Penkoske PA. Perinatal management of critical aortic valve stenosis diagnosed by fetal echocardiography. Br Heart J 1989;61:365–367.

Rowe RD, Freedom RM, Mehrizi A, et al. The neonate with congenital heart disease. Philadelphia: Saunders, 1981: 564–565.

Sharland GK, Chita SK, Fagg NLK, et al. Left ventricular dysfunction in the fetus: relation to aortic valve anomalies and endocardial fibroelastosis. Br Heart J 1991;66: 419–424.

Simpson JM, Sharland GK. Natural history and outcome of aortic stenosis diagnosed prenatally. Heart 1997;77: 205–210.

Stewart PA, Buis-Liem T, Verwey RA, et al. Prenatal ultrasonic diagnosis of familial asymmetric septal hypertrophy. Prenat Diagn 1986;6:249–256.

Turley K, Bove EL, Amato JJ, et al. Neonatal aortic stenosis. J Thorac Cardiovasc Surg 1990;99:679–684.

Wheller JJ, Hoiser DM, Teske DW, Craenen JM, Kilman JW. Results of operation for aortic valve stenosis in infants, children, and adolescents. J Thorac Cardiovasc Surg 1988; 96:474–477.

CHAPTER 43
Atrioventricular Canal Defect

► CONDITION

Atrioventricular (AV) canal defects are also known as atrioventricular septal defect, common atrioventricular canal, endocardial cushion defect, ostium primum atrial septal defect, and persistent ostium atrioventriculare commune. Complete AV canal defect consists of an unrestrictive atrial septal defect, an unrestrictive ventricular septal defect, and a single common atrioventricular valve. It occurs because of failure of development of the endocardial cushion during embryogenesis and persistence of the primitive single atrioventricular canal beyond 6 weeks of gestation. Although the AV canal defect may involve a wide spectrum of abnormalities of the atrial and ventricular septa and the AV valves, the complete form with associated AV valve regurgitation is the one that most commonly presents during the neonatal period (Chin et al. 1982).

AV canal defects can be partial or complete. With a partial AV canal defect, there are two separate AV orifices, with communication between two atria or between the left ventricle and the right atrium. While the right AV valve is usually normal, the left valve usually has three leaflets (Becker and Anderson 1981). With a complete AV canal defect, there is a defect in the inferior portion of the atrial septum and the superior portion of the ventricular septum, together with a single AV valve orifice, which usually has five valve leaflets. The anterior and posterior valve leaflets are inserted on the anterior and posterior surfaces of the ventricular septum, respectively; the degree of bridging of the anterior leaflet across the ventricular septum determines the type of defect (Rastelli et al. 1966). For type A complete AV canal defects, the anterior leaflet does not bridge the ventricular septum and is attached on both sides of the septum by chordae tendineae. For type B complete AV canal defects, the anterior leaflet some-what bridges the ventricular septum and is attached to the right ventricle by an anomalous papillary muscle. For type C complete AV canal defects, the anterior leaflet is not attached to the septum, and completely bridges it, being attached at either side by papillary muscles.

► INCIDENCE

Complete AV canal defect accounts for 1 to 5% of all cases of congenital heart disease (Rowe et al. 1981). In one series of 357 cases of congenital heart disease 13% were AV canal defects, almost 70% of which were of the complete type (Fontana and Edwards 1962). Familial clustering of AV canal defects has also been described (Disegni et al. 1985; Tennant et al. 1984). In two large population-based series, the incidence of endocardial cushion defect was 0.11 to 0.25 case per 1000 live births (Ferencz et al. 1985; Fyler et al. 1980).

► SONOGRAPHIC FINDINGS

Prenatal diagnosis of a complete AV canal defect is relatively straightforward, because a large defect or hole is easily visualized at the crux of the heart during diastole on the four-chamber view. This hole represents the defects in the inferior portion of the atrial septum, the superior portion of the ventricular septum, and the single AV valve orifice. In the normal four-chamber view of the heart, the tricuspid valve inserts more apically than the mitral valve, leading to an offset appearance at the crux of the heart. With an AV canal defect, this offset appearance may be lost, with both valves forming a straight line across the crux of the heart when closed.

Because the defect can be large, the cardiac conduction apparatus is frequently abnormal, resulting in an

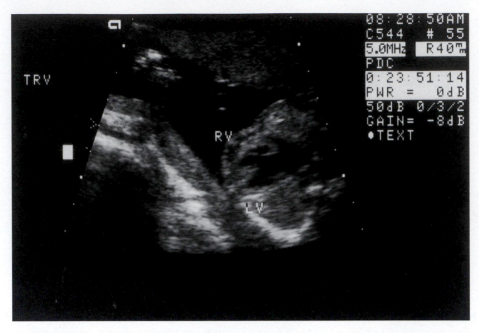

Figure 43-1. Prenatal sonographic image of a fetus with an atrioventricular canal defect. This fetus had heterotaxy syndrome. RV = right ventricle; LV = left ventricle.

increased frequency of bradyarrhythmias. In one series, 11 of 29 fetuses with AV canal defects also had complete heart block (Machado et al. 1988). In addition, all 11 of these fetuses also demonstrated features of the heterotaxy syndrome (Fig. 43-1) (see Chapter 49). Prenatal echocardiography should focus on the structure of the AV valve. The presence of a common leaflet at the level of the AV valve is suggestive of complete AV canal defect, while in its partial form the only abnormality may be a small defect in the inferior portion of the atrial septum (Romero et al. 1988).

Color and pulsed Doppler echocardiography may demonstrate turbulent systolic flow on the atrial side of the common AV valve because of significant valvular regurgitation (Fig. 43-2) (Barber and Chin 1990). The presence of significant valvular regurgitation can be quantified, and when present throughout systole, it may be predictive of hydrops fetalis (Gembruch et al. 1991). In contrast, valvular regurgitation confined to early systole is not associated with hydrops and may be an indicator of improved prognosis.

Prenatal sonography should also focus on excluding other abnormalities, such as malformations associated with aneuploidies or additional cardiac malformations. Sonographic markers associated with aneuploidy should be specifically sought, as approximately 50% of cases of AV canal defects have a chromosomal abnormality, the majority of which are due to trisomy 21 or 8p deletion (Machado et al. 1988). Additional cardiac malformations may be present in over 70% of cases, such as tetralogy of Fallot, coarctation, pulmonary stenosis, and double-outlet right ventricle (Machado et al. 1988). In

the Baltimore–Washington infant study, 336 children were identified with an endocardial cushion defect. Of these, 76% were identified as having a syndrome (78% of these had trisomy 21) (Carmi et al. 1992).

▶ DIFFERENTIAL DIAGNOSIS

The differential diagnosis for complete AV canal defects includes a large atrial or ventricular septal defect, or a single ventricle (Barber and Chin 1990). While complete AV canal defects can usually be easily distinguished from these lesions by prenatal echocardiography, differentiation from partial AV canal defects may be more problematic. Genetic considerations in the differential diagnosis include trisomy 21 (see Chapter 136) heterotaxy (Ivemark syndrome; see Chapter 49), Ellis–van Creveld sydrome (see Chapter 97). Holt–Oram syndrome, and CHARGE association.

▶ ANTENATAL NATURAL HISTORY

Few data are available on the antenatal natural history of isolated complete AV canal defects and none are available for partial forms of this condition. If chromosomal abnormalities are also present, the rate of intrauterine loss is significantly increased. The worst antenatal prognosis seems to be associated with complete forms of the AV canal defect, in which there is also significant regurgitation across the common AV valve. Such cases are mostly associated with hydrops fetalis

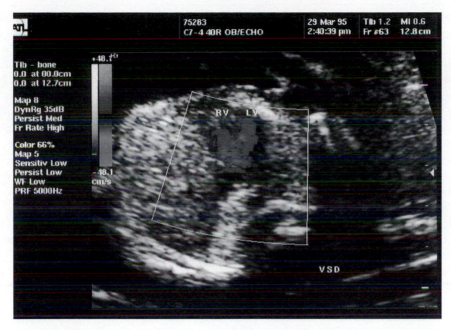

Figure 43-2. Color Doppler study in a fetus with AV canal defect, demonstrating turbulent flow and shunting within the heart. *(Photograph courtesy of Dr. Marjorie C. Treadwell.)* **See color plate.**

(Gembruch et al. 1991). The partial forms of the AV canal defect tend to present clinically after 1 month of postnatal life because volume overload does not occur until pulmonary vascular resistance has dropped significantly (Chin et al. 1982).

▶ MANAGEMENT OF PREGNANCY

If an AV canal defect is suspected on obstetric sonographic studies, a referral to a pediatric cardiologist or other specialist skilled in fetal echocardiography is recommended. Careful sonographic imaging for the presence of additional cardiac malformations is also recommended. Because of the strong correlation between AV canal defects and Down syndrome and the inability to detect Down syndrome with obstetric ultrasonography, all patients should be offered prenatal karyotype evaluation. Prenatal consultation with a pediatric cardiac team, (including cardiology, cardiothoracic surgery, and neonatology), may also be helpful for planning immediate neonatal intervention.

Early delivery is not recommended because a low birth weight carries a less favorable prognosis for neonatal cardiac surgery as compared with a higher birth weight. Delivery should take place under controlled circumstances at a tertiary-care center with an on-site pediatric cardiology team immediately available. The mode of delivery should be dictated by obstetric indications. However, the presence of hydrops may make vaginal delivery problematic because of soft-tissue dys-

tocia. Weighing the benefits of cesarean delivery to avoid dystocia against the very poor prognosis for infants with hydrops secondary to structural cardiac malformations may then constitute a dilemma.

▶ FETAL INTERVENTION

No fetal intervention has been described for prenatally diagnosed cases of AV canal defect.

▶ TREATMENT OF THE NEWBORN

Some infants with incomplete AV canal defect are detected during the newborn period but the majority are asymptomatic at birth. The presence of a complete AV canal defect usually results in symptoms at birth, such as a heart murmur. In other infants with complete AV canal, tachycardia, tachypnea, and failure to thrive develop during early infancy. The development of clinical symptoms prior to 3 months of age may be delayed because pulmonary vascular resistance remains high, which limits left-to-right shunting. If symptomatic presentation occurs prior to 3 months it is usually due to the presence of severe valvular regurgitation or additional cardiac malformations. Infants presenting with these symptoms need appropriate medical and surgical intervention to avoid the development of significant pulmonary hypertension. Left untreated, infants with complete AV canal defects have a 50% chance of survival beyond 6 months, and only a 30% chance of survival beyond 1 year (Berger et al. 1978).

Initial medical treatment of the newborn with a complete AV canal defect includes cardiorespiratory support and complete cardiac workup, including electrocardiography. The administration of digoxin to enhance myocardial contractility and diuretics to optimize preload is recommended (Barber and Chin 1990). Appropriate caloric supplementation is also recommended to make up for the high metabolic state associated with an intracardiac shunt and pulmonary edema. Two-dimensional echocardiography with pulsed and color Doppler studies should be performed soon after birth to confirm the cardiac malformation and to assess the morphology of the valve leaflets. With careful echocardiographic evaluation and optimal visualization of cardiac anatomy, cardiac catheterization and angiography may be avoided (Zellers et al. 1994).

▶ SURGICAL TREATMENT

Primary surgical repair of complete AV canal defect is usually performed electively between 3 and 6 months of age, or earlier if significant symptoms are present (Sand and Pacifico 1990). Delay beyond this time may expose the infant to significant risk for the development of pulmonary hypertension and eventually Eisenmenger syndrome. Correction of partial AV canal defects is performed electively during the first few years of life. Controversy exists regarding the role of pulmonary artery banding for temporary palliation for infants with complete AV canal defects and congestive heart failure, with some authors suggesting primary repair and others supporting the use of banding (Kirklin and Blackstone 1979; Silverman et al. 1983).

Primary repair of AV canal defects is facilitated by the establishment of cardiopulmonary bypass. Repair usually involves closure of the atrial septal defect with a patch of pericardium, closure of the interventricular defect with a Dacron patch, and attachment of the common AV valve leaflets to this patch. Care must be taken to avoid surgical injury to the AV node or bundle of His to prevent surgically induced complete heart block. The use of a double-patch technique may produce less distortion of the valve, although it may be possible to achieve similar results using a single patch and ventricular distention (Santos et al. 1986). The precise details of surgical repair, especially if additional cardiac malformations are present, are beyond the scope of this textbook but are easily available in the literature (Capouya and Laks 1991).

Poor prognostic factors for the surgical repair of AV canal defects include the presence of significant valvular regurgitation, poor overall functional capability, ventricular hypoplasia, presence of a ventricular septal defect, accessory valve orifice, or additional cardiac malformations (Studer et al. 1982). Mortality directly related to surgery is approximately 0.6% for partial and 2% for complete AV canal defects (Kirklin et al. 1986; Sand and Pacifico 1990). In another more recent series, overall operative mortality was 3.6% for complete AV canal defects (Tweddell et al. 1996). Higher operative mortality rates described in other series (up to 30%) may reflect different surgical techniques in earlier eras or the presence of additional complex cardiac malformations (Clapp et al. 1987).

▶ LONG-TERM OUTCOME

Long-term survival after surgical repair of AV canal defects is excellent. Almost 90% of survivors can be expected to be normally functioning at long-term follow-up, and survival at 12 years after surgery is approximately 85% (Sand and Pacifico 1990). Valve failure occurs in 10% of cases following repair, which may necessitate valve replacement.

Controversy exists about whether the presence of Down syndrome affects survival after surgical repair of AV canal defects. Caution is necessary in comparing outcomes following repair in infants with and without Down syndrome, as most infants with Down syndrome tend to have complete AV canal defects and an earlier tendency for pulmonary hypertension to develop as compared with chromosomally normal infants with AV canal defects. In one series comparing 47 cases of complete AV canal defects in chromosomally normal infants with 12 cases in infants with Down syndrome, there was a trend toward higher mortality in the Down syndrome group (Morris et al. 1992). However, in a larger series comparing 94 infants with Down syndrome with 127 chromosomally normal infants with AV canal defects, Down syndrome was not found to be an independent risk factor for adverse outcome, after controlling for disease severity (Rizzoli et al. 1992). In another series, infants with AV canal defects and Down syndrome did even better than chromosomally normal infants with AV canal defects (Vet and Ottenkamp 1989). In view of these findings, most pediatric cardiology centers do not treat infants with AV canal defects and Down syndrome any differently from the way they treat chromosomally normal infants.

▶ GENETICS AND RECURRENCE RISK

A strong correlation exists between the presence of AV canal defects and chromosomal abnormalities, particularly trisomy 21 and 8p deletion. If Down syndrome is also present, the recurrence risk is related more to the aneuploidy than to the structural cardiac defect. Familial clustering of isolated AV canal defects has also been described, which suggests the possibility of a single-gene defect. (Disegni et al. 1985; Tennant et al. 1984). The recurrence risk of AV canal defects in siblings of those affected ranges from 1.5 to 8.7% (Sanchez-Cascos 1978). In general, with one affected child, we quote a recurrence risk of 3%, and with two affected children we quote a recurrence risk of 10% (Nora and Nora 1988). The recurrence risk in offspring of chromosomally normal parents with AV canal defects is approximately 10% (Emanuel et al. 1983). This risk is higher when the mother has an AV canal defect as compared with the father being affected.

In a large study of 103 individuals with isolated AV canal defect, Digilio et al. (1993) found 4 of 111 siblings to be similarly affected (3.6%), 4 of 206 parents affected (1.9%), and 5 of 644 uncles and aunts affected (0.8%). None of the grandparents were affected. Prenatal diagnosis in a subsequent pregnancy is by fetal echocardigraphy.

REFERENCES

Barber G, Chin AJ. Volume loads except TAPVD. In: Long WA, ed. Fetal and neonatal cardiology. Philadelphia: Saunders, 1990:452–464.

Becker AE, Anderson RH. Pathology of congenital heart disease. London: Butterworths 1981.

Berger TJ, Blackstone EH, Kirklin JW, et al. Survival and probability of cure without and with operation in complete atrioventricular canal. Ann Thorac Surg 1978;27: 104–111.

Capouya ER, Laks H. Atrioventricular canal defects. Ann Thorac Surg 1991;51:860–863.

Carmi R, Boughman JA, Ferencz C. Endocardial cushion defect: further studies of "isolated" versus "syndromic" occurrence. Am J Med Genet 1992;43:569–575.

Chin AJ, Keane JF, Norwood WI. Repair of complete atrioventricular canal in infancy. J Thorac Cardiovasc Surg 1982;84:437–445.

Clapp SK, Perry BL, Farooki ZQ, et al. Surgical and medical results of complete atrioventricular canal: a ten year review. Am J Cardiol 1987;59:454–458.

Digilio MC, Marino B, Cicini MP, Giannotti A, Formigari R, Dallapiccola B. Risk of congenital heart defects in relatives of patients with atrioventricular canal. Am J Dis Child 1993;147:1295–1297.

Disegni E, Pierpont ME, Bass JL. Two-dimensional echocardiography in detection of endocardial cushion defect in families. Am J Cardiol 1985;55:1649–1652.

Emanuel R, Somerville J, Inns A, et al. Evidence of congenital heart disease in the offspring of parents with atrioventricular defects. Br Heart J 1983;49:144–147.

Ferencz C, Rubin JD, McCarter RJ, et al. Congenital heart disease: prevalence of live birth: the Baltimore-Washington infant study. Am J Epidemiol 1985;121: 31–36.

Fyler DC, Buckley LP, Hellenbrand W, et al. Report of the New England Regional infant cardiac program. Pediatrics 1980;65(suppl):375.

Fontana RS, Edwards JE. Congenital cardiac disease. a review of 357 cases studied pathologically. Philadelphia: Saunders, 1962.

Gembruch U, Knopfle G, Chatterjee M, et al. Prenatal diagnosis of atrioventricular canal malformations with up-to-date echocardiographic technology: report of 14 cases. Am Heart J 1991;121:1489–1497.

Kirklin JW, Blackstone EH. Management of the infant with complete atrioventricular canal. J Thorac Cardiovasc Surg 1979;78:32–34.

Kirklin JW, Blackstone EH, Bargeron LM, et al. The repair of AV canal defects in infancy. Int J Cardiol 1986;13: 333–360.

Machado MV, Crawford DC, Anderson RH, et al. Atrioventricular septal defect in prenatal life. Br Heart J 1988; 59:352–355.

Morris CD, Magilke D, Reller M: Down's syndrome affects results of surgical correction of complete atrioventricular canal. Pediatr Cardiol 1992;13:80–84.

Nora JJ, Nora AH. Update on counseling the family with a first-degree relative with a congenital heart defect. Am J Med Genet 1988;29:137–142.

Rastelli GC, Kirklin JW, Titus JL. Anatomic observations on complete form of persistent common atrioventricular canal with special reference to atrioventricular valves. Mayo Clin Proc 1966;41:296–308.

Rizzoli G, Mazzucco A, Maizza F, et al. Does Down syndrome affect prognosis of surgically managed atrioventricular canal defects? J Thorac Cardiovasc Surg 1992;104:945–953.

Romero R, Pilu G, Jeanty P, et al. Atrioventricular septal defects. In: Romero R, Pilu G, Jeanty P, Ghidini A, Hobbins JC, eds. Prenatal diagnosis of congenital anomalies. East Norwalk, CT: Appleton & Lange, 1988:144–147.

Rowe RW, Freedom RM, Mehrizi A, et al. The neonate with congenital heart disease. In: Rowe RW, Freedom RM, Mehrizi A, Bloom KR, eds. The neonate with congenital heart disease. Philadelphia: Saunders, 1981:373–396.

Sanchez-Cascos A. The recurrence risk in congenital heart disease. Eur J Cardiol 1978;7:197–210.

Sand ME, Pacifico AD. Repair of atrioventricular septal defects. In: Long WA, ed. Fetal and neonatal cardiology. Philadelphia: Saunders, 1990:780–788.

Santos A, Boucek M, Ruttenberg H, et al. Repair of atrioventricular septal defects in infancy. J Thorac Cardiovasc Surg 1986;91:505–510.

Silverman N, Levitsky S, Fisher E, et al. Efficacy of pulmonary banding in infants with complete AV canal. Circulation 1983;68(suppl 2):148–153.

Studer M, Blackstone EH, Kirklin JW, et al. Determinants of early and late results of repair of atrioventricular septal (canal) defects. J Thorac Cardiovasc Surg 1982;84:523–542.

Tennant SN, Hammon JW, Bender HW, et al. Familial clustering of atrioventricular canal defects. Am Heart J 1984; 108:175–177.

Twed
enc
fect
Vet T\
defe
Chil

A complete fetal survey should be performed, with special attention paid to the presence or absence of hydrops, indicated by pericardial or pleural effusions, ascites, or anasarca. Echocardiographic assessment should include measurement of ventricular escape rate and atrial rate. An atrial rate of less than 120 beats per minute (bpm) should raise the possibility of a missed structural heart defect. In addition, assessment of stroke volume, left ventricular ejection fraction, combined ventricular output, and the presence, or absence, of AV valvular insufficiency should be noted (Takomiya et al. 1989; Veille et al. 1990). Valvular insufficiency can be diagnosed by Doppler echocardiography. Peak systolic flow velocities in the ascending aorta and diastolic umbilical flow velocities should be assessed as indirect indicators of cardiac output, and should be measured as a basis for comparison with future echocardiograms.

Doppler ultrasound assessment of the umbilical artery has been used to estimate impedance to flow in the placental circulation. However, because calculations depend on the time taken for the velocity of flow to decay in diastole, the prolonged diastolic component in CHB limits the value of this technique (Olah et al. 1991, 1993). Complete absence or reversal of flow during diastole in CHB, however, has the same clinical significance as in cases in which the heart rate is normal (Olah et al. 1991). This form of sonographic assessment is thought to be particularly useful in CHB because of its association with anti-Ro antibodies and antibodies in connective-tissue disease, such as systemic lupus erythematosus, in which placental infarction and immunoglobulin deposition are frequently encountered (Guzman et al. 1987; Veille et al. 1990). Increases in placental resistance may be sufficient to precipitate cardiac decompensation, although no further slowing in the ventricular escape rate occurs.

Growth restriction may occur as a result of fetal CHB. Therefore, serial measurements of biparietal diameter and long bones should be performed at bimonthly intervals to assess fetal growth.

Measurement of the cardiothoracic ratio should also be performed by two-dimensional echocardiography as part of routine assessment (Palodini et al. 1990). An increase in the cardiothoracic index from the normal range may assist in predicting the extent of lung compression and possible pulmonary hypoplasia, as well as the severity of cardiac failure indicated by cardiac enlargement (Olah et al. 1993).

▶ DIFFERENTIAL DIAGNOSIS

When presented with a fetus with bradycardia, the differential diagnosis consists of heart block as a complication of structural heart disease, heart block in a struc-

▶ **TABLE 44-1.** STRUCTURAL HEART DEFECTS MOST COMMONLY ASSOCIATED WITH FETAL COMPLETE HEART BLOCK

Left atrial isomerism
Transposition of the great arteries
Atrioventricular septal defect
Pulmonic atresia
Anomalous pulmonary venous connection
Double-outlet right ventricle
Atrioventricular discordance
Absent right atrioventricular connection
Double-inlet ventricle
Right atrial isomerism
Pulmonic stenosis

turally normal heart (most often due to transplacental passage of maternal antibodies in connective tissue disease), and sinus bradycardia in a premorbid fetus. The most common structural defects seen in association with CHB are listed in Table 44-1. Although pregnant women with connective-tissue disease are at significantly increased risk of having a fetus with CHB, only 50% of fetuses with bradycardia are born to women with a history of collagen vascular disease (McCauliffe 1995; Petri et al. 1989). A fetus presenting with CHB may be the first manifestation of maternal collagen vascular disease.

A fetus diagnosed early in the development of heart block may present with irregular heart rhythm due to second-degree AV block. This may occur either as partial progressive AV block, the Wenckebach phenomenon, or as second-degree AV block in which the P–R interval is relatively fixed and the ratio of transmission may be 2:1, 3:1, 4:1, etc. Schmidt et al. (1991) have observed progression from normal sinus rhythm to second-degree block to CHB. Echocardiographic assessment is essential to diagnose fetal bradyarrhythmias accurately.

▶ ANTENATAL NATURAL HISTORY

While bradycardia is well tolerated by most fetuses, non-immune hydrops will develop in up to 25% as a result of cardiac decompensation (Carpenter et al. 1986; Crowley et al. 1985; Holzgreve et al. 1984; Kleinman et al. 1982; Machado et al. 1988; Stewart et al. 1983). In 90% of the cases associated with structurally normal hearts, the infant is born with neonatal lupus erythematosus (McCauliffe 1995; see "Treatment of the Newborn" which follows).

Fetal CHB usually presents during the second trimester in structurally normal hearts that have completed development. Although fetal CHB has been diagnosed as early as 17 weeks, it has a mean presentation at 26 weeks of gestation (Schmidt et al. 1991). There is some evidence to suggest that a progressive rise in transplacental passage of immunoglobulin occurs after 22 weeks of gestation, which correlates with progressive immune-mediated injury to the fetal conduction system (Stiehm 1975).

The first case of CHB in a fetus was reported in 1945 by Plante and Stevens. It was not long after this that McCuistion et al. (1954) suggested that transplacental passage of some factor present in maternal serum was responsible. An association between fetal CHB and maternal collagen vascular disease was similarly recognized some decades ago (Hagg 1957). Many years later, the association was made between fetal CHB and specific maternal antibodies circulating in numerous maternal collagen vascular diseases (Gross et al. 1989; McCreadie et al. 1990; Scott et al. 1983; Taylor et al. 1988; Watson et al. 1984; Weston et al. 1982). Antibodies to soluble ribonuclear proteins, anti-Ro (Sjögren syndrome antigen-A, SS-A) and anti-La (Sjögren syndrome antigen-B, SS-B) have been demonstrated in the serum of affected fetuses and their mothers (Franco et al. 1981; Kephart et al. 1981; Miyagowa et al. 1981). CHB in fetuses with structurally normal hearts is almost uniformly associated with the presence of anti-Ro or anti-La antibodies.

Anti-Ro and anti-La antibodies have been demonstrated to bind to fetal heart conduction tissue (Deng et al. 1987; Harsfield et al. 1991). The pathophysiology of CHB involves the transplacental passage of maternal autoantibody, anti-Ro, which binds to an antigen in the fetal heart conduction system with consequent inflammation and fibrosis. The fetal and neonatal heart contains the body's highest concentration of Ro antigen (Deng et al. 1987; Harley et al. 1985; Wolin et al. 1984). IgG deposits have been demonstrated in the cardiac tissues of affected infants (Litsey et al. 1985; Lee et al. 1987). Studies in vitro, using anti-Ro and anti-La antibodies, have demonstrated that anti-Ro antibodies selectively bind to newborn myocardium but not to adult myocardium and that this binding inhibits repolarization (Alexander et al. 1992).

Although it is thought that anti-Ro and anti-La antibodies play an important role in the pathogenesis of fetal CHB, some authors have suggested that there must be a cofactor (Taylor et al. 1988). The mothers of infants with CHB almost always have anti-Ro and anti-La antibodies. However, the majority of mothers with these antibodies have normal pregnancies, suggesting that a second factor is necessary for the development of CHB. It has been suggested that viral infections may initiate immune damage by influencing antigenic expression. Ro and La ribonucleoproteins may become immunogenic by forming complexes with viral genomes (Venables et al. 1983). Interestingly, an increased frequency of antibodies to cytomegalovirus has been observed in mothers of babies with CHB (Peckham et al. 1983; Taylor et al. 1988).

The majority of the fetuses with CHB tolerate the slower ventricular rate relatively well and progress to term without incident. But in 15 to 25% of fetuses with CHB nonimmune hydrops will develop and the fetus will die in utero or shortly after delivery. In a multicenter review, Schmidt et al. (1991) found that fetuses with structurally normal hearts and CHB had only a 14% survival rate, with ventricular heart rates of less than 55 bpm. We have seen no survivors with ventricular rates less than 50. The presence of nonimmune hydrops was a poor prognostic feature, with only a 15% survival rate. Similarly, when CHB complicated structural heart disease, the survival was only 14%. The development of AV valve incompetence is also a harbinger of fetal cardiac decompensation and nonimmune hydrops (Schmidt et al. 1991). AV valve incompetence appears to be due to distortion at the valve rings by progressive ventricular dilation at the slow ventricular rate. In the fetal-sheep model of CHB, slower ventricular rates cause progressive diastolic distention of the ventricles distorting the AV valve rings, resulting in regurgitation (Crombleholme et al. 1991). The AV valve incompetence can be immediately reversed by increasing the ventricular rate by a pacemaker, which reduces the diastolic ventricular distention. AV valve incompetence tends to precede the development of nonimmune hydrops because it results in venous hypertension and passive hepatic congestion, leading to pericardial and pleural effusions, ascites, and anasarca.

In addition to progressive destruction of the fetal conduction system by an inflammatory response to maternal autoantibody deposition, a generalized myocarditis may also be seen in fetal CHB. In these cases, antibody deposition occurs throughout the heart, and inflammatory reaction results in progressive myocardial decompensation. Subendocardial fibroelastosis may result, which can be an indicator of end-stage myocardial injury. These may appear as echogenic papillary muscles or areas of subendocardial myocardium.

▶ MANAGEMENT OF PREGNANCY

A woman with no previous history of collagen vascular disease who presents carrying a fetus with CHB should have a formal rheumatologic evaluation. On close questioning, these women often report dry eyes/mouth or arthralgia, which suggest collagen vascular disease (McCauliffe 1995). Although in most fetuses CHB is well tolerated, there is an increased incidence of obstetrical problems in mothers who have anti-Ro antibodies. The fetus should undergo a complete anatomic sonographic survey, including Doppler waveform studies of umbilical arterial diastolic flow. Echocardiography should be performed, not only to exclude structural heart disease, but to confirm AV dissociation and document the atrial and ventricular rates. In addition, assessment of ventricular contractility, presence or absence of increased myocardial echogenicity suggestive of subendocardial fibroblastosis, AV valve incompetence, and stroke volume should be noted and serve as a baseline for comparison with future studies. During the third trimester there may be progressive slowing of ventricular rate, and increased frequency of surveillance is indicated in fetuses with ventricular rates of less than 65 bpm. Heart rates less than 60 bpm should prompt twice-weekly ultrasound examinations to detect AV valve incompetence or early signs of nonimmune hydrops. Similarly, serial echocardiography is indicated to detect subtle changes in contractility, stroke volume, myocardial echogenicity, and onset of AV valve incompetence. Diastolic flow in the umbilical arteries is also a useful marker to follow because it indicates impedance to flow in the placental circulation. Increased resistance due to deposition of immune complexes in the placental bed may precipitate heart failure. Because of the progressive dilation of heart chambers, cardiothoracic ratios are indicators of possible pulmonary hypoplasia. Because of the lack of heart-rate variability, standard nonstress tests are not helpful, but the atrial rate does remain under autonomic control and can be assessed for validity.

The indications for delivery in fetal CHB include obvious signs of deteriorating cardiac status, with the subsequent development of nonimmune hydrops. The mode of delivery in fetal CHB is controversial. If the fetus is being delivered for signs of cardiac decompensation, the stress of vaginal delivery may cause further hemodynamic compromise (Palodini et al. 1990). In addition, detection of fetal distress in fetal CHB is very difficult. Some authors have delivered noncompromised fetuses with CHB vaginally, using continuous heart-rate monitoring and fetal blood sampling during labor (Olah et al. 1993). Some authors have advocated continuous monitoring of ventricular rate by scalp electrodes, atrial rate by external transducers, or fetal pulse oximetry by scalp probes or transcutaneous pCO_2 (Chan et al. 1990a, 1990b; Todras et al. 1989). Other authors have suggested continuous intrapartum echocardiography.

We recommend cesarean delivery for any fetus at more than 30 weeks of gestation with CHB and evidence of hemodynamic compromise, manifested by nonimmune hydrops, a ventricular rate of less than 55 bpm, AV valve insufficiency, or poor contractility. In fetuses in which CHB is well tolerated, vaginal delivery may be considered, but only if appropriate intrapartum monitoring is available. Delivery should be performed at a center with pediatric cardiologists and surgeons who are available for placement of either temporary transvenous or epicardial pacing leads.

▶ FETAL INTERVENTION

Numerous antenatal treatments, both medical and surgical, have been proposed in the management of the fetus with CHB. The medical therapies are divided into those intended to minimize the immunologic injury to the fetal heart and those geared toward increasing the ventricular rate.

The form of treatment used most often is administration of steroids to the mother to limit the fetal inflammatory response (Barclay et al. 1987; Bunyan et al. 1987; Fox and Hawkins 1990). Higher steroid levels are achieved in the fetus; therefore, dexamethasone is preferred over prednisone. Because of the fear of adverse side effects due to steroids, such as maternal diabetes, lowered resistance to infection, and poor wound healing, some authors have recommended against prophylactic treatment for anti-Ro antibody–positive mothers. However, once antibody-mediated damage to the fetal conduction system has occurred, it is permanent.

The use of intravenous γ-globulin in fetal CHB has been described. Intravenous γ-globulin is thought to bind circulating anti-Ro antibody in the maternal circulation to prevent transplacental passage, by increasing immune clearance of the antibody. It may also downregulate anti-Ro antibody production.

Plasmapheresis has also been recommended, to limit cardiac damage once pericardial effusion, heart enlargement, or conduction disturbance develops (Bunyan et al. 1987), but plasmapheresis cannot reverse fetal CHB once it is established (Heurman et al. 1985). Bunyan et al. (1988) have suggested that plasmapheresis be used prior to 20 weeks of gestation, before increased antibody passage occurs across the placenta. This requires plasmapheresis three times a week, in addition to steroid treatment. The use of plasmapheresis is based on the idea of removing maternal anti-Ro antibody and decreasing transplacental passage, but damage to the fetal conduction system is not reversed using this regimen. None of these immunologic strategies has any proven efficacy in preventing or reversing the consequences of fetal CHB due to anti-Ro antibodies.

Another approach to the medical management of fetal CHB has been to pharmacologically increase the fetal heart rate using maternal β-mimetic agents, such as terbutaline. Ritodrine and isoproterenol have also been used in attempts to accelerate the fetal heart rate (Carpenter et al. 1986; Martin et al. 1988; Schmidt et al. 1991). The responses to these agents have been variable, and no definite benefit has been proven (Crowley et al. 1985; Carpenter et al. 1986; Machado et al. 1988). In addition, doses sufficient to cause any increase in fetal ventricular rate are often poorly tolerated by the mother. Early cesarean delivery for temporary pacemaker placement has been associated with a mortality rate that approaches 80% (Kleinman et al. 1985; Martin et al. 1988).

The lack of effective medical treatment for the fetus with CHB and evidence of cardiac decompensation has prompted some groups to attempt pacing the fetal heart in utero. Carpenter et al. (1986) reported the first attempt at percutaneous ultrasound-guided transthoracic fetal heart pacing. In this case, the 22-week-old fetus was severely hydropic, and although the pacing wire was able to capture and pace the fetal heart, the fetus died within 3 hours. In an animal model of fetal CHB, Crombleholme et al. established the technique for pacemaker placement and in utero pacing to save the fetus from hydrops (Crombleholme et al. 1987, 1990, 1991). Based on this experimental work, Harrison and colleagues performed open fetal surgery for the placement of an epicardial pacing lead and insertion of a telemetrically programmable pulse generator. As in Carpenter's case, this fetus was severely hydropic, and although capture and pacing of the heart were achieved, the fetus died intraoperatively (Harrison et al. 1995).

In order for fetal cardiac pacing to be effective, appropriate case selection is essential. Fetuses without hydrops do not need cardiac pacing. Fetuses with advanced hydrops are unlikely to benefit from cardiac pacing. However, a fetus with CHB with ventricular escape rates of less than 55 bpm is at especially high risk. These fetuses should be followed closely for development of early signs of hydrops, such as pericardial or pleural effusion or AV valve insufficiency, which usually precedes hydrops. These fetuses are high risk, but still good candidates for fetal cardiac pacemaker placement. We favor open fetal surgery for fetal CHB, because a percutaneously placed pacing lead may become dislodged, causing cardiac tamponade, chorioamnionitis, or cord enlargement. The contraindications to open fetal surgery for pacemaker placement include uterine irritability, maternal illness, structural fetal heart disease, massive hydrops, or poor ventricular function associated with subendocardial fibroelastosis. We recommend that steroids be administered to the pregnant woman for all fetuses with CHB to minimize ongoing immune-mediated myocardial cardiac injury. The injury to the fetal conduction system is permanent and irreversible, but progressive myocarditis may be averted by maternal steroid treatment. Except for one anecdotal case, there are no data to support the use of plasmaphere-sis in fetal CHB. Similarly, β-mimetic agents may show a minor increase in fetal ventricular rate, but not enough to be clinically significant.

▶ TREATMENT OF THE NEWBORN

Neonatal lupus erythematosus (NLE) is a misnomer, as these newborns do not have systemic lupus erythematosus, but a constellation of clinical disorders associated with, and probably in part caused by, autoantibodies that are passively acquired by the fetus transplacentally (McCauliffe 1995). The majority of newborns with NLE exhibit cutaneous or cardiac disease, among other symptoms (Table 44-2).

In the absence of structural heart disease, the newborn with congenital CHB has NLE, which is associated with a distinctive skin rash of erythematous round eruptions due to antibody disposition on basal keratinocytes (McCauliffe 1995). This rash may be increased by light exposure, especially phototherapy for hyperbilirubinemia. Parents are advised to keep affected infants out of direct sunlight for the first 6 months of life, after which the NLE resolves. In addition to cardiac and dermatologic manifestations, NLE may present with thrombocytopenia or anemia, as well as hepatosplenomegaly, hepatitis or cholestasis, aseptic meningitis, myopathy, or myasthenia (McCauliffe 1995).

In the delivery room, an isoproterenol drip should be initiated as soon as intravenous access is secure. Steroids should be administered to prevent ongoing myocardial injury. Some neonatologists have performed exchange transfusions to eliminate circulating maternal antibody, but no data are available to evaluate its use. Cardiac pacing is the definitive treatment. If the child is unstable or delivered for cardiac decompensation, a transvenous or transthoracic temporary pacing lead should be placed. This may not be possible in a premature infant, in whom a left anterior thoracotomy for placement of temporary epicardial pacing leads should be performed until the infant is sufficiently large to undergo permanent placement of a cardiac pacemaker. If the fetus is hydropic, delivered for cardiac decompensation, or has a ventricular rate less than 55 bpm, some form of cardiac pacemaker should be placed urgently.

▶ **TABLE 44-2.** CLINICAL MANIFESTATIONS OF NEONATAL LUPUS ERYTHEMATOSUS

System	Description	Presentation
Cutaneous	Erythematous round, oval, and annular patches	Weeks to months after delivery. Resolves after 6 months, occasional residual pigmentation
Cardiac	Complete heart block, myocarditis, congestive heart failure	Usually third trimester, but as early as 17 weeks, invisible heart block
Hematologic	Thrombocytopenia, anemia, leukopenia	At birth, usually self-limited
Hepatic	Hepatomegaly, hepatitis, cholestasis	At birth, usually self-limited

The degree of heart block is permanent and if the heart is decompensating, medical therapy such as isoproterenol is unlikely to prevent progressive deterioration.

▶ LONG-TERM OUTCOME

The mortality rate for infants presenting in the newborn nursery with CHB is 25%. In a long-term follow-up study Vetter and Rashkind (1983) documented 90% survival after the neonatal period. Most deaths were due to pacemaker failure. These children need to be followed for the later development of rheumatologic disease. McCauliffe (1995) described seven patients with congenital CHB who went on to develop collagen vascular diseases, either systemic lupus erythematosus or Sjögren syndrome. Whether this is due to NLE is unknown. More likely, this represents familial predisposition or inheritance of an HLA type associated with collagen vascular disease.

▶ GENETICS AND RECURRENCE RISK

There is no known genetic predisposition for the development of fetal CHB. The woman who has previously had a fetus with neonatal lupus erythematosus is at greatest risk for recurrence. The manifestations of NLE tend to be the same in subsequent pregnancies. Petri et al. (1989) found that mothers of infants with NLE manifested by CHB had a 64% chance of a subsequent fetus being similarly affected. However, McCune et al. (1987) found only a 25% recurrence of CHB.

Women with a history of an autoimmune disorder and anti-Ro antibodies constitute the next highest risk category. Ramsey-Goldman et al. (1986) found that only 7.6% of infants born to mothers with SLE who had anti-Ro antibodies were affected by NLE. Among mothers with SLE but no anti-Ro antibodies, the incidence of NLE was only 0.6%. Normal women, or those with ill-defined symptoms who produce anti-Ro antibodies, are probably at even lower risk. Unfortunately, this latter category accounts for 50% of cases of NLE, which are impossible to identify before the fetus or newborn is symptomatic (McCauliffe 1995; Petri et al. 1989).

Olah et al. have defined four known risk factors: a previous child with CHB, a high titer of anti-Ro antibody (>1:16), presence of anti-La antibody in addition to anti-Ro antibody, and maternal HLA-DR3 (Olah et al. 1993).

REFERENCES

Alexander E, Beryan JP, Rovost TT, et al. Anti-Ro/SS-A antigens in the pathophysiology of congenital heart block in neonatal lupus syndrome, an experimental model. Arthritis Rheum 1992;35:176–189.

Allan LD, Anderson RH, Sullivan ID, et al. Evolution of fetal arrhythmias by echocardiography. Br Heart J 1983;50:240–245.

Allan LD, Crawford DC, Anderson RH, et al. Echocardiographic and anatomic correlates in fetal congenital heart disease. Br Heart J 1984a;52:542–548.

Barclay CS, French MAH, Ross LD, et al. Successful pregnancy following steroid therapy and plasma exchange in a woman with anti-Ro (SS-A) antibodies: case report. Br J Obstet Gynaecol 1987;94:369–371.

Bunyan JP, Rowley R, Swersky SH, et al. Complete congenital heart block: risk of occurrence and therapeutic approach to prevention. J Rheumatol 1988;15:1104–1108.

Bunyan JP, Swersky SH, Fox HE, et al. Intrauterine therapy for presumptive fetal myocarditis with acquired heart block due to systemic lupus erythematosus. Arthritis Rheum 1987;30:44–49.

Cameron AD, Walker JJ, Nimrod CA. Diagnosis and management of fetal cardiac dysrhythmia. Contemp Rev Obstet Gynaecol 1989;1:195–199.

Camm AJ, Bexton RS. Congenital CHB. Eur Heart J 1984;5(suppl A):115–117.

Carpenter RJ, Strasburger JF, Gorson A Jr., et al. Fetal ventricular pacing for hydrops secondary to complete AV block. J Am Coll Cardiol 1986;8:1434–1436.

Chan FY, Ghash A, Tang M, et al. Simultaneous pulsed Doppler velocimetry of fetal aorta and inferior vena cava: diagnosis of fetal congenital heart block: two case reports. Eur J Obstet Gynecol Reprod Biol 1990a;35:89–95.

Chan FY, Woo SK, Ghosh A, et al. Prenatal diagnosis of congenital fetal arrhythmias by simultaneous pulsed Doppler velocimetry of the fetal abdominal aorta and inferior vena cava. Obstet Gynecol 1990b;76:200–204.

Crawford D, Chapman M, Allan LD. The assessment of persistent bradycardia in prenatal life. Br J Obstet Gynaecol 1985;92:941–944.

Crombleholme TM, Harrison ML, Longaker MT, et al. CHB in fetal lambs. I. Technique and acute physiologic response. J Pediatr Surg 1990;25:587–593.

Crombleholme TM, Longaker MT, Langer JC, et al. CHB and AV-sequential pacing in fetal lambs: the atrial contribution to combined ventricular output in the fetus. Surg Forum 1989;40:268–270.

Crombleholme TM, Shiraishi H, Adzick NS, Langberg J, et al. A model of nonimmune hydrops on fetal lambs: CHB-induced hydrops fetalis. Surg Forum 1991;42:487–489.

Crowley DC, Dick M, Rayburn WF, et al. Two-dimensional M-mode echocardiographic evaluation of fetal arryhthmias. Clin Cardiol 1983;51:237–243.

Crowley DC, Dick M, Rayburn WF, et al. Two-dimensional and M-mode echocardiographic evaluation of fetal arryhthmias. Clin Cardiol 1985;8:1–6.

Deng JS, Blair LW Jr., Shen-Schwarz S, et al. Localization of Ro (SS-A) antigen in the cardiac conduction system. Arthritis Rheum 1987;30:1232–1238.

Devore GR, Siassi B, Platt LD. Fetal echocardiography. III. M-mode ultrasound. Am J Obstet Gynecol 1983;146:792–799.

Fox R, Hawkins DF. Fetal pericardial effusion in association with congenital heart block and maternal systemic lupus erythematosus: case report. Br J Obstet Gynaecol 1990; 97:636–640.

Franco HL, Weston WL, Peeble C, et al. Autoantibodies directed against sicca syndrome antigens in the neonatal lupus syndrome. J Am Assoc Dermatol 1981;4:67–72.

Gochberg SH. Congenital heart block. Am J Obstet Gynecol 1984;88:238–241.

Gross KR, Petty RE, Lum VL, et al. Maternal autoantibodies and fetal disease. Clin Exp Rheumatol 1989;7:651–657.

Guzman L, Avilos E, Ortiz R, et al. Placental abnormalities in systemic lupus erythamatosus: in-situ deposition of antinuclear antibodies. J Rheumatol 1987;14:924–929.

Hagg GR. Congenital, acute lupus erythematosus associated with subendocardial fibroblastomas. Am J Clin Pathol 1957;28:648–654.

Harley JB, Kaine JL, Fox OF, et al. Ro (SS-A) antibody and antigen in a patient with congenital CHB. Arthritis Rheum 1985;28:1321–1325.

Harrison MR: Fetal surgery. Western J Med 1993;159:341–349.

Harsfield AC, Venables PJ, Taylor PV, et al. Ro and La antigens and maternal anti-La idiotypes on the surface of myocardial fibers in congenital heart block. J Radiol 1991; 4:165–176.

Heurman E, Golezewski N. Maternal connective tissue disease and congenital heart block. N Engl J Med 1985; 312–329.

Holzgreve W, Curry CJR, Golbus MS, et al. Investigation of non–immune hydrops fetalis. Am J Obstet Gynecol 1984; 150:805–812.

Kephart DC, Hood AF, Provost T. Neonatal lupus erythematosus: new serologic finding. J Invest Dermatol 1981; 77:331–333.

Kleinman CS, Downerstein RL. Ultrasonic assessment of cardiac function in the intact human fetus. J Am Coll Cardiol 1985;7(suppl):843–845.

Kleinman CS, Downerstein RL, Devore GR, et al. Fetal echocardiography for the evaluation of fetal CHF. N Engl J Med 1982;306:568–575.

Kleinman CS, Evans MI. International Fetal Medicine and Surgery Society Fetal Cardiac Registry 1988.

Kleinman CS, Hobbins JC, Joffe CC, et al. Echocardiographic studies of the human fetus: prenatal diagnosis of congenital heart disease and cardiac dysrrhythmias. Pediatrics 1980;65:1059–1066.

Lee LA, Coulter S, Erver S, et al. Cardiac immunoglobulin deposition in congenital heart block associated with maternal anti-Ro autoantibodies. Am J Med 1987;83:793–796.

Litsey SE, Noonan JA, O'Connor WN, et al. Maternal connective tissue disease and congenital heart block: demonstration of immunoglobulin in cardiac tissue. N Engl J Med 1985;312:98–100.

Machado MVL, Tynan MJ, Curry PVL, et al. Fetal CHB. Br Heart J 1988;60:512–515.

Martin TC, Anios F, Olander DS, et al. Successful management of congenital AV block associated with hydrops fetalis. J Pediatr 1988;112:984–986.

McCauliffe DP. Neonatal lupus erythematosus: a transplacentally acquired autoimmune disorder. Semin Dermatol 1995;14:47–53.

McCreadie M, Celermajor J, Sholler G, et al. A case control study of congenital heart block: association to maternal antibodies to Ro (SS-A) and La (SS-B). Br J Rheumatol 1990;29:10–14.

McCue CM, Montakas ME, Tinglstod JB, et al. Congenital heart block in newborns of mothers with connective tissue disease. Circulation 1977;56:82–90.

McCuistion CH, Schoch EP. Possible discoid lupus erythematosus in a newborn infant. Arch Dermatol 1954;70: 782–785.

McCune AB, Weston WL, Lee LA. Maternal and fetal outcome in neonatal lupus erythematosus. Ann Intern Med 1987;106:518–523.

McHenry MM, Coyler GG. Congenital CHB in newborns, infants, children, and adults. Med Times 1969;97:113–123.

Michaelson M, Engle MA. Congenital CHB: an international study of the natural history. Pediatr Cardiol 1972;4: 87–101.

Miyagowa S, Katomura W, Yashiaka J, et al. Placental transfer of anti-cytoplasmic antibodies in annular erythema of newborns. Arch Dermatol 1981;717:569–572.

Olah KSJ, Brown JS, Gee H. Monitoring the fetus with congenital heart block—the use of the first-interval resistance index. J Perinatol Med 1991;19(suppl s):211.

Olah KSJ, Gee H. Antibody medicated complete congenital heart block in the fetus. PACE 1993;16:1872–1879.

Palodini D, Chit SK, Allan LD. Prenatal measurement of cardiothoracic ration in evaluation of heart disease. Arch Dis Child 1990;65:20–23.

Peckham CS, Chin KS, Coleman JC, et al. Cytomegalovirus infection in pregnancy: preliminary findings from a prospective study. Lancet 1983;1:1352–1355.

Petri M, Watson R, Hochberg MC. Anti-Ro antibodies and neonatal lupus. Rheum Dis Clin North Am 1989;15: 335–360.

Plante RK, Stevens RA. Complete AV block in a fetus: Case reports. Am Heart J 1945;30:615–618.

Ramsey-Goldman R, Ham D, Deng J, et al. Anti-SS-A antibodies and fetal outcome in maternal systemic lupus erythematosus. Arthritis Rheum 1986;29:1269–1273.

Schmidt KG, Ulmer HF, Silverman NH, et al. Perinatal outcome of fetal complete AV block: a multi-center experience. J Am Coll Cardiol 1991;17:1360–1366.

Scott JS, Maddison PJ, Taylor PV, et al. Connective tissue disease, antibodies to ribonucleoprotein and congenital heart block. N Engl J Med 1983;309:209–212.

Shenker L. Fetal cardiac arryhthmias. Obstet Gynecol Surv 1979;34:561–572.

Stewart PA, Tango HM, Wlodimiroff JW, et al. Arrhythmia and structural abnormalities of the fetal heart. Br Heart J 1983;50:550–554.

Stiehm EF. Fetal defense mechanisms. Am J Dis Child 1975; 129:438–443.

Takomiya O, Hata T, Kitao M. Fetal Doppler echocardiographic assessment of cardiac blood flow velocity in normal fetuses and those with congenital heart disease. Nippon Sanka Fujinka Gokkai Zasshi 1989;41:211–216.

Taylor PV, Scott JS, Gerlis LM, et al. Maternal antibodies against fetal cardiac antigens in congenital CHB. N Eng J Med 1988;315:667–672.

Teteris MJ, Chisholm JW, Ullery JC. Antenatal diagnosis of

congenital heart block: report of a case. Obstet Gynecol 1979;32:851–853.

Todras T, Proslitero P, Gaglioti P, et al. Conservative management of fetal beginning arrhythmia leading to persistent bradycardia. Eur J Obstet Gynecol Reprod Biol 1989; 34:211–215.

Veille JC, Sivakoff M, Nemeth M: Evaluation of the human fetal cardiac size and function. Am J Perinatol 1990;7: 54–59.

Venables PJW, Smith PR, Maini RN. Purification and characterization of the Sjögren's syndrome A and B antigens. Clin Exp Immunol 1983;54:731–738.

Vetter VL, Rashkind H. CHB and connective tissue disease. N Engl J Med 1983;309:236–238.

Watson RM, Lane AT, Barnett NK et al. Neonatal lupus erythematosus. Medicine (Baltimore) 1984;63:362–378.

Weston WL, Harmon C, Peeble C, et al. A serologic marker for lupus erythematosus. Br J Dermatol 1982;107: 377–382.

Wolin S, Steitz JA. The Ro small cytoplasmic ribonucleoproteins: identification of the antigenic protein and its binding site on the Ro RNAs. Proc Natl Acad Sci USA 1984; 81:1966–2000.

CHAPTER 45

Cardiomyopathy

► CONDITION

Cardiomyopathy refers to cardiac hypertrophy manifested by an increased interventricular septal size and/or free ventricular wall size in the absence of an increased cardiac load, accompanied by decreased cardiac function and by ventricular dilation (Michels et al. 1992). More broadly, cardiomyopathy is defined as a disease of the myocardium characterized by the presence of systolic or diastolic dysfunction or abnormal myocardial structure (Schwartz et al. 1996). The condition is rarely observed during fetal life.

Although a small subset of patients with the inherited form of hypertrophic cardiomyopathy present clinically during fetal life, fetuses with cardiomyopathy are more likely to have a broad spectrum of underlying pathophysiology. The traditional classification of cardiomyopathy as dilated or hypertrophic is helpful in deciding management strategies. In the fetus, dilated cardiomyopathy is more common than hypertrophic cardiomyopathy; causes for dilated cardiomyopathy include infectious disease, dysrhythmias, and carnitine deficiency. The most common cause of fetal hypertrophic cardiomyopathy is maternal diabetes.

► INCIDENCE

The incidence of hypertrophic cardiomyopathy is reportedly as high as 1 in 5000 adults (Watkins et al. 1995b). The incidence of adults with dilated cardiomyopathy in the United States and Europe is on the order of 2 to 8 cases per 100,000 individuals (Kelly and Strauss 1994). On the other hand, the diagnosis of fetal cardiomyopathy is extremely rare. In one retrospective review of 625 fetal echocardiograms, only 6 (1%) had evidence of dilated cardiomyopathy (Schmidt et al. 1989).

► SONOGRAPHIC FINDINGS

Relatively few reports of the prenatal diagnosis of fetal cardiomyopathy exist. These reports describe the diagnosis of fetal cardiomyopathy in one of three situations: a fetus that is the offspring of a diabetic mother, the fetus at risk for familial hypertrophic cardiomyopathy, and the fetus affected by a genetic syndrome that includes cardiomyopathy as one manifestation.

The heart in the offspring of the diabetic mother was described by Gutgesell et al. (1980), who studied 47 infants of diabetic mothers by echocardiography. In this study, 24 of the infants were clinically symptomatic. Five of these had marked septal hypertrophy with echocardiographic features that suggested left ventricular outflow obstruction. Five infants had hypertrophy of the right ventricular free wall. One symptomatic infant died from an unrelated bacterial infection. In the clinically asymptomatic infants, three were shown to have septal hypertrophy, two had right ventricular free wall hypertrophy and no patients had left ventricular outflow obstruction. None of the patients in the entire study had evidence of dilated or congestive cardiomyopathy, and all patients had resolution of their echocardiographic abnormalities during the first 6 months of life. This was the first report to suggest the use of echocardiography to follow cardiac changes occurring in infants of diabetic mothers. These alterations were shown to be due to an increased mass of myocardial nuclei and sarcoplasm in the hearts of infants of diabetic mothers, but they were self-limited.

Subsequently, fetuses in mothers who had well-controlled type I insulin-dependent diabetes were studied at 4-week intervals between 20 and 30 weeks of gestation by M-mode and Doppler echocardiographic studies (Rizzo et al. 1992). These investigators measured intraventricular septal thickness, left and right ventricular wall thickness, and the ratio between the peak velocities during the early passive ventricular filling and active atrial filling at the level of the atrioventricular valves. They also studied peak velocities and time to peak velocity at the level of the ascending aorta and pulmonary artery. The findings in the 14 fetuses of diabetic mothers were compared with those in 10 normal control fetuses. This study revealed that all indexes investigated increased linearly with advancing gestation. The fetuses in the diabetic mothers showed an accelerated increase in cardiac size occurring during the late second trimester, manifested by progressive thickening of the intraventricular septum and ventricular walls. These investigators demonstrated that strict control of maternal diabetes did not prevent the accelerated fetal cardiac growth and abnormal development of cardiac function, which was mainly manifested by impaired diastolic function (Rizzo et al. 1992). The study was followed by a related report that compared fetal echocardiographic indexes in fetuses of mothers with well-controlled insulin-dependent diabetes to normal fetuses during the second and third trimester (Gandhi et al. 1995). An increase in right ventricular shortening fraction was associated with global cardiac enlargement, which did not adversely affect myocardial contractility. These authors hypothesized that metabolically stable maternal diabetes may be associated with a mild but definite myocardial hypertrophy that affects the growth of the ventricular and septal walls (Gandhi et al. 1995). The echocardiographic changes associated with maternal diabetes are not, strictly speaking, a cardiomyopathy, but rather a self-limited cardiac hypertrophy. Only in extremely rare cases does the maternal diabetes result in systolic or diastolic cardiac dysfunction, progressing to congenital heart failure.

Although familial hypertrophic cardiomyopathy does not usually manifest with clinical symptoms until adolescence or early adulthood, at least one case of prenatal hypertrophic apical cardiomyopathy has been documented (Stewart et al. 1986). On the other hand, it is unclear how often prenatal diagnosis has been used for this condition, given that many young adults who have hypertrophic cardiomyopathy are unaware of it. Adult patients who are clinically symptomatic may not desire pregnancy or parenting. In one report, a 25-year-old primigravida was described with hypertrophic apical cardiomyopathy whose fetus had normal echocardiographic examinations at 19 and 21 weeks of gestation. At 27 weeks of gestation, two-dimensional and M-mode echocardiograms revealed a generalized fetal cardiac hypertrophy with a markedly thickened intraventricular septum. This was confirmed at 32 and 36 weeks of gestation but did not worsen throughout the rest of the pregnancy. The patient was studied postnatally and followed to age 15 months, when stable cardiac hypertrophy was observed (Stewart et al. 1986).

Genetic syndromes, such as Noonan syndrome, can present with hypertrophic cardiomyopathy. In a case report, a fetus with cystic hygroma and a normal karyotype, diagnosed postnatally with Noonan syndrome, was referred for fetal echocardiography at 23 weeks of gestation. A small primum atrial septal defect, increased echogenicity of the mitral valve, and modest hypertrophy of both ventricles were observed (Sonesson et al. 1992). In the same fetus, observed serially at 35 weeks of gestation, prominent hypertrophy of both ventricles was demonstrated. Retrospectively, these authors noted that the first sign of myocardial abnormality was observed in the diastolic filling of both ventricles. However, this may be a subtle finding, as all fetuses have abnormal diastolic filling boundaries as compared with infants.

In general, dilated cardiomyopathy is the more common presentation during fetal life. In a retrospective review of six cases of fetal dilated cardiomyopathy, Schmidt et al. (1989) made a sonographic diagnosis by numerous approaches, including the four-chamber, long-axis, short-axis, and aortic-arch views. Prenatal sonographic imaging was complemented by M-mode echocardiography for better definition of the motion patterns of the atrioventricular and semilunar valves (Schmidt et al. 1989). This group defined the right and left ventricular fractional shortening index (FS) as:

$$FS = (EDD - ESD) \times 100/EDD,$$

where EDD = the end-diastolic diameter of the ventricle and ESD = the end-systolic diameter of the ventricle. These investigators demonstrated that in five of the affected fetuses, the right ventricular fractional shortening index was less than 2 SD below the normal mean for gestational age, and in four, the left ventricular fractional shortening index was less than 2 SD below the normal mean. In addition, they observed significantly larger mean end-diastolic diameters. In affected fetuses, the fractional shortening decreased progressively during gestation while the chamber enlargement increased (Schmidt et al. 1989).

▶ DIFFERENTIAL DIAGNOSIS

The most important consideration in the differential diagnosis is to determine whether the cardiomyopathy is dilated or hypertrophic (Table 45-1). In dilated cardiomyopathy, the ventricle is thin-walled and dilated; mitral and or tricuspid regurgitation is also present (Figs. 45-1 and 45-2). The important potentially treatable conditions to be ruled out include dysrhythmias, infection, carnitine deficiency, and severe anemia (usually accompanied by hydrops fetalis). Viruses potentially involved in fetal cardiomyopathy include group B Coxsackie, echovirus, rubella, and herpes (Boston et al.

▶ **TABLE 45-1.** DIFFERENTIAL DIAGNOSIS OF FETAL CARDIOMYOPATHY

Dilated (more common)
Dysrhythmias
Infection
Carnitine deficiency
Severe anemia (with hydrops)
Familial
Hypertrophic
Maternal Diabetes
Inborn Errors of Metabolism
Noonan syndrome
Familial
Twin-Twin Transfusion

1994). Carnitine deficiency, although not directly diagnosable prenatally, should be considered, because postnatal treatment exists. Dilated cardiomyopathy is an important cause of adult morbidity and mortality, and it represents the leading indication for cardiac transplantation (Krajinovic et al. 1995). Familial transmission has been documented in a minimum of 20 to 25% of cases of dilated cardiomyopathy (Michels et al. 1992). In a review of six cases of fetal dilated cardiomyopathy, three had a positive family history for the condition (Schmidt et al. 1989).

As mentioned above, maternal diabetes is the most common reason for fetal hypertrophic cardiomyopathy. Occasionally, hypertrophic cardiomyopathy can be seen

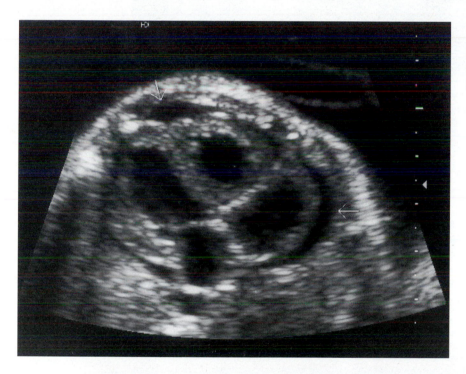

Figure 45-1. Antenatal four-chamber view of a fetal heart, demonstrating dilation of all four chambers. Arrows indicate the presence of a pericardial effusion.

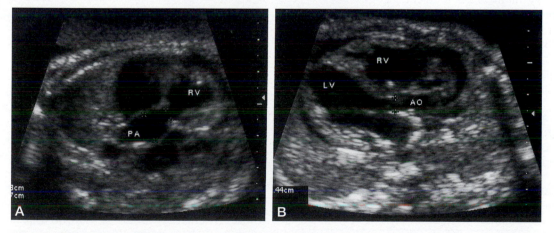

Figure 45-2. (A) Antenatal sonographic image of same fetus shown in Figure 45-1, demonstrating significant dilation of the pulmonary outflow tract. (B) Corresponding view of the left ventricular outflow tract, also showing dilation.

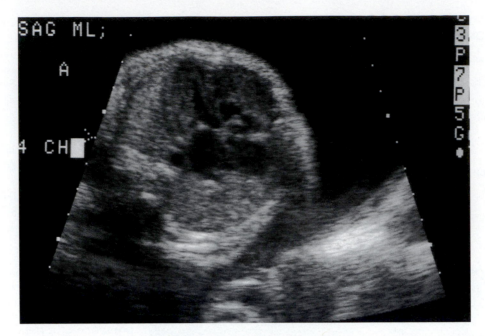

Figure 45-3. Antenatal four-chamber view of a fetal heart, demonstrating marked biventricular hypertrophy in a recipient of twin–twin transfusion.

▶ **TABLE 45-2.** METABOLIC CAUSES OF CARDIOMYOPATHY IN INFANCY

Storage Disorders
Glycogen storage disease, type II (Pompe disease)
Lysosomal glycogenosis without acid maltase deficiency
Glycogen storage disease, type III
Cardiac glycogenosis
GM1-gangliosidosis (-galactosidase deficiency)
GM2-gangliosidosis (Sandhoff disease)
Ethanolaminosis
Familial steatosis
Inborn Errors of Fatty Acid Oxidation
Carnitine transport defect
Carnitine-acyl carnitine translocase defect
Carnitine palmitoyltransferase II defect
Long- and medium-chain acyl coenzyme A (COA) dehydrogenase deficiencies
Long-chain 3-hydroxyacyl-coA dehydrogenase deficiency
Inborn Errors of Mitochondrial Oxidative Phosphorylation
Lethal infantile cardiomyopathy
Benign infantile mitochondrial myopathy and cardiomyopathy
Maternally inherited myopathy and cardiomyopathy
Inherited cardiomyopathy with multiple deletions of mitochondrial DNA
Myoclonic epilepsy and ragged red fiber disease (MERRF)
Mitochondrial myopathy, encephalopathy, lactic acidosis, and stroke-like episodes (MELAS)
Kearns-Sayre syndrome

Modified from Kohlschütter and Hausdorf 1986 and Kelly and Strauss 1994

in the recipient of a twin–twin transfusion (Fig. 45-3). Inborn errors of metabolism associated with infantile cardiomyopathy are listed in Table 45-2. These include storage disorders, such as Pompe disease (glycogen storage disease, type II). This autosomal recessive condition results in symmetric massive hypertrophy of individual muscle fibers due to infiltration with glycogen. Pompe disease is diagnosed histochemically by the presence of vacuolar myopathy with positive periodic acid–Schiff (PAS) staining and fiber reactivity for acid phosphatase. Frozen sections of liver reveal the absence of lysosomal acid α-glucosidase (Cottrill et al. 1987). For the sake of completeness, inborn errors of enzymes or transport proteins involved in mitochondrial β-oxidation of fatty acids are included in Table 45-2. Disorders of fatty acid oxidation are among the most common metabolic diseases known, with an incidence of 1 in 10,000 to 1 in 15,000 live births (Kelly and Strauss 1994). However, they generally become apparent only during a fasting episode associated with infection and are unlikely to be recognized during fetal life.

Single-gene disorders associated with hypertrophic cardiomyopathy include neurofibromatosis, Friedreich ataxia, LEOPARD syndrome (lentigines, echocardiographic abnormalities, ocular hypertelorism, pulmonary stenosis, abnormal genitalia, retardation of growth, deafness), and Noonan syndrome (Schwartz et al. 1996). Of these, Noonan syndrome is the only one that has been described during fetal life (Battiste et al. 1977; Sonesson et al. 1992).

Familial hypertrophic cardiomyopathy is character-ized clinically by myocardial hypertrophy, variation in the onset and severity of clinical symptoms, and an annual sudden-death rate of 2 to 4% (Jarcho et al. 1989). It is the most common cause of unexpected sudden death in apparently healthy young adults (Watkins et al. 1995b). Autopsy studies performed on patients who die from familial hypertrophic cardiomyopathy reveal pathognomonic myocyte and myofibrillar disarray (Jarcho et al. 1989; Watkins et al. 1995b). Familial hyper-trophic cardiomyopathy rarely presents during fetal life.

▶ ANTENATAL NATURAL HISTORY

Relatively little is known about the antenatal natural history of fetal cardiomyopathy. It is likely that more will be learned when fetuses are initially diagnosed by molecular analysis as carrying one of the inherited mutations for the condition. Subsequently, these fetuses can be studied by prenatal sonography to study clinical correlations. In a retrospective analysis of 625 women who underwent fetal echocardiography between the years of 1980 and 1987, 6 cases of dilated cardiomyopathy were identified. All had structurally normal hearts. Three of the 6 fetuses were referred for a positive family history of cardiomyopathy in siblings. Two of these fetuses had had initially normal echocardiographic examinations at 20 weeks of gestation. One fetus was noted to have reduced right ventricular function at 34 weeks of gestation and ultimately required heart transplantation at 5 months of age. The other fetus died at 1 week postpartum and on autopsy was found to have endocardial fibroelastosis of the left ventricle. A third fetus at risk for familial dilated cardiomyopathy was shown to have tricuspid regurgitation at 26 weeks of gestation. This progressed to right ventricular hypertrophy and severely reduced right ventricular function; this ultimately resulted in hydrops fetalis and death at 4 days of age. Hydrops fetalis manifested in 4 of the fetuses, and they were found to have reduced biventricular function on echocardiography. The overall prognosis was poor for this group of fetuses. Only 2 of the 6 fetuses survived; 1 of these infants survived with a heart transplant at 5 months of age.

▶ MANAGEMENT OF PREGNANCY

Fetuses in which cardiomyopathy is suspected should be referred to a center capable of performing fetal echocardiography to rule out structural heart disease. Ideally, this center should be able to serially monitor the fetal cardiac function, including repeated measurement of the ventricular fractional shortening index and

cardiac chambers, and rule out dysrhythmias such as supraventricular tachycardia and atrial flutter. It is important to rule out dysrhythmias, because they are treatable. If a high index of suspicion exists for an arrhythmia, 24-hour monitoring of the pregnant patient and fetus in the hospital is recommended. A targeted fetal sonographic study should be performed to identify any additional anomalies that could help in the diagnosis of a specific genetic syndrome. An attempt should be made to identify whether the mother has evidence of diabetes or infection.

It is important to obtain a complete family history, with specific questions directed toward sudden death in family members. Consideration should be given to performing echocardiography on both parents.

▶ FETAL INTERVENTION

If a dysrhythmia is diagnosed, medical treatment is indicated (see Chapters 44 and 54).

▶ TREATMENT OF THE NEWBORN

Infants born after a fetal diagnosis of cardiomyopathy need to be delivered in a center capable of newborn resuscitation and aggressive cardiac management. Symptomatic infants may have respiratory distress and require mechanical ventilation with oxygen administration. A chest x-ray film should be obtained to demonstrate cardiomegaly. An electrocardiogram should also be obtained. Infants with cardiomyopathy may have left ventricular hypertrophy with or without strain. If the electrocardiogram demonstrates giant QRS complexes in all leads with a shortened P–R interval, glycogen storage disorders may be considered (Kohlschütter and Hausdorf 1986). A complete physical examination is indicated. Additional anomalies or a dysmorphic facies may suggest a particular genetic disorder. If inborn errors of metabolism are suspected, observe the infant for evidence of enlargement of the liver, spleen, or tongue, with clinical evidence of seizures, skeletal changes, or corneal opacities. Workup should also include measurement of carnitine and acylcarnitine levels, as supplementation with carnitine will result in clinical improvement if a deficiency exists.

Further treatment for infants with dilated cardiomyopathy consists of administration of diuretics, and digoxin and afterload reduction if pulmonary edema develops. Hypertrophic cardiomyopathy is treated with calcium-channel blockers and β-blockers to relax the heart. It is our experience that infants of mothers with diabetes almost never require treatment, even when their hypertrophic cardiomyopathy is severe.

▶ SURGICAL TREATMENT

The only surgical treatment for severe dilated cardio-myopathy is heart transplantation. Specific surgical treatment of an underlying structural heart lesion is discussed in Chapters 42, 43, 46–48, 50–52, and 55–57.

▶ LONG-TERM OUTCOME

The natural history for 20 infants identified with cardiomyopathy during the first year of life has been described (Maron et al. 1982). Fourteen of the infants presented with a murmur that suggested evidence of outflow obstruction. For all these infants, the initial diagnosis was a suspected congenital cardiac malformation. Twelve of the 14 infants who presented with a murmur underwent cardiac catherization, which demonstrated substantial left and right ventricular outflow-tract obstruction, asymmetric hypertrophy of the ventricular septum relative to the left ventricular free wall, and a thickened interventricular septum. This study indicated that the onset of pulmonary edema during the first year of life was an unfavorable prognostic sign, as 9 of the affected 11 infants died. Several patients were treated with propranolol to decrease left ventricular outflow-tract obstruction, but the authors expressed caution regarding the negative inotropic effect on ventricular contractility, and recommended administration of diuretics as a conservative and safe regimen.

In Maron et al.'s report (1982), 6 of the 20 infants were documented to have a family history of dilated cardiomyopathy as demonstrated by at least one of the parents' having echocardiographic evidence of asymmetric septal hypertrophy. Although this report is almost two decades old, it does emphasize that the familial and genetic contribution is probably greater than was originally appreciated.

In another report, the clinical course of 63 consecutive infants and children who presented with idiopathic dilated cardiomyopathy was described (Burch et al. 1994). The age at diagnosis was 1 day to 15 years (median, 12 months), with follow-up occurring through 1 day to 13 years of life (median, 19 months). The survival of this group from clinical presentation onward was 79% at 1 year after diagnosis and 61% at 5 years after diagnosis. Predictors of adverse outcome in this group included the presence of a mural thrombus, a left ventricular end-diastolic pressure of greater than 20 mm Hg, and an age at presentation of greater than 2 years. In 36 of the 63 patients, left ventricular echocardiography showed a decline or no improvement. Of these 36, 17 died, and 3 required cardiac transplantation. In 16 of 63 patients, partial improvement was noted; 3 patients in this group died. In the group whose left ventricular function returned to normal (11 of 63),

all patients survived. These authors concluded that with no documentation of improvement in left ventricular echocardiographic dimensions or function, a poor prognosis exists, and these infants or children should be considered for cardiac transplantation.

▶ GENETICS AND RECURRENCE RISK

The majority of the metabolic causes of cardiomyopathy in infancy described in Table 45-2 are autosomal recessive conditions with a 25% recurrence risk. If a syndrome is diagnosed, the recurrence risk is that of the specific syndrome.

The genetics of isolated cardiomyopathy are increasingly being explained at the molecular level. Familial dilated cardiomyopathy has been described variously as a recessively inherited and X-linked (Berko and Swift 1987) condition, but in the majority of families, the disease is inherited as an autosomal dominant disorder with age-related penetrance (Krajinovic et al. 1995). Much progress has ensued recently regarding the understanding of the molecular basis of the hypertrophic cardiomyopathies. Approximately 50% of familial hypertrophic cardiomyopathies are due to mutations occurring in genes on chromosomes 1, 14, and 15, although other disease loci are known at chromosomes 11p13-q13, 7q3, and 9q13-q22 (Krajinovic et al. 1995; Watkins et al. 1995b). Approximately 30% of cases of familial hypertrophic cardiomyopathy and some sporadic cases are due to missense mutations in the cardiac β-myosin heavy-chain gene on chromosome 14q11. All these mutations are single-nucleotide substitutions that result in a change of a single amino acid in the globular head or the head–rod junction of the myosin heavy-chain molecule. These mutations are not null alleles. They act as dominant-negative alleles, which means that they result in the production of an alternative molecule that impairs cross-bridge cycling and interferes with the assembly of the sarcomere (Watkins et al. 1995a). Approximately 15% of cases are due to mutations occurring in the cardiac troponin T gene on chromosome 1q3. These mutations are associated with a poor prognosis and a high incidence of sudden death before age 35 years (Watkins et al. 1995a). Approximately 3% of cases of familial hypertrophic cardiomyopathy are due to mutations in the α-tropomyosin gene on chromosome 15q2. All these loci are important in specifying genes for a sarcomeric contractile protein.

Because of the substantial progress being made in the molecular mapping of genes that affect families with hypertrophic cardiomyopathy, presymptomatic diagnosis is now possible. The case history has been reported of a 24-year-old man diagnosed with a cardiac β-myosin heavy-chain gene mutation following identification of his affected sister. At the time of his diagnosis, his partner was expecting a child. He asked for DNA testing on his daughter shortly after her birth. She was diagnosed as carrying the same mutation. An ethical debate ensued as to the wisdom of identifying a healthy newborn infant as a carrier of this gene mutation (Ryan et al. 1995). The parents very strongly wanted this information so that they would be able to redirect the child's lifestyle to avoid energetic activities and to ensure regular medical and cardiac surveillance. Physicians argued against this diagnosis because of the future stigmatization of the child with regard to employment, life insurance, and loans. In addition, the question has been raised as to whether the presence of the mutation is equivalent to having clinical evidence of the disease. For this condition, the presence of the responsible gene is necessary but not sufficient for the development of clinical symptoms of cardiomyopathy. Clinical and ethical debate continues regarding the advisability of presymptomatic molecular diagnosis for this condition (Davis 1995).

REFERENCES

Battiste CE, Feldt RH, Lie JT. Congestive cardiomyopathy in Noonan's syndrome. Mayo Clin Proc 1977;52:661–664.

Berko BA, Swift M. X-linked dilated cardiomyopathy. N Engl J Med 1987;316:1186–1191.

Boston BA, DeGroff C, Hanna CE, Reller M. Reversible cardiomyopathy in an infant with unrecognized congenital adrenal hyperplasia. J Pediatr 1994;124:936–938.

Burch M, Siddiqi SA, Celemajer DS, Scott C, Bull C, Deanfield JE. Dilated cardiomyopathy in children: determinants of outcome. Br Heart J 1994;72:246–250.

Cottrill CM, Johnson GL, Noonan JA. Parental genetic contribution to mode of presentation in Pompe disease. Pediatrics 1987;79:379–381.

Davis J. Genetic testing for familial hypertrophic cardiomyopathy in newborn infants: ethical issues. BMJ 1995;310:858.

Gandhi JA, Zhang XY, Maidman JE. Fetal cardiac hypertrophy and cardiac function in diabetic pregnancies. Am J Obstet Gynecol 1995;173:1132–1136.

Gutgesell HP, Speer ME, Rosenberg HS. Characterization of the cardiomyopathy in infants of diabetic mothers. Circulation 1980;61:441–450.

Jarcho JA, McKenna W, Pare P, et al. Mapping a gene for familial hypertrophic cardiomyopathy to chromosome 14q1. N Engl J Med 1989;321:1372–1378.

Kelly DP, Strauss AW. Inherited cardiomyopathies. N Engl J Med 1994;330:913–919.

Kohlschütter A, Hausdorf G. Primary (genetic) cardiomyopathy in infancy. Pediatrics 1986;145:454–459.

Krajinovic M, Pinamonti B, Sinagra G, et al. Linkage of familial dilated cardiomyopathy to chromosome 9. Am J Hum Genet 1995;57:846–852.

Maron BJ, Tajik AJ, Ruttenberg HD, et al. Hypertrophic cardiomyopathy in infants: clinical features and natural history. Circulation 1982;65:7–17.

Michels VV, Moll PP, Miller FA, et al. The frequency of familial dilated cardiomyopathy in a series of patients with idiopathic dilated cardiomyopathy. N Engl J Med 1992;326:77–82.

Rizzo G, Arduini D, Romanini C. Accelerated cardiac growth and abnormal cardiac flow in fetuses of type I diabetic mothers. Obstet Gynecol 1992;80:369–376.

Ryan MP, French J, Al-Mahdawi S, Nihoyannopoulos P, Cleland JGF, Oakley CM. Genetic testing for familial hypertrophic cardiomyopathy in newborn infants. BMJ 1995;310:856–859.

Schmidt KG, Birk E, Silverman NH, Scagnelli SA. Echocardiographic evaluation of dilated cardiomyopathy in human fetus. Am J Cardiol 1989;63:599–605.

Schwartz ML, Cox GF, Lin AE, et al. Clinical approach to genetic cardiomyopathy in children. Circulation 1996;94:2021–2038.

Sonesson S-E, Fouron JC, Lessard M. Intrauterine diagnosis and evolution of a cardiomyopathy in a fetus with Noonan's syndrome. Acta Paediatr 1992;81:368–370.

Stewart PA, Buis-Liem T, Verwey RA, Wladimiroff JW. Prenatal ultrasonic diagnosis of familial asymmetric septal hypertrophy. Prenat Diagn 1986;6:249–256.

Watkins H, McKenna WJ, Thierfelder L, et al. Mutations in the genes for cardiac troponin T and alpha tropomyosin in hypertrophic cardiomyopathy. N Engl J Med 1995a;332:1058–1064.

Watkins H, Seidman JG, Seidman CE. Familial hypertrophic cardiomyopathy: a genetic model of cardiac hypertrophy. Hum Mol Genet 1995b;4:1721–1727.

CHAPTER 46

Coarctation of the Aorta

► CONDITION

Coarctation of the aorta refers to narrowing of a segment of the aorta along the aortic arch, usually near the origin of the ductus arteriosus (Fig. 46-1). The narrowed segment of the aorta can be of any length and can be preductal, juxtaductal, or postductal in location. The area of narrowing can be caused by a discrete soft-tissue shelf, or can be due to hypoplasia of a segment of the arch, leading to complete aortic-arch interruption. Previously, coarctation was divided into infantile and adult forms. The infantile form classically occurred in a preductal location, was associated with other cardiac malformations, and was more likely to be associated with neonatal congestive heart failure. The adult form classically occurred in juxtaductal or postductal locations and was associated with a better prognosis. This distinction now seems to be imprecise and is of little relevance, with both forms of coarctation presenting at various ages.

The pathogenesis of coarctation is unclear. It may be due to a developmental defect of the aortic arch,

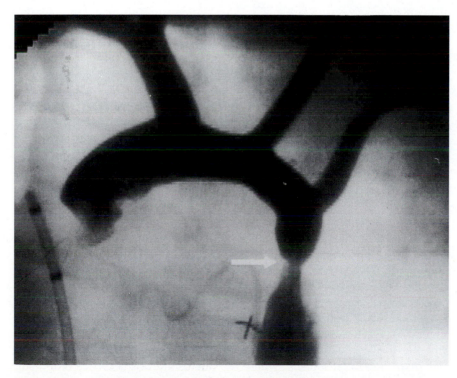

Figure 46-1. Postnatal ascending aortogram in a 6 month old infant. Arrow indicates site of severe coarctation of the aorta. *(Photograph courtesy of Dr. Ziyad Hijazi.)*

possibly because of failure of connection of the fourth and sixth bronchial arches to the descending aorta. Another possible mechanism is the development of abnormal blood flow patterns in utero, leading to decreased aortic-arch flow and increased flow in the pulmonary artery and ductus arteriosus. The consequence of this imbalance in flow may be the development of relative hypoplasia of the aortic arch. A third possible mechanism for the pathogenesis of coarctation is the presence of aberrant ductal tissue in the arch, leading to narrowing of the aortic arch after closure of the ductus (Whitley and Perry 1990).

Associated cardiac malformations are present in up to 90% of cases of coarctation, including bicuspid aortic valve, aortic stenosis or insufficiency, septal defects, transposition of the great vessels, double-outlet right ventricle, postnatal patent ductus arteriosus, and truncus arteriosus (Romero et al. 1988). Additional noncardiac malformations are present in 13% of cases (Campbell and Polani 1961). A strong association exists between Turner syndrome and coarctation, with 10% of Turner syndrome patients being affected (see Chapter 135).

▶ INCIDENCE

Coarctation of the aorta is present in 0.2 in 1000 live births (Ferencz et al. 1985). While there is a significant male preponderance for coarctation in the entire population, there appears to be an equal incidence in both genders at birth. Coarctation accounts for up to 8% of all cases of congenital heart disease.

▶ SONOGRAPHIC FINDINGS

Prenatal diagnosis of coarctation of the aorta using ultrasound examination is controversial. Some believe that it cannot be reliably diagnosed prenatally because in most cases the hemodynamic complications depend on closure of the ductus. Although it is true that coarctation of the aorta can be entirely a postnatal event, several series of prenatally diagnosed cases of coarctation have been documented (Allan et al. 1988; Sharland et al. 1994). An increased nuchal translucency measurement may be an early marker for aortic coarctation (Moselhi and Thilaganathan 1996).

Pathologic examination of fetuses with increased nuchal translucency thickness has demonstrated a high prevalence of cardiac defects and abnormalities of the great arteries. This has been shown in both trisomic and chromosomally normal fetuses (Hyett et al. 1995, 1996). In fetuses with trisomy 21, the aortic valve and ascending aorta are wider than in normal fetuses, while the aortic isthmus is narrower. In chromosomally normal fetuses the aorta is narrowed at both the level of the isthmus and immediately above the aortic valve.

Later in gestation, prenatal visualization of a shelf or discrete area of narrowing in the aortic arch is extremely difficult. However, if there is complete hypoplasia or arch interruption, Doppler evaluation may demonstrate a disturbance of flow. Prestenotic or poststenotic dilation of the aortic arch may also be present. Growth curves for the transverse aortic arch at various gestational ages have been published, with the suggestion that cases of coarctation are associated with measurements at or below the third percentile (Hornberger et al. 1992). However, no data are available on the reliability or sensitivity of these techniques for the prenatal diagnosis of coarctation.

Relative enlargement of the right ventricle and pulmonary artery, when compared with the left ventricle and aorta, may be more easily detectable signs consistent with coarctation. In one series of prenatally diagnosed dilation of the right ventricle and pulmonary artery, 18 of 24 fetuses had coarctation (Allan et al. 1988). Doppler visualization of reduced aortic blood flow was present in most cases of coarctation, but was also present in some normal fetuses. Discrepancy in the size of the ventricles, caused by relative hypoplasia of the left heart structures, has a poor positive predictive value for coarctation, with the false positive rate being higher after 34 weeks of gestation (Brown et al. 1997). Overall, 62% of cases of coarctation may have ventricular discrepancy recognizable on fetal echocardiograms. The higher false positive rate at later gestational ages may be due to the normal relative increase in right heart size as gestation advances (Sharland and Allan 1992). At present, no prenatal sonographic signs—taken either individually or in combination—can reliably distinguish true cases of coarctation from false positive results (Sharland et al. 1994).

▶ DIFFERENTIAL DIAGNOSIS

The main differential diagnosis for isolated coarctation of the aorta diagnosed prenatally is pulmonic stenosis, which may also present with a dilated right ventricle. However, in cases of pulmonic stenosis the pulmonary artery is small or hypoplastic as compared with the typically pulmonary arterial dilation seen with coarctation. Other cardiac malformations commonly coexist with coarctation, so their presence cannot exclude coarctation.

▶ ANTENATAL NATURAL HISTORY

The antenatal course of fetuses with coarctation of the aorta is usually benign, since the presence of an open ductus arteriosus carries blood supply from the heart to the aorta. However, in cases of severe coarctation or arch hypoplasia, progressive dilation of the right ventricle may result in right ventricular hypertrophy. The antenatal course may also be influenced by the presence of additional cardiac and noncardiac malformations, which frequently coexist with coarctation. As pregnancy advances, it is possible that isolated coarctation initially caused by a discrete shelf in early gestation may progress into complete arch hypoplasia (Allan et al. 1984). The prognosis for an individual fetus may therefore change as pregnancy progresses and the arch abnormality evolves. Congestive heart failure may occur early during the newborn period following closure of the ductus, especially in infants with an intact ventricular septum.

▶ MANAGEMENT OF PREGNANCY

If the diagnosis of coarctation is suspected on obstetric ultrasound evaluation, fetal echocardiography should be performed by an appropriately trained specialist to confirm the diagnosis and to evaluate for the presence of additional cardiac malformations. In addition, careful sonographic evaluation should be performed for other noncardiac abnormalities, such as diaphragmatic hernia or sonographic signs of Turner or DiGeorge syndrome. Because of the significant association with chromosomal abnormalities, karyotype evaluation should be offered, including fluorescence in situ hybridization analysis for chromosome 22 deletions. Pediatric cardiology and neonatology consultations should also be arranged to facilitate neonatal treatment.

Serial ultrasound evaluation during pregnancy is recommended because the appearance and severity of the coarctation may change as pregnancy advances. Progressive obstruction will be evidenced by increasing right ventricular dilation with hypertrophy and possibly congestive cardiac failure. It is rare for coarctation to require early delivery, as the presence of an open ductus during intrauterine life usually delays significant hemodynamic disturbances until after birth. Because there is no absolute indication for cesarean delivery with coarctation, the mode of delivery should be dictated by standard obstetric circumstances. Delivery should occur at a tertiary-care center, with the immediate availability of a pediatric cardiologist.

▶ FETAL INTERVENTION

No fetal intervention has been described for isolated coarctation of the aorta.

▶ TREATMENT OF NEWBORN

Immediate neonatal resuscitation is essential in the management of significant aortic coarctation. Medical stability depends on the presence of continued patency of the ductus arteriosus with a right-to-left shunt supporting systemic perfusion. Because hyperventilation and supplemental oxygen therapy reduce pulmonary vascular resistance, these interventions may reduce the right-to-left shunt, thereby reducing systemic perfusion. Supplemental oxygen therapy should therefore be avoided unless absolutely necessary and, when used, should be limited to 40 to 60% maximum fractional inspired oxygen (FiO_2).

Prostaglandin E_1 infusion should be started to maintain patency of the ductus in severe cases of aortic coarctation. This will improve perfusion of the lower body, increase urinary output, and improve metabolic acidosis (Whitley and Perry 1990). Prostaglandin E_1 infusion has been shown to improve surgical survival in left-sided obstructive congenital cardiac disease (Leoni et al. 1984). Diuresis and inotropic support with dopamine or dobutamine may be necessary if severe congestive cardiac failure develops.

Additional treatment of the newborn includes complete echocardiographic evaluation to confirm the diagnosis, to evaluate the severity of the coarctation, and to exclude any additional coexisting cardiac malformations. The involvement of a pediatric cardiologist and pediatric cardiac surgeon is essential.

The definitive neonatal treatment of coarctation is primary surgical repair. Balloon angioplasty has been advocated as an alternative to surgical repair, but it is associated with increased risks of restenosis at the site of coarctation. In addition, since most cases of coarctation presenting during the newborn period are complex, or demonstrate aortic hypoplasia, balloon angioplasty is often not possible (Whitley and Perry 1990). Isolated coarctation that is not symptomatic may be managed expectantly, with close surveillance of Doppler gradients across the area of narrowing or examination of the femoral pulse.

▶ SURGICAL TREATMENT

Surgical repair of symptomatic isolated coarctation of the aorta is generally delayed until at least 6 months of age, unless there is complete interruption of the aortic arch, which requires urgent correction (Beeman and Hammon 1990). The presence of poor peripheral perfusion or congestive heart failure refractory to initial medical therapy may prompt earlier primary surgical repair. The timing of surgery also depends on the diagnosis of additional cardiac malformations, with the presence of a coexisting ventricular septal defect often considered an indication for immediate operation.

The most common surgical procedure used to repair isolated coarctation of the aorta is a subclavian-flap aortoplasty (Beeman and Hammon 1990). Through a left thoracotomy, the left subclavian artery is ligated proximal to the vertebral artery and a flap is created from the proximal subclavian stump. The aorta is incised across the area of coarctation, and the flap is used to patch the defect in the aorta. Another similar technique is the patch aortoplasty, in which a patch of pericardium, rather than a subclavian flap, is used to close the aortic defect. The main complications associated with subclavian-flap aortoplasty are aneurysm formation at the flap site and weakening of the left arm with subclavian steal symptoms.

Other surgical approaches include resection of the area of coarctation with subsequent end-to-end anastomosis, or anastomosis of the descending aorta to the undersurface of the aortic arch. These approaches tend to be reserved for cases with large aortic diameters, because the recurrence rate for coarctation in such cases is increased. For cases of aortic-arch interruption, direct end-to-end anastomosis of the two aortic ends is performed by using an endogenous vessel or graft.

Operative mortality for primary repair of isolated coarctation is less than 5% and probably approaches zero (Beeman and Hammon 1990). Mortality increases with the presence of additional complex cardiac malformations and the presence of medical complications such as congestive heart failure, metabolic acidosis, and prolonged preoperative ventilation.

▶ LONG-TERM OUTCOME

Long-term survival after coarctation of the aorta depends on the presence of additional cardiac malformations. For isolated coarctation, 92% of patients are alive 15 years after repair, as compared with 81% with coexisting ventricular septal defect; 41% are alive at 3 years with more complex cardiac malformations (Kirklin and Barratt-Boyes 1986). Survival 25 years after repair has been estimated at 79% of affected individuals (Morris and Menashe 1991). Restenosis at the site of coarctation repair may occur in up to 50% of cases, depending on the type of correction (Beekman et al. 1981). However, some centers have reported extremely low rates of recurrence of the coarctation following subclavian-flap aortoplasty (Moulton et al. 1984). Aortic stenosis may also occur in up to 7% of cases following repair in infancy (Kirklin and Barratt-Boyes 1986).

▶ GENETICS AND RECURRENCE RISK

There is a strong association between Turner syndrome (45,X) and coarctation of the aorta, with 10% of patients with this syndrome also having coarctation. The occurrence of Turner syndrome is generally sporadic (see Chapter 135). In addition, coarctation has been described as part of the DiGeorge sequence. Inheritance patterns for most cases of coarctation of the aorta are considered polygenic. Estimates of recurrence risk for children with one parent diagnosed with coarctation range from 2.7 to 4.4%. The recurrence risk for siblings of an affected child is 2% (Nora and Nora 1988; Whitley and Perry 1990). The recurrence risk if two siblings are affected is 6% (Nora and Nora 1988). At least one familial cluster of coarctation of the aorta, possibly consistent with autosomal dominant inheritance, has also been described (Gerboni et al. 1993). In this family, four members of three generations had mild or severe coarction of the aorta, either isolated or in association with other congenital heart defects, Prenatal diagnosis was successfully performed in this family using fetal echocardiography, which at 26 weeks of gestation demonstrated severe narrowing of the aortic isthmus and hypoplastic left heart.

REFERENCES

Allan LD, Crawford DC, Tynan M. Evolution of coarctation of the aorta in intrauterine life. Br Heart J 1984;52:471–473.

Allan LD, Chita SK, Anderson RH, et al. Coarctation of the aorta in prenatal life: an echocardiographic, anatomical, and functional study. Br Heart J 1988;59:356–360.

Beeman SK, Hammon JW. Neonatal left ventricular outflow tract surgery. In: Long WA, ed. Fetal and neonatal cardiology. Philadelphia: Saunders, 1990:760–769.

Beekman RH, Rocchini AP, Behrendt DM, et al. Reoperation for coarctation of the aorta. Am J Cardiol 1981;48:1108–1114.

Brown DL, Durfee SM, Hornberger LK. Ventricular discrepancy as a sonographic sign of coarctation of the fetal aorta: how reliable is it? J Ultrasound Med 1997;16:95–99.

Campbell M, Polani PE. Etiology of coarctation of the aorta. Lancet 1961;1:473.

Ferencz C, Rubin JD, McCarter RJ, et al. Congenital heart disease: prevalence at live birth: the Baltimore-Washington infants study. Am J Epidemiol 1985;121:31–36.

Gerboni S, Sabatino G, Mingarelli R, et al. Coarctation of the aorta, interrupted aortic arch, and hypoplastic left heart syndrome in three generations. J Med Genet 1993;30:328–329.

Hornberger LK, Weintraub RG, Pesonen E, et al. Echocardiographic study of the morphology of the aortic arch in the human fetus. Circulation 1992;86:741–747.

Kirklin JW, Barratt-Boyes BG. Cardiac surgery. New York: Wiley, 1986:1036–1070.

Hyett J, Moscoso G, Nicolaides K. Increased nuchal translucency in trisomy 21 fetuses: relationship to narrowing of the aortic isthmus. Hum Reprod 1995;10:3049–3051.

Hyett J, Moscoso G, Papapanagiotou G, Perdu M, Nicolaides KH. Abnormalities of the heart and great arteries in chromosomally normal fetuses with increased nuchal translucency thickness at 11–13 weeks of gestation. Ultrasound Obstet Gynecol 1996;7:245–250.

Leoni F, Huhta JC, Douglas J, et al. Effect of prostaglandin on early surgical mortality in obstructive lesions of the systemic circulation. Br Heart J 1984;52:654–659.

Morris CD, Menashe VD. 25-year mortality after surgical repair of congenital heart defect in childhood: a population-based cohort study. JAMA 1991;266:3447–3452.

Moselhi M, Thilaganathan B. Nuchal translucency: a marker for the antenatal diagnosis of aortic coarctation. Br J Obstet Gynaecol 1996;103:1044–1045.

Moulton AL, Brenner JI, Roberts G, et al. Subclavian flap repair of coarctation of the aorta in neonates: realization of growth potential? J Thorac Cardiovasc Surg 1984;87:220–235.

Nora JJ, Nora AH. Update on counseling the family with a first-degree relative with a congenital heart defect. Am J Med Genet 1988;29:137–142.

Romero R, Pilu G, Jeanty P, et al. Coarctation and tubular hypoplasia of the aortic arch. In: Romero R, Pilu G, Jeanty P, Ghidini A, Hobbins JC, eds. Prenatal diagnosis of congenital anomalies. East Norwalk, CT: Appleton & Lange, 1988:171–173.

Sharland GK, Allan LD. Normal fetal cardiac measurements derived by cross-sectional echocardiography. Ultrasound Obstet Gynecol 1992;2:175.

Sharland GK, Chan KY, Allan LD. Coarctation of the aorta: difficulties in prenatal diagnosis. Br Heart J 1994;71:70–75.

Whitley HG, Perry I.W. Coarctation. In: Long WA, ed. Fetal and neonatal cardiology. Philadelphia: Saunders, 1990:477–486.

CHAPTER 47
Double-Outlet Right Ventricle

► CONDITION

Double-outlet right ventricle (DORV) is also known as the Taussig–Bing anomaly; it refers to a congenital cardiac malformation in which most of the pulmonary artery and the aorta arise from the right ventricle. Such an abnormality is generally compatible with life only when there is an additional malformation that allows blood flow from one side of the heart to the other, most commonly a ventricular septal defect (VSD).

Attempts have been made to define the malformation based on the relative area of each outflow tract arising from the right ventricle, with an anatomic threshold of 50% being used. The surgical definition of DORV requires that at least 90% of the area of the outflow tracts to arise from the right ventricle. The most commonly used definition requires one great artery to arise fully over the right ventricle and at least 50% of the other great artery to also originate from the right ventricle (Aoki et al. 1994). Therefore, cases of tetralogy of Fallot in which the majority of the aortic outflow tract arises from the right ventricle could also be defined as DORV. Such anomalies may arise because of arrest of normal rotation of the outflow tracts (Bostrom and Hutchins 1988).

Three types of DORV have been described. The most common is due to aortic outflow tract situated posterior to the pulmonary outflow tract, each spiralling around the other as they exit the heart (Romero et al. 1988). The Taussig–Bing heart is a subtype of DORV in which the aortic outflow tract ascends posterior to the pulmonary outflow tract in a parallel fashion. In the third type of DORV, the aortic outflow tract ascends anterior to the pulmonary outflow tract in a parallel fashion. DORV may also be classified based on the location of the VSD, either subaortic or subpulmonary.

Additional cardiac malformations are almost always present, with the most common being a VSD. Other co-existing cardiac malformations include atrial septal defect, atrioventricular canal defect, pulmonary stenosis, coarctation of the aorta, and anomalous venous return. Noncardiac malformations may also be present, including chromosomal abnormalities, such as trisomy 18 or 13, tracheoesophageal fistula, cardiosplenic syndrome, and orofacial clefting (Rowe et al. 1981; Wladimiroff et al. 1989).

► INCIDENCE

DORV is rare, and accounts for approximately 1% of all congenital cardiac malformations. However, this incidence may be higher if cases of tetralogy of Fallot that can also be defined as DORV are included. In one multicenter series, DORV accounted for 4.1% of all cases of prenatally diagnosed congenital heart disease (Paladini et al. 1996). The presence of preexisting maternal diabetes mellitus seems to be a significant risk factor for the development of DORV, with an odds ratio of 21.3 (Ferencz et al. 1990). The incidence of DORV ranges from 0.041–0.056 per thousand live births (Fyler et al. 1980; Ferencz et al. 1985).

► SONOGRAPHIC FINDINGS

Definitive prenatal sonographic diagnosis of DORV is difficult. There have been several cases of successful prenatal diagnosis made by careful examination of both the four-chamber cardiac view and the appearance of the outflow tracts. On the four-chamber view, a VSD is almost always present, either in a subpulmonary or a subaortic location. In DORV, both outflow tracts are visible arising from the right ventricle and are often in

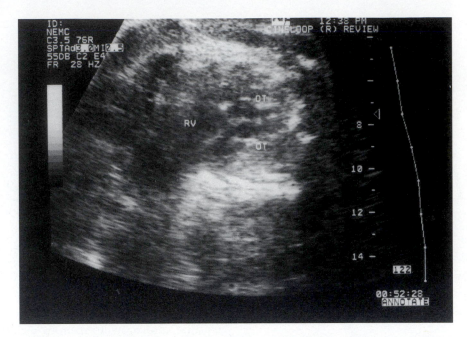

Figure 47-1. Prenatal sonographic image from a fetus with DORV, demonstrating parallel outflow tracts emanating from the right ventricle. RV = right ventricle; OT = outflow tract.

a side-by-side, or parallel, position (Fig. 47-1) (Stewart et al. 1985).

In one series of 24 fetuses with parallel outflow tracts, 7 were found to have transposition of the great arteries, while the remaining 17 had DORV (Allan 1997). In that series, most of the mothers were referred for fetal echocardiography because of an initial abnormal four-chamber cardiac view. In another series, 13 cases of DORV were correctly diagnosed by fetal echocardiography, 5 of which had an abnormal four-chamber cardiac view (Paladini et al. 1996). A transverse three-vessel view through the upper fetal mediastinum, demonstrating the main pulmonary artery, ascending aorta, and superior vena cava, may also be helpful in diagnosing DORV (Yoo et al. 1997). It appears clear, therefore, that maximal prenatal detection of DORV requires careful visualization of both the four-chamber view and the cardiac outflow tracts.

▶ DIFFERENTIAL DIAGNOSIS

Because DORV is almost always associated with additional cardiac malformations, a final diagnosis is often not possible until postnatal life. The prenatal sonographic appearance of DORV can be similar to that of tetralogy of Fallot (see Chapter 55) and transposition of the great arteries with a coexisting VSD (see Chapter 56). Indeed, the differentiation of some cases of DORV and tetralogy of Fallot may be based solely on the relative area of the aortic outflow tract that arises from the

right ventricle. The appearance of parallel great arteries, which is present in some subtypes of DORV, may aid in differentiation from tetralogy of Fallot, but does not help to differentiate from transposition of the great arteries.

▶ ANTENATAL NATURAL HISTORY

The antenatal natural history of DORV depends on the presence and nature of any additional cardiac or extracardiac malformations. For isolated DORV with a VSD, in utero development should be normal, and should not lead to congestive heart failure. In postnatal life, however, congestive heart failure may develop because the right ventricle provides both pulmonary and systemic circulation. In cases of DORV with pulmonary stenosis, in utero cardiac failure and hydrops may develop, but this is much more likely to occur during postnatal life as the ductus arteriosus closes.

In a series of 13 cases of DORV diagnosed prenatally, 7 resulted in elective termination of pregnancy, 3 in intrauterine fetal death, and 3 in live-born neonates (Paladini et al. 1996). There were 5 cases of chromosomal abnormalities in this series, 4 of which were trisomy 18 and 1 trisomy 16. Of the 3 cases of intrauterine death, 1 fetus had extracardiac malformations in addition to trisomy 18. It is not clear from this report if the other 2 fetuses that died in utero or the 3 live-born neonates had additional malformations. In a series of 24 fetuses with parallel great vessels, 17 of which had DORV, 22 had additional cardiac malformations, 8 had extracardiac anomalies, and 1 had trisomy 18 (Allan 1997). This series resulted in 6 terminations of pregnancy, 1 intrauterine fetal death, and 17 live-born neonates, 15 of whom required early surgical intervention.

▶ MANAGEMENT OF PREGNANCY

Following prenatal sonographic detection of DORV, fetal echocardiography should be performed to confirm the diagnosis and assess for additional cardiac malformations. In addition, a careful sonographic evaluation of extracardiac fetal anatomy is required to exclude orofacial clefting, tracheoesophageal fistula, and cardiosplenic syndrome. Because up to 40% of cases of DORV will have a chromosomal abnormality, most commonly trisomies 18 and 13, fetal karyotyping should also be offered. Careful genetic counseling is required to provide parents with a complete set of options for management of the pregnancy. Prenatal consultations with a neonatologist, geneticist, pediatric cardiologist, and pediatric cardiac surgeon are recommended to ensure timely and appropriate treatment during the newborn period.

In the absence of hydrops, there is no indication to alter management of the pregnancy, timing of delivery, or mode of delivery. Serial sonographic assessment to confirm appropriate fetal growth and absence of hydrops is recommended. The optimal management of the fetus with congenital heart disease and secondary hydrops fetalis is unclear. Mortality in such cases is usually very high (Kleinman et al. 1982), and it is uncertain if either early delivery or cesarean delivery will change the outcome. Delivery should occur in a tertiary-care center, with the immediate availability of a pediatric cardiologist and pediatric cardiac surgeon.

▶ FETAL INTERVENTION

No data on fetal intervention for DORV are available.

▶ TREATMENT OF NEWBORN

Initial care of the newborn with DORV depends on the presence of additional cardiac or extracardiac malformations. For example, if significant pulmonary stenosis is also present, a duct-dependent situation may exist, and the infant may benefit from prostaglandin infusion to maintain the patency of the ductus arteriosus (Allan 1997). In addition, initial treatment requires prompt postnatal evaluation by a pediatric cardiologist, with echocardiography, to confirm the prenatal diagnosis and to assess for the presence of additional cardiac malformations (Fig. 47-2).

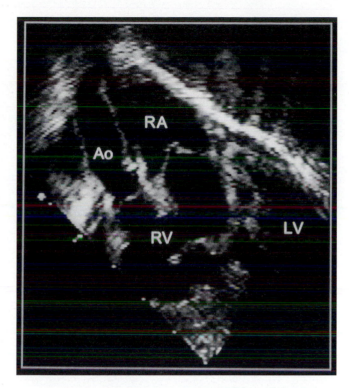

Figure 47-2. Subxiphoid long-axis transthoracic echocardiographic view of an infant with a variant of DORV. Both great vessels arise from the right ventricle in a side-by-side arrangement. RA = right atrium; LV = left ventricle; RV = right ventricle; Ao = aorto. *(Image courtesy of Dr. Jonathan Rhodes.)*

The presence of a VSD should be categorized as subaortic, subpulmonary, noncommitted, or doubly committed (Lev et al. 1972). Coronary-artery anatomy should be defined, and tricuspid-to-pulmonary-valve annular distance should be measured, as these have implications for surgical repair (Sakata et al. 1988). The treatment of the newborn with DORV requires early surgical intervention, which today usually involves a single primary repair procedure rather than an initial palliative procedure (Tchervenkov et al. 1995).

▶ SURGICAL TREATMENT

Contemporary data on operative mortality and reoperation rates suggest that repair of DORV should be performed early in infancy, thereby avoiding the need for additional palliation procedures (Aoki et al. 1994; Tchervenkov et al. 1995). The main principles behind surgical repair of DORV are to achieve an anatomic biventricular repair by connecting the left ventricle to the systemic circulation and to repair all associated cardiac lesions simultaneously (Tchervenkov et al. 1995).

Preoperative echocardiographic evaluation is crucial in planning the surgical approach to DORV. When the tricuspid-to-pulmonary-valve annular distance is greater than the diameter of the aortic anulus, intraventricular rerouting is the surgical procedure of choice in the repair of DORV with a coexisting VSD, particularly if the VSD is subaortic in location (Aoki et al. 1994). With this procedure, an intraventricular tunnel is created to take blood flow directly from the VSD to the aortic outflow tract, while maintaining the preexisting continuity of flow from the right ventricle to pulmonary outflow tract (Kirklin et al. 1964). A right ventricular outflow patch may be required to direct blood flow appropriately.

When the tricuspid-to-pulmonary-valve annular distance is small, or if the anatomy otherwise prevents an intraventricular rerouting procedure, other surgical techniques are performed, such as an arterial switch procedure, with blood flow taken directly from the VSD to the pulmonary outflow tract. If significant pulmonary stenosis is also present, or if coronary artery anatomy is abnormal, a conduit procedure may be needed, in which blood flow is directed from the VSD to the aortic outflow tract and a conduit is placed to channel blood flow from the right ventricle to the pulmonary artery (Rastelli-type procedure).

Immediate operative mortality following repair of DORV ranges from 8 to 11% (Aoki et al. 1994; Tchervenkov et al. 1995). Risk factors for early mortality include the presence of multiple VSDs, or aortic-arch obstruction (Kleinert et al. 1997).

▶ LONG-TERM OUTCOME

Long-term survival following surgical repair of DORV has been estimated to be from 73 to 88% at 5 to 8 years (Aoki et al. 1994; Serraf et al. 1991; Tchervenkov et al. 1995). The incidence of reoperation ranges from 26 to 42% (Aoki et al. 1994; Serraf et al. 1991). Reasons for reoperation include subaortic stenosis, subpulmonary stenosis, and the presence of a significant residual VSD. In another series, the probability of survival, free from reoperation, was calculated as 65% at 10 years (Kleinert et al. 1997). The presence of a noncommitted VSD was a significant risk factor for reoperation, while the presence of a subaortic VSD was protective against reoperation (Aoki et al. 1994). In one series, 95% of long-term survivors had no restriction on physical activities and required no cardiac medications (Tchervenkov et al. 1995).

▶ GENETICS AND RECURRENCE RISK

An association exists between DORV and both trisomies 13 and 18. The recurrence risk for these syndromes is extremely low, unless one parent is a balanced translocation carrier. In one consanguineous family, cardiac abnormalities, either tetralogy of Fallot or DORV with subaortic VSD and pulmonary stenosis, were found in three of four offspring (Bindewald et al. 1994). This implies the existence of a rare autosomal recessive syndrome involving DORV.

REFERENCES

Allan LD. Sonographic detection of parallel great arteries in the fetus. AJR Am J Roentgenol 1997;168:1283–1286.

Aoki M, Forbess JM, Jonas RA, et al. Result of biventricular repair for double-outlet right ventricle. J Thorac Cardiovasc Surg 1994;107:338–350.

Bindewald B, Ulner H, Muller U. Fallot complex: severe mental and growth retardation: a new autosomal recessive syndrome? Am J Med Genet 1994;50:173–176.

Bostrom MPG, Hutchins GM. Arrested rotation of the outflow tract may explain double-outlet right ventricle. Circulation 1988;77:1258–1265.

Ferencz C, Rubin JD, McCarter RJ, et al. Maternal diabetes and cardiovascular malformations: predominance of double outlet right ventricle and truncus arteriosus. Teratology 1990;41:319–326.

Ferencz C, Rubin JD, McCArter RJ, et al. Congenital heart disease: prevalence of live birth: the Baltimore-Washington infant study. Am J Epidemiol 1985;121:31–36.

Fyler DC, Buckley LP, Hellenbrand W, et al. Report of the New England Regional infant cardiac program. Pediatrics 1980;65(suppl):375.

Kirklin JW, Harp RA, McGoon DC. Surgical treatment of origin of both vessels from the right ventricle, including cases of pulmonary stenosis. J Thorac Cardiovasc Surg 1964;48:1026–1036.

Kleinert S, Sano T, Weintraub RG, et al. Anatomic features and surgical strategies in double-outlet right ventricle. Circulation 1997;96:1233–1239.

Kleinman CS, Donnerstein RL, DeVore GR, et al. Fetal echocardiography for evaluation of in utero congestive heart failure: a technique for study of nonimmune fetal hydrops. N Engl J Med 1982;306:568–575.

Lev M, Bharati S, Meng CCL, et al. A concept of double outlet right ventricle. J Thorac Cardiovasc Surg 1972;64:271–281.

Paladini D, Rustico M, Todros T, et al. Conotruncal anomalies in prenatal life. Ultrasound Obstet Gynecol 1996;8:241–246.

Romero R, Pilu, G, Jeanty P, et al. Double outlet right ventricle. In: Romero R, Pilu, G, Jeanty P, Ghidini A, Hobbins JC, eds. Prenatal diagnosis of congenital anomalies. East Norwalk, CT: Appleton & Lange, 1988:166–168.

Rowe RD, Freedom RM, Mehrizi A, et al. The neonate with congenital heart disease. 2nd ed. Philadelphia: Saunders, 1981.

Sakata R, Lecompte Y, Batisse A, et al. Anatomic repair of anomalies of ventriculoarterial connection associated with ventricular septal defect. I. Criteria of surgical decision. J Thorac Cardiovasc Surg 1988;95:90–95.

Serraf A, Lacour-Gayet F, Bruniaux J, et al. Anatomic repair of Taussig–Bing hearts. Circulation 1991;84:SIII200–SIII205.

Stewart PA, Wladimiroff JW, Becker AE. Early prenatal detection of double outlet right ventricle by echocardiography. Br Heart J 1985;54:340–342.

Tchervenkov CI, Marelli D, Beland MJ, et al. Institutional experience with a protocol of early primary repair of double-outlet right ventricle. Ann Thorac Surg 1995;60: S610–S613.

Wladimiroff JW, Stewart PA, Reuss A, et al. Cardiac and extra-cardiac anomalies as indicators for trisomies 13 and 18: a prenatal ultrasound study. Prenat Diagn 1989;9: 515–520.

Yoo SJ, Lee YH, Kim ES, et al. Three-vessel view of the fetal upper mediastinum: an easy means of detecting abnormalities of the ventricular outflow tracts and great arteries during obstetric screening. Ultrasound Obstet Gynecol 1997;9:173–182.

CHAPTER 48

Ebstein Anomaly

► CONDITION

Congenital downward displacement of the septal and posterior leaflets of the tricuspid valve is known as Ebstein anomaly. This downward displacement is associated with valvular dysplasia, resulting in tricuspid insufficiency (Schiebler et al. 1968). The displaced septal and posterior leaflets become adherent to the right ventricular walls, which may also be dysplastic. This results in division of the right ventricle into two segments, a proximal atrialized portion that forms a common enlarged chamber with the right atrium and a distal functional right ventricular chamber. Significant right atrial enlargement is common, and atrial septal defects or patent foramen ovale is commonly seen during neonatal life. Other cardiac malformations coexist with Ebstein anomaly in approximately one-third of cases (Celermajer et al. 1994). The most common additional malformations are pulmonary stenosis, pulmonary atresia with intact ventricular septum, ventricular septal defect, mitral-valve prolapse, aortic coarctation, patent ductus arteriosus, and right ventricular hypoplasia. Rarer coexisting malformations include tetralogy of Fallot, atrioventricular septal defect, aortic atresia, mitral dysplasia, and left ventricular diverticulum (Celermajer et al. 1994).

► INCIDENCE

The incidence of Ebstein anomaly in the general population is approximately 1 in 20,000 live births (Nora et al. 1974). It accounts for 0.3 to 0.6% of congenital heart defects in children and occurs equally in males and females (Rao 1990).

First-trimester maternal lithium ingestion has been implicated in the occurrence of Ebstein anomaly for over 20 years. Based on data from an international reg-

istry of mothers exposed to lithium during pregnancy it was suggested that the risk of Ebstein anomaly was 400 times greater in lithium-exposed infants than in the general population (Weinstein 1976). From the registry of 225 infants born to women treated with lithium during the first trimester, there was an 8% incidence of all cardiac malformations and a 2.7% incidence specifically of Ebstein anomaly.

Subsequent controlled studies have suggested that the actual risk of Ebstein anomaly is considerably less than originally estimated from population registries. A total of 2 cohort studies and 4 case–control studies did not demonstrate as high a risk of Ebstein anomaly as was suggested from population registries, although the precise magnitude of the risk of Ebstein anomaly following first-trimester lithium exposure is unclear (Cohen et al. 1994). It was estimated that first-trimester lithium exposure is associated with a 4 to 12% incidence of congenital anomalies, as compared with a general population risk of from 2 to 4%.

► SONOGRAPHIC FINDINGS

Prenatally, Ebstein anomaly is suggested by an abnormal four-chamber cardiac view, in which the right atrium appears grossly enlarged (Fig. 48-1). The tricuspid valve is displaced downward toward the apex and below the level of the atrioventricular junction. Dysplasia of the valve appears as abnormal thickening, nodularity, and irregularity of the leaflets. The right ventricular wall may become dysplastic and appear thin (Roberson and Silverman 1989). Pulsed and color Doppler evaluation may also demonstrate significant tricuspid regurgitation. As tricuspid regurgitation worsens, congestive heart failure may develop, leading to cardiac enlargement and eventually hydrops. On prenatal sonography, supraventricular

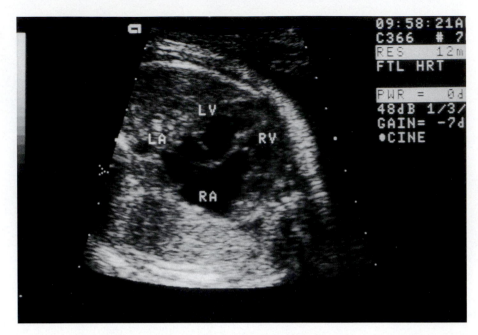

Figure 48-1. Antenatal four-chamber view of a fetal heart, demonstrating abnormally enlarged right atrium (RA) and downward displacement of tricuspid valve toward an abnormally small right ventricle. LA = left atrium; LV = left ventricle; RV = right ventricle.

tachycardia may also be noted in association with Ebstein anomaly (Sharf et al. 1983), and accessory conduction pathways resulting in Wolff–Parkinson–White syndrome may be common.

Prenatal sonographic diagnosis of Ebstein anomaly is accurate. In one series of 17 fetuses diagnosed prenatally with Ebstein anomaly, the diagnosis was confirmed postnatally in 15, either by autopsy, surgery, or neonatal imaging (Hornberger et al. 1991). In another series of 19 cases of prenatally identified tricuspid abnormalities, 6 of 10 cases of Ebstein anomaly were correctly diagnosed by fetal echocardiography. The remaining 4 were incorrectly described prenatally as valvular dysplasia without displacement (Oberhoffer et al. 1992).

► DIFFERENTIAL DIAGNOSIS

The sonographic detection of right atrial enlargement should prompt a search for abnormalities of the tricuspid and pulmonary valves. The differential diagnosis of Ebstein anomaly includes isolated tricuspid-valve dysplasia without significant downward displacement of valve leaflets. In its most severe form such valve dysplasia may represent an unguarded tricuspid-valve orifice. In each of these conditions, significant tricuspid regurgitation and cardiomegaly will most likely be present, but only in Ebstein anomaly will there be an abnormally located insertion site for the valve. However, the differentiation between Ebstein anomaly and tri-

cuspid dysplasia is largely academic; both conditions can present clinically with heart failure and additional cardiac malformations (Sharland et al. 1991).

Echocardiography should easily distinguish pulmonary stenosis, anatomic pulmonary atresia, tricuspid atresia, transposition of the great vessels, Uhl anomaly, and tetralogy of Fallot from Ebstein anomaly (Rao 1990). Uhl anomaly is an almost total absence of the myocardium of the right ventricle. With pulmonary stenosis or atresia, significant right ventricular hypertrophy should be visible, together with a small pulmonary artery. Functional pulmonary atresia with diminished pulmonary flow may occur secondary to Ebstein anomaly, tricuspid dysplasia, and tricuspid insufficiency; these may be difficult to differentiate without neonatal imaging (Rao 1990). In cases of tricuspid atresia, marked right atrial enlargement will be present, but forward flow across the site of the tricuspid valve will not be present. Uhl anomaly involves severe hypoplasia of the myocardium of the right ventricle, which may present with right atrial enlargement but with the tricuspid valve in a normal position (Benson et al. 1995).

► ANTENATAL NATURAL HISTORY

Infants with Ebstein anomaly diagnosed in utero have a significantly worse prognosis as compared with patients diagnosed later in childhood (Celermajer et al. 1994). In one series of 16 cases of Ebstein anomaly diagnosed prenatally, 11 were managed expectantly, 4 of which resulted in intrauterine death (Sharland et al. 1991). Another 6 infants died within 3 months of birth, with only 1 infant surviving. All of 6 fetuses with Ebstein anomaly followed sequentially with ultrasound examination had significant increases in cardiac size, as measured by cardiothoracic ratio, as pregnancy progressed (Sharland et al. 1991).

In a further series of 17 fetuses diagnosed prenatally with Ebstein anomaly, 14 were managed expectantly, and in this group there were 6 intrauterine deaths, 5 early neonatal deaths, and only 3 survivors (Hornberger et al. 1991). Eight of the 17 fetuses had pulmonary hypoplasia, and hydrops developed in 3. Therefore, the prognosis in prenatally diagnosed Ebstein anomaly is poor: one-third die in utero and only one-tenth survive the neonatal period.

▶ MANAGEMENT OF PREGNANCY

If the diagnosis of Ebstein anomaly is suspected after prenatal ultrasonography, the patient should be referred to a tertiary-care center for careful sonographic evaluation of fetal anatomy and fetal echocardiography to confirm the diagnosis and to exclude additional noncardiac malformations. However, no obvious pattern of extracardiac malformations has been described in association with Ebstein anomaly, and karyotypic abnormalities are rare (Siebert et al. 1989). In one series of 16 infants with Ebstein anomaly no karyotypic abnormalities were found (Ferencz et al. 1987). In another series of 16 fetuses with Ebstein anomaly, one case of Down syndrome was found (Roberson and Silverman 1989), and a further series of 17 fetuses with Ebstein anomaly included 1 fetus with trisomy 13 (Hornberger et al. 1991). Although some authors have suggested routine karyotyping for fetuses when the diagnosis of Ebstein anomaly is made (Romero et al. 1988), from a review of published series this diagnostic intervention does not seem to be justified for isolated Ebstein anomaly. Prenatal consultation with a pediatric cardiologist is recommended, and the option of termination of pregnancy should be provided.

Following prenatal diagnosis, serial evaluation with obstetric ultrasonography is recommended to confirm adequate fetal growth and to exclude the development of congestive heart failure. If hydrops develops, the option of early delivery may be considered; however, it is unclear that this will alter the expected high mortality rate (Romero et al. 1988). In the absence of hydrops there is no indication to alter obstetric management, including timing and route of delivery. Delivery should occur in a tertiary-care center, with the immediate availability of appropriately trained neonatologists, pediatric cardiologists, and pediatric cardiothoracic surgeons.

▶ FETAL INTERVENTION

No fetal intervention has been described following the prenatal diagnosis of Ebstein anomaly.

▶ TREATMENT OF THE NEWBORN

Many cases of Ebstein anomaly are completely asymptomatic and do not present until adolescence. By contrast, most cases diagnosed prenatally tend to have tricuspid regurgitation and cardiomegaly, which usually results in the development of congestive heart failure during the newborn period. Infants with Ebstein anomaly diagnosed in utero have a significantly worse overall prognosis as compared with patients diagnosed later in childhood (Radford et al. 1985).

Careful evaluation by a pediatric cardiologist is recommended during the immediate newborn period, including echocardiography, to confirm the diagnosis and to exclude the presence of additional cardiac malformations. For patients with arrhythmias such as Wolff–Parkinson–White syndrome, electrophysiologic mapping may also be required to localize any accessory conduction pathways. Clinical improvement of cyanosis is likely in many cases during the initial newborn period as pulmonary vascular resistance falls, thereby reducing right-to-left shunting of blood.

If severe hypoxemia is also present, infusion of prostaglandin E_1 to maintain patency of the ductus arteriosus may also improve pulmonary vascular flow. This requirement for prostaglandin infusion usually decreases as pulmonary vascular resistance continues to fall following delivery (Rao 1990). Treatment with diuretics and digoxin may also be needed if congestive heart failure is present, and lidocaine or procainamide may be needed if arrhythmias develop. Medical management of Ebstein anomaly is preferable during the neonatal period because of poor results with surgical repair (McFaul et al. 1976; Rao 1990)

▶ SURGICAL TREATMENT

Indications for surgical repair of Ebstein anomaly are unclear but include the presence of New York Heart Association functional class III or IV disease, severe or progressive cyanosis, paradoxical emboli, right ventricular outflow-tract obstruction, progressive cardiac enlargement, and development of atrial arrhythmias due to the presence of accessory conduction pathways (Danielson et al. 1992). Sudden death postoperatively can occur secondary to ventricular arrhythmias. Preoperative electrophysiologic studies, with prophylactic lidocaine therapy followed by procainamide for 3 months, is recommended to reduce this complication (Danielson et al. 1992).

Surgical technique for Ebstein anomaly involves repairing the tricuspid valve, which should be possible in up to 60% of cases (Danielson et al. 1992). Following median sternotomy and cardiopulmonary bypass, redundant right atrial tissue is excised and a patch closure of any atrial septal defect is performed. The portion of the right ventricle is plicated, and an annuloplasty is performed to narrow the tricuspid annulus, allowing the single anterior leaflet to function as a monocuspid valve. If the tricuspid valve cannot be repaired, complete valve replacement is performed. Corrections of associated anomalies are also made, such as relief of pulmonary stenosis and ablation of accessory conduction pathways (Danielson et al. 1992).

In the largest single series published to date, 189 patients with Ebstein anomaly underwent surgical repair (Danielson et al. 1992). There was a 7.3% incidence of early death within 30 days in the group who underwent valvuloplasty and a 5.8% incidence of early death in the group who underwent complete valve replacement.

Another approach to the surgical repair of Ebstein anomaly involves vertical plication of the right ventricle with reimplantation of the tricuspid-valve leaflets (Quaegebeur et al. 1991). In a series of 10 patients treated with this technique, 9 demonstrated significant clinical improvement and 8 showed diminished tricuspid regurgitation on echocardiography. One patient continued to have significant tricuspid regurgitation and required prosthetic valve replacement. All 10 patients in this series survived (Quaegebeur et al. 1991).

▶ LONG-TERM OUTCOME

The long-term outcome for Ebstein anomaly depends on the timing of clinical presentation and diagnosis. Patients diagnosed during the fetal and early neonatal periods almost always have severe disease, with tricuspid regurgitation and significant cardiomegaly. Up to 50% of infants diagnosed with Ebstein anomaly during the neonatal period die within the first year of life (Rowe et al. 1981).

In a series of 189 patients with Ebstein anomaly managed surgically, there were 10 late deaths, 4 of which were presumed secondary to arrhythmias and 3 of which were secondary to congestive cardiac failure (Danielson et al. 1992). Over 90% of survivors were in New York Heart Association functional class I or II, and 9 affected adult women had a total of 12 successful pregnancies. Four (3.6%) of the patients treated by valvuloplasty required subsequent tricuspid-valve replacement, in one case 14 years after the initial surgical repair.

In another series of 220 cases of Ebstein anomaly, actuarial survival was 67% at 1 year and 59% at 10 years of age (Celermajer et al. 1994). Significant predictors of death included severe tricuspid regurgitation at presentation, diagnosis in utero, and right ventricular outflow-tract obstruction. Of 155 survivors overall, 83% remained in New York Heart Association functional class I, and 67% required no ongoing medical therapy.

▶ GENETICS AND RECURRENCE RISK

Ebstein anomaly usually occurs as an isolated lesion or together with an additional cardiac malformation. It does not seem to occur with karyotypic abnormalities or as part of a recognizable genetic syndrome or association. Although most cases are sporadic, there have been several familial reports, including occurrence in two sisters born to consanguineous Sri Lankan parents (Donegan et al. 1968; Gueron et al. 1966; McIntosh et al. 1992). Estimates of recurrence risk suggest a 1% rate of recurrence if one previous sibling has been affected and a 3% rate of recurrence if two siblings have been affected (Nora and Nora 1988).

▶ REFERENCES

Benson CB, Brown DL, Roberts DJ. Uhl anomaly of the heart mimicking Ebstein anomaly in utero. J Ultrasound Med 1995;14:781–783.

Celermajer DS, Bull C, Till JA, et al. Ebstein anomaly: presentation and outcome from fetus to adult. J Am Coll Cardiol 1994;23:170–176.

Cohen LS, Friedman JM, Jefferson JW, et al. A reevaluation of risk of in utero exposure to lithium. JAMA 1994;271: 146–150.

Danielson GK, Driscoll DJ, Mair DD, et al. Operative treatment of Ebstein anomaly. J Thorac Cardiovasc Surg 1992; 104:1195–1202.

Donegan CC Jr, Moore MM, Wiley TM Jr, Hernandez FA, Green JR Jr, Schiebler GL. Familial Ebstein anomaly of the tricuspid valve. Am Heart J 1968;75:375–379.

Ferencz C, Rubin JD, McCarte RJ, et al. Cardiac and non-cardiac malformations: observations in a population-based study. Teratology 1987;35:367–378.

Gueron M, Hirsch M, Stern J, Cohen W, Levy MJ. Familial Ebstein anomaly with emphasis on the surgical treatment. Am J Cardiol 1966;18:105–111.

Hornberger LK, Sahn DJ, Kleinman CS, et al. Tricuspid valve disease with significant tricuspid insufficiency in the fetus: diagnosis and outcome. J Am Coll Cardiol 1991;17:167–173.

McFaul RC, Davis Z, Giuliani ER, et al. Ebstein malformation: surgical experience at the Mayo Clinic. J Thorac Cardiovasc Surg 1976;72:910–915.

McIntosh N, Chitayat D, Bardanis M, et al. Ebstein anomaly: report of a familial occurrence and prenatal diagnosis. Am J Med Genet 1992;42:307–309.

Nora JJ, Nora AH. Update on counseling the family with a first-degree relative with a congenital heart defect. Am J Med Genet 1988;29:137–142.

Nora JJ, Nora AH, Toews WH. Lithium, Ebstein anomaly and other congenital heart defects. Lancet 1974;1:594–595.

Oberhoffer R, Cook AC, Lang D, et al. Correlation between echocardiographic and morphological investigations of lesions of the tricuspid valve diagnosed during fetal life. Br Heart J 1992;68:580–585.

Quaegebeur JM, Sreeram N, Fraser AG, et al. Surgery for Ebstein anomaly: the clinical and echocardiographic evaluation of a new technique. J Am Coll Cardiol 1991;17:722–728.

Radford DJ, Graff RF, Neilson GH. Diagnosis and natural history of Ebstein anomaly. Br Heart J 1985;54:517–522.

Rao PS. Other tricuspid valve anomalies. In: Long WA, ed. Fetal and neonatal cardiology. Philadelphia: Saunders, 1990:541–550.

Roberson DA, Silverman NH. Ebstein anomaly: echocardiographic and clinical features in the fetus and neonate. J Am Coll Cardiol 1989;14:1300–1307.

Romero R, Pilu G, Jeanty P, et al. Ebstein anomaly. In: Romero R, Pilu G, Jeanty P, Ghidini A, Hobbins JC, eds. Prenatal diagnosis of congenital anomalies. Norwalk, CT: Appleton & Lange, 1988:149–151.

Rowe RD, Freedom RM, Mehrizi A, et al. The neonate with congenital heart disease. 2nd ed. Philadelphia: Saunders, 1981;515–528.

Schiebler GL, Gravenstein JS, Van Mierop LH. Ebstein anomaly of the tricuspid valve: translation of original description with comments. Am J Cardiol 1968;22:867–873.

Sharf M, Abinader EG, Shapiro I, et al. Prenatal echocardiographic diagnosis of Ebstein anomaly with pulmonary atresia. Am J Obstet Gynecol 1983;147:300–303.

Sharland GK, Chita SK, Allan LD. Tricuspid valve dysplasia or displacement in intrauterine life. J Am Coll Cardiol 1991;17:944–949.

Siebert JR, Barr M, Jackson JC, et al. Ebstein anomaly and extracardiac defects. Am J Dis Child 1989;143:570–572.

Weinstein MR. The International Register of Lithium Babies. Drug Information J 1976;10:94–100.

CHAPTER 49

Heterotaxy Syndrome

► CONDITION

Heterotaxy is defined as any arrangement of the body organs that deviates from complete situs solitus with levocardia and dextrocardiac loop (the normal arrangement) or from complete situs inversus with dextrocardia and a levocardiac loop. During development there is a failure to form symmetry along the left–right axis in the heterotaxy syndrome. This asymmetry is first manifested embryologically at 2 to 23 days of gestation, with looping of the cardiac tube to the right (Gutgesell 1990). During this same period, abdominal situs is determined (Chandra 1974). The 270-degree counterclockwise rotation of the intestine about the axis of the superior mesenteric artery is completed by 10 weeks of gestation. Because looping of the cardiac tube and intestinal rotation both occur during the fourth week of gestation, defects of the cardiac situs are frequently associated with abnormal intestinal rotation. Because development of the heart is dependent on the formation of a normal left–right relationship, heterotaxy is associated with congenital heart disease in the majority of cases (Chandra 1974; Gutgesell 1990).

There is a spectrum of defects in heterotaxy syndrome, varying from isolated levocardia with abdominal situs inversus or isolated dextrocardia with abdominal situs solitus to total absence of asymmetry along the left–right axis. The most significant forms of heterotaxy syndrome are seen in left isomerism (also known as the polysplenia syndrome) or right isomerism (also known as asplenia syndrome). The term *asplenia* originated from Ivemark's initial description of cardiac malformations associated with congenital asplenia (Ivemark 1955). Moller et al. (1967) subsequently described another syndrome, also with cardiac and visceral abnormalities, but because it was associated with multiple splenic masses, it was called "polysplenia syndrome."

These syndromes of cardiac and visceral anomalies represent visceral isomerism (Gray et al. 1994). The terms *dextroisomerism* (asplenia syndrome) and *levoisomerism* (polysplenia syndrome) have been suggested to better describe organ arrangements that are not limited to the spleen. Sapire et al. (1986) have described these syndromes in relation to anatomic features of the atria, as right atrial isomerism (asplenia syndrome) and left atrial isomerism (polysplenia syndrome). This distinction was suggested because the anatomic features of the atria more reliably reflect the visceral abnormalities than does the spleen. Usually asplenia occurs in right atrial isomerism and polysplenia occurs in left atrial isomerism, but discrepancies have been reported (Caruso and Becher 1979). In addition, each condition has been reported with both the presence of a normal spleen (Laman et al. 1967; Landing et al. 1971) and normal cardiac anatomy (Peoples et al. 1983). Left atrial isomerism accounts for most cases of "polysplenia syndrome" (Moller et al. 1967; Peoples et al. 1983; Rose et al. 1975; Van Mierop et al. 1972). Left atrial isomerism usually has absent right-sided organs and bilaterally placed organs. Both conditions have features of the left-sided organ. Polysplenia is usually manifested as multiple splenic masses along the greater curvature of the stomach. The combined weight of the splenic tissue is approximately equivalent to a normal spleen. Left atrial isomerism is usually associated with less severe cardiac anomalies and better survival than right atrial isomerism (Peoples et al. 1983; Sapire et al. 1986).

The organs most involved in left atrial isomerism are the lungs, liver, heart, and intestines. The lungs are symmetric images of the left lung with only two lobes. Each side has left-sided relationships between the pulmonary artery and the main-stem bronchi (Moller et al. 1967). The pulmonary artery courses over the top of and then behind the main-stem bronchus on both sides, as in a normal left lung. The bronchi branch in a pattern similar to the left tracheobronchial tree and there is no horizontal mirror minor fissure on the right because there are only two lobes.

The liver usually is abnormal in shape and position and typically has a central globular appearance, as it is symmetric. The gallbladder may be midline, hypoplastic, or absent. In 10% of the cases, biliary anomalies can also be seen (Peoples et al. 1983). Several cases of biliary atresia have been reported in left atrial isomerism (Teichberg et al. 1982).

The intestines demonstrate nonrotation or reverse rotation of the midgut loop. The initial 90-degree counterclockwise rotation occurs, but the final 180-degree rotation about the superior mesenteric artery does not occur. The result is that the small intestine is on the right side of the abdomen and the colon is on the left. In severe reverse rotation, the midgut rotates clockwise instead of counterclockwise. The result is that the duodenum lies inferior to the superior mesenteric artery and the transverse colon behind it. These rotational abnormalities are prone to proximal intestinal obstruction or midgut volvulus.

Cardiac anomalies in the left atrial isomerism can occur at every level of the heart (Moller et al. 1967; Peoples et al. 1983; Rose et al. 1975; Tommasi et al. 1981; Van Mierop et al. 1972). In 50% of the cases, there are bilateral venae cavae connecting to the superior posterior aspect of the ipsilateral atrium. In rare cases, a single superior vena cava (SVC) connects to the coronary sinus, but the coronary sinus is usually absent. In 65% of the cases, the infrahepatic inferior vena cava (IVC) is interrupted. The IVC above the renal veins connects to the azygous system. The hepatic veins connect directly to the floor of the atrium. Anomalous pulmonary venous connection occurs in 40% of the patients. This is usually partial, with the veins from each lung entering the ipsilateral atrium on the opposite sides of the midline. The atria each show features of the left atrium with a long narrow atrial appendage. The atrial septum is usually absent, with an ostium primum defect in 65% of the cases.

Peoples et al. (1983) reviewed the ventricular anatomy of 127 cases of left atrial isomerism and found that in 38 the ventricular septum was intact, in 80 a ventricular septal defect (VSD) was present, and in 9 there was a univentricular heart. The VSD was either a form of endocardial cushion defect or a VSD in one of the typical locations. The atrioventricular connection is ambiguous through either a common or two-leaflet valve (Tommasi et al. 1981). In a univentricular heart, there is usually a double-inlet ventricle to a chamber of right or left ventricular morphology.

The great vessels in the left atrial isomerism are concordant in 69% (Peoples et al. 1983). The remainder are equally divided between discordant atrioventricular connection and double-outlet ventricle (usually of the right, but sometimes double-outlet left ventricle can be seen). In 20% of the cases, the side of the aortic arch is opposite the side of the cardiac apex.

The pulmonary valve of the right ventricular outflow area is normal in 65% of the cases. In the remaining cases, the pulmonic valve is stenotic (20%) or atretic (10%) with isolated subpulmonic stenosis in the remainder. In the left side of the heart, Peoples et al. (1983) found obstructive lesions in 22% of cases. These included valvular or subvalvular aortic stenosis (11 cases), coarctation of the aorta (7), hypoplastic left heart, hypoplastic left ventricle (6), mitral stenosis (3), and cor triatriatum (1).

The asplenia syndrome is now best described, in terms of the visceral asymmetry, as right atrial isomerism. Although most patients will be asplenic, some patients will have a normal spleen or multiple spleens. These patients usually come to the attention of a pediatric cardiologist early in life, secondary to severe associated congenital heart disease. Although historically 90% of the patients with the asplenia syndrome died by 1 year of age, survival has significantly improved due to advances in cardiologic diagnosis, the use of prostaglandin E_1 in duct-dependent lesions, and improvements in cardiac surgery (Chang et al. 1993; Ivemark et al. 1955; Van Mierop et al. 1972).

In asplenia syndrome, there are multiple visceral abnormalities affecting the heart, lungs, liver, and gastrointestinal tract. The lungs are both trilobed and the pulmonary arterial relationships with the tracheobronchial tree may be obscured by proximal pulmonary atresia. The lungs often derive significant blood flow from systemic vessels. The liver occupies a central position in the upper abdomen with the globular transverse lie.

▶ INCIDENCE

It is difficult to estimate the incidence of heterotaxy. Prior to 1960, over 1700 cases of heterotaxy had been reported, but these were not population-based. Reports have estimated incidences of situs inversus totalis to be between 1 in 20,400 among patients seen at the Mayo Clinic between 1910 and 1947 (Mayo et al. 1949) and 1 in 10,100 among patients seen at Massachusetts General Hospital (Adams and Churchill 1947). Autopsy studies and radiographic screening have yielded higher incidences, in the range of 1 in 8900 to 1 in 770. One of the highest incidence was noted in a radiographic screening study for tuberculosis at 1 in 4400 (Francisco and Ongpin 1946). According to one report, asplenia is twice as common in males (Van Mierop et al. 1972).

► SONOGRAPHIC FINDINGS

The determination of visceral situs may be quite challenging for the ultrasonographer. Often, abnormal cardiac situs and a structural defect are detected simultaneously, raising the suspicion of heterotaxy. Certain cardiac defects are more commonly associated with heterotaxy syndrome. These include total anomalous pulmonary venous return, VSD, single ventricle, transposition of the great arteries, and dextrocardia in the asplenia syndrome. In polysplenia, bilateral SVC, absent or interrupted IVC, anomalous pulmonary venous return, dextrocardia, atrioventricular septal defect, transposition of great arteries, and double-outlet right ventricle are typical (Van Mierop et al. 1972). The sonographic findings distinguishing between polysplenia and asplenia are summarized in Table 49-1.

Detection of visceral sites can be difficult, as the liver may have a central position and the stomach bubble location may be right, left, or central (Fig. 49-1). In the asplenia syndrome, the relationship between the IVC and aorta is helpful in diagnosing heterotaxy. Huhta et al. (1982) noted in newborns that in asplenia syndrome the descending aorta and the IVC run on the same side of the spine, either to the right or left. The aorta is usually positioned posterior to the IVC. This relationship is best appreciated in a transverse cross section of the fetal abdomen below the diaphragm (Fig. 49-2). The IVC and aorta should then be followed proximally to the right atrium and descending thoracic aorta, respectively. The IVC is often interrupted in the polysplenia syndrome, with blood flow continued via communication though the azygos vein on either the left or right side of the spine. The aorta usually courses anterior to the spine in the midline. There is a good deal of overlap between these conditions, and identification of IVC and aorta on the same side of the spine has been described in both asplenia and polysplenia syndrome.

Echocardiographic assessment should attempt to identify the presence of right, left, or bilateral SVC and its connection to the atria. In bilateral SVCs, the left may connect to the coronary sinus or the left atrium. An attempt should be made to identify the pulmonary veins. In total anomalous pulmonary veins, if a venous connection is seen with situs ambiguous, then right atrial isomerism should be suspected. In contrast, partial anomalous venous connection to the right atrium suggests left atrial isomerism. In addition, the atrioventricular connection and ventriculoatrial connection should be determined.

► ANTENATAL NATURAL HISTORY

Little is known of the antenatal natural history of heterotaxy because it has been recognized prenatally only recently. Abnormal situs does not in itself pose adverse consequences for the fetus, with two notable exceptions. The prenatal as well as postnatal courses are thought to be determined primarily by the severity of the cardiac defect. Most structural heart defects associated with heterotaxy are well tolerated in utero. In cases in which heterotaxy results in intestinal malrotation, the risk of midgut volvulus exists. No case of prenatal midgut volvulus due to heterotaxy has been reported to date.

► MANAGEMENT OF PREGNANCY

In cases of suspected heterotaxy, obstetric management should include a detailed sonographic evaluation to delineate the extent of visceral abnormalities and situs as much as possible. Fetal echocardiography should be performed in all cases to determine the nature and severity of associated cardiac defects. Because of the

► **TABLE 49-1.** PRENATAL SONOGRAPHIC FINDINGS IN HETEROTAXY SYNDROMES

Finding	Polysplenia	Asplenia
Sidedness	Left	Right
Spleen	Present (multiple)	Absent
Gall Bladder	Absent	Present
Liver	Left or Right side	Midline
Heart Malformations	ASD, AVC, TGA, DORV	AVC, single ventricle, TGA, PS
Vena Cava	Interrupted IVC Bilateral SVC	Same side as aorta Bilateral SVC
Anomalous Pulmonary Venous Return	70% of cases	100% of cases
Sex Ratio	Equal in males and females	2 females : 1 male

KEY: ASD = atrial septal defect; AVC = atrioventricular canal defect; DORV = double-outlet right ventricle; IVC = inferior vena cava; PS = pulmonic stenosis; SVC = superior vena cava; TGA = transportation of great arteries.

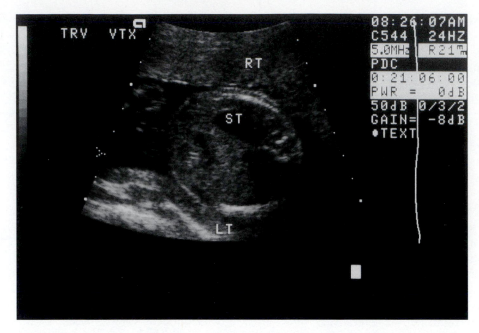

Figure 49-1. Antenatal sonographic image demonstrating the presence of the fetal stomach in right upper quadrant.

increased risk of associated chromosomal defects, we recommend that all fetuses with heterotaxy should undergo genetic amniocentesis.

Heterotaxy does not usually result in problems complicating the pregnancy and there is no indication for changing the mode or timing of delivery except for standard obstetrical indications. However, because of the potential for severe structural heart disease, referral for delivery in a tertiary-care center with neonatologists, pediatric cardiologists, and pediatric cardiac surgeons should be considered.

▶ FETAL INTERVENTION

There is no fetal intervention for heterotaxy.

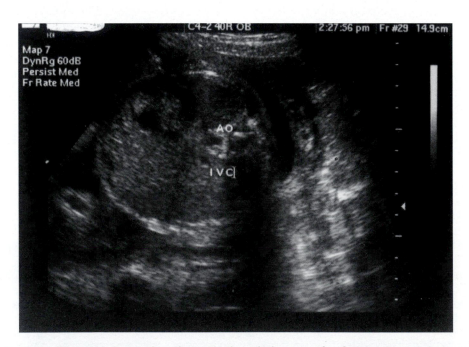

Figure 49-2. Transverse section through the abdomen of a fetus with total sinus inversus. The fetal right side is superior in this picture. Ao = aorta; IVC = inferior vena cava. *(Courtesy of Dr. Marjorie Treadwell.)*

▶ TREATMENT OF THE NEWBORN

Much of the initial treatment of the infant with heterotaxy will be dictated by the specific cardiac defect associated with it. The reader is referred to the chapters on structural heart disease (see Chapters 46–57). The newborn with heterotaxy should undergo plain abdominal radiography of the chest and abdomen to confirm a suspicion of heterotaxy. Postnatal echocardiography should be performed to confirm prenatal echocardiographic assessment and to define the anatomic defect. When the infant is stable for transport to the radiology suite, an upper gastrointestinal series and small-bowel follow-through should be performed to evaluate errors in intestinal fixation that may predispose to midgut volvulus (Fig. 49-3). In cases of asplenia, the newborn should be maintained on prophylactic penicillin and receive the pneumococcal vaccine.

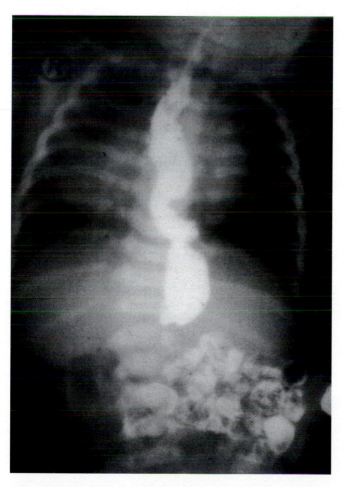

Figure 49-3. Postnatal contrast study in an infant with heterotaxy. Note that there is dextrocardia, vascular congestion, and situs ambiguous with the stomach lying centrally. The stomach is small and the liver fills the upper abdomen. *(Courtesy of Dr. Roy McCauley.)*

▶ LONG-TERM OUTCOME

The long-term outcome of children with heterotaxy is directly related to the severity of an associated cardiac anomaly.

▶ GENETICS AND RECURRENCE RISK

Heterotaxy occasionally occurs in families in a recurring pattern, suggestive of autosomal recessive, X-linked, or autosomal dominant inheritance. Alonso et al. (1995) recently reported six families with a pattern of recurrence suggestive of an autosomal dominant inheritance. Ferraro et al. (1997) studied a large family in which a gene for heterotaxy (HTX-1) was mapped to the 19-centiMorgan (cM) region in Xq24-q27.1. This same group has reported localizing HTX-1 to Xq26.2 and a submicroscopic deletion in Xq26, which is associated with familial situs ambiguous. Every pregnant patient who has had a fetus with heterotaxy should be evaluated by a medical geneticist to obtain a family history and to provide advice on the potential recurrence risks with subsequent pregnancies.

REFERENCES

Adams R, Churchill ED. Situs inversus, sinusitis and bronchiectosis. J Thorac Surg 1947;7:206–217.

Alonso S, Pierpoint ME, Radtke W, et al. Heterotaxia syndrome and autosomal dominant inheritance. Am J Med Genet 1995;56:12–15.

Caruso G, Becher AE. How to determine atrial situs? Considerations initiated by 3 cases of absent spleen with a discordant anatomy between bronchi and atria. Br Heart J 1979;41:359–367.

Chandra RS. Biliary atresia and other structural anomalies in the congenital polysplenia syndrome. J Pediatr 1974;85:649–655.

Chang J, Brueckner M, Touloukian RJ. Intestinal rotation and fixation abnormalities in heterotaxia: early detection and management. J Pediatr Surg 1993;28:1281–1285.

Ferraro GB, Gebbia M, Pilia G, et al. A submicroscopic deletion in Xq26 associated with familial situs ambiguous. Am J Med Genet 1997;61:395–401.

Francisco SA, Ongpin C. Situs inversus totalis: case discovered by X-ray among Filipinos. J Philip Med Assoc 1936;16:133–140.

Gray SW, Skandalakis JE, Ricketts R. Anomalies of situs and symmetry. In: Skandalakis JE, Gray SW, eds. Embryology for surgeons. 2nd ed. Baltimore: Williams and Wilkins, 1994;1052–1059.

Gutgesell HP. Cardiac malposition and heterotaxy. In: Garsen A, Brickner JT, McNamara IG, eds. The science and practice of pediatric cardiology, Malvern, PA: Lu & Folger 1990;1280–1303.

Huhta JC, Smallhorn JF, Macartney FJ. Two dimensional echocardiographic diagnosis of situs. Br Heart J 1982;48: 97–101.

Ivemark B. Implications of agenesis of the spleen on the pathogenesis of cono-truncus anomalies in childhood. Acta Paediatr Scand 1955;44(suppl 104):1–110.

Laman TE, Levine MS, Amplaz K, et al. "Asplenic syndrome" in association with rudimentary spleen. Am J Cardiol 1967;20:136–140.

Landing BH, Lawrence TY, Payne VC Jr, et al. Bronchial anatomy in syndromes with abnormal visceral situs: abnormal spleen and congenital heart disease. Am J Cardiol 1971;28:456–462.

Mayo CW, Rice RG. Situs inversus totalis: statistical review of data on seventy-six cases, special reference to diseases of the biliary tract. Arch Surg 1949;58:724–730.

Moller JH, Nakib A, Anderson RC, et al. Congenital cardiac disease associated with polysplenia: a development complex of bilateral "left-sidedness." Circulation 1967;36: 789–795.

Peoples WM, Moller JH, Edwards JE. Polysplenia: a review of 146 cases. Pediatr Cardiology 1983;4:129–135.

Rose V, Izukawa T, Moes CA. Syndromes of asplenia and polyspleni: a review of cardiac and non-cardiac malformations in 60 cases with special reference to diagnosis and prognosis. Br Heart J 1975;37:840–852.

Sapire DW, Ho YS, Anderson RA, et al. Diagnosis and significance of atrial isomerism. Am J Cardiol 1986;58: 342–346.

Teichberg S, Markowitz J, Silverberg M, et al. Abnormal cilia in a child with the polysplenia syndrome and extrahepatic biliary atresia. J Pediatr 1982;100:399–401.

Tommasi SM, Daliento L, Ho SY, et al. Analysis of atrioventricular junction, ventricular mass, and ventriculoarterial junction in 43 specimens and atrial isomerism. Br Heart J 1981;45:236–247.

Van Mierop LHS, Gessner IH, Schiebler GL. Asplenia and polysplenia syndrome. Birth Defects 1972;8:36–41.

CHAPTER 50

Truncus Arteriosus

▶ CONDITION

Truncus arteriosus (also known as common aorticopulmonary trunk, truncus arteriosus communis, and single-outlet heart), refers to a single large ventricular outflow tract arising from both right and left ventricles. This single large outflow tract, or truncus, gives rise to the coronary arteries, aorta, and pulmonary arteries.

In the original anatomic classification of Collett and Edwards (1949), four subtypes were described:

>Type I demonstrates a single pulmonary trunk arising from the truncus, which then subdivides into right and left pulmonary arteries.
>Type II demonstrates two pulmonary arteries arising directly from the posterior surface of the truncus.
>Type III demonstrates two pulmonary arteries arising from the lateral aspects of the truncus.
>Type IV demonstrates absent pulmonary arteries, but collateral arteries arising from the descending aorta supply the pulmonary vasculature.

Van Praagh and Van Praagh (1965) subsequently described a further classification system in which type A truncus is associated with a ventricular septal defect (VSD) and type B truncus is not associated with a VSD. Type A truncus is divided further into four subtypes, which closely resemble the classification of Collett and Edwards:

>Type A1 demonstrates a partially separated pulmonary trunk.
>Type A2 demonstrates two pulmonary arteries arising directly from the truncus.
>Type A3 demonstrates a single pulmonary artery arising from the truncus together with further collaterals arising from the descending aorta.
>Type A4 demonstrates significant arch anomalies in association with the truncus.

Almost 60% of cases of truncus are type I, based on the classification of Collett and Edwards, 35% are type II, 5% are type III, and a small minority are type IV (Bharati et al. 1974). In 65% of cases the single truncus seems to arise predominantly from the right ventricle, which may make differentiation from tetralogy of Fallot difficult. The truncus arises entirely from the right ventricle in 15% of cases, straddles the ventricular septum equally in a further 15% of cases, and arises mostly from the left ventricle in less than 5% of cases (Bharati et al. 1974). The single valve within the truncus is known as the truncal valve, and it is tricuspid in over 65% of cases, although the number of leaflets may range from two to five. Truncal-valve dysplasia is very common, although significant truncal stenosis is rare, occurring in only 5% of cases (Bharati et al. 1974). Truncal-valve regurgitation may be common, occurring in up to 40% of cases (Di Donato et al. 1985).

Associated cardiac malformations are common with truncus arteriosus; a VSD is present in the vast majority of cases. Right-sided aortic arch, atrial septal defect, abnormal origin of brachiocephalic vessels, aortic coarctation, atrioventricular canal defect, mitral atresia, and abnormal cardiac situs have all been described in association with truncus (Bharati et al. 1974). Extracardiac abnormalities include situs inversus, heterotaxy syndrome (see Chapter 49), DiGeorge sequence, and genitourinary anomalies (Bharati et al. 1974; Collett and Edwards 1949).

▶ INCIDENCE

Truncus arteriosus is a rare form of congenital heart disease, accounting for only 1.5% of all severe cardiac malformations seen during infancy (Fyler et al. 1980). Its incidence is estimated to be 3 in 100,000 live births and may be slightly more frequent in females. The incidence of truncus arteriosus may be increased 12-fold in the presence of pregestational diabetes mellitus in the mother (Ferencz et al. 1990).

▶ SONOGRAPHIC FINDINGS

Prenatal diagnosis of truncus arteriosus is possible with obstetric sonography and targeted fetal echocardiography. Visualization of the outflow tracts should demonstrate a single large ventricular outflow tract, overriding a VSD (Romero et al. 1988) (Fig. 50-1). The right ventricular outflow tract should be absent, and pulmonary arterial branches may be visible arising from the truncus or from the descending aorta. A distended coronary sinus may also be visible directly posterior to the left atrium (de Araujo et al. 1987). Diagnosis in utero may also be aided by the identification of additional anomalies, such as those involving the aortic arch, as well as by Doppler identification of truncal-valve regurgitation (Marasini et al. 1987). Truncus arteriosus may also lead to the development of congestive heart failure in utero, leading to the typical sonographic features of hydrops.

A transverse view through the upper fetal mediastinum, which normally contains the main pulmonary artery, ascending aorta, and superior vena cava, should demonstrate only two vessels in cases of truncus arteriosus (Yoo et al. 1997). The importance of visualization of the outflow tracts is evident from one series of six cases of prenatally diagnosed truncus arteriosus in which only two of the six cases were detected with the four-chamber cardiac view (Paladini et al. 1996). The remaining four cases were detected using a combination of four-chamber and outflow-tract views.

▶ DIFFERENTIAL DIAGNOSIS

Differentiation between truncus arteriosus and tetralogy of Fallot (see Chapter 55) with coexisting pulmonary atresia may be extremely difficult because both have virtually identical sonographic appearances. Visualization of pulmonary arteries arising from the back of the truncus and the presence of more than three leaflets in the truncal valve may aid in the correct diagnosis (Houston et al. 1981). Truncus arteriosus may also be difficult to differentiate from aorticopulmonary window, in which the clinical features of truncus are present, but without a VSD and with a normal pulmonary valve (Graham and Gutgesell 1990; Riggs and Paul 1982).

▶ ANTENATAL NATURAL HISTORY

Few reports of the antenatal natural history of truncus arteriosus are available. In one series of six cases diagnosed prenatally, three pregnancies were terminated, two cases resulted in neonatal death, and one fetus survived (Paladini et al. 1996). The antenatal development of hydrops is rare with truncus arteriosus, as the relatively high fetal pulmonary vascular resistance prevents the development of significant ventricular dysfunction.

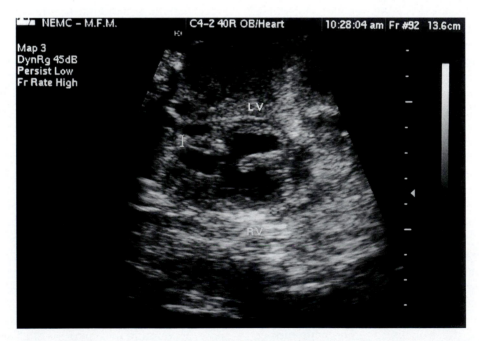

Figure 50-1. Prenatal sonographic image of a fetus with truncus arteriosus, demonstrating a large single outflow tract that appears to override the interventricular septum. LV = left ventricle; RV = right ventricle.

Immediately after delivery, however, the drop in pulmonary vascular resistance leads to significantly increased pulmonary flow, truncal-valve insufficiency, and ventricular dysfunction. Development of congestive heart failure in utero is likely only if significant truncal-valve dysplasia and obstruction are present.

▶ MANAGEMENT OF PREGNANCY

Once the diagnosis of truncus arteriosus is suspected on a prenatal sonographic image, referral to a tertiary-care center is recommended for a thorough targeted sonographic evaluation as well as fetal echocardiography by an appropriately trained specialist. Prospective parents should meet with a pediatric cardiologist. Attention should be paid to the potential presence of additional cardiac malformations, as well as the possibility of heterotaxy syndrome. It is unclear if a prenatal karyotype is indicated, as only small case series of truncus arteriosus are available for review. In one series, only 1 of 22 infants with truncus arteriosus had a chromosomal abnormality (Ferencz et al. 1987). In another series of 6 cases of truncus arteriosus, 1 infant was found to have trisomy 18 (Paladini et al. 1996). In addition, in one case report of prenatally diagnosed truncus arteriosus the fetus had trisomy 13 (de Araujo et al. 1987). Therefore, from a total of 29 cases (23 infants and 6 fetuses) of truncus arteriosus 3 cases, or almost 10%, had chromosomal abnormalities, which may be sufficient to warrant recommending invasive prenatal karyotype evaluation. Furthermore, DiGeorge syndrome is associated with conotruncal cardiac anomalies. DiGeorge syndrome can be diagnosed prenatally by use of a fluorescence in situ hybridization probe for chromosome 22q11 (Fig. 50-2). All patients undergoing prenatal karyotyping should have fluorescence in situ hybridization studies included for the 22q11 microdeletion. If a chromosome abnormality or DiGeorge syndrome is diagnosed, the prospective parents should meet with a medical geneticist.

After prenatal diagnosis, serial evaluation with obstetric ultrasonography is recommended to confirm adequate fetal growth and to exclude the development of congestive heart failure. Infants with this condition can deteriorate rapidly as pulmonary vascular resistance falls after birth. Therefore, delivery of the fetus with truncus arteriosus should occur at a tertiary-care center, with the immediate availability of a neonatologist, pediatric cardiologist, and pediatric cardiothoracic surgeon. The timing and route of delivery should not be changed by the diagnosis of truncus arteriosus. The onset of spontaneous labor should be awaited, and cesarean delivery should be reserved for standard obstetric indications. It is unclear if intervention with early or cesarean delivery is of any benefit when the diagnosis is com-

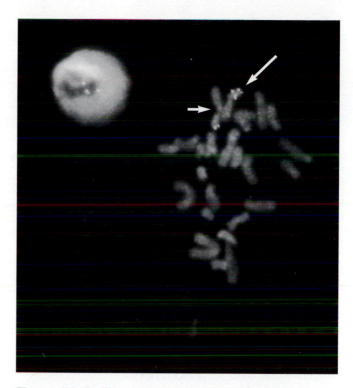

Figure 50-2. Fluorescence in situ hybridization studies using a DNA probe specific to DiGeorge region. The long arrow indicates chromosome 22 with distal flanking marker and presence of DiGeorge probe. The short arrow indicates the other chromosome 22 with distal flanking probe but absent DiGeorge probe. This is diagnostic for a microdeletion of chromosome 22. (Courtesy of Janet Cowan.)

plicated by the presence of hydrops. The prognosis in such cases is almost always poor, irrespective of obstetric interventions (Romero et al. 1988).

▶ FETAL INTERVENTION

No fetal intervention has been described following the prenatal diagnosis of truncus arteriosus.

▶ TREATMENT OF THE NEWBORN

Immediately following delivery, the newborn with truncus arteriosus should have an evaluation by a pediatric cardiologist, including an echocardiographic examination to confirm the diagnosis and to exclude the presence of additional cardiac malformations. If complete visualization of cardiac and major-vessel anatomy is not obtained with echocardiography, cardiac catheterization may be required, with particular attention paid to the branching pattern of the pulmonary arteries, the anatomy of the aorta, and the presence of truncal insufficiency (Graham and Gutgesell 1990).

Progressive congestive heart failure is likely to occur soon after delivery because pulmonary vascular resistance falls, often as early as 1 or 2 weeks after birth. Coronary-artery perfusion may also be compromised, which, in combination with postnatal increased myocardial oxygen demand, may predispose to subendocardial ischemia (Graham and Gutgesell 1990). To stabilize congestive heart failure during the newborn period, aggressive medical therapy is required, including the use of diuretics and digoxin. Medical therapy is often inadequate to prevent further deterioration of cardiac failure in these patients. Early intervention with definitive surgical repair may be the only option to prevent worsening cardiac failure and also to prevent the development of pulmonary hypertension secondary to increased pulmonary flow. Delaying surgical repair may also lead to the development of chronic ventricular dysfunction secondary to volume overload, which may compromise later repair (Graham 1982).

▶ SURGICAL TREATMENT

Surgical palliation of truncus arteriosus by means of pulmonary artery banding in an effort to reduce pulmonary flow and prevent the development of irreversible pulmonary hypertension has yielded disappointing results. In one series of 15 cases of pulmonary artery banding for truncus arteriosus during infancy the overall mortality rate was 73%, with all but one death occurring soon after surgery (Singh et al. 1976). Early definitive surgical repair of truncus arteriosus now seems to be the treatment of choice (Graham and Gutgesell 1990).

The standard surgical procedure for repair of truncus arteriosus involves placing a homograft between the right ventricle and the pulmonary artery and closing the VSD. This leaves the left ventricle in continuity with the truncus leading to the aorta. Hospital mortality for this procedure has been quoted as almost 30%, although the reported series often span a long period, include patients with many complicating factors, and use a valveless conduit (Di Donato et al. 1985; Spicer et al. 1984). More recent data, from a procedure in which a valved conduit was used, have demonstrated better results, with hospital mortality rates ranging from 11 to 17% of cases (Ebert et al. 1984; Pearl et al. 1992). Increased mortality occurs if significant truncal-valve insufficiency is present, and in such cases a truncal-valve replacement or truncal-valve repair is generally also performed (Elami et al. 1994). Other risk factors for early death include the presence of coronary-artery anomalies, interrupted aortic arch, and age greater than 100 days at repair (Hanley et al. 1993). In infants with simple truncus arteriosus repaired within the first 100 days of life the operative mortality was 0% (Hanley et al. 1993).

▶ LONG-TERM OUTCOME

The most common long-term complication following surgical repair of truncus arteriosus is the requirement for replacement of the right ventricle–pulmonary artery conduit because of body growth or development of pseudointimal proliferation within the conduit. Conduit replacement may be required in up to 60% of long-term survivors (Ebert et al. 1984). Reoperation may be associated with a further 4 to 7% risk of mortality (Pearl et al. 1992). Late deaths following contemporary surgical repair are uncommon, with only 3 late deaths in a series of 89 hospital survivors following repair; 2 of these 3 deaths were unrelated to the underlying cardiac condition (Ebert et al. 1984). The quality of life following surgical repair appears to be excellent, with 97% of patients in one series being very functional (Di Donato et al. 1985).

▶ GENETICS AND RECURRENCE RISK

Truncus arteriosus may occur as part of the spectrum of the DiGeorge sequence. In a series of 26 infants with truncus arteriosus, a high prevalence of facial dysmorphism, aortic-arch abnormalities, and immunodeficiency possibly consistent with DiGeorge sequence was noted (Radford et al. 1988). Familial clustering of truncus arteriosus is rare, with one case report of the abnormality recurring in a subsequent pregnancy and one case report of dizygotic twins concordant for the abnormality (Ferry et al. 1994; Lang et al. 1991). Generalized estimates of recurrence risk suggest a 1% rate of recurrence if one previous sibling has been affected and 3% if two siblings have been affected (Nora and Nora 1988). If chromosomal analysis was not performed prenatally, it should be performed postnatally with fluorescence in situ hybridization studies for a microdeletion of chromosome 22q11. In some cases, the microdeletion is inherited from one of the parents, who may not have cardiac disease. Diagnosis of DiGeorge syndrome in an infant necessitates study of the parental karyotypes before accurate recurrence risk counseling can be given.

REFERENCES

Bharati S, McAllister HA, Rosenquist GC, et al. The surgical anatomy of truncus arteriosus communis. J Thorac Cardiovasc Surg 1974;67:501–510.

Collett RW, Edwards JE. Persistent truncus arteriosus: a classification according to anatomic types. Surg Clin North Am 1949;29:1245–1270.

de Araujo LM, Schmidt KG, Silverman NH, et al. Prenatal detection of truncus arteriosus by ultrasound. Pediatr Cardiol 1987;8:261–263.

Di Donato RM, Fyfe DA, Puga FJ, et al. Fifteen-year experience with surgical repair of truncus arteriosus. J Thorac Cardiovasc Surg 1985;89:414–422.

Ebert PA, Turley K, Stanger P, et al. Surgical treatment of truncus arteriosus in the first 6 months of life. Ann Surg 1984;200:451–456.

Elami A, Laks H, Pearl JM. Truncal valve repair: initial experience with infants and children. Ann Thorac Surg 1994;57:397–402.

Ferencz C, Rubin JD, McCarter RJ, et al. Cardiac and noncardiac malformations: observations in a population-based study. Teratology 1987;35:367–378.

Ferencz C, Rubin JD, McCarter RJ, et al. Maternal diabetes and cardiovascular malformations: predominance of double outlet right ventricle and truncus arteriosus. Teratology 1990;41:319–326.

Ferry P, Massias C, Salzard C, et al. Recurrence of common truncus arteriosus: prenatal diagnosis of a case report. J Gynecol Obstet Biol Reprod 1994;23:696–700.

Fyler DC, Buckley LP, Hellenbrand WE, et al. Report of the New England Regional Cardiac Program. Pediatrics 1980; 65(suppl):375–461.

Graham TP. Ventricular performance in adults after operation for congenital heart disease. Am J Cardiol 1982;50: 612–620.

Graham TP, Gutgesell HP. Conotruncal abnormalities. In: Long WA, ed. Fetal and neonatal cardiology. Philadelphia: Saunders, 1990:561–570.

Hanley FL, Heinemann MK, Jonas RA, et al. Repair of truncus arteriosus in the neonate. J Thorac Cardiovasc Surg 1993;105:1047–1055.

Houston AB, Gregory NL, Murtagh E, et al. Two-dimensional echocardiography in infants with persistent truncus arteriosus. Br Heart J 1981;46:492–497.

Lang MJ, Aughton DJ, Riggs TW, et al. Dizygotic twins concordant for truncus arteriosus. Clin Genet 1991;39:75–79.

Marasini M, Cordone M, Zampatti C, et al. Prenatal ultrasonic detection of truncus arteriosus with interrupted aortic arch and truncal valve regurgitation. Eur Heart J 1987;8:921–924.

Nora JJ, Nora AH. Update on counseling the family with a first-degree relative with a congenital heart defect. Am J Med Genet 1988;29:137–142.

Paladini D, Rustico M, Todros T, et al. Conotruncal anomalies in prenatal life. Ultrasound Obstet Gynecol 1996;8: 241–246.

Pearl JM, Laks H, Drinkwater DC, et al. Repair of conotruncal abnormalities with the use of the valved conduit: improved early and midterm results with the cryopreserved homograft. J Am Coll Cardiol 1992;20:191–196.

Radford DJ, Perkins L, Lachman R, et al. Spectrum of DiGeorge syndrome in patients with truncus arteriosus: expanded DiGeorge syndrome. Pediatr Cardiol 1988;9: 95–101.

Riggs TW, Paul MH: Two-dimensional echocardiographic prospective diagnosis of common truncus arteriosus in infants. Am J Cardiol 1982;50:1380–1384.

Romero R, Pilu G, Jeanty P, et al. Truncus arteriosus. In: Romero R, Pilu G, Jeanty P, Ghidini A, Hobbins JC, eds. Prenatal diagnosis of congenital anomalies. Norwalk, CT: Appleton & Lange, 1988:168–171.

Singh AK, DeLeval MR, Pincott JR, et al. Pulmonary artery banding for truncus arteriosus in the first year of life. Circulation 1976;54(suppl):III17–III19.

Spicer RL, Behrendt D, Crowley DC, et al. Repair of truncus arteriosus in neonates with the use of a valveless conduit. Circulation 1984;70:126–129.

Van Praagh R, Van Praagh S. The anatomy of common aorticopulmonary trunk (truncus arteriosus communis) and its embryologic implications: a study of 57 necropsy cases. Am J Cardiol 1965;16:406–426.

Yoo SJ, Lee YH, Kim ES, et al. Three-vessel view of the fetal upper mediastinum: an easy means of detecting abnormalities of the ventricular outflow tracts and great arteries during obstetric screening. Ultrasound Obstet Gynecol 1997;9:173–182.

CHAPTER 51

Hypoplastic Left and Right Ventricles

► CONDITION

Hypoplastic Left Ventricle

Hypoplastic left ventricle, also known as hypoplastic left heart syndrome (HLHS), is a condition in which there is congenital hypoplasia of the left ventricle, atresia of the aortic and mitral valves, and hypoplasia of the aortic arch. Each of the components of HLHS may occur with varying degrees of severity, ranging from aortic stenosis with a small left ventricle to complete aortic and mitral atresia with a slit-like left ventricular remnant. Hypoplastic left ventricle and mitral atresia may also occur without aortic atresia, but such an anomaly is rare (Kiel 1990). The cause of HLHS is unknown, but it may be due to abnormal intracardiac streaming during weeks 5 to 8 of embryonic life (Harh et al. 1973). HLHS may also evolve during prenatal life from isolated severe aortic stenosis, which may result in decreased right-to-left shunting between the atria, and subsequent hypoplasia of the left ventricle (Sharland et al. 1991).

Associated cardiac anomalies are common with HLHS. Left-to-right shunting occurs in the newborn, returning oxygenated blood from the pulmonary veins through a patent foramen ovale into the right atrium. The right ventricle provides both pulmonary and systemic circulations, the latter through a patent ductus arteriosus with retrograde flow to the aortic arch and coronary vessels. The mitral valve is hypoplastic; the tricuspid valve is often large and regurgitant. The aortic outflow tract usually ends blindly below the coronary arteries, and the aortic valve and arch are hypoplastic. Coarctation of the aorta is present in 80% of cases (Hawkins and Doty 1984). Other associated cardiac anomalies include ventricular septal defect, aortic-arch interruption, and transposition of the great vessels (Kiel 1990). Central nervous system malformations have also been described in association with HLHS, including microcephaly, holoprosencephaly, and agenesis of the corpus callosum (Sanders et al. 1996).

Hypoplastic Right Ventricle

Hypoplastic right ventricle (HRV) is also known as pulmonary atresia with intact ventricular septum (PA:IVS). The normally formed right ventricle becomes hypoplastic, in association with pulmonary atresia, and occasionally tricuspid atresia. The competence of the tricuspid valve determines the size of the right ventricle, with type I HRV being associated with a competent valve and small ventricle and type II HRV being associated with an incompetent valve and normal or large right ventricle (Romero et al. 1988). Blood flows from the right to the left atria through the foramen ovale, and the left ventricle supplies both systemic and pulmonary circulations, the latter by retrograde flow through the ductus arteriosus. Additional cardiac malformations that may coexist include atrial and ventricular septal defects and transposition of the great vessels.

► INCIDENCE

Hypoplastic Left Ventricle

HLHS accounts for up to 9% of all cases of congenital heart disease, with an incidence of 1 in 10,000 live births (Kiel 1990). Twice as many males as females are affected.

Hypoplastic Right Ventricle

Hypoplastic right ventricle is extremely rare, accounting for only 1 in 144,000 live births and for less than 3% of all cases of congenital heart disease diagnosed during the first year of life (Fyler et al. 1980).

▶ SONOGRAPHIC FINDINGS

Hypoplastic Left Ventricle

HLHS is generally easy to detect prenatally by means of the standard four-chamber cardiac view. This should demonstrate an inequality in ventricle size, with the left ventricular cavity often appearing as a small remnant to the left of the right ventricle (Fig. 51-1) (Silverman et al. 1984). The left ventricular wall may be hypocontractile or immobile and may also appear echogenic (Kluckow et al. 1993). The apex of the left ventricle will usually end more proximally than the right ventricular apex, and the ventricular cavity may be in a globular shape rather than in the normal elliptical shape. The right ventricular cavity is often enlarged, and the left atrium is usually small, with left-to-right bowing of the interatrial septum (Sanders et al. 1996). The aortic outflow tract will be atretic, with hypoplasia of the ascending aorta. However, the aortic arch and descending aorta should be visible because of retrograde filling through the ductus arteriosus. Doppler echocardiography may also be helpful in demonstratiing a lack of antegrade flow into the left ventricle, abnormal flow

through the foramen ovale, and retrograde flow in the ascending aorta (Blake et al. 1991).

Even though these findings should be detectable at 18 to 20 weeks of gestation, it is possible that isolated aortic stenosis may evolve over time into HLHS, so that the typical features of HLHS may not become visible until the third trimester (Sharland et al. 1991). The detection rate of prenatal ultrasonography for HLHS is unclear in the general population, although in one series, 28% of all cases of HLHS were detected prenatally (Montana et al. 1996). However, the positive predictive value of prenatal ultrasonography for HLHS is high, with up to 95% of cases of prenatally diagnosed HLHS confirmed on postnatal examination (Chang et al. 1991).

Hypoplastic Right Ventricle

Prenatal diagnosis of hypoplastic right ventricle is relatively straightforward if there is a significant disproportion in size between the two ventricular cavities (Fig. 51-2) (McGahan et al. 1991). However, if the right ventricle is normal in size, prenatal diagnosis may be extremely difficult, relying on the identification of isolated pulmonary atresia (Romero et al. 1988). While the right ventricular cavity is usually very small, the right ventricular wall is often hypertrophied (Grundy et al. 1987). Although adequate visualization of the right ventricular outflow tract may be difficult, Doppler echocardiography may demonstrate absence of flow across the pulmonary valve. As with HLHS, the diagnosis of hypoplastic right ventricle may not be clear at an initial second-trimester

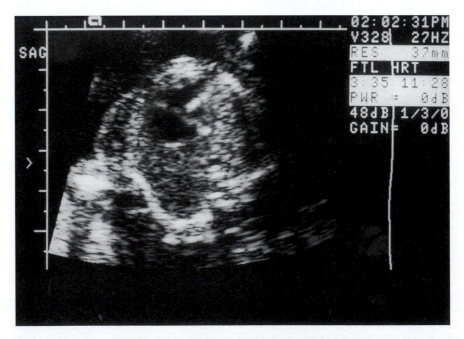

Figure 51-1. Prenatal sonographic image of the low-chamber cardiac view in a fetus with hypoplastic left heart syndrome, demonstrating a very small left ventricle in comparison with the size of the right ventricle.

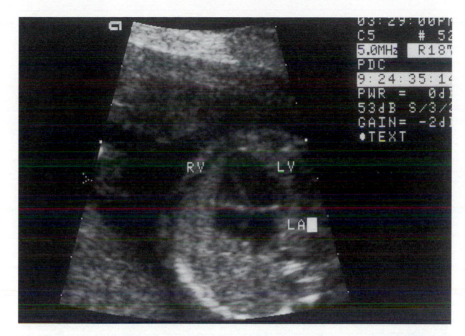

Figure 51-2. Antenatal low-chamber cardiac view in a fetus with hypoplastic right heart syndrome, demonstrating a disproportionally small right ventricle. RV= right ventricle; LV = left ventricle; LA = left atrium.

ultrasound examination, but instead may evolve over time so that true hypoplasia may not be visible until late in the third trimester (Hornberger et al. 1996).

▶ DIFFERENTIAL DIAGNOSIS

Hypoplastic Left Ventricle

Other conditions that should be included in the differential diagnosis of HLHS include left-sided cardiac masses, aortic stenosis, and univentricular heart (Sanders et al. 1996). Large cardiac masses, such as rhabdomyomas (see Chapter 53), may completely obliterate the left ventricular cavity, thus mimicking HLHS. However, normal ventricular dimensions will be present, and Doppler echocardiography should demonstrate normal flow through the mitral and aortic valves (Fig. 51-3). Severe aortic stenosis may be difficult to differentiate from HLHS because complete obliteration of the left ventricle may occur as the stenosis worsens (see Chapter 42). It is possible that aortic stenosis in early fetal life may actually progress to hypoplastic left ventricle as gestation advances (Sharland et al. 1991). Differentiation should be possible based on Doppler echocardiography demonstrating antegrade flow in the ascending aorta with aortic stenosis, as compared with retrograde flow in HLHS. Univentricular heart is a condition in which the entire atrioventricular junction is connected to a single ventricle. There is little agreement on the precise definition of univentricular heart, which makes prenatal differentiation difficult.

Hypoplastic Right Ventricle

The differential diagnosis of hypoplastic right ventricle is similar to that for HLHS and includes right-sided cardiac masses, pulmonary stenosis, and univentricular heart. Doppler echocardiography may be helpful in demonstrating absence of antegrade flow through the pulmonary valve, therefore confirming the presence of complete pulmonary atresia.

▶ ANTENATAL HISTORY

Hypoplastic Left Ventricle

Hypoplastic left heart syndrome may evolve in utero from critical aortic stenosis (Kluckow et al. 1993; Sharland et al. 1991). The precise antenatal natural history of HLHS is therefore very variable. This malformation has several degrees of severity, ranging from critical aortic stenosis with normal left ventricular size to complete atresia of the aortic and mitral valves with near absence of the left ventricle. In the vast majority of cases diagnosed prior to 24 weeks of gestation, termination of pregnancy is elected. In a series of 77 cases of HLHS diagnosed prior to 24 weeks, 72 resulted in termination of the pregnancy (Allan et al. 1991).

Expectant management of prenatally diagnosed HLHS is associated with a poor prognosis. In 1 series of 20 cases of prenatally diagnosed HLHS, 9 pregnancies were terminated (Blake et al. 1991). Four of the 11 expectantly managed pregnancies resulted in intrauterine

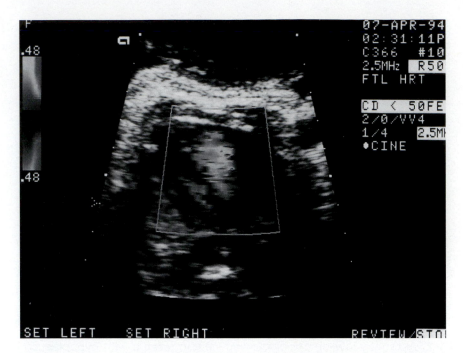

Figure 51-3. Doppler study from a fetus with hypoplastic left and right ventricles. Doppler studies are helpful in working through the differential diagnosis. *(Courtesy of Dr. Marjorie C. Treadwell.)* **See color plate.**

fetal death, 7 resulted in live births, and 5 of these 7 infants died within 1 week of birth. Intra-uterine congestive heart failure may occur with HLHS because of right ventricular overload. In 1 series, nonimmune hydrops developed in 4 of 20 cases of prenatally diagnosed HLHS. Only 1 of these cases resulted in a liveborn infant, following administration of digoxin to the mother (Blake et al. 1991).

Hypoplastic Right Ventricle

Congestive heart failure can often develop in utero with hypoplastic right ventricle because of significant tricuspid regurgitation. However, there are no large series of prenatally diagnosed hypoplastic right ventricle that allow accurate prediction of antenatal history.

Hypoplastic Right Ventricle

No fetal intervention has been described for the management of hypoplastic right ventricle.

▶ MANAGEMENT OF PREGNANCY

Hypoplastic Left Ventricle

Following prenatal diagnosis of HLHS, a careful sonographic fetal anatomy survey is recommended to exclude additional cardiac and extracardiac malformations. This evaluation should include a search for sonographic markers of Turner syndrome and trisomies 13, 18, and 21. Fetal echocardiography should be performed by an appropriately trained specialist to confirm the diagnosis and to exclude other cardiac malformations. Invasive fetal testing for karyotype analysis is recommended because of the association between HLHS and chromosomal abnormalities. Chromosomal abnormalities were found in 2 of 85 cases of HLHS in infants in one study (Ferencz et al. 1987) and in 9 of 83 cases in a later study, including trisomies 13, 18, and 21 (Natowicz et al. 1988). In a series of 20 cases of HLHS diagnosed prenatally, one fetus also had trisomy 13 and 2 had Turner syndrome (Blake et al. 1991). Referral for prenatal consultation with a pediatric cardiologist, and cardiothoracic surgeon is also recommended.

If the diagnosis is made prior to fetal viability, termination of pregnancy may be offered because of the significant neonatal mortality and surgical morbidity. If expectant management is desired, sonographic surveillance to confirm appropriate fetal growth and to evaluate for the development of fetal hydrops is recommended. If fetal hydrops occurs, the prognosis deteriorates further, and the optimal management of such pregnancies is uncertain. Administration of digoxin to the mother has been reported for fetal hydrops secondary to HLHS in a twin pregnancy (Blake et al. 1991). Delivery should occur at a tertiary-care center, with the immediate availability of a neonatologist, pediatric cardiologist, and cardiothoracic surgeon. There is no indication to alter the timing or method of delivery based on the prenatal diagnosis of HLHS. In one series of 13 cases of HLHS, all spontaneous or induced labors resulted in normal vaginal deliveries, and there was only one case of an abnormal fetal heart rate pattern (Jackson et al. 1991). Routine labor management therefore does not need to be modified when the fetus has HLHS.

Hypoplastic Right Ventricle

As with HLHS, following the prenatal diagnosis of hypoplastic right ventricle a careful sonographic fetal anatomy survey is recommended to exclude additional cardiac and extracardiac malformations. Fetal echocardiography should be performed by an appropriately trained specialist to confirm the diagnosis and to exclude other cardiac malformations. It is unclear if invasive fetal testing for karyotype analysis is needed, because in one series of 48 cases of tricuspid or pulmonary atresia there were no chromosomal abnormalities (Ferencz et al. 1987). There may be a higher prevalence of chromosomal abnormalities in fetuses with prenatally diagnosed right ventricular hypoplasia, although there are no series available to confirm the need for karyotype analysis.

Referral for prenatal consultation with a pediatric cardiologist and cardiothoracic surgeon is also recommended. If the diagnosis is made prior to fetal viability, termination of pregnancy may be offered because of the significant neonatal mortality and surgical morbidity. If expectant management is desired, sonographic surveillance to confirm appropriate fetal growth and to evaluate for the development of fetal hydrops is recommended. If fetal hydrops occurs, the prognosis deteriorates further, and the optimal management of such pregnancies is uncertain. Delivery should occur at a tertiary-care center, with the immediate availability of a neonatologist, pediatric cardiologist, and cardiothoracic surgeon. There is no indication to alter the timing or method of delivery based on the prenatal diagnosis of hypoplastic right ventricle.

▶ FETAL INTERVENTION

Hypoplastic Left Ventricle

The only fetal intervention that has been described for HLHS is maternal administration of digoxin in a case of HLHS complicated by nonimmune hydrops (Blake et al. 1991). In utero balloon dilation has been described for critical aortic stenosis (see Chapter 42), but if the stenosis has progressed to the development of HLHS it is unlikely that such an intervention will be of any benefit.

▶ TREATMENT OF THE NEWBORN

Hypoplastic Left Ventricle

All infants with HLHS will die soon after birth without surgical intervention. For many years the options for surgery were limited and, when available, the outcome from surgical intervention was very poor. Because of this poor prognosis, comfort care without aggressive resuscitation efforts has become a common method of treatment for infants with HLHS. The provision of comfort measures only has been challenged recently as more centers become skilled in surgical palliation of HLHS and as survival from such surgery has improved (O'Kelly and Bove 1997). Decisions regarding the aggressiveness of treatment for newborns with HLHS should be made during the antenatal period, and, depending on the results from the local pediatric cardiothoracic surgery center, such decisions should include options for surgical intervention and provision of only comfort care (Thwaites 1997).

Following delivery of an infant with HLHS, supplemental oxygen should be administered judiciously so as to avoid significant reduction in pulmonary vascular resistance, which may decrease the amount of blood shunted across the ductus arteriosus. The infant should be transported to a neonatal intensive care unit, and prostaglandin E_1 infusion should be started as soon as feasible to maintain patency of the ductus arteriosus. Other supportive measures that are essential include correction of metabolic acidosis and use of inotropic agents, such as dopamine, to maintain adequate cardiac output. If inadequate atrial communication is present, efforts to maximize cardiac output by balloon atrial septostomy may be considered during the initial resuscitative efforts (Kiel 1990).

Postnatal consultation with a pediatric cardiologist should be obtained promptly, and echocardiography should be performed to confirm the prenatal diagnosis and to exclude additional cardiac malformations. Echocardiography should document patency of the ductus, presence of coarctation, size of an atrial septal defect, and presence of significant tricuspid regurgitation (Sanders et al. 1996). Consultation with a pediatric cardiothoracic surgeon should then be obtained to decide on timing and method of surgical intervention.

Hypoplastic Right Ventricle

As with HLHS, care should be taken with the administration of supplemental oxygen to an infant with hypoplastic right ventricle, so as to avoid significant reduction in pulmonary vascular resistance, which may decrease the amount of blood shunted across the ductus arteriosus. The infant should be transported to a neonatal intensive care unit, and prostaglandin E_1 infusion should be started as soon as possible to increase blood flow across the ductus arteriosus. If inadequate atrial communication is present, balloon atrial septostomy may be considered to maximize cardiac output during the initial treatment phase. Consultation with a pediatric cardiologist should be obtained promptly, and echocardiography should be performed to confirm the prenatal diagnosis and to exclude additional cardiac malformations. Echocardiography should document patency of the ductus, size of the right ventricular cavity, and size of the tricuspid annulus. Consultation with a pediatric cardiothoracic surgeon should then be obtained to decide on timing and method of surgical intervention.

▶ SURGICAL TREATMENT

Hypoplastic Left Ventricle

All infants with HLHS will require surgical intervention to permit postnatal survival. Contraindications to surgery include a decision by parents to receive comfort care only or the presence of significant hemodynamic instability, such as severe hypoperfusion, metabolic acidosis, or coagulopathy. These conditions should be aggressively corrected prior to surgical intervention. Two surgical choices are present for infants with HLHS: the Norwood three-stage procedure and neonatal cardiac transplantation.

The Norwood procedure is a complex operation, the precise surgical details of which are beyond the scope of this chapter. The first of the three stages is performed as soon as possible after birth and after initial medical stabilization. This first stage involves ligation of the ductus arteriosus, anastomosis of the transected proximal pulmonary artery to the ascending aorta, and an atrial septectomy (Beeman and Hammon 1990). This maximizes intra-atrial mixing of blood and maintains adequate pulmonary-to-systemic blood flow. In addition, pulmonary blood flow is controlled by constructing a Blalock–Taussig shunt, which anastomoses the subclavian to the pulmonary arteries. If this first stage of palliation is successful, the subsequent two stages are planned as a Fontan-type procedure at 6 to 24 months of age. This consists of an anastomosis from the right atrium to the right pulmonary artery, followed by construction of an atrial baffle to direct systemic venous return to the pulmonary circulation and pulmonary venous return to the tricuspid valve and aorta (Beeman and Hammon 1990).

The results for the Norwood procedure are variable, depending on the institution, operator experience, and modifications to the procedure to account for anatomic variations. The greatest surgical mortality seems to be related to the first stage of the Norwood procedure, with recent surgical mortality rates ranging from 23 to 46% for this first stage (Forbess et al. 1995; Kern et al. 1997). Among 23 patients who completed the second stage of the Norwood procedure, there was only 1 death, and among 12 patients who completed the third stage there was 1 further death (Kern et al. 1997). In one of the largest series from a single center, 120 of 158 patients survived the first stage of surgery, 103 of 106 patients subsequently survived the second stage, and 53 of 62 survived the final stage of the Norwood procedure (Bove and Lloyd 1996).

The alternative surgical management for HLHS is neonatal cardiac transplantation. This may require an initial interventional procedure to stent the ductus arteriosus or to enlarge the interatrial communication. In the largest series of cardiac transplantations as a primary treatment for HLHS, 176 infants were listed for transplantation, 34 of whom (19%) died during the waiting period (Razzouk et al. 1996). Of the 142 infants who underwent successful transplantation in this series, the median age at surgery was 26 days and there was a 9% operative mortality rate.

Hypoplastic Right Ventricle

The choice of surgical procedure for right ventricular hypoplasia depends on the size of the tricuspid valve and the presence of right ventricula–dependent coronary circulation. Because of the significant anatomic variation between patients there is no agreement on a single best surgical approach to right ventricular hypoplasia. Management should be individualized for each infant depending on size and function of the right ventricle as well as on the presence of other abnormalities. Surgical procedures that have been recommended include pulmonary valvotomy, right ventricular outflow-tract reconstruction, or systemic-to-pulmonary shunts using a Fontan or Blalock–Taussig procedure (Armstrong 1995). Depending on the anatomic variation with right ventricular hypoplasia, the operative mortality may range from 27 to 50% (DeLeval et al. 1982).

▶ LONG-TERM OUTCOME

Hypoplastic Left Ventricle

The long-term outcome for infants with HLHS has improved in recent years, with modifications to the original Norwood procedure. In one series of 53 infants operated on from 1990 to 1996 the 5-year actuarial survival was 61% (Kern et al. 1997). In one of the largest series of Norwood procedures from a single center, 5-year actuarial survival was 58% from an initial cohort of 158 infants (Bove and Lloyd 1996). The 5-year actuarial survival for primary neonatal cardiac transplantation was 76% from another initial cohort of 176 infants with HLHS

(Razzouk et al. 1996). However, in this cohort, half of these late deaths were due to organ rejection, and approximately 4% required retransplantation. Although long-term outcome may appear better after transplantation compared with the Norwood procedure, this is tempered by the short supply of suitable neonatal donor hearts and the long-term need for medications to manage organ rejection.

Both survival and long-term outcome data for infants with HLHS should include neurodevelopmental information and quality-of-life outcomes. In one series of 11 survivors of staged repair of HLHS, 64% had major developmental disabilities (Rogers et al. 1995). Conversely, in another series of 14 survivors of pediatric heart transplantation for HLHS or cardiomyopathy, only 1 had a significant neurologic deficit (Lynch et al. 1994). More data are needed to adequately assess the long-term neurologic and quality-of-life outcome for infants following surgical management of HLHS.

Hypoplastic Right Ventricle

Few series are available describing the long-term outcome following surgery for hypoplastic right ventricle. In one series of 17 infants who were treated with both pulmonary valvotomy and systemic–pulmonary shunt, the long-term survival rate was 53% (Moulton et al. 1979). In another series of 60 patients with hypoplastic right ventricle, 5-year actuarial survival was only 36% (DeLeval et al. 1982).

▶ GENETICS AND RECURRENCE RISK

Hypoplastic Left Ventricle

The inheritance pattern for HLHS is not clear, and in the majority of cases it occurs sporadically. HLHS has been reported as an autosomal recessive condition, which would imply a recurrence risk as high as 25% (Grobman and Pergament 1996; Shokeir 1971). Other reports suggest HLHS is inherited in a polygenic pattern, with a recurrence risk of only 2% if one previous sibling was affected (Brownell and Shokeir 1976). The recurrence risk increases to 6% if two previous siblings have been affected by HLHS (Nora and Nora 1988). In another series, a recurrence risk of 13.5% has been quoted for HLHS (Boughman et al. 1987). It is possible that different subsets of HLHS may have different patterns of inheritance, which may explain the wide range of recurrence risks quoted for HLHS (Brenner et al. 1989). If a chromosome abnormality is documented, the recurrence risks are related to the chromosomal findings.

Hypoplastic Right Ventricle

Hypoplastic right ventricle occurs in a sporadic pattern. No recurrence risk data are available for counseling parents with a previously affected infant.

REFERENCES

Allan LD, Cook A, Sullivan I, et al. Hypoplastic left heart syndrome: effects of fetal echocardiography on birth prevalence. Lancet 1991;337:959–961.

Armstrong BE. Congenital cardiovascular disease and cardiac surgery in childhood: Part 1. Cyanotic congenital heart defects. Curr Opin Cardiol 1995;10:58–67.

Beeman SK, Hammon JW. Neonatal left ventricular outflow tract surgery. In: Long WA, ed. Fetal and neonatal cardiology. Philadelphia: Saunders, 1990:760–769.

Blake DM, Copel JA, Kleinman CS: Hypoplastic left heart syndrome: prenatal diagnosis, clinical profile, and management. Am J Obstet Gynecol 1991;165:529–534.

Boughman JA, Berg KA, Astemborski JA, et al. Familial risks of congenital heart defect assessed in a population-based study. Am J Med Genet 1987;26:839–849.

Bove EL, Lloyd TR. Staged reconstruction for hypoplastic left heart syndrome: contemporary results. Ann Surg 1996;224:387–395.

Brenner JI, Berg KA, Schneider DS, et al. Cardiac malformations in relatives of infants with hypoplastic left-heart syndrome. Am J Dis Child 1989;143:1492–1494.

Brownell LG, Shokeir MHK. Inheritance of hypoplastic left heart syndrome: further observations. Clin Genet 1976;9:245–249.

Chang AC, Huhta JC, Yoon GY, et al. Diagnosis, transport, and outcome in fetuses with left ventricular outflow tract obstruction. J Thorac Cardiovasc Surg 1991;102:841–848.

DeLeval M, Bull C, Stark J, et al. Pulmonary atresia and intact ventricular septum: surgical management based on a revised classification. Circulation 1982;66:272–280.

Ferencz C, Rubin JD, McCarter RJ, et al. Cardiac and noncardiac malformations: observations in a population-based study. Teratology 1987;35:367–378.

Forbess JM, Cook N, Roth SJ, et al. Ten-year institutional experience with palliative surgery for hypoplastic left heart syndrome: risk factors related to stage I mortality. Circulation 1995;92:II262–II266.

Fyler DC, Buckley LP, Hellenbrand WE, et al. Report of the New England Regional Cardiac Program. Pediatrics 1980;65:375–461.

Grobman W, Pergament E. Isolated hypoplastic left heart syndrome in three siblings. Obstet Gynecol 1996;88:673–675.

Grundy H, Burlbaw J, Gowdamarajan R, et al. Antenatal detection of hypoplastic right ventricle with fetal M-mode echocardiography: a report of two cases. J Reprod Med 1987;32:301–304.

Harh JY, Paul MH, Gallen WJ, et al. Experimental production of hypoplastic left heart syndrome in the chick embryo. Am J Cardiol 1973;31:51–56.

Hawkins JA, Doty DB. Aortic atresia: morphologic characteristics affecting survival and operative palliation. J Thorac Cardiovasc Surg 1984;88:620–626.

Hornberger LK, Need L, Benacerraf BR. Development of significant left and right ventricular hypoplasia in the second and third trimester fetus. J Ultrasound Med 1996;15:655–659.

Jackson GM, Ludmir J, Castelbaum AJ, et al. Intrapartum course of fetuses with isolated hypoplastic left heart syndrome. Am J Obstet Gynecol 1991;165:1068–1072.

Kern JH, Hayes CJ, Michler RE, et al. Survival and risk factor analysis for the Norwood procedure for hypoplastic left heart syndrome. Am J Cardiol 1997;80:170–174.

Kiel EA. Aortic valve obstruction. In: Long WA, ed. Fetal and neonatal cardiology. Philadelphia: Saunders, 1990: 465–476.

Kluckow MR, Cooper S, Sholler GF. Prenatal diagnosis of hypoplastic left heart syndrome. Aust NZ J Obstet Gynaecol 1993;33:135–139.

Lynch BJ, Glauser TA, Canter C, et al. Neurologic complications of pediatric heart transplantation. Arch Pediatr Adolesc Med 1994;148:973–979.

McGahan JP, Choy M, Parrish MD, et al. Sonographic spectrum of fetal cardiac hypoplasia. J Ultrasound Med 1991; 10:539–546.

Montana E, Khoury MJ, Cragan JD, et al. Trends and outcomes after prenatal diagnosis of congenital cardiac malformations by fetal echocardiography in a well defined birth population, Atlanta, Georgia 1990–1994. J Am Coll Cardiol 1996;28:1805–1809.

Moulton AL, Bowman FO, Edie RN, et al. Pulmonary atresia with intact ventricular septum: sixteen–year experience. J Thorac Cardiovasc Surg 1979;78:527–536.

Natowicz M, Chatten J, Clancy R, et al. Genetic disorders and major extracardiac anomalies associated with the hypoplastic left heart syndrome. Pediatrics 1988;82: 698–706.

Nora JJ, Nora AH. Update on counseling the family with a first-degree relative with a congenital heart defect. Am J Med Genet 1988;29:137–142.

O'Kelly SW, Bove EL. Hypoplastic left heart syndrome: terminal care is not the only option. BMJ 1997;314:87–88.

Razzouk AJ, Chinnock RE, Gundry SR, et al. Transplantation as a primary treatment for hypoplastic left heart syndrome: intermediate-term results. Ann Thorac Surg 1996;62:1–8.

Rogers BT, Msall ME, Buck GM, et al. Neurodevelopmental outcome of infants with hypoplastic left heart syndrome. J Pediatr 1995;126:496–498.

Romero R, Pilu G, Jeanty P, et al. Hypoplastic right ventricle. In: Romero R, Pilu G, Jeanty P, Ghidini A, Hobbins JC, eds. Prenatal diagnosis of congenital anomalies. Norwalk, CT: Appleton & Lange, 1988:155–156.

Sanders RC, Blackmon LR, Hogge WA, et al. Hypoplastic left heart syndrome. In: Sanders RC, Blackmon LR, Hogge WA, Wulfsberg EA, eds. Structural fetal abnormalities: the total picture. St. Louis: Mosby, 1996:73–75.

Sharland GK, Chita SK, Fagg NLK, et al. Left ventricular dysfunction in the fetus: relation to aortic valve anomalies and endocardial fibroelastosis. Br Heart J 1991;66:419–424.

Shokeir MHK. Hypoplastic left heart syndrome: an autosomal recessive disorder. Clin Genet 1971;2:7–14.

Silverman NH, Enderlein MA, Golbus MS. Ultrasonic recognition of aortic valve atresia in utero. Am J Cardiol 1984; 53:391–392.

Thwaites R. Hypoplastic left heart syndrome: quality of life is also important. BMJ 1997;314:1414.

CHAPTER 52

Pulmonic Stenosis and Atresia

▶ CONDITION

The term *pulmonic stenosis* refers to narrowing of the right ventricular outflow tract; *pulmonic atresia* implies complete occlusion of the right ventricular outflow tract. Pulmonic atresia, when associated with an intact ventricular septum, is also known as hypoplastic right ventricle and is described in detail in Chapter 51. Pulmonic atresia with coexistent ventricular septal defect is generally considered as part of the spectrum of tetralogy of Fallot and is described in detail in Chapter 55. Pulmonic stenosis usually results from fusion of the three cusps of the pulmonary valve. Other causes of pulmonic stenosis include narrowing of the infundibular portion of the right ventricular outflow tract, hypoplasia of the pulmonary artery, or pulmonary-valve dysplasia, in which the valve leaflets are thickened and immobile. Pulmonary artery hypoplasia may occur in association with Williams syndrome or with congenital rubella syndrome (Gutgesell 1990). Pulmonary valve dysplasia may occur in association with Noonan syndrome, which has a phenotype similar to Turner syndrome, but a normal karyotype (Mendez and Opitz 1985).

Pulmonic stenosis may lead to right ventricular hypertrophy, a decrease in right ventricular chamber size, and poststenotic dilation of the pulmonary artery (Romero et al. 1988). Poststenotic dilation of the pulmonary artery is rarely present in utero and usually takes several months of neonatal life to develop (Gutgesell 1990). In cases of critical pulmonic stenosis, hypoplasia of the right ventricular cavity may occur together with hypertrophy of the ventricular wall and dilation of the right atrium. In such cases, neonates usually have an interatrial communication through either a patent foramen ovale or a secundum atrial septal defect. Other associated cardiac defects that may be seen with pulmonic stenosis include ventricular septal defect, total

anomalous pulmonary venous return, and aortic stenosis (Romero et al. 1988).

▶ INCIDENCE

Pulmonic stenosis is a relatively common congenital cardiac defect, and in many mild forms the diagnosis may not be made until late in childhood. The incidence of congenital pulmonic stenosis is approximately 1 in 1500 live births (Mitchell et al. 1971). This lesion may account for 5% to 10% of all pediatric cardiology patients at tertiary-care centers (Gutgesell 1990).

▶ SONOGRAPHIC FINDINGS

Prenatal sonographic features of congenital pulmonic stenosis include decreased size of the right ventricular chamber, thickening of the right ventricular walls, right atrial enlargement, increased diameter of the pulmonary artery, thickening of the pulmonary valve, and incomplete valvular opening (Fig. 52-1). However, several of these features may be extremely difficult, if not impossible, to demonstrate reliably with two-dimensional echocardiography in the fetus. Duplex and color flow Doppler sonography may be used in the prenatal diagnosis of pulmonic stenosis to demonstrate poststenotic turbulence of flow in the pulmonary artery as well as significant tricuspid regurgitation. The demonstration of reversed flow across the fetal ductus is also suggestive of severe pulmonic stenosis or atresia and in one study was found in all 7 fetuses with this prenatal diagnosis (Mielke et al. 1997).

The ability of routine prenatal sonography to detect pulmonic stenosis or atresia in unselected populations seems limited. In the largest study evaluating the

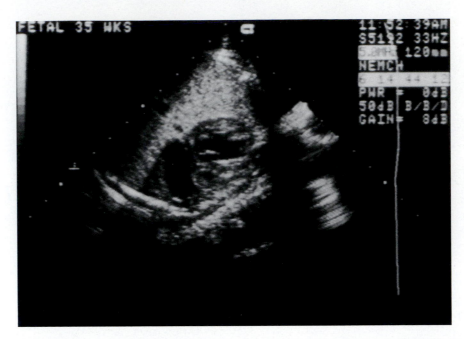

Figure 52-1. Prenatal sonographic image at 35 weeks of gestation, demonstrating pulmonic atresia with intact ventricular septum.

prenatal detection rates for various congenital cardiac malformations, only 9 of 180 cases of pulmonic stenosis or atresia were detected prenatally (Montana et al. 1996). In another series of 11,984 fetuses examined by prenatal sonography, there were 19 cases of pulmonic stenosis or atresia of varying severity, only two of which were detected prenatally (Tegnander et al. 1995). However, if the diagnosis of pulmonic stenosis or atresia is made by targeted prenatal sonography, it appears to be accurate, with all 7 cases in 1 series confirmed on postnatal examination (Mielke et al. 1997). In another series of 12 cases of prenatally diagnosed pulmonic stenosis or atresia, the four-chamber view was abnormal in all cases, and 10 of the 12 cases were confirmed on postnatal examination (Hornberger et al. 1994). Another problem in prenatal diagnosis of pulmonic stenosis is the possibility of late appearance of the typical sonographic features, which may lead to the diagnosis being missed during an 18- to 20-week fetal anatomy survey (Todros et al. 1988).

▶ DIFFERENTIAL DIAGNOSIS

Differentiation of pulmonic stenosis from pulmonic atresia through the use of prenatal sonography is difficult, with the only reliable feature allowing differentiation being the presence of antegrade pulmonary blood flow in pulmonic stenosis. In cases of pulmonic stenosis without documented antegrade pulmonary flow it may be impossible to differentiate prenatally between stenosis and atresia (Hornberger et al. 1994). Tetralogy of Fallot should be considered in the differential diagnosis of all cases of pulmonic stenosis or atresia. Hypertrophy of the right ventricular walls is almost always present in both isolated pulmonic stenosis and tetralogy of Fallot. The presence of a ventricular septal defect and an overriding aorta, together with the sonographic features of pulmonic stenosis should be sufficient to lead to the diagnosis of tetralogy of Fallot.

▶ ANTENATAL NATURAL HISTORY

Pulmonic stenosis may evolve in utero, leading to hypoplasia of the right ventricle or to worsening tricuspid regurgitation and congestive heart failure or hydrops (Romero et al. 1988). Few data are available describing the antenatal natural history of pulmonic stenosis or atresia. In a series of 222 cases of prenatally diagnosed cardiac malformations that were managed expectantly, there were 4 cases of pulmonic stenosis and 9 cases of pulmonic atresia (Sharland et al. 1990). All 4 fetuses with pulmonic stenosis survived through the neonatal period. However, 2 of the 9 fetuses with pulmonic atresia died in utero, and 2 more died during the neonatal period. In another series of 3 fetuses with pulmonic stenosis and 3 with pulmonic atresia managed expectantly, 1 fetus with pulmonic atresia died in utero (Smythe et al. 1992).

► MANAGEMENT OF PREGNANCY

Following prenatal diagnosis of pulmonic stenosis or atresia, careful assessment of the remainder of the fetal anatomy survey is recommended to rule out associated cardiac and noncardiac malformations. Fetal echocardiography should be performed by an appropriately trained specialist to confirm the prenatal diagnosis and to exclude additional cardiac malformations such as ventricular septal defect, total anomalous pulmonary venous return, and aortic stenosis. Referral for prenatal consultation with a pediatric cardiologist and neonatologist is recommended.

Invasive testing to evaluate the fetal karyotype is generally recommended for most cases of prenatally diagnosed cardiac malformations, although the incidence of chromosomal abnormalities with isolated pulmonic stenosis or atresia is low. In 1 series of 105 infants with pulmonic stenosis there was only 1 abnormal karyotype (Ferencz et al. 1987). In another series of 7 fetuses with pulmonic stenosis or atresia, 1 fetus had a balanced translocation that was also present in the mother (Mielke et al. 1997). In a further series of 3 fetuses with pulmonary atresia and ventricular septal defect, 1 fetus had trisomy 13 (Paladini et al. 1996).

Following confirmation of diagnosis, termination of pregnancy may be considered for eligible patients. For expectantly managed patients, the fetus should be monitored with serial ultrasound examinations to confirm appropriate fetal growth and to detect early signs of hydrops. There is no reason to alter timing or mode of delivery based on a prenatal diagnosis of isolated pulmonic stenosis; therefore, in these cases the delivery plan should be for standard obstetric indications. Delivery of fetuses with critical pulmonic stenosis or pulmonic atresia should occur at a tertiary-care center, with the immediate availability of a neonatologist and pediatric cardiologist.

► FETAL INTERVENTION

No fetal intervention has been described following the prenatal diagnosis of pulmonic stenosis or atresia.

► TREATMENT OF THE NEWBORN

Most infants with mild-to-moderate pulmonic stenosis are asymptomatic during the newborn period. Those with severe stenosis or atresia present with congestive heart failure, cyanosis, and severe hypoxia (Fig. 52-2). If critical pulmonic stenosis or pulmonic atresia has been diagnosed during the antenatal period, maintenance of a patent ductus arteriosus may be during the newborn period. Maintenance of a patent ductus arteriosus can be achieved by starting a prostaglandin E_1 infusion, and limiting oxygen supplementation to

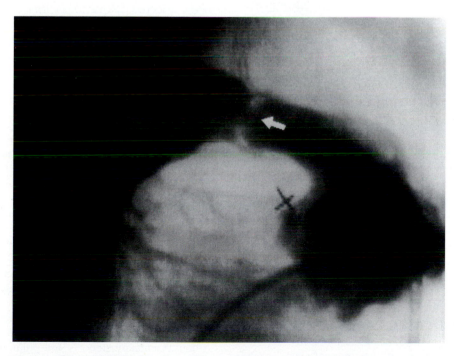

Figure 52-2. Lateral projection of a right ventricular angiogram in a symptomatic 1-day-old newborn with severe pulmonary valve stenosis. Arrow indicates the narrowed valve. *(Courtesy of Ziyad Hijazi, MD.)*

maintain reasonably normal perfusion. Immediately following delivery the neonate should be evaluated by a pediatric cardiologist. Echocardiography should be performed to confirm the diagnosis, assess the severity of stenosis, and rule out additional cardiac malformations. Medical stabilization may require the use of diuretics and digitalis.

Newborns with critical pulmonic stenosis may be treated with right-sided cardiac catheterization and balloon pulmonary valvuloplasty. By positioning a balloon across the pulmonary valve and inflating to 100 lb per square inch (psi) for 10 seconds, a significant decrease in pressure gradient across the valve can be achieved (Lababidi 1990). Such balloon dilation has been used safely in a series of 23 infants with pulmonic stenosis, with good short-term and medium-term relief of stenosis (Sullivan et al. 1985). In that series of 23 infants and children with pulmonic stenosis, repeat pulmonary valve dilation was required on only four occasions. However, there are insufficient data to define precisely which infants are treated best by balloon valvuloplasty and which infants will require surgical valvotomy.

▶ SURGICAL TREATMENT

Surgical approaches to critical pulmonic stenosis include transarterial pulmonary valvotomy, closed transventricular pulmonary valvotomy, and open pulmonary valvotomy using cardiopulmonary bypass. The need for surgical treatment of pulmonic stenosis depends on the pressure gradient across the pulmonary valve. With gradients of less than 25 mm Hg, 5% of children require surgery; 20% of those with gradients of 25 to 49 mm Hg and 76% of those with gradients of 50 to 79 mm Hg require surgical treatment (Hayes et al. 1993).

The most commonly performed surgical procedure is a closed transventricular pulmonary valvotomy, with or without a modified Blalock–Taussig shunt from the subclavian to the pulmonary artery (Coles and Trusler 1990). Following thoracotomy or sternotomy, a stab incision is made in the right ventricular wall and a valvulotome, or Hegar dilator, is inserted to open the pulmonary valve. In 1 series of 16 infants less than 3 months of age who had critical pulmonic stenosis, 14 survived following closed transventricular valvotomy, and all survivors demonstrated clinical improvement (Srinivasan et al. 1982).

▶ LONG-TERM OUTCOME

Late results after treatment of pulmonic stenosis seem favorable. Estimates of 25-year actuarial survival range from 90 to 95% (Hayes et al. 1993; Morris and Menashe 1991). In a series of 14 infants who survived closed transventricular pulmonary valvotomy for critical pulmonic stenosis 2 required repeat surgery, 1 needing open valvotomy for restenosis and 1 needing closure of a secundum atrial septal defect (Srinivasan et al. 1982). It seems that in the majority of patients, adequate growth of the right ventricle and pulmonary annulus occurs following surgical repair. If the infundibular portion of the right ventricular outflow tract is hypoplastic on initial evaluation, the requirement for late reoperation to repair residual stenosis increases significantly and may be as high as 50% at 10 years postoperatively (Coles and Trusler 1990).

▶ GENETICS AND RECURRENCE RISK

Pulmonic stenosis may occur as part of Williams syndrome, which may also involve supravalvular aortic stenosis, developmental delay, and unusual facies. Williams syndrome is due to the deletion of one copy of the elastin gene on chromosome 7. Pulmonic stenosis may also occur as part of Noonan syndrome. Both Williams and Noonan syndromes generally occur sporadically. At least one case report describing familial clustering of cases of pulmonic stenosis has also been reported (Manetti et al. 1990). Without a history suggestive of a mendelian or chromosomal disorder, the recurrence risk for a couple with one previously affected child having another child with pulmonic stenosis is 2% but is increased to 6% if two previous children have been affected (Nora and Nora 1988). The chance of having an affected infant if the mother has pulmonic stenosis is 4–6.5%, but if the father is affected, it is only 2% (Nora and Nora 1988).

REFERENCES

Coles JG, Trusler GA. Neonatal surgery for critical pulmonary stenosis. In: Long WA, ed. Fetal and neonatal cardiology. Philadelphia: Saunders, 1990:770–773.

Ferencz C, Rubin JD, McCarter RJ, et al. Cardiac and noncardiac malformations: observations in a population-based study. Teratology 1987;35:367–378.

Gutgesell HP. Pulmonary valve abnormalities. In: Long WA, ed. Fetal and neonatal cardiology. Philadelphia: Saunders, 1990:551–560.

Hayes CJ, Gersony WM, Driscoll DJ, et al. Second natural history study of congenital heart defects. Circulation 1993; 87(suppl 2):I28–I37.

Hornberger LK, Benacerraf BR, Bromley BS, et al. Prenatal detection of severe right ventricular outflow tract obstruction: pulmonary stenosis and pulmonary atresia. J Ultrasound Med 1994;13:743–750.

Lababidi Z. Neonatal catheter palliations. In: Long WA, ed. Fetal and neonatal cardiology. Philadelphia: Saunders, 1990:702–713.

Manetti A, Favilli S, Mandorla S, et al. Familial pulmonary stenosis: considerations on genetic aspects. G Ital Cardiol 1990;20:726–728.

Mendez HMM, Opitz JM. Noonan syndrome: a review. Am J Med Genet 1985;21:493–506.

Mielke G, Steil E, Kendziorra H, et al. Ductus arteriosus-dependent pulmonary circulation secondary to cardiac malformations in fetal life. Ultrasound Obstet Gynecol 1997;9:25–29.

Mitchell SC, Korones SB, Berendes HW. Congenital heart disease in 56,109 births: incidence and natural history. Circulation 1971;43:323–332.

Montana E, Khoury MJ, Cragan JD, et al. Trends and outcomes after prenatal diagnosis of congenital cardiac malformations by fetal echocardiography in a well defined birth population, Atlanta, Georgia 1990–1994. J Am Coll Cardiol 1996;28:1805–1809.

Morris CD, Menashe VD. 25-year mortality after surgical repair of congenital heart defect in childhood: a population-based cohort study. JAMA 1991;266:3447–3452.

Nora JJ, Nora AH. Update on counseling the family with a first-degree relative with a congenital heart defect. Am J Med Genet 1988;29:137–142.

Paladini D, Rustico M, Todros, T, et al. Conotruncal anomalies in prenatal life. Ultrasound Obstet Gynecol 1996;8: 241–246.

Romero R, Pilu G, Jeanty P, et al. Pulmonic stenosis. In: Romero R, Pilu G, Jeanty P, Ghidini A, Hobbins JC, eds. Prenatal diagnosis of congenital anomalies. Norwalk, CT: Appleton & Lange 1988:173–175.

Sharland GK, Lockhart SM, Chita SK, et al. Factors influencing the outcome of congenital heart disease detected prenatally. Arch Dis Child 1990;65:284–287.

Smythe JF, Copel JA, Kleinman CS. Outcome of prenatally detected cardiac malformations. Am J Cardiol 1992;69: 1471–1474.

Srinivasan V, Konyer A, Broda JJ, et al. Critical pulmonary stenosis in infants less than three months of age: a reappraisal of closed transventricular pulmonary valvotomy. Ann Thorac Surg 1982;34:46–50.

Sullivan ID, Robinson PJ, Macartney FJ, et al. Percutaneous balloon valvuloplasty for pulmonary valve stenosis in infants and children. Br Heart J 1985;54:435–441.

Tegnander E, Eik-Nes SH, Johansen OJ, et al. Prenatal detection of heart defects at the routine fetal examination at 18 weeks in a non-selected population. Ultrasound Obstet Gynecol 1995;5:372–380.

Todros T, Presbitero P, Gaglioti P, et al. Pulmonary stenosis with intact ventricular septum: documentation of development of the lesion echocardiographically during fetal life. Int J Cardiol 1988;19:355–362.

tachycardias, premature extrasystoles, and ventricular tachycardia (Mehta 1993). Two theories have been proposed to account for the development of these dysrhythmias. One is that the rhabdomyomas consist of an overgrowth of Purkinje cells, which may be capable of impulse conduction (Mehta 1993). The more prevalent hypothesis is that the arrhythmias develop as a result of disruption of conduction tissue by tumor growth within the intraventricular septum (Groves et al. 1992). In summary, the antenatal natural history can be compromised by the development of dysrhythmias, right or left ventricular outflow-tract obstruction, valvular insufficiency, myocardial dysfunction due to tumor infiltration, hydrops, and death (Green et al. 1991).

Intracardiac rhabdomyomas are composed of large muscle fibers that contain prominent vacuoles that histologically give them a spider web or honeycomb appearance (Ostör and Fortune 1978; Thibault and Manuelidis 1970).

▶ MANAGEMENT OF PREGNANCY

Any pregnant patient with a positive family history of tuberous sclerosis should have serial prenatal sonographic examinations with detailed attention to the fetal heart, central nervous system, and kidneys (Platt et al. 1987). Fetal echocardiography is recommended. Early delivery is indicated if there is a suggestion that the cardiac tumor is compromising cardiac function (Chitayat et al. 1988). Administration of digoxin to the mother is indicated if supraventricular tachycardia is the cause of the hydrops as opposed to outflow-tract obstruction.

If an intracardiac rhabdomyoma is demonstrated in a fetus with no known history of tuberous sclerosis, genetic counseling is indicated. A genetic counselor and/or medical geneticist should meet with the family to obtain a detailed three-generation pedigree. Primary and secondary criteria for the diagnosis of tuberous sclerosis are listed in Table 53-1. Of note is that the majority of primary criteria (only one abnormality required for diagnosis) are not applicable to the fetus. The combination of a positive family history and fetal cardiac rhabdomyoma allows a presumptive diagnosis of tuberous sclerosis. Alternatively, a fetus identified with cardiac rhabdomyoma and renal cysts but a negative family history will also have a presumptive diagnosis of tuberous sclerosis. When a positive family history exists and a rhabdomyoma is found in the fetus, the fetus can be diagnosed as being affected. The question of termination of the pregnancy can be discussed with the family at this point. If the family history is negative, the parents should be counseled that they can undergo a series of diagnostic tests to determine if one of them has a very mild, previously unsuspected form of tuberous sclerosis (see "Genetics and Recurrence Risk"). With the finding of a fetal cardiac rhabdomyoma, the diagnosis is still very likely to be tuberous sclerosis, and this condition should be discussed thoroughly with the family (Journel et al. 1986). Fetal karyotyping is not indicated for this condition. On the other hand, DNA diagnosis by linkage analysis is available if there are other affected family members. No indication exists at present to perform an amniocentesis to obtain fetal DNA on the first affected family member, but umbilical cord blood should be collected and stored. This will ensure that DNA from an affected individual is available and will obviate the need to perform venipuncture on an infant.

▶ FETAL INTERVENTION

There are no fetal interventions for rhabdomyoma indicated at present.

▶ TREATMENT OF THE NEWBORN

The fetus with an intracardiac rhabdomyoma should be delivered at a tertiary-care center, and a neonatologist should be present at the delivery because of the risk of the development of dysrhythmias. Ideally, the infant should be delivered in a center where pediatric cardiologists are also available. In addition to a complete

▶ **TABLE 53-1.** DIAGNOSTIC CRITERIA FOR TUBEROUS SCLEROSIS

Primary Criteria (only 1 required for diagnosis)	Secondary Criteria (2 required for diagnosis)
Facial angiofibroma (adenoma sebaceous)	Positive family history
Ungual fibromas	Cardiac rhabdomyoma
Cortical tubers (at autopsy)	Bilateral renal angiomyolipomata or cysts
Subependymal hamartoma	Single retinal hamartoma
Multiple retinal hamartoma	Shagreen patch
Fibrous plaque on forehead	Hypopigmented macules
	Infantile spasms

Source: Fryer AE, Connor JM, Povey S, et al. Evidence that the gene for tuberous sclerosis is on chromosome 9. Lancet 1977;1:659–661.

physical examination, the newborn should have a chest x-ray examination, electrocardiography, four-extremity blood pressure measurement, and postnatal echocardiography. Additional diagnostic studies should include postnatal renal sonography to look for the presence of renal cysts (Saguem et al. 1992).

In some studies, magnetic resonance imaging (MRI) is considered superior to CT examination for the postnatal diagnosis of cortical tubers because MRI provides better soft-tissue contrast without exposure to ionizing radiation. White-matter tubers are readily identified within the white matter or cortical gyri. These tubers are sclerotic areas that exist throughout the cerebral hemispheres. They are the result of malformations of neuronal and glial elements characterized by decreased neurons and increased glia, and abnormal heterotopic cells (Truhan and Filipek 1993). MRI has been used to demonstrate the presence of cortical, subcortical, and subependymal tumors in a 3-week-old infant (Christophe et al. 1989). These abnormalities were more completely and clearly seen on the T_1-weighted MR images as opposed to CT images. To our knowledge, MRI has not yet been used antenatally to look for the presence of cortical tubers.

▶ SURGICAL TREATMENT

Surgical intervention should be restricted to cases with significant hemodynamic obstruction or life-threatening arrhythmias (Smythe et al. 1990). Because the natural history of these tumors is that they regress postnatally, a nonoperative approach with careful postnatal follow-up is recommended when possible.

▶ LONG-TERM OUTCOME

Previous reports in the medical literature have emphasized a poor prognosis for fetuses or neonates affected with intracardiac rhabdomyomas. These include a reported 33% mortality rate during the first week of life and an 80% mortality rate during the first year of life (Green et al. 1981). Since approximately 60% of patients with tuberous sclerosis have asymptomatic rhabdomyomas, a more variable prognosis is likely to exist. As stated earlier, the natural history of the rhabdomyomas is that they regress and that the cardiac volume increases, so the prognosis should be reasonably good (Webb et al. 1993). Fetuses in whom symptoms of hydrops or dysrhythmias develop antenatally do have an increased risk of mortality.

Concerns regarding long-term outcome are mainly focused on the developmental and health consequences of tuberous sclerosis. The long-term outcome for patients with tuberous sclerosis is extremely variable and can range from completely normal intelligence to severe mental retardation. The prevalence of mental retardation in an unbiased sample of patients with tuberous sclerosis is 38% (Webb et al. 1993). Understandably, most parents are concerned about the risk for the development of seizures and mental retardation. There is a high likelihood that infants affected with tuberous sclerosis will have infantile spasms. For infants in whom seizures develop within the first year of life, there is a higher likelihood of mental retardation. It has been suggested that there is a correlation between the presence of cortical tubers and the severity of mental retardation (Kwiatkowski and Short 1994). Other health consequences of tuberous sclerosis include renal angiomyolipomas, pulmonary lymphangiomyomas, seizure disorders, and multiple skin findings that could be considered a cosmetic issue.

▶ GENETICS AND RECURRENCE RISK

The most likely cause for rhabdomyoma is tuberous sclerosis, which is inherited as a single gene with an autosomal dominant pattern of inheritance. Previously, most scientists thought that there was a high rate of spontaneous mutation for this condition, on the order of 60% of cases (Kwiatkowski and Short 1994). Results of MRI in parents of affected children, however, suggest that the percentage of cases due to spontaneous mutations has been overestimated (Christophe et al. 1989). The penetrance for known cases of tuberous sclerosis is on the order of 90 to 95%, but one of the characteristics of this condition is that there is extraordinary variability in the expression of the phenotype. For example, an affected parent of normal intelligence can have an affected child with severe mental retardation. Although the inheritance pattern is classically described as autosomal dominant, several families have also been described with two affected children being born to normal parents. It is now appreciated that the incidence of somatic or gonadal mosaicism for a mutation in one of the tuberous sclerosis genes is as high as 10% (Verhoef et al. 1999). There have also been several cases of discordance of expression in monozygotic twins, which raises the question of an imprinting affect (Kwiatkowski and Short 1994).

If a fetal rhabdomyoma is documented in the setting of a negative family history, both parents should undergo a through clinical and radiologic examination for the diagnosis of tuberous sclerosis. The suggested workup includes a dermatologic examination under ultraviolet light, a CT scan, and MRI study of the brain (Roach et al. 1991), as well as renal sonography to look for the presence of angiomyolipomas or cysts.

There are two distinct genes involved in the causation of tuberous sclerosis, TSC1 and TSC2 (Jones et al.

1999). Approximately half of cases have a single gene linked to the ABO blood group locus at chromosome 9 band q34 (Fryer et al. 1987). The other half of cases have a different gene at chromosome 16 band p13 near the adult polycystic kidney disease gene. This gene product has been identified and named tuberin, a 198-kd protein of unknown function (European Chromosome 16 Tuberous Sclerosis Consortium 1993). Both of the genes that cause tuberous sclerosis, TSC1 and TSC2, function as tumor suppressors.

In the future, prenatal diagnosis for this condition will likely be DNA-based. For families with a positive family history of tuberous sclerosis, DNA linkage studies should ideally be performed prior to contemplation of pregnancy. It would be useful to know prior to conception whether the affected families' gene maps to chromosome 9 or chromosome 16. A comprehensive mutation analysis of the genes TSC1 and TSC2 was able to characterize mutations in 120 of 150 (80%) of cases studied (Jones et al. 1999). Mutation analysis of affected individuals' DNA must be performed prior to a subsequent pregnancy in order to facilitate DNA-based diagnosis of chorionic villi in the first trimester. For families that have not undergone mutation analysis, prenatal diagnosis for tuberous sclerosis consists of serial prenatal sonographic examinations. As previously discussed, this has limitations, because definitive diagnosis can occur only during the late second trimester. The availability of DNA diagnosis is eagerly awaited, because this would allow families the opportunity to know the results of prenatal diagnosis as early as the first trimester.

REFERENCES

Abushaban L, Denham B, Duff D. Ten year review of cardiac tumours in childhood. Br Heart J 1993;70:166–169.

Barth PG, Stam FC, Harten JJ. Tuberous sclerosis and dysplasia of the corpus callosum: case report of their combined occurrence in a newborn. Acta Neuropathol 1978; 42:63–64.

Blethyn J, Jones A, Sullivan B. Prenatal diagnosis of unilateral renal disease in tuberous sclerosis. Br J Radiol 1991; 64:161–164.

Bordarier C, Lellouch-Tubiana A, Robain O. Cardiac rhabdomyoma and tuberous sclerosis in three fetuses: a neuropathological study. Brain Dev 1994;16:467–471.

Brackley KJ, Farndom PA, Weaver JB, Dow DJ, Chapman S, Kilby MD. Prenatal diagnosis of tuberous sclerosis with intracerebral signs at 14 weeks' gestation. Prenat Diagn 1999;19:575–579.

Calhoun BC, Watson PT, Hegge F. Ultrasound diagnosis of an obstructive cardiac rhabdomyoma with severe hydrops and hypoplastic lungs: a case report. J Reprod Med 1991; 36:317–319.

Chitayat D, McGillivray BC, Diamant S, Wittmann BK, Sandor GG. Role of prenatal detection of cardiac tumours

in the diagnosis of tuberous sclerosis—report of two cases. Prenat Diagn 1988;8:577–584.

Christophe C, Bartholome J, Blum D, et al. Neonatal tuberous sclerosis: US, CT, and MR diagnosis of brain and cardiac lesions. Pediatr Radiol 1989;19:446–448.

Coates TL, McGahan JP. Fetal cardiac rhabdomyomas presenting as diffuse myocardial thickening. J Ultrasound Med 1994;13:813–816.

Deeg KH, Viogt HJ, Hofbeck M, Singer H, Kraus J. Prenatal ultrasound diagnosis of multiple cardiac rhabdomyomas. Pediatr Radiol 1990;20:291–292.

DeVore GR, Hakim S, Kleinman CS, Hobbins JC. The in utero diagnosis of an interventricular septal cardiac rhabdomyoma by means of real-time directed, M-mode echocardiography. Am J Obstet Gynecol 1982;143: 967–969.

European Chromosome 16 Tuberous Sclerosis Consortium. Identification and characterization of the tuberous sclerosis gene on chromosome 16. Cell 1993;75:1305–1315.

Fryer AE, Connor JM, Povey S, et al. Evidence that the gene for tuberous sclerosis is on chromosome 9. Lancet 1977;1:659–661.

Gava G, Buoso G, Beltrame GL, Memo L, Visentin S, Cavarzerani A. Cardiac rhabdomyoma as a marker for the prenatal detection of tuberous sclerosis: case report. Br J Obstet Gynaecol 1990;97:1154–1157.

Green KW, Bors-Koefoed R, Pollack P, Weinbaum PJ. Antepartum diagnosis and management of multiple fetal cardiac tumors. J Ultrasound Med 1991;10:697–699.

Groves AM, Fagg NL, Cook AC, Allan LD. Cardiac tumours in intrauterine life. Arch Dis Child 1992;67:1189–1192.

Jones AC, Shyamsundar MM, Thomas MW et al. Comprehensive mutation analysis of TSC1 and TSC2 and phenotypic correlations in 150 families with tuberous sclerosis. Am J Hum Genet 1999;64:1305–1315.

Journel H, Roussey M, Plais MH, Milon J, Almange C, LeMarec B. Prenatal diagnosis of familial tuberous sclerosis following detection of cardiac rhabdomyoma by ultrasound. Prenat Diagn 1986;6:283–289.

Kwiatkowski DJ, Short MP. Tuberous sclerosis. Arch Dermatol 1994;130:348–354.

Mehta AV. Rhabdomyoma and ventricular preexcitation syndrome: a report of two cases and review of literature. Am J Dis Child 1993;147:669–671.

Muller L, de Jong G, Falck V, Hewlett R, Hunter J, Shires J. Antenatal ultrasonographic findings in tuberous sclerosis. S Afr Med J 1986;69:633–638.

Platt LD, Devore GR, Horenstein J, Pavlova Z, Kovacs B, Falk RE. Prenatal diagnosis of tuberous sclerosis: the use of fetal echocardiography. Prenat Diagn 1987;7:407–412.

Ostör AG, Fortune DW. Tuberous sclerosis initially seen as hydrops fetalis: report of a case and review of the literature. Arch Pathol Lab Med 1978;102:34–39.

Roach ES, Kerr J, Mendelsohn D, Laster DW, Raeside C. Detection of tuberous sclerosis in parents by magnetic resonance imaging. Neurology 1991;41:262–265.

Saguem MH, Laarif M, Remadi S, Bozakoura C, Cox JN. Diffuse bilateral glomerulocystic disease of the kidneys and multiple cardiac rhabdomyomas in a newborn: relationship with tuberous sclerosis and review of the literature. Pathol Res Pract 1992;188:367–373.

Smythe JF, Dyck JD, Smallhorn JF, Freedom RM. Natural history of cardiac rhabdomyoma in infancy and childhood. Am J Cardiol 1990;66:1247–1249.

Thibault JH, Manuelidis EE. Tuberous sclerosis in a premature infant: report of a case and review of the literature. Neurology 1970;20:139–146.

Truhan AP, Filipek PA. Magnetic resonance imaging. Its role in the neuroradiologic evaluation of neurofibromatosis, tuberous sclerosis, and Sturge-Weber syndrome. Arch Dermatol 1993;129:219–226.

van Oppen AC, Brelau-Siderius EJ, Stoutenbeek P, Pull Ter Gunne AJ, Merkus JM. A fetal cystic neck mass associated with maternal tuberous sclerosis: case report and literature review. Prenat Diagn 1991;11:915–920.

Verhoef S, Bakker L, Tempelnars AM, et al. High rate of mosaicism in tuberous sclerosis complex. Am J Hum Genet 1999;64:1632–1637.

Webb DW, Thomas RD, Osbourne JP. Cardiac rhabdomyomas and their association with tuberous sclerosis. Arch Dis Child 1993;68:367–370.

CHAPTER 54

Tachyarrhythmias

▶ CONDITION

Fetal tachyarrhythmias detected in utero include irregular cardiac rhythm resulting from isolated extrasystoles, supraventricular tachycardia, and atrial flutter. The most common of the above arrhythmias is an irregular cardiac rhythm resulting from isolated extrasystoles (Kleinman 1986; Silverman et al. 1985). Most of these extrasystoles originate in the atria and resolve spontaneously (Kleinman 1986; Reed et al. 1987). An increased frequency of premature beats has been attributed to the maternal use of caffeine, tobacco, and alcohol (De Vore 1984). Although premature atrial or ventricular contractions have not been considered a risk factor for anomalies in the past, more recent reports suggest that a fetal structural cardiac abnormality may be found in up to 2% of such cases (Beall and Paul 1986; Reed 1991).

Supraventricular tachycardia is the most common serious dysrhythmia detected prenatally (Bergmans et al. 1985; Kleinman et al. 1985a). The majority of supraventricular tachycardias are considered to be re-entrant dysrhythmias and are identified by a fetal heart rate of more than 200 beats per minute (bpm) with one-to-one atrial-to-ventricular activity (Fig. 54-1) (Simpson and Marx 1994). Paroxysmal supraventricular tachycardia may also occur as part of the Wolff–Parkinson–White syndrome, together with a short P–R interval, prolonged QRS, and presence of a delta wave on electrocardiogram. Typically, supraventricular tachycardia has not been associated with congenital heart disease; however, in 5 to 10% of cases, structural cardiac abnormalities can be found (Beall and Paul 1986; Reed 1989). The presence of structural heart disease in addition to supraventricular tachycardia is associated with a poor fetal outcome (Bergmans et al. 1985).

Fetal atrial flutter has been diagnosed and reported less commonly than supraventricular tachycardia (Klein-man 1986). The atrial rate in flutter can be estimated between 300 and 500 bpm with a variable ventricular response dependent on the degree of atrioventricular block (Fig. 54-2). Fetal atrial flutter has a poor prognosis, due in part to its association with structural heart disease (in up to 20% of cases) and with the development of hydrops fetalis (Kleinman 1986; Reed 1991; Simpson and Marx 1994).

In contrast to benign arrhythmias such as isolated extrasystoles, fetal dysrhythmias have the potential for serious sequelae. It has been well described that fetuses with tachyarrhythmias have decreased cardiac output and are at risk for hydrops fetalis (Reed 1989; Reed et al. 1987). Protracted supraventricular tachycardia can lead to cardiac failure in a matter of days (Allan 1984). The exact mechanism for the development of cardiac failure and hydrops remains unclear. The progression to hydrops in utero seems to follow right heart failure with tricuspid regurgitation and right ventricular dilatation, signifying impending decompensation (Allan et al. 1983; Chao et al. 1992; Gembruch et al. 1993). It has been postulated that either passive liver congestion associated with cardiac failure or decreased hepatic perfusion from decreased cardiac output may result in hypoalbuminemia, leading to decreased oncotic pressure and transudation of fluid into interstitial spaces (Johnson et al. 1992). Pericardial and pleural effusions, fetal ascites, and subcutaneous edema are probably late manifestations of cardiac decompensation.

▶ INCIDENCE

Arrhythmias are identified in approximately 1% of all fetuses; however, the actual incidence of fetal arrhythmias is expected to be higher because a significant proportion of them can be intermittent or resolve spontaneously

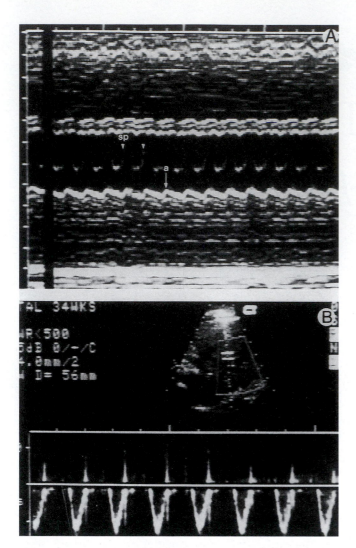

Figure 54-1. (A) M-mode echocardiogram in a fetus in supraventricular tachycardia as shown by an atrial contraction rate (a) and excursion of the septum primum (sp) at a rate of 240 bpm. (B) Doppler echocardiogram of ascending aortic velocities from the same fetus showing a ventricular rate of 240 bpm. *(Reprinted, with permission, from Simpson LL, Marx GR. Diagnosis and treatment of structural fetal cardiac abnormality and dysrhythmia. Semin Perinatol 1994;18:215–227.)*

(Reed 1989; Simpson and Marx 1994). The most common and clinically significant tachyarrhythmias identified in utero are supraventricular tachycardia and atrial flutter.

▶ SONOGRAPHIC FINDINGS

Ultrasound evaluation should include a complete fetal survey and a survey of the cardiac anatomy to confirm absence of structural malformations. The incidence of abnormal cardiac anatomy varies with the type of

arrhythmia. The fetus should also be examined for evidence of hydrops as defined by fluid collections in the pericardium, the pleural spaces, ascites, or skin edema. Amniotic fluid may also be increased. An increase in fetal cardiac size or wall thickness may be an indication of abnormal cardiac hemodynamics (Reed 1989).

Echocardiography, including M-mode assessment and Doppler analysis, is an important tool in the diagnosis and evaluation of fetal dysrhythmias (De Vore et al. 1983; Kleinman et al. 1980; Silverman et al. 1985). The atrial and corresponding ventricular activity can be viewed by two-dimensional echocardiography and the rates determined by placement of the M-mode cursor perpendicular to the atrial and ventricular walls. M-mode echocardiography can also be used to identify pericardial effusions and to measure wall thickness, chamber size, and fractional shortening (see Figs. 54-1 and 54-2). Doppler evaluation of atrioventricular and semilunar valve flows can be used to time the ventricular contractions (Strasburger et al. 1986). The hemodynamic effects of a dysrhythmia are assessed by determining the size and function of the four chambers, the magnitude of the semilunar and atrioventricular flow velocity integrals, and the presence of mitral or tricuspid regurgitation or nonimmune hydrops fetalis. Color flow mapping may also be used to identify flow disturbances. The approach to the ultrasound evaluation of arrhythmias is summarized in Table 54-1.

▶ DIFFERENTIAL DIAGNOSIS

The differential diagnosis of fetal tachyarrhythmias includes benign isolated extrasystoles and more significant dysrhythmias such as atrial flutter and supraventricular tachycardia. M-mode echocardiography is useful in differentiating these conditions, as described above.

▶ TABLE 54-1. EVALUATION OF ARRHYTHMIAS

Type of Study	Findings
Two-dimensional ultrasound examination	Anatomy
	Chamber dilatation
	Hydrops
M-mode	Type of arrhythmia
	Pericardial effusion
	Hypertrophy/dilatation
Doppler	Flow disturbances (regurgitation)
	Volume flow
Color flow	Flow disturbances

Reproduced, with permission, from Reed KL. Fetal arrhythmias: etiology, diagnosis, pathophysiology, and treatment. Semin Perinatol 1989;13:294–304.

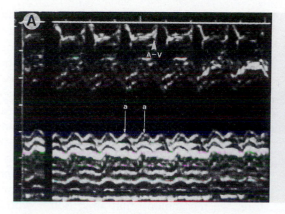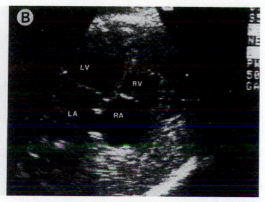

Figure 54-2. (A) Fetus in atrial flutter as shown by an atrial contraction rate of 480 bpm (arrowhead labeled A-V for atrioventricular valve opening). (B) Four-chamber view in the same fetus in atrial flutter showing dilated right atrium and pericardial effusion (arrow). LA = left atrium; LV = left ventricle; RV = right ventricle; RA = right atrium. *(Reprinted, with permission, from Simpson LL, Marx GR. Diagnosis and treatment of structural fetal cardiac abnormality and dysrhythmia. Semin Perinatol 1994;18:215–227.)*

▶ ANTENATAL NATURAL HISTORY

Premature atrial and ventricular contractions are considered to be benign and do not require treatment. However, it has been reported that a sustained tachyarrhythmia may subsequently develop in up to 1% of fetuses with premature beats (Kleinman 1986).

The natural history of isolated in utero supraventricular tachycardia remains unclear. Although intermittent supraventricular tachycardia may be of no clinical significance, sustained supraventricular tachycardia may be life-threatening (Bergmans et al. 1985; Southall et al. 1980). Spontaneous resolution of supraventricular tachycardia has been reported (Newburger and Keane 1979; Santulli 1990). Complete resolution of protracted supraventricular tachycardia with subsequent normal fetal development has been observed (Simpson et al. 1997). In a small series of isolated fetal supraventricular tachycardia, hydrops developed in only 1 of 9 cases managed conservatively without medical therapy (Simpson et al. 1997). Interestingly, the fetus in which signs of hydrops developed had intermittent supraventricular tachycardia at a rate of 200 bpm occurring less than 50% of the time. In the remaining 8 fetuses in which hydrops did not develop, 5 had intermittent episodes of supraventricular tachycardia occurring less than 50% of the time and 2 had more sustained supraventricular tachycardia occurring between 50 and 75% of the time. Spontaneous resolution of the supraventricular tachycardia in these remaining 8 fetuses occurred within 10 days of diagnosis, with no recurrence in the antepartum or newborn period. Antiarrhythmic agents were not administered to these 8 mothers or their infants, who were all delivered at term. However, sustained supraventricular tachycardia can be associated with the development of congestive heart failure and hydrops and the potential for fetal death.

The presence of structural heart disease in association with fetal supraventricular tachycardia has been reported to have a poor outcome (Bergmans et al. 1985). However, a case of fetal supraventricular tachycardia and congenital heart disease has been observed in an infant, who is now 3 years old, without any recurrence of the dysrhythmia after surgery for a double-inlet single left ventricle, subaortic stenosis and coarctation of the aorta (Simpson et al. 1995).

Although rapid progression to fetal hydrops can occur with sustained supraventricular tachycardia of 24 to 48 hours' duration, signs of cardiac failure will not develop in all fetuses (Kleinman et al. 1985a; Newburger and Keane 1979). In approximately 25% of cases, there seems to be no associated hemodynamic compromise. However, 55 to 60% of fetuses with supraventricular tachycardia will have evidence of cardiac decompensation in utero or during the newborn period (Bergmans et al. 1985; Newburger and Keane 1979). At the time of diagnosis of supraventricular tachycardia, Kleinman (1986) detected hydrops fetalis in 16 of 18 cases. Fortunately, even in the presence of cardiac failure, supraventricular tachycardia has a favorable prognosis (Kleinman 1986). In utero medical treatment can result in conversion to normal sinus rhythm within 48 hours (Sarno et al. 1989). Conversion to sinus rhythm seems to occur more easily in the absence of fetal hydrops (Kleinman et al. 1985a). It has also been shown that because of impaired placental transfer of antiarrhythmic agents, fetuses with hydrops could require 2 to 3 weeks of therapy before converting to normal sinus rhythm (Maxwell et al. 1988). Atrial flutter seems to have a poor in utero prognosis, with two of three fetuses with atrial flutter and associated hydrops dying in one series (Kleinman 1986; Simpson and Marx 1994).

▶ MANAGEMENT OF PREGNANCY

The typical presentation of fetal tachyarrhythmia involves the auscultation of a rapid fetal heart rate in an asymptomatic woman at a routine prenatal visit. Such a finding should prompt a thorough prenatal evaluation, including a detailed ultrasound examination for fetal anatomy, growth, and biophysical status, in addition to an echocardiogram with M-mode and Doppler evaluation to characterize the arrhythmia fully and evaluate its impact on myocardial function. The latter studies are generally performed in consultation with a pediatric cardiologist. The finding of structural cardiac abnormalities in 5 to 10% of cases of supraventricular tachycardia reaffirms the need for careful anatomic assessment of the fetal heart (Beall and Paul 1986; Reed 1989).

In the absence of additional structural cardiac malformation, it is well accepted that in utero medical therapy or delivery, or both, is appropriate in cases of fetal supraventricular tachycardia with evidence of hemodynamic compromise. Gestational age is a significant factor in deciding appropriate intervention. In one series, use of digoxin alone or digoxin with verapamil or propranolol achieved in utero control in 13 of 14 cases of supraventricular tachycardia with associated hydrops (Kleinman et al. 1985b). Higher doses of digoxin are often necessary to achieve therapeutic levels because of the variable absorption, large volume of distribution, and rapid clearance associated with pregnancy. Conversion to sinus rhythm seems to occur more easily in the absence of fetal hydrops (Kleinman et al. 1985a). This may be because of impaired placental transfer of antiarrhythmic agents in hydropic fetuses (Maxwell et al. 1988). In a retrospective study of 11 cases of supraventricular tachycardia and 4 cases of atrial flutter with hydrops, a median of 12.5 days was required for in utero conversion to sinus rhythm, as compared with a median of 3 days in the absence of hydrops (van Engelen et al. 1994). In this series, indications were that flecainide was more effective than digoxin in achieving rhythm control.

We recommend digoxin for first-line therapy of isolated fetal tachyarrhythmia, with procainamide or flecainide reserved for second-line treatment when delivery is not desirable because of gestational age and when conversion to normal sinus rhythm with digoxin has been unsuccessful. Successful in utero conversion from supraventricular tachycardia to atrial flutter with a variable ventricular response after maternal administration of digoxin has been described (Simpson et al. 1995). Atrial flutter has been found to be more difficult to treat successfully in utero, and this is partly responsible for the reported poor prognosis associated with this dysrhythmia (Simpson and Marx 1994). In one series, antiarrhythmics were effective for in utero control of supraventricular tachycardia in 88% of cases, as compared with 66% of cases of atrial flutter (van Engelen et al. 1994). Although second-line antiarrhythmic agents may be tried, elective preterm delivery may be necessary in cases of supraventricular tachycardia alternating with atrial flutter that are refractory to digoxin. On the basis of the adverse outcomes reported in the literature, we recommend that atrial flutter with or without hydrops be promptly treated with an antiarrhythmic if delivery is not a reasonable option because of gestational age (Simpson et al. 1995).

In contrast, in the absence of hydrops or hemodynamic compromise, conservative management without medical therapy may be a reasonable option for fetuses with supraventricular tachycardia. Spontaneous resolution of protracted supraventricular tachycardia with subsequent normal fetal development has been observed (Bergmans et al. 1985; Simpson et al. 1997; Stewart et al. 1983). A review of the literature has identified seven cases of supraventricular tachycardia that converted to normal sinus rhythm spontaneously during parturition, with no recurrences after delivery (Bergmans et al. 1985). It is postulated that vagal stimulation during delivery slows conduction through the atrioventricular node, resulting in conversion to normal sinus rhythm.

Close follow-up of cases of isolated fetal supraventricular tachycardia without hydrops is warranted because of the potential for hydrops if conservative management without medical therapy is undertaken. Initially, daily assessments with ultrasound and fetal echocardiography are necessary. The interval between fetal evaluations can be extended, and resolution of the supraventricular tachycardia has been documented with individualization of follow-up thereafter. This regimen requires a reliable and compliant patient. If frequent evaluations are not possible or if compliance is questionable, medical therapy with antiarrhythmics is more appropriate.

When supraventricular tachycardia is diagnosed, the perinatologist and pediatric cardiologist together formulate a treatment plan (Simpson and Marx 1994). Initially the fetus is assessed by the perinatologist for any signs of biophysical compromise. A detailed sonographic examination to determine fetal growth, development, and biophysical status is performed, with careful examination for the presence of pericardial, pleural, or abdominal fluid. The pediatric cardiologist then confirms the atrial and ventricular rate of contraction, atrial and ventricular size and function, and the presence and magnitude of atrioventricular-valve regurgitation. Aortic and pulmonary flow-velocity integrals are determined during episodes of tachycardia and episodes of normal sinus rhythm. Immediate medical therapy is undertaken if there are signs of hemodynamic compromise, fetal distress, or hydrops fetalis. In all other cases, the mother is admitted to hospital and the fetus is monitored for 24 hours to determine the duration of the dysrhythmia. Expectant management without immediate medical therapy is considered if there are no signs of compromise, if the fetal tachycardia is not sustained, and if the patient is compliant (Simpson and Marx 1994).

When fetal supraventricular tachycardia is persistent despite digoxin, and the gestational age precludes delivery, an additional antiarrhythmic drug should be tried. Procainamide, flecanide, quinidine, verapamil, propranolol, and amiodarone have all been given for fetal tachyarrhythmias, with variable success (Bergmans et al. 1985; Kleinman et al. 1985b; Wladimiroff and Stewart 1985). Unlike digoxin, however, these drugs can be associated with significant toxicity to the mother and fetus. Both procainamide and quinidine have the potential for proarrhythmic effects in the fetus and gastrointestinal toxicity in the mother (Kleinman et al. 1985a). Verapamil has been associated with cardiac decompensation and sudden fetal demise (Epstein et al. 1985; Owen et al. 1988). Intrauterine growth restriction and subsequent neonatal bradycardia and hypoglycemia have been observed with the use of propranolol (Gladstone et al. 1975; Rubin 1981). Amiodarone can be considered for more protracted dysrhythmias, but both maternal and fetal thyroid dysfunction are potential complications. At our institution, flecanide or procainamide are most commonly used as the second-line treatment when delivery is not desirable. Procainamide can be administered orally or intravenously to the mother, and serum levels can be closely monitored. Procainamide has a short half-life, which is an important characteristic if maternal or fetal toxicity is experienced. Delivery is planned at term when conversion to normal sinus rhythm is successful, or sooner if conversion fails to occur and there is evidence of cardiac decompensation or fetal compromise.

When the diagnosis of fetal tachyarrhythmia is first made at term, medical therapy may be used in order to facilitate a trial of labor and possible vaginal delivery (Silverman et al. 1985). Vaginal delivery should be possible in most cases; however, when conversion to normal sinus rhythm is unsuccessful or hydrops is present, delivery by cesarean section may be more appropriate. Intrapartum fetal monitoring may not be reliable with supraventricular tachycardia, and the fetus with hydrops may not tolerate labor. Intermittent sonographic surveillance of fetal well-being may be necessary in such cases.

▶ FETAL INTERVENTION

For fetuses with evidence of hemodynamic compromise or hydrops prior to term, treatment of the rhythm disturbance is accomplished by administering anti-arrhythmic medications to the mother. This approach is described in detail in the section for management of pregnancy. Maternal administration of digoxin, flecanide, procainamide, quinidine, and verapamil have been successfully used.

If an adequate trial of maternal medical therapy fails despite appropriate drug levels and time for effect, direct fetal therapy may be considered. This may be achieved by direct intravenous infusion of digoxin or amiodarone into the umbilical vein. Amiodarone may be helpful in this regard due to its prolonged duration of action.

In very rare cases, direct fetal intramuscular injection of medications may be possible, but this approach should be considered less optimal than direct fetal intravascular infusion (Hallak et al. 1991; Weiner and Thompson 1988). Direct fetal therapy should be reserved for the preterm fetus that has evidence of heart failure and has not responded to maternally administered therapy. In one case, supraventricular tachycardia at 24 weeks of gestation was successfully controlled with direct fetal therapy after more traditional transplacental therapy with digoxin, verapamil, and procainamide had failed (Weiner and Thompson 1988). In this case report the fetus received 70 μg of digoxin in three divided doses administered intramuscularly over a period of 24 hours. In a further case, a 25-week-old fetus with severe hydrops fetalis secondary to supraventricular tachycardia was successfully treated with fetal intramuscular injections of digoxin together with maternal digoxin (Hallak et al. 1991). Fetal umbilical blood sampling had revealed poor placental transfer of digoxin even after 2 weeks of therapeutic maternal levels.

▶ TREATMENT OF THE NEWBORN

Because 50% of infants have a relapse of tachycardia after birth, it is important to assess the neonatal rate with an electrocardiogram (van Engelen et al. 1994). Neonatal echocardiography should also be performed to confirm the absence of structural cardiac malformation and to evaluate cardiac function. Cardioversion, transvenous atrial overdrive pacing, or antiarrhythmic drugs have been used postnatally to convert the heart rate of infants who have tachycardia at birth to normal sinus rhythm (van Engelen et al. 1994). In the absence of hemodynamic instability, it is reasonable to either observe neonates closely without medical therapy, or begin prophylactic medical therapy for up to one year.

▶ SURGICAL TREATMENT

No surgical treatments for tachyarrhythmias have been described.

▶ LONG-TERM OUTCOME

In a group of 51 cases presenting with fetal tachycardia, 50% of all surviving infants had a relapse of tachycardia after birth (van Engelen et al. 1994). Relapse appeared to be more common in those with atrial flutter; 60% of infants with fetal atrial flutter had a relapse, as compared with 42% of infants with fetal supraventricular tachycardia. In the group of 33 infants with supraventricular tachycardia, a re-entry mechanism could be seen on the electrocardiogram in 8 cases: 4 with Wolff–Parkinson–White syndrome and 4 with permanent junctional reciprocating tachycardias. At 1 month of age, 78% of the patients with a history of fetal supraventricular tachycardia or atrial flutter were receiving antiarrhythmic drugs, usually digoxin, and sometimes in combination with propranolol, verapamil, or flecainide either for recurrent tachycardia or as prophylaxis. At 3 years of age, 14% were taking antiarrhythmic drugs (van Engelen et al. 1994). Of the 3 patients who were still receiving medications, 1 had Wolff–Parkinson–White syndrome and 2 had permanent junctional reciprocating tachycardia. The need for drug therapy seems to diminish as childhood advances, with re-entry tachycardia proving to be the most therapy-resistant form before and after birth as well as during later childhood.

▶ GENETICS AND RECURRENCE RISK

We are unaware of any reported cases of a recurrence of fetal arrhythmias in subsequent pregnancies. An exception is Wolff–Parkinson–White syndrome, which involves paroxysmal supraventricular tachycardia and has a well-documented familial occurrence (Harnischfeger 1959).

REFERENCES

Allan LD. Cardiac ultrasound of the fetus. Arch Dis Child 1984;59:603–604.

Allan LD, Anderson RH, Sullivan ID, et al. Evaluation of fetal arrhythmias by echocardiography. Br Heart J 1983;50:240–245.

Beall MH, Paul RH. Artifacts, blocks, and arrhythmias: confusing nonclassical heart rate tracings. Clin Obstet Gynecol 1986;29:83–94.

Bergmans MGM, Jonker GJ, Kock HCLV. Fetal supraventricular tachycardia: review of the literature. Obstet Gynecol Surv 1985;40:61–68.

Chao RC, Ho ESC, Hsieh KS. Fetal atrial flutter and fibrillation: prenatal echocardiographic detection and management. Am Heart J 1992;124:1095–1098.

De Vore GR. Fetal echocardiography—a new frontier. Clin Obstet Gynecol 1984;27:359–377.

De Vore GR, Siassi B, Platt LD. Fetal echocardiography. III. The diagnosis of cardiac arrhythmias using real-time-directed M-mode ultrasound. Am J Obstet Gynecol 1983;146:792–799.

Epstein ML, Kiel EA, Victorica BE. Cardiac decompensation following verapamil therapy in infants with supraventricular tachycardia. Pediatrics 1985;75:737–740.

Gembruch U, Redel DA, Bald R, et al. Longitudinal study in 18 cases of fetal supraventricular tachycardia: Doppler echocardiographic findings and pathophysiologic implications. Am Heart J 1993;125:1290–1301.

Gladstone GR, Hordof A, Gersony WM. Propranolol administration during pregnancy: effect on the fetus. J Pediatr 1975;86:962–964.

Hallak M, Neerhof MG, Perry R, et al. Fetal supraventricular tachycardia and hydrops fetalis: combined intensive, direct, and transplacental therapy. Obstet Gynecol 1991;78:523–525.

Harnischfeger WW. Hereditary occurrence of the pre-excitation (Wolff-Parkinson-White) syndrome with re-entry mechanism and concealed conduction. Circulation 1959;19:28–40.

Johnson P, Sharland G, Allan LD, et al. Umbilical venous pressure in nonimmune hydrops fetalis: correlation with cardiac size. Am J Obstet Gynecol 1992;167:1309–1313.

Kleinman CS. Prenatal diagnosis and management of intrauterine arrhythmias. Fetal Ther 1986;1:92–95.

Kleinman CS, Copel JA, Weinstein EM, et al. In utero diagnosis and treatment of fetal supraventricular tachycardia. Semin Perinatol 1985a;2:113–129.

Kleinman CS, Copel JA, Weinstein EM, et al. Treatment of fetal supraventricular tachyarrhythmias. J Clin Ultrasound 1985b;13:265–273.

Kleinman CS, Hobbins JC, Jaffe CC, et al. Echocardiographic studies of the human fetus: prenatal diagnosis of congenital heart disease and cardiac dysrhythmias. Pediatrics 1980;65:1059–1066.

Maxwell DJ, Crawford DC, Curry PVM, et al. Obstetric importance, diagnosis, and management of fetal tachycardias. BMJ 1988;297:107–110.

Newburger JW, Keane JF. Intrauterine supraventricular tachycardia. J Pediatr 1979;95:780–786.

Owen J, Colvin EV, Davis RO. Fetal death after successful conversion of fetal supraventricular tachycardia with digoxin and verapamil. Am J Obstet Gynecol 1988;158:1169–1170.

Reed KL. Fetal arrhythmias: etiology, diagnosis, pathophysiology, and treatment. Semin Perinatol 1989;13:294–304.

Reed KL. Introduction to fetal echocardiography. Obstet Gynecol Clin North Am 1991;18:811–822.

Reed KL, Sahn DJ, Marx GR, et al. Cardiac doppler flows during fetal arrhythmias: physiologic consequences. Obstet Gynecol 1987;70:1–6.

Rubin PC. Beta-blockers in pregnancy. N Engl J Med 1981;305:1323–1326.

Santulli TV. Fetal echocardiography: assessment of cardiovascular anatomy and function. Clin Perinatol 1990;17:911–940.

Sarno AP, Masaki DI, Platt LD, et al. Fetal heart rate monitoring casebook: peripartum management of fetal supraventricular tachycardia. J Perinatol 1989;9:351–354.

Silverman NH, Enderlein MA, Stanger P, et al. Recognition of fetal arrhythmias by echocardiography. J Clin Ultrasound 1985;13:255–263.

Simpson LL, Marx GR. Diagnosis and treatment of structural fetal cardiac abnormality and dysrhythmia. Semin Perinatol 1994;18:215–227.

Simpson LL, Marx GR, D'Alton ME. Management of supraventricular tachycardia in the fetus. Curr Opin Obstet Gynecol 1995;7:409–413.

Simpson LL, Marx GR, D'Alton ME. Supraventricular tachycardia in the fetus: conservative management in the absence of hemodynamic compromise. J Ultrasound Med 1997;16:459–464.

Southall DP, Richards J, Hardwick RA, et al. Prospective study of fetal heart ate and rhythm patterns. Arch Dis Child 1980;55:506–511.

Stewart PA, Tonge HM, Wladimiroff JW. Arrhythmia and structural abnormalities of the fetal heart. Br Heart J 1983;50:550–554.

Strasburger JF, Huhta JC, Carpenter RJ, et al. Doppler echocardiography in the diagnosis and management of persistent fetal arrhythmias. J Am Coll Cardiol 1986;7:1386–1391.

van Engelen AD, Weijtens O, Brenner JI, et al. Management outcome and follow-up of fetal tachycardia. J Am Coll Cardiol 1994;24:1371–1375.

Weiner CP, Thompson MIB. Direct treatment of fetal supraventricular tachycardia after failed transplacental therapy. Am J Obstet Gynecol 1988;158:570–573.

Wladimiroff JW, Stewart PA. Treatment of fetal cardiac arrhythmias. Br J Hosp Med 1985;34:134–140.

CHAPTER 55

Tetralogy of Fallot

► CONDITION

Tetralogy of Fallot is a cardiac malformation that comprises ventricular septal defect (VSD), right ventricular outflow-tract obstruction, aorta overriding the interventricular septum, and right ventricular hypertrophy. This malformation presumably occurs because of unequal division of the conotruncus or incorrect alignment of the ascending aorta during embryogenesis (Romero et al. 1988). This condition exists in a wide spectrum of severity, ranging from mild right ventricular outflow-tract obstruction to complete pulmonic atresia, and aortic override ranging from minimal to 75% (Pinsky and Arciniegas 1990). In addition, the hypoplasia may involve simply the infundibulum of the right ventricle or it may also involve the pulmonary valve or pulmonary arteries. The VSD is most often in a superior or perimembranous location, and it is usually large and nonrestrictive. The diameter of the aortic root is generally inversely proportional to that of the pulmonary artery, so that in cases of pulmonic atresia the aorta is very wide, with over 50% committed to the right ventricle (Graham and Gutgesell 1990).

In general, tetralogy of Fallot does not cause significant intrauterine hemodynamic compromise for the fetus because of similarities in the pressure between the systemic and pulmonary circulations. Right ventricular hypertrophy is therefore usually not seen until after birth. In cases of tetralogy with complete absence of the pulmonary valve, significant regurgitation may cause congestive cardiac failure in utero and ultimately, hydrops (Romero et al. 1988). Following birth, the closure of the ductus arteriosus, together with the narrowed right ventricular outflow tract, results in development of a significant right-to-left shunt. This leads to blood flow bypassing the pulmonary bed, resulting in hypoxemia in the systemic circulation. Because the right ventricular outflow-tract obstruction is fixed, the degree

of right-to-left shunt is almost entirely dependent on the systemic vascular resistance (Graham and Gutgesell 1990). In times of low systemic resistance, such as during exercise, fever, or following feeding, the right-to-left shunt becomes more pronounced, which leads to cyanotic spells in the child. These can be treated by knee–chest positioning and by the use of peripheral vasoconstrictors.

Additional abnormalities that may coexist with tetralogy of Fallot include chromosomal abnormalities such as trisomies 13, 18, and 21, syndromes such as velocardiofacial, and associations such as CHARGE and VATER (Sanders et al. 1996). In 1 series, 3 of 6 cases (50%) of prenatally diagnosed tetralogy were associated with trisomy 18 (Crawford et al. 1988). In another series of prenatally diagnosed cardiac malformations 3 of the 18 fetuses (17%) with tetralogy and known karyotype had trisomy 13 (Paladini et al. 1996). In a series of 138 live-born infants with tetralogy, 17 (12%) had chromosomal abnormalities (Ferencz et al. 1987).

► INCIDENCE

Tetralogy of Fallot is one of the most common congenital cardiac malformations, occurring in approximately 2 in 10,000 live births (Graham and Gutgesell 1990). It accounts for 5 to 10% of congenital cardiac defects diagnosed in live-born infants (Fyler et al. 1980; Ferencz et al. 1987).

► SONOGRAPHIC FINDINGS

Because right ventricular hypertrophy does not generally develop in utero, and visualization of fetal right ventricular outflow tract obstruction is difficult, the prenatal diagnosis of tetralogy of Fallot relies on the

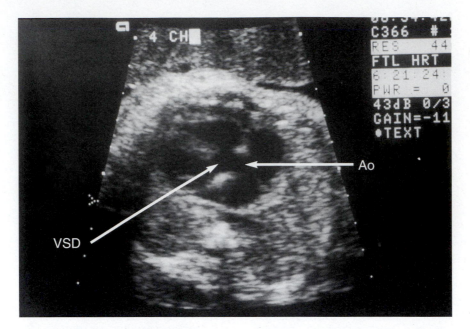

Figure 55-1. Antenatal sonographic image of a fetus with tetralogy of Fallot, demonstrating the aortic outflow tract overriding the VSD. Ao = aorta.

demonstration of the aortic outflow tract overriding a VSD at the interventricular septum (Fig. 55-1) (Romero et al. 1988). The demonstration of a VSD with overriding aorta may be performed as early as 14 weeks of gestation with the aid of transvaginal sonography (Bronshtein et al. 1990). Because of the difficulties in visualizing small perimembranous VSDs with prenatal sonography, the diagnosis of tetralogy may be missed on a standard four-chamber view of the heart. This emphasizes the importance of careful visualization of the cardiac outflow tracts during prenatal sonography. In 1 series of 22 fetuses with tetralogy, the four-chamber view was abnormal in only 1 case (Paladini et al. 1996). The VSD is best imaged by a demonstration of discontinuity between the interventricular septum and the aortic outflow tract in the left parasternal long-axis view rather than by a standard four-chamber cardiac view (DeVore et al. 1988). Color Doppler sonography may also be helpful in demonstrating flow from the right ventricle, across the VSD and into a dilated aortic root (Anderson et al. 1994).

Additional features that may assist in the prenatal diagnosis of tetralogy include the right ventricle being slightly larger than the left, a relatively small pulmonary artery, a dilated aortic root, and axis deviation (Fig. 55-2) (Sanders et al. 1996). In fetuses with tetralogy, the aortic-root diameter is increased as compared with other biometric parameters, such as the biventricular diameter (DeVore et al. 1988). However, the presence of a normal pulmonary artery:aorta ratio does not exclude tetralogy; in many cases the pulmonary artery narrowing may not become apparent until late in gestation (Lee et al. 1995).

In some cases of tetralogy with absence of the pulmonary valve, the pulmonary outflow tract may even appear massively dilated (Liang et al. 1997). Polyhydramnios may also be present in cases of tetralogy with absent pulmonary valve, as the massively dilated pulmonary artery may cause tracheobronchial and esophageal compression that leads to an apparent increase in amniotic fluid volume (Callan and Kan 1991).

The usefulness of screening ultrasonography for prenatal detection of tetralogy is unclear. In 1 study, 13 of the 20 cases (65%) of tetralogy were detected prenatally when careful screening obstetric sonography took place (Kirk et al. 1997). By contrast, in another study only 9 of 66 cases (14%) of tetralogy were detected using fetal echocardiography (Montana et al. 1996).

▶ DIFFERENTIAL DIAGNOSIS

Cardiac malformations that should be included in the differential diagnosis of tetralogy of Fallot include pulmonic atresia with a VSD (see Chapter 52), truncus arteriosus, (see Chapter 50) and double-outlet right ventricle (see Chapter 47). Doppler echocardiography may be helpful in confirming the presence of pulmonic atresia as opposed to narrowing of the right ventricular outflow tract, which is more typically seen with tetralogy. The differentiation of truncus arteriosus from tetralogy with coexisting pulmonic atresia is very difficult, with both having almost identical antenatal sonographic appearances. Visualization of more than three leaflets in a truncal valve may help differentiate these

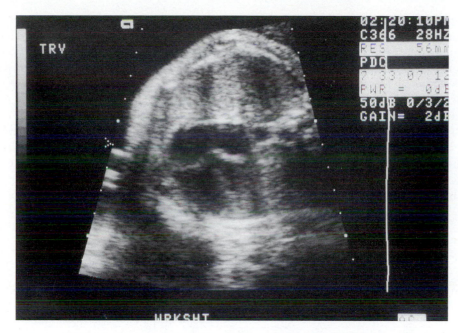

Figure 55-2. Axis deviation in a case of tetralogy of Fallot.

two conditions (see Chapter 50). It may be necessary to base differentiation of tetralogy from some cases of double-outlet right ventricle solely on the relative area of the aortic outflow tract that arises from the right ventricle (see Chapter 47).

▶ ANTENATAL NATURAL HISTORY

In general, since the pressures in the pulmonary and systemic circulations are similar, tetralogy of Fallot does not cause intrauterine hemodynamic instability. An exception would be tetralogy with absent pulmonary valve, in which significant regurgitation may lead to hydrops (Romero et al. 1988). In addition, if a major chromosomal abnormality is also present, such as trisomy 13 or 18, there will be a considerably increased risk of intrauterine death. As a general rule, the antenatal natural history of isolated tetralogy of Fallot is relatively uneventful. However, there have been reports of progression of the degree of pulmonic stenosis associated with tetralogy as gestation progresses, which would suggest that fetuses diagnosed with tetralogy should be followed serially as pregnancy continues (Hornberger et al. 1995).

In 1 series of 22 cases of prenatally diagnosed tetralogy of Fallot, 9 pregnancies (41%) were terminated, no cases resulted in intrauterine death, 6 infants (27%) died during the neonatal period, and 7 infants (32%) survived (Paladini et al. 1996). In another series of 11 cases of prenatally diagnosed tetralogy, 2 pregnancies (18%) were terminated, no cases resulted in

intrauterine death, 6 infants (55%) died during the postnatal period, and 3 infants (27%) survived (Smythe et al. 1992).

▶ MANAGEMENT OF PREGNANCY

Following prenatal diagnosis of tetralogy of Fallot a careful sonographic fetal anatomy survey is recommended to exclude additional complex cardiac malformations, such as absence of the pulmonary valve. A sonographic search for extracardiac malformations should also be performed. In particular, malformations associated with the major autosomal trisomies, CHARGE, and VATER should be excluded (Sanders et al. 1996). Fetal echocardiography should be performed by an appropriately trained specialist to confirm the diagnosis and to exclude other cardiac malformations.

Invasive fetal testing for karyotype analysis is recommended following the prenatal diagnosis of tetralogy, because in reported series the incidence of chromosomal abnormalities ranges from 12 to 50% (Crawford et al. 1988; Ferencz et al. 1987). If a karyotype is performed, additional fluorescence in situ hybridization (FISH) studies for chromosome 22q11 microdeletions that comprise the CATCH 22 syndrome should also be carried out (Trainer et al. 1996). Referrals for prenatal consultation with a pediatric cardiologist and cardiothoracic surgeon are also recommended.

If the diagnosis is made before fetal viability, termination of pregnancy may be offered because of the significant neonatal mortality and surgical morbidity in this condition. If expectant management is desired, sonographic surveillance to confirm appropriate fetal growth and to evaluate for the development of fetal hydrops is recommended, especially if additional cardiac malformations such as absence of the pulmonary valve are present. If fetal hydrops occurs, the prognosis is poor; the optimal management of such pregnancies is unknown. Delivery should occur at a tertiary-care center, with the immediate availability of a neonatologist, pediatric cardiologist, and cardiothoracic surgeon. There is no indication to alter the timing or method of delivery based on the prenatal diagnosis of tetralogy of Fallot.

► FETAL INTERVENTION

No fetal intervention has been described for tetralogy of Fallot.

► TREATMENT OF THE NEWBORN

The presence of cyanosis in a newborn with tetralogy of Fallot suggests that significant right ventricular outflow-tract obstruction is present. In such cases, or if there is any other reason to suspect ductal dependence, prostaglandin E_1 infusion should be started to maintain patency of the ductus arteriosus. When oxygen supplementation is required, care should be taken to limit the inspired fraction of oxygen so as to avoid significant reduction in pulmonary vascular resistance, which may decrease the amount of blood shunted across the ductus arteriosus. The infant should be transported to a neonatal intensive care unit as soon as possible.

Consultation with a pediatric cardiologist should be obtained promptly and echocardiography performed to confirm the prenatal diagnosis and to exclude additional cardiac malformations. The degree of pulmonary arterial obstruction should be assessed, which may require the use of cardiac catheterization. Cardiac catheterization is useful in delineating the coronary arterial anatomy, the degree of pulmonary artery narrowing, the anatomy of the pulmonary arterial branches and aorta, and the extent of the VSD (Graham and Gutgesell 1990). Further medical management in the neonatal intensive care unit will include maintenance of adequate oxygenation and treatment of metabolic acidosis and congestive heart failure. If assisted ventilation, oxygen supplementation, and prostaglandin E_1 infusion cannot maintain adequate oxygenation, consultation with a pediatric cardiothoracic surgeon should be obtained to decide on timing and method of surgical intervention, such as a palliative shunt procedure or definitive repair (Sanders et al. 1996).

Some neonates with tetralogy of Fallot do not have significant cyanosis, may have minimal right ventricular outflow-tract obstruction, and may not be dependent on a patent ductus arteriosus. Such infants generally do not require prostaglandin E_1 infusion, provided they can maintain adequate oxygenation, even after spontaneous closure of the ductus arteriosus. In these cases, cardiac catheterization can generally be delayed until 3 to 6 months of age, with surgical repair planned for soon after onset of symptoms or electively at 18 to 24 months of age (Pinsky and Arciniegas 1990). However, in over 70% of infants with tetralogy symptoms develop sufficient to warrant surgical intervention within the first year of life (Castaneda and Jonas 1990).

► SURGICAL TREATMENT

Debate still exists on the timing of surgical repair for tetralogy of Fallot and the role of palliative shunting procedures prior to definitive correction. Infants with isolated tetralogy of Fallot and favorable anatomy generally receive complete primary repair soon after the onset of symptoms or within the first year of life. Infants with more complex tetralogy, such as hypoplasia of the pulmonary arteries or anomalous coronary arterial anatomy, are initially treated with a systemic-to-pulmonary shunt followed by final repair at 18 to 24 months of age (Pinsky and Arciniegas 1990). As surgical techniques advance, the age at which complete primary repair is performed continues to decrease (Castaneda and Jonas 1990).

Primary repair of tetralogy of Fallot requires cardiopulmonary bypass and a median sternotomy approach (Castaneda and Jonas 1990). The infundibulum of the right ventricular outflow tract is incised, and the incision is carried up to the bifurcation of the pulmonary artery. Thickened or dysplastic pulmonary valve leaflets are usually excised. A Dacron patch is used to close the VSD and a patch of pericardium is used to augment the right ventricular outflow tract and pulmonary artery. If a patent foramen ovale or patent ductus arteriosus is present, these are also closed at this time. For the few patients who are not candidates for complete primary repair, the most commonly performed palliative procedure is a Blalock–Taussig systemic-to-pulmonary shunt, in which the subclavian artery is anastomosed to the pulmonary artery.

The operative mortality rate for primary repair of tetralogy of Fallot during infancy has improved, with mortality quoted as 14% in 1979 but subsequently improved to 3% in 1990 (Touati et al. 1990; Tucker et al. 1979). At one center, of 467 infants who underwent surgery for tetralogy of Fallot, there were only 16 (3.4%)

early postoperative deaths (Pinsky and Arciniegas 1990). In another series at one center, of 366 infants who had complete correction of tetralogy, using a 6- to 8-kg weight cutoff for surgical eligibility, the operative mortality rate was only 0.5% (Karl et al. 1992). Operative mortality now appears to be most affected by the presence of complex cardiac anatomy or an abnormal metabolic state, rather than infant age or weight (Castaneda and Jonas 1990).

► LONG-TERM OUTCOME

A study of the long-term outcome of 163 patients who survived complete repair of tetralogy of Fallot demonstrated a 90% 30-year actuarial survival rate, with 94% of survivors in either New York Heart Association functional class I or II (Murphy et al. 1993). However, up to 12% of patients who survive surgical correction may have unsatisfactory results, and reoperation may be required for those with residual right ventricular outflow-tract obstruction or residual VSD (Pinsky and Arciniegas 1990). Other long-term complications include the development of pulmonary valve insufficiency and arrhythmias, possibly leading to sudden death.

► GENETICS AND RECURRENCE RISK

Tetralogy of Fallot has been described with velocardiofacial syndrome, DiGeorge syndrome, and the CHARGE and VATER associations (Sanders et al. 1996). In addition, tetralogy has been described with trisomies 13, 18, and 21. Chromosome 22q11 microdeletions that are seen as part of the CATCH 22 syndrome have been noted in many infants with tetralogy, being present in 21% of infants with tetralogy in one series (Trainer et al. 1996).

The recurrence risk for tetralogy of Fallot is 2.5% if 1 previous sibling has been affected and increases to 8% if 2 previous siblings have been affected (Nora and Nora 1988). If the mother has tetralogy, the recurrence risk for her offspring is 2.5%. If the father is affected, the recurrence risk for his offspring is 1.5% (Nora and Nora 1988).

REFERENCES

Anderson CF, McCurdy CM, McNamara MF, et al. Case of the day. 8. Diagnosis: Color Doppler aided diagnosis of tetralogy of Fallot. J Ultrasound Med 1994;13:341–342.

Bronshtein M, Siegler E, Yoffe N, et al. Prenatal diagnosis of ventricular septal defect and overriding aorta at 14 weeks' gestation, using transvaginal sonography. Prenat Diagn 1990;10:697–702.

Callan NA, Kan JS. Prenatal diagnosis of tetralogy of Fallot with absent pulmonary valve. Am J Perinatol 1991;8: 15–17.

Castaneda AR, Jonas RE. Neonatal repair of tetralogy of Fallot. In: Long WA, ed. Fetal and neonatal cardiology. Philadelphia: Saunders, 1990:774–779.

Crawford DC, Chita SK, Allan LD. Prenatal detection of congenital heart disease: factors affecting obstetric management and survival. Am J Obstet Gynecol 1988;159: 352–356.

DeVore GR, Siassai B, Platt LD. Fetal echocardiography. VIII. Aortic root dilation—a marker for tetralogy of Fallot. Am J Obstet Gynecol 1988;159:129–136.

Ferencz C, Rubin JD, McCarter RJ, et al. Cardiac and noncardiac malformations: observations in a population-based study. Teratology 1987;35:367–378.

Fyler DC, Buckley LP, Hellenbrand WE, et al. Report of the New England Regional Cardiac Program. Pediatrics 1980; 65(suppl):375–461.

Graham TP, Gutgesell HP. Conotruncal abnormalities. In: Long WA, ed. Fetal and neonatal cardiology. Philadelphia: Saunders, 1990:561–570.

Hornberger LK, Sanders SP, Sahn DJ, et al. In utero pulmonary artery and aortic growth and potential for progression of pulmonary outflow tract obstruction in tetralogy of Fallot. J Am Coll Cardiol 1995;25:739–745.

Karl TR, Sano S, Pornviliwan S, et al. Tetralogy of Fallot: favorable outcome of a non-neonatal transatrial, transpulmonary repair. Ann Thorac Surg 1992;54:903–907.

Kirk JS, Comstock CH, Lee W, et al. Sonographic screening to detect fetal cardiac abnormalities: a 5-year experience with 111 abnormal cases. Obstet Gynecol 1997;89: 227–232.

Lee W, Smith RS, Comstock CH, et al. Tetralogy of Fallot: prenatal diagnosis and postnatal survival. Obstet Gynecol 1995;86:583–588.

Liang CC, Tsai CC, Hsieh CC, et al. Prenatal diagnosis of tetralogy of Fallot with absent pulmonary valve accompanied by hydrops fetalis. Gynecol Obstet Invest 1997;44: 61–63.

Montana E, Khoury MJ, Cragan JD, et al. Trends and outcomes after prenatal diagnosis of congenital cardiac malformations by fetal echocardiography in a well defined birth population. Atlanta, Georgia 1990–1994. J Am Coll Cardiol 1996;28:1805–1809.

Murphy JG, Gersh BJ, Mair DD, et al. Long-term outcome in patients undergoing surgical repair of tetralogy of Fallot. N Engl J Med 1993;329:593–599.

Nora JJ, Nora AH. Update on counseling the family with a first-degree relative with a congenital heart defect. Am J Med Genet 1988;29:137–142.

Paladini D, Rustico M, Todros T, et al. Conotruncal anomalies in prenatal life. Ultrasound Obstet Gynecol 1996;8: 241–246.

Pinsky WW, Arciniegas E. Tetralogy of Fallot. Pediatr Clin North Am 1990;37:179–192.

Romero R, Pilu G, Jeanty P, et al. Tetralogy of Fallot. In Romero R, Pilu G, Jeanty P, Ghidini A, Hobbins JC, eds.

Prenatal diagnosis of congenital anomalies. Norwalk, CT: Appleton & Lange, 1988:157–160.

Sanders RC, Blackmon LR, Hogge WA, et al. Tetralogy of Fallot. In: Sanders RC, Blackmon LR, Hogge WA, Wulfsberg EA,eds. Structural fetal abnormalities: the total picture. St. Louis: Mosby, 1996:81–83.

Smythe JF, Copel JA, Kleinman CS. Outcome of prenatally detected cardiac malformations. Am J Cardiol 1992;69: 1471–1474.

Touati GD, Vouhe PR, Amodeo A, et al. Primary repair of tetralogy of Fallot in infancy. J Thorac Cardiovasc Surg 1990;99:396–403.

Trainer AH, Morrison N, Dunlop A, et al. Chromosome 22q11 microdeletions in tetralogy of Fallot. Arch Dis Child 1996;74:62–63.

Tucker WY, Turley K, Ullyot DJ, et al. Management of symptomatic tetralogy of Fallot in the first year of life. J Thorac Cardiovasc Surg 1979;78:494–501.

CHAPTER 56

Transposition of Great Vessels

► CONDITION

Transposition of the great arteries (TGA) may be either complete or corrected. Complete TGA is also known as d-transposition, simple transposition, or atrioventricular concordance with ventriculoarterial discordance. This anomaly probably occurs because of failure of the aorticopulmonary septum to follow a spiral course during embryogenesis, resulting in the aorta arising from the right ventricle and the pulmonary artery arising from the left ventricle (de la Cruz et al. 1981). Atrial septal defect (ASD) and ventricular septal defect (VSD) are commonly seen with complete TGA and may also be associated with pulmonary artery obstruction. Complete TGA usually causes no significant hemodynamic compromise in utero, but rapid deterioration occurs soon after birth in those cases without sufficient mixing of the right- and left-sided circulations.

By contrast, corrected TGA refers to the connection of the right atrium to the morphologic left ventricle, which connects to the pulmonary artery, while the left atrium connects to the morphologic right ventricle and then to the aorta. This anomaly is also known as l-transposition, or atrioventricular discordance with ventriculoarterial discordance. Because both right and left cardiac blood flow follow their intended paths from systemic to pulmonary and back to systemic circulations, this anomaly effectively cancels itself out (Romero et al. 1988). While the right atrium empties into the anatomic right ventricle, this ventricle is in fact the morphologic left ventricle with a transposed pulmonary artery as its outflow tract. Similarly the left atrium empties into the anatomic left ventricle, which is in fact the morphologic right ventricle, connected to a transposed aorta. Physiologically it might be expected that this anomaly would not lead to hemodynamic compromise; however, because of a frequent association with VSD, pulmonic stenosis,

conduction defects, and atrioventricular valve abnormalities, significant neonatal morbidity and mortality may occur.

► INCIDENCE

TGA accounts for 10% of all infants born with congenital cardiac defects, representing approximately 2 in 10,000 live births (Fyler et al. 1980).

► SONOGRAPHIC FINDINGS

Complete TGA is recognized on prenatal sonography by careful visualization of the cardiac outflow tracts. The normal crossover of the pulmonary artery and aorta is not seen, and the outflow tracts appear to run parallel to each other. Each outflow tract should be followed to its branches to positively differentiate the pulmonary artery from the aorta (Figs. 56-1 and 56-2). The pulmonary trunk should be visible arising from the posterior ventricle, bifurcating into the left and right pulmonary arteries and ductus arteriosus. The aorta is visible arising anterior to the pulmonary artery and connecting to the aortic arch with brachiocephalic vessels.

Prenatal sonographic diagnosis of corrected TGA is extremely difficult because the ventricular outflow tracts may appear to arise correctly from the anatomic right and left ventricles. Sonographic diagnosis relies on the demonstration of parallel outflow tracts, with absence of the normal crossover (Morelli et al. 1996). In addition, the morphologic appearance of the anatomic left ventricle is more suggestive of a right ventricle, with a moderator band and triangular-shaped ventricular cavity. A normal left ventricular cavity should not

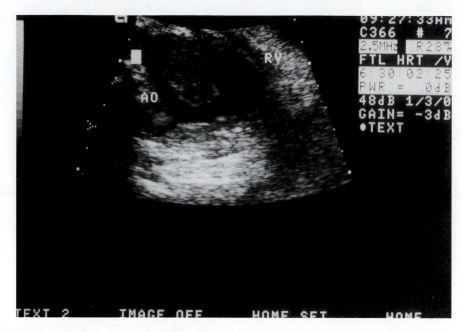

Figure 56-1. Prenatal sonogram of a fetus with TGA, demonstrating the right ventricle and its outflow tract, which when followed shows distally the aorta (AO) and branching vessels to the fetal head.

demonstrate a moderator band and should be elliptical, rather than triangular, in shape.

Prenatal sonography is an important means of diagnosing or excluding additional coexisting cardiac malformations. VSD may be present in 50% of cases of TGA and, when found, is commonly accompanied by subvalvular pulmonic stenosis (Schiebler et al. 1961).

As a result of interference with the conduction apparatus of the heart, arrhythmias are common, with complete heart block found in 4 of 21 fetuses with corrected TGA (Gembruch et al. 1989). Other cardiac malformations that may be detectable include ventricular hypoplasia and coarctation of the aorta (Santoro et al. 1997). The presence of situs inversus may also

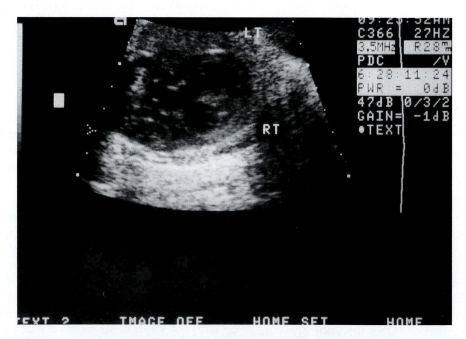

Figure 56-2. Prenatal sonogram of the same fetus shown in Figure 56-1 demonstrating the left ventricle and its outflow tract (LT). This tract, when followed, showed the pulmonary arteries. RT = right ventricular outflow tract.

be found in the presence of corrected TGA (Abossolo et al. 1996).

The usefulness of sonography as a tool in the prenatal diagnosis of TGA is unclear. In 1 series of screening sonograms of 11,894 fetuses, none of the 4 cases of TGA were detected prenatally (Tegnander et al. 1995). In another series of 50 infants operated on for TGA, 17 (34%) were successfully diagnosed prenatally through the use of obstetric sonography (Lupoglazoff et al. 1997). In addition, in another recent series of 111 congenital cardiac abnormalities, 5 of the 8 cases (63%) of TGA were detected on prenatal screening sonography (Kirk et al. 1997). In a review of all congenital cardiac malformations in one geographical area, only 5 of the 80 cases (6%) of TGA were detected prenatally (Montana et al. 1996).

▶ DIFFERENTIAL DIAGNOSIS

One of the most difficult congenital cardiac anomalies to differentiate from TGA is double-outlet right ventricle, especially when TGA is accompanied by a VSD (Sanders et al. 1996). Careful attention should be paid to any potential straddling or overriding of atrioventricular valves. The Taussig–Bing heart, a variant of double-outlet right ventricle in which the aortic and pulmonary outflow tracts ascend in a parallel fashion, may mimic the appearance of TGA (see Chapter 47).

▶ ANTENATAL NATURAL HISTORY

In general, both complete and corrected forms of TGA are well tolerated by the fetus in utero because both ventricles pump into the systemic circulation. However, the presence of additional cardiac malformations, such as VSD or pulmonic stenosis, may alter the antenatal natural history, potentially leading to the development of congestive heart failure, or hydrops, in utero. Deterioration in hemodynamic status can be expected soon after birth, especially when there is no communication between right and left sides of the heart to allow adequate mixing of blood.

In 1 series of 6 fetuses with TGA diagnosed prenatally, 1 pregnancy was terminated, and the remaining 5 resulted in live births; 2 of these infants died during the neonatal period (Smythe et al. 1992). In another series evaluating the outcome of various prenatally diagnosed cardiac malformations, all 3 fetuses with TGA survived (Sharland et al. 1990). More recently, in 23 cases of prenatally diagnosed TGA, 6 pregnancies (26%) were terminated, 3 (13%) fetuses died in utero, 8 (35%) died during the neonatal period, and 6 (26%) survived (Paladini et al. 1996).

▶ MANAGEMENT OF PREGNANCY

Following prenatal diagnosis of TGA, a careful sonographic fetal anatomy survey is recommended to exclude additional cardiac malformations, such as VSD, pulmonic stenosis, aortic coarctation, and arrhythmias. A sonographic search for extracardiac malformations should also be performed, although in general such abnormalities are rarely found with TGA. Fetal echocardiography should be performed by an appropriately trained specialist to confirm the diagnosis and to exclude other cardiac malformations. Invasive fetal testing for karyotype analysis is recommended following the prenatal diagnosis of most cardiac malformations, although the incidence of chromosomal abnormalities is likely to be very low. In 1 series of 23 cases of prenatally diagnosed TGA, chromosomal analysis was normal in the 21 cases in which karyotype was known (Paladini et al. 1996). Referral for prenatal consultation with a pediatric cardiologist and cardiothoracic surgeon is also recommended.

If the diagnosis is made prior to fetal viability, termination of pregnancy may be offered because of the significant neonatal mortality and surgical morbidity. If expectant management is desired, sonographic surveillance to confirm appropriate fetal growth and to evaluate for the development of fetal hydrops is recommended, especially if additional cardiac malformations such as VSD and pulmonic stenosis are present. If fetal hydrops occurs, the prognosis deteriorates further; the optimal management of such pregnancies is uncertain. Delivery should occur at a tertiary-care center, with the immediate availability of a neonatologist, pediatric cardiologist, and cardiothoracic surgeon. There is no indication to alter the timing or method of delivery based on the prenatal diagnosis of TGA.

▶ FETAL INTERVENTION

No fetal intervention has been described for the obstetric or prenatal management of TGA.

▶ TREATMENT OF THE NEWBORN

The condition of most infants with isolated complete TGA will deteriorate soon after birth, resulting in death, without surgical intervention. Following delivery, care should be taken with the administration of supplemental oxygen so as to avoid significant reduction in pulmonary vascular resistance, which may decrease the amount of blood shunted across the ductus arteriosus. The infant should be transported to a neonatal intensive care unit and, if cyanosis is present, prostaglandin

E$_1$ infusion should be started to maintain patency of the ductus arteriosus.

Consultation with a pediatric cardiologist should be obtained promptly, and echocardiography should be performed to confirm the prenatal diagnosis and to determine the absence of additional cardiac malformations. Patency of both ventricular outflow tracts should be assessed, and the coronary arterial anatomy should be mapped in preparation for surgical repair. When an intact ventricular septum exists and when inadequate atrial communication is present, balloon atrial septostomy may be needed during the initial resuscitation to maximize oxygenation of systemic blood (Graham and Gutgesell 1990). Such balloon atrial septostomy may be performed either during cardiac catheterization or using echocardiographic guidance. This usually results in sufficient bidirectional shunting of blood to improve the systemic oxygen content. Occasionally, atrial septostomy is insufficient to improve systemic oxygenation, which may be secondary to inadequate atrial defect size, abnormal ventricular compliance, elevated pulmonary vascular resistance, or left ventricular outflow-tract obstruction (Graham and Gutgesell 1990). Consultation with a pediatric cardiothoracic surgeon should then be obtained to decide on the timing and method of surgical intervention, such as surgical atrial septostomy or arterial switch procedure.

Infants with TGA and a coexisting large VSD are usually stable initially, and then after a few weeks of life congestive heart failure occurs. These infants account for less than 25% of all cases of TGA. Such patients can usually be treated medically, with digoxin and diuretics, before surgical repair is considered. However, delay in surgical repair beyond the end of the third month of life may lead to the development of abnormal pulmonary vascular resistance, which occurs earlier in infants with TGA and VSD as compared with infants with left-to-right shunts without TGA (Graham and Gutgesell 1990).

▶ SURGICAL TREATMENT

Surgical repair is indicated for all infants with complete TGA and is generally best performed soon after birth, often within the first 2 weeks of life. Initial procedures, such as the Senning or the Mustard operation, were designed to physiologically correct cardiac blood flow through the use of the atrial septum or a baffle to redirect vena caval return to the left ventricle and pulmonary venous return to the right ventricle. However, such atrial repairs were associated with high operative mortality as well as significant late complications (Castaneda and Mayer 1990). Subsequently, an anatomic repair, known as the arterial switch procedure, has been devised, and involves dividing the pulmonary artery with reanasto-

mosis to the right ventricular outflow tract, and dividing the aorta with reanastomosis to the left ventricular outflow tract. To be successful this procedure must be done early in neonatal life, before the left ventricle adapts to the lower-pressure pulmonary circulation that would prevent it being able to subsequently support the systemic circulation.

Arterial switch repair is performed through a median sternotomy incision and with cardiopulmonary bypass (Castaneda and Mayer 1990). The aorta is transected distal to the origin of the coronary arteries. The coronary arteries are then excised and transposed to the origin of the pulmonary artery from the left ventricle. The pulmonary artery is then transected distal to this coronary artery connection but proximal to the bifurcation, and is reanastomosed to the original right ventricular outflow-tract stump. Similarly, the aorta is reanastomosed to the left ventricular outflow-tract stump. This results in complete anatomic repair of the great vessels and coronary arteries.

The operative mortality rate for the arterial switch repair is between 5 and 8%, with a 1 month survival of 84% (Kirklin et al. 1992). Risk factors for perioperative death include the presence of multiple VSDs, anomalous coronary-artery anatomy, additional cardiac malformations, and long aortic cross-clamp time. In another series of 432 arterial switch procedures performed in a single center at an average of 3 days of life, the operative mortality rate was 8%, with anomalous coronary-artery anatomy being the only identified risk factor for early death (Serraf et al. 1993).

▶ LONG-TERM OUTCOME

Overall long-term results for TGA suggest a 60% actuarial survival at 15 years of age (Morris and Menashe 1991). Long-term results specifically for the atrial switch repair (Senning or Mustard procedures) suggest that up to 10% die while waiting for surgery, but of those operated on, 80% are alive after 20 years (Kirklin et al. 1990). There seems to be a progressive decline in the prevalence of normal sinus rhythm in these patients, which may account for sudden late deaths. Although atrial switch survivors can live normal active lives, exercise testing is generally subnormal (Kirklin et al. 1990).

Survival data on long-term outcome following the arterial switch repair is not readily available because it has been in use for less than 20 years. Five-year survival following the arterial switch repair was 82% in one multicenter series, with almost all survivors in New York Heart Association functional class I (Kirklin et al. 1992).

The long-term fate of the coronary arteries is unclear, as there may be significant kinking or compression following the arterial switch procedure. Surveillance with echocardiography and myocardial scintigraphy is therefore recommended for survivors to detect early ventricular ischemia (Kaplan and Allada 1992). In one series of 58 children with coronary-artery surveillance following the arterial switch procedure, 8% had evidence of late coronary-artery complications (Bonnet et al. 1996). Delayed repair of TGA may be associated with progressive impairment of cognitive function (Newburger et al. 1984).

► GENETICS AND RECURRENCE RISK

Almost all cases of TGA occur as isolated cardiac malformations with normal karyotype (Paladini et al. 1996). Risk of recurrence has been estimated as 1.5% if 1 prior sibling has been affected, and this may increase to 5% with 2 prior affected siblings (Nora and Nora 1988).

REFERENCES

Abossolo T, Alessandri JL, Saltet A, et al. In utero diagnosis of situs inversus abnormalities: a case of prenatal diagnosis of visceral situs inversus with corrected transposition of great vessels. J Gynecol Obstet Biol Reprod 1996;25: 267–273.

Bonnet D, Bonhoeffer P, Piechaud JF, et al. Long-term fate of the coronary arteries after the arterial switch operation in newborns with transposition of the great arteries. Heart 1996;76:274–279.

Castaneda AR, Mayer JE. Neonatal repair of transposition of the great arteries. In: Long WA, ed. Fetal and neonatal cardiology. Philadelphia: Saunders, 1990:789–795.

de la Cruz MV, Arteaga M, Espino-Vela J, et al. Complete transposition of the great arteries: types and morphogenesis of ventriculoarterial discordance. Am Heart J 1981; 102:271–281.

Fyler DC, Buckley LP, Hellenbrand WE, et al. Report of the New England Regional Cardiac Program. Pediatrics 1980; 65(suppl):375–461.

Gembruch U, Hansmann M, Redel DA, et al. Fetal complete heart block: antenatal diagnosis, significance and management. Eur J Obstet Gynecol Reprod Biol 1989;31:9–22.

Graham TP, Gutgesell HP. Conotruncal abnormalities. In: Long WA, ed. Fetal and neonatal cardiology. Philadelphia: Saunders, 1990:561–570.

Kaplan S, Allada V. Evolution of therapy for D-transposition of the great arteries. Circulation 1992;86:1654–1656.

Kirk JS, Comstock CH, Lee W, et al. Sonographic screening to detect fetal cardiac anomalies: a 5-year experience with 111 abnormal cases. Obstet Gynecol 1997;89: 227–232.

Kirklin JW, Colvin EV, McConnell ME, et al. Complete transposition of the great arteries: treatment in the current era. Pediatr Clin North Am 1990;37:171–177.

Kirklin JW, Blackstone EH, Tchervenkov CI, et al. Clinical outcome after the arterial switch operation for transposition: patient, support, procedural, and institutional risk factors. Circulation 1992;86:1501–1515.

Lupoglazoff JM, Lhosmot JP, Azancot A, et al. Has prenatal diagnosis of transposition of great vessels changed its prognosis? Arch Mal Coeur Vaiss 1997;90:667–672.

Montana E, Khoury MJ, Cragan JD, et al. Trends and outcomes after prenatal diagnosis of congenital cardiac malformations by fetal echocardiography in a well defined birth population. Atlanta, Georgia 1990–1994. J Am Coll Cardiol 1996;28:1805–1809.

Morelli PJ, Kimball TR, Witt SA, et al. Echocardiographic considerations in demonstrating complex anatomy of criss-cross atrioventricular valves and discordant atrioventricular and ventriculoarterial relations. J Am Soc Echocardiogr 1996;9:727–729.

Morris CD, Menashe VD: 25-year mortality after surgical repair of congenital heart defect in childhood: a population-based cohort study. JAMA 1991;266:3447–3452.

Newburger JW, Silbert AR, Buckley LP, et al. Cognitive function and age at repair of transposition of the great arteries in children. N Engl J Med 1984;310:1495–1499.

Nora JJ, Nora AH. Update on counseling the family with a first-degree relative with a congenital heart defect. Am J Med Genet 1988;29:137–142.

Paladini D, Rustico M, Todros T, et al. Conotruncal anomalies in prenatal life. Ultrasound Obstet Gynecol 1996; 8:241–246.

Romero R, Pilu G, Jeanty P, et al. Corrected transposition of the great arteries. In: Romero R, Pilu G, Jeanty P, Ghidini A, Hobbins JC, eds. Prenatal diagnosis of congenital anomalies. Norwalk, CT: Appleton & Lange, 1988: 164–166.

Sanders RC, Blackmon LR, Hogge WA, et al. Transposition of the great arteries. In: Sanders RC, Blackmon LR, Hogge WA, Wulfsberg EA, eds. Structural fetal abnormalities: the total picture. St. Louis: Mosby, 1996:84–86.

Santoro G, Masiello P, Baldi C, et al. Corrected transposition of the great arteries with isolated aortic coarctation: in utero echocardiographic diagnosis. Pediatr Cardiol 1997; 18:396–398.

Schiebler GL, Edwards JE, Burchell HB, et al. Congenital corrected transposition of the great vessels: a study of 33 cases. Pediatrics 1961;27:851.

Serraf A, Lacour-Gayet F, Bruniaux J, et al. Anatomic correction of transposition of the great arteries in neonates. J Am Coll Cardiol 1993;22:193–200.

Sharland GK, Lockhart SM, Chita SK, et al. Factors influencing the outcome of congenital heart disease detected prenatally. Arch Dis Child 1990;65:284–287.

Smythe JF, Copel JA, Kleinman CS. Outcome of prenatally detected cardiac malformations. Am J Cardiol 1992;69: 1471–1474.

Tegnander E, Eik-Nes SH, Johansen OJ, et al. Prenatal detection of heart defects at the routine fetal examination at 18 weeks in a non-selected population. Ultrasound Obstet Gynecol 1995;5:372–380.

CHAPTER 57

Atrial and Ventricular Septal Defects

► CONDITION

Atrial Septal Defect

Atrial septal defect (ASD) refers to a congenital malformation in the development of the interatrial septum. In embryonic life, the interatrial septum begins as a septum primum, growing from the atrial walls to the endocardial cushions, which contains a temporary opening known as the foramen primum (Romero et al. 1988a). Subsequently, a septum secundum grows on the right side of the septum primum and contains a normal opening known as the foramen ovale. The lower part of the septum primum forms a flap valve for this foramen ovale. Soon after birth, increased left atrial pressure closes this flap, normally resulting in complete closure of the foramen ovale by 3 months of life.

Three different types of ASDs are possible, depending on the location within the heart (Romero et al. 1988a). An inlet ASD is located near the entrance of the superior vena cava; a secundum ASD occurs in the body of the interatrial septum; a primum or outlet ASD is located near the atrioventricular junction and usually behaves similarly to an AV canal defect (see Chapter 43). Secundum ASDs typically occur because of absence of the foramen ovale flap valve. ASDs usually cause no hemodynamic effects in utero because of the normal right-to-left shunting of blood across the patent foramen ovale. If an ASD persists after birth it may allow for a left-to-right shunt, which can result in congestive heart failure or pulmonary hypertension.

Ventricular Septal Defect

Ventricular septal defect (VSD) refers to a congenital malformation in the development of the interventricular septum. VSDs can occur in the muscular or membranous portions of the septum. Muscular VSDs may be further subdivided into inlet, trabecular, or infundibular defects (Soto et al. 1980). VSDs may also be classified as being either subvalvular or muscular (Capelli et al. 1983). Subvalvular VSDs are directly related to the atrioventricular or semilunar valves, without interposed muscle between the defect and the valve cusps. Such subvalvular defects may be further subclassified as inlet, subtricuspid, subaortic, subpulmonary, or double-committed subarterial, in which the defect is below the pulmonary and aortic valves. Muscular VSDs are bordered on all sides by muscle and are not directly related to the valves. Such defects may be further subclassified as being apical, central, or outlet in location. Most of these VSD types can be defined by echocardiography, although it is important to realize that small muscular defects can be missed by sonography during both the prenatal and the postnatal periods (Capelli et al. 1983).

VSDs usually cause no hemodynamic effects in utero because of the similarity in pressures between the right and left sides of the heart during prenatal life. Most VSDs are also asymptomatic immediately following birth. If the VSD persists after birth it may allow for a left-to-right shunt, which can result in congestive heart failure or pulmonary hypertension.

► INCIDENCE

Atrial Septal Defect

Because of the difficulties in differentiating ASDs from asymptomatic patency of the foramen ovale, the precise incidence of ASD is difficult to establish. A patent foramen ovale may be present in up to 30% of normal adults. ASDs comprise 7.5% of all congenital cardiac malformations (Ferencz et al. 1987). In one population series, the incidence of ASD was 6 in 10,000 total births (Mitchell et al. 1971).

Ventricular Septal Defect

VSDs are the most common single congenital cardiac malformation, accounting for 26% of all structural cardiac abnormalities (Ferencz et al. 1987). In one population series, the incidence of VSD was 2 in 10,000 total births (Mitchell et al. 1971). However, with the increasing use of prenatal and neonatal echocardiography, the birth incidence of VSDs seems to be much higher than previously suggested. In one series, 5% of all newborns were found to have an isolated muscular VSD (Roguin et al. 1995). In addition, VSDs are frequently found in association with other cardiac malformations, such as tetralogy of Fallot and transposition of the great vessels.

► SONOGRAPHIC FINDINGS

Atrial Septal Defect

Prenatal sonographic diagnosis of ASD is problematic because the differentiation between a normal patent foramen ovale and true ASD may be difficult. The foramen ovale normally increases in size linearly with advancing gestational age (Phillippos et al. 1994). Large defects of the septum secundum are visualized as dropout of echoes at the level of the interatrial septum (Romero et al. 1988a). If an apical four-chamber view is used it may be difficult to confirm an intact interatrial septum. For adequate visualization, the ultrasound probe should be perpendicular to the septum, which can be achieved through the use of a subcostal approach to the four-chamber view (Romero et al. 1988a).

The accuracy of sonographic screening for prenatal detection of ASD is poor. In a series of 7459 fetuses who were screened at 18 weeks of gestation, there were 10 ASDs, none of which were identified prenatally (Tegnander et al. 1995). In another series, only 5% of the 761 ASDs that were present in a single large population were detected prenatally (Montana et al. 1996).

Ventricular Septal Defect

As with an ASD, prenatal sonographic diagnosis of a VSD can be difficult because it relies on visualization of dropout of echoes at the level of the interventricular septum, which is best achieved using a subcostal approach to the four-chamber view. In order to con-

firm an intact interventricular septum, the septum should also be visualized by means of a long-axis view of the left and right ventricles, together with an apex-to-base sweep along the short axis of the heart (Romero et al. 1988b). Small membranous VSDs are still commonly missed on prenatal sonography, despite adequate views of all parts of the interventricular septum. In addition, artifactual areas of hypoechogenicity in the septum during the apical four-chamber view may give the false impression of a VSD; therefore a true VSD is confirmed only when it is visible in at least two different planes (Romero et al. 1988b). Color Doppler sonography may also be used to demonstrate flow across the area of defect (Fig. 57-1) (Sanders et al. 1996).

The accuracy of prenatal sonographic screening for VSDs is poor. In a series of 7459 fetuses who were screened at 18 weeks of gestation, there were 53 VSDs, none of which were identified prenatally (Tegnander et al. 1995). In another series, only 5% of the 486 VSDs present in a single large population were detected prenatally (Montana et al. 1996). The accuracy of targeted fetal echocardiography for prenatal detection of isolated VSDs is also poor. In one series of targeted fetal echocardiograms, only 4 (31%) of 13 ASDs or VSDs were correctly identified (Benacerraf et al. 1987). In another series of fetal echocardiograms, there were 29 VSDs, 19 (66%) of which were correctly identified; the vast majority of these were associated with other more complex cardiac malformations (Crawford et al. 1988). In one further series, only 11 (44%) of 25 isolated VSDs were correctly identified prenatally, with small and moderate-sized VSDs the most likely to be missed (Kirk et al. 1997).

► DIFFERENTIAL DIAGNOSIS

Atrial Septal Defect

The main differential diagnosis to consider following the prenatal diagnosis of an ASD is the possibility of a normal patent foramen ovale.

Ventricular Septal Defect

As with ASD, it is important to consider a normal interventricular septum in all cases following the prenatal diagnosis of VSD because false positive diagnoses are possible, especially if the septum is visualized by means of an apical four-chamber view. Other diagnoses to consider include the presence of additional, more complex cardiac malformations that may involve a VSD, such as tetralogy of Fallot, transposition of the great vessels, double-outlet right ventricle, and tricuspid atresia (Fig. 57-2).

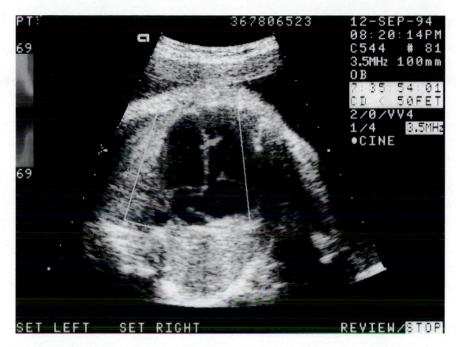

Figure 57-1. Fetal cardiac image using color Doppler sonography, which clearly demonstrates flow across the ventriculoseptal defect. See color plate.

▶ ANTENATAL HISTORY

Atrial Septal Defect

In the majority of cases, an isolated ASD will not cause any significant hemodynamic compromise in utero be-cause of the normal right-to-left shunting of blood across the patent foramen ovale. It is also possible for ASDs to close spontaneously in utero, although the exact frequency of this occurrence is unclear because the accuracy of prenatal diagnosis of isolated ASD is so poor.

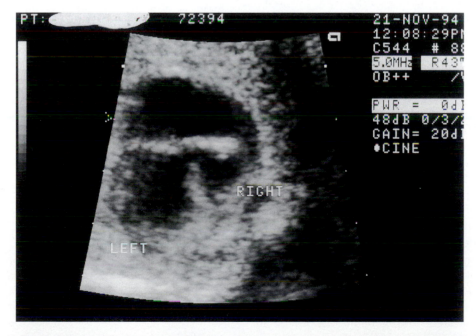

Figure 57-2. Ventricular septal defect in a fetus with tricupsid atresia. Note the rela-tive hypoplasia of the right ventricle. *(Courtesy of Dr. Marjorie Treadwell.)*

Ventricular Septal Defect

As with ASDs, almost all isolated VSDs cause no significant hemodynamic compromise in utero; the pressures in both ventricles are similar, so shunting of blood between ventricles is not a problem. Many isolated VSDs, especially small muscular types, close spontaneously, either in utero or soon after birth (Nir et al. 1994). In 1 series, 26 (74%) of 35 isolated VSDs diagnosed prenatally closed spontaneously before birth, and there was no correlation between the size of the defect and probability of closure (Orie et al. 1994). In another series, 89% of all muscular VSDs were asymptomatic and resulted in spontaneous closure within 1 to 10 months of neonatal life (Roguin et al. 1995). However, because prenatal diagnosis of VSDs is so poor, it is possible that VSDs successfully diagnosed in utero may be larger and may represent a group that has a more unfavorable prognosis.

In 1 series of 14 fetuses with VSDs diagnosed prenatally, 6 (43%) were terminated, 2 (14%) died in utero, 1 (7%) died postnatally, and 5 (36%) survived (Smythe et al. 1992). In another series of 19 fetuses with VSDs diagnosed prenatally, 1 (5%) died in utero, 10 (53%) died postnatally, and 8 (42%) survived (Sharland et al. 1990).

▶ MANAGEMENT OF PREGNANCY

Atrial Septal Defect

Following prenatal diagnosis of an ASD, a careful sonographic fetal anatomy survey is recommended to exclude additional complex cardiac malformations. A sonographic search for extracardiac malformations should also be performed. Fetal echocardiography should be performed by an appropriately trained specialist to confirm the diagnosis and to exclude other cardiac malformations. Invasive fetal testing for karyotype analysis is recommended following the prenatal diagnosis of ASD because the incidence of chromosomal abnormalities may be up to 10% (Ferencz et al. 1987). Referral for prenatal consultation with a pediatric cardiologist is also recommended.

If expectant management is desired, sonographic surveillance to confirm appropriate fetal growth and to evaluate for the development of fetal hydrops is recommended, although the chances of significant hemodynamic disturbances occurring in utero are extremely low with isolated ASD. Although delivery need not necessarily occur at a tertiary-case center if the ASD is isolated and uncomplicated, arrangements should be in place for a prompt careful examination of the infant soon after delivery and for referral to a pediatric cardiol-ogist during the newborn period. There is no indication to alter the timing or method of delivery based on the prenatal diagnosis of isolated ASD.

Ventricular Septal Defect

Following prenatal diagnosis of a VSD, a careful sonographic fetal anatomy survey is recommended to exclude additional complex cardiac malformations, such as tetralogy of Fallot, transposition of the great vessels, or double-outlet right ventricle. Although most VSDs diagnosed after birth are isolated, the majority of prenatally diagnosed VSDs occur in association with more complex cardiac malformations (Crawford et al. 1988). A sonographic search for extracardiac malformations should also be performed. Fetal echocardiography should be performed by an appropriately trained specialist to confirm the diagnosis and to exclude other cardiac malformations.

Invasive fetal testing for karyotype analysis is recommended following the prenatal diagnosis of VSD because the incidence of chromosomal abnormalities may be up to 18%, although in 1 series of 7 prenatally diagnosed VSDs, 5 (71%) were associated with aneuploidy (Ferencz et al. 1987; Paladini et al. 1993). Referral for prenatal consultation with a pediatric cardiologist is also recommended.

Elective termination of pregnancy may be considered by some patients, especially if the VSD is part of a more complex cardiac malformation. However, the chances of spontaneous closure, both in utero and postnatally, should be emphasized before a decision on terminating the pregnancy is made. If expectant management is desired, sonographic surveillance to confirm appropriate fetal growth and to evaluate for the development of fetal hydrops is recommended, although the chances of significant hemodynamic disturbances occurring in utero are extremely low with isolated VSD.

Even though delivery need not necessarily occur at a tertiary-care center if the VSD is isolated and uncomplicated, arrangements should be in place for a prompt, careful examination of the infant soon after delivery and for referral to a pediatric cardiologist during the early newborn period. If there is a suspicion that the VSD may be large and may become clinically significant soon after birth, consideration should be given to delivery in a tertiary-care center. There is no indication to alter the timing or method of delivery based on the prenatal diagnosis of isolated VSD.

▶ FETAL INTERVENTION

No fetal intervention has been described for the prenatal management of either isolated ASD or VSD.

► TREATMENT OF THE NEWBORN

Atrial Septal Defect

Almost all infants with isolated ASD are asymptomatic at the time of delivery and do not require any alteration to usual neonatal care or resuscitation practices. A careful physical examination is mandatory to confirm hemodynamic stability immediately following delivery and again during the neonatal period. Consultation with a pediatric cardiologist should be obtained promptly and echocardiography performed to confirm the prenatal diagnosis and to rule out additional cardiac malformations.

Ventricular Septal Defect

Most infants with isolated VSD are asymptomatic at the time of delivery and do not require any alteration to usual neonatal care or resuscitation practices. A careful physical examination is mandatory to confirm hemodynamic stability immediately following delivery and again during the neonatal period. Consultation with a pediatric cardiologist should be obtained promptly and echocardiography performed to confirm the prenatal diagnosis and to rule out additional cardiac malformations.

Infants with large, membranous VSDs tend to become progressively more symptomatic during the first months of life as the pulmonary vascular resistance falls and left-to-right shunting increases. This can lead to right ventricular failure, which may require digitalis, fluid restriction, and diuretics (Sanders et al. 1996). The use of hydralazine to achieve afterload reduction may also decrease the left-to-right shunt. As pulmonary vascular congestion worsens, lung compliance decreases, and such infants have difficulty feeding, which may require caloric supplementation or tube feedings.

► SURGICAL TREATMENT

Atrial Septal Defect

Most infants with an isolated ASD will remain completely asymptomatic during the first decade of life. Initially, there is a fall in pulmonary vascular resistance at the time of birth, which leads to left-to-right shunting of blood across the ASD. However, because of the distensibility of the ventricles during infancy, this shunt leads to progressive distention of the right ventricle rather than a sudden increase in pulmonary blood flow. In general, this situation persists throughout the second decade of life, at which time pulmonary artery blood flow increases significantly, leading to symptoms of right heart failure. In addition, as pulmonary flow increases, pulmonary vascular resistance can increase again, even-tually leading to Eisenmenger syndrome, which results from cyanosis due to right-to-left shunting of blood.

The rate of spontaneous closure of isolated ASDs is 22% for infants less than 1 year, 33% for children aged 1 to 2 years, and 3% for children older than 4 years (Cockerham et al. 1983). Because of the risks of heart failure and pulmonary hypertension, it has been recommended that children with significant ASDs that persist beyond 4 years of age undergo elective surgical closure of the defect (Cockerham et al. 1983). Surgical repair is generally performed on cardiopulmonary bypass, through a median sternotomy incision, and by the use of pericardium or prosthetic material to close the defect (Merrill and Bender 1985). The operative mortality rate for this procedure is currently less than 1% (Ward 1994).

Because of the limitations of most of the studies of the natural history of isolated ASD, it has also been argued that only children with symptomatic ASDs should be offered surgical repair (Ward 1994). There are virtually no good data on the natural history of asymptomatic children with ASDs because almost none of these children will have a diagnosis, so it is difficult to warrant routine surgical repair in the asymptomatic state. In addition, ASDs diagnosed prenatally may represent yet another patient group with a completely different natural history during childhood.

Ventricular Septal Defect

The majority of isolated VSDs tend to close spontaneously, and therefore the most common indication for surgical repair of a VSD is failure of medical treatment of a symptomatic patient. Other indications for surgical repair include pulmonary hypertension, aortic insufficiency, recurrent respiratory infections, persistent failure to thrive, and prior bacterial endocarditis. Most infants who become symptomatic from a VSD tend to demonstrate congestive heart failure at 1 to 2 months of life. If maximal medical treatment fails to relieve symptoms, definitive primary surgical repair should be performed. The repair is usually done by means of cardiopulmonary bypass, through a right atrial approach and the use of a Dacron patch to close the defect (Merrill and Bender 1985). Operative mortality currently should be less than 5%.

Controversy exists about whether all asymptomatic VSDs should be surgically repaired. In one series of 141 patients with restrictive VSDs, elective surgical repair was performed, with no operative mortality, and the authors concluded that the accepted indications for VSD closure should be expanded (Backer et al. 1993). However, given that there is a 50% chance that a small VSD will close spontaneously by 5 years of age and an 80% chance that it will close by adolescence, it is difficult to recommend elective surgical repair in childhood for small asymptomatic VSDs (Waldman 1993).

▶ LONG-TERM OUTCOME

Atrial Septal Defect

The long-term outcome following surgical repair for isolated ASD is excellent, with a 92%, 25-year actuarial survival (Morris and Menashe 1991). It is possible that right ventricular enlargement and arrhythmias may persist postoperatively, but the long-term consequences of these conditions are unclear (Merrill and Bender 1985). Almost all patients have a normal life span and a normal level of activity following surgical repair of ASD.

Ventricular Septal Defect

The long-term outcome following surgical repair for isolated VSD is also excellent, with an 86%, 25-year actuarial survival (Morris and Menashe 1991). The risk of bacterial endocarditis remains significant following surgical repair of VSD, although it is twice as likely to occur before VSD closure than subsequently (Waldman 1993). The majority of patients have a normal life span and normal level of activity following surgical repair of VSD.

▶ GENETICS AND RECURRENCE RISK

Atrial Septal Defect

Almost all cases of ASD are sporadic in occurrence. The recurrence risk if 1 previous sibling has an ASD is 2.5%; this increases to 8% if 2 previous siblings were affected (Nora and Nora 1988). If the mother has an ASD, the recurrence risk for offspring is 4%; the recurrence risk is only 1.5% if the father has an ASD (Nora and Nora 1988).

Ventricular Septal Defect

Almost all cases of VSD are sporadic in occurence. The recurrence risk if 1 previous sibling has a VSD is 3%; this increases to 10% if 2 previous siblings were affected (Nora and Nora 1988). If the mother has a VSD, the recurrence risk for offspring is 6% to 10%; the recurrence risk is only 2% if the father has a VSD (Nora and Nora 1988).

REFERENCES

Backer CL, Winters RC, Zales VR, et al: Restrictive ventricular septal defect: how small is too small to close? Ann Thorac Surg 1993;56:1014–1019.

Benacerraf BR, Pober BR, Sanders SP. Accuracy of fetal echocardiography. Radiology 1987;165:847–849.

Capelli H, Andrade JL, Somerville J. Classification of the site of ventricular septal defect by 2-dimensional echocardiography. Am J Cardiol 1983;51:1474–1480.

Cockerham JT, Martin TC, Gutierrez ER, et al. Spontaneous closure of secundum atrial septal defect in infants and young children. Am J Cardiol 1983;52:1267–1271.

Crawford DC, Chita SK, Allan LD. Prenatal detection of congenital heart disease: factors affecting obstetric management and survival. Am J Obstet Gynecol 1988;159:352–356.

Ferencz C, Rubin JD, McCarter RJ, et al. Cardiac and noncardiac malformations: observations in a population-based study. Teratology 1987;35:367–378.

Kirk JS, Comstock CH, Lee W, et al. Sonographic screening to detect fetal cardiac abnormalities: a 5-year experience with 111 abnormal cases. Obstet Gynecol 1997;89: 227–232.

Merrill WH, Bender HW. The surgical approach to congenital heart disease. Curr Prob Surg 1985;22:1–55.

Mitchell SC, Korones SB, Berendes HW. Congenital heart disease in 56,109 births: incidence and natural history. Circulation 1971;43:323–332.

Montana E, Khoury MJ, Cragan JD, et al. Trends and outcomes after prenatal diagnosis of congenital cardiac malformations by fetal echocardiography in a well defined birth population, Atlanta, Georgia, 1990–1994. J Am Coll Cardiol 1996;28:1805–1809.

Morris CD, Menashe VD. 25-year mortality after surgical repair of congenital heart defect in childhood: a population-based cohort study. JAMA 1991;266:3447–3452.

Nir A, Driscoll DJ, Edwards WD. Intrauterine closure of membranous ventricular septal defects: mechanism of closure in two autopsy specimens. Pediatr Cardiol 1994; 15:33–37.

Nora JJ, Nora AH. Update on counseling the family with a first-degree relative with a congenital heart defect. Am J Med Genet 1988;29:137–142.

Orie J, Flotta D, Sherman FS. To be or not to be a VSD. Am J Cardiol 1994;74:1284–1285.

Paladini D, Calabro R, Palmieri S, et al. Prenatal diagnosis of congenital heart disease and fetal karyotyping. Obstet Gynecol 1993;81:679–682.

Phillipos EZ, Robertson MA, Still KD. The echocardiographic assessment of the human fetal foramen ovale. J Am Soc Echocardiog 1994;7:257–263.

Roguin N, Du Z, Barak M, et al. High prevalence of muscular ventricular septal defect in neonates. J Am Coll Cardiol 1995;26:1545–1548.

Romero R, Pilu G, Jeanty P, et al. Atrial septal defects. In: Romero R, Pilu G, Jeanty P, Ghidini A, Hobbins JC, eds. Prenatal diagnosis of congenital anomalies. Norwalk, CT: Appleton & Lange, 1988a:139–141.

Romero R, Pilu G, Jeanty P, et al. Ventricular septal defects. In: Romero R, Pilu G, Jeanty P, Ghidini A, Hobbins JC, eds. Prenatal diagnosis of congenital anomalies. Norwalk, CT: Appleton & Lange, 1988b:141–144.

Sanders RC, Blackmon LR, Hogge WA, et al. Transposition of the great arteries. In Sanders RC, Blackmon LR, Hogge WA, Wulfsberg EA, eds. Structural fetal abnormalities: the total picture. St. Louis: Mosby, 1996:81–83.

Sharland GK, Lockhart SM, Chita SK, et al. Factors influencing the outcome of congenital heart disease detected prenatally. Arch Dis Child 1990;65:284–287.

Smythe JF, Copel JA, Kleinman CS. Outcome of prenatally detected cardiac malformations. Am J Cardiol 1992;69: 1471–1474.

Soto B, Becker AE, Moulaert AJ, et al. Classification of ventricular septal defects. Br Heart J 1980;43:332.

Tegnander E, Eik-Nes SH, Johansen OJ, et al. Prenatal detection of heart defects at the routine fetal examination at 18 weeks in a non-selected population. Ultrasound Obstet Gynecol 1995;5:372–380.

Waldman JD. Why not close a small ventricular septal defect? Ann Thorac Surg 1993;56:1011–1102.

Ward C. Secundum atrial septal defect: routine surgical treatment is not of proven benefit. Br Heart J 1994;71:219–223.

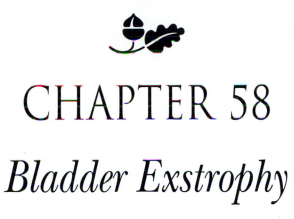

CHAPTER 58

Bladder Exstrophy

▶ CONDITION

Exstrophy of the bladder has been recognized for centuries, but it was not until the 19th century that surgical correction was first attempted (Hall et al. 1953). The first attempts at diversion of urine into the colon were made in 1850, and the first successful closure of bladder exstrophy was performed in 1862 (Canning et al. 1996). In contrast to patients with cloacal exstrophy that have other unrelated abnormalities, infants with bladder exstrophy have defects confined to the bladder, abdominal wall, perineum, genitalia, and bony pelvis.

At birth the diagnosis of bladder exstrophy is easily made by the presence of characteristic findings. The bladder plate protrudes immediately beneath the umbilical cord (Fig. 58-1). The rectus muscles are divergent due to separated pubic bones. There is an outward rotation of the innominate bones and eversion of the pubic rami (Sponsellor et al. 1991). The phallus is short, with a dorsal urethral plate, splayed glans, and dorsal chordee. In females, the mons pubis, clitoris, and labia are separated and the vaginal orifice may be dis-

placed anteriorly. Bilateral inguinal hernias are commonly seen at birth because of the large internal and external inguinal ring caused by the splaying of the rectus musculature and lack of obliquity of the inguinal canal. Hussman et al. (1990) reported that 56% of males and 15% of females have inguinal hernias. In a report by Peppas et al. (1995) in patients presenting with hernia within 1 year of primary closure, 10 to 53% of the hernias were incarcerated.

In bladder exstrophy the umbilical cord inserts low on the abdomen and the anus and scrotum tend to be more anteriorly placed than normal (see Fig. 58-1). Although the rectus abdominus muscles insert normally at the pubic tubercles, the diastasis of the pubic symphysis and lateral displacement of the iliac bones causes splaying of the rectus muscles. This lateral displacement of the rectus muscles widens the inguinal canal, predisposing to indirect inguinal hernias in these patients (Connor et al. 1989; Hussman et al. 1990; Stringer et al. 1994). Because the bladder is external, the peritoneal reflection is deeper in the pelvis than normal and the ureters course deeply through the pelvis and enter the

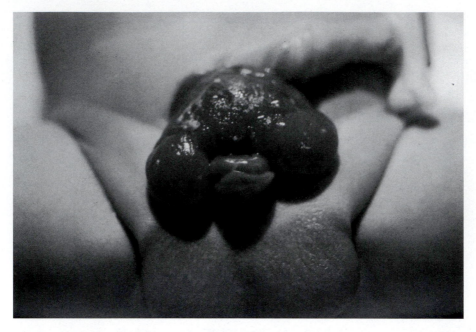

Figure 58-1. Newborn male infant with bladder exstrophy, demonstrating the presence of a low umbilical cord with a protruding bladder plate and a short penis with a splayed glans.

bladder with almost no submucosal tunnel, which predisposes them to vesicoureteral reflux (Nisonson and Lattimer 1968).

The penis in males with bladder exstrophy is short and broad because of pubic bone separation, which prevents the midline joining of the corpora cavernosa (see Fig. 58-1). The overall length of the corpora cavernosa is shortened but reasonable length may be obtained with epispadias repair from the deep corporal bodies (Woodhouse et al. 1984). There is usually a marked dorsal chordee and the penile curvature is compounded by shorter dorsal tunica albuginea. Females with bladder exstrophy have a hemiclitoris on each side of the bladder and the vaginal orifice may be duplicated and displaced anteriorly (Damario et al. 1994). The uterus may be duplicated, but the fallopian tubes and ovaries are usually normal.

All patients with bladder exstrophy have some degree of pubic diastasis, with the hips rotated outward. Many patients have a waddling gait in early childhood, but long-term hip or gait problems are rare.

In normal development the cloacal membrane occupies the infraumbilical position of the abdominal wall, and this bilaminar membrane is infiltrated by mesenchyme to form the lower abdominal musculature. The genital folds fuse superiorly to form the genital tubercle. The most widely accepted theory for the cause of exstrophy is based on the work of Muecke (1964), in chick embryos. In this model, overgrowth or persistence of a thickened cloacal membrane results in truncated mesenchymal migration. Later rupture of the membrane

without the mesenchymal reinforcement results in exstrophy. Bladder exstrophy results if the rupture occurs after the descent of urorectal septum. If rupture occurs in the absence of the urorectal septum, then cloacal exstrophy occurs. The prenatal sonographic observation by Langer et al. of an intact cloacal membrane that subsequently ruptured during the second trimester suggests that the presence or absence of the urorectal septum and not timing of membrane rupture distinguishes bladder exstrophy from cloacal exstrophy (Langer et al. 1992).

▶ INCIDENCE

A broad range of incidences have been reported for bladder exstrophy, from 1 in 3000 to 1 in 50,000 live births (Lattimer et al. 1996; Sanders 1996). Rickham estimated the incidence of bladder exstrophy at 1 in 10,000 live births (Rickham 1960). The International Clearinghouse for Birth Defects Monitoring Systems estimated the incidence of bladder exstrophy at 3.3 in 100,000 live births (Lancaster 1987). All reports have consistently shown a male predominance, which, derived from multiple series, averages 2.3 : 1 (Bennett 1973; Harvard et al. 1951; Higgins 1962; Jeffs et al. 1982). Individual reports exist that describe a male predominance as high as 5 : 1 or 6 : 1 (Ives et al. 1980; Lancaster 1987). There are no estimates available for the prenatal incidence of bladder exstrophy.

While no definite teratogenic effect has been demonstrated, there is a slightly increased risk of bladder exstrophy with maternal progestin use (Blickstein et al. 1991). Also, a single case of bladder exstrophy has been reported in the child of a user of lysergic acid diethylamide. A slightly increased risk of bladder exstrophy has been observed in mothers less than 20 years of age (Lancaster 1987).

▶ SONOGRAPHIC FINDINGS

The prenatal sonographic diagnosis of bladder exstrophy is based on the association of several findings, including inability to visualize the bladder, presence of a mass on the anterior abdominal wall in the suprapubic region, small penis with an anteriorly displaced scrotum, low umbilical-cord insertion, and splayed iliac crests (Barth et al. 1990; Bronshtein et al. 1993; Gearhart et al. 1995a; Jaffe et al. 1990; Meizner et al. 1986; Mirk et al. 1986; Pinette et al. 1996; Richards et al. 1992). The fetal bladder is most easily identified between the umbilical arteries, using color Doppler sonography. If completely empty, the bladder may not be seen, but since it normally fills and empties every 5 to 15 minutes, persistent observation should identify the normal bladder (Gearhart et al. 1995a). However, the normal bladder may not be imaged if there is a lack of urine production, either due to bilateral renal agenesis or bilateral multicystic dysplastic kidneys.

All of the features of bladder exstrophy may not be seen in every patient. In the report by Gearhart et al. (1995), in 17 fetuses with prenatal sonographic examinations in whom a retrospective diagnosis of bladder exstrophy could be made, not every feature was present. In 71% of cases there was persistent nonvisualization of the fetal bladder. In only 47% of cases was a persistent lower abdominal-wall mass or bulge seen. A very small penis with an anteriorly displaced scrotum was seen in 57% of fetuses. Even less commonly appreciated was the low umbilical-cord insertion (29%) and abnormal widening of the iliac crests (18%).

In a female, the clitoris is bifocal and there are widely separated labia, but this may be difficult to discern sonographically.

▶ DIFFERENTIAL DIAGNOSIS

The differential diagnosis of bladder exstrophy includes cloacal exstrophy, omphalocele, and gastroschisis. However, the lower abdominal-wall bulge with low cord insertion immediately cephalad to the exstrophied bladder usually allows its identification. The kidneys are usually normal in bladder exstrophy. In contrast, in cloacal exstrophy, unilateral renal agenesis is common, as is hydronephrosis. In addition, there is often prolapse of the ileum through the cloaca to form the "elephant trunk" deformity (see Chapter 60). Myelomeningocele and omphalocele are also commonly associated with cloacal exstrophy. Rarely, a small omphalocele may be seen in bladder exstrophy (Gearhart et al. 1989). The lower abdominal-wall bulge or soft-tissue mass in cloacal exstrophy is usually larger and more heterogeneous than in bladder exstrophy (Pinette et al. 1996).

▶ ANTENATAL NATURAL HISTORY

Although few prospectively diagnosed cases of bladder exstrophy have been reported, review of retrospective cases suggests that this diagnosis has no implications for the pregnancy. These are usually isolated sporadic anomalies, without increased risk for intrauterine death, or neonatal compromise at birth.

▶ MANAGEMENT OF PREGNANCY

Once there is a diagnosis of bladder exstrophy, an attempt to completely define the anomaly should be made. The position of the abdominal-wall bulge and umbilical-cord insertion, sex of the fetus, and the size and position of the penis should be determined. If the sex of the fetus is in doubt, genetic amniocentesis may be indicated to help counsel the parents and plan the postnatal reconstruction. Prenatal consultation with a pediatric urologist is extremely helpful in advising parents about the reconstructive procedures that will be necessary and about the long-term prognosis. There is no need to alter the delivery plan, and cesarean section should be reserved for obstetrical indications. Because bladder closure is best accomplished during the first 3 days of life, delivery in a tertiary-care center with pediatric urologists and anesthesiologists is preferred, but transportation of the newborn to a pediatric center is also possible.

▶ FETAL INTERVENTION

There are no fetal interventions for bladder exstrophy.

▶ TREATMENT OF THE NEWBORN

In the management of bladder exstrophy, staged functional reconstruction and urinary diversion are the two most commonly employed strategies. Urinary diversion is usually undertaken only when reconstruction is unavailable or repeated attempts at functional reconstruction have failed. Gender reassignment is almost never necessary, given modern reconstructive techniques, and is reserved for rare cases in which no other option is available. The staged functional reconstruction is undertaken with specific goals for each stage. During the newborn period, the goal is bladder closure with protection of the upper urinary tract, and preservation for later continent reconstruction. In the second stage, at about 1 year of age in the male, the goal is to optimize genital structure and function and to increase bladder outlet resistance to foster growth of the bladder. In the final stage of functional reconstruction, undertaken at about 4 years of age, the goal is to achieve urinary continence.

▶ SURGICAL TREATMENT

The most commonly used technique for bladder closure involves the conversion of an exstrophied bladder to an incontinent epispadias (Gearhart and Jeffs 1989b, 1990 a and b; Jeffs et al. 1982). An incision circumscribes the exstrophied bladder extending distal to the verumontanum on both sides of the prostatic urethra, resulting in a wide plate of bladder neck and prostatic urethra. The bladder is completely mobilized and the corpora cavernosa directed off the inferior pubic cavernosa with care to preserve the neurovascular bundles. The corpora cavernosa are approximated in the midline. The neourethra, with or without paraexstrophy flaps, is tubularized. Ureteral stents suprapubic to the vesicostomy site are exteriorized prior to closing the bladder. The pelvic ring is closed by a nonabsorbable monofilament suture. The midline abdominal defect is then closed by approximation of the rectus fascia and skin. Pubic approximation is possible during the first days of the life, without osteotomy. After staged reconstruction, all patients should be maintained on prophylactic antibiotics because of the high incidence of vesicoureteral reflux. Although most children will have vesicoureteral reflux, it is unusual for them to require an antireflux procedure before subsequent bladder-neck reconstruction.

The second stage of functional reconstruction, undertaken between 6 and 12 months of age, focuses on phallic reconstruction. Epispadias repair and urethroplasty not only reconstruct the phallus, but also result in increased outflow resistance and enhanced bladder capacity (Gearhart et al. 1989a). The goals of epispadias repair are to provide length for the phallus and to release the dorsal chordee (Gearhart et al. 1990a; Hendren 1979; Hinman 1958). In addition, the urethra is reconstructed to place the meatus at the tip of the glans penis (Kajbafzadeh et al. 1995; Mitchell et al. 1996; Ransley et al. 1989).

The last stage of functional reconstruction in bladder exstrophy is undertaken at about 4 years of age (Perlmutter et al. 1991). It is important that the child's bladder capacity be at least 60 ml in order to have func-

tional capacity following bladder-neck reconstruction (Jeffs et al. 1982). The Young–Dees–Leadbetter technique remains the most commonly used technique to reconstruct the bladder neck (Gearhart et al. 1990b; Leadbetter 1964; Marshall et al. 1949; Woodhouse et al. 1984). The ureters are reimplanted in a cephalad position in either a cross-trigonal or cephalotrigonal procedure to prevent vesicoureteral reflux (Brock et al. 1998; Canning et al. 1990). Next, the posterior bladder mucosa is tubularized over a Foley catheter to create a neourethra, and the muscular layer of bladder is closed over the neourethra to create a new bladder neck. If capacity is inadequate, bladder augmentation is then performed (McLaughlin et al. 1995). The bladder neck and urethra are then sutured to the undersurface of the pubis.

Urinary diversion is reserved for patients who have inadequate anatomy for reconstruction at birth or when attempts at reconstruction have failed. Among the most commonly employed technique is the ureterosigmoidostomy, which allows continence, and with nonrefluxing ureterocolonic anastomoses, protection of the upper urinary tracts. However, long-term hyperchloremic metabolic acidosis, ureteral obstruction, and colonic malignancy are possible complications. Ileal conduits are not considered suitable for urinary diversion in children due to long-term complications. A colon conduit may be an alternative, with fewer long-term complications than ileal conduits. Once a child achieves anal continence, anastomosis of the colon conduit to the rectosigmoid can be performed.

▶ LONG-TERM OUTCOME

One report reviewed the experience at the Johns Hopkins Hospital with 87 patients treated for exstrophy of the bladder (Lakshmanan et al. 1998). The age at follow-up ranged from 8 months to 22 years. Bladder-neck reconstruction was performed in 58 of 87 patients, with 47 (81%) continent of urine. Among the remaining 11 patients, 4 were less than 6 months from bladder-neck repair, 2 were lost to follow-up, 1 was diverted, 1 awaits bladder augmentation, 2 have had bladder augmentation, and 1 is totally incontinent of urine. The average time to continence during the day ranged from 3 months to 5 years (mean, 2 years), and to nighttime continence, a mean of 4 years. Other centers have reported continence rates in the 69 to 71% range with bladder-neck reconstruction (Lottman et al. 1996; Jones et al. 1993; Mollard et al. 1994).

Patients who do not achieve continence within 1 to 2 years of bladder-neck reconstruction seldom have sufficient continence over time (Gearhart 1998). These patients may require remedial approaches, including repeat bladder-neck reconstruction, often with concomitant bladder augmentation. The majority of patients in whom initial bladder-neck reconstruction fails need bladder augmentation (Gearhart et al. 1994,1995b).

There may be significant psychologic consequences to this anomaly and the results of reconstructive procedures. Ben-Chaim et al. (1996) reported the results of a diagnostic psychiatric questionnaire and interview with 20 patients with bladder exstrophy and their parents. Behavioral, social, and school competency problems were experienced by 70% of the adolescents and 33% of the school-aged children. In nearly 70% of the participants, concern was present about the sexual function or disfigurement. The mechanics of sexual intercourse and anxiety about the appearance and adequacy of their genitalia were perceived as barriers to relationships by both adults and adolescents.

The issue of sexual function, fertility, and self-esteem become more important long-term issues for children born with bladder exstrophy who undergo reconstruction. Ben-Chaim et al. (1996) reported the results of an anonymous questionnaire and chart review in 20 adult patients (16 men and 4 women). Of the 20, 6 were married (4 men, 2 women), 2 men have fathered children, and 1 woman has had two children. Ten of the 16 men ejaculate a volume of 2 ml, with history of retrograde ejaculation in 6. Semen analysis was performed in 4 men, with an average ejaculate volume of 0.4 ml with azoospermia in 3 and oligospermia in 1. All patients experienced normal erections, but were unsatisfactory in 7 because of a small penis, and 12 of 16 experienced satisfactory orgasms. Stein et al. (1994) have suggested that in males, bladder-neck reconstruction may be performed at the expense of fertility. Fertility in males is of secondary concern in reconstructive surgery of the urethra and bladder neck. Erectile and sexual function are well preserved but patients are bothered by small penile length and dorsal chordee. In contrast, females appear to have normal fertility, sexuality, and sexual function (Gearhart 1998). However, uterine prolapse after pregnancy and delivery is common and is thought to be due to intrinsic weakness of the pelvic floor (Krisiloff et al. 1978). Uterine prolapse is less common after early pelvic closure with osteotomy (Jeffs et al. 1982). Rectal prolapse occurs frequently in untreated patients, possibly due to bladder mucosal irritation-induced straining. This disappears with bladder closure (Jeffs et al. 1982).

Adenosarcoma of the bladder occurs in patients with bladder exstrophy approximately 400 times more commonly than in the normal population (Kanzari et al. 1974; Krishnansetty et al. 1988). It is the most common bladder tumor occurring in patents with untreated bladder exstrophy (Davillas et al. 1991) and has been reported in adults who had bladder closure after infancy (Facchini et al. 1987). While bladder malignancy has yet to be reported in patients who had bladder closure at birth, long-term monitoring with cytologic evaluation is recommended (Canning et al. 1996).

▶ GENETICS AND RECURRENCE RISK

Bladder exstrophy, in general, is a rare sporadic anomaly. However, there are families at increased risk for recurrence. Of 2500 index cases, Shapiro et al. (1984) found 9 affected siblings with a risk of a second affected family member of 3.6%. The risk to offspring of a patient with bladder exstrophy is estimated at 1.4%, and the risk of 2 affected siblings is about 1% (Carter 1984).

REFERENCES

Barth R, Filly RA, Sondheimer FK. Prenatal sonographic findings in bladder exstrophy. J Ultrasound Med 1990;9: 359–361.

Ben-Chaim J, Jeffs RD, Reiner WG, et al. The outcome of adult exstrophy patients. J Urol 1996;155:1251–1256.

Bennett AH. Exstrophy of the bladder treated by uretero-sigmoidostomies. Urology 1973;2:165–169.

Blickstein I, Katz Z. Possible relationship between bladder exstrophy and epispadias with progestins taken during early pregnancy. Br J Urol 1991;68: 105–108.

Brock JW, O'Neill JA. Bladder exstrophy. In: O'Neill JA, Rowe MI, Grosfeld JL, Fonkalsud EW, Coran AG, eds. Pediatric surgery. 5th ed. St. Louis: Mosby-Year Book, 1998:1709–1725.

Bronshtein M, Bar-Hava I, Blumenfeld Z. Differential diagnosis of the nonvisualized fetal urinary bladder by transvaginal sonography in the early second trimester. Obstet Gyncol 1993;82:490–493.

Canning DA, Koo HP, Duckett JW. Anomalies of the bladder and cloaca. In: Gillenwater JY, Grayhack JT, Howard SS, Duckett JW (eds): Adult and Pediatric Urology, 3rd ed. Mosby Year–book Inc, St. Louis, 1996:2445–2488.

Canning DA, Gearhart JP, Jeffs RD. Cephalotrigonal reimplant as an adjunct to bladder neck reconstruction. Presented at the American Urologic Association Annual Meeting. New Orleans, May 1990.

Carter CO. The genetics of urinary tract malformations. J Genet Hum 1984;32:23–27.

Connor JP, Hensle TW, Lattimer JK, et al. Long-term follow up of 207 patients with bladder exstrophy: an evaluation in treatment. J Urol 1989;142:793–797.

Damario MA, Carpenter SE, Jones H Jr, et al. Reconstruction of the external genitalia in females with bladder exstrophy. Int J Gynecol Obstet 1994;44:245–250.

Davillas N, Thanos A, Kiakatas J, et al. Bladder exstrophy complicated by adenocarcinoma. Br J Urol 1991;68: 107–111.

Facchini V, Gadducci A, Colombi L, et al. Carcinoma developing in bladder exstrophy: case report. B J Obstet Gynaecol 1987;94:795–798.

Gearhart JP. Bladder exstrophy and urinary continence. In: Stringer MD, Oldhorn KT, Mouriquand PDE, Howard ER, eds. Pediatric surgery and urology: long-term outcomes. Philadelphia: Saunders, 1998:540–548.

Gearhart JP, Ben-Chaim J, Jeffs RD, et al. Criteria for the prenatal diagnosis of classic bladder exstrophy. Obstet Gynecol 1995a;85:961–964.

Gearhart JP, Jeffs RD. Bladder exstrophy: increase in capacity following epispadias repair. J Urol 1989a;142:525–530.

Gearhart JP, Jeffs RD. Management and treatment of classic bladder exstrophy. In: Ashcroft KW, ed. Pediatric urology. Philadelphia: Saunders, 1990a.

Gearhart JP, Jeffs RD. Reconstruction of the lower urinary tract. Dial Pediatr Urol 1990b;13:4–12.

Gearhart JP, Jeffs RD. State of the art reconstructive surgery for bladder exstrophy at the Johns Hopkins Hospital. Am J Dis Child 1989b;143:1475–1479.

Gearhart JP, Peppas DS, Jeffs RD. The application of continent urinary stomas to bladder augmentation or replacement in the failed exstrophy reconstruction. Br J Urol 1995b;75:87–91.

Hall EG, McCandless AE, Richham PP. Vesicointestinal fissure with diphallus. Br J Urol 1953;25:219–221.

Harvard BM, Thompson GJ. Congenital exstrophy of the urinary bladder: late results of treatment by the Coffey-May method of ureterointestinal anastomosis. J Urol 1951;65:223–227.

Hendren WH. Penile lengthening after previous repair of epispadias. J Urol 1979;12:527–531.

Higgins CC. Exstrophy of the bladder: report of 158 cases. Am Surg 1962;28:99–106.

Hinman R. A method of lengthening and repairing the penis in exstrophy of the bladder. J Urol 1958;79:237–242.

Hussman DA, McLorie GA, Churchill BM, et al. Inguinal pathology and its association with classic bladder exstrophy. J Pediatr Surg 1990;25:332–336.

Ives E, Coffey R, Carter CO. A family study of bladder exstrophy. J Med Genet 1980;17:139–143.

Jaffe R, Schoenfeld A, Ovadia J. Sonographic findings in the prenatal diagnosis of bladder exstrophy. Am J Obstet Gynecol 1990;162:675–678.

Jeffs RD, Guice SL, Oesch J. The factors in successful exstrophy. J Urol 1982;127:974–980.

Jones JA, Mitchell ME, Rink RC. Improved results using a modification of the Young-Dees-Leadbetter bladder neck repair. Br J Urol 1993;71:555–559.

Kajbafzadeh AM, Duffy PG, Ransley PG. The evolution of penile reconstruction in epispadias repair: a report of 180 cases. J Urol 1995;154:858–862.

Kanzari SJ, Majid A, Ortega AM, et al. Exstrophy of the urinary bladder complicated by adenocarcinoma. Urology 1974;3:496–501.

Krishnansetty RM, Rao MK, Hines CR, et al. Adenocarcinoma and dysfunctional urterosigmoidostomy. J Ky Med Assoc 1988;86:409–413.

Krisiloff M, Puchner PJ, Tretter W, et al. Pregnancy in women with bladder exstrophy. J Urol 1978;119:478–483.

Lakshmanan Y, Peppas DS, Gearhart JP, et al. Bladder exstrophy: a 21 year experience with functional recon-struction in 87 consecutive patients followed from birth. Urology (in press).

Lancaster PAL. Epidemiology of bladder exstrophy: a communication from the International Clearinghouse for Birth Defects Monitoring Systems. Teratology 1987;36:221–227.

Langer JC, Brennan B, Lappalainen RE, et al. Cloacal exstrophy: prenatal diagnosis before rupture of the cloacal membrane. J Pediatr Surg 1992;27:1352–1355.

Lattimer JK, Smith MJK. Exstrophy closure: a follow up on 70 cases. J Urol 1996;95:356–362.

Leadbetter GW. Surgical correction of total urinary incontinence. J Urol 1964;91:261–265.

Lottman H, Melin Y, Beze-Beyrie P, et al. Is it possible to achieve continence with spontaneous voiding? A retrospective study of 57 cases. Presented at the European Society of Pediatric Urology meeting, London, March 22, 1996.

McLaughlin KP, Rink RC, Adams MC, et al. Stomach in combination with other intestinal segments in pediatric lower urinary tract reconstruction. J Urol 1995;154:1162–1168.

Marshall VF, Marchetti AA, Krantz KE. The correction of stress incontinence by simple vesicourethral suspension. Surg Gynecol Obstet 1949;88:509–513.

Meizner I, Bar-Ziv J. Prenatal ultrasonic diagnosis of anterior abdominal wall defects. Eur J Obstet Gynecol Reprod Biol 1986;22:217–224.

Mirk P, Calisti A, Fileni A. Prenatal sonographic diagnosis of bladder exstrophy. J Ultrasound Med 1986;5:291–293.

Mitchell ME, Bagli DJ. Complete penile disassembly for epispadias repair: the Mitchell technique. J Urol 1996;155:300–305.

Mollard P, Mouriquard PDE, Buttein X. Urinary continence after reconstruction of classical bladder exstrophy (73 cases) Br J Urol 1994;73:298–301.

Muecke EC. The role of the cloacal membrane in exstrophy: the first successful experimental study. J Urol 1964;92:659–665.

Nisonson I, Lattimer J. How well can the exstrophied bladder work? J Urol 1968;99:622–627.

Peppas DS, Connolly JA, Jeffs RD, et al. Prevalence and repair of inguinal hernias in children with classic bladder exstrophy. J Urol 1995;154:1901–1905.

Perlmutter AD, Weinstein MD, Reitelman C. Vesical neck reconstruction in patients with epispadias-exstrophy complex. J Urol 1991;146:613–615.

Pinette MG, Pan YQ, Pinette SG, et al. Prenatal diagnosis of fetal bladder and cloacal exstrophy by ultrasound: a report of three cases. J Reprod Med 1996;41:132–134.

Ransley PG, Duffy PG, Wollin M: Bladder exstrophy closure and epispadias. In: Spitz L, Nixon HH, eds. Operative surgery: paediatric surgery. 4th ed. Edinburgh: Butterworths, 1989.

Richards DS, Langham M Jr, Mahaffey SM. The prenatal ultrasonographic diagnosis of cloacal exstrophy. J Ultrasound Med 1992;11:507–510.

Rickham PP. Vesicointestinal fissure. Arch Dis Child 1960;35:967–971.

Sanders RC. Exstrophy of the bladder. In: Sanders AC, Blackman LR, Hogge WA, Wulfsberg EA, eds. Structural fetal abnormalities: the total picture. St. Louis: Mosby-Year Book, 1996:91–92.

Shapiro E, Lepor H, Jeffs RD. The inheritance of the exstrophy-epispadias complex. J Urol 1984;132:308–312.

Sponsellor PD, Bisson CS, Gearhart JP, et al. The anatomy of the pelvis in the exstrophy complex. J Bone Joint Surg Am 1991;153:487–495.

Stein R, Stockle M, Fisch M, et al. The fate of the adult exstrophy patient. J Urol 1994;152:1413–1417.

Stringer MD, Duffy PG, Ransley PG. Inguinal hernias associated with bladder exstrophy. Br J Urol 1994;73:308–312.

Woodhouse C, Kallett M. Anatomy of the penis and its deformities in exstrophy and epispadias. J Urol 1984;132:1122–1126.

CHAPTER 59

Body-Stalk Anomaly

▶ CONDITION

Body-stalk anomaly is a severe abdominal-wall defect that results from abnormalities in the development of the cephalic, caudal, and lateral embryonic body folds. This maldevelopment results in the absence or shortening of the umbilical cord with the abdominal organs lying outside the abdominal cavity and directly attached to the placenta (Shalev et al. 1995). Body-stalk anomaly was first described by Kermauncr in 1906 in a newborn with an abdominal-wall defect consisting of an amniotic sac that contained viscera; the anterior wall of the sac was directly attached to the placenta and there was no umbilical cord. Other than the references given in text-books of pathology, body-stalk anomaly was not appreciated in the general obstetric literature until the report of Lockwood and colleagues in 1986.

After gastrulation, the embryo consists of a three-layered, flat, oval germinal disk. The rapid growth of the embryo, especially along the sagittal axis causes the germinal disk to curve. Through circumferential folding, the embryo becomes cylindrical. As a result of this process, the body of the embryo closes, the body stalk forms, and an intraembryonic coelom (peritoneal cavity) separates from an extraembryonic coelom (chorionic cavity) (Giacoia 1992). The amniotic cavity, which is initially located dorsal to the germinal disk, grows rapidly and eventually encircles the fetus, obliterates the chorionic cavity, and envelops the umbilical cord. The abnormality in the folding process prevents this obliteration of the chorionic cavity and formation of the umbilical cord. Without an umbilical cord, the fetus becomes directly attached to the placental chorionic plate. This body-stalk anomaly consists of a sac of amnion–mesoderm that contains the displaced abdominal organs (Giacoia 1992).

Causes proposed for body-stalk defect include early amnion rupture with direct mechanical pressure and amniotic bands (see Chapter 101), vascular disruption of the early embryo, or an abnormality in the germinal disk that leads to the formation of an anomalous amniotic cavity. In the early-amnion-rupture theory, the abdominal-wall and spinal defects could be secondary to the passage of the lower half of the fetal body into the coelomic cavity through the defect in the amniotic sac. The fetus has no room to move and remains practically attached to the placenta. Limb amputations and encephalocele could be secondary to the entrapment of the fetal skull and/or limbs in the coelomic cavity (Daskalakis et al. 1997). Alternatively, early generalized compromise of embryonic blood flow could lead to a failure of closure of the ventral body wall and persistence of the coelomic cavity (Van Allen et al. 1987). This could also lead to a rupture of an unsupported amnion and formation of amniotic bands.

▶ INCIDENCE

Body-stalk anomaly is the rarest and most severe of the abdominal-wall defects. The incidence of body-stalk anomaly in a population of Scottish patients identified by abnormal maternal serum screening results was 1 in 14,273 (Mann et al. 1984). The incidence of body-stalk anomaly in a Hawaiian birth defects registry that encompassed the years 1986–1997 was 0.32 per 10,000 births (Forrester and Merz 1999). Recently, an increased incidence of body-stalk anomaly was noted in a population of first-trimester fetuses studied for nuchal translucency thickness. In this first-trimester population, the incidence of body-stalk anomaly was between 10 in 4116 cases and 14 in 106,727 cases (Daskalakis et al. 1997; Souka et al. 1998). Several case reports exist of body-stalk anomaly and limb–body-wall complex in association with monozygotic twinning and with maternal cocaine abuse (Martinez et al. 1994; Viscarello et al. 1992).

▶ SONOGRAPHIC FINDINGS

The criteria for the diagnosis of body-stalk anomaly in the first trimester include demonstration of abdominal organs in the extraembryonic coelom and a short umbilical cord with only two vessels (Ginsberg et al. 1997). The diagnosis may be more difficult to make during the second trimester than during the first because of the presence of severe oligohydramnios. During the second trimester, Goldstein et al. (1989) suggested that body-stalk anomaly should be strongly considered when there is a body-wall defect, skeletal abnormalities, and the umbilical cord is absent or very rudimentary (Figs. 59-1 and 59-2).

In a multicenter project of screening for chromosomal defects by fetal nuchal translucency thickness and maternal age, 14 of 106,727 fetuses examined had a body-stalk anomaly (Daskalakis et al. 1997). During the first trimester, the ultrasonographic features observed included a major abdominal-wall defect, severe kyphoscoliosis, and short umbilical cord. In all of the cases observed, the upper part of the fetal body was in the amniotic cavity and the lower part was in the coelomic cavity. The nuchal translucency thickness was above the 95th percentile in 10 of the 14 cases, but the fetal karyotype was normal in 12 of the 14 fetuses evaluated. These authors suggested that early amnion rupture before obliteration of the coelomic cavity is a possible cause of the syndrome (Daskalakis et al. 1997).

Multiple case reports have described the prenatal sonographic diagnosis of body-stalk anomaly (Giacoia 1992; Ginsberg et al. 1997; Jauniaux et al. 1990; Lockwood 1986; Shalev et al. 1995; Takeuchi et al. 1995). An additional helpful sonographic finding is the presence of scoliosis, which is observed in about 75% of cases (Ginsberg et al. 1997). Scoliosis is thought to be due to the absence of thoracolumbar and paraspinal muscles on the ipsilateral side of the abdominal-wall defect. In addition, it is thought that fetal hyperextension and direct attachment to the placenta, which limit fetal movement, result in skeletal anomalies.

▶ DIFFERENTIAL DIAGNOSIS

The differential diagnosis for body-stalk anomaly includes isolated omphalocele, isolated gastroschisis, short umbilical cord syndrome (Miller et al. 1981), and limb–body-wall complex. Some authors consider body-stalk anomaly to be a severe form of amniotic band syndrome (see Chapter 101) (Takeuchi et al. 1995). Amniotic bands are present in 40% of cases of body-stalk anomaly. In addition, some of the limb defects that can be associated with body-stalk anomaly can be attributed to amniotic bands.

Limb–body-wall complex is included in the spectrum of defects seen in the early-amnion-rupture sequence. Two phenotypes are thought to exist in limb–

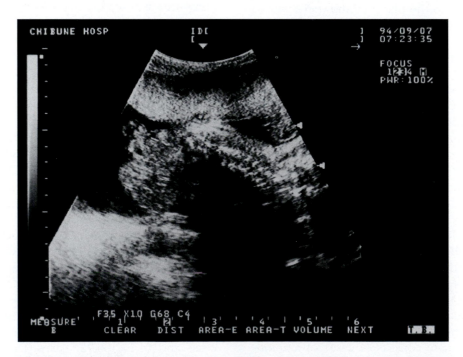

Figure 59-1. Longitudinal sonographic image of a fetus with body-stalk anomaly, demonstrating severe kyphoscoliosis of the lower spine. *(Reprinted, with permission, from Takeuchi K, Fujita I, Nakajima K, Kitagaki S, Koketsu I. Body stalk anomaly: prenatal diagnosis. Int J Gynecol Obstet 1995;51:49–52.)*

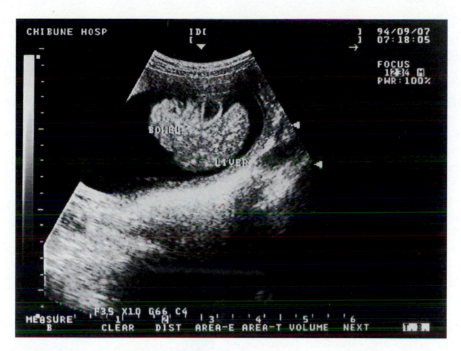

Figure 59-2. Coronal sonographic image of the fetus in Figure 59-1, with body-stalk anomaly demonstrated a 5-by-6-cm mass with a covering membrane that contained stomach, liver, and bowel. *(Reprinted, with permission, from Takeuchi K, Fujita I, Nakajima K, Kitagaki S, Koketsu I. Body stalk anomaly: prenatal diagnosis. Int J Gynecol Obstet 1995;51:49–52.*

body-wall complex. In the first one, craniofacial defects, amniotic bands, and/or adhesions are seen. In the second phenotype, urogenital abnormalities, anal atresia, abdominal placental attachment, and a persistent embryonic coelom are seen. The overlap between body-stalk anomaly, limb–body-wall complex, and a severe form of amniotic band syndrome can be confusing. In a complete review of the limb–body-wall complex, Van Allen et al. (1987) stated that the diagnosis of limb–body-wall complex is based on the presence of two of three of the following: exencephaly or encephalocele with facial clefts, thoracoschisis and/or abdominoschisis, and a limb defect. In an evaluation of fetuses with limb–body-wall complex, 24 of 25 cases studied by Van Allen et al. had associated internal structural defects. In 85% of these cases there was evidence of persistence of the extraembryonic coelom by examination of the placenta. The abnormalities observed in this group of fetuses and data from experimental models support vascular disruption during 4 to 6 weeks of gestation as the cause for limb–body-wall complex.

Martínez-Frías (1997) disagreed with Van Allen et al.'s definition of limb–body-wall complex. He stated that an infant with encephalocele, facial clefts, and limb defects could be considered as having limb–body-wall complex. Martínez-Frías argued that the presence of abdominal-wall defect with a variable spectrum of associated anomalies (with or without limb deficiencies), should be called body-wall complex. He distinguished

body-wall complex from the amniotic band sequence without body-wall defects, but included amniotic band sequence with body-wall defects in the category of body-wall complex.

Further adding to the confusion is that the epidemiology of body-stalk anomaly and limb–body-wall complex is similar. Both malformations have been associated with cocaine abuse. Both conditions are associated with young maternal age, and inheritance is sporadic, with normal karyotypes (Negishi et al. 1998).

With regard to sonographic diagnosis, it is helpful to remember that body-stalk anomaly is not associated with craniofacial or limb anomalies.

▶ ANTENATAL NATURAL HISTORY

The discrepancy in the prevalence of body-stalk anomaly between 10 to 14 weeks of gestation and 17 to 19 weeks of gestation suggests that body-stalk anomaly is associated with a high incidence of spontaneous abortion early in the second trimester (Daskalakis et al. 1997).

The patterns of malformations associated with body-stalk anomaly depend on the degree of abnormal development of each of the four major embryonic folds. Associated anomalies observed in cases of body-stalk anomaly include colonic atresia, agenesis of the colon, intestinal atresia, cloacal exstrophy, vaginal atresia, agenesis of the uterus and gonads, absent external genitalia, hypoplastic kidneys, absent diaphragm, spina bifida, and dysplastic thorax.

► MANAGEMENT OF PREGNANCY

If the diagnosis of body-stalk anomaly is suspected, the pregnant patient should be referred to a tertiary-care center capable of anatomic sonographic diagnosis. The diagnosis of body-stalk anomaly is generally reliable. The major issue is to be certain that the sonographic abnormality observed is not isolated omphalocele or gastroschisis, which would carry a reasonably normal prognosis. If the diagnosis of body-stalk anomaly is certain, chromosomal analysis is not indicated, as all reported cases have been associated with a normal karyotype. If the diagnosis of body-stalk anomaly is made, termination of pregnancy should be offered, as the condition is uniformly fatal in a newborn. A further complication of pregnancy is that abnormal fetal presentation is common and cesarean delivery may be indicated to allow delivery of an intact fetus. Infants who are born alive with body-stalk anomaly die shortly after birth.

► FETAL INTERVENTION

There are no fetal interventions indicated for body-stalk anomaly.

► TREATMENT OF THE NEWBORN

In the rare setting of the limited postnatal survival of an affected newborn with body-stalk anomaly, only comfort care is indicated. The condition is uniformly fatal (Fig. 59-3).

► SURGICAL TREATMENT

There are no surgical treatments indicated for body-stalk anomaly.

► LONG-TERM OUTCOME

Fetuses with body-stalk anomaly do not survive.

► GENETICS AND RECURRENCE RISK

All cases of body-stalk anomaly reported in the literature have been sporadic. The pregnant patient should be advised that there is no increased recurrence risk in

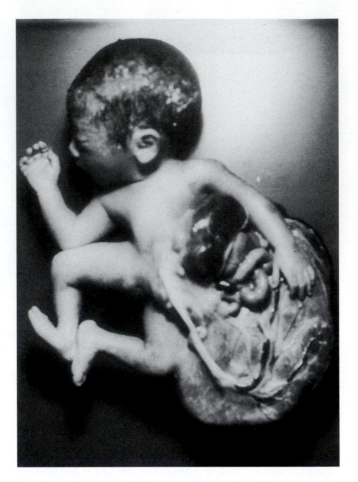

Figure 59-3. Postmortem photograph of the same fetus shown in Figures 59-1 and 59-2, demonstrating a large omphalocele in continuity with the placenta and a very short umbilical cord. *(Reprinted, with permission, from Takeuchi K, Fujita I, Nakajima K, Kitagaki S, Koketsu I. Body stalk anomaly: prenatal diagnosis. Int J Gynecol Obstet 1995;51:49–52.)*

subsequent pregnancies. However, an increased incidence of body-stalk anomaly in monozygotic twins has been reported (Shih et al. 1996). This is probably due to an early embryonic cleavage disorder and is thought to represent a gradual transition from monoamniotic twins to conjoined twins. The development of body-stalk anomaly is therefore an intrinsic part of the twinning process and should not carry an increased recurrence risk.

REFERENCES

Daskalakis G, Sebire NJ, Jurkovic D, Snijders RJM, Nicolaides KH. Body stalk anomaly at 10–14 weeks of gestation. Ultrasound Obstet Gynecol 1997;10:416–418.

Forrester MB, Merz RD. Epidemiology of abdominal wall defects, Hawaii, 1986–1997. Teratology 1999;60:117–123.

Giacoia GP. Body stalk anomaly: congenital absence of the umbilical cord. Obstet Gynecol 1992;80:527–529.

Ginsberg NE, Cadkin A, Strom C. Prenatal diagnosis of body stalk anomaly in the first trimester of pregnancy. Ultrasound Obstet Gynecol 1997;10:419–421.

Goldstein I, Winn HN, Hobbins JC. Prenatal diagnostic criteria for body stalk anomaly. Am J Perinatol 1989;6: 84–85.

Jauniaux E, Vyas S, Finlayson C, Moscoso G, Driver M, Campbell S. Early sonographic diagnosis of body stalk anomaly. Prenat Diagn 1990;10:127–132.

Kermauner F. Die Missbildungen des Rumpfes: In: Schwalbe E, Gruben GB, eds. Morphologie der Mißbildungen des Menschen and der Tiere. 3rd ed. Jena, Germany: Gustav Fisher 1906:41–85.

Lockwood CJ, Scioscia AL, Hobbins JC. Congenital absence of the umbilical cord resulting from maldevelopment of embryonic body folding. Am J Obstet Gynecol 1986;155: 1049–1051.

Mann L, Ferguson-Smith MA, Desai M, Gibson AA, Raine PA. Prenatal assessment of anterior and abdominal wall defects and their prognosis. Prenat Diagn 1984;4:427–435.

Martinez JM, Fortuny A, Comas C, et al. Body stalk anomaly associated with maternal cocaine abuse. Prenat Diagn 1994;14:669–672.

Martínez-Frías ML. Clinical and epidemiological characteristics of infants with body wall complex with and without limb deficiency. Am J Med Genet 1997;73:170–175.

Miller ME, Higginbottom D, Smith DW. Short umbilical cord: its origin and relevance. Pediatrics 1981;67:618–621.

Negishi H, Yaegashi M, Kato EH, Yamada H, Okuyama K, Fujimoto S. Prenatal diagnosis of limb-body wall complex. J Reprod Med 1998;43:659–664.

Shalev E, Eliyahu S, Battino S, Weiner E. First trimester transvaginal sonographic diagnosis of body stalk anomaly. J Ultrasound Med 1995;14:641–642.

Shih J-C, Shyu M-K, Hwa S-L, et al. Concordant body stalk anomaly in monozygotic twinning-early embryo cleavage disorder. Prenat Diagn 1996;16:467–470.

Souka AP, Snijders RJM, Novakov A, Soares W, Nicolaides KH. Defects and syndromes in chromosomally normal fetuses with increased nuchal translucency thickness at 10–14 weeks of gestation. Ultrasound Obstet Gynecol 1998;11:391–400.

Takeuchi K, Fujita I, Nakajima K, Kitagaki S, Koketsu I. Body stalk anomaly: prenatal diagnosis. Int J Gynecol Obstet 1995;51:49–52.

Van Allen MI, Curry C, Gallagher L. Limb-body wall complex. I. Pathogenesis. Am J Med Genet 1987;28:529–548.

Viscarello RK, Ferguson DD, Nores J, Hobbins JC. Limb-body wall associated with cocaine abuse: further evidence of cocaine's teratogenicity. Obstet Gynecol 1992;80:523–526.

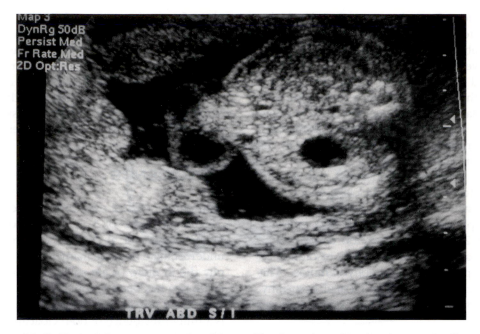

Figure 60-3. Prenatal sonogram of a fetus with cloacal exstrophy demonstrating several sonographic features of cloacal exstrophy. In this image, seen in transverse at the level of the umbilical-cord insertion, the lower-abdominal-wall defect and omphalocele membrane are evident.

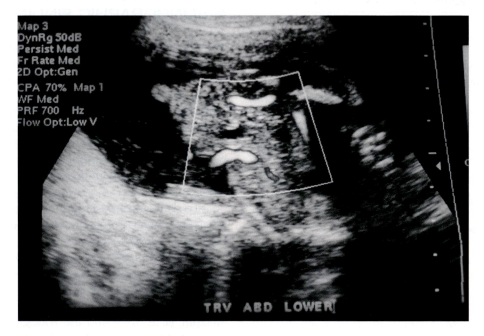

Figure 60-4. A lower-abdominal transverse image in the same fetus seen in Figure 60-3, in which no bladder is seen between the umbilical arteries, which appear bright white in this black-and-white version of a color Doppler image, and the elephant-trunk deformity caused by prolapse of the ileum is also seen.

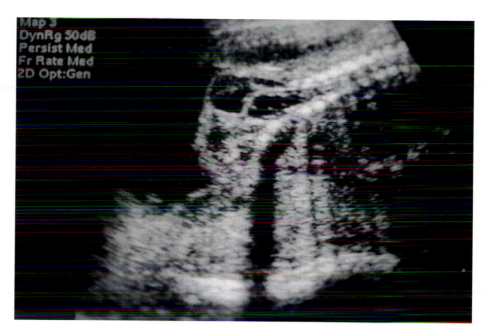

Figure 60-5. The same fetus as in Figures 60-3 and 60-4 is seen in sagittal section of the spine, demonstrating the large sacral myelomeningocele.

not done prospectively, this report has helped to define sonographic features of cloacal exstrophy that may allow early prenatal diagnosis (Figs. 60-3 to 5). These sonographic features may assist the sonographer in distinguishing cloacal exstrophy from other midline anterior-abdominal-wall defects.

▶ DIFFERENTIAL DIAGNOSIS

The differential diagnosis of cloacal exstrophy includes bladder exstrophy (see Chapter 58), omphalocele (see Chapter 63), gastroschisis (see Chapter 62), amniotic band syndrome (see Chapter 101), and the limb–body-wall complex. The sonographic features of each of these allows it to be distinguished from cloacal exstrophy. In bladder exstrophy, there is a small soft-tissue mass on the surface of the abdominal wall and no normal-appearing bladder, omphalocele, spinal abnormalities or club feet. Omphaloceles are usually more cephalad on the abdomen and lack other features of cloacal exstrophy. The loops of intestine floating free in the amniotic fluid in gastroschisis usually can be easily distinguished from the omphalocele of cloacal exstrophy, even with loops of intestine floating in ascitic fluid.

The amniotic band syndrome and limb–body-wall complex usually lack the lower abdominal omphalocele and myelomeningocele and a normal bladder can usually be seen in the pelvis. Cases of limb–body-wall complex usually have large gastropleuroschisis with distorted spine.

▶ ANTENATAL NATURAL HISTORY

Because of the rarity of cloacal exstrophy, and the even rarer prenatal diagnoses of these cases, little is known about its antenatal natural history. In the cases studied by Meizner et al. (1995), 4 of the 6 developed polyhydramnios, which may predispose to preterm labor and delivery. The cause of polyhydramnios in cloacal exstrophy is not known. There appears to be an increased incidence of intrauterine fetal death and stillbirth in cloacal exstrophy.

▶ MANAGEMENT OF PREGNANCY

The mother carrying a fetus in which cloacal exstrophy is suspected should be referred to a tertiary-care center for prenatal sonographic evaluation. If the features of cloacal exstrophy cannot be completely defined sonographically, fetal magnetic resonance imaging (MRI) may be indicated. If the diagnosis is made prior to 24 weeks of gestation, the parents should be offered pregnancy termination. If the parents decide to proceed with the pregnancy, amniocentesis should be considered to determine the genetic sex of the fetus. However, even if the karyotype is 46,XY, female gender reassignment is almost always necessary due to the inadequacy of phallic development, which makes reconstruction as a male impossible. The parents should be counseled about the nature of this complex anomaly by a team consisting of a pediatric surgeon, pediatric urologist, pediatric neurosurgeon, neonatologist,

fascial closure. The hospitalization in these infants may be prolonged by several weeks.

Inguinal hernias will develop in most infants with gastroschisis because of increased intraabdominal pressure. Occasionally, incisional hernias seen as bulging from attenuated fascia at the closure site will require remedial surgery months or years later. There are no long-term sequelae from gastroschisis if there is no associated hypoperistalsis syndrome.

▶ GENETICS AND RECURRENCE RISK

Gastroschisis has been generally considered a sporadic event, with a multifactorial cause, but there have been reports of familial recurrence (Hershey et al. 1989; Lowry and Baird 1982; Salinar et al. 1979). Torfs et al. (1991) described a 4.3% sibling recurrence rate in a population-based study. A 4.3% recurrence risk implies a mixture of genetic predisposition with environmental factors. In 1 study, Torfs and Curry (1993) found only 6 published reports of familial occurrence of gastroschisis. A single-gene defect is unlikely for this condition. Families should receive genetic counseling regarding recurrence risk. They should be offered MSAFP testing and prenatal sonography in future pregnancies.

REFERENCES

Amoury RA, Beatty EC, Wood WI, et al. Histology of the intestine in human gastroschisis relationship to intestinal malfunction: dissolution of the "peel" and its ultrastructural characteristics. J Pediatr Surg 1988;23:950–956.

Amoury RA, Holder TM. Gastroschisis complicated by intestinal atresia. Surgery 1977;82:373–381.

Bair JH, Russ PD, Pretorius DH. Fetal omphalocele and gastroschisis: a review of 24 cases. Am J Radiol 1986;147:1047–1051.

Baird PA, MacDonald EC. An epidemiologic study of congenital malformations of the anterior abdominal wall in more than half a million consecutive live births. Am J Hum Genet 1981;33:470–478.

Bond SJ, Harrison MR, Filly RA, et al. Severity of intestinal damage in gastroschisis: correlation with prenatal sonographic findings. J Pediatr Surg 1988;23:520–525.

Bowerman R, Aulla N, Ginsberg H. High resolution sonographic identification of fetal midgut herniation into the umbilical cord: differentiation from fetal anterior abdominal wall defects. J Ultrasound in Med 1988;109(suppl):7.

Brock DJ, Barron L, Duncan P, et al. Significance of elevated mid-trimester maternal plasma AFP values. Lancet 1979;1:1281.

Bryant MS, Tepas JJ, Mollitt DL, et al. The effect of initial operative repair on the recovery of intestinal function in gastroschisis. Am Surg 1985;55:210.

Calzolari E, Volpato S, Bianchi F, et al. Omphalocele and gastroschisis: a collaborative study of five Italian congenital malformation registries. Teratology 1993;47:47–55.

Caniano DA, Brokaw B, Ginn-Pease ME. An individualized approach to the management of gastroschisis. J Pediatr Surg 1990;25:287–300.

Caplan MS, MacGregor SN. Perinatal management of congenital diaphragmatic hernia and anterior abdominal wall defects. Clin Perinatol 1989;16:917.

Carlan SJ, Knuppel RA, Perez J, et al. Antenatal fetal diagnosis and maternal transport gastroschisis. Clin Pediatr 1990;29:378.

Carpenter MW, Curci MR, Dibbins AW, et al. Perinatal management of ventral wall defects. Obstet Gynecol 1984;64:646.

Colombani PM, Cunningham MD. Perinatal aspects of omphalocele and gastroschisis. Am J Dis Child 1977;131:1386.

Coughlin JP, Drucker DE, Jewell MR et al. Delivery room repair of gastroschisis. Surgery 1993;114:822–827.

Crandall BF, Robinson L, Grau P. Risks associated with an elevated maternal serum alpha-fetoprotein level. Am J Obstet Gynecol 1991;165:581–586.

Crawford RAF, Ryan G, Wright VM, et al. The importance of serial biophysical assessment of fetal well being in gastroschisis. Br J Obstet Gynaecol 1992;99:899–902.

Cyr DR, Mack LA, Schoenecker SA, et al. Bowel migration in the normal fetus: US detection. Radiology 1986;161:119–121.

DeLorenzo M, Yazbeck S, Ducharme JC. Gastroschisis: a 15-year experience. J Pediatr Surg 1987;22:710–712.

deVries PA. The pathogenesis of gastroschisis and omphalocele. J Pediatr Surg 1980;15:245.

Duhamel B. Embryology of exomphalos and allied malformations. Arch Dis Child 1963;38:142.

Egenaes J, Bjerkedal T. Forekomst av gastroschisis og omfalocele i Norge 1967–1979. Tidsskr Nor Laegeforen 1982;102:172–176.

Ein SH, Rubin SZ. Gastroschisis: primary closure or silo pouch. J Pediatr Surg 1980;15:549.

Ein SH, Superina R, Bagwell C, et al. Ischemic bowel after primary closure for gastroschisis. J Pediatr Surg 1988;23:728–730.

Ewigman BG, Crane JP, RADIUS Study Group. Effect of prenatal ultrasound screening on perinatal outcome. N Engl J Med 1993;329:821–827.

Fonkalsrud EW. Selective repair of neonatal gastroschisis based on degree of visceroabdominal disproportion. Surgery 1980;139:138.

Glick PL, Harrison MR, Adzick NS, et al. The missing link in the pathogenesis of gastroschisis. Pediatr Surg 1985;20:406–409.

Goldbaum G, Daling J, Milham S. Risk factors for gastroschisis. Teratology 1990;42:397–403.

Goldfine C, Haddow JE, Knight GJ, et al. Amniotic fluid alpha-fetoprotein and acetylcholinesterase measurements in pregnancies associated with gastroschisis. Prenat Diag 1989;8:697–700.

Gornall P. Management of intestinal atresia complicating gastroschisis. J Pediatr Surg 1989;24:522–525.

Green JJ, Hobbins JC. Abdominal ultrasound examination of the first-trimester fetus. Am J Obstet Gynecol 1988;159:165–175.

Gutenberger JE, Miller DL, Dibbins AW, et al. Hypogammaglobulinemia and hypoalbuminemia in neonates with ruptured omphaloceles and gastroschisis. J Pediatr Surg 1973;8:353–359.

Guzman ER. Early prenatal diagnosis of gastroschisis with transvaginal ultrasonography. Am J Obstet Gynecol 1990;162:1253–1254.

Haddow JE, Palomaki GE, Holman MS. Young maternal age and smoking during pregnancy as risk factors for gastroschisis. Teratology 1993;47:225–228.

Hemmenki K, Saloniemi I, Kyronen P, et al. Gastroschisis and omphalocele in Finland in the 1970's: prevalence at birth and its correlates. J Epidemiol Commun Health 1982;36:289–293.

Hershey DW, Haesslein HC, Marr CC, et al. Familial abdominal wall defects. Am J Med Genet 1989;34:174.

Hill LM, Breckle R, Gehrking WC. Prenatal detection of congenital malformations by ultrasonography. Am J Obstet Gynecol 1985;151:44–50.

Hoyme HE, Jones MC, Jones KL. Gastroschisis: abdominal wall disruption secondary to early gestational interruption of the omphalomesenteric artery. Semin Perinatol 1983;7:294–298.

Killam WP, Miller RC, Seeds JW. Extremely high maternal serum alpha-fetoprotein levels at second-trimester screening. Obstet Gynecol 1991;78:257.

King DR, Savrin R, Boles ET. Gastroschisis update. J Pediatr Surg 1980;15:553.

Kirk EP, Wah RH. Obstetric management of the fetus with omphalocele or gastroschisis: a review and report of 112 cases. Am J Obstet Gynecol 1983;146:512.

Klein M, Kluck P, Tibboel D, et al. The effect of fetal urine on the development of the bowel in gastroschisis. J Pediatr Surg 1983;18:47.

Knott PD, Colley NV. Can fetal gastroschisis always be diagnosed prenatally? Prenat Diagn 1987;7:607–610.

Langer JC, Longaker MT, Crombleholme TM, et al. Etiology of intestinal damage in gastroschisis. I. Effects of amniotic fluid exposure and bowel constriction in a fetal lamb model. J Pediatr Surg 1989;24:992–997.

Langer JC, Bell JG, Castillo RO, et al. Etiology of intestinal damage in gastroschisis. II. Timing and reversibility of histological changes, mucosal function, and contractility. J Pediatr Surg 1990;25:1122–1126.

Langer JC, Khanna J, Caco C, et al. Prenatal diagnosis of gastroschisis: development of objective sonographic criteria for predicting outcome. Obstet Gynecol 1993;81:53–56.

Larson JM, Pretorius DH, Budorick NE, et al. Value of maternal serum alpha-fetoprotein levels of 5.0 MoM or greater and prenatal sonography in predicting fetal outcome. Radiology 1993;189:77–81.

Lenke RR, Hatch EI. Fetal gastroschisis: a preliminary report advocating the use of cesarean section. Obstet Gynecol 1986;67:395.

Lenke RR, Persutte WH, Nemes J. Ultrasonographic assessment of intestinal damage in fetuses with gastroschisis: is it of clinical value? Am J Obstet Gynecol 1990;163:995–998.

Lewinsky RM, Jonson JM, Lao TT, et al. Fetal gastroschisis associated with monosomy 22 mosaicism and absent cerebral diastolic flow. Prenat Diagn 1990;10:605–608.

Lewis DF, Towers CV, Garite TH, et al. Fetal gastroschisis and omphalocele: is cesarean section the best mode of delivery? Am J Obstet Gynecol 1990;163:773–775.

Lindham S. Omphalocele and gastroschisis in Sweden 1965–1976. Acta Paediatr Scand 1981;70:55–60.

Lowry RB, Baird PA. Familial gastroschisis and omphalocele. Am J Hum Genet 1982;34:517–518.

Luck SR, Sherman JO, Raffensperger JG, et al. Gastroschisis in 106 consecutive newborn infants. Surgery 1985;98:677.

McKeown T, McMahon B, Record RG. An investigation of 69 cases of exomphalos. Am J Hum Genet 1953;5:168–175.

Mann L, Ferguson-Smith MA. Prenatal assessment of anterior abdominal wall defects and their prognosis. Prenatal Diag 1984;14:427.

Martinez-Frias ML, Prieto SL, Zaplana J. Epidemiological study of gastroschisis and omphalocele in Spain. Teratology 1984;29:337–382.

Mayer T, Black R, Matlak ME, et al. Gastroschisis and omphalocele. Ann Surg 1980;192:783.

Mercer S, Mercer B, D'Alton MA, et al. Gastroschisis: ultrasonographic diagnosis, perinatal embryology, surgical and obstetric treatment and outcomes. Can J Surg 1988;31:25.

Molenaar JC, Tibboel D. Gastroschisis and omphalocele. World J Surg 1993;17:337–341.

Moore KL, Persaud TVN. The developing human: clinically oriented embryology. 5th ed. Philadelphia: Saunders, 1993.

Moore T, Stokes GF. Gastroschisis. Surgery 1953;33:112–120.

Moore TC. Gastroschisis with antenatal evisceration of intestines and urinary bladder. Ann Surg 1962;157:263.

Moore TC. The role of labor in gastroschisis bowel thickening and prevention by elective pre-term and pre-labor cesarean section. Pediatr Surg Int 1992;7:256–259.

Moretti M, Khoury A, Rodriquez J, et al. The effect of mode of delivery on the perinatal outcome in fetuses with abdominal wall defects. Am J Obstet Gynecol 1990;163:833–838.

Muraji T, Tsugawa C, Nishijima E, et al. Gastroschisis: a 17-year experience. J Pediatr Surg 1989;24:343–345.

Nicholls G, Upadhyaya V, Gornall P, et al. Is specialist center delivery of gastroschisis beneficial? Arch Dis Child 1993;69:71–73.

Nicolaides KH, Snijders RJM, Cheng HH, et al. Fetal gastrointestinal and abdominal wall defects: associated malformations and chromosomal abnormalities. Fetal Diagn Ther 1992;7:102–115.

Novotny A, Klein RJ, Boeckman CR: Gastroschisis: an 18-year review. J Pediatr Surg 1993;28:650–652.

Nyberg DA, Mahony BS, Pretorius DH. Diagnostic ultrasound of fetal anomalies. Yearbook Medical Publisher, Chicago, 1993; 385–432.

Oh KS, Dorst JP, Dominguez R, et al. Abnormal intestinal motility in gastroschisis. Radiology 1978;127:457–460.

Oldham KT, Coran AG, Drongowski RA, et al. The development of necrotizing enterocolitis following repair of gastroschisis: a surprisingly high incidence. J Pediatr Surg 1988;23:945–949.

O'Neill JA, Grosfeld JL. Intestinal malfunction after antenatal exposure of viscera. Am J Surg 1974;127:129–132.

Paidas M, Crombleholme TM, Robertson FM. Prenatal diagnosis and management of the fetus with an abdominal wall injury. Semin Perinatol 1994;18(3):182–195.

Palomaki GE, Hill LE, Knight GJ, et al. Second-trimester maternal serum alpha-fetoprotein levels in pregnancies associated with gastroschisis and omphalocele. Obstet Gynecol 1988;71:906.

Paulozzi LJ. Seasonality of omphalocele in Washington state. Teratology 1986;33:133–134.

Pokorny WJ, Harberg, FJ, McGill CW. Gastroschisis complicated by intestinal atresia. J Pediatr Surg 1981;16:261.

Redford RHA, McNay MB, Whittle MJ. Gastroschisis and exomphaloceles: precise diagnosis by mid-pregnancy ultrasound. Br J Obstet Gynaecol 1985;92:54.

Roeper PJ, Harris J, Lee G, et al. Secular rates and correlates for gastroschisis in California (1968–1977). Teratology 1987;35:203–210.

Romero R, Pilu G, Jeanty P, et al. The abdominal wall: prenatal diagnosis of congenital anomalies. Norwalk, CT: Appleton & Lange, 1988.

Rosendahl H, Kivinen S. Antenatal detection of congenital malformations by routine ultrasonography. Obstet Gynecol 1989;73:947.

Royner BD, Richards D. Growth retardation in fetuses with gastroschisis. J Ultrasound Med 1977;16:13–16.

Salinar CF, Bartoshefsky L, Othersen HB, et al. Familial occurrence of gastroschisis. Am J Dis Child 1979;133:514–517.

Sawin R, Glick P, Schaller R, et al. Gastroschisis wringer clamp: a safe, simplified method for delayed primary closure. J Pediatr Surg 1992;27:1346–1348.

Schmidt D, Rose E, Greenberg F. An association between fetal abdominal wall defects and elevated levels of human chorionic gonadotropin in mid-trimester. Prenat Diag 1993;13:9–12.

Schuster S. A new method for the staged repair of large omphaloceles. Surg Gynecol Obstet 1967;125:261–266.

Sermer M, Benzie RJ, Pitson L, et al. Prenatal diagnosis and management of congenital defects of the anterior abdominal wall. Am J Obstet Gynecol 1987;156:308–312.

Shah R, Woolley MM. Gastroschisis and intestinal atresia. J Pediatr Surg 1991;26:788–790.

Shaw A. The myth of gastroschisis. J Pediatr Surg 1975;10:235–244.

Sipes SL, Weiner CP, Sipes DR, et al. Gastroschisis and omphalocele: does either antenatal diagnosis or route of delivery make a difference in perinatal outcome? Obstet Gynecol 1990a;76:195–199.

Sipes SL, Weiner CP, Wiliamson RA, et al. Fetal gastroschisis complicated by bowel dilation: an indication for imminent delivery? Fetal Diagn Ther 1990b;5:100.

Stiller RJ, Haynes, de Regt R, et al. Elevated maternal serum alpha-fetoprotein concentration and fetal chromosomal abnormalities. Obstet Gynecol 1990;75:994.

Stoodley N, Sherma A, Noblett H, et al. Influence of place of delivery on outcome of babies with gastroschisis. Arch Dis Child 1993;69:71–73.

Stringel G. Large gastroschisis: primary repair with Gore-Tex patch. J Pediatr Surg 1993;28:653–655.

Stringel G, Filler RM. Prognostic factors in omphalocele and gastroschisis. J Pediatr Surg 1978;14: 515–519.

Tibboel D, Raine P, McNee M, et al. Developmental aspects of gastroschisis. J Pediatr Surg 1986a;21:865–869.

Tibboel D, Vermey-Keers C, Kluck P, et al. The natural history of gastroschisis during fetal life: development of the fibrous coating on the bowel loops. Teratology 1986b;33:267–272.

Timor-Tritsch IE, Warren WB, Peisner DB, et al. First trimester midgut herniation: a high-frequency transvaginal sonographic study. Am J Obstet Gynecol 1989;161:831–833.

Torfs C, Curry C, Roeper P. Gastroschisis. J Pediatr 1990;116:1.

Torfs CP, Curry CJR. Familial cases of gastroschisis in a population-based registry. Am J Med Genet 1993;45:465–467.

Van Allen MI. Fetal vascular disruptions: mechanisms and some resulting birth defects. Pediatr Annu 1981;10:31–50.

Walkinshaw SA, Renwick M, Hebisch G, et al. How good is ultrasound in the detection and evaluation of anterior abdominal wall defects? Br J Radiol 1992;65:298–301.

Werler MM, Mitchell AA, Shapiro S. First trimester maternal medication use in relation to gastroschisis. Teratology 1992b;45:361–367.

Yaster M, Scherer TLR, Stone MM, et al. Prediction of successful primary closure of congenital abdominal-wall defects using intraoperative measurements. J Pediatr Surg 1989;24:1217–1220.

Zivkovle SM. Repair of gastroschisis using umbilical cord as patch. J Pediatr Surg 1991;26:1179–1180.

CHAPTER 63

Omphalocele

▶ CONDITION

Omphalocele is a defect in the ventral abdominal wall characterized by an absence of abdominal muscles, fascia, and skin. The defect is covered by a membrane consisting of peritoneum and amnion and can vary in size from a few centimeters to most of the ventral abdominal wall. Unlike gastroschisis, in omphalocele, the umbilical cord inserts into this membrane at a location far from the abdominal wall (deVries 1980). The defect is thought to be caused by an abnormality that occurs during the process of body infolding at 3 to 4 weeks of gestation (Dimmick and Kalouset 1992). At that time, 3 folds occur simultaneously, and each is associated with a distinct type of omphalocele. Cephalic folding defects result in a high or epigastric omphalocele. An example of this is pentalogy of Cantrell (see Chapter 64), which consists of an epigastric omphalocele, anterior diaphragmatic defect, sternal cleft, pericardial defect, and associated intracardiac defects (Cantrell et al. 1958). A defect in lateral folding results in the classic omphalocele (Fig. 63-1) with a midabdominal defect. A defect in caudal folding results in a low or hypogastric omphalocele as seen in bladder or cloacal exstrophy (see Chapters 58 and 60) (Duhamel 1963; Meller et al. 1989). The spectrum of severity of abdominal-wall abnormalities can vary from a small umbilical hernia to a large defect with extrusion of the abdominal viscera.

▶ INCIDENCE

The incidence of omphalocele ranges from approximately 1 in 4000 to 1 in 7000 live births (Baird et al. 1981;

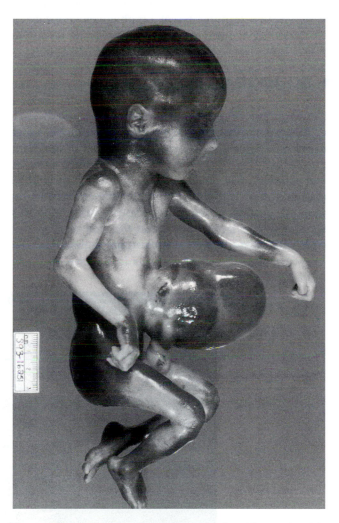

Figure 63-1. Classic appearance of a 22-week-old fetus with omphalocele due to defect in lateral folding. *(Courtesy of Dr. Joseph Semple.)*

syndromic diagnosis. Peripheral vascular access should be established and intravenous fluids given. Mechanical ventilation is frequently necessary, especially postoperatively, when abdominal contents replaced into a small abdominal cavity impede diaphragmatic occlusion and lung expansion. Antibiotics are generally given postoperatively. Initial treatment of the newborn is directed toward preoperative stabilization.

▶ SURGICAL TREATMENT

The surgical approach to the treatment of omphalocele has changed considerably over the past four decades. Until 1965, the only approach for the treatment of omphalocele was the skin-flap technique described by Gross (1948). The principal disadvantage of this technique was the creation of a large disfiguring ventral hernia that ultimately required reoperation. This is usually not an insurmountable problem, and success has been reported for repair of these hernias. Considerable time (usually 6 months to 2 years, but sometimes longer) can lapse between initial surgery and final correction of the hernia (Swartz et al. 1985). If at all possible, primary fascial closure is the preferred method of repair because of a lower incidence of sepsis, bilary obstruction, and fistula and a reduced number of operations and rate of mortality in patients who undergo this repair (Fig. 63-4) (Aaronson et al. 1977; Robin and Ein 1976; Sauter et al. 1991; Canty et al. 1983; Mabogunje

and Mahour 1984). For very large omphaloceles, a staged reduction using a prosthetic silo is preferred (Allen and Wrenn 1969; Othersen and Smith 1986; Schuster 1967). This procedure consists of suturing a Silastic mesh to the rim of fascial defect, which then covers the herniated contents of the omphalocele (Fig. 63-5). This technique consists of paralysis with neuromuscular blocking agents, enlargement of the fascial defect, and gradual stretching of the abdominal wall. Nonoperative (conservative) approaches to the treatment of omphalocele have also been successful, but have the disadvantages noted above as well as prolonged hospitalization (Hatch et al. 1987; Mobogunje and Mahour 1984). As long as the omphalocele membrane is intact, wrapping the newborn with elastic-bandage wraps will gradually reduce the size of the omphalocele and enlarge the peritoneal cavity. A delayed primary repair can be performed after a period of days to weeks. We have found this approach particularly useful in premature infants with giant omphaloceles. It may also be helpful in cases of giant omphalocele with associated pulmonary hypoplasia.

Although the presence of multiple associated anomalies accounts for the majority of deaths in cases of omphalocele, respiratory complications also account for a significant percentage of the morbidity and mortality due to this lesion (Paidas et al. 1994). Newborns with omphalocele, particularly giant omphalocele, have a high incidence of respiratory insufficiency and chest-wall deformity. Some evidence suggests that impaired

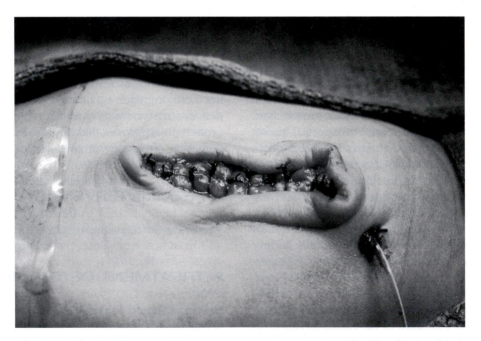

Figure 63-4. Intraoperative postclosure appearance of newborn abdomen after primary omphalocele repair. The umbilical artery has been transposed to a right-lower-quadrant site for umbilical artery catheter placement for arterial blood pressure monitoring.

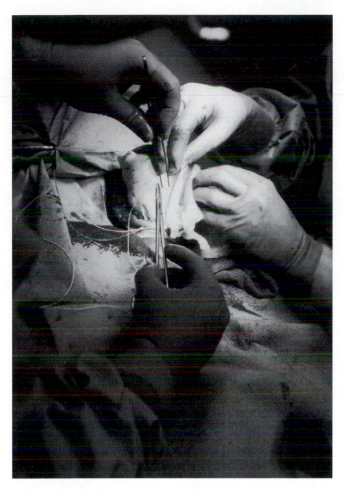

Figure 63-5. Silo repair of omphalocele.

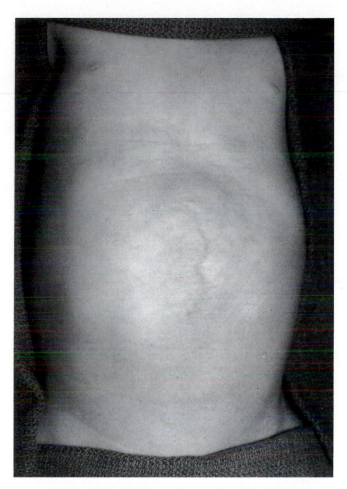

Figure 63-6. Abdominal appearance 1 year after primary repair of a large omphalocele. Note the absence of a normal umbilicus.

lung growth and pulmonary hypoplasia may even be evident antenatally (Argyle 1989; Hershenson et al. 1985; Thompson et al. 1993).

Neonates may require prolonged mechanical ventilation because of the need for positive pressure to expand a chest compressed by a large abdominal mass. Bronchopulmonary dysplasia and chronic lung disease are potential long-term complications.

▶ LONG-TERM OUTCOME

Even with primary repair of omphalocele, a protracted stay in the newborn nursery can be anticipated. Under the best circumstances, except for hernias of the umbilical cord, some period of mechanical ventilation following omphalocele repair is required. In some cases of giant omphaloceles, there may be underlying pulmonary hypoplasia, which complicates ventilatory management. Following extubation most infants have feeding difficulties because of the prolonged period

without oral stimulation and poor coordination of sucking and swallowing. In addition, many infants have high respiratory rates following omphalocele repair. Because of the compromised diaphragmatic excursion and chest-wall motion, these infants maintain this minute ventilation by shallow, rapid breathing patterns. This rapid breathing often interferes with suckling, and gavage feeding may be necessary.

As mentioned previously, the anomalies associated with omphalocele will have a major impact on outcome. This is especially true of chromosomal and cardiac defects. As survival rates of patients with omphalocele increase, more outcome data will become available, particularly with respect to other aspects that have an impact on the quality of life (Fig. 63-6). Preliminary studies suggest that there are higher rates of behavioral problems and musculoskeletal abnormalities in children with abdominal-wall defects (Ginn-Pease et al. 1991; Loder and Guiboux 1993). There is one reported case of successful pregnancy in adulthood following the staged-repair procedure for a large omphalocele (Ein and Bernstein 1990).

▶ GENETICS AND RECURRENCE RISK

The recurrence risk depends on the cause of the omphalocele. If the fetus has a chromosomal abnormality due to aneuploidy, such as trisomy 18, the recurrence risk is 1% or the age-related maternal risk, whichever is higher. Familial cases of Beckwith–Wiedemann syndrome may have as high as a 50% recurrence risk. Nonsyndromal (isolated) omphalocele is generally considered to be a sporadic event, with a negligible recurrence risk. However, at least 17 cases of familial omphalocele have been described (DiLiberti 1982; Osuna et al. 1996; Pryde et al. 1992). Most of these families appear to transmit the gene as an autosomal dominant. In one asymptomatic patient, five consecutive pregnancies by two different nonconsanguineous partners were complicated by fetuses with isolated omphalocele (Pryde et al. 1992).

REFERENCES

Aaronson IA, Eckstein HB. The role of Silastic prosthesis in the management of gastroschisis. Arch Surg 1977;112:297–302.

Allen RG, Wrenn EL. Silon as a sac in the treatment of omphalocele and gastroschisis. J Pediatr Surg 1969;4:3–8.

Ardinger HH, Williamson RA, Gant S. Association of neural tube defects with omphalocele in chromosomally normal fetuses. Am J Med Genet 1987;27:135–142.

Argyle JC. Pulmonary hypoplasia in infants with giant abdominal wall defects. Pediatr Pathol 1989;9:43–55.

Baird PA, MacDonald EC. An epidemiologic study of congenital malformations of the anterior abdominal wall in more than half a million consecutive live births. Am J Hum Genet 1981;33:470–478.

Benacerraf BR, Saltzman DH, Estroff JA, et al. Abnormal karyotype of fetuses with omphalocele: prediction based on omphalocele contents. Obstet Gynecol 1990;75:317.

Brooke DJ, Banon L, Duncan P, et al. Significance of elevated mid-trimester maternal plasma AFP values. Lancet 1979;1:1281–1282.

Brown DL, Emerson DS, Schulman LP, Carson SA. Sonographic diagnosis of omphalocele during 10th week of gestation. AJR Am J Roentgenol 1989;153:825–826.

Bryker CR, Breg WR. Penatology of Cantrell. In: Buyse ML, ed. Birth defects encyclopedia. Cambridge, MA: Blackwell Scientific, 1990:1375–1377.

Cameron G, McQuown DS, Modanlon HD, et al. Intrauterine diagnosis of an omphalocele by diagnostic ultrasound. Am J Obstet Gynecol 1978;131:821–823.

Cantrell JR, Haller JA, Ravitch MM. A syndrome of congenital defects involving the abdominal wall, sternum, diaphragm, pericardium, and heart. Surg Gynecol Obstet 1958;107:602.

Canty TG, Collins DL. Primary fascial closure in infants with gastroschisis and omphalocele: a superior approach. J Pediatr Surg 1983;18:707.

Carpenter MW, Curci MR, Dibbins AW, et al. Perinatal management of ventral wall defects. Obstet Gynecol 1984;64:646.

Cohen MM, Ulstrom R. Beckwith-Wiedemann syndrome. In: Bergsma G, ed. Birth defects compendium. 2nd ed. New York: Liss, 1979:140–144.

Copel JA, Pilu G, Kleinman CS. Congenital heart disease and extracardiac anomalies: associations and indications for fetal echocardiography. Am J Obstet Gynecol 1986; 154:1121–1132.

Craigo SD, Gillieson MS, Cetrulo CL. Pentalogy of Cantrell. In: Department of Radiology Staff, eds. The fetus. Vol. 2, Nashville: Vanderbilt University, 1992:3.

Crawford DC, Chapman MG, Allan LD. Echocardiography in the investigation of anterior abdominal wall defects in the fetus. Br J Obstet Gynaecol 1985;92:1034–1036.

deVries PA. The pathogenesis of gastroschisis and omphalocele. J Pediatr Surg 1980;15:245–249.

DiLiberti JH. Familial omphalocele: analysis of risk factors and case report. Am J Med Genet 1982;13:263–268.

Dimmick JE, Kalouset DE, eds. Developmental pathology of the embryo and fetus. Philadelphia: Lippincott, 1992: 527–529.

Duhamel B. Embryology of exomphalos and allied malformations. Arch Dis Child 1963;38:142.

Ein SH, Bernstein A. A 24-year follow-up of a large omphalocele: from silon pouch to pregnancy. J Pediatr Surg 1990;25:1190–1193.

Geijn EJ, Vugt JMG, Sollie JE. Ultrasonographic diagnosis and perinatal management of fetal abdominal wall defects. Fetal Diagn Ther 1991;6:2–10.

Getachew MM, Goldstein RB, Edge V, et al. Correlation between omphalocele contents and karyotypic abnormalities: sonographic study in 37 cases. AJR Am J Roentgenol 1991;158:133–136.

Ghidini A, Sirtori M, Romero R, Hobbins JC. Prenatal diagnosis of pentalogy of Cantrell. J Ultrasound Med 1988; 7:567.

Gilbert WM, Nicolaides KH. Fetal omphalocele: associated malformations and chromosomal defects. Obstet Gynecol 1987;70:633–635.

Ginn-Pease ME, King DR, Tarnowski KJ, et al. Psychosocial adjustment and physical growth in children with imperforate anus or abdominal wall defects. J Pediatr Surg 1991; 26:1129–1135.

Greenwood RD, Rosenthal A, Nadas AS. Cardiovascular malformations associated with omphalocele. J Pediatr 1974;85:818–821.

Greenwood D, Sommer A, Rosenthal A, et al. Cardiovascular abnormalities in the Beckwith-Wiedemann syndrome. Am J Dis Child 1977;131:293.

Gross RE. A new method for surgical treatment of large omphaloceles. Surgery 1948;24:277–292.

Hasan S, Hermansen MC. The prenatal diagnosis of ventral abdominal wall defects. Am J Obstet Gynecol 1986;155: 842–845.

Hatch EI, Baxter R. Surgical options in the management of large omphaloceles. Am J Surg 1987;153:449–453.

Hershenson MC, Brouillette RT, Klemka L, et al. Respiratory insufficiency in newborns with abdominal wall defects. J Pediatr Surg 1985;20:348–353.

Hsieh TT, Lai YM, Liou JD, et al. Management of the fetus with an abdominal wall defect: experience of 31 cases. J Formosa Med Assoc 1989;88:469–473.

Hughes MD, Nyberg DA, Mack LA, et al. Fetal omphalocele: prenatal US detection of concurrent anomalies and other predictors of outcome. Radiology 1989;173:371–376.

Killam WP, Miller RC, Seeds JW. Extremely high maternal serum alpha-fetoprotein levels at second-trimester screening. Obstet Gynecol 1991;78:257–267.

Kirk EP, Wah RH: Obstetric management of the fetus with omphalocele or gastroschisis: a review and report of one hundred twelve cases. Am J Obstet Gynecol 1983;512–517.

Lafferty PM, Emmerson AJ, Fleming PJ, et al. Anterior abdominal wall defects. Arch Dis Child 1989;64:1029–1031.

Lewis DF, Towers CV, Garite TJ, et al. Fetal gastroschisis and omphalocele: is cesarean section the best mode of delivery? Am J Obstet Gynecol 1990;163:773–775.

Lindham S. Omphalocele and gastroschisis in Sweden 1965–1976. Acta Paediatr Scand 1981;70:55–60.

Loder RT, Guiboux JP. Musculoskeletal involvement in children with gastroschisis and omphalocele. J Pediatr Surg 1993;28:584–590.

Mabogunje OA, Mahour GH. Omphalocele and gastroschisis–trends in survival across two decades. Am J Surg 1984;148:679–686.

McKeown T, McMahon B, Record RG. An investigation of 69 cases of exomphalos. Am J Hum Genet 1953;5:168–175.

Meller JL, Reyes HM, Loeff DS. Gastroschisis and omphalocele. Clin Perinatol 1989;16:113.

Molenaar JC, Tibboel D. Gastroschisis and omphalocele. World J Surg 1993;17:337–341.

Moretti M, Khoury A, Rodriquez J, et al. The effect of mode of delivery on the perinatal outcome in fetuses with abdominal wall defects. Am J Obstet Gynecol 1990;163:833–838.

Nicolaides KH, Snijders RJM, Cheng HH, et al. Fetal gastrointestinal and abdominal wall defect: associated malformations and chromosomal abnormalities. Fetal Diagn Ther 1992;7:102–115.

Nyberg DA, Fitzsimmons J, Mack LA, et al. Chromosomal abnormalities in fetuses with omphalocele—significance of omphalocele contents. J Ultrasound Med 1989;8:299–308.

Osuna A, Lindham S. Four cases of omphalocele in two generations of the same family. Clin Genet 1976;9:354–356.

Othersen HB, Smith CD. Pneumatic reduction bag for treatment of gastroschisis and omphalocele. Ann Surg 1986;203:512–516.

Paidas MJ, Crombleholme TM, Robertson FM. Prenatal diagnosis and management of the fetus with an abdominal-wall defect. Semin Perinatol 1994;18:196–214.

Palomaki GE, Hill LE, Knight GJ, et al. Second trimester maternal serum screening alpha-fetoprotein levels in pregnancies associated with gastroschisis and omphalocele. Obstet Gynecol 1988;71:906–909.

Pryde PG, Greb A, Isada NB, et al. Familial omphalocele: considerations in genetic counseling. Am J Med Genet 1992;44:624–627.

Redford RHA, McNay MB, Whittle MJ. Gastroschisis and exomphaloceles: precise diagnosis by mid-pregnancy ultrasound. Br J Obstet Gynaecol 1985;92:54–59.

Robin SZ, Ein SH. Experience with 55 silon pouches. J Pediatr Surg 1976;11:803–807.

Romero R, Pilu G, Jeanty P, et al. Omphalocele: prenatal diagnosis of congenital anomalies. Appleton & Lange, Norwalk, 1988:220–223.

Salinar CF, Bartoshefsky L, Othersen HB, et al. Familial occurrence of gastroschisis. Am J Dis Child 1979;133:514–517.

Sauter ER, Falterman KW, Arensman RM. Is primary repair of gastroschisis and omphalocele always the best operation? Am Surg 1991;57:142–144.

Schuster SR. A new method for the staged repair of large omphaloceles. Surg Gynecol Obstet 1967;125:837–850.

Sermer M, Benzie RJ, Pitson L, et al. Prenatal diagnosis and management of congenital defects of the anterior abdominal wall. Am J Obstet Gynecol 1987;156;308–312.

Sipes SL, Weiner CP, Sipes DR, et al. Gastroschisis and omphalocele: does either antenatal diagnosis or route of delivery make a difference in perinatal outcome? Obstet Gynecol 1990a;76:195–199.

Sipes SL, Weiner CP, Williamson RA, et al. Fetal gastroschisis complicated by bowel dilation: an indication for imminent delivery? Fetal Diagn Ther 1990b;5:100–105.

Sotelo A. Neoplasms associated with Beckwith-Wiedemann syndrome. Perspect Pediatr Pathol 1977;3:255–259.

Spitz L, Bloom KR, Milner S, et al. Combined anterior abdominal wall, sternal, diaphragmatic, pericardial, and intracardiac defects: a report of 5 cases and their management. H Pediatr Surg 1975;10:491–496.

Stiller RJ, Haynes R, deRegt R, et al. Elevated maternal serum alpha-fetoprotein concentration and fetal chromosomal abnormalities. Obstet Gynecol 1990;75:994–999.

Swartz KR, Harrison MW, Campbell JR, et al. Ventral hernia in the treatment of omphalocele and gastroschisis. Ann Surg 1985;3:347–350.

Toyama WM: Combined congenital defects of the anterior abdominal wall, sternum, diaphragm, pericardium, and heart: a case report and review of the syndrome. Pediatrics 1972;50:778–780.

Tucci M, Bard H: The associated anomalies that determine prognosis in congenital omphaloceles. Am J Obstet Gynecol 1990;13:1646–1649.

CHAPTER 64

Pentalogy of Cantrell

▶ CONDITION

Pentalogy of Cantrell is an unusual form of abdominal-wall defect that consists of five associated anomalies, including: (1) midline epigastric abdominal wall defect, (2) defect of the lower sternum, (3) deficiency of the anterior diaphragm, (4) defect in the diaphragmatic pericardium, and (5) intracardiac defects. This constellation of anomalies was first described by Cantrell et al. (1958), hence, the term pentalogy of Cantrell, although it has also been referred to as the Cantrell–Haller–Ravitch syndrome and peritoneal pericardial diaphragmatic hernia. Although pentralogy of Cantrell has been used interchangeably with ectopia cordis, in their original description Cantrell et al. (1958) were careful to distinguish between these two anomalies (see Chapter 61).

Cantrell suggested that the defects in this syndrome fell into two groups by mechanism of embryologic development. In the first group, a developmental failure of mesoderm results in diaphragmatic, pericardial, and intracardiac defects. The diaphragmatic defect is a failure of the transverse septum to develop. The pericardial defect arises from the somatic mesoderm immediately adjacent to the region of the same layer from which the transverse septum develops. Defective development of one but not the other of these structures is possible only with highly specific loss of somatic mesoderm. This is rarely seen in pentalogy of Cantrell, and these defects occur together in most patients. The intracardiac lesions result from abnormal development of the epimyocardium, which is derived from the splanchnic mesoderm. While the resulting intracardiac defects vary, almost all include defects of the cardiac septa.

The second group of defects results from failure of the ventral migration of the periprimordial structures and include the sternal defect and the epigastric omphalocele. All elements of the sternum are present, and

the costocartilages connect with the cartilaginous plates, which represent the paired sternal anlagen with variable degrees of fusion. The sternal defect results not from an absence of sternal primordia but from the failure of paired sternal anlagen to complete migration. A similar failure of migration results in the abdominal-wall defect. The normal layers of the ventral abdominal wall are present, but there is a lack of ventral migration of the myotomes. These patients have structurally normal rectus abdominus muscles that correctly attach to the pubic symphysis, but deviate laterally as they run cephalad to insert into the costal margins at the midclavicular line. This lack of migration is thought to be due to a defective development of the paramedian mesoderm.

The heart in pentalogy of Cantrell is normally positioned within the chest. In contrast, ectopia cordis is characterized by abnormal position of the heart outside of the chest (see Chapter 61). This becomes confusing, as classification systems for ectopia cordis list three types: cervical, thoracic, and thoracoabdominal, which is the same as pentalogy of Cantrell. Ectopia cordis may encompass partial or complete sternal defects, and invariably includes intracardiac anomalies, but does not include the pericardial, diaphragmatic, and abdominal-wall defects seen in the pentalogy of Cantrell. Kanagusuntheram and Verzin (1962) suggested that ectopia cordis occurs as a result of excessive pericardial coelom formation and subsequent destruction of the transverse septum with rupture of the anterior body wall at 6 weeks of gestation (Kanagusuntheram and Verzin 1962). Ravitch (1986) has suggested that the high frequency of major intrinsic cardiac defects with true ectopia cordis indicates that there is a primary defect in the splanchnic mesoderm responsible for cardiac development.

The primitive thoracic wall consists of somatopleura covering the ventral wall of the pericardial cavity. The ectodermal layer of the somatopleura forms the skin, but the remainder of the components of the body wall derive from invading dorsal mesoderm during the sixth week of gestation. The sternum appears as two parallel condensations of mesenchyme, the lateral sternal bands. A median cranial condensation, the presternum, appears independently. The lateral sternal bands fuse with the presternum cranially and with the tips of the ribs laterally. During the seventh week, the sternal bands begin fusing at their cephalic end and proceed caudally and cease by the ninth or tenth week.

▶ INCIDENCE

The pentalogy of Cantrell is a rare association of anomalies with only approximately 90 cases having been reported (Craigo et al. 1992). Males and females are affected equally. Due to the rarity of this condition, its incidence is difficult to estimate. Carmi et al. (1993) reported five cases of pentalogy of Cantrell ascertained through the Baltimore–Washington population based study of infants with congenital cardiovascular malformations, and estimated a regional prevalence of 5.5 cases for 1 million live-born infants.

▶ SONOGRAPHIC FINDINGS

The most obvious feature of pentalogy of Cantrell is the epigastric omphalocele (Fig. 64-1). There are reported

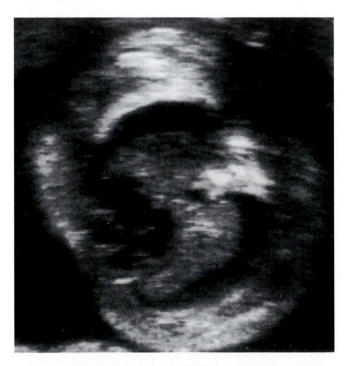

Figure 64-1. Prenatal sonographic image showing the transverse thoracic view of a fetus with pentalogy of Cantrell. The anterior chest-wall defect— epigastric omphalocele with the heart in the cephalad portion of the defect—can be appreciated.

cases with diastasis rectus without an omphalocele, which may be difficult to diagnose prenatally. The anterior diaphragmatic and pericardial defects are difficult, if not impossible, to discern sonographically. The three features of the pentalogy that may be most easily detected include the epigastric omphalocele, lower sternal defects, and intracardiac defects (Romero et al. 1988; Craigo et al. 1992).

Even if no other structural defects can be found, any fetus with an epigastric omphalocele should be evaluated for pentalogy of Cantrell, with particular attention paid to possible associated cardiac defects. The abdominal-wall defect in pentalogy of Cantrell may vary from a very large omphalocele containing stomach, liver, and apex of the heart to only widely displaced rectus abdominus muscles with skin covering the other defects and a ventral hernia.

The heart in the pentalogy of Cantrell is positioned within the fetal chest (Fig. 64-2). If the heart is located outside the fetal chest, this indicates ectopia cordis (see Chapter 61). Even though positioned within the chest, there is a subtle shift in the cardiac axis in pentalogy of Cantrell. The heart is normally oriented horizontally, with the apex to the left. However, in this syndrome the apex is oriented vertically, with the apex at the superior edge of the abdominal-wall defect. Usually, but not invariably, the heart in the pentalogy of Cantrell has intracardiac anomalies. The most commonly observed is a ventricular septal defect (Table 64-1).

In addition to the 5 anomalies that constitute the pentalogy of Cantrell, other anomalies have been reported to be associated. Care should be taken to adequately visualize the fetal spine and hands, as vertebral and digital anomalies are often seen, including kyphoscoliosis and clinodactyly. Likewise, a detailed inspection of the fetal head and face should be performed to exclude potentially associated craniofacial anomalies, including encephalocele, cleft lip, microphthalmia, and low-set ears (Fox et al. 1988; Ghidini et al. 1988). In addition, a two-vessel cord, absent left lung, cloacal exstrophy, and fetal ascites have all been observed in cases of pentalogy of Cantrell (Baker et al. 1984; Goncalves et al. 1994 ; Toyama et al. 1972). Egan et al. (1993) have reported a case of pentalogy of Cantrell associated with sirenomelia in a monozygotic twin. They suggested that anterior midline ventral-wall defects may be caused by either monozygotic twinning or vascular dysplasia. Similarly, a vascular steal phenomenon is thought to cause sirenomelia (see Chapter 87). They suggested that a common cause for these defects, that is, an alteration in vascular development, may be responsible. Carmi et al. (1992) found that 3 of their 5 patients had associated cleft lip with or without cleft palate. In a review of the literature on pentalogy of Cantrell and the various combinations of the anomalies within the spectrum, they suggested that pentalogy

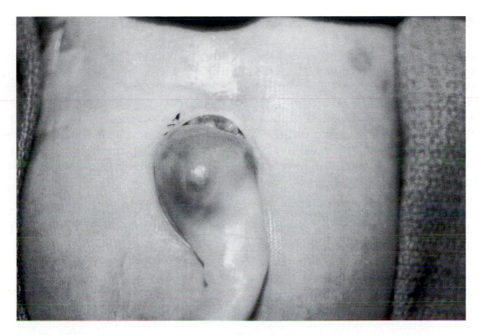

Figure 64-2. Postnatal appearance of the fetus in Figure 64-1. The epigastric omphalocele is apparent, with separation of the omphalocele membrane from the skin at the superior aspect of the abdominal-wall defect. The heart can be seen in the space between the skin and separated omphalocele membrane.

of Cantrell defines a specific midline ventral developmental field. Cleft lip with or without cleft palate and encephalocele tend to associate specifically with ventral midline anomalies within the spectrum of pentalogy of Cantrell. The authors speculated that these associations might be due either to previously observed tendencies or to specific occurrences of certain combinations of midline defects, or they may represent defined subunits of the midline developmental field (Carmi et al. 1992; Martin et al. 1992).

▶ DIFFERENTIAL DIAGNOSIS

The differential diagnosis in pentalogy of Cantrell includes simple omphalocele, ectopia cordis, amniotic band syn-

▶ **TABLE 64-1.** INTRACARDIAC ANOMALIES IN PENTALOGY OF CANTRELL

	Percent
Ventriculoseptal defect	37.5
Atrioseptal defect	20
Pulmonic stenosis	12.5
Tetralogy of Fallot	7.5
Left ventricular diverticulum	7.5
Anomalous venous return (caval)	7.5
Tricuspid atresia	2.3
Truncus arteriosus	2.3
Anomalous venous return (pulmonary)	2.3

drome, and the body-stalk anomaly (see Chapters 59, 61, 63, and 101).

▶ ANTENATAL HISTORY

Our understanding of the antenatal history of pentalogy of Cantrell is limited not only by the rarity of this syndrome, but also by the few cases that have been diagnosed prenatally. According to one report, fewer than 90 cases have been reported (Craigo et al. 1992). None of the anomalies in pentalogy of Cantrell if seen in isolation are associated with an adverse outcome or with in utero fetal death. Even the intracardiac anomalies most often seen in the pentalogy of Cantrell do not affect fetal survival. Ghidini et al. (1988) reported 10 cases from Yale in which there were no survivors. However, 5 of these pregnancies were terminated electively and the other 5 died postnatally. The authors did not distinguish between pentalogy of Cantrell and ectopia cordis, however. The prognosis for ectopia cordis is quite different and significantly worse than for pentalogy of Cantrell. This is a common error in reports of pentalogy of Cantrell, which adversely affects outcome and leads to an overly pessimistic prognosis once the pentalogy of Cantrell has been diagnosed. The overall prognosis in pentalogy of Cantrell is more closely correlated with the severity of the intracardiac defect and other associated anomalies not part of the pentalogy (Paidas et al. 1994).

Carmi R, Parvari R, Weinstein J. Mapping of an X-linked gene for ventral midline defects (the TAS gene). Am J Hum Genet 1993;53(suppl):A984. abstract.

Carpenter MW, Curci MR, Gibbins AW, et al. Perinatal management of ventral wall defects. Obstet Gynecol 1984;64: 646–650.

Craigo S, Gillieson MS, Cetrulo CL, et al. Pentalogy of Cantrell. Fetus 1992;3:7598–7601.

Egan JF, Petrikovsky BM, Vintzileos AM, et al. Combined pentalogy of Cantrell and sirenomelia: a case report with speculation about a common etiology. Am J Perinatol 1993;10:327–329.

Fox JE, Gloster ES, Mirchandovi R. Trisomy 18 with Cantrell pentalogy in a stillborn infant. Am J Med Genet 1988;31: 391–394.

Ghidini A, Sirtori M, Romero R, et al. Prenatal diagnosis of pentalogy of Cantrell. J Ultrasound Med 1988;7:567–570.

Goncalves LF, Jeanty P. Ultrasound evaluation of fetal abdominal wall defects in Callen PW, ed. Ultrasonography in obstetrics and gynecology. Philadelphia: Saunders, 1994:371–388.

Kanagusuntheram R, Verzin JA. Ectopia cordis in man. Thorax 1962;17:159–167.

Lafferty PM, Emerson AJ, Fleming PJ, et al. Anterior abdominal-wall defects. Arch Dis Child 1989;64:1029–1031.

Martin RA, Cunniff C, Erickson L, et al. Pentalogy of Cantrell and ectopia cordia, a familial developmental field complex. Am J Med Genet 1992;42:839–841.

Paidas M, Crombleholme TM, Robertson FM. Prenatal diagnosis and management of the fetus with an abdominal wall defect. Sem Perinatol 1994;18:196–214.

Parvari R, Carmi R, Weissenbach J, et al. Refined genetic mapping of X-linked thoracoabdominal syndrome. Am J Med Genet 1996;61:401–402.

Parvari R, Weinstein Y, Ehrlich S, et al. Linkage localization of the thoracoabdominal syndrome (TAS) gene to Xq 25-26. Am J Med Genet 1994;49:431–434.

Ravitch MM. The chest wall. In: Welch KJ, Randolph JG, Rovitch MM, O'Neill JA, Rowe MI eds. The chest wall in pediatric surgery. 4th ed. Chicago: Year Book, 1986: 563–568.

Romero R, Pilu G, Jeanty P, et al. Omphalocele. Prenatal diagnosis of congenital anomalies. Norwalk, CT: Appleton & Lange, 1988:220–223.

Sermer M, Benzie RJ, Piston L, et al. Prenatal diagnosis and management of congenital defects of the anterior wall. Am J Obstet Gynecol 1987;156:308–312.

Sipes SL, Weiner CP, Williamson RA, et al. Gastroschisis and omphalocele: does either antenatal diagnosis or route of delivery make a difference in perinatal outcome? Obstet Gynecol 1990;76:195–199.

Toyama WM. Combined congenital defects of the anterior abdominal wall, sternum, diaphragm, pericardium and heart: a case report and review of the syndrome. Pediatrics 1972;50:778–782.

CHAPTER 65

Anorectal Atresia (Imperforate Anus)

► CONDITION

Imperforate anus has been recognized since antiquity but has only been treatable in all its forms in the latter half of this century. The first surgical anoplasty for a low-type imperforate anus was performed by Amussat in Paris in 1835. The next significant advance did not occur until the work of Stephens, who described a combined sacral and abdominal-perineal approach based on cadaveric dissections, and highlighted the importance of the puborectolia sling (Stephens 1953). The modern approach to reconstruction of imperforate anus was pioneered by deVries and Pena in 1982 with the posterior sagittal approach to the whole spectrum of anorectal malformations using the posterior sagittal anorectoplasty (PSARP) (deVries and Pena 1982; Pena and deVries 1982).

Anomalies of the anus and rectum have usually been explained on the basis of an arrest of the caudal descent of the urorectal septum toward the cloacal membrane between 4 and 8 weeks of gestation (Fitzgerald and Fitzgerald 1994). At 4 to 6 weeks the cloacal membrane becomes partitioned into the anterior urogenital sinus and the posterior anorectum by the cranial to caudal growth of mesoderm-derived urorectal septum. The urorectal septum fuses with the cloacal membrane at what then becomes the perineal body (Paidas and Pena 1996). The mesoderm-derived urorectal septum is composed of the midline Tournex fold and two lateral Rathke folds. The lower third of the anal canal is derived from the ectoderm of the anal pit. Fusion of the hindgut mesoderm with the ectoderm occurs at the dentate line. Failure of Rathke folds to develop results in arrest of the inferior urorectal septum, resulting in a rectourethral fistula in the male and a persistent cloaca in the female. This arrest in Rathke folds usually occurs just below the paramesonephric duct, but a more caudal arrest in Rathke folds could result in a high rectovaginal fistula in a female. Failure of both Rathke and Tourneaux folds in males results in rectovesicular fistulas at the bladder neck. In the female it is more likely to result in cloacal anomaly or duplicated vagina and uterus (Paidas and Pena 1996). The malalignment of Tourneaux and Rathke folds may also result in rectourethral fistula in males and vestibular fistula in females. Isolated imperforate anus without a fistula occurs from failure of the anal pit to form, and despite normal descent of Tourneaux and Rathke folds, the lack of an ectodermal anal pit results in imperforate anus. Failure of the anal membrane to resorb or incomplete resorption despite formation of the anal pit results in rectal atresia or stenosis, respectively. Defects in mesoderm at the level of the perineal body are thought to result in perineal fistula.

As many as 50% of cases of anorectal malformations have associated anomalies (Table 65-1). Spinal or skeletal anomalies are present in 50% of cases, genitourinary anomalies in 58%, tracheoesophageal fistula in 10%, and cardiac anomalies in 5% (Sanders 1996).

▶ INCIDENCE

The incidence of imperforate anus is approximately 1 in 5000 live births (Kiely and Pena 1998; Stephens and Smith 1971). Most reports note a male preponderance of between 55 and 65% of cases (Kiely and Pena 1998; Stephens 1953; Weinstein 1965). Imperforate anus has been linked to maternal diabetes mellitus, thalidomide exposure, and ethanol intake.

▶ SONOGRAPHIC FINDINGS

It is unusual to make a diagnosis of imperforate anus on a prenatal sonographic examination. Sanders (1996) has noted that the anus can be seen in the normal fetus as an echogenic dot on a transverse view at the level of the genitalia. He notes that this dot is absent in cases of perforate anus. The reliability of the absence of this echogenic dot is unknown. It likely represents the echogenic sphincter complex, which may be present even if there is imperforate anus. More commonly, a dilated distal colon may be observed in the fetal pelvis (Guzman et al. 1995) (Fig. 65-1). Several authors have reported intraluminal colonic calcifications in imperforate anus (Grant et al. 1990; Sholen et al. 1983; Bean et al. 1978). This is presumed to be due to urine refluxing via the associated rectourethral fistula and precipitating as calcified meconium. There are a number of sonographically detectable abnormalities that may be seen in association with imperforate anus, including renal agenesis, renal dysplasia, horseshoe kidney, uterine duplications, cardiovascular, central venous system, and gastrointestinal and skeletal system anomalies. Imperforate anus may also occur as part of the VACTERL association. When associated with esophageal atresia, increased amniotic fluid volume and an absent stomach bubble may be noted. Imperforate anus occurs in trisomies 18 and 21; sonographic features of these syndromes should be ruled out (see Chapters 132 and 134).

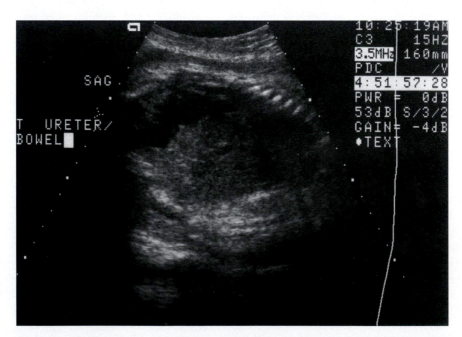

Figure 65-1. Prenatal sonographic image of a fetus who was diagnosed at birth with imperforate anus. Mild colonic distention was noted prenatally.

▶ DIFFERENTIAL DIAGNOSIS

The main differential diagnosis for anorectal atresia includes colonic atresia, Hirschsprung disease, meconium plug syndrome (Nyberg et al. 1987), and distal small-bowel atresia (Vermesch et al. 1986), hydrometrocolpos, ovarian cyst, obstructive uropathy, megacystic-microcolon hypoperistalsis syndrome, urachal cyst, and persistent cloaca (Paidas and Pena 1996). Harris et al. (1987) reviewed sonographic features of 12 cases of anorectal atresia and found evidence of bowel dilatation in the distal colon in 5 of the 12 cases. The features of distal bowel obstruction become more obvious as the fetus approaches term. The earliest reported prenatal diagnosis of imperforate anus is 29 weeks' gestation.

Because of the distal level of obstruction, some authors found it unusual that any degree of bowel dilatation was detectable and blamed the rectourethral or rectovesical fistula as a cause of bowel dilatation (Goldstein 1994).

▶ ANTENATAL HISTORY

Only a few cases of imperforate anus have been diagnosed prenatally (Bean et al. 1978; Harris et al. 1987; Rant et al. 1990; Guzman et al. 1995; Nyberg et al. 1987). If isolated, finding of anorectal atresia should not have any direct bearing on the outcome of the pregnancy. If seen as part of the VACTERL association, however, polyhydramnios may appear after 28 weeks' gestation if associated esophageal atresia is present (Greenwood et al. 1975; Smith et al. 1988).

▶ FETAL INTERVENTION

There are no fetal interventions for imperforate anus.

▶ MANAGEMENT OF PREGNANCY

A fetus in which imperforate anus is suspected should undergo a targeted sonographic examination to rule out associated anomalies. In particular, a detailed examination of the genitourinary tract is indicated because of the possibility of associated renal agenesis, renal dysplasia, and horseshoe kidney. Careful examinations of the central nervous system and spine, as well as the gastrointestinal tract, are indicated. Because of the increased risk of structural heart disease, an echocardiogram should be obtained. Because there is also an increased incidence of aneuploidy, especially trisomies 18 and 21, amniocentesis for karyotype analysis is recommended. The nature of this anomaly does not alter the indications for delivery, and vaginal delivery should be planned except when standard obstetric indications suggest cesarean delivery. Because the child will require immediate postnatal evaluation and treatment, delivery in a tertiary-care center with pediatric radiologists, surgeons, and dysmorphologists available is advisable. Because of the complex nature of this anomaly and the extensive nature of the reconstructive surgery, prenatal consultation with a pediatric surgeon is recommended.

▶ TREATMENT OF THE NEWBORN

The newborn with imperforate anus should be expeditiously evaluated to rule out serious potential associated malformations. Plain chest, abdominal, and pelvic radiographs should be obtained to exclude vertebral anomalies and assess the sacrum, which has a direct bearing on the prognosis in imperforate anus. An abdominal ultrasound examination should be obtained to evaluate the genitourinary tract and the level of the rectal pouch (Willital 1971).

Once the infant's respiratory status has been assessed, a nasogastric tube should be passed into the stomach to exclude the presence of esophageal atresia. The infant's perineum should be inspected to confirm imperforate anus, and look for signs of low imperforate anus or rectoperineal fistula (Fig. 65-2). The adequacy of the sphincter complex can be crudely evaluated by eliciting a reflex contraction by gently scraping the perineum with a swab.

The infant should receive nothing orally and should receive intravenous fluids until the evaluation is complete and a decision is made to proceed with perineal anoplasty in low lesions or colostomy for intermediate and high lesions. An echocardiogram should be obtained, as cardiovascular anomalies occur in 12 to 22% of infants with imperforate anus (Boocock and Donnai 1987; Greenwood et al. 1975; Templeton and Ditesheim 1985). Duodenal obstruction due to either atresia or to malrotation occurs in 1 to 2% of cases (Greenwood et al. 1975; Partridge and Gough 1961). Hirschsprung disease also occurs in association with imperforate anus (Kiesewetter et al. 1965; Wangensteen and Rice 1930).

A flat perineum with missing sacral segments on the pelvic radiograph and poor contraction following perineal scratch suggests a high imperforate anus. In males, passage of meconium via the urethra suggests an intermediate or high lesion. Meconium passing through a perineal fistula suggests a low imperforate anus. After 24 hours, air should have reached the distal rectum. A plain lateral radiograph can be obtained with the body prone and the hips raised, a modification of the so-called invertogram (Narasimharao et al. 1983). A gap of 1 cm or more between the rectum and

COLOR PLATE

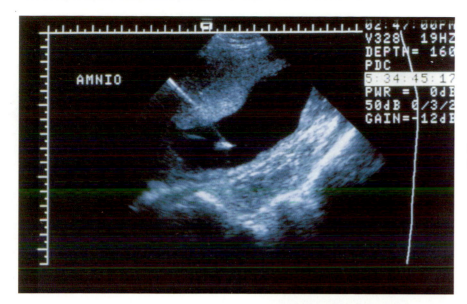

Figure 2-2. Ultrasound image of amniocentesis.

Figure 2-9. Ultrasound image of the same case shown in Figure 2-8, demonstrating the use of color Doppler to enhance visualization of the umbilical cord.

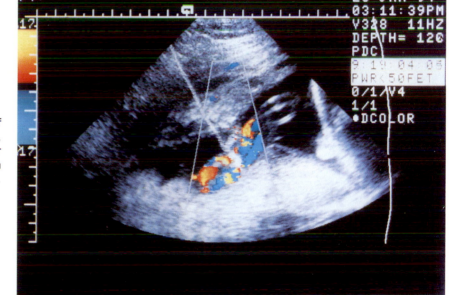

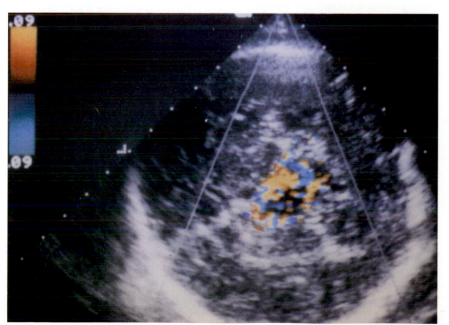

Figure 22-2. Doppler color flow studies demonstrating the presence of prominent convoluted vessels within the cystic lesion shown in Figure 22-1. *(Reprinted, with permission, from Doren M, Tercanli S, Holzgreve W. Prenatal sonographic diagnosis of a vein of Galen aneurysm: relevance of associated malformations for timing and mode of delivery. Ultrasound Obstet Gynecol 1995;6:287–289.)*

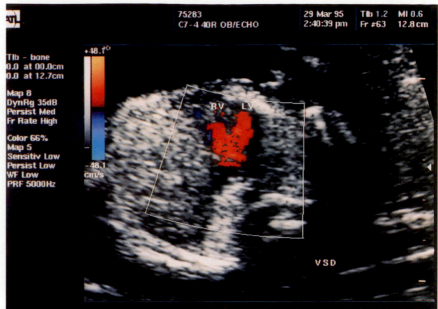

Figure 43-2. Color Doppler study in a fetus with AV canal defect, demonstrating turbulent flow and shunting within the heart. *(Photograph courtesy of Dr. Marjorie C. Treadwell.)*

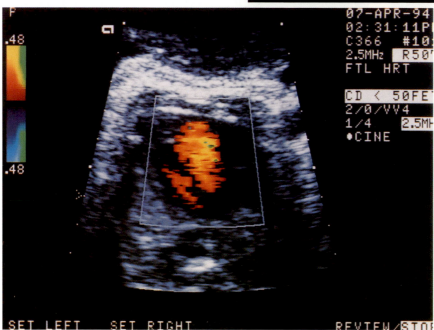

Figure 51-3. Doppler study from a fetus with hypoplastic left and right ventricles. Doppler studies are helpful in working through the differential diagnosis. *(Courtesy of Dr. Marjorie C. Treadwell.)*

Figure 57-1. Fetal cardiac image using color Doppler sonography, which clearly demonstrates flow across the ventriculoseptal defect.

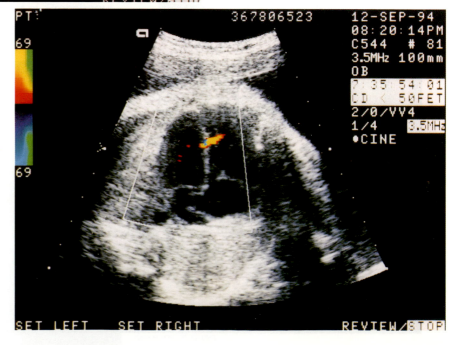

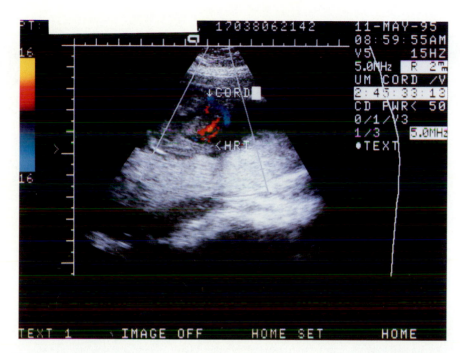

Figure 61-2. Color flow doppler image of a fetus with ectopia cordis. This fetus was found to have severe associated intra-cardiac abnormalities and subsequently died in utero.

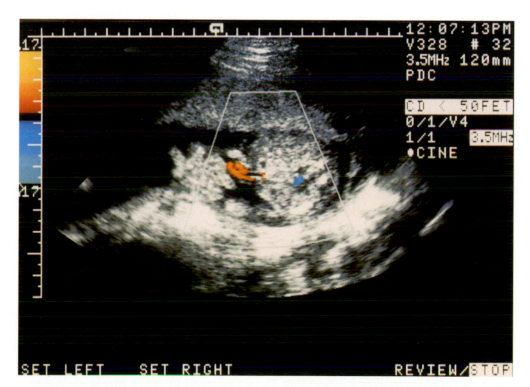

Figure 62-2. Color flow Doppler image in a fetus with gastroschisis, demonstrating a small defect with herniated midgut.

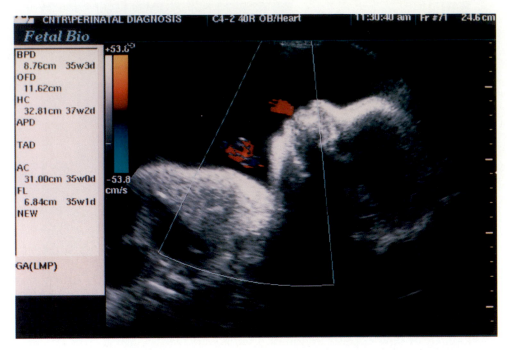

Figure 69-2. Color flow Doppler study demonstrating fetal vomiting in a case of duodenal atresia.

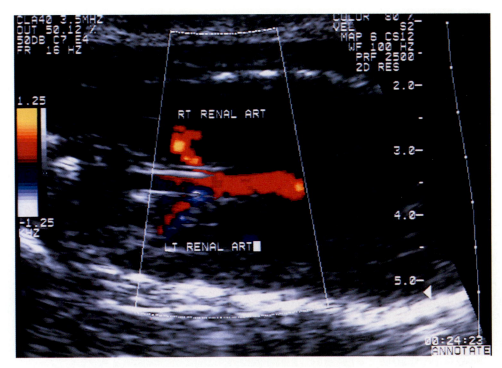

Figure 86-3. Color Doppler sonographic study demonstrating the presence of two normal renal arteries coming off the fetal aorta.

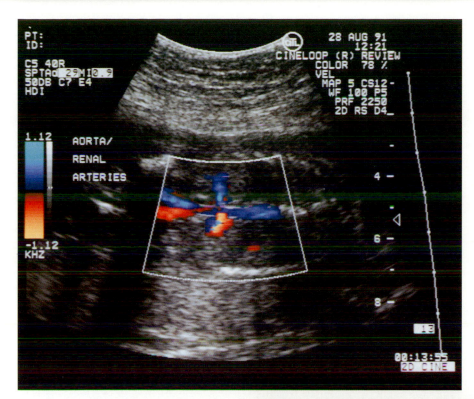

Figure 87-4. Color flow Doppler image demonstrating presence of two renal arteries. The demonstration of two normal renal arteries makes the diagnosis of sirenomelia unlikely.

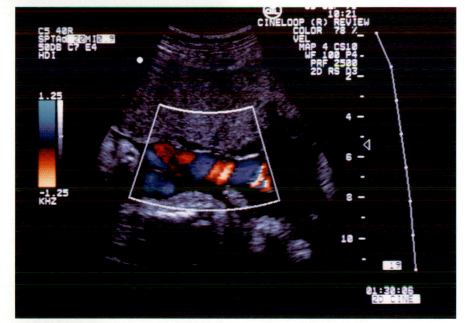

Figure 109-1. Color Doppler velocimetry studies showing the normal coiling of the umbilical cord.

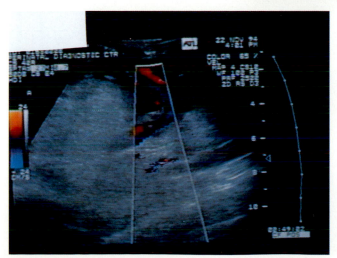

Figure 109-2. Color Doppler velocimetry studies demonstrating a straight umbilical cord. Note the lack of coiling as compared with Figure 109-1.

Figure 110-1. Color Doppler study demonstrating the presence of two umbilical arteries and one umbilical vein.

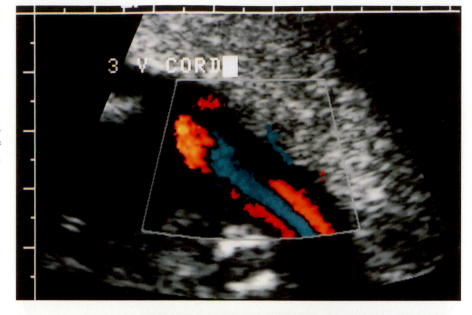

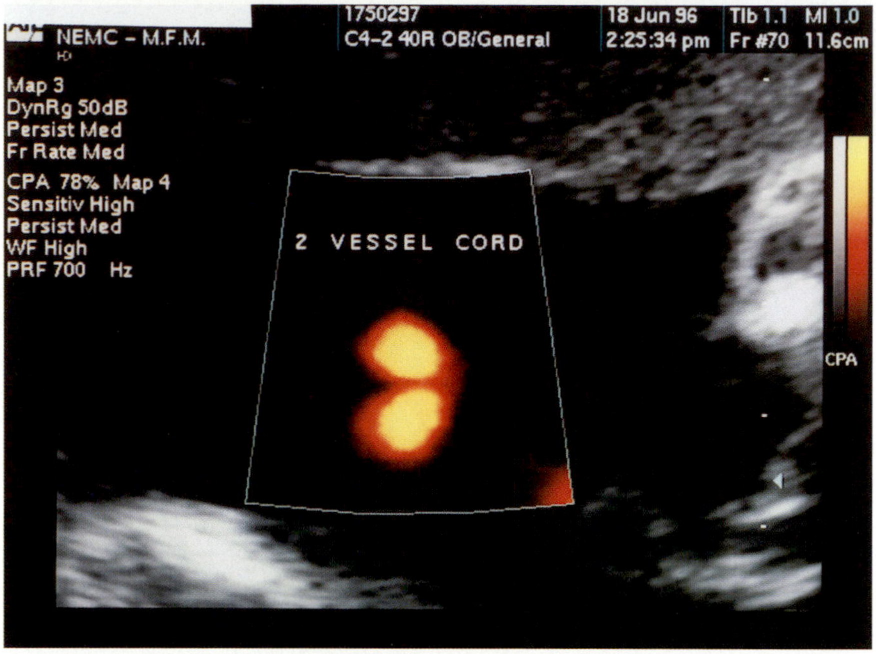

Figure 110-2. Cross-sectional view of the umbilical cord demonstrating the presence of two umbilical vessels.

Figure 110-3. Longitudinal view of the umbilical arteries at the bifurcation of the aorta, demonstrating the presence of a single umbilical artery. BL = bladder.

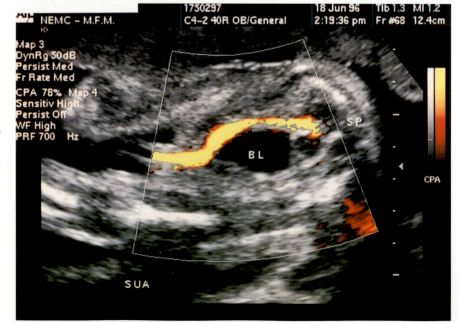

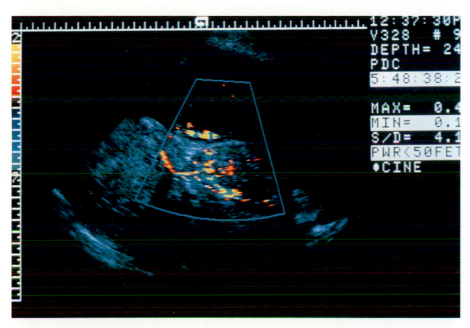

Figure 116-3. Color flow Doppler study of the same fetus shown in Figure 116-1 demonstrating the vascularity of the tumor.

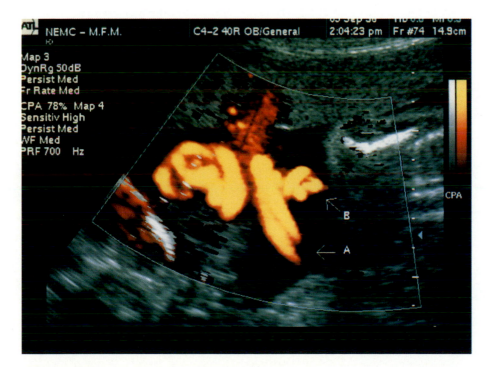

Figure 122-1. Power Doppler imaging of entangled umbilical cords in a case of monoamniotic twins.

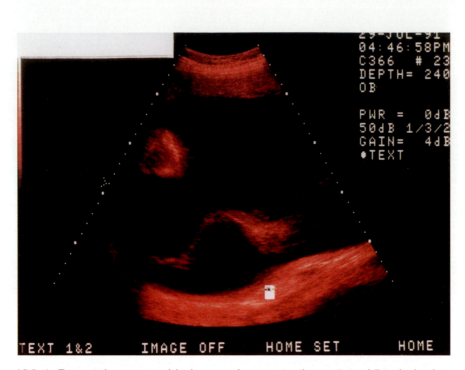

Figure 123-1. Prenatal sonographic image demonstrating a "stuck" twin in the upper left section of the image and the co-twin in a sac with polyhydramnios.

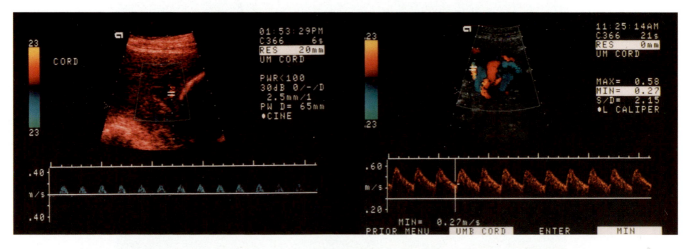

Figure 123-2. Composite ultrasound images demonstrating absent end diastolic flow in the umbilical artery of the donor stuck twin and normal flow velocity waveforms in the recipient fetus.

CHAPTER 66

Choledochal Cyst

► CONDITION

Choledochal cysts are rare congenital cystic dilations of the biliary tree first recognized by Vater in 1723. These cystic dilations of the biliary tract have been classified by the portion of the biliary tree affected. The most common form consists of fusiform dilation of the common bile duct (Fig. 66-1). Type I choledochal cyst accounts for 85 to 90% of all cases. All cases of choledochal cyst that have been diagnosed prenatally, to date, have been of the type I variety (Bancroft et al. 1994). The less common forms of choledochal cyst include: diverticulum of the common bile duct (Type II), which are intraduodenal or intrapancreatic; choledochocele (Type III); multiple extrahepatic cysts with or without intrahepatic cysts (Type IV); and Caroli's disease, which consists of single or multiple intrahepatic cysts associated with hepatic fibrosis and a normal extrahepatic biliary tree (type V) (Caroli et al. 1958).

The wall of a choledochal cyst is usually thickened with dense connective tissue interlaced with strands of smooth-muscle fibers associated with some inflammatory reaction (O'Neill et al. 1987). Normal biliary mucosal lining is absent, although sparse islands of columnar epithelium and microscopic bile ducts within the wall may be seen. In older patients, stones may be seen within the choledochal cyst or within intrahepatic ducts (Bhagat and Chaudhrey 1989; Landing 1974). Most newborns with choledochal cysts have complete biliary obstruction at the level of the duodenum, which has been likened to a form of biliary atresia (Landing 1974; Vergnes et al. 1990). Approximately 60% of choledochal cysts detected prenatally were found postnatally to have complete obstruction of the distal bile duct (Bancroft et al. 1994). Liver histology in infants with choledochal cysts is usually normal, but may show mild bile-duct proliferation consistent with chronic biliary obstruction (Hanai et al. 1967). Rare cases have been reported with coexistence of choledochal cysts and congenital hepatic fibrosis (Mall et al. 1974; Murray-Lyon et al. 1973, Orenstein and Whittington 1982; Ramirez et al. 1989; Yamaguchi 1980). Although malignancies, usually adenosquamous or small-cell carcinomas, have been reported in association with choledochal cysts, these lesions occur only after decades of chronic inflammation and recurrent cholangitis, and have not been reported in an infant or a child (Joseph 1980).

Theories regarding the cause of choledochal cyst disease have evolved from abnormalities in the early stages of embryonic development, to congenital weakness of the wall combined with distal obstruction, to the "common channel" hypothesis (O'Neill et al. 1987). Some authors have suggested that choledochal cysts result from embryologic abnormalities in the growth of hepatic diverticulum, and support their assertion by the frequently observed associated anomalies of duplications, gallbladder agenesis, and duodenal atresia (Barlow et al. 1976; Martin and Rowe 1979). Miyano et al. (1980) have emphasized that weakness of the choledochal wall results primarily from obstruction of the distal duct during fetal development. Spitz (1977) was able to produce cystic dilatation of the common bile duct in neonatal lambs by ligation of the distal common bile duct. In contrast, only dilatation of the gallbladder occurred in their adult controls. The cause of distal common-bile-duct obstruction in choledochal cyst has been variously suggested to be due to congenital stenosis, persistence of epithelial membrane, abnormal valves, or neuromuscular incoordination of the sphincter (Ito et al. 1984). Kusanoki et al. (1988) suggested that the obstruction may be due to aganglionosis of the distal bile duct, similar to Hirshsprung's disease of the colon.

Todani et al. (1977) noted that the majority of patients with choledochal cyst have an anomalous arrangement of the pancreatic or biliary duct system in which the pancreatic duct enters at an abnormal angle proximal

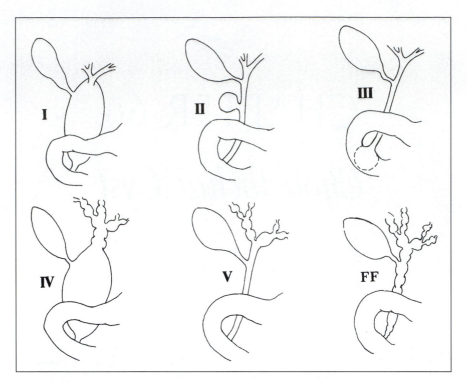

Figure 66-1. Classification scheme of choledochal cysts. Type I is the most common form, with cystic dilation of the extrahepatic bile ducts but normal intrahepatic ducts. Type II is a cystic diverticulum of the common bile duct. Type III is a diverticulum of the distal common bile duct, or choledochocele. Both Types II and III are rare. Type IV is the second most common form, with cystic dilation of both the extrahepatic and intrahepatic ducts. Type V, or Caroli's disease, has cystic dilation of the intrahepatic ducts but relatively normal extrahepatic ducts. In forme fruste (FF), the extrahepatic ducts are diseased but have only mild or negligible cystic dilation and the intrahepatic ducts have cystic dilation. *(Reprinted, with permission, from Ashcraft KW, Holder TM. Pediatric surgery. Philadelphia: Saunders, 1993:486.)*

to the circular muscle fibers of the ampulla of Vater (Giordani et al. 1984; Todani et al. 1977). They suggested this arrangement would permit reflux of pancreatic enzymes containing trypsin upward into the common bile duct, resulting in damage to the duct wall in utero (Oguchi et al. 1988).

Rustad and Lilly (1987) noted that the "long common channel" that results from an anomalous pancreaticobiliary junction is quite common and seen in up to 50% of patients with biliary disorders other than choledochal cyst. In addition, choledochal cyst has been diagnosed as early as 15 weeks of gestation, well before the development of pancreatic exocrine function (Schroeder et al. 1989). This raises doubts about the common-channel theory as the cause for choledochal cyst disease.

▶ INCIDENCE

Choledochal cyst is a rare congenital anomaly with an estimated occurrence of 1 case in every 2 million live births (Dewbury et al. 1980). It is more common in females in all ethnic groups, with a ratio of 2.5:1, which some have suggested may indicate it is a sex-linked defect (Alonzo-Lej et al. 1959; Kim 1981). Asian populations, particularly Chinese and Japanese, have a much higher incidence of choledochal cyst than any other race.

▶ SONOGRAPHIC FINDINGS

The characteristic sonographic finding in fetal choledochal cyst is a simple anechoic cyst in the upper abdomen in close proximity to the porta hepatis (Fig. 66-2). Rarely, the cyst can be imaged in continuity with the bifurcation of the right and left hepatic ducts or joined by the cystic duct from the gallbladder (Fig. 66-3). Elrad et al. (1985) were the first to describe finding dilated ducts leading into a cystic mass that was later confirmed to be a choledochal cyst (Frank et al. 1981). It may be difficult to distinguish a choledochal cyst from gallbladder duplication, duodenal atresia, mesenteric

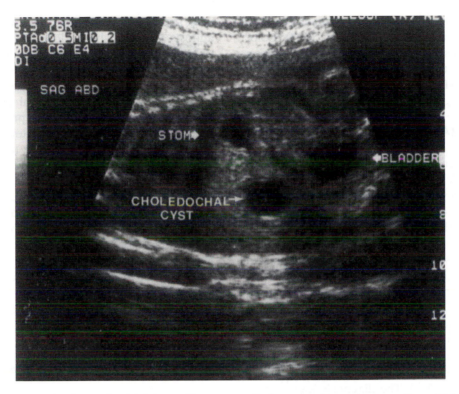

Figure 66-2. A 17-week-old fetus with an anechoic mass in porta hepatis, which postnatal evaluation confirmed to be a type I choledochal cyst. *(Reprinted, with permission, from Gallivan EK, Crombleholme TM, D'Alton ME, et al. Early prenatal diagnosis of choledochal cyst. Prenat Diagn 1996;16:934–937. Copyright John Wiley & Sons Limited. Reproduced with permission.)*

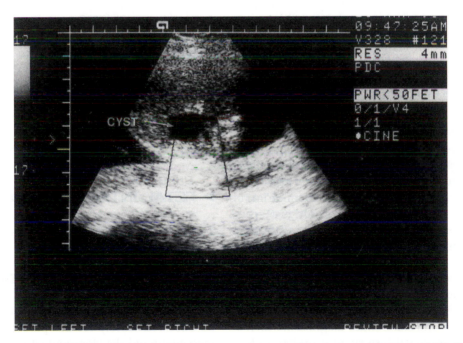

Figure 66-3. Color flow Doppler imaging in the same fetus shown in Figure 66-2 can be used to show the cyst's relationship to the hepatic artery and portal vein. *(Reprinted, with permission, from Gallivan EK, Crombleholme TM, D'Alton ME, et al. Early prenatal diagnosis of choledochal cyst. Prenat Diagn 1996;16:934–937. Copyright John Wiley & Sons Limited. Reproduced with permission.).*

more cases are identified, no estimate of their incidence can be made. Unlike cholelithiasis in children or adults, there is no apparent sex predominance for fetal cholelithiasis.

▶ SONOGRAPHIC FINDINGS

Fetal gallstones are seen as echogenic foci within the lumen of the gallbladder, with associated distal shadowing (Fig. 67-1). Brown et al. (1992) have also included echogenic foci within the gallbladder's lumen with either no associated distal shadowing or "comet-tail" or V-shaped artifact. However, echogenic foci without associated distal shadowing more likely represents biliary sludge due to calcium bilirubinate. It is important to distinguish intraluminal calcifications due to fetal gallstones from intrahepatic calcifications, calcified hemangiomas or hamartomas in the liver, or intraabdominal calcifications due to meconium peritonitis. The best sonographic confirmation is seeing the echogenic foci with associated distal shadowing clearly within the echolucent gallbladder lumen (see Fig. 67-1). Sepulveda et al. (1995) reported 8 cases of cholecystomegaly, in which 3 were found to have aneuploidy (2 trisomy 18, 1 trisomy 13). While they suggested that cholecystomegaly may be a sonographic marker of aneuploidy, Petrikovsky and Klein (1995) challenged this view. They suggested that the cholecystomegaly may have been due to gallstones or sludge and did not represent a new marker for aneuploidy.

▶ DIFFERENTIAL DIAGNOSIS

Several lesions associated with calcifications may be mistaken for gallstones. Calcifications may be seen in the fetal liver within hematomas, hemangiomas, or hamartomas. Calcifications may also be seen in the right upper quadrant as the result of meconium peritonitis, calcified adrenal cyst, hematoma, or neuroblastoma (see Chapters 74 and 114). Calcifications may occur within the lumen of the colon in cases of imperforate anus with rectourethral fistula as a result of urine reflux into rectal lumen (Miller et al. 1988). These calcifications may be seen proximally to the transverse colon. Hematomas and polyps within the wall of the gallbladder are echogenic but do not cause acoustic shadowing (Durrell et al. 1984).

▶ ANTENATAL NATURAL HISTORY

Although fewer than 35 cases of fetal gallstones have been reported, some aspects of the antenatal natural history have been established. The diagnosis of fetal gallstones has no adverse consequences for the pregnancy. It requires no alteration in the delivery plan and is not associated with fetal loss. Despite recognized associations with gallstones postnatally, few prenatally diagnosed cases have had risk factors for gallstones, with the exception of a single case of hereditary spherocytosis (Beretsky and Lonkin 1983; Brown et al. 1992). Similarly, predisposing factors, other than pregnancy,

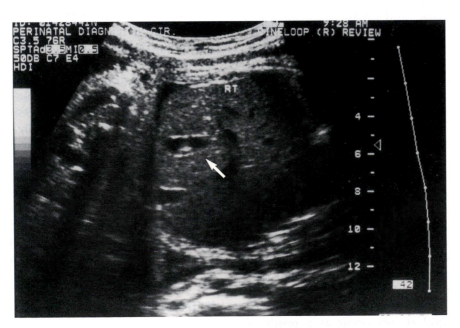

Figure 67-1. Ultrasound of a fetus at 24 weeks of gestation demonstrating dilated gallbladder and an echogenic gallstone with acoustic shadowing (arrow). *(Reprinted, with permission, from Robertson FM, Crombleholme TM, Paidis M, et al. Prenatal diagnosis and management of gastrointestinal anomalies. Semin Perinatol 1994;18:182–195.)*

were identified rarely in mothers, the most common maternal risk factor being a history of gallstones (Brown et al. 1992). In 1 case there had been placental abruption with placental hematoma and it was suggested that a possible pigment load might predispose to fetal gallstones (Brown et al. 1992).

Stasis of bile within the gallbladder has been shown to be a critical factor in the pathogenesis of gallstones of any type. Bile stasis is thought to be an important causative factor in gallstone formation during pregnancy (Braverman et al. 1980). It is possible that the hormonal influences predisposing to maternal bile stasis and gallstone formation may affect their fetuses similarly.

Estrogen is a recognized risk factor for gallstones and its levels are known to increase in pregnancy from 14 to 40 weeks (Beischer and Brown 1972). Estrogen is known to increase cholesterol secretion in bile and depress bile acid synthesis (Cotran et al. 1989). This progressive rise in estrogen levels during the later trimesters may account for fetal cholelithiasis being observed only in the third trimester.

Infants diagnosed prenatally with gallstones appear to have no clinical sequelae. If echogenic foci are associated with distal shadowing, 20% resolve postnatally, but 62% resolve if associated with comet-tail shadowing, and 75% resolve if associated with no distal shadowing (Brown et al. 1992). The remainder of infants with cholelithiasis appear to be asymptomatic. However, awareness of fetal cholelithiasis is important because symptoms referable to the biliary tract may be difficult to diagnose in infants and children. Only awareness of gallstones as a potential cause of symptoms will allow prompt recognition and treatment and minimal morbidity (Jacir et al. 1986).

▶ MANAGEMENT OF PREGNANCY

The diagnosis of fetal gallstones has no implications for the management of the pregnancy. A detailed history should be obtained for risk factors for maternal cholelithiasis. In addition, the mother should have an ultrasound examination to screen for the presence of gallstones.

▶ FETAL INTERVENTION

There are no fetal interventions for cholelithiasis.

▶ TREATMENT OF THE NEWBORN

The newborn with a prenatal diagnosis of fetal cholelithiasis should have a postnatal ultrasound examination performed during the newborn period. In healthy term infants, sonographic observation alone is indicated unless symptoms develop. The diagnosis of acute or chronic cholelithiasis may be difficult in an infant, but should be suspected with vomiting, irritability, or ileus. Gallstones associated with predisposing risk factors that are detected during the newborn period resolve spontaneously in 75% of cases with elimination of these risk factors—for example, by treatment with diuretics or total parenteral nutrition. It is unclear if gallstones with distal shadowing on an ultrasound examination performed in utero will spontaneously resolve during infancy. The only data on this come from Brown et al. (1992), who observed spontaneous resolution in 40% of cases of fetal gallstones when associated with acoustic shadowing. The higher rate of spontaneous resolution they observed when echogenic foci were present without acoustic shadowing may have been because they were "sludge" rather than true gallstones.

▶ SURGICAL TREATMENT

In asymptomatic infants diagnosed with fetal gallstones we currently recommend observation only. If gallstones are radiopaque, periodic plain radiographs may be obtained to observe for spontaneous resolution. If stones are radiolucent, sonographic surveillance is recommended. We have a low threshold for performing cholecystectomy, as symptoms of acute or chronic cholecystitis in infants are often vague and nonspecific, and once it is symptomatic, acute cholecystitis is associated with a high rate of complications (Brill et al. 1982).

In infants undergoing abdominal surgery for other indications, such as pyloric stenosis or intestinal atresia, we recommend a cholecystectomy, as it can be performed with little additional morbidity.

▶ LONG-TERM OUTCOME

The awareness of cholelithiasis in an infant leads to early intervention once symptoms referable to the gallbladder develop. Asymptomatic gallstones require no intervention. There are no long-term sequelae associated with a diagnosis of fetal cholelithiasis.

▶ GENETICS AND RECURRENCE RISK

There are no data on risk of recurrence of cholelithiasis in subsequent pregnancies. If maternal risk factors for cholelithiasis are present, such as a history of hemolytic anemia or of gallstones, a prenatal ultrasound examination during the third trimester is indicated to screen for an affected fetus. Hereditary spherocytosis is inherited as an autosomal dominant disorder. If the family

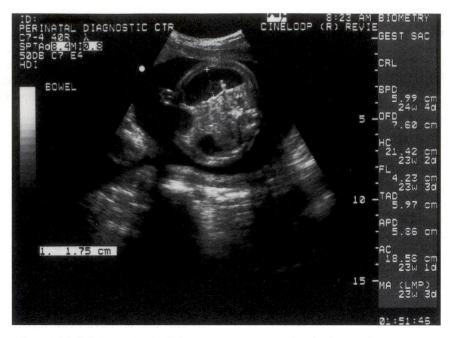

Figure 68-1. Fetal sonographic image demonstrating multiple dilated loops of intestine due to an isolated decending colonic atresia.

atresia may be extremely difficult to make with certainty. The sonographic image in colonic atresia is multiple dilated loops of bowel (Fig. 68-1). It may be difficult to distinguish dilated loops of small bowel from dilated loops of colon. Polyhydramnios is an un-usual finding in isolated colonic atresia and should raise suspicions about a more proximal intestinal obstruction. Perforation may occur proximal to the atresia, with resulting ascites and meconium peritonitis (Fig. 68-2).

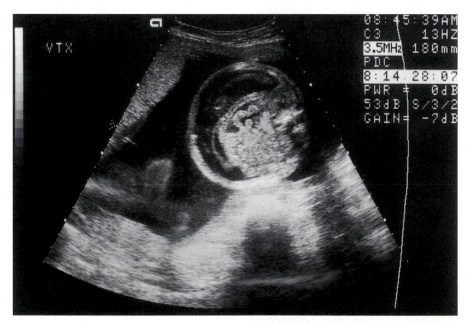

Figure 68-2. Sonographic examination of the same fetus in Figure 68-1 performed 2 weeks later, demonstrating decompression of the loops of intestine but with the new finding of fetal ascites. This was proven to be due to proximal perforation above the descending colonic atresia with secondary meconium peritonitis.

▶ DIFFERENTIAL DIAGNOSIS

The differential diagnosis of these sonographic findings includes anorectal atresia and Hirschsprung's disease (see Chapters 65 and 72).

▶ ANTENATAL NATURAL HISTORY

Half of colonic atresias occur proximal to the splenic flexure and half occur distal to it (Coran and Eraklis 1969). Atresia of the colon proximal to the splenic flexure is more likely to be associated with loss of proximal colon. Atresia distal to the splenic flexure is less likely to result in loss of bowel length. This difference appears to be related to the watershed nature of the blood supply to the colon at the splenic flexure. The atresias occurring in the colon vary from luminal webs to full mesenteric defects. The rarity of colonic atresia and the lack of prospective prenatally diagnosed cases of colonic atresia limits our understanding of its antenatal natural history. We do not believe that this diagnosis has any adverse implications for the pregnancy, and because associated anomalies are less frequent, the overall prognosis is excellent.

▶ MANAGEMENT OF PREGNANCY

Because of the potential for associated anomalies, when colonic atresia is suspected the fetus should undergo detailed sonographic examination with special attention to skeletal anomalies and the four-chamber view of the heart. If cardiac anatomy is poorly seen, fetal echocardiography should be performed. There is no indication for karyotype analysis in fetuses in which colonic atresia is suspected, except as indicated by maternal age or if seen in association with anomalies known to be associated with chromosomal abnormalities, such as omphalocele. Colonic atresia is not associated with prematurity, and this diagnosis has no implications for timing or mode of delivery. However, because of the need for radiographic evaluation and surgery during the immediate postnatal period, we recommend delivery in a tertiary-care center, with pediatric surgeons, pediatric radiologists, and neonatologists available.

▶ FETAL INTERVENTION

There are no fetal interventions for colonic atresia.

▶ TREATMENT OF THE NEWBORN

In the nursery, the infant with colonic atresia will show abdominal distention and either fail to pass meconium or pass only a small amount. Plain abdominal radiographs will demonstrate multiple loops of dilated bowel with air-fluid levels consistent with obstruction. A sump-style nasogastric tube should be passed for intestinal decompression and venous access obtained for volume resuscitation. Due to the distal location of the obstruction, fluid can be sequestered within more proximal loops of bowel. Antibiotics should be started and a pediatric surgical consultation obtained.

A plain radiograph of colonic atresia may be indistinguishable from a more proximal intestinal atresia or meconium ileus. Because of this differential diagnosis, a barium enema should be performed. In cases of meconium ileus, surgery may be avoided if Gastrografin enema is successful in relieving the obstruction. In colonic atresia, a microcolon is noted distal to the site of obstruction. Perforation of the microcolon has been reported during barium enema for colonic atresia (Sturim and Teinberg 1966).

▶ SURGICAL TREATMENT

In the past, survival was rare for cases of colonic atresia not diagnosed during the first 3 days of life. Most morbidity and mortality associated with colonic atresia occurs in unrecognized cases. Once a diagnosis has been made and the infant has been volume-resuscitated, surgery should be performed. The procedure is determined by the nature and location of the atresia and the physiologic status of the infant. Previously, a primary anastomosis was performed for right-sided atresias because newborns often did not tolerate ileostomy well. Conversely, because colostomy was well-tolerated in newborns, this was the preferred procedure in left-sided atresias. Currently, we favor resection, or tapering enteroplasty of the dilated proximal colon with primary anastomosis in colonic atresias of either the left or right colon. In infants who may be compromised by other factors, such as sepsis or severe respiratory distress, we perform a proximal colostomy or ileostomy with closure at a later date when the infant is more stable. Current means of nutritional support have diminished concerns about ileostomy in a newborn.

▶ LONG-TERM OUTCOME

Because of the rarity of isolated colonic atresia, most reported series are small and encompass several decades of observations. Experience with this unusual lesion, as well as marked improvements in supportive care, have improved survival, which currently is greater than 90% (Bowles et al. 1976; Powell and Raffensperger 1982). Deaths usually occur only as a result of associated congenital anomalies or a marked delay in the recognition of the colonic atresia (Philapart et al. 1986). In most historical reviews, deaths usually occurred prior to the 1970s because of preoperative colonic perforation. Delayed function of the distal colonic segment has been observed in several patients and occasionally required intravenous nutritional support. In such cases, a biopsy to detect the presence of ganglion cells is appropriate to exclude distal aganglionosis consistent with Hirschsprung's disease (Currie et al. 1983; Wolloch and Dintsman 1976). Occasionally, contrast enemas obtained in patients who have undergone surgery for correction of colonic atresia will demonstrate persistent tapering of the distal segment. In the absence of symptoms, this radiographic feature is of no concern.

▶ GENETICS AND RECURRENCE RISK

We are aware of one case report of a family in which congenital colonic atresia was present in two maternal half brothers and their maternal uncle (Benawra et al. 1981). The pattern of inheritance was consistent with autosomal dominance with reduced penetrance or was X-linked. A familial syndrome of pyloric atresia associated with small-bowel and colonic atresia has also been described (Guttman et al. 1973). In general, however, recurrence of colonic atresia is rare.

REFERENCES

Benawra R, Puppala BL, Mangurten HH, Booth C, Bassuk A. Familial occurrence of congenital colonic atresia. J Pediatr 1981;99:435–436.

Bowles ET, Vassy LE, Ralston M. Atresia of the colon. J Pediatr Surg 1976;11:69–75.

Coran AG, Eroklis AJ. Atresia of the colon. Surgery 1969;65: 828–831.

Currie ABM, Hemalatha AH, Doraiswomy NV, et al. Colonic atresia associated with Hirschsprung's disease. J R Coll Surg Edinb 1983;28: 31–34.

Gaub OC. Congenital stenosis and atresia of the intestinal tract above the rectum: with a report of an operated case of atresia of the sigmoid in an infant. Trans Am SA 1922; 40:582–590.

Guttman FM, Braun P, Garance PH, et al. Multiple atresias involving the gastrointestinal tract from the stomach to rectum. J Pediatr Surg 1973;8:633–640.

Jackman S, Brereton RJ. A lesson in intestinal atresias. J Pediatr Surg 1988;23:852–853.

Johnson JF, Dean BL. Hirschsprung's disease co-existing with colonic atresia. Pediatr Radiol 1981;11: 97–98.

Louw JH, Barnard CN. Congenital intestinal atresia: observations on its origin. Lancet 1955;2:1065–1068.

Philippart AI: Atresis, stenosis, and other obstructions of the colon. In: Welch KJ, Randolph JG, Rovitch MM, O'Neill Jr, JA, Rowe MI, eds. Pediatric surgery. 4th ed. Chicago: Year Book Medical Publishers 1986;984–985.

Potts WJ. Congenital atresia of the intestine and colon. Surg Gynecol Obstet 1947;85:14–18.

Powell RW, Raffensperger JG. Congenital colonic atresia. J Pediatr Surg 1982;17:166–170.

Rescorla FJ, Grosfeld JL. Intestinal atresia and stenosis: analysis of survival in 120 cases. Surgery 1985;98: 668–676.

Robertson FR, Crombleholme TM, Paidas M, et al. Prenatal diagnosis and management of gastrointestinal anomalies. Semin Perinatol 1994;18:196–214.

Sturim HS, Teinberg JL. Congenital atresia of the colon. Surgery 1966;59:458–464.

Touloukian RJ. Diagnosis and treatment of jejunoileal atresia. World J Surg 1993a;17:310–317.

Touloukian RJ. Intestinal atresia and stenosis. In: Ashcroft KW, Holder TM, eds. Pediatric surgery. 2nd ed. Philadelphia: Saunders 1993b:305–319.

Wolloch Y, Dintsman M. Colonic atresia associated with Hirschsprung's disease. Isr J Med Sci 1976;12:202–207.

CHAPTER 69

Duodenal Atresia

► CONDITION

Duodenal atresia, or stenosis, is a leading cause of intestinal obstruction in newborns and one of the most common gastrointestinal anomalies that can be diagnosed prenatally. At 1 month of gestation, the lumen of the duodenum is thought to be obliterated by proliferating epithelium. This solid core of epithelium undergoes vacuolization and recanalization, restoring the lumen. Failure of recanalization of the solid stage is thought to result in duodenal atresia or stenosis. Atresia is more common than stenosis and occurs in approximately 70% of cases (Bowden et al. 1967; Skandalakis et al. 1994). Skandalakis et al. (1994) have described 3 types of duodenal atresia. The most common duodenal anomaly (69% of cases) is membranous mucosal atresia (type I) with an intact muscular wall. The proximal duodenum is ballooned out while the duodenum distal to the atresia is narrowed. This mucosal membrane may take on the shape of a "wind sock" due to peristalsis and increased proximal intraluminal pressure (Rowe et al. 1968). The origin of the wind-sock membrane is usually intimately associated with the ampulla of Vater. A type II duodenal atresia is rare (2% of cases) and has a short fibrous cord connecting the two ends of the atretic duodenum. Type III duodenal atresia has a complete separation between the two ends of the duodenum and can be associated with biliary-tract anomalies in 6% of cases (Knechtle and Filston 1990; Jona and Berlin et al. 1976; Reid 1973a and b). Duodenal stenosis accounts for the remaining 23% of cases. These anatomic relations are rarely evident sonographically. An annular pancreas occurs in 20 to 30% of patients with duodenal atresia or stenosis (Fonkalsrud et al. 1969; Reid 1973a and b; Wesley et al. 1977). The developmental relationship between annular pancreas and duodenal atresia and stenosis is unclear.

An annular pancreas can produce extrinsic compression and result in stenosis, but it is more commonly associated with an intrinsic obstruction due to complete atresia (Merrill and Raffensperger 1976).

► INCIDENCE

Duodenal stenosis or atresia occurs in approximately 1 in 10,000 live births (Fonkalsrud et al. 1969). In most cases the condition is sporadic, although Fonkalsrud has described an autosomal dominant pattern of inheritance (Fonkalsrud 1979).

► SONOGRAPHIC FINDINGS

Prenatal sonographic diagnosis of duodenal obstruction has been made as early as 20 weeks of gestation (Hancock and Wiseman 1989). The majority of cases, however, are not diagnosed until the third trimester. The most common indication for sonography is uterine size greater than dates due to polyhydramnios, which is present in up to 53% of cases (Farrant et al. 1981; Girvan and Stephens 1974). Prenatal sonography may show the characteristic "double bubble" sign (Fig. 69-1) that represents the dilated fluid-filled stomach and proximal duodenum (Balcar et al. 1984; Langer et al. 1989). Although occasionally seen earlier, duodenal atresia is not usually diagnosed prior to 24 weeks of gestation. If the fetus has recently vomited (Fig. 69-2), or in cases of stenosis in which sufficient amounts of amniotic fluid pass the obstruction, these features may be subtle or absent (Bowie and Clair 1982). If the diagnosis of duodenal atresia or stenosis is suspected, serial ultrasound examination may be required to prove the diagnosis. Because 30% of patients with duodenal atresia will have

in infants with type III defects. Adeyemi (1988) has identified an association between duodenal atresia, partial situs inversus, and right-sided diaphragmatic hernia through the foramen of Bochdalek. This is an extremely rare condition known as multiple organ malrotation syndrome (MOMS) (Adeyemi 1988).

▶ MANAGEMENT OF PREGNANCY

If duodenal atresia is suspected, the fetus should undergo genetic amniocentesis, because of the high incidence of associated chromosomal anomalies. Fetal echocardiography should also be performed to evaluate possible associated congenital heart anomalies, even in the presence of a normal karyotype. Early detection of associated anomalies may influence decisions regarding continuation of the pregnancy. Although of uncertain clinical value, amniotic fluid bile acid concentration has been found to be markedly elevated in intestinal obstruction (Deleze et al. 1977). Abnormal bile acid concentration has been described in 2 patients with polyhydramnios, 1 whose baby had duodenal atresia and the other ileal atresia. While the amniotic fluid bilirubin and amylase concentrations were normal, the bile acid concentrations were 30.3 and 83.1 μmol per liter (normal, 1.2 to 2.4 μmol per liter) respectively (Deleze et al. 1977). Studies of experimentally created intestinal obstruction showed no differences in amniotic fluid values of bilirubin, amylase, or lipase from controls (Toulakian 1977).

Duodenal atresia is complicated by polyhydramnios in 17 to 53% of cases (Farrant et al. 1981; Girvan and Stephens 1974; Hancock and Wiseman 1989). Polyhydramnios can contribute to the development of preterm labor. Forty-three percent of affected infants are premature and may be small for gestational age (Jolleys 1981). We recommend a prenatal pediatric surgical consultation with parents to help alleviate anxiety and to provide answers to questions concerning postnatal intervention. Delivery should be planned in a center with appropriate neonatal and pediatric surgical support.

▶ FETAL INTERVENTION

There are no fetal interventions for duodenal atresia.

▶ TREATMENT OF THE NEWBORN

In the delivery room, the newborn with duodenal atresia should have immediate nasogastric decompression to prevent aspiration of gastric contents and gastric perforation. The gastric aspirate will usually be bile-stained, since 85% of cases of duodenal obstruction are distal

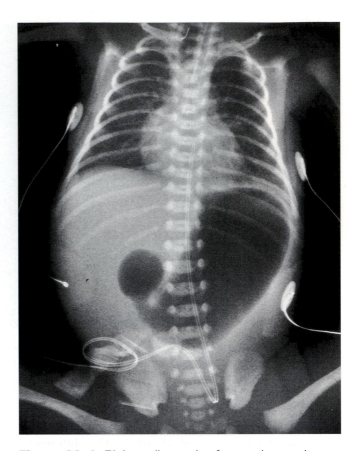

Figure 69-4. Plain radiograph of a newborn, showing dilated stomach and proximal duodenum with lack of air distal to the obstruction.

to the entry of the bile ducts. Failure to decompress the stomach will result in bilious vomiting shortly after birth. Intravascular fluid deficit should be corrected with intravenous fluid administration. Nasogastric fluids should be replaced volume for volume, and attention should be paid to electrolyte and acid–base abnormalities induced by large proximal gastrointestinal fluid losses. Abdominal radiography will verify tube placement and confirm the diagnosis in cases of duodenal atresia. The classic double bubble sign is seen with absence of gas in the rest of the bowel (Fig. 69-4). In cases of duodenal stenosis, the high-grade partial obstruction may allow gas to pass into the small bowel, and the clinical presentation may be indistinguishable from that of bowel rotation with midgut volvulus or high jejunal obstruction. In such cases, or whenever there is doubt about the diagnosis, an emergency radiographic contrast study should be performed to exclude malrotation with midgut volvulus (Fig. 69-5).

▶ SURGICAL TREATMENT

The surgical reconstruction is usually performed on the day of delivery after the infant is assessed for the

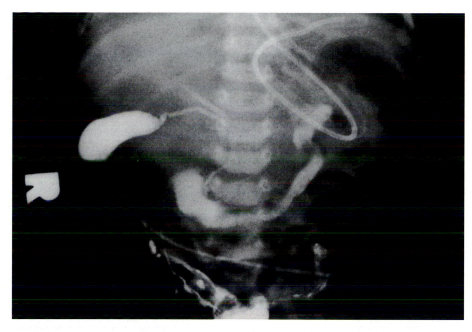

Figure 69-5. Upper gastrointestinal contrast study demonstrating displaced but patent duodenal sweep due to a large duodenal duplication. *(Reprinted, with permission, from Malone F, Crombleholme TM, Nores J, et al. Pitfalls of the "double bubble" sign: a case of congenital duodenal duplication. Fetal Diagn Ther 1997;12:298–300.)*

presence or absence of associated anomalies and appropriate volume resuscitation and correction of electrolyte disturbances has occurred. The most common site of obstruction in both duodenal atresia and stenosis is in the second portion of the duodenum adjacent to the ampulla of Vater. In duodenal atresia, there is usually an intrinsic web causing the obstruction. Although some have advocated excision of this web, risk of injury to the ampulla of Vater has prompted most surgeons to bypass this obstruction. This is most commonly done by either a duodenoduodenostomy or a duodenojejunostomy. In cases of stenosis, one must be certain to exclude the presence of a wind-sock deformity. Once the proximal duodenum is opened, a Foley catheter can be passed distally, and the inflated balloon can then be withdrawn. In a wind-sock deformity, the membrane can be delivered and safely excised. In 1 to 3% of cases, a second more distal obstruction by an intrinsic web may be detected by this technique. In cases of gross dilatation of the proximal duodenum, it should be tapered or imbricated to prevent stasis, bacterial overgrowth, and complications of blind-loop syndrome (Grosfeld et al. 1993). Because of the risk of late blind-loop syndrome, we avoid duodenojejunostomy. In most instances, we employ a transverse proximal duodenum to longitudinal distal duodenal, or diamond-shaped anastomosis (Kimura 1977; Kimura et al. 1990) (Fig. 69-5). We perform a proximal imbricating duodenal enteroplasty to prevent late complications of megaduodenum (Table 69-2). Because of chronic in utero ob-

struction, transient proximal dysmotility prevents initiation of normal feeding for 10 to 14 days postoperatively. A transanastomotic nasojejunal feeding tube is passed that allows enteral alimentation until proximal gastroduodenal motility returns. Breast milk can be used often, supplemented by formula as needed.

During the past 25 years, there has been steady improvement in the survival of babies with duodenal atresia, from 68% in 1968 to 95% in 1991 (Fonkalsrud et al. 1969; Hancock and Wiseman 1989; Stauffer and Schwoebel 1998). The majority of deaths today occur in infants with associated complex congenital heart defects (Hancock and Wiseman 1989). The improvement in survival, although certainly due in part to advances in neonatal, anesthetic, and surgical care, may also reflect prenatal selection. While often diagnosed after 24 weeks of gestation, duodenal atresia is increasingly

▶ **TABLE 69-2.** LATE COMPLICATIONS OF DUODENAL ATRESIA AND STENOSIS

Megaduodenum
Dysmotility
Duodenogastric reflux
Gastritis
Peptic ulcer
Gastroesophageal reflux
Choledochal cyst
Cholelithiasis
Cholecystitis

CHAPTER 71
Hepatic Calcifications

▶ CONDITION

Fetal hepatic calcifications can be divided into three main categories: peritoneal, parenchymal, and vascular. Peritoneal hepatic calcifications present as calcified masses on the surface of the fetal liver. Most commonly, this is due to meconium peritonitis resulting from in utero bowel rupture. Meconium peritonitis is the most common cause of fetal abdominal calcifications (Lince et al. 1985) (see Chapter 74). Parenchymal calcifications are due to the presence of intrauterine infection or tumor. Fetal tumors may be primary in the liver or metastatic, presenting as a complex mass with areas of increased echogenicity and possible shadowing. Fetal tumors encompass both benign and malignant varieties, including hemangioendotheliomas, hamartomas, and hepatoblastomas. Parenchymal calcifications appear as scattered nodules, with additional evidence of other affected organs. The most common in utero infections that can cause fetal calcifications include varicella and the TORCH agents (Fig. 71-1). Finally,

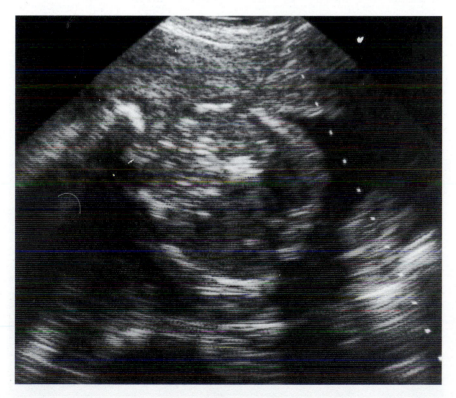

Figure 71-1. Transverse scan through abdomen of a fetus with varicella infection demonstrating multiple areas of intraparenchymal calcification. *(Reprinted, with permission, from Drose JA, Dennis MA, Thickman D. Infection in utero: US findings in 19 cases. Radiology 1991;178:369–374.)*

hepatic calcifications due to vascular abnormalities result from calcified portal or hepatic venous clots, which are due to hypoperfusion or thromboembolism (Bronshtein and Blazer 1995; Nguyen and Leonard 1986).

▶ INCIDENCE

With the increased utilization of prenatal sonographic screening, fetal hepatic calcifications are detected prenatally more frequently than they are observed in newborn infants. In 1 study, evidence of hepatic calcifications was noted in 14 of 24,600 fetuses, an incidence of 1 in 0.05% of screened fetuses (Bronshtein and Blazer 1995). In a population of 1500 spontaneously aborted fetuses, 33 were demonstrated to have hepatic calcification, an incidence of 2.2% in this abnormal patient population (Hawass et al. 1990). In the 33 affected fetuses, 17 hepatic calcifications were demonstrated in the first trimester and 16 in the second trimester.

▶ SONOGRAPHIC FINDINGS

Fetal hepatic calcifications can be detected by the beginning of the second trimester of pregnancy (Fig. 71-2). Bronshtein and Blazer (1995) reported their 8-year experience in extensive targeted sonographic screening for fetal abnormalities in 24,600 consecutive pregnancies, which included hepatic calcifications. Of these, 19,700 were studied by vaginal sonography between 14 and 16 weeks of gestation, and 4900 were studied by transabdominal sonography between 18 and 26 weeks of gestation. Hepatic calcification was identified in 14 fetuses; of these, 12 had one or two areas of focal calcifications. One fetus had evidence of 4 different foci of calcifications. In 1 fetus, there were diffuse hepatic, peritoneal, and intestinal calcifications. The diagnosis of fetal hepatic calcification was made in these fetuses between 15 and 26 weeks of gestation. No correlation was seen between the number or location of calcifications and the occurrence of malformations or eventual outcome for the child. Of the 14 affected fetuses, 13 had persistent hepatic calcifications noted on serial sonographic scans. In 1 case initially diagnosed at 15 weeks of gestation, calcifications resolved by 24 weeks. 4 fetuses had associated anomalies, which included 2 cases of trisomy 18, 1 case of dwarfism and hydronephrosis, and 1 case of polyhydramnios and bowel calcifications. This last fetus died in utero at 32 weeks of gestation and no autopsy was performed. Of the remaining 10 fetuses, all were normal at birth with no sequelae of the calcifications. In a more recent study, Koopman and Wladimiroff (1998) reported their experience with 7 fetuses with intrahepatic hyperechogenic foci. 1 case of trisomy 18 was identified. Another case had associated encephalocele and unilateral renal agenesis. Outcome was normal in 5 fetuses with isolated intrahepatic findings.

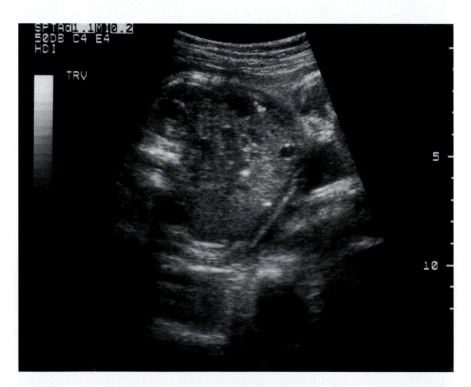

Figure 71-2. Transverse abdominal scan showing fewer, more punctate, areas of intraparenchymal calcifications. This is the more commonly seen fetal presentation.

▶ DIFFERENTIAL DIAGNOSIS

The differential diagnosis of hepatic calcifications due to peritoneal problems includes meconium peritonitis (see Chapter 74) and ruptured hydrometrocolpos. The differential diagnosis of parenchymal calcifications includes infectious causes, specifically herpes simplex virus type II, varicella–zoster (Taylor et al. 1993), rubella, cytomegalovirus, echovirus 11, syphilis (Kogutt 1991), and toxoplasmosis (Shackelford and Kirks 1977). The primary tumors likely to cause parenchymal fetal calcification include hemangioma, hemangioendothelioma, hamartoma, teratoma, and hepatoblastoma. Mestastatic neuroblastoma also can cause fetal hepatic calcifications (Friedman et al. 1981). Intrahepatic vascular calcification can be due to portal venous thromboemboli (Blanc et al. 1967; Friedman et al. 1981), hepatic venous thrombi, ischemic necrosis secondary to vascular insufficiency, and subcapsular hematomas, which can be due to hydrops or fetal chromosomal abnormalities (Buxton et al. 1991). Fetal hepatic calcifications have been described in a set of monozygotic twins, most likely due to a thrombotic event (Richards et al. 1988). Fetal hepatic calcifications have been postulated to be a secondary effect of cordocentesis in a fetus with trisomy 9 (Satge et al. 1994). It is hypothesized that the calcifications are due to placentofetal embolization from chorionic vein thrombi or intravascular clotting caused by maternal release of thromboplastin. Both of these events are more common in aneuploid fetuses.

▶ ANTENATAL NATURAL HISTORY

In what is admittedly a biased study, Hawass et al. (1990) detected hepatic calcifications in 33 of 1500 products of conception that were spontaneously miscarried. Of the 33 cases, calcified hepatic venous thrombi were demonstrated in 18. In 12 cases, calcified portal venous thrombi were documented. In only 2 of the cases were parenchymal calcifications documented, and 1 case showed mixed findings. In this patient population, 85% of fetuses had associated anomalies. The most common finding was intraluminal meconium calcifications (seen in 27% of fetuses), cystic hygroma (seen in 18% of fetuses), and bony metaphyseal defects (seen in 18% of fetuses) (Hawass et al. 1990). It is unclear whether severe fetal illness or hypoperfusion predisposed the fetus to calcification of the hepatic or portal veins. Since this population spontaneously miscarried, these findings cannot be generalized to a population of pregnant women with continuing pregnancies. Because the 3 affected fetuses with associated anomalies in Bronshtein and Blazer's study (1995) were terminated, no information is available about the antenatal natural history for those conditions. One of the 14 fetuses with calcifications did spontaneously miscarry, but no autopsy

was performed. The remaining 10 fetuses were normal and had no abnormalities in the natural history.

▶ MANAGEMENT OF PREGNANCY

Recommendations for follow-up of fetal hepatic calcifications include a targeted sonographic examination to look for associated anomalies. Bronshtein and Blazer (1995) recommend serial sonographic studies, even though the fetal hepatic calcifications persisted in 13 of their 14 affected cases. Thus, their recommendations for serial sonographic studies is unclear, because their data seem to indicate that once the calcifications are demonstrated, they persist throughout the pregnancy. For fetuses identified with hepatic calcifications, an amniocentesis should be performed for fetal karyotyping as well as obtaining amniotic fluid for cytomegalovirus culture. In addition, maternal serologic samples should be obtained for infection with toxoplasmosis, rubella, cytomegalovirus, and herpes. It is important to document cytomegalovirus because if it is present, the risk of preterm delivery is increased, and the fetus is at risk for hearing damage and developmental abnormalities (Watt-Morse et al. 1995). If the fetal karyotype is normal, serology is negative, and cytomegalovirus culture is negative, the overall prognosis for the fetus is excellent (Bronshtein and Blazer 1995).

However, if fetal hepatic calcifications are associated with an intrahepatic mass, an effort should be made to determine the underlying cause, because the presence of a hepatic tumor has potentially adverse implications for outcome of pregnancy. If multiple areas of intraparenchymal calcification are demonstrated, the adrenal glands and sympathetic chain should be examined sonographically to rule out primary neuroblastoma (see Chapter 114). The recommended site and route of delivery depends on the underlying cause of the calcifications. If the antenatal workup has been completely within normal limits, delivery can take place in the community hospital. If, however, other abnormalities have been detected and prolonged postnatal workup requiring pediatric specialists is anticipated, the delivery should occur in a tertiary-care center to keep the mother and baby together.

▶ FETAL INTERVENTION

There are no fetal interventions for hepatic calfications.

▶ TREATMENT OF THE NEWBORN

In the newborn, an infectious cause for hepatic calcifications should be documented in the absence of relevant prenatal studies. For example, if amniotic fluid was not cultured for cytomegalovirus, a urine culture for cytomegalovirus should be obtained during the newborn period. Similarly, cultures for newborn TORCH titers should be sent. A complete and detailed physical examination to rule out features suggestive of genetic or chromosomal abnormalities is indicated. If antenatally the calcifications were suspected to be due to meconium peritonitis, consideration should be given to obtaining a plain abdominal film to follow postnatal passage of air throughout the bowel and to rule out intestinal perforation. Consideration should be given to performing abdominal sonography on the newborn infant to determine if the calcifications are still present after birth. If the calcifications are parenchymal, suggesting the presence of tumor, postnatal imaging studies may include abdominal computed tomographic (CT) scanning or magnetic resonance imaging (MRI). If the pattern of calcifications appear to suggest a vascular accident in utero, consideration should be given to obtaining liver-function tests in the infant.

▶ LONG-TERM OUTCOME

Determining long-term prognosis requires knowledge of the location and configuration of calcifications plus the presence or absence of other lesions or anomalies (Nguyen and Leonard 1986). The long-term outcome will be related to the underlying cause, if determined, of the hepatic calcifications. Bronshtein and Blazer's 1995 study provided reassuring information that of the 10 fetuses with negative cultures, normal karyotype, and absence of additional sonographic abnormalities all were confirmed as normal at birth. The gestational age at delivery for these infants was between 37 and 41 weeks, and all were appropriately developed for gestational age. At 4 months to 4.5 years of postnatal life, all of these children were healthy and thriving. Because of this information, parents who have undergone full prenatal testing with completely normal results can, in general, be reassured that the outcome for their fetuses will be good.

▶ GENETICS AND RECURRENCE RISK

The only genetic conditions that have been reported in association with fetal hepatic calcifications are trisomies 9 and 18. We have observed 2 cases of trisomy 21 with hepatic calcifications. The recurrence risk associated with these conditions is the maternal age–related risk, or 1%, depending on which of these is the greater number.

▶ REFERENCES

Blanc WA, Berdon WE, Baker DH, Wigger HJ. Calcified portal vein thromboemboli in newborn and stillborn infants. Radiology 1967;88:287–292.

Bronshtein M, Blazer S. Prenatal diagnosis of liver calcifications. Obstet Gynecol 1995;86:739–743.

Buxton PJ, Maheswaran P, Dewbury KC, Moore IE. Neonatal hepatic calcification in subcapsular haematoma with hydrops fetalis. Br J Radiol 1991;64:1058–1060.

Drose JA, Dennis MA, Thickman D. Infection in utero: US findings in 19 cases. Radiology 1991;178:369–374.

Friedman AP, Haller JO, Boyer B, Cooper R. Calcified portal vein thromboemboli in infants: radiography and ultrasonography. Radiology 1981;140:381–382.

Hawass ND, El Badawi MG, Fantani JA, Al-Meshari A, Makanjoula D, Edress YB. Foetal hepatic calcification. Pediatr Radiol 1990;20:528–535.

Kogutt MS. Hepatic calcifications presumably due to congenital syphilis. AJR Am J Roentgenol 1991;156:634–635.

Koopman E, Wladimiroff JW. Fetal intrahepatic hyperechogenic foci: prenatal ultrasound diagnosis and outcome. Prenat Diagn 1998;18:339–342.

Lince DM, Pretorius DH, Manco-Johnson ML, Manchester D, Clewell WH. The clinical significance of increased echogenicity in the fetal abdomen. AJR Am J Roentgenol 1985;145:683–686.

Nguyen DL, Leonard JC. Ischemic hepatic necrosis: a cause of fetal liver calcification. AJR Am J Roentgenol 1986;147:596–597.

Richards DS, Cruz AC, Dowdy KA. Prenatal diagnosis of fetal liver calcifications. J Ultrasound Med 1988;7:691–694.

Satge D, Gasser B, Geneix A, Malet P, Stoll C. Hepatic calcifications in a fetus with trisomy 9 that underwent cordocentesis. Prenat Diagn 1994;14:303–306.

Shackelford GD, Kirks DR. Neonatal hepatic calcification secondary to transplacental infection. Radiology 1977;122:753–757.

Taylor WG, Walkinshaw SA, Thomson MA. Antenatal assessment of neurological impairment. Arch Dis Child 1993;68:604–605.

Watt-Morse ML, Laifer SA, Hill LM. The natural history of fetal cytomegalovirus infection as assessed by serial ultrasound and fetal blood sampling: a case report. Prenat Diagn 1995;15:567–570.

CHAPTER 72

Hirschsprung's Disease

► CONDITION

Hirschsprung's disease is one of the most common causes of intestinal obstruction in newborns (Kleinhaus and Boley 1993). It usually presents as a low intestinal obstruction without sepsis. In the least severe cases, delayed passage of meconium may be the only abnormality (Potter 1989). In more severe cases, the neonate presents with abdominal distention and bilious or feculent vomiting, in addition to failure to pass meconium. In its most serious form, infants present with overwhelming sepsis due to enterocolitis; a smaller number will present with peritonitis from perforation of a normal intestine proximal to the aganglionic segment. The age at diagnosis varies considerably, but half of the cases are diagnosed during the newborn period, 75% within 3 months and 80% within the first year of life (Ikeda and Goto 1984; Rowe et al. 1995).

Hirschsprung's disease is characterized by severe constipation due to functional colonic obstruction with megacolon. The condition bears the name of Harold Hirschsprung, who in 1888 described the autopsy findings of two infants who died with congenital megacolon. While at least 12 cases had been reported prior to 1888, Hirschsprung's complete description of the clinical and postmortem findings resulted in his name becoming attached to the condition. Hirschsprung focused his attention on the dilated hypertrophied megacolon, but the underlying abnormality was not determined until 1920, when Dalla Valle reported the absence of ganglion cells in Auerbach plexus in the nondilated transition zone. The absence of ganglion cells in the distal nondilated segment involves Auerbach plexus (myenteric), Henle plexus (deep submucosal), and Meissner plexus (submucosal) (Skandalakis and Gray 1994). The dilated proximal segment of colon ends in a funnel-shaped transition zone, which tapers into the narrowed,

patent, but functionally obstructed distal segment. This distal segment is usually normal in caliber and appears narrow only compared to the proximal megacolon (Fig. 72-1). The peristalsis of the proximal normal colon tends to dilate the proximal aganglionic segment, and so the transition zone is part of the aganglionic segment.

The abnormal innervation in Hirschsprung's disease always extends proximally from the anus, including the internal sphincter (Puri 1996). Histologically,

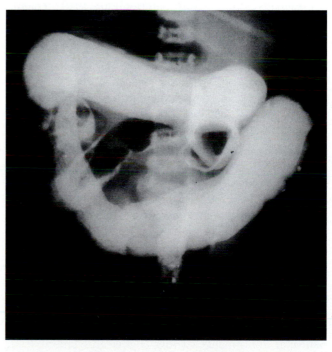

Figure 72-1. Barium enema radiograph from an infant with Hirschsprung's disease. The dilated proximal bowel is the segment of bowel with normal ganglion cells. Note the narrow rectum and wide sigmoid. *(Courtesy of Dr. R. S. McCauley.)*

in the absence of ganglion cells there are hypertrophied parasympathetic nerve bundles in the submucosa and between the muscular layers of the bowel. The parasympathetic (cholinergic) and sympathetic (adrenergic) nervous systems innervate the normal colon. The parasympathetic system is excitatory to the colon and inhibits the internal sphincter. Conversely, the sympathetic nervous system inhibits the colon and excites the internal sphincter. In addition, the colon normally receives intrinsic innervation via purinergic, serotonergic, and peptidergic systems (Nirasawa et al. 1986). Ganglion cells receive impulses from both cholinergic fibers and intrinsic nonadrenergic inhibitory fibers. In Hirschsprung's disease the extrinsic innervation is present with increased cholinergic and adrenergic fibers, but the intrinsic innervation is absent (no purinergic, serotonergic, or peptidergic fibers). In Hirschsprung's disease the wave of relaxation that normally precedes each propulsive peristaltic wave does not occur. In addition, the normal reflex relaxation of the internal sphincter following rectal distention does not occur.

The ganglion cells coordinate intrinsic and extrinsic impulses, and in their absence a functional obstruction results. Absence of the intrinsic nervous system is the underlying neurophysiologic abnormality in Hirschsprung's disease.

During embryonic life, neurenteric ganglion cells migrate from the neural crest to the upper end of the alimentary tract and then follow vagal fibers caudad (Dereymaeker 1943; Van Campenhout 1946; Yntema and Hammond 1947). Ganglion cells can be seen in the proximal small bowel by 7 weeks of gestation, and the rectum by 12 weeks of gestation (Okamoto and Ueda 1967). Why ganglionic migration stops is unknown. It is not due to failure of vagal fibers to innervate the bowel. Postganglionic fibers from normal ganglia proximal to affected segments and preganglionic parasympathetic vagal fibers that fail to connect with ganglion cells continue to elongate (Bodian et al. 1951; Kamijo et al. 1953; Nixon 1964).

Megacolon is not always due to Hirschsprung's disease. It is now recognized that several anomalies of the myenteric plexus may produce a similar clinical presentation to Hirschsprung's disease, including neuronal loss, abnormal nerves, and intestinal neuronal dysplasia (Puri and Wester 1998; Scharli and Sossai 1998). Several reports have appeared describing a clinical presentation that is indistinguishable from Hirschsprung's disease in which ganglia were present but there was either hypoganglionosis, immature ganglia, or other neuronal abnormalities (Burghaighis and Emery 1971; Munakata et al. 1978; Tanner et al. 1976).

The internal sphincter is involved in all cases, but the proximal extent of aganglionosis varies. The rectosigmoid is involved in about half of patients, and an additional 15% have involvement of the splenic flexure

or hepatic flexure or have total colonic Hirschsprung's disease. In 8% of the cases, aganglionosis may extend to the small bowel (Bickler 1992). Rare cases of discontinuous aganglionic segments with normal functioning intervening bowel have been reported (Anderson and Chandra 1986; Seldenrijk et al. 1986; Skandalakis and Gray 1994; Sprinz et al. 1961).

▶ INCIDENCE

The incidence figures quoted for Hirschsprung's disease have increased from the earliest report by Hautau in 1960 of 1 in 41,200, as a result of greater appreciation of the spectrum of disease. The incidence of Hirschsprung's disease today is now thought to be 1 in 5000 live births, second only to pyloric stenosis as a cause of intestinal obstruction in newborns (Passarge 1967). There is no racial predilection, and males are more commonly affected than females, with a ratio of approximately 4:1 (Kleinhaus et al. 1979; Sherman et al. 1989). The number of females with Hirschsprung's disease has varied from 5 to 22% of cases (Bodian et al. 1949; Keefer and Mokrohisky 1954; Richardson and Brown 1962). These incidence figures are based on live births. It is unknown if Hirschsprung's disease is associated with lethal malformations, as aganglionosis often cannot be recognized grossly at autopsy of a fetus or newborn because dilation and hypertrophy have not yet developed.

Numerous anomalies are associated with Hirschsprung's disease. Two percent of patients with aganglionosis have Down syndrome (Passarge 1967). Coran et al. (1978) noted that 26% of their patients had associated anomalies, including congenital heart disease, Smith–Lemli–Opitz syndrome, and multiple renal anomalies. Other large series have confirmed this finding, with 16 to 32% of patients having one or more associated anomalies. Except for Down syndrome and anomalies of the genitourinary tract, there is no consistent pattern (Lister 1977; Passarge 1967; Seldenrijk et al. 1986) (Table 72-1).

▶ SONOGRAPHIC FINDINGS

The sonographic findings of Hirschsprung's disease are nonspecific and rare. Hirschsprung's disease has been suspected or diagnosed prenatally in only three cases (Eliyahu et al. 1994; Vernesh et al. 1986; Wrobleski and Wesselhoeft 1979). The combination of polyhydramnios, diffuse and progressive fetal-bowel distention, and increased abdominal circumference raises the possibility of fetal Hirschsprung's disease (Fig. 72-2). Some have argued that because most cases occur in term infants, and cases are rarely symptomatic within the first 24 hours, Hirschsprung's disease does not occur prenatally.

▶ **TABLE 72-1.** HIRSCHSPRUNG'S DISEASE:
ASSOCIATED ANOMALIES

Chromosomal Abnormalities
  Trisomies 18, 21, and 22
  Turner syndrome
  Ring 13 chromosome
  45,X/46,XX/47,XXX mosaicism
Gastrointestinal anomalies
  Intestinal malrotation
  Atresias of colon, ileum, duodenum, esophagus
  Imperforate anus
  Colonic diverticulosis
Anomalies of cardiovascular, urinary, skeletal systems
Syndromes and other associations
  Ondine's curse
  Waardenburg syndrome
  Schwachman syndrome
  Smith–Lemli–Opitz syndrome
  Neurofibromatosis
  Familial neuroblastoma
  Achondroplasia
  Diastrophic dysplasia
  Multiple endocrine neoplasia, type I

Adapted from Bemmick JE 1992.

The three reported cases challenge this view, as Hirschsprung's disease can present at least in the third trimester of gestation. However, these cases resulted from total colonic aganglionosis, and presented with small-bowel dilation and polyhydramnios. The majority of cases, however, involve the rectosigmoid region and are unlikely to result in polyhydramnios. Given the absorption of amniotic fluid that occurs in the ileum and colon proximal to this region, functional obstruction at this level would also not be expected to cause bowel dilation.

Another sonographic finding that has been suggested as a possible sign of fetal Hirschsprung's disease is echogenic bowel (Wrobleski and Wesselhoeft 1979). However, no case of Hirschsprung's disease has been diagnosed based solely on the sonographic finding of echogenic bowel.

▶ **DIFFERENTIAL DIAGNOSIS**

The sonographic findings of bowel dilation associated with polyhydramnios suggests a differential diagnosis including jejunal, ileal, or colonic atresia or stenosis, persistent cloaca, meconium ileus, and imperforate anus (Table 72-2). The prenatal sonographic features of bowel atresias, especially ileal or colonic, can be indistinguishable from Hirschsprung's disease. Atresias are a more common cause of fetal small-bowel obstruction, however. The sonographic features of persistent cloaca should distinguish it from Hirschsprung's disease. In neonates, perforation of the colon proximal to the aganglionic segment can occur. This has not been reported prenatally, but would be expected to present with sonographic features of meconium peritonitis such as intraabdominal calcifications, ascites, or pseudocyst formation. In the

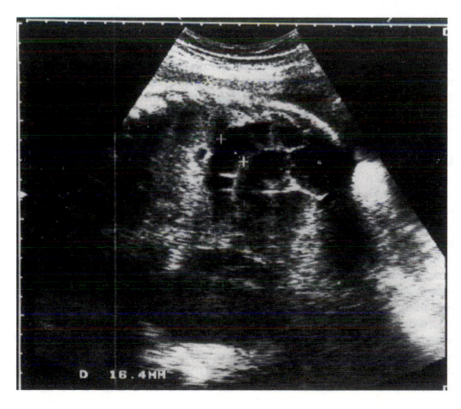

Figure 72-2. Prenatal sonographic image of a fetus at 26 weeks of gestation demonstrating multiple dilated bowel loops. On the second day of postnatal life a barium enema was suggestive of Hirschsprung's disease. *(Reprinted, with permission, from Eliyahu S, Yanai N, Blondheim O, et al. Sonographic presentation of Hirschsprung's disease: a case of an entirely aganglionic colon and ileum. Prenat Diagn 1994;14:1170–1172.)*

Soave introduced the endorectal pullthrough in 1964, with subsequent modification by Boley (1984). The major difference between Soave's procedure and Swenson's is that the dissection of the rectum is performed in a submucosal plane protecting the pelvic innervation. The ganglionated bowel is pulled through the aganglionic muscular rectal cuff and anastomosed at the dentate line. The aganglionic muscular rectal cuff is split in the posterior midline to prevent interference with normal function of the pullthrough.

Recently, many pediatric surgeons have begun performing a definitive pullthrough procedure at the time of diagnosis without preliminary colostomy, with good results (So et al. 1988; Teitelbaum and Coran 1998). This is, of course, limited to infants with no evidence of enterocolitis. Georgeson et al. (1995) have also reported success with a laparoscopic Swenson procedure without need for preliminary colostomy. This approach not only avoids colostomy, but is associated with more rapid postoperative recovery and discharge from the hospital. In newborns with a transition zone at the distal descending colon or more distal a primary transanal Soave procedure can be performed which avoids even laparoscopy. This approach allows the infant to be discharged within 2 to 3 days of the procedure (Albanese et al. 1999; Langer et al. 1999).

► LONG-TERM OUTCOME

The longest follow-up information available for patients with Hirschsprung's disease who have undergone pullthrough procedures was reported by Swenson et al. in 1985. The long-term functional results were excellent, with no cases of impotence or urinary incontinence, and a 1.4% incidence of chronic fecal soiling. Normal bowel habits were experienced by 89.7% of these patients. However, these results have not been reproduced by other surgeons performing Swenson's operation. This has led to the more common use of the Soave or Duhamel procedures. Currently, similar long-term results are routinely anticipated with these other procedures.

► GENETICS AND RECURRENCE RISK

There is good evidence for a genetic predisposition to Hirschsprung's disease. Siblings of female index patients have 360 times the risk of developing Hirschsprung's disease than that of the general population (recurrence risk, 7.2%). Siblings of male index patients have a risk of the disease 130 times that of the general population (recurrence risk, 2.6%). The proportion of affected siblings also increases when the index patient has a "long" aganglionic segment extending beyond the sigmoid colon (Carter et al. 1981; Duhamel 1964; Passarge 1967; Raffensperger 1990; Swenson 1950).

It is estimated that mutations in the RET proto-oncogene may account for as many as 20% of cases of Hirschsprung's disease (Martucciello and Holschneider 1998). The association with Down syndrome and other chromosomal abnormalities also suggests a genetic component to the cause of some cases of Hirschsprung's disease. Trisomy 21 is the most common chromosomal abnormality occurring in Hirschsprung's disease, occurring in 4.5 to 16% of cases (Puri 1993; Polley and Coran 1986). Other chromosomal abnormalities associated with Hirschsprung's disease include partial trisomy of 22q11 and 11q23 (Beedgen et al. 1986); deletion of 2p22 in combination with the reciprocal translocation (Webb et al. 1988); trisomy 18 mosaicism (Passarge 1973); interstitial deletions of 13q (Bottani et al. 1991; Kiss and Osztovics 1989; Lamont et al. 1989) and 10q (Fewtrell et al. 1994; Luo et al. 1993; Martucciello et al. 1992).

Familial cases of Hirschsprung's disease have been described. Richardson and Brown (1962) reviewed 54 cases in 21 families, including 1 family in which 5 of 6 sons from the same mother, but with 3 different fathers, had Hirschsprung's disease. Bodian et al. (1951) estimated the probability of producing a second male sibling with the disease at 20%. In a large Texas cohort Reyna described 6 affected members in a 54-member, 5-generation pedigree. He suggested autosomal dominant inheritance with variable expression of the phenotype. The incidence of familial Hirschsprung's disease, however, is only on the order of 3 to 7% of total cases (Reyna 1994). Klein (1964) suggested that males and females are equally affected with long aganglionic segments, but males are frequently affected with short-segment aganglionosis. They estimated the probability of a second child with Hirschsprung's disease to be 5% if male, but less than 1% if female, with an overall risk of 4% for short-segment cases. The risk for either sex following birth of a child with long-segment Hirschsprung's disease, however, is 12.5% (Klein 1964).

Complex segregation analysis performed on multiple families seems to indicate two different patterns of inheritance in Hirschsprung's disease. For families in which there is long-segment aganglionosis extending beyond the sigmoid colon, the mode of inheritance appears to be autosomal dominant, with variable expression of the phenotype. For families affected by short-segment aganglionosis, the inheritance pattern is either multifactorial or due to a recessive gene with very low penetrance (Badner et al. 1990).

A gene for long-segment familial Hirschsprung's disease has been mapped to chromosome 10q11.2 (Angrist et al. 1993; Edery et al. 1994). Tight linkage occurs between this gene and the RET proto-oncogene. Point mutations in the RET proto-oncogene have been demonstrated in families with both long- and short-segment aganglionosis, suggesting that the two forms of Hirschsprung's disease are due to mutations at the same locus (Edery et al. 1994). In addition to RET as a major susceptibility gene for Hirschsprung's disease, genetic studies have identified other susceptibility genes including the ligand for RET, the glial-cell-line–derived neurotrophic factor (GNNF) (Angrist et al. 1996; Ivanchuk et al. 1996; Solomon et al. 1996), and the endothelin B receptor (EDNRB) and its ligand endothelin-3 (Edery et al. 1996; Hofstra et al. 1996; Pieffenberger et al. 1996). These susceptibility genes do not account for the etiology of aganglionosis in many patients, especially sporadic cases. A search continues for other candidate susceptibility genes (Kusafuha and Puri 1998).

REFERENCES

Albanese CT, Jennings RW, Smith B, et al: Perineal one-stage pull-through for Hirschsprung's disease. J Pediatr Surg 1999;34:377–500.

Aldridge RT, Campbell PE. Ganglion cell distribution in the normal rectum and anal canal: a basis for the diagnosis of Hirschsprung's disease by anorectal biopsy. J Pediatr Surg 1968;3:475–478.

Anderson KD, Chandra R. Segmental aganglionosis of the appendix. J Pediatr Surg 1986;21:852–854.

Angrist M, Kauffman E, Slaugenhaupt SA, et al. A gene for Hirschsprung's disease (megacolon) in the pericentromeric region of human chromosome 10. Nat Genet 1993;4:351–356.

Angrist M, Bolk S, Halushka M, et al. Germline mutations in glial cell line-derived neurotrophic factor (GDNF) and RET in a Hirschsprung disease patient. Nat Genet 1996; 14:341–344.

Badner JA, Sieber WK, Garver KL, Chakravarti A. A genetic study of Hirschsprung disease. Am J Hum Genet 1990;46: 568–580.

Beedgen B, Natzenadel W, Querfeld U, et al. Partial trisomy 22 and 11 due to paternal 11:22 translocation associated with Hirschsprung's disease. Eur J Pediatr 1986;145: 229–232.

Bickler SW. Long-segment Hirschsprung's disease. Oral Surg 1992;127: 1047–1051.

Bodian M, Carter CO, Ward BCH. Hirschsprung's disease (with radiological observations). Lancet 1951;1:302–309.

Bodian M, Stephans FD, Ward BCH. Hirschsprung's disease and idiopathic megacolon. Lancet 1949;1:6–11.

Boley SJ. A new operative approach to total colonic aganglionoisis. Surg Gynecol Obstet 1984;159:481–484.

Bottani A, Xie Y, Binkert F, et al. A case of Hirschsprung's disease with a chromosome 13 microdeletion, del (13) (q32.3q33.2): potential mapping of onc disease locus. Hum Genet 1991;87:718–750.

Burghaighis AC, Emery JL. Functional obstruction of the intestine due to neurologic immaturity. Prog Pediatr Surg 1971;13: 37–52.

Carter CO, Evans K, Hickman V. Children of those treated surgically for Hirschsprung's disease. J Med Genet 1981; 18:87–90.

Coran AG, Behrendt DM, Weintraub WH, et al., eds. Surgery of the neonate. Boston: Little, Brown 1978:171–178.

Dalla Valle A. Richerche istologische su di un caso di megacolon congenitao. Pediatrics 1920;28:740–752.

Dereymaeker A. Recherches expérimentales sur l'origine du systéme nerveux entérique chez l'embryon de poulet. Arch Biol (Paris) 1943;54:359–375.

Duhamel B. A new operation for the treatment of Hirschsprung's disease. Arch Dis Child 1964;39:116–121.

Edery P, Attie T, Amiel J, et al. Mutation in the endothelin-3 gene in Waardenberg-Hirschsprung's disease (Shah-Waardenberg syndrome). Nat Genet 1996;12:442–444.

Edery P, Pelet A, Mulligan LM, et al. Long segment and short segment familial Hirschsprung's disease: variable clinical expression of the RET locus. J Med Genet 1994; 31:602–606.

Eliyahu S, Yanai N, Blondheim O, et al. Sonographic presentation of Hirschsprung's disease: a case of an entirely aganglionic colon and ileum. Prenat Diagn 1994;14: 1170–1172.

Fewtrell M, Tram P, Thomson A, et al. Hirschsprung's disease associated with deletion of chromosome 10 (q11.2 q21.2): a further link with the neurocristopathies? J Med Genet 1994;31:325–327.

Georgeson KE, Fuenfer MM, Hardin WD. Primary laparoscopic pull through for Hirschsprung's disease in infants and children. J Pediatr Surg 1995;30:1017–1022.

Hautau ER. Congenital malformations in infants born to Michigan residents in 1958. Mich Med 1960;59:1833–1836.

Hirschsprung H. Folle von engoborener pylorusstenose beobochtet bei Sauglingen. Jahresber Kinderheilkd 1888; 27:61–64.

Hofstra RMW, Osinga J, Tan-Sindhunata G, et al. A homozygous mutation in the endothelin-3 gene associated with a combined Waardenberg type 2 and Hirschsprung phenotype (Shah-Waardenburg syndrome). Nat Genet 1996;12: 445–447.

Holschneider AM, Kellner E, Steibel P, et al. The development of anorectal continence and its significance in the diagnosis of Hirschsprung disease. J Pediatr Surg 1976;11: 151–154.

Ikeda K, Goto S. Diagnosis and treatment of Hirschsprung's disease in Japan: an analysis of 1628 patients. Ann Surg 1984;199:400–405.

Ivanchuk S, Myers S, Eng C, et al. De novo mutation of GDNF ligand or the RET/GDNFR-x receptor complex in Hirschsprung's disease. Hum Mol Gen 1996;5:2023–2026.

Kamijo K, Hiatt RB, Koelle GB. Congenital megacolon: a comparison of the spastic and hypertrophied segments with respect to cholinesterase activities and sensitivities to acetylcholine, DFP, and the barium ion. Gastroenterology 1953;24:173.

Keefer GP, Mokrohisky JF. Congenital megacolon (Hirschsprung's disease). Radiology 1954;63:157–175.

Kiss P, Osztovics M. Association of 13q deletion and Hirschsprung's disease. J Med Genet 1989;26:793–794.

Klein D. Un nouveau pas franchi dans le pronostic genetique do la maladie de Hirschsprung (megacolon congenital). J Genet Hum 1964;13:233–235.

Kleinhaus S, Boley SJ. Hirschsprung's disease. In: Wyllie R, Hyams JS, eds. Pediatric gastrointestinal disease. Philadelphia: Saunders, 1993:698–705.

Kleinhaus S, Boley SJ, Sheran M, et al. Hirschsprung's disease: a survey of the members of the surgical section of the American Academy of Pediatrics. J Pediatr Surg 1979; 14:588–597.

Parents of patients who have been identified as having cystic fibrosis in association with the jejunoileal atresia should be advised regarding the 25% risk of recurrence. DNA-based prenatal diagnosis is available in subsequent pregnancies.

In general, parents of patients with jejunoileal atresia and stenosis should receive genetic counseling.

REFERENCES

Ahlgren LS. Apple peel jejunal atresia. J Pediatr Surg 1987; 22:451–453.

Al-Awadi SA, Ferag TI, Naguib K, Cushieri A, Issa M. Familial jejunal atresia with "apple peel" variant. J R Soc Med 1981;74:499–503.

Arnal-Monreal F, Pombo F, Capdevila-Puerta A. Multiple hereditary gastrointestinal atresias: a study of a family. Acta Paediatr Scand 1983;72:773–778.

Damato N, Filly RA, Goldstein RB, et al. Frequency of fetal anomalies in sonographically detected polyhydramnios. J Ultrasound Med 1993;12:11–15.

de Lorimier AA, Fonkalsrud EW, Hays DM. Congenital atresia and stenosis of the jejunum and ileum. Surgery 1969; 65:819–827.

de Lorimier AA, Harrison MR. Intestinal plication in the treatment of atresia. J Pediatr Surg 1983;18:734–736.

Dickson JAS. Apple peel small bowel: an uncommon variant of duodenal and jejunal atresia. J Pediatr Surg 1970; 5:595–597.

Dimmick JE, Hardwick DF. Gastrointestinal system and exocine pancreas. In: Dimmick JE, Kalousek DK, eds. Developmental pathology of the embryo and fetus. New York: Lippincott, 1992:523–524.

Goldstein I, Reece EA, Yarkoni S, et al. Growth of the fetal stomach in normal pregnancies. Obstet Gynecol 1987;70: 641.

Grosfeld JL, Balantine TV, Shoemaker R: Operative management of intestinal atresia and stenosis based on pathologic findings. J Pediatr Surg 1979;14:368–375.

Guttman FM, Braun P, Garance PH, et al. Multiple atresias and a new syndrome of hereditary multiple atresias involving the gastrointestinal tract from stomach to rectum. J Pediatr Surg 1973;8:633–638.

Guttman FM, Braum P, Bensousson AL. The pathogenesis of intestinal atresia. Surg Gynecol Obstet 1975;141:203–206.

Kirkinen P, Jouppila P. Prenatal ultrasonic findings in congenital chloride diarrhea. Perinat Diagn 1984;4:457.

Langer JC, Khanna J, Caco C, et al. Prenatal diagnosis of gastroschisis: Description of objective sonographic criteria for predicting outcome. Obstet Gynecol 1993;81:53–56.

Louw JH, Barnard CN. Congenital intestinal atresia: observation on its origin. Lancet 1955;2:1065.

Martin LW, Zerella JT. Jejuno-ileal atresia: a proposed classification. J Pediatr Surg 1976;11:399–403.

Muller F, Frot JC, Aubry MC, et al. Meconium ileus in cystic fibrosis fetuses. Lancet 1984;1:223.

Muller F, Dommergues M, Ville Y, et al. Amniotic fluid digestive enzymes: diagnostic value in fetal gastrointestinal obstructions. Prenat Diagn 1994;14:973–979.

Nixon HH, Tawes R. Etiology and treatment of small intestinal atresia: analysis of a series of 127 jejunoileal atresias and comparison with 62 duodenal atresias. Surgery 1971; 69:41–46.

Nyberg DA, Mack LA, Patten RM, et al. Fetal bowel: normal sonograph findings. J Ultrasound Med 1987;6:3.

Rescorla FJ, Grosfeld JL. Intestinal atresia and stenosis: analysis of survival in 120 cases. Surgery 1985;98:668–675.

Richwood AMK. A case of ileal atresia and ileocutaneous fistula caused by amniocentesis. J Pediatr 1977;91:312–314.

Robertson FM, Crombleholme TM, Paidas M, et al. Prenatal diagnosis and management of gastrointestinal anomalies. Semin Perinatol 1994;18:182–195.

Romero R, Pike G, Jeanty P, et al. Bowel obstruction in prenatal diagnosis of congenital anomalies. In: Romero R, Pike G, Jeanty P, Ghidini A, Hobbins JC, eds. Prenatal diagnosis of congenital anomalies. Norwalk CT: Appleton & Lange, 1988:239–243.

Rowe MI, O'Neill JA Jr, Grosfeld JL, et al. Intestinal atresia and stenosis. In: Rowe MI, O'Neill JA Jr, Grosfeld, JL, Fonkalsrud EW, Coron AG, eds. Essentials of pediatric surgery. St. Louis: Mosby, 1995:508–514.

Santulli TV, Chin CC, Schullinger JN. Management of congenital atresia of the intestine. Am J Surg 1970;119:152.

Seashore JH, Collins FS, Markowitz RI. Familial apple peel jejunal atresia: surgical, genetic, and radiographic aspects. Pediatrics 1987;80:540–542.

Swift PGF, Driscoll IB, Vowles KDJ. Neonatal small bowel obstruction associated with amniocentesis. BMJ 1979;1: 720–721.

Therkelson AJ, Rohder H. Intestinal atresia caused by second trimester amniocentesis. Br J Obstet Gynecol 1981;88:559–561.

Touloukian RJ. Diagnosis and treatment of jejunoileal atresia. World J Surg 1993;17:310–319.

Wallenburg HSC, Wladimoroff VW. The amniotic fluid. Polyhydramnios and oligohydramnios. J Perinat Med 1977;5: 193–205.

Zerella JT, Martin LW. Jejunal atresia with absent mesentery and helical ileum. Surgery 1976;80:550–553.

CHAPTER 74

Meconium Peritonitis

▶ CONDITION

Perforation of the bowel that occurs antenatally leads to a sterile chemical peritonitis referred to as meconium peritonitis. The peritonitis can be localized or diffuse and can lead to a fibrotic reaction with intraperitoneal calcifications. The clinical manifestations of meconium peritonitis depend on its underlying cause, timing, and whether or not the perforation heals spontaneously. The spectrum of disease ranges from asymptomatic intraabdominal calcifications to giant cystic meconium peritonitis (Dirkes et al. 1995; Robertson et al. 1994). Meconium peritonitis has been associated with intestinal atresia or stenosis, meconium ileus, internal hernia, bowel ileus, intussusception, gastroschisis, Meckel diverticulum, and cytomegalovirus infection (Petrikovsky et al. 1993; Pletcher et al. 1991).

The presence of associated anomalies is unusual and depends on the underlying cause of meconium peritonitis. Up to 15 to 40% of neonates with meconium peritonitis have cystic fibrosis (Park and Grand 1981; Payne and Nielsen 1983). However, in prenatally diagnosed meconium peritonitis, cystic fibrosis is reported to be the cause in only 8% of cases (Dirkes et al. 1995; Foster et al. 1987). This apparent discrepancy may be due to the increased sensitivity of prenatal sonographic imaging in detecting abdominal calcification, as compared with postnatal plain films (Williams et al. 1984).

▶ INCIDENCE

Meconium peritonitis occurs in approximately 1 in every 35,000 live births (Olson et al. 1982; Pan et al. 1983).

▶ SONOGRAPHIC FINDINGS

A spectrum of findings may be observed on prenatal sonographic examination. The most consistent finding is abdominal calcifications, which are present in 85% of cases (Fig. 74-1A). Conversely, meconium peritonitis is the most common cause of fetal intraabdominal calcifications. The sonographic criteria used for the diagnosis of meconium peritonitis include intraabdominal calcifications that cause acoustic shadowing not caused by solid organ, intraluminal, intravascular, biliary, or tumor calcifications. Other findings include polyhydramnios, fetal ascites, and bowel dilatation in 50% and 27% of cases, respectively (Foster et al. 1987). The presence of dilated bowel, cysts, or ascites usually predicts complicated meconium peritonitis that will require postnatal surgical intervention. Dirkes et al. (1995) divided sonographically diagnosed cases of fetal intraabdominal calcifications into simple and complex categories. Simple meconium peritonitis has isolated calcifications seen without any bowel dilatation, meconium pseudocysts, ascites, or polyhydramnios (see Fig. 74-1A). Intraabdominal calcifications in association with any of these features is classified as complex meconium peritonitis (see Fig. 74-1B).

While not sufficient for a diagnosis, meconium peritonitis often starts as echogenic bowel that goes on to perforate with subsequent formation of intraperitoneal calcifications (see Chapter 70). Serial sonography is indicated to follow this progression. Similarly, simple meconium peritonitis may evolve into complex meconium peritonitis with the development of bowel dilatation, meconium pseudocyst, ascites, or polyhydramnios (Dirkes et al. 1995).

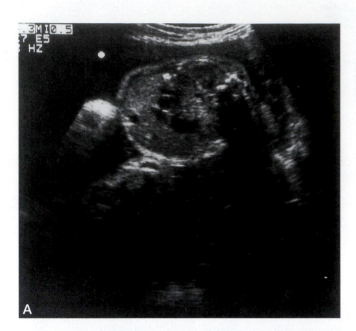
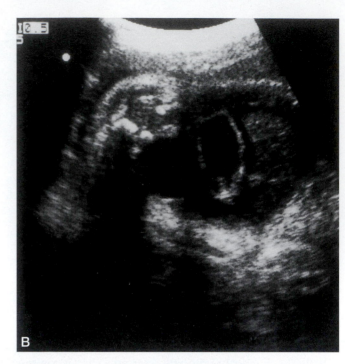

Figure 74-1. (A) Prenatal sonographic image demonstrating isolated intraperitoneal calcifications with acoustic shadowing. This represents a case of simple meconium peritonitis. (B) In contrast, this fetus has intraperitoneal calcifications with an associated meconium pseudocyst and ascites. This is an example of complex meconium peritonitis. *(Reprinted, with permission, from Dirkes K, Crombleholme TM, Jacir NN, et al. Prenatal natural history of meconium peritonitis diagnosed in utero. J Pediatr Surg 1995;30: 979–982.)*

► DIFFERENTIAL DIAGNOSIS

The differential diagnosis of meconium peritonitis includes fetal gallstones, hepatic calcifications, calcifications within hemangiomas, hematomas, and tumors such as dermoid, hepatoblastoma, neuroblastoma and teratoma. Calcifications may also be observed in congenital infections such as cytomegalovirus and toxoplasmosis. Intraluminal calcification may also occur from reflux of urine into the colon in imperforate anus with retro-urethral fistula.

► ANTENATAL NATURAL HISTORY

The natural history of meconium peritonitis diagnosed in utero is markedly different from meconium peritonitis diagnosed in the newborn nursery. The overall mortality rate in antenatal reports is 11 to 14% (Chabulinski et al. 1992; Dirkes et al. 1995; Foster et al. 1987). This differs markedly from the mortality rates of 40 to 50% in postnatal series (Park and Grand 1981; Payne and Nielsen 1983; Tibboel et al. 1986). A major factor in the survival of patients with meconium peritonitis is the underlying cause. Tibboel et al. (1986) found that primary intestinal obstruction was present in 53% of 1084

neonatal cases of meconium peritonitis reviewed and reported a 54% mortality rate among their own 22 cases (Tibboel et al. 1986). Brugman et al. (1979) reported a 62% mortality rate in cases of meconium peritonitis that were associated with obstruction caused by atresia.

Prenatally diagnosed meconium peritonitis differs from postnatally diagnosed meconium peritonitis in reduced morbidity, lower incidence of cystic fibrosis, and an overall better prognosis (Chabulinski et al. 1992; Dirkes et al. 1995; Dunne et al. 1983). It is clear that ultrasound examination is more sensitive in detecting intraabdominal calcifications, and this may account for more cases with less severe meconium peritonitis being detected in utero (Dunne et al. 1983; Foster et al. 1987; Williams et al. 1984). Asymptomatic calcifications in hernia sacs, scrotal masses, and the abdomen are common incidental findings detected postnatally (Berdon et al. 1967; Gunn et al. 1978; Marchildon 1978; Thompson et al. 1973). These asymptomatic patients may have had bowel perforations in utero that sealed spontaneously and represent the postnatal equivalent of simple meconium peritonitis. Estroff et al. (1992) reported a case of fetal ascites that resolved, leaving abdominal calcifications that were asymptomatic at birth. Because many cases are clinically silent, neonatal series of meconium peritonitis are skewed by sicker infants with more severe meconium peritonitis and a higher attendant morbidity and mortality rate (Dirkes et al. 1995). The natural history of meconium peritonitis diagnosed in utero more clearly reflects the entire spectrum of the disease (Dirkes et al. 1995).

▶ MANAGEMENT OF PREGNANCY

Fetal abdominal calcifications detected by prenatal ultrasound examination should prompt an effort to determine whether these represent biliary, vascular, intraluminal, solid organ, or tumor calcifications or the true intraabdominal calcification of meconium peritonitis. Intrahepatic calcifications are discussed in Chapter 71. The presence of associated findings, such as dilated loops of bowel, meconium pseudocysts, ascites, and polyhydramnios should be excluded. Because these findings may develop later in gestation, serial sonography is advisable. In the absence of the findings that characterize complex meconium peritonitis, an excellent prognosis can be anticipated, and delivery in a community setting can be safely recommended (Dirkes et al. 1995). Even in simple meconium peritonitis, however, a postnatal abdominal radiographic examination should be obtained, and if normal, feedings can be initiated.

In cases of meconium peritonitis in which associated abnormalities such as bowel dilatation, meconium cysts, ascites, or polyhydramnios are prenatally diagnosed there is a 50% chance that surgical intervention will be required during the newborn period (Dirkes et al. 1995). Consideration should be given to delivery of the infant with complex meconium peritonitis in a tertiary-care center.

Although the reported incidence of cystic fibrosis in neonatal meconium peritonitis ranges from 15 to 40%, three of the patients reported by Dirkes et al. (1995) had normal sweat tests and the remaining patients had no clinical manifestations of cystic fibrosis. Other prenatal series of meconium peritonitis have reported only an 8% incidence of cystic fibrosis (Boureau and Pat 1974; Chabulinski et al. 1992; Finkel and Slovis 1982; Foster et al. 1987; Park and Grand 1981). Why meconium peritonitis associated with cystic fibrosis most commonly produces peritoneal calcification is unknown. Finkel and Slovis (1982) postulated that pancreatic enzymes, which are deficient in 80% of patients with cystic fibrosis, may be necessary for calcification to occur (Boureau and Pat 1974). Conversely, Foster et al. (1987) speculated that the thick tenacious nature of meconium in cystic fibrosis precludes free spillage into the peritoneum.

Sonographic detection of meconium peritonitis can alert the obstetrician to a fetus potentially at risk for complications from obstruction, perforation, pseudocyst formation, ascites, and polyhydramnios that may pre-cipitate preterm labor and premature delivery. Pediatric surgical consultation may be helpful in providing counseling about the overall favorable prognosis in cases of prenatally diagnosed meconium peritonitis. In cases of complex meconium peritonitis, the parents can be advised of a more guarded prognosis, with a 50% chance of surgical intervention during the neonatal period. Parental DNA testing to define the fetal risk for cystic fibrosis may be appropriate in cases of meconium peritonitis (Robertson et al. 1994). This can be performed by a referral laboratory on blood samples or mouth swabs from the parents. If both parents are carriers and the pregnancy is at less than 24 weeks of gestation, fetal testing for cystic fibrosis mutations may be indicated if termination of the pregnancy is an option for the parents. If an amniocentesis is being performed for other reasons, consideration should be given to testing amniocytes for mutations seen in cystic fibrosis.

▶ FETAL INTERVENTION

There are no fetal interventions in meconium peritonitis.

▶ TREATMENT OF THE NEWBORN

The infant should undergo abdominal examination immediately after delivery and an abdominal radiograph and ultrasound study of the abdomen should be obtained to confirm the prenatal findings (Fig. 74-2). An upper gastrointestinal study with small-bowel follow-through using water-soluble contrast may be necessary to confirm or exclude perforation, stenosis, atresia, or meconium pseudocysts (Fig. 74-3). Postnatal treatment is directed by the underlying cause of meconium peritonitis. Abdominal radiography will confirm intraabdominal calcification and demonstrate the presence or absence of cystic lesions or intestinal obstruction. Asymptomatic neonates with calcifications and otherwise normal plain abdominal radiographs and abdominal sonographic examinations may be cautiously observed and fed. If dilated bowel, meconium cysts, or ascites are present, nasogastric decompression and intravenous fluids should be administered. Associated anomalies should be evaluated and surgical correction performed when the infant is stable. A sweat chloride test or testing for DNA mutations should be performed during the postoperative period to exclude or definitively diagnose cystic fibrosis in all cases of meconium peritonitis. DNA analysis is preferable in newborns presenting with gastrointestinal symptoms. If DNA analysis reveals the presence of a mutation in the cystic fibrosis transmembrane regulator gene, sweat testing is unnecessary, as some mutations have been found in patients with normal sweat tests (Highsmith et al. 1994).

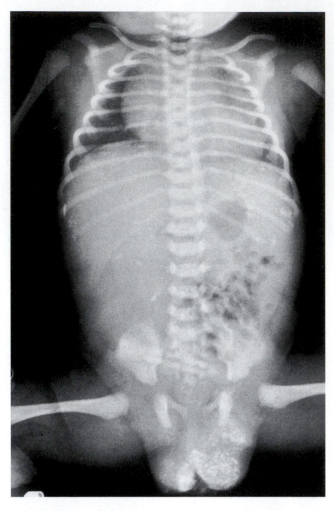

Figure 74-2. Plain abdominal radiograph in a newborn demonstrating intraabdominal calcifications, particularly over the dome of the liver and in the scrotum.

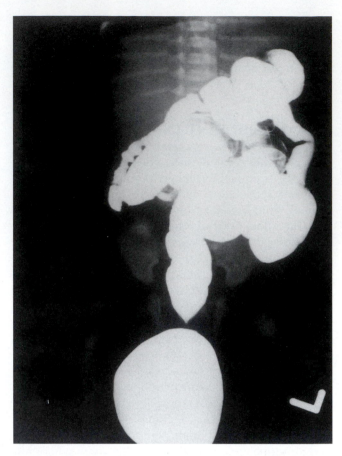

Figure 74-3. Upper gastrointestinal contrast study with small-bowel follow-through demonstrating extraabdominal contrast in a meconium pseudocyst in the right lower quadrant.

► **SURGICAL TREATMENT**

The infant with complex meconium peritonitis will require surgical intervention in 50% of cases (Dirkes et al. 1995). The indications for surgery include intestinal perforation with ascites, meconium pseudocyst, intestinal atresia or stenosis, or volvulus. Surgical exploration for complications of meconium peritonitis may be extremely difficult because of the intense inflammatory reaction that occurs within the peritoneal cavity (Fig. 74-4). Because of this and bacterial contamination of the peritoneal cavity, cases of meconium peritonitis complicated by perforation or meconium pseudocyst are best managed by resection and enterostomy. In cases of volvulus, the nonviable intestine is resected and proximal and distal stomas are created. In cases involving the proximal intestine, long-term venous access can be obtained to provide parenteral nu-

tritional support until gastrointestinal continuity can be established.

► **LONG-TERM OUTCOME**

The long-term outcome of infants with meconium peritonitis depends on the underlying cause. In fetuses with simple meconium peritonitis, the prognosis is excellent. In complex meconium peritonitis, the prognosis relates to the underlying cause of the perforation. In isolated meconium peritonitis, without cystic fibrosis, Hirschsprung's disease, or intestinal pseudo-obstruction, the prognosis is excellent. In infants with cystic fibrosis or chronic pseudo-obstruction, however, the prognosis is more guarded.

► **GENETICS AND RECURRENCE RISK**

There is no known risk of recurrence for isolated meconium peritonitis. However, the approximately 8% of

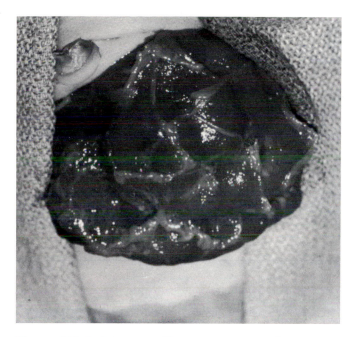

Figure 74-4. Intraoperative appearance of meconium peritonitis in a newborn with a perforated colon. Note the adhesions, which are the results of an inflammatory reaction that occurred in utero.

antenatally diagnosed cases with cystic fibrosis are at a 25% risk for recurrence in subsequent pregnancies.

REFERENCES

Berdon WE, Baker DH, Becker J et al. Scrotal masses in healed meconium peritonitis. N Engl J Med 1967;277: 585–587.

Boureau M, Pat D. Valeur diagnostique des calcifications intraperitoneales au cours de la peritonite meconiale. J Parisiennes Pediatr 1974;9:149–152.

Brugman SM, Bjelland JJ, Thomassin JE, et al. Sonographic findings with radiologic correlation in meconium peritonitis. J Clin Ultrasound 1979;7:305–306.

Chabulinski K, Deutinger J, Bernaschek G. Meconium peritonitis: extrusion of meconium and different sonographical appearances in relation to the stage of the disease. Prenat Diagn 1992;12:631–636.

Dirkes K, Crombleholme TM, Jacir NN, et al. Prenatal natural history of meconium peritonitis diagnosed in utero. J Pediatr Surg 1995;30:979–982.

Dunne M, Haney P, Sun CCJ. Sonographic features of bowel perforation and calcific meconium peritonitis in utero. Pediatr Radiol 1983;13:231–233.

Estroff JA, Bromley B, Benacerraf BR. Fetal meconium peritonitis without sequelae. Pediatr Radiol 1992;22:277–278.

Finkel LI, Slovis TL. Meconium peritonitis, intraperitoneal calcifications and cystic fibrosis. Pediatr Radiol 1982;12: 92–93.

Foster MA, Nyberg DA, Mahoney BS et al. Meconium peritonitis: Prenatal sonographic findings and their clinical significance. Radiology 1987;165:661–665.

Gunn LC, Ghianzoli OG, Gardner HG. Healed meconium peritonitis presenting as a reducible scrotal mass. J Pediatr 1978;92:847–849.

Highsmith WE, Burch LH, Zhou Z, et al. A novel mutation in the cystic fibrosis gene in patients with pulmonary disease but normal sweat chloride concentrations. N Engl J Med 1994;331:974–980.

Marchildon MB. Meconium peritonitis and spontaneous gastric perforations. Clin Perinatol 1978;5:79–81.

Olson MM, Luck SR, Lloyd-Still J, et al. Spectrum of meconium disease in infancy. J Pediatr Surg 1982;17:479–481.

Pan EY, Chen LY, Yang JZ, et al. Radiographic diagnosis of meconium peritonitis: a report of 200 cases including 6 fetal cases. Pediatr Radiol 1983;13:199–205.

Park RW, Grand RJ. Gastrointestinal manifestation of cystic fibrosis: a review. Gastroenterology 1981;81:1143–1161.

Payne RM, Nielsen AM. Meconium peritonitis. Am Surg 1983;28:224–231.

Petrikovsky B, Konigberg K, Pletcher B. Meconium peritonitis mimicking urinary ascites. Fetus 1993;3(6):9–12.

Pletcher BA, Williams MK, Mulinos R, et al. Intrauterine cytomegalovirus infection presenting as fetal meconium peritonitis. Obstet Gynecol 1991;78:903–905.

Robertson FM, Crombleholme TM, Paidas MJ, et al. Prenatal diagnosis and management of gastrointestinal anomalies. Semin Perinatol 1994;18:182–195.

Thompson RB, Rosen DI, Gross DM. Healed meconium peritonitis presenting as an inguinal mass. J Urol 1973; 110:364–366.

Tibboel D, Gaillard JLJ, Molenaar JC. The importance of mesenteric vascular insufficiency in meconium peritonitis. Hum Pathol 1986;17:411–416.

Williams J, Nathan RO, Worthen NJ, et al. Sonographic demonstration of the progression of meconium peritonitis. Obstet Gynecol 1984;64:822–826.

overproduction, such as acne, a deep voice, or the development of hirsutism during pregnancy. A complete family history should be obtained, with specific questions asked regarding history of infertility in family members, prior cases of ambiguous genitalia, neonatal deaths, or consanguinity (Meyers-Seifer and Charest 1992). Antenatal workup and treatment of the fetus with ambiguous genitalia is best performed in the setting of a multidisciplinary team that includes specialists in pediatric endocrinology, genetics, neonatology, pediatric urology, and surgery, and psychology. It is recommended, however, that only one member of the team communicate with the family. We recommend that a prenatal karyotype be obtained to determine the genetic sex, as well as to rule out the presence of associated chromosomal abnormalities. It is our recommendation, however, that the parents be told only that the karyotype is normal or abnormal, and not be told the genetic sex. The parents should be informed that definitive gender assignment may not be possible until 2 to 3 days after birth. It is our experience that if parents are told the fetal sex chromosome results antenatally that they psychologically "bond" to the chromosomal gender. Because some fetuses with a 46,XY karyotype cannot be raised as males, we prefer not to tell the parents antenatally that the chromosome results were male. We also recommend that fetuses with ambiguous genitalia be delivered in a tertiary-care center, to avoid confusion on the admitting papers and birth certificate because when the sex of rearing differs from the sex assignment at birth, parents experience a lot of difficulties with changing medical records and the birth certificate. Therefore, we recommend delivery in a tertiary-care center and admitting the baby to the newborn intensive care unit or special care nursery as "baby," not "baby boy" or "baby girl."

At the time of amniocentesis, amniotic fluid should be analyzed for the presence of 7-dehydrocholesterol. This metabolite is normally quite low in amniotic fluid; elevated levels are strongly suggestive of Smith–Lemli–Opitz syndrome (Irons et al. 1999). Furthermore, amniotic fluid cells should be saved as a source of DNA for mutational analysis of the 21-hydroxylase gene.

▶ FETAL INTERVENTION

In families known to be at risk for affected fetuses with congenital adrenal hyperplasia, prenatal diagnosis for chromosomal sex and DNA analysis can be performed as early as 10 weeks of gestation by chorionic villus sampling (CVS). If the fetus is diagnosed as female and affected with congenital adrenal hyperplasia, consideration can be given to giving the mother corticosteroids antenatally to prevent masculinization of an affected female fetus.

A review of 403 at-risk pregnancies evaluated at the New York Cornell Medical Center diagnosed 84 fetuses with classical 21-hydroxylase deficiency (21-OHD) (Carlson et al. 1999). Of these 52 were female. In 23 affected female fetuses, dexamethasone administered to the mother at or before 10 weeks of gestation was effective in reducing virilization. No significant or permanent side effects were noted in the mothers or the fetuses, indicating that dexamethasone treatment is safe. Treated newborns did not differ in weight, length, or head circumference from untreated affected newborns (Carlson et al 1999). In addional, successful prenatal treatment of an affected female with congenital adrenal hyperplasia due to 11β hydroxylase deficiency has also been described (Cerame et al. 1999).

Smith–Lemli–Opitz syndrome, a disorder of cholesterol metabolism, can present *in utero* with growth restriction and ambiguous genitalia. Postnatal treatment with cholesterol supplementation improves plasma sterol levels and enhances growth and development. In one reported case, antenatal treatment of a fetus with Smith–Lemli–Opitz syndrome by administration of fresh frozen plasma (cholesterol level = 219mg/dl) via repeated transfusions resulted in improved fetal cholesterol levels and increased fetal red cell volume (Irons et al. 1999).

▶ TREATMENT OF THE NEWBORN

Parents of an affected fetus or infant with ambiguous genitalia should be told that their infant has a sex that is incompletely developed and has yet to be determined (Izquierdo and Glassberg 1993). The major considerations in the treatment of the newborn include: (1) to rule out life-threatening processes, (2) to determine the sex of rearing and gender identity, (3) to plan for surgery if necessary, (4) to plan for as normal pubertal development and fertility as possible, and (5) to provide genetic counseling. The affected newborn with ambiguous genitalia should be admitted to a tertiary-care nursery capable of providing diagnostic tests and treatment. The infant's blood pressure should be checked. Physical examination of the genital area should include a measurement of the phallus length as precisely as possible along the dorsum of the stretched penis from the pubic ramus to the tip of the glans (a measurement of 2.5 cm is 2.5 SD below the mean at term) (Meyers-Seifer and Charest 1992). Although the clitoris reaches a term size at 27 weeks of gestation, the penis continues to grow until full term. On physical examination, an attempt should be made to palpate gonads. If they are palpable, are they symmetric and is the position above or below the inguinal ring? The infant should be specifically examined for the presence of hypospadias and/or chordee. An assessment should be made of the labioscrotal folds for the degree of fusion (see Fig. 76-4). The perineum should be examined for the presence of a urethra, vagina, vaginal pouch, or urogenital sinus. A rectal examination should be performed to try to palpate the uterus (Meyers-Seifer and Charest 1992). A complete physical examination should be obtained to look for the presence of other abnormalities. A clinical geneticist can help in this regard.

The initial blood work recommended includes serum electrolytes, glucose, and cholesterol, serum 17-hydroxyketosteroids, and a chromosome analysis, if it was not performed antenatally. The use of the buccal smear is no longer recommended. Fluorescence in situ hybridization studies using X- and Y-chromosome–specific probes on nondividing cells is equally rapid and more accurate.

Additional studies that can be performed during the newborn period include urogenital sinography, which will outline the urethral and vaginal anatomy, magnetic resonance imaging of the pelvic region, and abdominal sonography. Kutteh et al. (1995) studied 100 term infants with the external genitalia covered. A neonatal uterus was identified in 47 of 50 female infants (sensitivity, 94%). The absence of the uterus correctly predicted 49 of 50 male infants (specificity, 98%). Most of the time the neonatal uterus demonstrated the typical linear echo of the endometrial cavity. The only false positive was a distended bowel that was incorrectly identified as a uterus. These authors recommended that the bedside determination of the presence of the uterus was important in the initial studies regarding gender assignment, as infants who have a uterus will almost always be assigned as a female.

Infants with ambiguous genitalia who require medical treatment during the newborn period include those with congenital adrenal hyperplasia, who are treated with adrenogenital steroids. This prevents potentially life-threatening urinary salt wasting and dehydration. In addition, it arrests virilization and permits normal growth and development of normal female secondary sex characteristics, menstruation, and fertility. In males who are undermasculinized due to 5α-reductase deficiency, an elevated plasma testosterone : dihydrotestosterone ratio is seen after human chorionic gonadatropin (hCG) stimulation. The diagnostic test is the presence of diminished 5α-reductase activity in skin fibroblasts, usually in the setting of a positive family history. Infants affected with 5α-reductase deficiency who are 46,XY should be assigned as male and given topical dihydrotestosterone therapy. This will enlarge the phallus and allow eventual repair of the hypospadias (Al-Attia et al. 1993).

It is beyond the scope of this chapter to thoroughly discuss all of the underlying enzyme abnormalities that can cause ambiguous genitalia. However, female pseudohermaphrodites with 21-hydroxylase deficiency and 3β-hydroxysteroid dehydrogenase deficiency will have hyperkalemia and hyponatremia. Male pseudohermaphrodites with cholesterol side-chain cleavage defects and 3β-hydroxysteroid dehydrogenase defects will also have hyperkalemia and hypokalemia. Female pseudohermaphrodites with 11β-hydroxylase deficiency and male pseudohermaphrodites with 17α-hydroxylase deficiency will have hypokalemia. Diagnoses of most of these inborn errors of metabolism rely on the demonstration of the elevated immediate precursor in the affected infant's serum.

▶ SURGICAL TREATMENT

For the overmasculinized female, clitoral recession, labioscrotal reduction, and vaginoplasty can be performed between 2 and 5 months of age. Male pseudohermaphrodites who are assigned a female gender can undergo a clitoral reduction, vaginoplasty, gonadectomy, and removal of wolffian ducts if surgery is elected. These patients will require estrogen at puberty (Izquierdo and Glassberg 1993). Pseudohermaphrodites who are assigned as male can undergo correction of the hypospadias at about 1 year of age. At this time, if indicated, the testes can be placed into the scrotum. Some of these patients will require hCG stimulation during the newborn period and testosterone therapy at puberty. In patients with gonadal dysgenesis, the dysgenetic gonads are prone to neoplasia and should be removed. For patients who are true hermaphrodites, it is recommended that the tissue that is contrary to the sex of rearing be removed. For example, in patients being raised as female, testes and wolffian duct structures should be removed.

▶ LONG-TERM OUTCOME

The majority of patients with ambiguous genitalia are heterosexual based on the sex of rearing at the time of adulthood (Hurtig 1992). Four key considerations have been identified for the successful adjustment of the child to his or her gender (McGillivray 1992):

1. The parents should resolve any uncertainty about the sex of rearing of the child as soon as possible after birth.
2. Genital reconstruction should be undertaken as soon as possible to ensure a consistent response to the child by parents, caretakers, observers, and self.
3. Properly timed hormonal and surgical intervention should occur prior to and during puberty.
4. The patient should eventually be informed about his or her condition at an age-appropriate time.

It is important to recognize that the recommendations given in this chapter follow traditional medical guidelines. Until recently, sex assignment in the newborn was based on phallic size in the male, potential fertility in the female, and cosmetic appearance of the reconstructed genitalia. Increasing attention is being paid to long-term psychological difficulties experienced by adults who encountered conflict between the appearance of their surgically reconstructed external genitalia and their sexual identity (Reiner 1999). Furthermore, several groups of adult patients currently advocate that genitalia should be left ambiguous permanently. Support groups such as the Intersex Society of North America and the Androgen Insensitivity Support Group can serve as clearinghouses of information for prospective parents (Warne et al. 1998). Unfortunately, no published study to date has adequately addressed the quality of life of adults who remain intersexual, but pilot surveys are being developed (Schober, 1999).

▶ GENETICS AND RECURRENCE RISK

The genetics of many of the conditions that result in ambiguous genitalia are given in Table 76-2. Patients with mixed gonadal dysgenesis secondary to a mitotic nondisjunction do not have an increased risk of recurrence in subsequent pregnancies (McGillivray 1992).

Partial androgen insensitivity is familial and is now known as the Reifenstein syndrome. The androgen receptor gene has been mapped to Xq11-12. Defects in the androgen receptor are responsible for approximately 50 to 70% of males with pseudohermaphroditism (Lumbroso et al. 1994). With molecular analysis of this gene, it is now known that the main mechanism that causes androgen insensitivity syndrome is a single nucleotide change that introduces a premature stop codon or an amino acid substitution into the coding sequence of the androgen receptor gene. Over 100 point mutations have been reported in this gene (Lobaccaro et al. 1994).

It is of interest that the gene abnormality in the 5α-reductase deficiency, inherited as an autosomal recessive disorder, causes abnormal sexual development only in 46,XY homozygotes. Heterozygous 46,XY males are apparently completely normal. In addition, 46,XX homozygotes with 5α-reductase deficiency are completely normal and fertile (al-Attia et al. 1993). Several Santo Domingan families have been described in the literature with this condition (al-Attia et al. 1993).

It is important to make an accurate diagnosis of the underlying cause of the ambiguous genitalia, as the genetic bases for many of these conditions are now known and prenatal diagnosis is available for subsequent pregnancies. In particular, prenatal treatment is available for the congenital adrenal hyperplasia and Smith–Lemli–Opitz syndromes. Therefore, it is important to rule out these diagnoses in the family of a fetus that presents with ambiguous genitalia.

▶ TABLE 76-2. INHERITANCE PATTERNS OF DISORDERS KNOWN TO CAUSE AMBIGUOUS GENITALIA

Female pseuodhermaphroditism	
Congenital adrenal hyperplasia	Autosomal recessive
Male pseudohermaphroditism	
Testosterone synthetic defects	Autosomal recessive
Leydig-cell hypoplasia	Autosomal recessive
5α-reductase deficiency	Autosomal recessive
Androgen insensitivity syndrome	X-linked
Gonadal disorders	
Gonadal dysgenesis	
46,XY	Sporadic and familial
45,X/46,XY	Sporadic
True hermaphroditism	Sporadic, rarely familial
46,XX/69,XXY	Sporadic

Modified from Meyer-Seifer CH, Charest NJ. Diagnosis and management of patients with ambiguous genitalia. Semin Perinatol 1992;16:332–339.

REFERENCES

Aarskog D. Syndromes and genital dysmorphology. Horm Res 1992;2:82–85.

al-Attia HM, Bakir AM, Butt NJ. Aspects of 5-alpha reductase deficiency, a review. Acta Clin Belg 1993;48:195–201.

Ali QM. Determination of fetal sex by ultrasound: state of the art. East Afr Med J 1992;69:703–706.

Benacerraf BR, Saltzman DH, Mandell J. Sonographic diagnosis of abnormal fetal genitalia. J Ultrasound Med 1989; 8:613–617.

Bronshtein M, Riechler A, Zimmer EZ. Prenatal sonographic signs of possible fetal genital anomalies. Prenat Diagn 1995;15:215–219.

Carlson AD, Obeid JS, Kanellopoulou N, Wilson RC, New MI. Congenital adrenal hyperplasia: update on prenatal diagnosis and treatment. J Steroid Biochem Mol Biol 1999;69:19–29.

Cerame BI, Newfield RS, Pascoe L, et al. Prenatal diagnosis and treatment of 11 beta-hydroxylase deficiency congenital adrenal hyperplasia resulting in normal female genitalia. J Clin Endocrinol Metab 1999;84:3129–3134.

Cooper C, Mahony BS, Bowie JD, Pope II. Prenatal ultrasound diagnosis of ambiguous genitalia. J Ultrasound Med 1985;4:433–436.

de Elejalde BR, de Elejalde MM, Heitman T. Visualization of the fetal genitalia by ultrasonography: a review of the literature and analysis of its accuracy and ethical implications. J Ultrasound Med 1985;4:633–639.

Griffin JE. Androgen resistance—the clinical and molecular spectrum. N Engl J Med 1992;326:611–618.

Hurtig AL. The psychosocial effects of ambiguous genitalia. Comp Ther 1992;18:22–25.

Irons MB, Nores J, Stewart TL, et al. Antenatal therapy of Smith–Lemli–Opitz syndrome. Fetal Diagn Ther 1999;14:133–137.

Izquierdo G, Glassberg KI. Gender assignment and gender identity in patients with ambiguous genitalia. Urology 1993;42:232–242.

Kutteh WH, Santos-Ramos R, Ermel LD. Accuracy of ultrasonic detection of the uterus in normal newborn infants: implications for infants with ambiguous genitalia. Ultrasound Obstet Gynecol 1995;5:109–113.

Lobaccaro JM, Lumbroso S, Poujol N, Belon C, Sultan C. Molecular genetics of androgen insensitivity syndromes. Cell Mol Biol 1994;40:301–308.

Lumbroso S, Lobaccaro JM, Belon C, et al. Molecular prenatal exclusion of familial partial androgen insensitivity (Reifenstein syndrome). Eur J Endocrinol 1994;130:327–332.

Mandell J, Bromley B, Peters CA, Benacerraf BR. Prenatal sonographic detection of genital malformations. J Urol 1995;153:1994–1996.

McGillivray BC. Genetic aspects of ambiguous genitalia. Pediatr Clin North Am 1992;39:307–317.

Meyers-Seifer CH, Charest NJ. Diagnosis and management of patients with ambiguous genitalia. Semin Perinatol 1992;16:332–339.

Natsuyama E. Sonographic determination of fetal sex from twelve weeks of gestation. Am J Obstet Gynecol 1984;149:748–757.

Reiner WG. Assignment of sex in neonates with ambiguous genitalia. Curr Opin Pediatr 1999;11:363–365.

Schober JM. Quality-of-life studies in patients with ambiguous genitalia. World J Urol 1999;17:249–252.

Sivan E, Koch S, Reece EA. Sonographic prenatal diagnosis of ambiguous genitalia. Fetal Diagn Ther 1995;10:311–314.

Warne GL, Zajac JD, MacLean HE. Androgen insensitivity syndrome in the era of molecular genetics and the Internet: a point of view. J Pediatr Endocrinol Metab 1998;11:3–9.

Wheeler PG, Weaver DD, Obeime MO, Vance GH, Bull MJ, Escobar LF. Urorectal septum malformation sequence: report of thirteen additional cases and review of the literature. Am J Med Genet 1997;73:456–462.

CHAPTER 77
Echogenic Kidneys

▶ CONDITION

There are some conditions that render the renal parenchyma echogenic on ultrasound examination. While increased renal echogenicity can be a normal variant in children, it has been associated with nephrotic syndrome, glomerulonephritis, and renal dysplasia (Brenbridge et al. 1986; Kraus et al. 1990; Krensky et al. 1983; Cramer et al. 1986). Premature infants also have an increased incidence of increased renal echogenicity (Benacerraf 1998). While increased echogenicity is a subjective assessment, kidneys that are brighter than liver are considered to be echogenic. This becomes a potential indicator of fetal disease because of the association of this finding with chromosomal abnormality, adult and infantile polycystic kidney disease, Pearlman syndrome, Beckwith–Wiedemann syndrome, and cytomegalovirus infection. The cause of the increased echogenicity of the kidney in these conditions is unknown.

▶ INCIDENCE

No data are available to estimate the incidence of echogenic kidneys in the fetus, in either normal fetuses or those with underlying pathology.

▶ SONOGRAPHIC FINDINGS

The kidneys should be considered to be echogenic if the reflectivity of the renal parenchyma is greater than the reflectivity of the liver (Fig. 77-1). Once identified, it is important to note other possible associated findings that would aid in the differential diagnosis. It is important to look for other sonographic features that are associated with aneuploidy, especially trisomy 13, including ventriculomegaly, holoprosencephaly, agenesis of the corpus callosum, cleft lip or palate, cyclasia, or microphthalmia. Because of the association of echogenic kidneys with cytomegalovirus infection, attention should be paid to the presence of intracranial calcifications, echogenic bowel, ascites, hydrops, or cardiomegaly (Choong et al. 1993). If the possible renal abnormalities seen with echogenic kidneys (including severe obstructive uropathy at any level from the bladder outlet to the ureteropelvic junction) occur during the second trimester, they can result in increased echogenicity from renal dysplasia. The kidneys in adult and infantile polycystic kidney disease can also be echogenic, but they are usually much larger than normal and may lack normal renal architecture and have severe associated oligohydramnios (see Chapter 85).

▶ DIFFERENTIAL DIAGNOSIS

As noted above, it is important to remember that increased renal echogenicity is a normal variant and there may be no underlying pathology. The differential diagnosis of echogenic kidneys includes cytomegalovirus infection, aneuploidy, particularly trisomy 13, other chromosomal abnormalities such as partial trisomy 10, adult and infantile forms of polycystic kidney disease, and renal dysplasia secondary to obstructive uropathy.

▶ ANTENATAL NATURAL HISTORY

What is known about the antenatal history of echogenic kidneys is based on two small retrospective reports. Chitty et al. (1991) reported 5 fetuses with enlarged echogenic kidneys in which the amniotic fluid volume

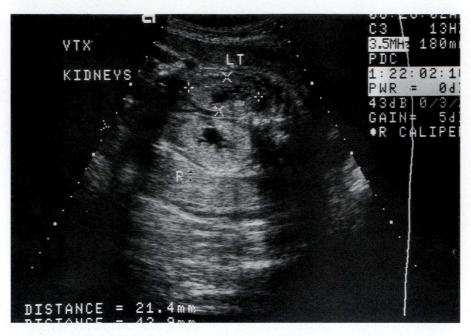

Figure 77-1. Prenatal sonographic image from a fetus at 28 weeks of gestation demonstrating the presence of bilateral echogenic kidneys.

was preserved. The causes of renal echogenicity in their cases included infantile or autosomal recessive polycystic kidney disease, adult or autosomal recessive polycystic kidney disease, trisomy 13, Pearlman syndrome, and cystic renal dysplasia. Estroff et al. (1991) reported their experience with 19 patients with echogenic kidneys in which the process was bilateral in 14 and unilateral in 5. This group excluded cases of renal dysplasia induced by obstructive uropathy as a cause of increased echogenicity. Surprisingly, only 21% of these fetuses proved to be normal at birth. Five fetuses (26%) did not survive because of associated oligohydramnios in cases of infantile polycystic kidney disease or bilateral multicystic dysplastic kidneys. There was a 53% survival rate in this series. However, all infants had abnormalities, including unilateral renal dysplasia, unilateral multicystic dysplastic kidney and hydronephrosis. The most important prognostic factor in this report was the presence or absence of oligohydramnios. If the amniotic fluid volume is preserved and the fetus is otherwise normal except for echogenic kidneys of uncertain cause the prognosis is good but the infant will be expected to have nonlethal renal disease. In contrast, in cases of echogenic kidneys associated with oligohydramnios the survival rate is dismal (Benacerraf et al. 1998).

▶ MANAGEMENT OF PREGNANCY

The sonographic detection of echogenic kidneys indicates the need for a targeted fetal anatomy scan to be performed to evaluate potentially associated conditions. In particular, it is important to evaluate the amniotic fluid volume and genitourinary tract for signs of obstructive uropathy or features of adult or infantile polycystic kidney disease. In addition, features of cytomegalovirus infection should be sought. Because of reported cases of chromosomal abnormality associated with echogenic kidney, we recommend that a genetic amniocentesis be performed (Chitty et al. 1991; Estroff et al. 1991). Because of the prognostic significance of the development of oligohydramnios in patients with echogenic kidneys, serial scans are indicated. Estroff et al. (1991) noted that echogenic kidneys associated with moderate to severe oligohydramnios have an extremely poor postnatal outcome. In contrast, normal amniotic fluid volume in a fetus with echogenic kidney was associated with a good prognosis. The most important aspect of management of a pregnancy in which echogenic kidneys are detected is to appropriately counsel the parents and systematically exclude potential causes. TORCH titers should be obtained. A family history is essential to rule out polycystic kidney disease. In addition, maternal and paternal renal ultrasound examinations should be performed, due to the high prevalence of adult polycystic kidney disease in the general population (see Chapter 82). The infantile or recessive form of polycystic kidney disease is more commonly observed prenatally, and a fetus with large echogenic kidneys is more likely to have the infantile form if both parents have normal renal ultrasound examinations.

Decisions regarding mode and site of delivery can be deferred until a definitive diagnosis is made or serial scans have demonstrated oligohydramnios or preserved amniotic fluid volume.

▶ FETAL INTERVENTION

There are no fetal interventions for echogenic kidneys.

▶ TREATMENT OF THE NEWBORN

The newborn noted to have echogenic kidneys in utero should undergo careful postnatal examination to exclude potential underlying causes. If a karyotype has not been obtained prenatally it should be done postnatally. A renal ultrasound examination should be obtained to assess the size and echogenicity of the kidney. If hydronephrosis of any degree is detected, the infant should also undergo voiding cystoureterography (VCUG) and a diuretic renal scan to assess function and to evaluate for obstruction and vesicoureteral reflux (see Chapters 78 and 79). By 36 to 48 hours of postnatal age the newborn's serum creatinine and blood urea nitrogen levels should reflect the infant's renal function. The newborn's blood pressure should be carefully monitored in cases of adult or autosomal dominant polycystic kidney disease (Cole et al. 1997) (see Chapter 82).

▶ LONG-TERM OUTCOME

No specific data are available on the long-term outcome for fetuses diagnosed with echogenic kidneys. As this is a sonographic finding and not a specific etiologic diagnosis, the reader is referred to chapters on the specific underlying diagnoses, including polycystic kidneys (see Chapter 85), hydronephrosis (see Chapters 78, 79, and 80), multicystic dysplastic kidneys (see Chapter 82), and trisomy 13 (see Chapter 126).

▶ GENETICS AND RECURRENCE RISK

The risk of recurrence of echogenic kidney depends on whether the underlying cause is sporadic (cytomegalovirus infection, trisomy 13, Beckwith–Wiedemann syndrome) or has a recognized pattern of inheritance. Infantile polycystic kidney disease is inherited as an autosomal recessive condition, and there is a 25% chance that a subsequent pregnancy will be affected, while the adult form of autosomal dominant polycystic kidney disease has a 50% chance of affecting subsequent fetuses. It is not known what percentage of affected fetuses will present in utero with echogenic kidneys in a subsequent pregnancy. However, in autosomal dominant polycystic kidney disease, families should have blood samples collected for DNA analysis prior to a subsequent pregnancy (Breuning et al. 1990). Once a mutation has been identified in a specific family, prenatal DNA diagnosis is available as early as 10 weeks via chorionic villi sampling (see Chapter 82).

REFERENCES

Benacerraf BR. Increased renal echogenicity. Ultrasound of fetal syndromes. New York: Churchill Livingstone, 1998: 422–429.

Brenbridge AN, Chevalier RL, Kaiser DL. Increased renal cortical echogenicity in pediatric renal disease: histopathologic correlations. J Clin Ultrasound 1986;14: 595–600.

Breuning MH, Snijewint FGM, Sauerverse JG, et al. Two step procedure for early diagnosis of polycystic kidney disease with polymorphic DNA markers on both sides of the gene. J Med Genet 1990;27:614–617.

Chitty LS, Griffin DR, Johnson P, et al. The differential diagnosis of enlarged hyperechogenic kidneys with normal or increased liquor volume: report of five cases and review of the literature. Ultrasound Obstet Gynecol 1991;1: 115–121.

Choong KKL, Gruenwald SM, Hodson EM. Echogenic fetal kidneys in cytomegalovirus infection. J Clin Ultrasound 1993;21:128–132.

Cole BR, Conley SB, Stapleton B. Polycystic kidney disease in the first year of life. J Pediatr 1997;11:695–699.

Cramer BC, Jequier S, deChadarvian JP. Factors associated with renal parenchymal echogenicity in the newborn. J Ultrasound Med 1986;5:633–638.

Estroff JA, Mandell J, Benacerraf BR. Increased renal parenchymal echogenicity in the fetus: importance and clinical outcome. Radiology 1991;181:135–139.

Kraus RA, Gaisie G, Young LW. Increased renal parenchymal echogenicity: causes in pediatric patients. Radiographics 1990;10:1009–1018.

Krensky AM, Reddish JM, Littlewood Tiele R. Causes of increased renal echogenicity in pediatric patients. Pediatrics 1983;72:840–846.

CHAPTER 78

Hydronephrosis: Minimal

▶ CONDITION

Hydronephrosis is the most common abnormality reported on prenatal sonographic screening (Blyth et al. 1993; Thomas 1990). The vast majority of cases are mild, so-called physiologic hydronephrosis, which are of no clinical significance. Numerous theories have been proposed to try to account for this common finding. In the past, one popular theory was that mild fetal hydronephrosis resulted from changes in maternal hydration. However, Hoddick et al. (1985) demonstrated that the degree of maternal hydration had no significant influence on fetal urinary tract dilation. These findings were subsequently confirmed by Allen et al. (1987). Other potential causes suggested for mild dilation of the fetal urinary tract include transient obstruction, vesicoureteral reflux, and natural kinks and folds in the ureter that may occur during development (Homsy et al. 1986; Najmaldin et al. 1990; Zerrin et al. 1993). The hormonal milieu of the fetus may influence the renal pelvic diameter. Maternal hydronephrosis commonly occurs during pregnancy because of the influence of progesterone, a known smooth-muscle relaxant. It has been suggested that maternal progesterone may also be responsible for mild fetal upper urinary tract dilatation (Cendron et al. 1994).

Distinguishing physiologic fetal renal pelvic distention from significant or pathologic hydronephrosis is a challenge that requires accurate prenatal sonography and follow-up evaluation. Renal pelvic distention may range in anterior/posterior (AP) diameter from 3 to 11 mm in up to 18% of normal fetuses studied after 24 weeks of gestation (Hoddick et al. 1985). Because fetal hydronephrosis is so common, Arger et al. (1985) proposed criteria to help distinguish abnormal renal pelvic dilatation. They suggested that a pelvic diameter of >10 mm or a ratio of the AP pelvic diameter to the AP renal diameter >0.5 indicated significant fetal hy-

dronephrosis (Fig. 78-1). These criteria were subsequently modified by addition of caliectasis as an additional indicator of significant hydronephrosis (Kleiner et al. 1987). This study suggested that caliectasis may be an even more sensitive and reliable indicator for predicting pathologic hydronephrosis than simple pelviectasis (Fig. 78-2). Renal pelvic dilatation less than these criteria for pathologic hydronephrosis is considered minimal fetal hydronephrosis. Morin et al. (1996) defined minimal hydronephrosis as renal pelvic dilatation >4 but <10 mm in a fetus that was less than 24 weeks of gestation (Fig. 78-3).

▶ INCIDENCE

When a number of clinical studies are pooled, the calculated incidence of detectable dilatation of the fetal urinary tract approaches 1 in 100 pregnancies (Thomas 1990). However, difficulties in assessing the true incidence of pathologic fetal hydronephrosis stem from the high incidence of physiologic hydronephrosis and the limitations of criteria used to define pathologic urinary tract dilatation (Gruppe 1987). The overall incidence of congenital hydronephrosis in a large-scale maternal–fetal screening program in Sweden was 0.17% (Helin and Persson 1986). This figure was lower than the one reported (0.76%) in Britain, in a well-designed prospective study using antenatal ultrasonography at a specific time during pregnancy (Livero et al. 1989). In many of these cases, however, a large number of the fetuses displayed what would be considered physiologic hydronephrosis, in other words, the so-called minimal pyelectasis. Follow-up studies in patients diagnosed with prenatal hydronephrosis showed that only 1 in 500 fetuses required prenatal or postnatal intervention for hydronephrosis (Thomas 1990).

REFERENCES

Allen KS, Arger PH, Mennuti M, et al. Effects of maternal hydration on fetal pyelectasis. Radiology 1987;163: 807–809.

Arant BS. Neonatal adjustments to extra-uterine life. In: Edelmann CM Jr, ed. Pediatric kidney disease. 2nd ed. Boston: Little, Brown, 1992:1015–1042.

Arger PH, Coleman BG, Mintz MC, et al. Routine fetal genitourinary tract screening. Radiology 1985;156:485–489.

Avni EF, Rodesch F, Shulman CC. Fetal uropathy: diagnostic pitfalls and management. J Urol 1985;134:921–926.

Berman DJ, Maizels M. The role of urinary obstruction in the genesis of renal dysplasia. J Urol 1983;128:1091–1098.

Blane CE, Koff SA, Bowerman RA, et al. Nonobstructive fetal hydronephrosis: sonographic recognition and therapeutic implications. Radiology 1983;147:95–99.

Blyth B, Snyder HM, Duckett JW. Antenatal diagnosis and subsequent management of hydronephrosis. J Urol 1993; 149:693–698.

Bronshtein M, Yoffe N, Brandes JM, et al. First and early second trimester diagnosis of fetal urinary tract anomalies using transvaginal sonography. Prenat Diagn 1990;10: 653–666.

Cendron M, D'Alton ME, Crombleholme TM. Prenatal diagnosis and management of the fetus with hydronephrosis. Semin Perinatol 1994;18:163–181.

Daucher JN, Mandell J, Lebowitz RL. Urinary tract infection in infants in spite of prenatal diagnosis of hydronephrosis. Pediatr Radiol 1992;22:401–404.

D'Alton ME, DeCherney AH. Prenatal diagnosis. N Engl J Med 1993;328:114–120.

Dejter SW, Gibbons MD. The fate of infant kidneys with fetal hydronephrosis but initially normal postnatal sonography. J Urol 1989;142: 661–663.

Duckett JW. When to operate on neonatal hydronephrosis. Urology 1993;42:617–619.

Glazer GM, Filly RA, Callen PW. The varied sonographic appearance of the urinary tract in the fetus and newborn with urethral obstruction. Radiology 1982;144: 563–568.

Golbus MS, Harrison MR, Filly RA, et al. Prenatal diagnosis and treatment of fetal hydronephrosis. Semin Perinatol 1983;7:102–107.

Gordon I, Dhillon HK, Gatanah H, et al. Antenatal diagnosis of pelvic hydronephrosis: assessment of renal function and drainage as a guide to management. J Nucl Med 1991;32:1649–1654.

Gruppe WE. The dilemma of intrauterine diagnosis of congenital renal disease. Pediatr Clin North Am 1987;34: 629–637.

Harrison MR, Adzick NS. The fetus as a patient: surgical considerations. Ann Surg 1991;213:279–291.

Harrison MR, Filly RA. The fetus with obstructive uropathy: pathophysiology, natural history, selection and treatment. In: Harrison MR, Golbus MS, Filly RA, eds. The unborn patient: prenatal diagnosis and treatment. 2nd ed. Philadelphia: Saunders, 1991:328–393.

Harrison MR, Golbus MS, Filly RA, et al. Fetal surgery for congenital hydronephrosis. N Engl J Med 1982;306: 591–593.

Helin I, Persson PH. Prenatal diagnosis of urinary tract abnormalities by ultrasound. Pediatrics 1986;78:879–883.

Hoddick WK, Filly RA, Mahony BS, et al. Minimal fetal renal pyelectasis. J Ultrasound Med 1985;4:85–87.

Homsy YL, Williot P, Danais S. Transitional neonatal hydronephrosis: fact or fantasy? J Urol 1986;136:339–341.

Kleiner B, Callen PW, Filly RA. Sonographic analysis of the fetus with ureteropelvic junction obstruction. AJR Am J Roentgenol 1987;148:359–365.

Koff SA. Pathophysiology of ureteropelvic junction obstruction: clinical and experimental observations. Urol Clin North Am 1990;17:263–272.

Livero LN, Brookfield DSK, Egginton JA, et al. Antenatal ultrasonography to detect fetal renal abnormalities: a prospective screening program. BMJ 1989;298:1421–1423.

Mahoney BS, Filly RA, Callen PW, et al. Sonographic evaluation of fetal renal dysplasia. Radiology 1984;152: 143–149.

Morin L, Cendron M, Crombleholme TM, et al. Minimal hydronephrosis in the fetus: clinical significance and implications for management. J Urol 1996;155:2047–2049.

Najmaldin A, Burge DM, Atwell JD. Fetal vesicoureteral reflux. Br J Urol 1990;65:403–406.

Noe NH, Magill HL. Progression of mild ureteropelvic junction obstruction in infancy. Urology 1987;30:348–351.

Patten RM, Mack LA, Wang KY, et al. The fetal genitourinary tract. Radiol Clin North Am 1990;28:115–130.

Reznick VM, Kaplan GW, Murphy JL, et al. Follow-up of infants with bilateral renal disease detected in utero. Am J Dis Child 1988;142:453–456.

Scott JES, Renwick M. Antenatal diagnosis of congenital abnormalities in the urinary tract. Br J Urol 1987;62: 295–299.

Thomas DFM. Fetal uropathy. Br J Urol 1990;66:225–231.

Watson AR, Readett D, Nelson CS, et al. Dilemmas associated with antenatal detected urinary tract abnormalities. Arch Dis Child 1988;63:719–722.

Zerrin JM, Ritchey ML, Chang ACH. Incidental vesicoureteral reflux in neonates with antenatally detected hydronephrosis and other renal abnormalities. Pediatr Radiol 1993; 187:157–160.

CHAPTER 79

Hydronephrosis: Ureteropelvic Junction Obstruction

▶ CONDITION

Obstruction at the ureteropelvic junction (UPJ) is the most common cause of neonatal hydronephrosis (Lebowitz and Griscom 1986). Because 85 to 90% of affected newborns appear entirely normal on physical examination at birth, prenatal recognition permits treatment of a condition that may have gone unrecognized for years (Grignon et al. 1986). This form of hydronephrosis is characterized by obstruction to the flow of urine from the renal pelvis to the ureter. There have been numerous causes proposed for UPJ obstruction but no clear cause is established in most cases of this form of obstructive uropathy. Among the suggested causes are intrinsic valves at the UPJ, abnormally thickened or oriented muscular bands at the UPJ, high insertion of the ureter on the renal pelvis, anomalous crossing bands or vessels at the UPJ, ischemia, and segmental ureteral dismotility (Hendren et al. 1980; Johnston et al. 1977; Kelalis et al. 1971; Maizels and Stephens 1980; Williams and Karlaftis 1966). In the majority of cases, however, a patent UPJ is found at the time of surgical correction. The obstruction appears to be more functional than mechanical.

While the pathogenesis of UPJ obstruction is poorly understood, some aspects of the prenatal history are known. Complete obstruction at the UPJ before 8 to 10 weeks of gestation results in severe dysplastic changes in the developing kidney (McGrory 1980; Potter 1976; Sanders and Hartman 1984; Scholtmeijer and van der Harten 1975). The result is a multicystic dysplastic kidney (see Chapter 82). In contrast, incomplete UPJ obstruction that occurs during the first or second trimester does not result in multicystic dysplastic kid-

ney but may result in variable degrees of renal dysplasia, in addition to pelvicaliceal dilatation. In contrast, UPJ obstruction that occurs during the third trimester may result in marked pelvicaliceal dilatation, but usually does not cause renal dysplasia.

The diagnosis of UPJ obstruction in the fetus is based on pelvicaliceal dilatation that exceeds proposed criteria for minimal fetal hydronephrosis (see Chapter 78). Specifically, an anterior-posterior (AP) pelvic diameter of the renal pelvis ≥10 mm or the presence of caliectasis (Arger et al. 1985; Kleiner et al. 1987). To distinguish UPJ obstruction from other causes of obstructive uropathy, there must also be pelvic dilatation and an absence of findings suggestive of obstructive uropathy at a lower level, such as ureterectasis, vesicomegaly, ectopic ureterocele, and dilated posterior urethra. Although UPJ obstruction is, in large part, a diagnosis of exclusion, ultrasound examination has proven reliable in determining the level of obstruction (Kleiner et al. 1987).

▶ INCIDENCE

The overall incidence of genitourinary defects diagnosed by prenatal ultrasound examination has been estimated to be between 0.2 and 0.9%. The incidence of UPJ obstruction is estimated at 0.001% with a male:female ratio of 2:1. In newborns the left side is affected in almost two thirds of cases. Bilateral UPJ obstruction is seen postnatally in only 15% of cases (Johnston et al. 1977) but may be more common in prenatally diagnosed cases, as observed by Flake et al. (1986).

▶ SONOGRAPHIC FINDINGS

In unilateral UPJ obstruction the renal pelvis and infundibulum are dilated (Fig. 79-1). Dilation of the calices may also be seen. The anterior to posterior pelvis:kidney ratio is greater than 50% (Arger et al. 1985). The following findings are not seen in UPJ obstruction: dilated ureter, ectopic ureterocele, dilated or thickened urinary bladder, or a dilated posterior urethra. In more severe cases of UPJ obstruction only a single fluid-filled structure may be seen. This is the dilated pelvis with only a thin rim of cortex around it (Fig. 79-2) (Mahony 1994). In even more severe cases, the renal pelvis may be dilated into an abdominal cyst in which not even a rim of renal parenchyma is seen. These UPJ obstructions can reach significant size, distending the fetal abdomen and elevating the diaphragm (Jaffe et al. 1987). In rare instances, both the infundibulum and the renal pelvis are stenotic and only caliceal dilation is seen (Lucaya et al. 1984). In the most severe form of UPJ obstruction, the collecting system can rupture, with the formation of a perinephric urinoma. It is unusual to have salvageable renal function in a kidney with a perinephric hematoma (Adzick et al. 1985; Callen et al. 1983; Friedland et al. 1983; Harrison and Filly 1991). In unilateral UPJ obstruction, the contralateral kidney produces a normal volume of amniotic fluid and the bladder fills and empties normally, even in cases in which the UPJ obstruction has resulted in renal dysplasia. It is important to recognize that UPJ obstruction may be seen frequently in association with contralateral multicystic dysplastic kidney or renal agenesis. Either condition, in association with high-grade UPJ obstruction, may produce profound oligohydramnios (Mahony 1994).

Bilateral UPJ obstruction is present in 15 to 50% of cases, depending on the series reported (Flake et al. 1986; Kleiner et al. 1987). Fortunately, the involvement is often asymmetric and severe bilateral obstruction is rare. However, as reported by Flake et al. up to 5% mortality can be seen with bilateral UPJ obstruction, which progresses to oligohydramnios and secondary pulmonary hypoplasia.

UPJ obstruction paradoxically results in polyhydramnios in up to 25% of cases (Kleiner et al. 1987). The pathophysiology of the polyhydramnios is uncertain but is thought to be due to hyperfiltration occurring in the partially obstructed kidneys.

▶ DIFFERENTIAL DIAGNOSIS

The differential diagnosis of UPJ obstruction includes all other causes of hydronephrosis, including vesicoureteral reflux, megaureter, obstructed duplicated collecting system, and bladder-outlet obstruction (Table 79-1). A detailed sonographic evaluation of the kidneys should differentiate the anatomic level of obstruction causing hydronephrosis. Bladder-outlet obstruction,

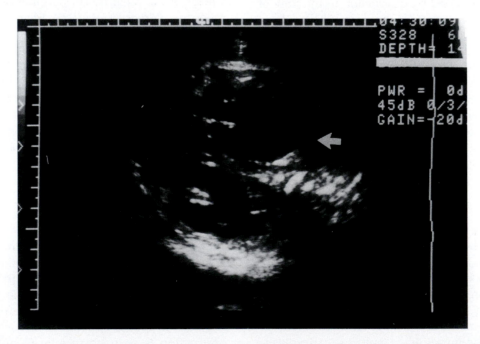

Figure 79-1. Sonogram at 24 weeks of gestation in coronal section of the fetal kidneys demonstrating characteristic features of UPJ obstruction affecting both kidneys with markedly dilated renal pelvis and calices. *(Reprinted, with permission, from Cendron M, D'Alton ME, Crombleholme TM. Prenatal diagnosis and management of the fetus with hydronephrosis. Semin Perinatol 1994;18:163–181.)*

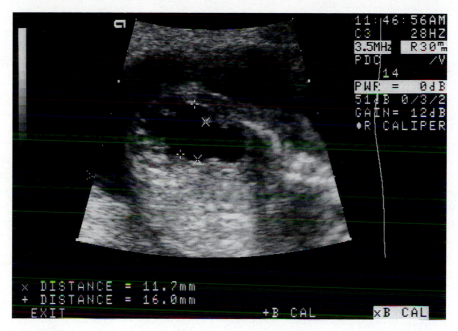

Figure 79-2. Sagittal section of fetal kidney with UPJ obstruction demonstrating markedly dilated renal pelvis and calices and thinning of the cortex.

whether due to urethral atresia or posterior urethral valves, should be associated with vesicomegaly with a thick and often trabeculated bladder wall. Cases of ureterovesical obstruction, such as megaureter, are distinguished by the lack of vesicomegaly, with a dilated tortuous ureter extending from the renal pelvis to the ureterovesical junction. A duplex collecting system frequently results in hydronephrosis due to obstruction at the site of the ureteral insertion, often at an ectopic site. This may occur in association with a ureterocele (see

Chapter 81). In such cases, the ureter is uniformly dilated up the superior pole of the kidney, which may have cystic dysplastic changes from long-standing high-grade obstruction.

Vesicoureteral reflux may occur in association with UPJ obstruction and may be difficult to distinguish from UPJ obstruction as a cause of hydronephrosis. One sonographic observation that is helpful in distinguishing between these two diagnoses is observing the degree of pelvic dilation that occurs with bladder emptying. UPJ obstruction is minimally affected by voiding; however, vesicoureteral reflux is usually evidenced by marked fluctuations in the size of the ureter and renal pelvis associated with bladder contraction.

► **TABLE 79-1.** CAUSES OF FETAL
HYDRONEPHROSIS

Bilateral hydronephrosis
  Supravesical obstruction
    Bilateral UPJ junction obstruction
    Bilateral ureterovesical junction obstruction
  Infravesical obstruction
    Posterior urethral valves
    Urethral atresia
    Obstructing ureterocele
  Vesicoureteral reflux (bilateral, usually high-grade)
  Prune belly syndrome
  Megacystis–megaureter complex
Unilateral hydronephrosis
  UPJ obstruction
  Ureterovesical junction obstruction
  Multicystic dysplastic kidney
  Megaureter (nonobstructing, nonrefluxing) (may be
    bilateral)
  Renal duplication (may be bilateral)
  Dilated loop of bowel

► **ANTENATAL NATURAL HISTORY**

The most important determinants of the outcome of UPJ obstruction in the fetus are the gestational age at onset, severity of obstruction, and whether the UPJ obstruction is unilateral or bilateral. In early gestation, high-grade obstruction at the ureteropelvic junction that occurs during the first trimester results in a multicystic dysplastic kidney. We have sonographically observed the progression from early UPJ obstruction to multicystic dysplastic kidney. In UPJ obstruction that occurs during the second trimester, the fetal kidneys are at risk for renal dysplasia and compromised renal function at birth. In contrast, UPJ obstruction that occurs during the last trimester rarely causes renal dysplasia, even in cases of high-grade obstruction. This vulnerability of the developing kidney to obstruction-induced dysplasia likely reflects the effect of increased pressure during the nephrogenic phase of renal development between 20 and 30 weeks of gestation (Harrison and Filly 1991).

In some cases, pelvicaliceal dilatation due to UPJ obstruction resolves during gestation. In the series reported by Flake et al. (1986), 2 cases resolved. One was a case of unilateral UPJ obstruction and one was a case of bilateral UPJ obstruction.

Our understanding of the prenatal history of UPJ obstruction is still evolving. UPJ obstruction is usually thought to be a benign condition. Flake et al. (1986) challenged this view with their results of a review of 28 fetuses referred to a fetal treatment center with prenatally diagnosed UPJ obstruction in 44 kidneys. This series was unusual in that over half the cases were bilateral, as compared with the usually quoted lower rates of 5 to 20% (Hendren et al. 1980; Johnston et al. 1977; Kelalis et al. 1971; Williams and Karlaftis 1966). These were isolated sonographic findings in asymptomatic pregnant women in 19 of the 28 cases. However, polyhydramnios, preterm labor, intrauterine growth restriction, vaginal bleeding, and twin gestation prompted ultrasound examination in the remaining 9 cases. All but 5 newborns required surgical intervention postnatally, ranging from nephrostomy to pyeloplasty, ureteroureterostomy, or nephrectomy. Nongenitourinary anomalies were noted in 5 of the 28 fetuses. There was a 5% mortality rate in this series, with all deaths occurring in cases of bilateral UPJ obstruction (Flake et al. 1986).

Progression during gestation in the degree of hydronephrosis in cases of UPJ obstruction is a reliable predictor of the need for postnatal surgical decompression. Harrison and Filly (1991) felt that progression was more likely in bilateral UPJ obstruction. However, the degree of hydronephrosis seen in utero does not always correlate with postnatal parenchymal function.

Polyhydramnios may be seen in 25 to 33% of cases of UPJ obstruction (Flake et al. 1986; Kleiner et al. 1987). Polyhydramnios has been described in association with impaired renal function and bilateral obstruction (Laing et al. 1984; Hadlock et al. 1981; Henderson et al. 1980). It has been suggested that polyhydramnios occurring in UPJ obstruction is due to impaired renal concentrating ability, resulting in higher urine output (Harrison and Filly 1991).

While the prognosis in unilateral UPJ obstruction is usually excellent, there is a high incidence of genitourinary abnormalities in the contralateral side. These abnormalities may range from multicystic dysplasia to vesicoureteral reflux. However, because there is usually a normally functioning kidney on the contralateral side, amniotic fluid volume is maintained and there is no adverse affect on outcome of pregnancy and neonatal survival. Even in cases in which renal dysplasia complicates UPJ obstruction, there is often a compensatory increase in renal mass and function in the contralateral kidney (Sauer et al. 1986).

The prognosis in bilateral UPJ obstruction is somewhat more guarded. There is a 5% mortality associated with high-grade bilateral UPJ obstruction (Flake et al. 1986). In addition, fetuses with bilateral UPJ obstruction are at increased risk for polyhydramnios, progression in the degree of obstruction, and oligohydramnios in the most severe cases. While unilateral UPJ obstruction is an indication for postnatal genitourinary evaluation, it usually has few implications for the management of the pregnancy. In contrast, fetuses with bilateral UPJ obstruction should undergo serial sonographic assessments of the degree of dilation, renal parenchymal changes, and amniotic fluid volume.

In the series by Flake et al. (1986), oligohydramnios developed in 4 fetuses with bilateral UPJ obstruction, prompting early delivery. All 4 were delivered at 32 to 35 weeks of gestation and underwent pyeloplasty during the neonatal period, with normal renal function after repair. Nineteen of the 23 patients underwent pyeloplasty. Seven pyeloplasties were performed in cases of unilateral UPJ obstruction, with evidence of impaired function in the kidney. All had improved or stable function following pyeloplasty. Twelve pyeloplasties were performed in 9 patients with bilateral UPJ obstruction. In 5 of the 9, renal function was abnormal but became normal after pyeloplasty. An indication of the severity of UPJ obstruction in this group of patients is the 9 nephrectomies performed, either for multicystic dysplastic kidneys, perinephric urinomas or kidneys with no demonstrable renal function on preoperative diuretic renal scan.

▶ MANAGEMENT OF PREGNANCY

The fetus diagnosed with UPJ obstruction should have a prompt referral for detailed sonographic assessment to confirm the diagnosis, evaluate associated genitourinary abnormalities, and possible associated nongenitourinary abnormalities. There is an overall increased incidence of chromosomal abnormalities in cases of obstructive uropathy, and consideration should be given to amniocentesis for karyotype analysis. It is important to perform a level 2 scan to exclude other associated renal and extrarenal anomalies such as horseshoe kidney, multicystic dysplastic kidney, as well as diaphragmatic hernia, hydrocephalus, and congenital cystic adenomatoid malformation (Harrison and Filly 1991).

Pregnant women carrying a fetus suspected of having UPJ obstruction should be referred to a pediatric surgeon or pediatric urologist for prenatal consultation. In cases of isolated UPJ obstruction, a favorable prognosis can be anticipated, and routine obstetric care can be performed with planned postnatal genitourinary evaluation. In cases of bilateral UPJ obstruction or unilateral UPJ obstruction associated with either multicystic dysplastic kidney or renal agenesis, serial sonographic examinations at least every 2 to 3 weeks should be performed to evaluate progression in obstruction and development of oligohydramnios or polyhydramnios.

▶ FETAL INTERVENTION

In unilateral UPJ obstruction there is no indication for fetal intervention. However, in high-grade bilateral UPJ obstruction or unilateral UPJ obstruction associated with a multicystic dysplastic or renal agenesis, consideration may be given to fetal intervention. Fetuses with bilateral high-grade UPJ obstruction associated with a contralateral multicystic dysplastic kidney or renal agenesis that presents after 30 weeks of gestation should be considered for steroid administration and early delivery (Flake et al. 1986; Harrison and Filly 1991). Cases that present prior to 30 weeks of gestation may be candidates for evaluation for fetal intervention. Prognostic evaluation consists of direct sampling of fetal urine. Laboratory values associated with a good prognosis include a fetal urine sodium of less than 100 Meq per liter, chloride of less than 90 meq per liter and an osmolarity of less than 210 mOsm per liter, and a β_2-microglobulin of less than 4 mg per liter (Cendron et al. 1994; Crombleholme et al. 1990; Mandelbrot et al. 1991). Laboratory values for fetal urine electrolytes above these limits are associated with a poor postnatal prognosis.

Fetuses with bilateral high-grade UPJ obstruction, complicated by oligohydramnios, in which a good prognostic profile was obtained by direct renal pelvic tap for fetal urine electrolyte analysis, may be candidates for intervention. Placement of a Rocket catheter into the renal pelvis under ultrasound guidance may restore amniotic fluid volume and prevent ongoing damage to the obstructed kidney.

▶ TREATMENT OF THE NEWBORN

Once a fetus has been found on prenatal ultrasound examination to have a significant degree of hydronephrosis, careful follow-up should be planned to ensure proper postnatal treatment. At the time of the initial prenatal diagnosis of hydronephrosis, parental counseling is recommended. A team approach is extremely helpful to inform the parents and to help them understand the implications of this prenatal diagnosis (Cendron et al. 1994).

Every newborn with a prenatal diagnosis of hydronephrosis should undergo a detailed physical examination at birth for signs of sequelae from obstructive uropathy. Monitoring of the urinary output within the first 24 to 48 hours is unreliable. Failure to void during the first 2 days after birth may reflect normal fluid shifts or may be the first sign of a significant functional urologic abnormality (Arant 1992). The differential diagnosis in the neonate who does not void within the first 48 hours includes obstructive uropathy, renal failure, neurogenic bladder, and the effects of maternal medication (Arant 1992). However, most patients with an obstruction will void, albeit with a weak stream, within the first 2 days of life. Serum electrolyte, blood urea nitrogen, and creatinine levels measured within the first day of life are a reflection of maternal renal function via placental exchange. It is best to wait at least 24 hours to measure these values. The most helpful test in the initial evaluation of the newborn with prenatally diagnosed hydronephrosis is an ultrasound examination of the abdomen, including the bladder. Timing of the postnatal ultrasound examination depends on the degree of prenatal hydronephrosis (Dejter and Gibbons 1989). If severe dilation of the renal pelvis has been detected antenatally, then early ultrasound evaluation should be performed so as to permit early intervention. Otherwise, ultrasound examination can be postponed for 3 to 7 days in order to let the physiologic diuresis that usually occurs in the first 48 hours of life resolve (Arant 1992). If the initial postnatal renal ultrasound examination is normal, the evaluation should be pursued with a repeat study in 3 to 4 weeks. Fifty percent of neonates with UPJ and vesicoureteral reflux who were diagnosed antenatally with hydronephrosis have a normal upper urinary tract at the time of the first postnatal ultrasound examination (Dejter and Gibbons 1989).

Mild cases of hydronephrosis can be treated conservatively with observation, and may warrant only one or two ultrasound examinations during the postnatal period. It is rare for mild dilation of the upper-urinary tract to progress. In cases in which other findings are seen, such as cortical thinning, or upper-tract dilation with a normal bladder, voiding cystourethrography (VCUG) should be performed to evaluate for the presence of vesicoureteral reflux (VUR). If VUR is noted, then a renal nuclear medicine scan 99 technetium-diethylenetriaminepentaacetic (DTPA) or mercaptoacetyltriglycine (MAGIII) will be helpful in documenting function of the kidneys. If no evidence of reflux is noted on VCUG, then a MAGIII with furosemide should be obtained to evaluate the upper-urinary tract for a possible UPJ obstruction. If UPJ obstruction is noted, treatment is determined by the severity of the obstruction. In severe UPJ obstruction, in which a kidney shows 35% or less function, pyeloplasty should be performed. In the cases in which mild to moderate obstruction is noted, and the kidney has more than 35% function, observation alone may be indicated, with a repeat ultrasound examination in 3 months. A repeat renal scan will help to assess changes in renal function. As stated earlier, there is growing evidence to suggest that a mild degree of UPJ obstruction may not be functionally significant and does not warrant surgical intervention (Koff 1990; Gordon et al. 1991; Duckett 1993).

If prenatal ultrasound examination shows a multicystic dysplastic kidney, a VCUG and a renal scan should be obtained. These studies confirm the lack of function in the affected kidney and rule out any abnormalities in the contralateral kidney (Flack and Bellinger 1993).

Surgical intervention at birth is required in cases in which a severe obstruction will jeopardize renal function. This applies most often to cases of posterior urethral valves, obstructing ureterocele, and severe UPJ obstruction affecting a solitary kidney. Emergency surgical treatment is seldom warranted. Reconstruction of the urinary tract should not be attempted until the newborn has stabilized from a medical standpoint and has been fully evaluated. Temporary decompression of the urinary tract in cases of severe UPJ obstruction can be achieved by placement of a nephrostomy tube until definitive repair of the urinary tract can be accomplished. In the presence of a solitary kidney, every attempt should be made to ensure adequate drainage so as to not further jeopardize renal function.

Finally, current recommendations in treating the neonate with prenatally diagnosed hydronephrosis include the administration of prophylactic antibiotics, usually a penicillin derivative. In the past, most patients with hydronephrosis presented with a urinary-tract infection later in life. The incidence of urinary-tract infection in the setting of prenatally diagnosed hydronephrosis has not been thoroughly evaluated, but one study found that 3% of patients being evaluated radiologically during the first 6 months of life were found to have a positive culture from a catheterized specimen (Dacher et al. 1992).

▶ LONG-TERM OUTCOME

The long-term outcome of UPJ obstruction depends on whether it is unilateral or bilateral and if there is an underlying renal dysplasia. In the absence of renal dysplasia, renal function often returns to base-line levels following pyeloplasty. In cases in which UPJ obstruction has caused dysplastic changes, compensatory hypertrophy in the normal contralateral kidney ensures an excellent prognosis. However, in cases of contralateral multicystic dysplastic kidney or renal agenesis, renal dysplasia induced by UPJ obstruction will lead to progressive renal insufficiency and ultimately renal failure necessitating renal transplantation. This later group of patients requires follow-up with a pediatric nephrologist as well as a pediatric urologist.

▶ GENETICS AND RECURRENCE RISK

In general, VUR has a high familial incidence. It is thought to be an autosomal dominant condition with reduced penetrance (Devriendt et al. 1998). Multiple case reports suggest inheritance of a gene that specifically predisposes to UPJ obstruction. These include affected identical twin females, a mother and two children, and multiple siblings in different families (Buscemi et al. 1985; Cohen et al. 1978; Sidebottom and Sadlowski 1984). In 1 report, histocompatability typing of a family with 15 members and a history of UPJ stenosis suggested that the renal malformation and histocompatability haplotype were linked (Senger et al. 1979). More recently, study of a large affected kindred using DNA linkage markers on the short arm of chromosome 6 concluded that there was no linkage between the presence of ureteral abnormalities and the HLA genes (Klemme et al. 1998).

Whether inheritance of UPJ obstruction is dominant or multifactorial, it is clear that siblings are at increased risk for uropathology. In 1 study, 37 siblings of 20 probands with UPJ obstruction were evaluated with intravenous pyelography and VCUG. Fourteen of the 37 (38%) had some form of uropathology that required subsequent therapy (Dwoskin 1979). This author recommended that siblings of children with UPJ obstruction be investigated for uropathology regardless of age or sex.

Prenatal sonographic examination in subsequent pregnancies is indicated due to as much as a 50% recurrence risk.

REFERENCES

Adzick NS, Harrison MR, Flake AW. Urinary extravasation in the fetus with obstructive uropathy. J Pediatr Surg 1985; 20:608–614.

Arger PH, Coleman BG, Mintz MC, et al. Routine fetal genitourinary tract screening. Radiology 1985;156:485–489.

Arant BS. Neonatal adjustment of extrauterine life. In: Edelmann CM Jr, ed. Pediatric kidney disease. 2nd ed. Boston: Little, Brown, 1992;1015–1042.

Buscemi M, Shanske A, Mallet E, Ozoktay S, Hanna MK. Dominantly inherited ureteropelvic junction. Urology 1985;26:568–571.

Callen PW, Bolding P, Filly RA, et al. Ultrasonographic evaluation of fetal paranephric pseudocysts. J Ultrasound Med 1983;2:309–313.

Cendron M, D'Alton ME, Crombleholme TM. Prenatal diagnosis and management of the fetus with hydronephrosis. Semin Perinatol 1994;18:163–181.

Cohen B, Goldman SM, Kopilnick M, Khurana AV, Salik JO. Ureteropelvic junction obstruction: its occurrence in 3 members of a single family. J Urol 1978;120:361–364.

Crombleholme TM, Harrison MR, Golbus MS, et al. Fetal intervention in obstructive uropathy: prognostic indicators and efficacy of intervention. Am J Obstet Gynecol 1990; 162:1239–1244.

Dacher JN, Mandell J, Lebewitz RL. Urinary tract infection in infants in spite of prenatal diagnosis of hydronephrosis. Pediatr Radiol 1992;22:401–403.

Dejter SW, Gibbons MD. The fate of infant kidneys with fetal hydronephrosis but initially normal postnatal sonography. J Urol 1989;142:661–663.

Devriendt K, Gorenen P, VanEsch H, et al. Vesico-ureteral reflux: a genetic condition? Eur J Pediatr 1998;157: 265–271.

Duckett JW. When to operate on neonatal hydronephrosis. Urology 1993;42:617–619.

Dwoskin Y. Ureteropelvic junction obstruction and sibling uropathology. Urology 1979;13:153–154.

Flack CE, Bellinger MF. The multicystic dysplastic kidney and contralateral vesicoureteral reflux: protection of the solitary kidney. J Urol 1993;150:1873–1874.

Flake AW, Adzick NS, Harrison MR, et al. Ureteropelvic junction obstruction. J Pediatr Surg 1986;21:1058–1064.

Friedland G, Filly RA, Goris M, et al. Uroradiology: an integrated approach. New York: Churchill-Livingstone, 1983.

Gordon I, Dhillon HK, Gatanah H, et al. Antenatal diagnosis of pelvic hydronephrosis: assessment of renal function and drainage as a guide to management. J Nucl Med 1991;32:1649–1654.

Grignon A, Filiatrault D, Homsy YL, et al. Ureteropelvic junction stenosis: antenatal sonographic diagnosis, postnatal investigation and follow-up. Radiology 1986;160: 649–654.

Hadlock FP, Peter RL, Carpenter R, et al. Sonography of fetal urinary tract anomalies. AJR Am J Roentgenol 1981; 137:261–267.

Harrison MR, Filly RA. The fetus with obstructive uropathy: pathophysiology, natural history, selection and treatment. In: Harrison MR, Golbus MS, Filly RA, eds. The unborn patient: prenatal diagnosis and treatment. 2nd ed. Philadelphia: Saunders, 1991;328–393.

Henderson SC, VanKolkin RJ, Rahotzoh M. Multicystic kidney with hydramnios. J Clin Ultrasound 1980;8:249–255.

Hendren WH, Radhakishnan J, Middleton AW. Pediatric pyeloplasty. J Pediatr Surg 1980;15:133–141.

Jaffe R, Abramowitz J, Fejgin M, et al. Giant fetal abdominal cyst: ultrasonic diagnosis and management. J Ultrasound Med 1987;6:45–50.

Johnston JH, Evans JP, Glassbert KI, et al. Pelvic hydronephrosis in children: a review of 219 personal cases. J Urol 1977;117:97–103.

Kelalis PP, Culp OS, Stickler GB, et al. Uretopelvic obstruction in children: Experience with 109 cases. J Urol 1971; 706:418–424.

Kleiner B, Callen PW, Filly RA. Sonographic analysis of the fetus with ureteropelvic junction obstruction. Am J Radiol 1987;148:359–365.

Klemme L, Fish AJ, Richs R, et al. Familial ureteral abnormalities syndrome: genomic mapping, clinical findings. Pediatr Nephrol 1998;12:349–356.

Koff SA. Pathophysiology of ureteropelvic junction obstruction: clinical and experimental observations. Urol Clin North Am 1990;17:263–272.

Laing VD, Burke VC, Wing VW, et al. Post-partum evaluation of fetal hydronephrosis: optimal timing for follow-up sonography. Radiology 1984;152:423–424.

Lebowitz RL, Griscom NT. Neonatal hydronephrosis— 146 cases. Radiol Clin North Am 1986;7:275–282.

Lucaya J, Enriquez G, Delgado R, et al. Infundibulopelvic stenosis in children. AJR Am J Roentgenol 1984;142: 471–476.

Mahony BS. Ultrasound evaluation of the fetal genitourinary tract. In: Callen PW, ed. Ultrasonography in obstetrics and gynecology. 3rd ed. Philadelphia: Saunders, 1994: 389–419.

Maizels M, Stephens FD. Valves of the ureter as a cause of primary obstruction of the ureter: anatomic, embryologic, and clinical aspects. J Urol 1980;123:742–745.

Mandelbrot L, Dumez Y, Muller F, et al. Prenatal prediction of renal function in fetal obstructive uropathies. J Perinat Med 1991;19:283–287.

McGrory WW. Regulation of renal functional development Urol Clin North Am 1980;7:243–252.

Potter EL. Kidneys, ureters, urinary bladder, and urethra. In: Potter EL, Craig JM, eds. Pathology of the fetus and neonate. 3rd ed. Chicago: Year Book, 1976:434–473.

Sanders RC, Hartman DS. The sonographic distinction between neonatal multicystic kidney and hydronephrosis. Radiology 1984;151:621–627.

Sauer L, Glick RL, Adzick NS, et al. Compensatory renal growth following nephrectomy in fetal lambs. Surg Forum 1986;37:648–651.

Scholtmeijer RT, van der Harten JJ. Unilateral multicystic kidney and contralateral hydronephrosis in the newborn. Br J Urol 1975;47:176–181.

Senger DP, Rashid A, Wolfish NM. Familial urinary tract anomalies: association with the major histocampatibility complex in man. J Urol 1979;121:194–197.

Sidebottom RA, Sadlowski RW. Bilateral ureteropelvic junction obstructions in newborn identical twins. Urology 1984;24:379–381.

Williams DI, Karlaftis CM. Hydronephrosis due to pelvi-ureteric obstruction in the newborn. Br J Urol 1966;38: 138–146.

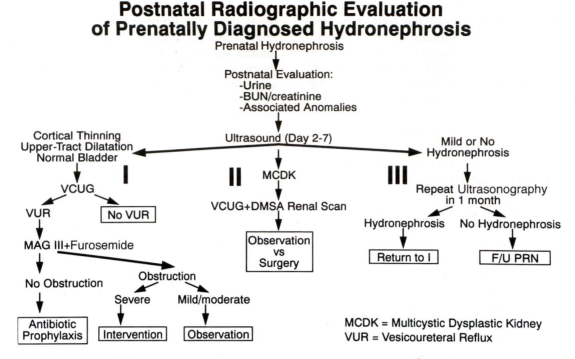

Figure 80-2. Algorithm for the postnatal evaluation of fetal hydronephrosis. MCDK = multicystic dysplastic kidney; VUR = vesicoureteral reflux; VCUG = voiding cystourethrography; F/U PRN = follow up as needed.

urine composition normally becomes progressively hypotonic between 16 and 21 weeks and may become even slightly more hypotonic late in gestation as a result of tubular maturation and increased fetal glomerular filtration rate (Glick et al. 1985; Nicolini et al. 1992). Glick et al. (1985) observed that fetuses with congenital hydronephrosis and normal renal function after birth had hypotonic urine but those with poor function produced urine that was isotonic. Similar observations were made in fetuses with hydronephrosis but good renal and pulmonary function evaluated postnatally by Weinstein and McFaydon and their colleagues (McFaydon et al. 1983; Weinstein et al. 1982).

It is uncertain why the fetus produces isotonic urine in the presence of long-standing obstruction. It has been suggested that dysplastic changes may alter tubular function sufficiently to prevent the resorption of Na and Cl. Rappaport et al. (1960) suggested that the stagnant urine may equilibrate with serum. The fluid aspirated from the fetus with severe obstructive uropathy may also present fluid produced by bladder urothelium.

In order to develop more sensitive fetal renal function tests, Glick et al. (1985) used bladder catheterization to evaluate 20 fetuses with obstructive uropathy. The fetuses who subsequently had a poor outcome were all "salt wasters" and those who had a good outcome had hypotonic urine. On the basis of this study, prognostic criteria for renal function at birth in congenital hydronephrosis were proposed (Table 80-2).

These results were questioned by other groups, who reported that these prognostic criteria did not accurately predict the renal function at birth. Wilkins et al. (1987) reported results using these prognostic criteria in nine cases of fetal obstructive uropathy. The criteria were accurate in predicting a poor outcome, as all four patients died and three of the four had evidence of renal dysplasia. In the fetuses with a predicted good prognosis, four of the five had poor renal function and the only patient with a good outcome underwent in utero decompression with a vesicoamniotic shunt.

The reports questioning the utility of the fetal urine electrolyte levels as prognostic criteria prompted a reevaluation in a series of 40 fetuses with bilateral hydronephrosis. Crombleholme et al. (1991) retrospectively assigned fetuses to the good prognostic group only if they had a Na <100, Cl <90, osmolarity <210,

▶ **TABLE 80-2.** PROGNOSTIC CRITERIA IN OBSTRUCTIVE UROPATHY

Sonography	No Cortical Cyst, Normal Echogenicity
Na	<100 mEq per liter
Cl	<90 mEq per liter
Osm	<210 mEq per liter
Ca	<2 mmol per liter
PO$_4$	<2 mmol per liter
β_2-microglobulin	<2 mg per liter

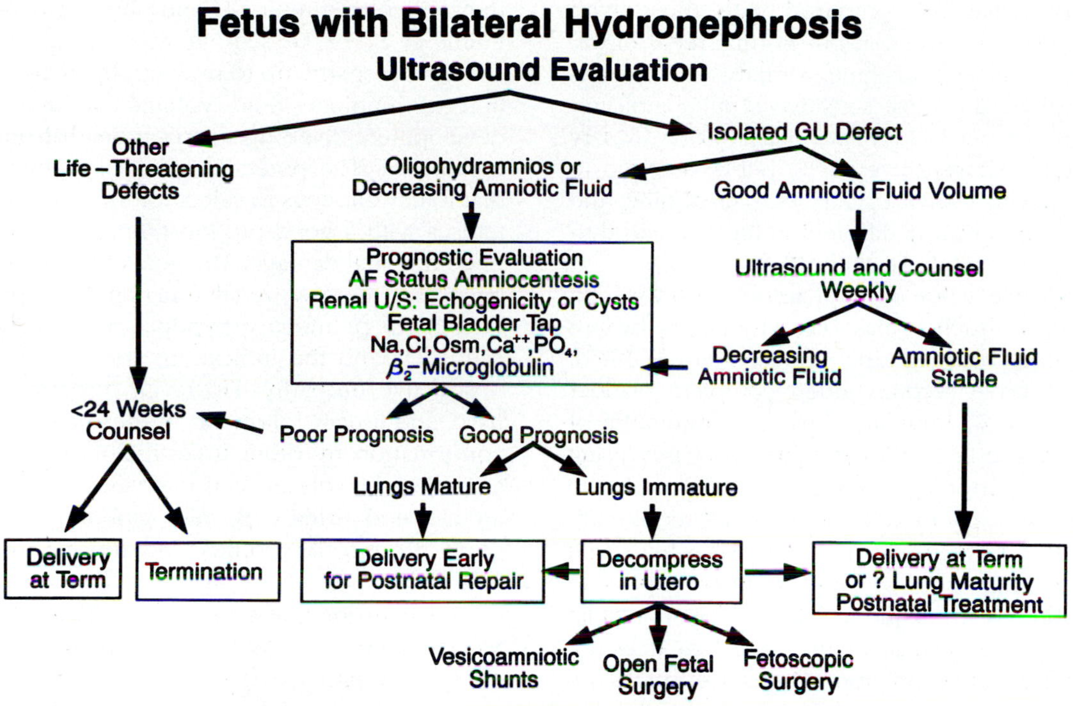

Fetus with Bilateral Hydronephrosis
Ultrasound Evaluation

Other Life–Threatening Defects

Isolated GU Defect

Oligohydramnios or Decreasing Amniotic Fluid

Good Amniotic Fluid Volume

Prognostic Evaluation
AF Status Amniocentesis
Renal U/S: Echogenicity or Cysts
Fetal Bladder Tap
Na,Cl,Osm,Ca^{++},PO$_4$,
β_2-Microglobulin

Ultrasound and Counsel Weekly

Decreasing Amniotic Fluid

Amniotic Fluid Stable

<24 Weeks Counsel

Poor Prognosis   Good Prognosis

Lungs Mature   Lungs Immature

Delivery at Term

Termination

Delivery Early for Postnatal Repair

Decompress in Utero

Delivery at Term or ? Lung Maturity Postnatal Treatment

Vesicoamniotic Shunts   Open Fetal Surgery   Fetoscopic Surgery

Figure 80-3. Algorithm for the perinatal management of the fetus with bladder-outlet obstruction. GU = genitourinary; AF = amniotic fluid.

and there was no sonographic evidence of dysplasia (Fig. 80-3). Fetuses were assigned to the poor prognosis group if even one criterion was met. There was a statistically significant difference in survival in the good versus the poor prognosis group (81 versus 12.5%) even excluding terminations (87 versus 30%). These prognostic criteria were intended as a means to select fetuses for in utero intervention. They accurately select the fetuses who have sufficient renal function to have a favorable outcome if decompressed in utero. If the fetal obstruction is unrelieved, the renal function is likely to deteriorate despite a favorable prognostic profile. Fetal obstructive uropathy is a dynamic process, and experimental studies in fetal lambs have demonstrated that the severity of renal damage from obstruction depends on the timing, duration, and severity of the obstruction (Glick et al. 1983, 1984; Harrison et al. 1981a, 1983). The fetal urine electrolytes obtained at 20 to 24 weeks of gestation may only reflect the renal function at the time they are assayed. In fact, Nicolini et al. (1992) have demonstrated by serial fetal bladder aspirations the worsening urinary electrolyte profile and renal function in fetuses with obstructive uropathy in which the obstruction was untreated. In the report from Wilkins et al. (1987), the fetuses in the favorable group had unrelieved obstruction and progression in their renal deterioration. The one fetus that was successfully decompressed in utero had a good outcome.

These prognostic criteria for in utero intervention in obstructive uropathy have become widely used and

are being more appropriately applied as selection criteria for intervention. However, Nicolini et al. (1992) have pointed out that one potential problem with these criteria is that they fail to take into account the gestational age of the fetus and that threshold values were established in fetuses with obstructive uropathy and not normal fetuses. The effect of gestational age on fetal urine electrolytes is most marked prior to 21 weeks of gestation, becoming progressively more hypotonic and then remaining relatively stable throughout the remainder of gestation. The criteria proposed by Glick et al. (1995) were selected to establish the threshold for a poor prognosis as 2 SD from the mean value of the patients with a good prognosis. This does skew the criteria toward including potentially compromised fetuses into the good-prognosis group. But as the results reported by Crombleholme et al. (1991) confirm, this has not resulted in the treatment of fetuses with irrevocably compromised renal function. In fact, overly stringent selection criteria for intervention as proposed by Nicolini et al. (1992) may exclude many potentially salvageable fetuses from treatment.

In addition to the use of fetal urine Na, Cl, and osmolarity other groups have suggested the addition of urine Ca^{++}, PO$_4$, and β_2-microglobulin to assess fetal renal function. Nicolini et al. (1992) studied fetal urine creatinine, urea, and electrolytes, notably Ca^{++}, Na, and PO$_4$, in a group of 24 fetuses with obstructive uropathy and 26 normal controls. They found that the urinary Ca^{++} and Na were significantly higher in fetuses with renal dysplasia as compared with those with lower urinary tract obstruction but normal renal histology or normal clinical outcome. Urinary Ca^{++} levels were found to be the most sensitive (100%) indicator of renal dysplasia but lacked specificity (60%). Urinary Na was slightly less sensitive (87%) but was found to be the most specific (80%). Urinary PO_4, creatinine, and urea were not significantly different in fetuses with dysplastic kidneys versus those without dysplasia.

The predictive value of fetal urine electrolytes in bladder-outlet obstruction has been found to be enhanced by serial bladder taps (Johnson et al. 1995). Johnson et al. have recommended complete bladder drainage at 48- to 72-hour intervals for a minimum of three taps to best establish a clear pattern of increasing or decreasing hypertonicity. While values clearly in the normal range on initial bladder tap may not require additional bladder taps to establish a prognosis, a fetus with elevated values may show a clear trend of improving electrolyte values with sequential taps. The sequential taps are thought to clear stagnant urine that may not accurately reflect renal function (Qureshi et al. 1996).

It has been observed that obstructive uropathy due to posterior urethral valves has a long natural history (Harrison and Adzick 1991; Parkhouse et al. 1988). Renal failure may not develop for years in a newborn with posterior urethral valves. A fetus with obstructive uropathy, and a favorable prognostic profile, and who has normal amniotic fluid is currently not considered a candidate for in utero decompression. A small number of fetuses diagnosed with hydronephrosis were observed to have findings consistent with obstructive uropathy, a favorable prognostic profile, and normal amounts of amniotic fluid, but progressive renal insufficiency subsequently developed during infancy despite good renal function initially. We thus have lacked criteria that allow us to identify a fetus with obstructive uropathy and a good prognostic profile who, despite the presence of normal amniotic fluid volume, is at risk for ongoing renal damage. Muller et al. (1993) reported the use of fetal urinary β_2-microglobulin as a predictor of postnatal renal function at 1 year of age. They reported that 17 of 40 patients with normal amniotic fluid volume and a good prognostic profile had a creatinine level of >0.56 mg per liter at 1 year of age. This value was selected as the threshold since it was 2 SD from the mean creatinine of normal 1-year-olds. In this group of patients, the β_2-microglobulin was found to be significantly elevated as compared with patients with the same prognostic profile but with a creatinine of <0.56 mg per liter at 1 year of age. β_2-Microglobulin may allow us to identify fetuses at risk for renal damage by unrelieved obstruction even though their amniotic fluid has not diminished.

Our current approach to in utero treatment for obstructive uropathy is to intervene in fetuses with a good prognostic profile only for decreasing amniotic fluid or frank oligohydramnios (Cendron et al. 1994; Crombleholme et al. 1991) (see Fig. 80-3). Fetal therapy of obstructive uropathy up to now has been aimed at restoration of amniotic fluid volume to allow pulmonary development, averting neonatal death from pulmonary hypoplasia. The potential utility of β_2-microglobulin is that it may allow us to select for in utero therapy among fetuses with a good prognostic profile those at risk for ongoing renal damage. The goal of this treatment would be preservation of renal function as opposed to prevention of pulmonary hypoplasia. This would significantly expand the indications for fetal intervention in obstructive uropathy. However, this report is preliminary, and longer follow-up of these children as well as confirmation by other investigators will be necessary to define the role of fetal intervention in the setting of an elevated urinary β_2-microglobulin in fetuses with good prognostic profiles and normal amniotic fluid volume.

One major question that is difficult to address in fetal treatment of obstructive uropathy is assessing the efficacy of prenatal decompression. In a report of a large experience with vesicoamniotic shunts at a single institution, Johnson et al. (1995) described the outcome in 55 fetuses who underwent shunt placement. Unfortunately, this was a heterogeneous group of patients with good- and poor-prognosis patients with a range of diagnoses including posterior urethral valves, prune belly, urethral atresia, and a variety of other anomalies. In the group with posterior urethral valves the postnatal survival was 60%. Of note is that the incidence of an elevated nadir creatinine level >1 mg per deciliter in the first year of life was 33%. Coplen et al. (1996) in a review of prenatal intervention for lower urinary tract obstruction from five reported series found an overall survival rate of only 48% and a catheter-related complication rate of 45%. In the report by Crombleholme et al. (1991), in both the good-prognosis and poor-prognosis groups survival was greater in fetuses who were decompressed in utero as opposed to those who were not decompressed. In the group of 10 fetuses with a poor prognosis, 3 were electively terminated, there were 4 neonatal deaths from pulmonary hypoplasia or renal dysplasia, and 3 survived. All 3 survivors had restoration of normal amniotic fluid levels, but renal failure developed in 2 of the 3 and they have undergone renal transplantation. Among the 14 patients with no intervention, there were no survivors (11 terminations and 3 neonatal deaths from pulmonary hypoplasia).

In the good-prognosis group of 9 fetuses, 1 was electively terminated, and there were no deaths, leaving 8 neonatal survivors. One infant died at 9 months of age from unrelated causes, with normal renal function. Of the 7 patients in the good-prognosis group who were not treated, 5 survived and 2 died after birth. Renal failure later developed in 2 of the survivors. The incidence of oligohydramnios in the good-prognosis group was 7 of 16. All 6 patients with oligohydramnios who had fetal intervention survived. The 1 patient with oligohydramnios that was untreated died at birth of pulmonary hypoplasia.

When in utero intervention restores amniotic fluid volume, neonatal death from pulmonary hypoplasia is averted. When oligohydramnios develops during the canalicular stage of lung development (16 to 24 weeks) the fetus usually has pulmonary hypoplasia precluding survival. In the group of fetuses reported by Crombleholme et al. (1991), there was a preponderance of oligohydramnios in the poor-prognosis group (23 of 24 as compared with 7 of 16 in the good-prognosis group). Fetuses from the good-prognosis group appear to survive as a result of fetal treatment in the face of variable rates of oligohydramnios. In the good-prognosis group, 6 of the 7 fetuses with oligohydramnios had intervention and all 6 survived with normal renal function. However, the seventh patient with oligohydramnios, who was not treated, died at birth of pulmonary hypoplasia. Uncorrected oligohydramnios was associated with a 100% neonatal mortality. Normal or restored amniotic fluid volume was associated with a 94% survival (Crombleholme et al. 1991).

In utero decompression appears to prevent neonatal death from pulmonary hypoplasia, but the effect on renal function is less clear. The development of postnatal renal failure in two infants who were not treated because amniotic fluid volume remained normal raises a question about treating obstructed fetuses before oligohydramnios develops. Because renal development or maldevelopment is complete at birth, relief of obstruction in infancy or childhood may not prevent the progression to end-stage renal failure (Warshaw et al. 1982).

The severity of renal dysplasia at birth depends on the timing and severity of obstruction before birth (Adzick et al. 1987; Glick et al. 1984). Experimental work suggests that relief of obstruction during the most active phase of nephrogenesis (20 to 30 weeks of gestation) may obviate further damage and allow normal nephrogenesis to proceed (Blyth et al. 1993; Bronshtein et al. 1990; Patten et al. 1990; Thomas 1990). One fetus in this series evaluated at 18 weeks of gestation had a favorable prognostic profile, but because the amniotic fluid level was normal, it was not a candidate for intervention. While the sonographic appearance of the kidneys was normal at 18 weeks of gestation, postnatal sonography suggested renal dysplasia and chronic renal insufficiency developed.

The maternal morbidity of vesicoamniotic shunts was minimal but there was a high incidence of chorioamnionitis—in 3 of 21 procedures. However, all cases of chorioamnionitis were early in the experience, before the routine use of prophylactic antibiotics and during a period when long-term (4 to 16 hours) bladder catheterization rather than aspiration was used for fetal urine sampling (Crombleholme et al. 1991; Glick et al. 1985). Among the five open cases of fetal surgery there was no fetal morbidity or mortality, but preterm labor was observed in each mother requiring aggressive tocolytic therapy (Crombleholme et al. 1988).

Harrison et al. (1981) first proposed the concept of in utero decompression in a report of poor outcome in 13 fetuses with obstructive uropathy. This same group subsequently reported the first case of vesicoamniotic shunting for obstructive uropathy using a "Harrison" double pig-tail catheter. Other groups quickly followed suit, and in a 1986 report of the International Fetal Surgery Registry, 62 fetuses had been treated by percutaneous vesicoamniotic shunts (Manning et al. 1986). The overall survival was only 48%; the survival rate was 76% in cases due to posterior urethral valves. The procedure-related mortality rate in the registry was 3%. There were several problems with this early experience with vesicoamniotic shunts. Many fetuses were treated inappropriately prior to the development of selection criteria. Secondly, many cases were assessed by indwelling fetal bladder catheters for several hours, which along with the lack of prophylactic antibiotics, predisposed to chorioamnionitis. In addition, as noted by Glick et al. (1985), multiple shunt insertions are often necessary because of shunt occlusion, or dislodgment. Iatrogenic "gastroschisis" has also been reported when trochars used for insertion lacerated the abdominal wall during placement of vesicoamniotic shunts (Manning et al. 1986) (Fig. 80-4). Rodeck has reported experience with the KCH catheter, which appears to function better than the Harrison catheter (Rodeck et al. 1988). The utility of vesicoamniotic shunts is limited, however, by the brief duration of decompression, risk of infection, catheter obstruction or dislodgment, fetal injury during placement, and potentially inadequate decompression of the fetal urinary tract. These factors make vesicoamniotic shunting inappropriate for early-gestation decompression of the urinary tract.

The presence of oligohydramnios in the second-trimester fetus with bilateral hydronephrosis due to bladder-outlet obstruction is uniformly fatal (Crombleholme et al 1991; Glick et al. 1985). Vesicoamniotic shunts are inadequate to treat these cases, and Harrison has reported his experience with open fetal surgery in eight cases (Crombleholme et al. 1988a, 1991; Harrison et al. 1991). Six of the eight treated were delivered by cesarean section at 32 to 35 weeks of gestation. Four of the six had restoration of amniotic fluid levels by the procedure and had no evidence of pulmonary hypoplasia. The other two fetuses died postnatally of severe pulmonary hypoplasia because of persistent oligohydramnios due to renal dysplasia. They displayed long-standing oligohydramnios prior to treatment and suffered pulmonary hypoplasia despite intervention. These cases would be excluded from treatment by current selection criteria. There were two stillbirths; one

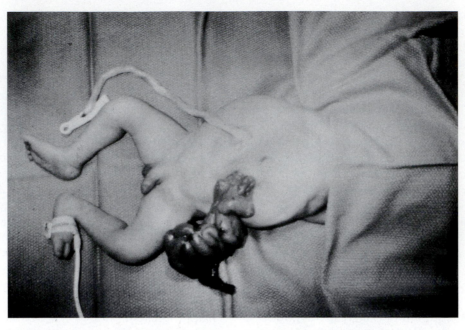

Figure 80-4. Newborn with iatrogenic gastroschisis due to herniation of viscera through the abdominal-wall defect created by attempted vesicoamniotic shunt placement. *(Courtesy of Burton Harris, M.D.)*

pregnancy was terminated (by parental request) because of cloacal anomaly, and the other when the mother discontinued tocolytic therapy.

Three of the four survivors have had no evidence of renal insufficiency during follow-up of up to 8 years. Progressive renal insufficiency developed in the fourth patient, requiring renal transplantation at 5 years of age; the child was doing well 4 years after transplantation.

Open fetal surgery for fetal vesicostomy to relieve bladder-outlet obstruction is technically feasible and has been successful in restoring amniotic fluid dynamics and preventing death from pulmonary hypoplasia. However, this is achieved at potentially significant risk to mother and fetus in the form of preterm labor precipitated by hysterotomy. Creation of a fetoscopic vesicocutaneous fistula may avoid many of the complications of open fetal surgery and creation of a vesicoamniotic fistula provides more reliable decompression than vesicoamniotic shunts. This technique was developed in fetal lambs in Harrison's laboratory, and application of this technique in human fetuses with obstructive uropathy, although unsuccessful, has been reported (Estes and Harrison 1992; Quintero et al. 1997).

▶ TREATMENT OF THE NEWBORN

Once a fetus has been found on prenatal ultrasound to have a significant degree of hydronephrosis, careful follow-up should be planned to ensure proper treatment postnatally. At the time of the initial prenatal diagnosis of hydronephrosis, parental counseling is recommended. A team approach is extremely helpful to inform the parents and to help them understand and cope with the diagnosis and understand the postnatal evaluation (see Figure 80-2).

Any newborn with a prenatal diagnosis of hydronephrosis should undergo a physical examination at birth. Monitoring of the urinary output within the first 24 to 48 hours is unreliable. Failure to void during the first two days after birth may reflect normal fluid shifts or may be the first sign of a significant urologic anomaly. In the neonate who does not void within the first 48 hours, the differential diagnosis of anuria includes obstructive uropathy, renal failure, urogenic bladder, and the effects of maternal medication. However, most patients with an obstructive process will void, albeit with a weak stream, within the first 2 days of life. Serum electrolytes, blood urea nitrogen, and creatinine levels measured within the first day of life are a reflection of maternal renal function via placental exchange. It is best to wait 24 hours to measure these levels. The most helpful test in the initial evaluation of the newborn with prenatally diagnosed hydronephrosis is ultrasonography of the abdomen including a scan of the bladder. Timing of the ultrasonography depends on the degree of prenatal hydronephrosis. If severe dilatation of the renal pelvis has been detected antenatally, then early ultrasound evaluation should be performed so as to permit early intervention. Otherwise, ultrasound examination can be postponed for 3 to 7 days in order to let the diuresis that occurs during the first 48 hours of life to resolve (Arant 1992). If the initial postnatal renal ultrasound is normal, the evaluation should be pursued, with a repeat ultrasound in 3 to 4 weeks. There is a high incidence (50% of lesions, such as ureteropelvic junction obstruction (UPJ) and vesicoureteral reflux) diagnosed in neonates with antenatal diagnosis of hydronephrosis that have a normal upper urinary tract at the time of the first ultrasound (Detjer and Gibbons 1989).

Mild cases of hydronephrosis can be watched and may warrant only one or two ultrasounds during the postnatal period (see Fig. 80-2). It is rare for mild dilatation of the upper urinary tract to progress. In cases in which other findings are seen, such as cortical thinning, upper-tract dilatation, and a normal bladder, voiding cystourethrography (VCUG) should be performed. If there is reflux, then a renal scan 99 technetium-diethylenetriaminpentaacetic acid (DTPA) or mercaptoacetyltriglycine (MAG III) will be helpful in documenting function of the kidneys. If no evidence of reflux is noted by VCUG, then a MAG III with furosemide should be obtained to evaluate possible UPJ obstruction. If UPJ obstruction is noted, treatment is determined by the severity of the obstruction. In severe UPJ obstruction, in which a kidney shows 35% or less function, pyeloplasty should be performed. In cases in which mild to moderate obstruction is noted and the kidney has more than 35% function, observation alone may be indicated, with repeat ultrasonography in 3 months. A repeat renal scan will help to assess changes in renal function. As stated earlier, there is growing evidence to suggest that a mild degree of UPJ obstruction may resolve and may not warrant surgical intervention (see Chapter 79).

If prenatal ultrasound reveals a multicystic dysplastic kidney, a VCUG and renal scan should be obtained. These studies confirm the lack of function in the affected kidney and rule out any abnormalities in the contralateral kidney (Flack and Bellinger 1993).

▶ SURGICAL TREATMENT

Surgical intervention at birth is required in cases when a severe obstruction will jeopardize renal function. This applies most often to cases of posterior urethral valves, obstructing ureterocele, and severe UPJ obstruction affecting a solitary kidney. Emergency surgical treatment is seldom warranted. Reconstruction of the urinary tract should not be attempted until the newborn has stabilized from a medical standpoint and has been fully evaluated. Drainage of the urinary tract can provide decompression by placement of either a ureteral catheter, suprapubic catheter, or a nephrostomy tube until definitive repair of the urinary tract can be accomplished.

Posterior urethral valves and obstructing ureterocele are amenable early to endoscopic treatment but may require further surgical intervention once the child has stabilized and grown. In the presence of a solitary kidney, every attempt should be made to ensure adequate drainage so as to not further jeopardize renal function.

▶ LONG-TERM OUTCOME

Reports in the urologic literature in the late 1970s and early 1980s reviewing experience with posterior urethral valves in newborns were notable for the lack of respiratory problems encountered. In contrast, more recently Nakayama et al. (1986) reported 11 cases of posterior urethral valves, clinically evident at birth, in which five of the infants died. Three died within hours of birth due to respiratory insufficiency and two survived their respiratory insufficiency only to die from renal failure within 3 weeks. Of the six survivors, four had severe respiratory problems requiring prolonged ventilatory support. In addition to the two infants who died early from renal failure, three others developed renal failure despite urinary diversion. Only two of the patients in this series had normal renal function after reconstruction of their urinary tracts.

Clinical experience suggests that the pulmonary and renal consequences of bladder obstruction will vary with the severity of the obstruction. The degree of obstruction will determine the volume of amniotic fluid, the extent of pulmonary hypoplasia, and the dysplastic effects of obstruction on the developing kidney. High-grade bladder-outlet obstruction causes megacystis, bilateral hydronephrosis, and oligohydramnios, which results in pulmonary hypoplasia and postnatal respiratory insufficiency. In addition to pulmonary hypoplasia and renal dysplasia, fetal urethral obstruction produces a wide variety of deformations, including Potter facies, limb abnormalities such as club foot and hip dislocation, and abnormal abdominal-wall muscular development (prune belly). Less-severe obstruction may permit enough urine output to allow sufficient pulmonary development for survival. Despite adequate pulmonary development for survival, partial high-grade obstruction may result in renal dysplasia, bladder dysfunction, and irreversible renal failure. Milder forms of obstruction may have normal pulmonary development and mild renal insufficiency or normal renal function. This broad spectrum of severity of fetal obstructive uropathy presents a diagnostic and therapeutic challenge: which cases are severe enough to warrant prenatal intervention, which should be delivered early to prevent ongoing renal damage, and which are best managed postnatally at term?

Freedman et al. (1997) have reported on the long-term outcome of 14 patients who underwent vesicoamniotic shunting for obstructive uropathy. This was

fetal cystoscopy and endoscopic fulguration of posterior urethral valves. Am J Obstet Gynecol 1995;172:206–209.

Qureshi F, Jacques SM, Seifman B, et al. In utero fetal urine analysis and renal histology do correlate with outcome in fetal obstructive uropathies. Fetal Diagn Ther 1996;11: 306–312.

Rappaport A, Nicholson TF, Yendt ER. Movement of electrolytes across the wall of the urinary bladder in dogs. Am J Physiol 1960;198:191–194.

Risdon RA. Renal dysplasia: a clinico-pathological study of 76 cases. J Clin Pathol 1975;24:57.

Rubenstein M, Meyer R, Berstein J. Congenital abnormalities of the urinary system: a postmortem survey of developmental anomalies and acquired congenital lesions in a children's hospital. J Pediatr 1961;58:356–362.

Stramm E, King G, Thickman D. Megacystis-microcolon–intestinal hypoperistalsis syndrome: prenatal identification in siblings and review of the literature. J Ultrasound Med 1991;10:599–604.

Thomas DFM, Gordon AC. Managment of prenatally diagnosed uropathies. Arch Dis Child 1989;64:6268–673.

Thomas DFM. Fetal uropathy. Br J Urol 1990;66:225–231.

Warshaw BI, Edelbrock HH, Ettinger RB. Progression to end stage renal disease in children with obstructive uropathy. J Pediatr 1982;100:182–188.

Weinstein L, Anderson CF, Finley PR, et al. The in utero management of urinary outflow tract obstruction. J Clin Ultrasound 1982;10:465–468.

Wigglesworth JS, Desai R. Effects on lung growth of cervical cord section of the rabbit fetus. Early Hum Dev 1979; 3:57–63.

Wigglesworth JS, Desai R. Is fetal respiratory function a major determinant for survival? Lancet 1982;1:564–567.

Wilkins IA, Chitkara U, Lynch L, et al. The nonpredictive value of fetal urine electrolytes: preliminary report of outcomes and correlations with pathologic diagnosis. Am J Obstet Gynecol 1987;157:694–698.

Winter RM, Knowles SA. Megacystis-microcolon–intestinal hypoperistalsis syndrome: confirmation of autosomal recessive inheritance. J Med Genet 1986;23:360–364.

Wladimiroff JW. Effect of furosemide on fetal urine production. Br J Obstet Gynaecol 1975;82:221–229.

Woodhouse CR, Reilly JM, Bahadur G, et al. Sexual function and fertility in patients treated for posterior urethral valves. J Urol 1989;142:586–588.

Young HH, Frantz WA. Congenital obstruction of the posterior urethra. J Urol 1919;3:289–365.

CHAPTER 81

Ectopic Ureterocele

▶ CONDITION

A ureterocele is a cystic dilatation that occurs at the distal end of the ureter at its junction with the bladder. Simple ureteroceles are those that are located in the normal location of the ureteral orifice in the trigone of the bladder. Simple ureteroceles are more commonly detected in adults and usually are associated with a single collecting system. Simple ureteroceles are rarely associated with the upper-pole ureter of a complete duplication of the collecting system. Simple uretero-celes may be associated with a varying degree of obstruction, but this is not significant in most patients. In ectopic ureterocele the ureteral orifice is located in an ectopic position, usually distal to the trigone. Ectopic ureterocele is associated with a duplex collecting system. Ectopic ureterocele is also associated with an increased incidence of duplication in the contralateral kidney. The ureterocele may vary in size, from a tiny cystic lesion within the submucosal ureter, to that of a large cystic balloon-like structure that fills the bladder. The size of these ureteroceles may fluctuate from one examination to the next. Histologically, the ureterocele is covered by the mucosa of the bladder and lined by the mucosa of the ureter, with varying degrees of attenuated smooth-muscle bundles and connective tissue between the two layers of mucosa.

Several theories have been proposed to account for the embryonic development of a ureterocele. In one theory, a membrane covering the ureteral orifice persists for a long period, leading to the development of the ureterocele (Chwalle 1927). In another theory, a ureterocele forms as a result of a stimulus to an expansion that transforms the bladder into a globular cap, creating an expanded thin-walled distal ureter (Stephens 1971). Lastly, a localized embryonic arrest has been hypothesized as the cause of the ureterocele (Tokunaka et al. 1981).

Ectopic ureterocele has been classified anatomically by Stephens (1958, 1983). In this classification scheme, stenotic ectopic ureterocele is characterized by a small stenotic orifice and accounts for approximately 40% of cases. In sphincteric ectopic ureterocele, the orifice of the ureterocele is within the internal sphincter and accounts for an additional 40% of cases. In sphincteric ectopic ureterocele the ureteral orifice may be of normal caliber or may be enlarged and may open either in the posterior urethra in males or distal to the external sphincter in females. Sphincterostenotic ectopic ureterocele accounts for approximately 5% of cases. The stenotic orifice of this type of ectopic ureterocele is located within the urethral floor. There are other rarer types of ectopic ureterocele, including cecoureterocele, in which the lumen extends distal to the level of the orifice as a long tongue or cecum; blind ectopic ureterocele, in which there is no orifice so that the ureter is completely obstructed; and nonobstructive ectopic ureterocele, in which the orifice is enlarged within the bladder.

In complete ureteral duplication, the ureter draining the upper-pole moiety usually opens caudal and medial to the ureter draining the lower-pole moiety. When a duplex system is found to be present on one side there is contralateral duplication in approximately 50% of the cases. This occurs far more frequently in females and can potentially result in bladder-outlet obstruction if the ureterocele is sufficiently large. The orifice of the ureterocele is usually obstructed either by stenosis or because it opens at the level of the urogenital diaphragm and is obstructed by the closed bladder neck. Not only can the ureterocele cause obstruction of the ureter from which it arises, but the ureterocele can also result in obstruction of the ureter draining the lower-pole moiety, placing the entire kidney at risk. In ectopic ureterocele the upper-pole moiety is commonly dysplastic and has poor or no function because

with the long-term follow-up needed to detect hypertension or malignant transformation. If long-term follow-up is in question, nephrectomy should be considered.

The issue of nephrectomy rests on the potential development of hypertension or malignant transformation. In the past 30 years there have only been 12 cases of malignancy associated with MCDK, only 6 of which occurred in children (Manzoni and Caldamone 1998; Minevich et al. 1996; Oddone et al. 1994; Raffensperger et al. 1986). All 6 pediatric patients had Wilms' tumor, while 5 adults had renal-cell carcinoma and 1 adult had mesothelioma.

As of 1995, no renal tumor had developed in patients with MCDK reported to the Multicystic Kidney Registry of the Section of Urology of the American Academy of Pediatrics (Wacksman 1995). Similarly, during the past 30 years there have been only 24 cases of hypertension that arose as a result of MCDK (Andretta et al. 1995; Angermeier et al. 1992; Elder et al. 1995; Manzoni and Caldamone 1998; Patterson and Klauber 1996; Susskind et al. 1989; Webb et al. 1997). In 13 of these cases, the hypertension responded to nephrectomy. The long-term data on malignant transformation and hypertension is meager and may not support routine prophylactic nephrectomy, but long-term surveillance is necessary in this group of patients at risk.

▶ GENETICS AND RECURRENCE RISK

Isolated MCDKs are usually sporadic, with no risk of recurrence in subsequent pregnancies. However, there have been familial cases whose defects range from bilateral renal agenesis to hydronephrosis, with an autosomal dominant pattern of inheritance and a 50% chance of a subsequent pregnancy being affected. MCDKs can also be seen as part of numerous syndromes (see Table 82-1). Features of the genetic syndromes should be sought and excluded, as they may be associated with a specific recurrence risk.

REFERENCES

Ambrose SS, Gould RA, Trulock TS, et al. Unilateral multicystic renal disease in adults. J Urol 1982;128:366–369.

Andretta F, Aragova F, Talenti F, et al. Il sene multicistico. Urol Pediatr 1995;1:31–38.

Angermeier KW, Kay R, Levin H. Hypertension as a complication of multicystic dysplastic kidney. Urology 1992;39:55–58.

D'Alton ME, Romero R, Grannum P, et al. Antenatal diagnosis of renal anomalies with ultrasound. IV. Bilateral multicystic kidney disease. Am J Obstet Gynecol 1986;154:532–537.

DeKlerk D, Marshall FF, Jeffs RD. Multicystic dysplastic kidney. J Urol 1977;118:306–310.

Elder J, Hladky D, Salzman AA. Outpatient nephrectomy for nonfunctioning kidneys. J Urol 1995;154:712–715.

Gaugh DCS, Postlewaite RJ, Lewis MA, et al. Multicystic renal dysplasia diagnosed in the antenatal period: a note of caution. Br J Urol 1995;76:244–248.

Gordon AC, Thomas DF, Arthur RJ, et al. Multicystic dysplastic kidney: Is nephrectomy still appropriate? J Urol 1988;140:1231–1234.

Greene LF, Feinzaig W, Dahlin DC. Multicystic dysplasia of the kidney with special reference to the contralateral kidney. J Urol 1971;105:482–486.

Hartman GE, Smolik LM, Shochat SJ. The dilemma of the multicystic dysplastic kidney. Am J Dis Child 1986;140:925–929.

Hashimoto BE, Filly RA, Callen PW. Multicystic dysplastic kidney in utero: changing appearance on ultrasound. Radiology 1986;159:107–111.

Holloway WR, Weinstein SH. Percutaneous decompression: treatment for respiratory distress secondary to multicystic dysplastic kidney. J Urol 1990;144:113–117.

Kaplan BS. Genesis, dysplasia, and cystic disease. In: O'Neill JA, Rowe MI, Grosfeld JL, Funkalsrud EW, Caran AG, eds. Pediatric surgery. 5th ed. St. Louis: Mosby Year Book, 1998:1575–1582.

Kleiner B, Filly RA, Mack L, et al. Multicystic dysplastic kidney: observations of contralateral disease in the fetal population. Radiology 1986;161:27–31.

Langino LA, Martin LW. Abdominal masses in the newborn infant. Pediatrics 1958;21:396–560.

Mahony BS. Ultrasound evaluation of the fetal genitourinary system. In: Callen PW, ed. Ultrasonography in obstetrics and gynecology. 3rd ed. Philadelphia: Saunders, 1994:389–419.

Manzoni G, Caldamone AA. Multicystic kidney. In: Stinger MD, Oldham KT, Maurequand PDE, Howard ED, eds. Pediatric surgery and urology: long term outcomes. Philadelphia: Saunders, 1998:632–641.

Minevich E, Wooksman J, Phipps L, et al. The importance of accurate diagnosis and early close follow up in patients with suspected MCDK. Presented at the 65th annual meeting of the American Academy of Pediatrics, Boston, October 1996.

Oddone M, Marino C, Sergi CE, et al. Wilms' tumor arising in a multicystic dysplastic kidney. Pediatr Radiol 1994;24:236–240.

Patterson BA, Klauber GT. Prognosis for children born with multicystic dysplastic kidneys. Br J Urology 1996;77(suppl 1):18. abstract.

Raffensperger J, Abousleiman A. Abdominal masses in children under one year of age. Surgery 1968;63:514–517.

Resnick J, Vernier RL. Cystic disease of the kidney in the newborn infant. Clin Perinatol 1981;8:375–379.

Rickwood AMK, Anderson PAM, Williams MPL. Multicystic renal dysplasia detected by prenatal ultrasonography: natural history and results of conservative management. Br J Urol 1992;69:538–540.

Rizzo N, Gabrielli S, Pilu G, et al. Prenatal diagnosis and obstetrical management of multicystic kidney disease. Prenat Diagn 1987;7:109–113.

Romero R, Pilu G, Jeanty P, et al. Multicystic kidney disease in prenatal diagnosis of congenital anomalies. East Norwalk, CT: Appleton & Lange, 1988:270–274.

Sanders RC, Hartman DS. The sonographic distinction between neonatal multicystic kidney and hydronephrosis. Radiology 1984;151:621–625.

Sanders RC. Multicystic dysplastic kidney. In: Sanders RC, Blackman LR, Hagge WA, Wolfsberg ED, eds. Structural fetal abnormalities: the total picture. St. Louis: Mosby Year Book, 1996:100–102.

Schwartz J. An unusual unilateral multicystic kidney in an infant. J Urol 1929;35:259–263.

Spence HM. Congenital unilateral multicystic kidney. J Urol 1955;74:693–697.

Stiller RJ, Pinto M, Heller C, et al. Oligohydramnios associated with bilateral multicystic dysplastic kidneys: prenatal diagnosis at 15 weeks' gestation. J Clin Ultrasound 1988;16:436–441.

Susskind MR, Kim KS, King LR. Hypertension and multicystic kidney. Urology 1989;34:362–366.

Wacksman J. Editorial comment. J Urol 1995;154:714–715.

Webb NJA, Lewis MA, Bruce J, et al. Unilateral multicystic dysplastic kidney: the case for nephrectomy. Arch Dis Child 1997;76:31–34.

CHAPTER 83
Ovarian Cysts

▶ CONDITION

Ovarian cysts arise from ovarian follicles. The primary stimulus for follicular development is follicle-stimulating hormone (FSH) secreted by the fetal pituitary, but maternal estrogens and placental human chorionic gonadotropin (hCG) also contribute to follicle growth in utero (Pryse-Davies and Dewhurst 1971). Primary follicles can be seen as early as the 20th week of gestation, and graafian follicles first appear during the 7th month (Peters et al. 1978; Pryse-Davies and Dewhurst 1971). At birth, maternal estrogen and hCG levels decrease sharply, and FSH production is decreased by the inhibitory mechanism of the hypothalamus–pituitary–ovarian axis (Grumbach and Kaplan 1975). This decrease in circulating estrogen and hCG levels at birth usually precludes the formation of simple ovarian cysts during childhood.

Ovarian cysts develop from mature follicles in hormonally active ovaries and are therefore most often seen after puberty. The cause of fetal ovarian cysts is unclear but is most likely stimulation of the fetal ovaries by fetal gonadotropins, maternal estrogens, and placental chorionic gonadotropin. The increased incidence of ovarian cysts seen in infants of mothers with diabetes mellitus, rhesus sensitization, and preeclampsia—conditions that are associated with excessive levels of serum chorionic gonadotropins (DeSa 1975; Nussbaum et al. 1988)—supports this pathogenesis. The association with fetal hypothyroidism has also been reported (Jafri et al. 1984). However, in most cases the cysts are detected in otherwise normal pregnancies (Sakala et al. 1991). It is most common for fetal ovarian cysts to be unilateral; however, bilateral ovarian cysts have been reported. In the review by Sakala et al. (1991) of 65 cases, 62 (95%) were unilateral, whereas 3 were bilateral.

▶ INCIDENCE

Ovarian and genital abnormalities account for 20% of all newborn abdominal masses, second only to those of urinary-tract origin (Griscom 1965; Wilson 1982). The first report of prenatal diagnosis of a fetal ovarian cyst was by Valenti et al. (1975); subsequently, over 300 cases of prenatally diagnosed ovarian cysts have been reported. Kirkinen and Jouppila (1985) reported 8 ovarian cysts detected antenatally in 21,000 pregnancies, for an incidence of 1 in 2625. DeSa (1975) found small follicular cysts in 113 (34%) of 332 stillborn fetuses and neonatal deaths. The cysts were defined as cystic structures lined by recognizable granulosa epithelium, with the greatest diameter in excess of 1 mm on microscopical section.

▶ SONOGRAPHIC FINDINGS

The following criteria are used to identify fetal ovarian cysts using ultrasound examination:

1. The presence of a cystic structure, usually located on one side of the fetal abdomen.
2. Identification of normal genitourinary tract (kidneys, ureter, and bladder).
3. Identification of a normal gastrointestinal tract (stomach, small and large bowel).
4. Female fetus.

Two types of cysts have been described: a simple cyst that is completely anechoic (Fig. 83-1) and complicated cysts containing internal echoes and fluid levels, internal septations, or anechoic areas intermixed with echogenic foci (Fig. 83-2). The antenatal diagnosis of an echogenic cyst is an accurate sonographic indicator

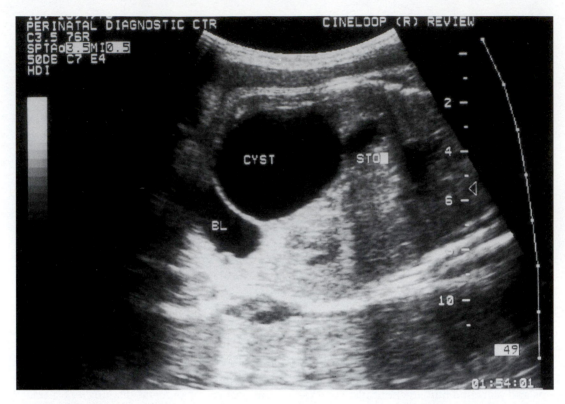

Figure 83-1. Ultrasound image demonstrating an anechoic cyst. This represents a simple ovarian cyst. BL = bladder; STO = stomach.

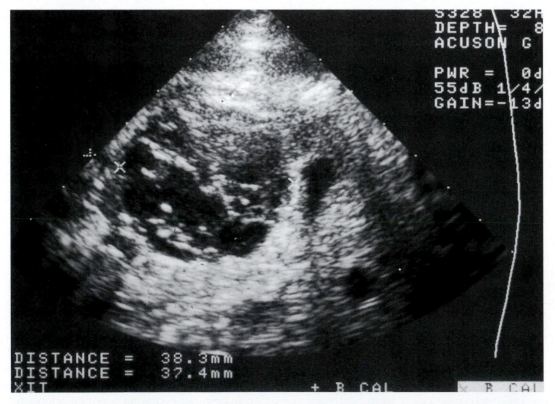

Figure 83-2. Ultrasound image of a complicated ovarian cyst, demonstrating internal echoes and anechoic areas interspersed with echogenic foci.

of ovarian torsion. In several series of echogenic cysts detected prenatally, postnatal surgery has confirmed the diagnosis (Brandt et al. 1991; Giorlandino et al. 1994; Meizner et al. 1991; Nussbaum et al. 1988).

The distinction between a pathologic cyst and a physiologic, mature follicle is based on size alone, with cysts >2 cm considered pathologic (Grapin et al. 1987). Cysts may vary in size from 2-by-2 cm to 8-by-11 cm in diameter (Grapin et al. 1987).

▶ DIFFERENTIAL DIAGNOSIS

The diagnosis of a fetal ovarian cyst is usually presumptive because mesenteric cysts, urachal cysts, or enteric duplications cannot be ruled out with absolute certainty. Factors more indicative of a fetal ovarian cyst include bilaterality, echogenicity, and cyst septations. Most cysts are benign; although ovarian neoplasms have been reported, they are extremely rare (Croitoru et al. 1991). Confirmation of normal kidneys and bladder will reduce the potential to confuse renal cysts or a posterior valve with persistent distention of the bladder as an ovarian cyst.

▶ ANTENATAL NATURAL HISTORY

Most cases of fetal ovarian cysts have been reported after 28 weeks of gestation (Brandt et al. 1991). Fewer cases have been reported during the second trimester, beginning as early as 19 weeks (Meizner et al. 1991). The size of most cysts remains unchanged in utero. A few cases have been reported to resolve in utero completely (Rizzo et al. 1989; McKeever and Andrews 1988). Polyhydramnios is present in approximately 18% of cases and is more commonly seen with cysts >6 cm (Sakala et al. 1991). The mechanism of the polyhydramnios has been suggested to be due to partial bowel obstruction secondary to compression by a large cyst (Carlson and Griscom 1972).

Anechoic cysts have the potential to become complex cysts, with the presence of echogenicity, fluid levels, and internal echoes (Fig. 83-3). The presence of these sonographic findings is usually an indicator that the cyst has undergone torsion. The incidence of antenatal torsion documented in a large series of cases is 40%. Torsion is the most common complication of prenatally diagnosed ovarian cysts. It is more common in large cysts (Nussbaum et al. 1988) but has occurred in cysts as small as 2 cm (Grapin et al. 1987). Of the cysts that remain anechoic in utero, a significant proportion, approximately 50%, will undergo spontaneous resolution after birth. There is an ongoing risk of torsion during the neonatal period that underscores the need for neonatal follow-up.

With the exception of a report of congenital hypothyroidism (Jafri et al. 1984) all other series report no associated congenital anomalies. The natural history of

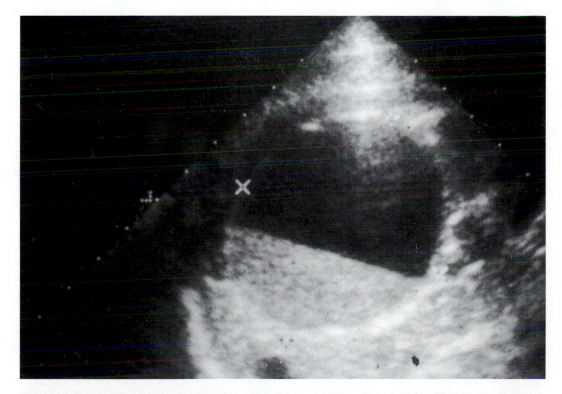

Figure 83-3. Ultrasound image of a cyst demonstrating fluid levels. This is another example of a complicated ovarian cyst.

▶ **TABLE 83-1.** ANTENATAL HISTORY OF OVARIAN CYSTS

Reference	Number	Unilateral/ Bilateral	Size (cm)	Spontaneous Resolution Prenatally	Evidence of Torsion Prenatally
D'Addario et al. 1990	27	23/2	2.8–7	11/23	11/27
Brandt et al. 1991	27	25/2	2.0–8	NR	6/27
Nussbaum et al. 1988	11	11/11	2.5–10	0/11	8/11
Meizner et al. 1991	15	NR	Mean, 5.41; with torsion mean, 4.33 without torsion	0/15	6/15
Giorlandino et al. 1994	42	41/42	Range not reported	0/42	18/42

NR = not reported.

all series with more than 10 cases reported is summarized in Table 83-1.

▶ MANAGEMENT OF PREGNANCY

Amniocentesis for karyotype is not indicated because there is no associated risk of aneuploidy, in excess of the background risk for the patient. No specialized antenatal fetal surveillance testing is necessary unless it is for other obstetric reasons. If a cyst is diagnosed to be echogenic, referral to pediatric surgery or adolescent gynecology is appropriate because all such cysts will require removal during the postnatal period owing to torsion. Delivery should occur in a center with appropriate pediatric surgical expertise available. Premature delivery is not indicated. Previous recommendations for cesarean section were based on anecdotal cases of poor outcomes for neonates with ovarian cysts that ruptured or caused soft-tissue dystocia. In the most recent series, vaginal delivery has been performed, and cesarean section was reserved for obstetric indications.

▶ FETAL INTERVENTION

The indications for fetal intervention in ovarian cysts remain undefined. It is our opinion that to prevent complications and subsequent oophorectomy, in utero aspiration of cysts >4 cm should be considered. Valenti et al. (1975) reported in utero aspiration for a 7-by-9-cm ovarian cyst with the intent of preventing intrapartum rupture. Landrum et al. (1986) reported aspiration of an 8-by-11-cm cyst in a 31-week-old fetus, ostensibly to prevent pulmonary hypoplasia. Pulmonary hypoplasia from a pelvic mass is unlikely, especially at 31 weeks. Aspiration to prevent in utero torsion and preserve ovarian tissue is a more appropriate goal (Fig. 83-4) (Crombleholme et al. 1997). In a review of seven cases of fetal ovarian cyst, indications for prenatal decompression include size >4cm, the presence of a

"wandering" mass, or rapid enlargement of a cystic mass. Analysis of the aspirated fluid reveals high levels of progesterone and testosterone, which are helpful in confirming the diagnosis (Crombleholme et al. 1997).

Giorlandino et al. (1990) have reported a case of an ovarian cyst treated by cyst aspiration and sclerosis with tetracycline. Although this treatment was successful, the use of tetracycline as a sclerosing agent in the fetus is not advised. Subsequently, Giorlandino et al. (1994) reported 4 cases of successful in utero cyst aspiration for cysts ranging from 5 to 8 cm in diameter with an 18-gauge needle. Cytologic evaluation of the aspirated fluid showed the presence of cyst-lining epithelial cells. No neonatal surgery was required.

D'Addario et al. (1990) reported in utero aspiration in two cases. One cyst ruptured during the aspiration, and both cases required neonatal surgery. No other details were reported. Of the 20 cases reported describing this type of management there have been no perinatal complications attributed to the intervention.

The disadvantages cited to prenatal aspiration of cysts are the limited published experience, the accuracy of differential diagnosis and the possibility that a choledochal cyst could be mistakenly aspirated, and that aspiration may be less likely to be effective in utero because of continued hormonal stimulation (Brandt et al. 1991). Cyst aspiration is not recommended for echogenic cysts. This sonographic finding indicates that the cyst has already undergone ovarian torsion; thus cyst aspiration would be of no benefit.

▶ TREATMENT OF THE NEWBORN

After delivery the neonate should have an ultrasound examination to confirm the antenatal diagnosis. If the postnatal scan demonstrates the presence of an echogenic cyst, surgery should be performed. Surgery usually consists of oophorectomy, because in most cases no viable ovarian tissue can be seen (Fig. 83-5) (Brandt et al. 1991). The pathologic reports of most reported

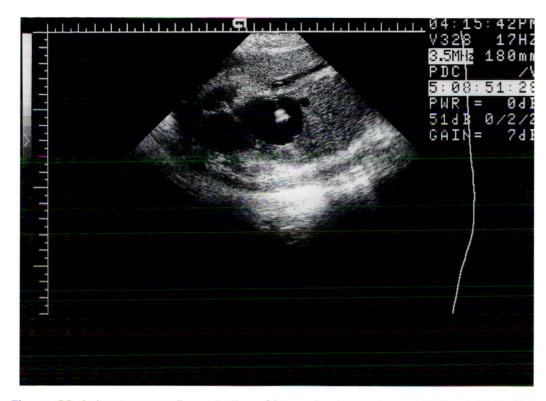

Figure 83-4. In utero needle aspiration of large simple ovarian cyst. *(Reprinted, with permission, from Crombleholme TM, Craigo SD, Garmel SH, D'Alton ME. Fetal ovarian cyst decompression to prevent torsion. J Pediatr Surg 1997;32:1447–1449.)*

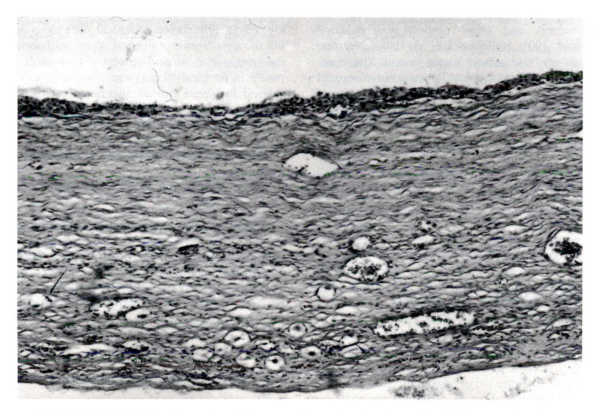

Figure 83-5. Histologic specimen from ovarian cyst demonstrating follicles in the cyst wall. *(Reprinted, with permission, from Holzgreve et al. Arch Obstet Gynecol 1989;245: 135–138.)*

program and are clean; 9 patients have a permanent colostomy; 7 young children soil and their parents have elected further treatment; and 5 have undergone surgery too recently to evaluate. In terms of urinary continence, 83 of 141 patients void spontaneously, 40 of 141 need to catheterize to empty their bladders, 4 have urinary diversions, and 1 has a continent diversion. Five other patients have urinary incontinence and will require further surgery. Eight patients have undergone surgery too recently to judge urinary continence. In Hendren's series, 24 patients were adults, of whom 14 were married, 17 have had coitus, and 6 have had children. Five adult women delivered their children by cesarean section and one by vaginal delivery (Greenberg and Hendren 1997).

▶ GENETICS AND RECURRENCE RISK

Persistent cloaca is a complex embryologic anomaly that is sporadic, with no increased risk of recurrence.

REFERENCES

Canning DA, Koo HP, Duckett JW. Anomalies of the bladder and cloaca. Pediatr Urol 1998:2445–2488.

deVries PA, Pena A. Posterior sagittal anorectoplasty. J Pediatr Surg 1982;17:638–642.

Gray SW, Skandalakis JE, eds. Embryology for surgeons. Philadelphia: Saunders, 1972.

Greenberg JA, Hendren WH. Vaginal delivery after cloacal malformation repair: a case report. Obstet Gynecol 1997; 90:666–667.

Hendren WH. Cloaca, the most severe degree of imperforate anus. Ann Surg 1998;228:331–346.

Hendren WH. Urogenital sinus and anorectal malformation: experience with 22 cases. J Pediatr Surg 1980;15: 628–641.

Hubbard A, Pena A. Total urogenital mobilization: an easier way to repair cloacas. J Pediatr Surg 1997; 32:263–268.

Pena A, deVries PA. Posterior sagittal anorectoplasty: important technical considerations and new applications. J Pediatr Surg 1982;17:696–711.

Rich MA, Brock WA, Pena A. Spectrum of genitourinary malformations in patients with imperforate anus. Pediatr Surg Int 1988;3:110–113.

Sato Y, Pringle KC, Bergman RA, et al. Congenital anorectal anomalies: MR imaging. Radiology 1988;168:157–162.

Stephens FD, Smith ED. Anorectal malformations in children. Chicago: Year Book, 1971.

CHAPTER 85

Polycystic Kidney Disease

► CONDITION

Polycystic kidney disease (PKD) is an inherited disorder with diffuse involvement of both kidneys. Aside from the presence of the cysts, there is no evidence of renal dysplasia. Multiple renal cysts frequently coexist with lesions in other viscera, especially the liver (Kaplan et al. 1989a). A renal cyst is defined as an enclosed sac or nephron segment lined by epithelial cells dilated to more than 200 μm. A cystic kidney is a kidney with three or more cysts present. Cystic kidney disease is the illness caused by a cystic kidney (Kaplan et al. 1989a).

As early as 1902, it was known that the age distribution of cystic renal disease had two peaks: one close to birth and the other between 30 and 60 years of age (Kaplan et al. 1989b). In general, the use of the term *polycystic kidney disease* is restricted to single-gene disorders: autosomal dominant PKD (traditionally known as adult-onset) and recessively inherited PKD (traditionally known as the infantile form). Since the 1970s, physicians have understood that the adult form can also present during infancy. In the recessive form of PKD, generalized dilatation of the collecting tubules exists, whereas in dominant PKD, cysts develop in localized segments of the kidney anywhere along the nephron (Kaplan et al. 1989a).

The dominantly inherited form of PKD (ADPKD) is a highly penetrant nephropathy with variable clinical expression that presents mainly during adulthood, but the disease can also occur at any other time during life. In ADPKD progressive asymptomatic enlargement of both kidneys occurs with a gradual decline in renal function. Ultrasonography can detect renal cysts in 56% of affected patients during the first decade of life, 80% during the second decade of life, and almost 100% of individuals by the third decade of life (Michaud et al. 1994). The infantile presentation of the adult onset form of PKD was not appreciated until 1971 (Shokeir 1978).

Bilateral PKD can be attributed to two genetically determined conditions. The so-called infantile form of PKD is inherited as an autosomal recessive condition. The cystic dilations are fusiform and arranged radially throughout the kidney. The cysts are due to dilations of the distal convoluted tubules and collecting ducts. Concomitant cystic hepatic involvement is observed. Among survivors, hepatic fibrosis, cirrhosis, and portal hypertension occur.

The recessively inherited form of polycystic disease (ARPKD) manifests during the neonatal period with respiratory distress or during early infancy with renal insufficiency. There is a wide variation in clinical course (Wisser et al. 1995). The renal involvement in ARPKD is invariably bilateral and largely symmetrical. It is always associated with generalized portal and interstitial fibrosis of the liver (Romero et al. 1984; Zerres et al. 1988). In 1971, Blyth and Ockenden subdivided patients with ARPKD into four groups according to the proportion of dilated renal tubules present. The perinatal classification was associated with the onset of renal failure in utero or at birth and resulted in perinatal or neonatal death. These patients had at least 90% involvement of the renal tubules. The neonatal presentation resulted in a smaller kidney size and mild hepatic fibrosis, but these patients died within 1 year and had 60% of their kidneys affected. The infantile presentation resulted in clinical symptoms by the age of 3 to 6 months, moderate hepatic fibrosis, and hepatosplenomegaly with progressive chronic renal failure, and systemic and portal hypertension. These patients had 25% of their kidneys affected. The latest presentation was the juvenile-onset, which occurred between 6 months and 1 year of age and had only 10% of the kidney affected (Blyth and Ockenden 1971).

From the perspective of prenatal diagnosis and neonatal presentation, the adult form of PKD is rarer—it usually presents during the fourth to fifth decade of

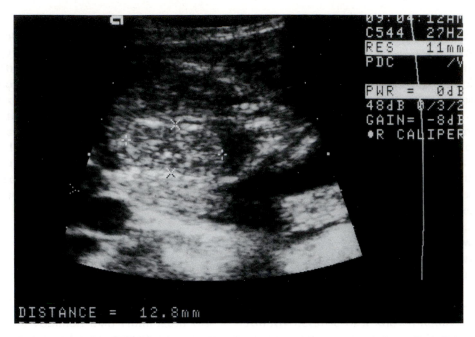

Figure 85-2. Prenatal sonographic image demonstrating increased echogenicity and multiple small cysts in a fetus with Meckel–Gruber syndrome.

series of branching divisions of the ureteral bud, forming the renal pelvis and major calices around 12 to 14 weeks of gestation. This branching reaches its maximum at 22 weeks of gestation but continues until 34 to 36 weeks of gestation, when the kidney is fully formed (Bronshtein et al. 1990). Pathogenesis of kidney diseases result from one of six causes (Bronshtein et al. 1990):

1. Failure of union between primitive collecting ducts and nephrons
2. Failure of involution of the first generation of nephrons
3. Obstruction of urine flow at the level of the pelvis, urethra, or bladder outlet
4. Intratubular obstruction
5. Abnormalities of the tubular wall and supporting tissues
6. Adrenocortical maternal steroid ingestion

PKD is characterized by enlargement of renal cysts, interstitial fibrosis, and gradual loss of normal renal tissue in association with progressive deterioration of renal function. In one study, apoptotic DNA fragmentation was detected in polycystic kidneys from five patients with renal failure (Woo 1995). Apoptotic cells were demonstrated in glomeruli, cyst walls, and both cystic and noncystic tubules of the polycystic kidneys. These authors hypothesize that apoptotic loss of renal tissue may be associated with progressive deterioration

▶ **TABLE 85-1.** CONDITIONS ASSOCIATED WITH RENAL CYSTS

Chromosomal abnormalities	Other
Trisomy 8 mosaic	Beckwith–Wiedmann syndrome
Trisomy 13	Noonan syndrome
Trisomy 18	Goldenhar syndrome
Triploidy	Lissencephaly
Turner syndrome (45,X)	
Single-gene disorders	
Ehlers–Danlos syndrome	
Orofacial digital syndrome	
Zellweger syndrome	
Tuberous sclerosis	
Lawrence–Moon–Biedl syndrome	
Multiple acyl CoA dehydrogenase defect	
Meckel–Gruber syndrome	
Acromandibular–renal syndrome	

of renal function that occurs in patients with PKD. The specific findings in ARPKD, consisting of large, coarsely hyperechoic kidneys, are thought to be secondary to the presence of innumerable microscopic cortical and medullary cysts. The interfaces of these cysts provide increased echogenicity.

ADPKD is the only form of cystic disease that involves a collecting tubule as well as the nephron. Normal and abnormal nephrons are intermixed (Pretorius et al. 1987). In ADPKD, cysts occur in only 1 to 2% of renal tubules, but it is thought that the affected abnormal nephrons enlarge steadily until they compress and distort the normal parenchyma to the point of causing impaired renal function (Grantham 1988). Michaud et al. (1994) reported on three cases of ADPKD and performed a literature review. Of 32 affected fetuses, 28 had prenatal sonographic manifestations of disease or siblings with early onset of disease. Pathologic studies demonstrated that the cysts could be found in newly formed nephrons or in more mature nephrons of the deep cortex. The glomeruli were predominantly affected in the fetus. These authors hypothesized that cysts develop in most patients with ADPKD during fetal life and that the rate at which these cysts increase in size determines the clinical severity of the disease (Michaud et al. 1994).

► MANAGEMENT OF PREGNANCY

The diagnosis of fetal renal cystic disease mandates complete ascertainment of the family history. It is also recommended that both parents have a renal ultrasound examination performed because of the high prevalence of the ADPKD gene in the general population. Due to the higher prevalence of ARPKD in the prenatally diagnosed population, a fetus with bilateral renal enlargement and echogenicity is more likely to have ARPKD if both parents have normal ultrasound examinations. However, caution must be observed, due to the apparent false positive diagnoses of ARPKD reported in the literature (Lilford et al. 1992). Several authors have described additional diagnostic testing to help with determination of the underlying cause. For example, Tsuda et al. (1994) diagnosed ARPKD in a fetus at risk by measuring hourly fetal urine production. This was reduced in an affected fetus as compared with a normal fetus. Magnetic resonance imaging (MRI) has been performed at 25 weeks of gestation in a fetus diagnosed with bilateral enlarged hyperechogenic kidneys, oligohydramnios, and a small bladder at 22 weeks of gestation. The MRI revealed corticomedullary differentiation but could not demonstrate the presence of renal cysts. The kidneys were noted to be massively increased in size with a very high water content in the renal parenchyma (Nishi et al. 1991). Nicolini et al. (1992) aspirated fetal urine

from 21 large cystic renal masses in 18 fetuses diagnosed between 20 and 35 weeks of gestation. They demonstrated that urinary concentrations of sodium, calcium, and phosphate were significantly higher in the multicystic group as compared with the hydronephrotic group. They concluded that reabsorption of phosphate was impaired in multicystic kidneys.

In the absence of the demonstration that one of the parents is affected with ADPKD, counseling regarding expected prognosis can be difficult. Even when one of the parents is known to have ADPKD, the short-, mid-, and long-term prognoses for fetuses in whom renal cysts are demonstrated early in life is unknown (Journel et al. 1989). In the past, fetuses diagnosed with ARPKD were given a dismal prognosis; however, increasing information from the pediatric literature indicates that general health and lifespan for these infants are better than was previously thought. For a presumed diagnosis of ARPKD, the prospective parents should have a complete discussion with a pediatric nephrologist and neonatologist regarding the extent of resuscitation for the affected newborn. Delivery should be planned to occur in a tertiary-care center, due to the expected problems with respiratory insufficiency, potential for air leak secondary to oligohydramnios and hypertension.

► FETAL INTERVENTION

There are no fetal interventions for polycystic kidney disease.

► TREATMENT OF THE NEWBORN

Newborns with ARPKD often receive minimal intervention because poor respiratory and renal outcomes are anticipated. In 1995, Bean et al. described two unrelated infants with ARPKD whose respiratory failure was successfully treated with surfactant and mechanical ventilation. Of interest was the fact that the massive kidney size restricted gastrointestinal capacity and limited feeding and growth. In these two cases, unilateral nephrectomy allowed improved feedings. Both patients had their caloric intake supplemented by nightly feedings by gastrostomy tube, to give a caloric equivalent of 120 to 130 kcal per kilogram of body weight per day. Both patients required long-term medications for treatment of hypertension; however, both exhibited normal neurodevelopment for age at 4 years 9 months and 19 months of follow-up. Both of these patients required minimal hospitalization after the neonatal period.

Aggressive neonatal resuscitation is controversial for ARPKD. Despite intervention, many patients die after birth because of respiratory compromise. Those who survive have progressive renal insufficiency and hepatic fibrosis, and will ultimately need renal transplantation. All of these issues must be discussed with the prospective parents.

Fetuses affected with ADPKD have far fewer symptoms and are unlikely to present with spontaneous pneumothorax, oligohydramnios, or liver or spleen enlargement (Cole et al. 1997). In the absence of severe oligohydramnios, standard resuscitation and neonatal supportive treatment are appropriate for infants with ADPKD.

▶ SURGICAL TREATMENT

The only surgical treatment available for these conditions is unilateral nephrectomy or renal transplantation. At New England Medical Center, we have performed unilateral nephrectomy on an emergency basis for an infant with ARPKD because the rapid and massive enlargement of the right kidney compressed the inferior vena cava and seriously impeded venous blood return to the heart (Figs. 85-3 and 85-4).

▶ LONG-TERM OUTCOME

A critical milestone for PKD appears to be survival past the first few months of age. Kaplan et al. (1989b) reviewed the clinical features in 55 cases of ARPKD. Of the 24 patients who presented during the neonatal pe-

riod, 12 (50%) survived beyond 2 years of age. These authors performed an actuarial analysis and showed that once a patient survived beyond 1 year of age, the projected chance of survival beyond 15 years of age was 78%. This data is in agreement with that of Cole et al. (1987), who performed a retrospective survey of 48 patients with PKD who survived the first month and were seen before 1 year of age. These authors indicated that most children diagnosed with PKD who survived the first months of life live for many years. The majority of all affected children require long-term antihypertensive therapy for persistent problems with high blood pressure.

What is not clearly known, however, is the prognosis for fetuses with the dominant form of PKD who are identified antenatally. In a review of 13 prenatal diagnoses of ADPKD, Pretorius et al. (1987) showed that 10 of 13 infants were alive at the time of follow-up. Three were dead because of elective termination of pregnancy, sepsis, or respiratory distress syndrome associated with hyaline-membrane disease. Of the 10 surviving children, 8 had normal renal function at the time of follow-up. There is some indication that the neonatal detection of ADPKD correlates with development of hypertension and renal failure in early childhood. However, it is unclear what the fetal presentation of ADPKD implies for future symptoms (Journel et al. 1989).

A review of the literature suggests that fetuses with severe oligohydramnios are unlikely to survive the perinatal period. Improvements in neonatal care permit moderate to severely affected infants with ARPKD to survive the perinatal period. Survival beyond 1 month

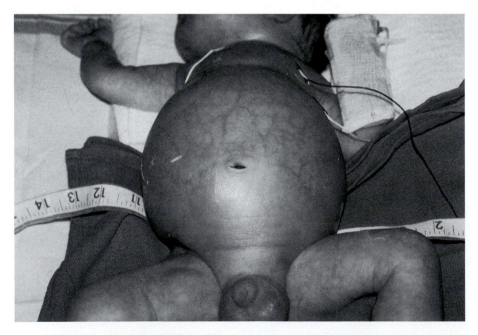

Figure 85-3. A neonate with ARPKD. Massive and rapid enlargement of the right kidney compressed the inferior vena cava, which necessitated emergency nephrectomy.

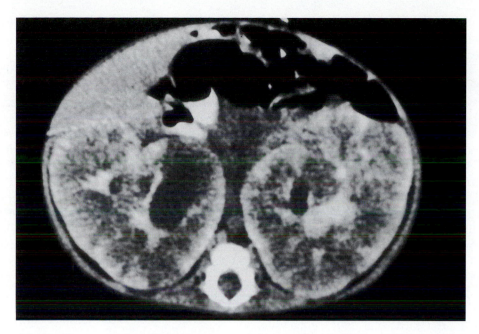

Figure 85-4. Postnatal CT scan from same infant in Figure 85-3 showing bilateral presence of multiple cysts in enlarged kidneys.

of life generally indicates the propensity for long-term survival in affected infants with ARPKD. These children require long-term medication and close medical follow-up; however, the literature does not indicate that they spend their entire lives in the hospital. The long-term prognosis for children affected with the dominantly inherited form of PKD is good because in childhood they are more mildly affected. Their clinical situation is also complicated by the fact that in most cases, one of their parents also has the disease, and they may therefore be more likely to continue the pregnancy.

▶ GENETICS AND RECURRENCE RISK

Several authors have discussed the difficulties associated with the dual identification of both fetus and parent affected with ADPKD. In Pretorius's study (1987) only 5 of 13 parents were aware of their disease prior to pregnancy. The diagnosis of renal cystic disease in the fetus and young infant should trigger an investigation of the family history. Sonography should be performed on the parents. In ADPKD, however, the severity of parental involvement does not predict either the severity of the child's involvement or the age at onset of symptoms (Michaud et al. 1994). It is well known that difficulties exist in genetic counseling for ADPKD. In one study, 23% of subjects were aware of the hereditary nature of the disease, only 18% had genetic counseling, and 9% had family members examined by sonography (Journel et al. 1989). Fertility is not reduced in ADPKD.

Because it is difficult to distinguish between ADPKD

and ARPKD on sonographic examination and many young parents who have ADPKD are normal on sonographic examination, most geneticists believe that DNA diagnosis is more reliable for prenatal detection of the affected fetus. Fortunately, much recent investigative activity has been directed toward mapping the various genes associated with ARPKD and ADPKD.

ARPKD appears to be genetically homogeneous (Guay-Woodford et al. 1995). ARPKD is caused by a single gene with multiple mutant alleles. This accounts for the relatively high phenotypic concordance within families, as well as the broad range of phenotypes evident among different families. The ARPKD gene was mapped to chromosome 6p21-cen in 1994 (Zerres et al. 1994). Most of the families analyzed in this initial report, however, had a milder clinical phenotype compatible with survival beyond infancy. In 1995, Guay-Woodford et al. confirmed and extended Zerres et al.'s findings by performing linkage analysis in families that manifested the severe perinatal lethal form of ARPKD. They narrowed the interval for the gene to 6p21.1-p12 and confirmed that ARPKD results from a single mutant gene.

In contrast, ADPKD is genetically heterogeneous. At least three genes are known to cause ADPKD (Grantham 1995). ADPKD-1 maps to chromosome 16p13.3 and is responsible for 85% of cases. ADPKD-2 has been mapped to chromosome 4q13-q23 (Peters et al. 1993). It has been postulated that a third gene, ADPKD-3, may be responsible for a small minority of cases, but its chromosomal location is unknown. Spontaneous mutations occur in less than 10% of cases of ADPKD (Gabow 1993).

DNA linkage analysis in ADPKD was first demonstrated in 1985, when Reeders et al. described a DNA marker located near the α-globin gene cluster on chromosome 16 that was co-inherited with ADPKD. The existence of a second gene causing ADPKD was first suspected in 1988 (Kimberling et al. 1988; Romeo et al. 1988). Peters et al. (1993) reported the assignment of a second gene for ADPKD to chromosome 4. Of interest is that patients who do not have ADPKD-1 seem to be diagnosed at an older age, are less likely to have hypertension, live longer, and have fewer renal cysts present at the time of diagnosis. This indicates phenotypic and well as genotypic heterogeneity for ADPKD (Ravine et al. 1992). The first DNA-based prenatal diagnosis of ADPKD was performed in 1986 by Reeders et al.

The ADPKD-1 gene was cloned and sequenced in 1994 (European Polycystic Kidney Disease Consortium 1994). It is a very large gene whose protein product is called "polycystin," which is a glycoprotein of about 4300 amino acid residues (Harris et al. 1995). Polycystin-1 is a cell–cell matrix interaction protein. It is important for production and maintenance of renal tissue and connective tissue in other organs. It is also expressed in arterial smooth muscle (Griffin et al. 1997). This explains the multisystem nature of the disease. Large sections of the gene are duplicated at separate locations on chromosome 16, and all of these segments of DNA are transcriptionally active. Most ADPKD-1 mutations have been detected in the single copy 3' end of the gene, but a group of patients with deletion of PKD-1 and the adjacent tuberous sclerosis 2 gene (with severe infantile PKD) have been characterized (Harris et al. 1995). In the typical patients with adult-onset ADPKD-1, small deletions, splicing defects, or a nonsense mutation have been detected in the 3' end of the gene. In each case, a transcript is produced by the mutant gene. Rarely, large deletions that disrupt, or completely delete, the PKD-1 gene are detected. In every case these mutations also disrupt the adjacent tuberous sclerosis gene. ADPKD-2 has also been cloned and sequenced. Both PKD-1 and PKD-2 code for novel proteins (van Adelsberg 1999). Polycystin-1 is a receptor and similarities between the polycystins and calcium channel subunits suggest that these proteins are subunits of a novel channel.

Families at risk for either ARPKD or ADPKD should have blood samples collected for DNA analysis prior to contemplating a future pregnancy. For both of these conditions, it is necessary to establish the linkage phase of the DNA markers by performing haplotyping on the index family. For ADPKD, due to the genetically heterogeneous nature of the disorder, there should be enough affected family members tested to determine whether the disease is due to ADPKD-1, ADPKD-2, or other genes (Breuning et al. 1990). To date, the largest review of prenatal DNA analysis in families at risk of ARPKD reviewed 65 diagnoses (Zerres et al. 1998). In the majority of the requesting families, the index child was deceased; DNA was extracted from paraffin-embedded tissue. In 4 of the 65 cases, a recombination event occurred between flanking markers and no diagnosis was possible. Forty-three fetuses were diagnosed correctly as unaffected. In 18 fetuses, homozygosity for the disease-associated haplotype was demonstrated. Pathologic changes consistent with ARPKD were seen as early as 13 weeks of gestation in 2 fetuses, both of which were terminated. This study showed that haplotype-based prenatal testing is feasible and reliable in pregnancies at risk for ARPKD (Zerres et al. 1998). Once a mutation has been identified in a specific family, prenatal DNA diagnosis is available as early as 10 weeks of gestation via chorionic villus sampling. DNA diagnosis is recommended for definitive prenatal diagnosis over prenatal sonographic diagnosis, which can be nonspecific.

REFERENCES

Bean SA, Bednarek FJ, Primack WA. Aggressive respiratory support and unilateral nephrectomy for infants with severe perinatal autosomal recessive polycystic kidney disease. J Pediatr 1995;127:311–314.

Blethyn J, Jones A, Sullivan B. Prenatal diagnosis of unilateral renal disease in tuberous sclerosis. Br J Radiol 1991; 64:161–164.

Blyth H, Ockenden BG. Polycystic disease of kidneys and liver presenting in childhood. J Med Genet 1971;8:257–284.

Bronshtein M, Yoffe N, Brandes M, Blumenfeld Z. First- and early second-trimester diagnosis of fetal urinary tract anomalies using transvaginal sonography. Prenat Diagn 1990;10:653–666.

Breuning MH, Snijdewint FGM, Dauwerse JG, et al. Two step procedure for early diagnosis of polycystic kidney disease with polymorphic DNA markers on both sides of the gene. J Med Genet 1990;27:614–617.

Cole BR, Conley SB, Stapleton B. Polycystic kidney disease in the first year of life. J Pediatr 1997;111:693–699.

Estroff JA, Mandell J, Benacerraf BR. Increased renal parenchymal echogenicity in the fetus: importance and clinical outcome. Radiology 1991;181:135–139.

European Polycystic Kidney Disease Consortium. The polycystic kidney disease 1 gene encodes a 14kb transcript and lies within a duplicated region on chromosome 16. Cell 1994;77:881–894.

Gabow P. Autosomal dominant polycystic kidney disease. N Engl J Med 1993;329:332–342.

Griffin MD, Torres VE, Grande JP, Kumar R. Vascular expression of polycystin. J Am Soc Nephrol 1997;8:616–626.

Grantham JJ. Polycystic kidney disease—an old problem in a new context. N Engl J Med 1988;319:944–946.

Grantham JJ. Polycystic kidney disease—there goes the neighborhood. N Engl J Med 1995;333:56–58.

Guay-Woodford LM, Muecher G, Hopkins D, et al. The severe perinatal form of autosomal recessive polycystic kidney disease maps to chromosome 6p21.1-p12: implications for genetic counseling. Am J Hum Genet 1995;56:1101–1107.

Harris PC, Ward CJ, Peral B, Hughes J. Autosomal dominant polycystic kidney disease: molecular analysis. Hum Mol Genet 1995;4:1745–1749.

Jeffrey S, Saggar-Malik AK, Economides DL, Blackmore SE, MacDermot KD. Apparent normalization of fetal renal size in autosomal dominant polycystic kidney disease (PKD1). Clin Genet 1998;53:303–307.

Journel H, Guyott C, Barc RM, Belbeosch P, Quemener A, Jouan H. Unexpected ultrasonographic prenatal diagnosis of autosomal dominant polycystic kidney disease. Prenat Diagn 1981;9:663–671.

Kaplan BS, Kaplan P, Rosenberg HK, Lamothe E, Rosenblatt DS. Polycystic kidney diseases in childhood. J Pediatr 1989a;115:867–880.

Kaplan BS, Kaplan JF, Shah V, Dillon MJ, Barratt M. Autosomal recessive polycystic kidney disease. Pediatr Nephrol 1989b;3:43–49.

Kimberling WJ, Fain PR, Kenyon JB, Goldgar D, Sujansky E, Gabow PA. Linkage heterogeneity of autosomal dominant polycystic kidney disease. N Engl J Med 1988;319:913–918.

Lilford RJ, Irving HC, Allibone EB: A tale of two prior probabilities—avoiding false positive antenatal diagnosis of autosomal recessive polycystic kidney disease. Br J Obstet Gynaecol 1992;99:216–219.

Luthy DA, Hirsch JH. Infantile polycystic kidney disease: observations from attempts at prenatal diagnosis. Am J Med Genet 1985;20:505–517.

MacDermot KD, Saggar-Malik AK, Economides DL, Jeffrey S. Prenatal diagnosis of autosomal dominant polycystic kidney disease (PKD1) presenting in utero and prognosis for very early onset disease. J Med Genet 1998;35:13–16.

McHugo JM, Shafi MI, Rowlands D, Weaver J. Prenatal diagnosis of adult polycystic kidney disease. Br J Radiol 1988;61:1072–1074.

Michaud J, Russo P, Grignon A, et al. Autosomal dominant polycystic kidney disease in the fetus. Am J Med Genet 1994;51:240–246.

Nicolini U, Vaughan JI, Gisk NM, Dhillon HK, Rodeck CH. Cystic lesions of fetal kidney: diagnosis and prediction of postnatal function by fetal urine biochemistry. J Pediatr Surg 1992;27:1451–1454.

Nishi T, Iwasaki M, Yamato M, Nakano R. Prenatal diagnosis of autosomal recessive polycystic kidney disease by ultrasonography and magnetic resonance imaging. Acta Obstet Gynecol Scand 1991;70:615–617.

Peters DJM, Spruit L, Saris JJ, et al. Chromosome 4 localization of a second gene for autosomal dominant polycystic kidney disease. Nat Genet 1993;5:359–362.

Pretorius DH, Lee E, Manco-Johnson ML, Weingast GSR, Sedman AB, Gabow PA. Diagnosis of autosomal dominant polycystic kidney disease in utero and in the young infant. J Ultrasound Med 1987;6:249–255.

Ravine D, Walker RG, Gibson RN, et al. Phenotype and genotype heterogeneity in autosomal dominant polycystic kidney disease. Lancet 1992;340:1330–1334.

Reeders ST, Breuning MH, Davies KE, et al. A highly polymorphic DNA marker linked to adult polycystic kidney disease on chromosome 16. Nature 1985;317:542–544.

Reeders ST, Zerres K, Gal A, et al. Prenatal diagnosis of autosomal dominant polycystic kidney disease with a DNA probe. Lancet 1986;1:6–8.

Romeo G, Devoto M, Costa G, et al. A second genetic locus for autosomal dominant polycystic kidney disease. Lancet 1988;2:8–10.

Romero R, Cullen M, Jeanty P, et al. The diagnosis of congenital renal anomalies with ultrasound. II. Infantile polycystic kidney disease. Am J Obstet Gynecol 1984;150:259–262.

Shokeir MHK. Expression of "adult" polycystic renal disease in the fetus and newborn. Clin Genet 1978;14:61–72.

Tsuda H, Matsumoto M, Imanaka M, Ogita S. Measurement of fetal urine production in mild infantile polycystic kidney disease—a case report. Prenat Diagn 1994;14:1083–1085.

van Adelsberg JS. The role of the polycystins in kidney development. Pediatr Nephrol 1999;13:454–459.

Wapner RJ, Kurtz AB, Ross RD, Jackson LG. Ultrasonographic parameters in the prenatal diagnosis of Meckel syndrome. Am J Obstet Gynecol 1981;57:388–392.

Wisser J, Hebisch G, Froster U, et al. Prenatal sonographic diagnosis of autosomal recessive polycystic kidney disease (ARPKD) during the early second trimester. Prenat Diagn 1995;15:868–871.

Woo D. Apoptosis and loss of renal tissue in polycystic kidney diseases. N Engl J Med 1995;333:18–25.

Zerres K, Hansmann M, Mallmann R, Gembruch U. Autosomal recessive polycystic kidney disease: problems of prenatal diagnosis. Prenat Diagn 1988;8:215–229.

Zerres K, Mucher G, Bachner L, et al. Mapping of the gene for autosomal recessive polycystic kidney disease (ARPKD) to chromosome 6p21-cen. Nat Genet 1994;7:429–432.

Zerres K, Mucher G, Becker J, et al. Prenatal diagnosis of autosomal recessive polycystic kidney disease (ARPKD): molecular genetics, clinical experience, and fetal morphology. Am J Med Genet 1998;76:137–144.

Zerres K, Weiss H, Bulla M, Roth B. Prenatal diagnosis of an early manifestation of autosomal dominant adult type polycystic kidney disease. Lancet 1992;2:988.

CHAPTER 86

Renal Agenesis

► CONDITION

Renal agenesis is the congenital absence of one or both kidneys due to the complete failure of the kidney to form. The syndrome of renal agenesis, severe oligohydramnios, amnion nodosum, flattened face, low-set and floppy ears, bilateral pulmonary hypoplasia, and perinatal death was first described by Potter in 1946.

Renal agenesis is a developmental anomaly that occurs at 4 to 6 weeks of embryonic life (Kaffe et al. 1977). Normal renal embryogenesis requires that three events take place—the ureteric buds must arise bilaterally from mesonephric (wolffian) ducts; subsequently, bilateral metanephric blastema must form from mesoderm in the caudal region of the nephrogenic cord; and finally, ureteric buds must grow, contact, and invaginate the metanephric blastema, thereby inducing differentiation of the blastema into two mature kidneys (Wax et al. 1994). Failure of the metanephros to develop results in complete absence of the kidney. This can be due to either nonexistence of the ureteral bud or failure of the ureteral bud to develop from the wolffian duct.

In unilateral renal agenesis, there is complete absence of the kidney on one side, with compensatory hypertrophy on the contralateral side. Most cases of unilateral renal agenesis are due to lack of induction of the metanephric blastema by the ureteral bud, but some cases of absent kidney may be due to in utero regression of a multicystic dysplastic kidney (see Chapter 82) (Mesrobian et al. 1993). In cases of unilateral renal agenesis, compensatory hypertrophy of the remaining kidney occurs prenatally. This has been demonstrated by Hartshorne et al. (1991), who performed a retrospective analysis of 20 fetuses who died with unilateral renal agenesis. Total renal mass was measured and was shown to comprise 82.7% of the weight of both kidneys removed from control fetuses at the same gesta-

tional age. Had prenatal compensatory hypertrophy not occurred, the total renal mass would have been only 50% of control values (Hartshorne et al. 1991). It is of biologic interest that in unilateral renal agenesis, symmetrical hypertrophy of all nephron components occurs during prenatal life, when the placenta clears all metabolic waste products. These authors hypothesized that it is the change in renal mass, rather than abnormality in function, that triggers compensatory growth of the contralateral kidney. This may be due to an as yet uncharacterized renotropic humoral growth factor (Hartshorne et al. 1991).

► INCIDENCE

The incidence of bilateral renal agenesis is 1 in 3000 births (Cardwell 1988; Droste et al. 1990). The incidence of bilateral renal agenesis is 1 in 240 stillbirths (Whitehouse and Mountrose 1978). Bilateral renal agenesis is 2.5 times more common in males than in females. Bilateral renal agenesis is also more common in twins as compared with singletons. Some authors have postulated a common cause for twinning and the development of renal agenesis (Roodhooft et al. 1984). An increased incidence of bilateral renal agenesis is not associated with advanced maternal age or maternal illness. Unilateral renal agenesis occurs in 1 in 500 to 1 in 1300 live births, although many cases are clinically silent (Bronshtein et al. 1995). In one study, the missing kidney was nearly always the left one (Hartshorne et al. 1991) but in another study of 46 consecutive cases of unilateral renal agenesis, the right kidney was absent in 19 of 46 individuals (Cascio et al. 1999). The true incidence of unilateral agenesis is likely to be even greater because this abnormality can be asymptomatic throughout life.

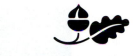

CHAPTER 87

Sirenomelia

▶ CONDITION

Sirenomelia, also known as "mermaid syndrome," has been noted since the Greco-Roman period. Initially described in the medical literature by Rocheus in 1542 (Murphy et al. 1992), the condition is characterized by a single lower extremity, with the concomitant presence of severe anomalies of the urogenital and gastrointestinal system. Although historical and mythologic accounts portray sirens and mermaids as females, the majority of patients with sirenomelia are male (deJonge et al. 1984). In all likelihood the confusion originated as a result of the fact that most patients with sirenomelia had no obvious external genitalia.

It is often stated that sirenomelia is characterized by apparent fusion of the lower limbs. This terminology is embryologically incorrect because *fusion* refers to two processes joining after breakdown of intervening epithelia. *Merging* is the more correct term, because it does not imply intervening breakdown of epithelium. Sirenomelia, therefore, is a syndrome of merging, malrotation, and dysgenesis of the lower extremities (Kapur et al. 1991). In 1865, Förster classified sirenomelia into three groups according to the number of feet present (van Zalen-Sprock et al. 1995). In symelia apus, the most common of the three conditions, both legs are merged completely into a single lower extremity. Both feet are absent or rudimentary. On radiographic studies, only one femur is present; there are no fibulae and one or two tibulae. In symelia unipus, one foot is present, and up to 10 toes also may be seen (see Fig. 87-1). In this type of sirenomelia, two femora, two tibia, and two fibulae are present. In symelia dipus, two distinct feet are present, although generally they are malrotated, and often give the appearance of fins. In 1961, Duhamel coined the term *caudal regression syndrome* and first recognized an association between caudal regression

and lower-extremity abnormalities. He noted the presence of additional associated anomalies in sirenomelia, including sacral agenesis, anorectal atresia, renal agenesis, single umbilical artery, and ambiguous genitalia (Duhamel 1961).

The cause of sirenomelia is still debated. Most agree that the site of injury to the embryo is the caudal mesoderm (Murphy et al. 1992). Sirenomelia probably results from a localized insult to the caudal end of the developing embryo between 13 and 22 days of development (Hoyme 1988). By 23 days of embryonic age, the prospective limb bud regions normally assume a lateral position, separated by allantoic structures. If the lower extremity remains unipodal, the insult must have occurred prior to this point in gestation (Stevenson et al. 1986). Two theories have been developed to explain the occurrence of sirenomelia: vascular and caudal injury. In 1927, Kampmeier reviewed 52 cases of sirenomelia, and was the first to note the constant finding of a single umbilical artery. He postulated that the single umbilical artery was very important in the etiology of the sirenomelia, and that a vascular abnormality would affect the allantoic circulation with subsequent abnormal development of caudal elements. More recently, Talamo et al. (1982) performed postmortem arteriography on an infant with sirenomelia and documented a persistent vitelline artery and a dorsal hypoplastic distal aorta. They demonstrated that the femoral arteries ran anteriorly and posteriorly along the single femur, rather than in the normal orientation of right and left. They thought that this demonstrated a failure of rotation during early embryonic life and supported the pathogenetic concept of limb-bud merging and malrotation after damage to the posterior axis mesoderm. Stevenson et al. (1986) dissected the abdominal vasculature in 11 cases of sirenomelia and documented the common feature of a single large artery arising from high

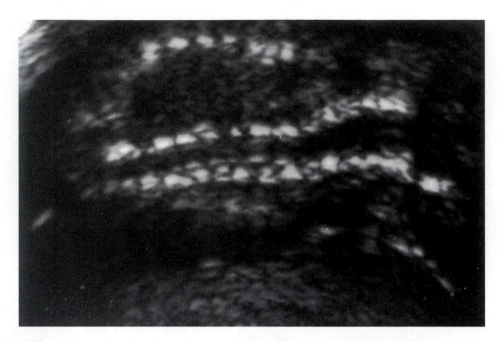

Figure 87-3. Sonographic image of scoliosis and abnormal vertebrae seen in a case of sirenomelia. This antenatally obtained image corresponds to the radiograph shown in Figure 87-1B. *(Reprinted, with permission, from Van Zalen-Sprock MM, Van Vugt JMG, Van Der Harten JJ, Van Geijn HP. Early second-trimester diagnosis of sirenomelia. Prenat Diagn 1995;15:171–177.)*

were notable for the fact that despite the presence of bilateral renal agenesis, the amniotic fluid volume was only slightly decreased as compared with normal fetuses at the same gestational age. A larger series of 11 cases of sirenomelia diagnosed prenatally noted oligohydramnios as a universal finding. In only 5 of 11 cases (45%) was the correct diagnosis made prenatally. The remaining cases were diagnosed as bilateral renal agenesis. Significant additional anomalies noted included cardiovascular defects (36%), abdominal-wall defects (36%), severe scoliosis (45%), and other skeletal deformities (90%) (Sirtori et al. 1989). Sonographic features that permit the correct antenatal diagnosis of sirenomelia include consideration of the diagnosis whenever bilateral renal agenesis is demonstrated, demonstration of persistently opposed lower extremities, and observation of a single hypoplastic foot with absent fibulae (Kapur et al. 1991).

▶ DIFFERENTIAL DIAGNOSIS

Sirenomelia should be considered in the setting of severe oligohydramnios. Other considerations in the differential diagnosis include isolated bilateral renal agenesis, which is 11 times more common than sirenomelia (Wright and Christopher 1982) (see Chapter 86). Color flow Doppler studies may be of benefit in imaging the renal arteries when bilateral renal agenesis is suspected

(see Fig. 87-4) (Sepulveda et al. 1998). Magnetic resonance imaging has also been suggested as a helpful adjunct to characterize sirenomelia in the setting of oligohydramnios (Fitzmorris-Glass et al. 1989; Twickler et al. 1993).

▶ ANTENATAL NATURAL HISTORY

Most patients with sirenomelia have bilateral renal agenesis. Consequently, oligohydramnios begins during the second trimester, when the kidneys would normally be producing fetal urine. Uterine size may be smaller than the gestational dates indicate. The consequences of severe oligohydramnios eventually manifest during the third trimester, and include pulmonary hypoplasia and Potter facies. There is an increased risk of spontaneous pregnancy loss with this condition. Sirenomelia occurs in 4 in 1000 pregnancies that are spontaneously lost (Malinger et al. 1987).

▶ MANAGEMENT OF PREGNANCY

When sirenomelia is suspected antenatally, consideration should be given to obtaining a fetal radiograph to look for the bony abnormalities seen in the lower merged extremity (Wright and Christopher 1982) (see Fig. 87-1B). If there is concern about inability to visualize

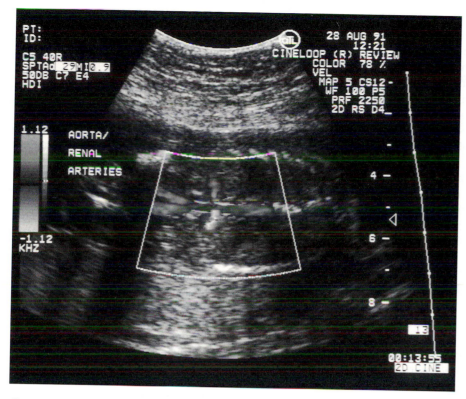

Figure 87-4. Color flow Doppler image demonstrating presence of two renal arteries. The demonstration of two normal renal arteries makes the diagnosis of sirenomelia unlikely. See color plate.

the fetal bladder, amnioinfusion should be considered (Langer et al. 1996). Maternal furosemide administration is no longer recommended because of the high incidence of false positive results. In the setting of severe oligohydramnios, chromosome studies from amniocytes may be very difficult to obtain, and their indication is debatable. Over 300 cases of sirenomelia have been reported in the literature, and the majority have had normal chromosome studies. Only two cases of chromosomal abnormalities have been reported, and in each case the abnormal chromosomes were obtained from specific organ tissue. In one case, chromosome studies were performed on pericardial tissue; they revealed mosaicism for a tandem duplication of the long arm of chromosome 1—46,XX/46,XX, dir dup (1) (q12 → qter) (Stevenson et al. 1986). In the other case, a fibroblast culture was obtained from the abnormal lower limb of an infant with sirenomelia. Metaphase spreads from this culture had a 6-fold increase in chromosomal breaks and a 23-fold increase in abnormal chromosome associations. There were multiple quadriradials observed that involved nonhomologous chromosomes. In contrast, fibroblasts obtained from a skin biopsy from the normal upper limb of the same patient had a normal karyotype (Sprague et al. 1970). Despite these intriguing findings, postnatal karyotyping in a confirmed case of sirenomelia is not indicated.

▶ FETAL INTERVENTION

There are no fetal interventions indicated for sirenomelia.

▶ TREATMENT OF THE NEWBORN

In the past, sirenomelia was considered uniformly fatal due to the known association with other major anomalies, including bilateral renal agenesis. Since 1989, however, there have been two reports of survivors with this condition. Lethality in this condition is due to the associated visceral anomalies that determine prognosis. If adequate renal function is present, survival outside the womb is possible. Savader et al. (1989) described the first survivor with this condition. This patient was noted to have fusion of the lower extremity to the level of the heels with a normal anus and kidneys, a normal heart, and single umbilical artery and transposition of the external genitalia and urethral opening. Postnatal magnetic resonance imaging confirmed the presence of distinct epiphyseal ossification centers and well-developed normal anatomic muscle groups that would permit future separation of the lower extremities. Subsequently, Murphy et al. (1992) described a patient who was diagnosed at 29 weeks of gestation and not expected to survive. Cesarean delivery was performed at term. The

study of collagen in the tissue and in chondrocytes cultured in agarose. Am J Med Genet 1994;49:439–446.

Glenn LW, Teng SSK. In utero sonographic diagnosis of achondrogenesis. J Clin Ultrasound 1985;13:195–198.

Godfrey M, Keene DR, Blank E, et al. Type II achondrogenesis-hypochondrogenesis: morphologic and immunohistopathologic studies. Am J Hum Genet 1988; 43:894–903.

Golbus MS, Hall BD, Filly RA, Poskanzer LB. Prenatal diagnosis of achondrogenesis. J Pediatr 1977;91:464–466.

Graham D, Tracey J, Winn K, Corson V, Sanders RC. Early second trimester sonographic diagnosis of achondrogenesis. J Clin Ultrasound 1983;11:336–338.

Jaeger HJ, Schmitz-Stolbrink A, Hulde J, Novak M, Roggenkamp K, Mathias K. The boneless neonate: a severe form of achondrogenesis type I. Pediatr Radiol 1994;24: 319–321.

Jimenez RB, Holmes LB, Kaiser JS, Weber AL. Achondrogenesis. Pediatrics 1973;51:1087–1090.

Lachman RS, Rappaport V. Fetal imaging in the skeletal dysplasias. Clin Perinatol 1990;17:703–722.

Mahony BS, Filly RA, Cooperberg PL. Antenatal sonographic diagnosis of achondrogenesis. J Ultrasound Med 1984;3:333–335.

Meizner I, Barnhard Y. Achondrogenesis type I diagnosed by transvaginal ultrasonography at 13 weeks' gestation. Am J Obstet Gynecol 1995;173:1620–1622.

Orioli IM, Castilla EE, Barbosa-Neto JG. The birth prevalence rate for the skeletal dysplasias. J Med Genet 1986; 23:328–332.

Ornoy A, Sekeles E, Smith P, Simkin A, Kohn G. Achondrogenesis type I in three sibling fetuses: scanning and transmission electron microscopic studies. Am J Pathol 1976;82:71–84.

Pretorius DH, Rumack CM, Manco-Johnson ML, et al. Specific skeletal dysplasias in utero: sonographic diagnosis. Radiology 1986;159:237–242.

Rimoin DL. International nomenclature of constitutional diseases of bone. J Pediatr 1978;93:614–616.

Rimoin DL. Molecular defects in the chondrodysplasias. Am J Med Genet 1996;63:106–110.

Saldino RM. Lethal short-limbed dwarfism: achondrogenesis and thanatophoric dwarfism. Am J Roentgenol Radium Ther Nucl Med 1971;112:185–197.

Smith WL, Breitweiser TD, Dinno N. In utero diagnosis of achondrogenesis type I. Clin Genet 1981;19:51–54.

Soothill PW, Vuthiwong C, Rees H. Achondrogenesis type II diagnosed by transvaginal ultrasound at 12 weeks' gestation. Prenat Diagn 1993;13:523–528.

Superti-Furga A, Hästbacka J, Wilcox WR, et al. Achondrogenesis type IB is caused by mutations in the diastrophic dysplasia sulphate transporter gene. Nat Genet 1996;12: 100–102.

Tongsong T, Srisomboon J, Saudasna J. Prenatal diagnosis of Langer-Saldino achondrogenesis. J Clin Ultrasound 1995;23:56–58.

van der Harten HJ, Brons JT, Dijkstra PF, et al. Achondrogenesis-hypochondrogenesis: the spectrum of chondrogenesis imperfecta: a radiological, ultrasonographic, and histopathologic study of 23 cases. Pediatr Pathol 1988;8:571–597.

Wenstrom KD, Williamson RA, Hoover WW, Grant SS. Achondrogenesis type II (Langer-Saldino) in association with jugular lymphatic obstruction sequence. Prenat Diagn 1989;9:527–532.

Whitley CB, Gorlin RJ. Achondrogenesis: new nosology with evidence of genetic heterogeneity. Radiology 1983; 148:693–698.

CHAPTER 89

Achondroplasia

► CONDITION

Achondroplasia is the most common form of short-limbed dwarfism. The condition has been recognized since ancient times. A person with achondroplasia may have served as an artistic model for depictions of the Egyptian god, Bes, who was the protector of children (Hecht 1990). The term achondroplasia, meaning total absence of cartilage, was first used by Parrot in 1878 (Scott 1976). Although this is not correct in a pathologic sense, the designation is commonly accepted.

► INCIDENCE

The incidence of achondroplasia is 1 in 26,000 live births (Oberklaid et al. 1979). Earlier studies that indicated an incidence of as high as 1 in 10,000 births probably included other causes of short-limbed dwarfism. Over 80% of cases are sporadic as opposed to familial (Shiang et al. 1994). Advanced paternal age is correlated with an increased incidence of new mutations resulting in achondroplasia (Murdoch et al. 1970).

► SONOGRAPHIC FINDINGS

Virtually all of the bones in the body are affected by achondroplasia. Postnatal radiographic studies of the lumbar spine, pelvis, and cranial regions permit definitive diagnosis (Fig. 89-1). Antenatally, diagnosis is complicated by a relatively normal appearance until the early second trimester. The most consistent sonographic finding is shortening of the long bones, particularly the femur, occurring between 21 and 27 weeks of gestation (Fig. 89-2) (Kurtz et al. 1986). The overall shape of the femurs is within normal limits. Initially, a normal

relationship of biparietal diameter to femur is present, but these measurements become progressively asynchronous over time (Filly et al. 1981). Additional findings that have been described during the second trimester include large head (macrocrania), abnormal facial profile due to frontal bossing (Fig. 89-3), protuberant abdomen, and trident-shaped hand (Fig. 89-4) (Cordone et al. 1993). For prenatal diagnosis in the setting of a parent affected with achondroplasia, the fetus is considered to be affected if the length of the long bones is less than the third percentile or if polyhydramnios is present (Elejalde et al. 1983; Lattanzi and Harger 1982). If both parents are unaffected, prenatal diagnosis is more challenging. A fetus in which long bone growth is initially normal but then drops below the 10th percentile during the third trimester needs to be serially evaluated for the possibility of achondroplasia or hypochondroplasia. Hypochondroplasia is considered to be an allele of achondroplasia, with less severe clinical manifestations.

► DIFFERENTIAL DIAGNOSIS

The most likely diagnosis for a fetus with shortened long bones is that the fetus is normal or has intrauterine growth restriction that is not due to a skeletal dysplasia. However, the differential diagnosis includes chromosomal abnormalities as well as other types of dwarfism, some of which may be lethal at birth. An important prenatal finding that distinguishes achondroplasia from some of the other skeletal dysplasias is the initially normal first- and second-trimester long-bone measurements.

Other considerations in the differential diagnosis include diastrophic dysplasia, a recessively inherited form of short-limbed dwarfism, with the additional findings

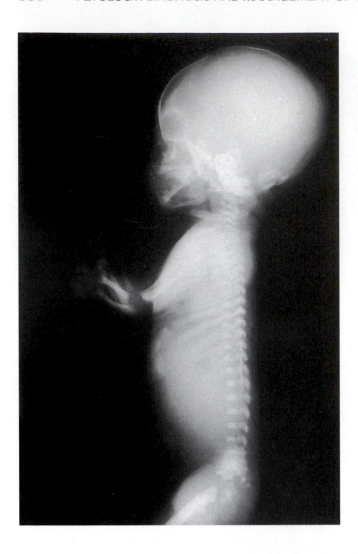

Figure 89-1. Postnatal radiograph of a patient with achondroplasia demonstrating flattened vertebral bodies with increased intervertebral space, cupped anterior ends to ribs, and hypoplastic midfacial bones. *(Reprinted, with permission, from Cordone M, Lituania M, Bocchino G, Passamonti U, Toma P, Camera G. Ultrasonographic features in a case of heterozygous achondroplasia at 25 weeks' gestation. Prenat Diagn 1993;13:400, Copyright 1993 John Wiley & Sons, Ltd. Reprinted, with permission, of John Wiley & Sons, Ltd.)*

of thickening of the external ear and the characteristic "hitch-hiker" thumbs (see Chapter 93). In achondrogenesis, a lethal, recessively inherited condition, there is deficient ossification of the vertebral bodies. As compared with achondroplasia, a greater discrepancy between head size and trunk exists in achondrogenesis (see Chapter 88). In chondroectodermal dysplasia (Ellis–van Creveld syndrome), progressive distal shortening of the extremities and postaxial polydactyly are present (see Chapter 94). In addition, congenital heart malformations are present in 50% of cases. In hypochondroplasia, the major findings are short stature and an increased upper- to lower-body-segment ratio. The facial features are within normal limits.

▶ ANTENATAL NATURAL HISTORY

Little is known about the antenatal natural history of achondroplasia. Distortion in bone growth is due to

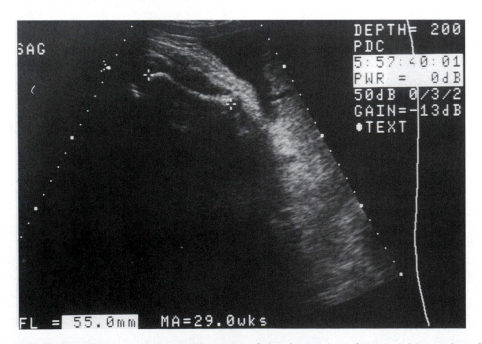

Figure 89-2. Shortening (<5%) and bowing of the femur in a fetus at 29 weeks of gestation with heterozygous achondroplasia.

Figure 89-3. Antenatal facial profile of the fetus in Figs. 89-1 and 89-2 demonstrating frontal bossing, depressed nasal bridge, and an elongated philtrum. *(Reprinted, with permission, from Cordone M, Lituania M, Bocchino G, Passamonti U, Toma P, Camera G. Ultrasonographic features in a case of heterozygous achondroplasia at 25 weeks' gestation. Prenat Diagn 1993;13:398, Copyright 1993 John Wiley & Sons, Ltd. Reprinted, with permission, of John Wiley & Sons, Ltd.)*

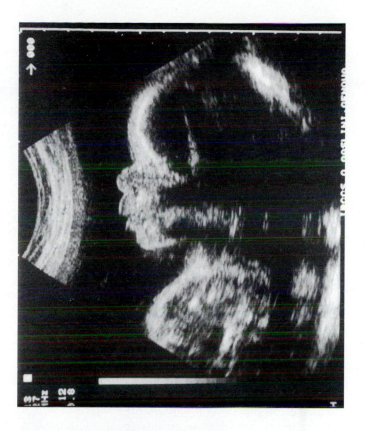

retardation in endochondral bone formation (Kurtz et al. 1986). Membranous bone formation occurs at a normal rate (Murdoch et al. 1970). The abnormality in achondroplasia is confined to cartilage, and consists of a failure of interstitial cells to proliferate. Bones that are initially formed from cartilage, such as the long bones of the extremities, bones at the base of the skull, and vertebral bodies, are affected by this condition.

In histologic studies of bone and cartilage from patients with achondroplasia, morphology is normal (Rimoin et al. 1976). The arrangement of rows and columns of cells is regular and well organized. The rate of endochondral ossification is reduced, and this contrasts with the normal periosteal ossification. This disparity results in periosteal bone extending beyond the

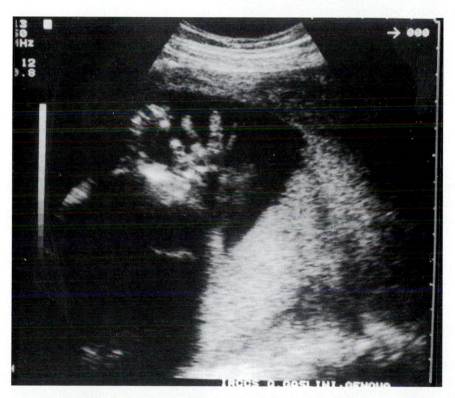

Figure 89-4. Prenatal sonogram of fetal hand at 25 weeks of gestation demonstrating relatively short phalanges and trident-like appearance. *(Reprinted, with permission, from Cordone M, Lituania M, Bocchino G, Passamonti U, Toma P, Camera G. Ultrasonographic features in a case of heterozygous achondroplasia at 25 weeks' gestation. Prenat Diagn 13: 397, Copyright 1993 John Wiley & Sons, Ltd. Reprinted, with permission, of John Wiley & Sons, Ltd.)*

growth plate, and gives the appearance of short squat bones with cupped ends. Ultrastructural studies are also generally normal. The only abnormalities demonstrated have been a relative increase in the number of dead cells surrounded by microscars that contain focal aggregations of collagen fibrils (Rimoin et al. 1976).

▶ MANAGEMENT OF PREGNANCY

For an unaffected mother, the antenatal course for this condition is usually benign. When achondroplasia is suspected, serial sonography may be useful to determine if macrocrania is developing, which may necessitate cesarean delivery.

For the mother affected with achondroplasia, special problems include increased incidence of fetal wastage, preeclampsia, and dyspnea on exertion and at rest. Cesarean delivery is mandatory for cephalopelvic disproportion secondary to marked pelvic contracture (Lattanzi and Harger 1982).

The cloning of the gene responsible for achondroplasia, fibroblast growth factor receptor 3 (*FGFR3*), (Shiang et al. 1994) allows DNA-based prenatal diagnosis. This is especially important for couples in which both partners are affected. In this situation, there is a 25% chance that the fetus will inherit the two mutant genes, resulting in homozygous achondroplasia. This condition is associated with a very high incidence of fetal and neonatal death. In one report, first-trimester DNA diagnosis has been described in a couple at risk for homozygous achondroplasia (Bellus et al. 1994).

▶ FETAL INTERVENTION

In recent years, fetal chromosome analysis has been increasingly performed for short fetal bones due to the concerns of possible trisomy 21 (see Chapter 134). In the setting of a fetus with short bones and a normal karyotype, amniotic fluid cells may be used as a source of fetal DNA to test for *FGFR3* mutations. If a *FGFR3* mutation is found, this would provide a definitive cause for the short fetal stature.

▶ TREATMENT OF THE NEWBORN

Most newborn infants with achondroplasia do not require special medical treatment and can be treated in the regular nursery. In fact, 75% of cases of achondroplasia are missed at birth. According to one study, even at 1 year of age, only 60% of cases are diagnosed (Saleh and Burton 1991). For infants with achondroplasia, the main issues are definitive diagnosis and coordination of subspecialty care. All infants with a suspected diagnosis of achondroplasia should have radiographs taken of the long bones.

The salient clinical findings of achondroplasia in the newborn include short stature of the rhizomelic type. This means that the proximal arms and legs are relatively more shortened than the distal segments of the extremities. However, the short stature may be mild or even absent. Horton et al. (1978) have shown that the range of birth length in newborns with achondroplasia overlaps the normal population. Mean growth velocity is also normal during the first year of life. It is after the first year that growth velocity drops significantly. Other features of achondroplasia during the newborn period may include macrocrania, frontal bossing, and midface hypoplasia with coarsened facial features. The lumbar lordosis that is apparent later in life is rarely appreciated at birth. Cognitive development, socialization, speech, and language milestones are achieved normally, but initial gross motor milestones may be delayed (Scott 1976). The muscular hypotonia responsible for delayed motor development disappears spontaneously at 4 to 6 years of age. The general pediatric recommendations for health supervision for children with achondroplasia have been summarized (Committee on Genetics, American Academy of Pediatrics 1995).

A serious potential problem in achondroplasia is cervicomedullary junction compression due to a small foramen magnum. This can result in occipitocervical pain, ataxia, incontinence, or the more serious complication of apnea and sudden infant death (Pauli et al. 1984). The foramen magnum is narrowed in a transverse direction (Hecht et al. 1989). Magnetic resonance imaging (MRI) studies in five affected patients have demonstrated the discrepancy between the size of the brain stem and the foramen magnum (Thomas et al. 1988). In addition, hydrocephalus is frequently found due to anatomic abnormalities in the occipital bone that produce intracranial venous hypertension. It has been hypothesized that obstruction at the jugular foramen elevates intracranial venous pressure, resulting in decreased absorption of cerebrospinal fluid into the sagittal sinus, producing a communicating hydrocephalus (Thomas et al. 1988).

Approximately 10% of patients with achondroplasia have respiratory complications due to foramen magnum compression (Stokes et al. 1983; Thomas et al. 1988). It is recommended that computed tomographic (CT) or MRI scanning be performed in conjunction with somatosensory evoked potentials to screen for this problem (Reid et al. 1987). Although posterior fossa decompression and atlantal laminectomy represent major surgical intervention, symptoms have been reported to improve postoperatively (Ryken and Menezes 1994). The increased mortality seen in achondroplasia (Hecht et al. 1987) is due primarily to this brain-stem compression and it affects children less than 4 years old.

▶ SURGICAL TREATMENT

The orthopedic deformities in achondroplasia consist of bowing of the legs, hyperlordosis, and spinal stenosis. In about 25% of cases, the bowing of the legs is treated with corrective osteotomies of the tibia. This surgery is usually performed between 3 and 10 years of age. Although spinal stenosis is universal, only in relatively few cases does it cause cauda equina syndrome, which manifests as a lower-motor-neuron flaccid paralysis. This becomes evident during very late adolescence or adulthood and requires a decompressive laminectomy. The most severe but least common orthopedic problem is thoracolumbar kyphosis, which can cause paraplegia earlier in childhood. This requires aggressive spinal surgery.

Surgical therapies currently being optimized may also significantly improve the cosmetic aspects of achondroplasia. Craniofacial surgery is possible to advance midfacial bones and correct severe dental malocclusion (Denny et al. 1992). Recombinant human growth hormone given to patients with achondroplastic dwarfism at doses of 0.3 mg per kilogram of body weight per week moderately increased overall height velocity, particularly in the short term. There were no untoward effects, particularly with regard to worsening of the degree of spinal stenosis (Horton et al. 1992). Further clinical trials are in progress to more fully assess long-term safety and efficacy of growth hormone in this condition. More recent evidence indicates that it is only velocity and not ultimate height that increases.

Leg lengthening has received much attention as a means of improving height and appearance for patients with achondroplasia (Fig. 89-5). The surgery is painful; it should be performed on only adolescents; and it may take up to 2 years to complete (Saleh and Burton 1991).

▶ LONG TERM OUTCOME

The long-term consequences of achondroplasia are cervicomedullary compression, spinal stenosis, restrictive and obstructive lung disease, otitis media, and tibial bowing (Hunter et al 1998). Mental development is generally normal.

Standard growth curves exist to assess normal growth for children with achondroplasia (Horton et al. 1978). The average adult height for an affected male is 52 inches (129 cm) and an affected female 48.6 inches (122 cm). The average adult weight for a male is 120 lb (55kg), and a female 100 lb (45kg) (Murdoch et al. 1970; Scott 1976). Obesity is common (Hecht et al. 1988). In sporadic cases, parental height does not significantly influence the dwarf's adult height (Murdoch et al. 1970; Scott 1976).

Further medical problems for children with achondroplasia include recurrent ear infections and conductive

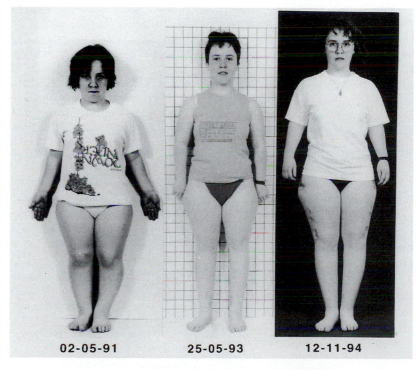

02-05-91   25-05-93   12-11-94

Figure 89-5. Patient with achondroplasia demonstrating cosmetic effects of multiple leg-lengthening operations over an almost 4-year period. *(Courtesy of Professor Michael Saleh, Sheffield Children's Hospital, Sheffield, United Kingdom.)*

and sensorineural hearing loss. Patients with achondroplasia have specific structural changes of the temporal bone, although it is unclear how these changes relate to hearing loss (Shohat et al. 1993). For many patients dental crowding necessitates orthodontic treatment.

The intelligence quotient is normal for individuals with achondroplasia. One study compared 20 adults affected with achondroplasia with siblings of the same sex and found that the mean number of years of formal education were comparable for each group. Females, more than males, have a significantly lower occupational level as compared with their sisters (Roizen et al. 1990). It was questioned whether this was due to a self-esteem problem that was more profound in females. The psychiatric aspects of achondroplasia have also been studied. In general, patients with achondroplasia had achieved satisfactory life adjustment and had secure identities as "little people" (Brust et al. 1976). The functional health status of adults with achondroplasia, as measured by the short form 36, is not drastically reduced in comparison with the general United States population (Mahomed et al. 1998).

▶ GENETICS AND RECURRENCE RISK

Achondroplasia is inherited as an autosomal dominant condition. Fifty percent of an affected parent's offspring will also have achondroplasia. The phenotype is 100% penetrant, which means that all offspring who carry the gene will express the full clinical appearance of achondroplasia. As stated earlier, the majority of cases are due to new mutations. Murdoch (1970) studied 148 patients with achondroplasia. Thirty-one (21%) had one or both parents affected, whereas 117 cases (79%) had no family history of the condition. It should be noted, however, that several cases of gonadal mosaicism have been described in which normal parents have given birth to multiple affected children (Fryns et al. 1983).

The gene involved in achondroplasia was localized to chromosome 4, band p16.3 in 1994. (LeMerrer et al. 1994). The gene involves coding sequences for fibroblast growth factor receptor 3 (*FGFR3*). At least nine different heparin-binding fibroblast growth factors are known. All of them have pleiotropic effects on different cell types and have quite different patterns of expression during development. Evidence that the *FGFR3* gene was a good "candidate" gene for achondroplasia included the fact that *FGFR3* mRNA is found in the central nervous system and all of the prebone cartilage structures of the mouse (Shiang et al. 1994).

In a landmark study, Shiang and coworkers (1994) demonstrated point mutations in the DNA of 15 of 16 individuals studied with achondroplasia. The mutations all occurred at nucleotide 1138 and resulted in the substitution of an arginine residue for a glycine at position 380 of the mature protein, which is in the transmembrane domain of *FGFR3*. This work has been validated and extended by other investigators, who have also shown that all achondroplasia mutations studied result in the same substitutions at the same amino acid of the transmembrane domain of the *FGFR3* protein (Bellus et al. 1994; Rousseau et al. 1994). The homogeneous nature of these mutations in achondroplasia is unprecedented for an autosomal dominant disorder. This may explain the phenotypic similarity between all patients with achondroplasia. Based on these results, rapid polymerase chain reaction–based prenatal diagnosis is now available for the condition (Bellus et al. 1994). DNA testing is relatively straightforward because the mutations involved are minimal in number, and they create new recognition sites for restriction endonucleases (Francomano 1995). In sporadic cases of achondroplasia, the FGFR3 mutation is exclusively paternal in origin (Wilin et al. 198).

It is now known that achondroplasia is only one of the four diseases caused by mutations in the *FGFR3* gene. The other three are hypochondroplasia and thanatophoric dysplasia (see Chapter 100), and severe achondroplasia with developmental delay and acanthosis nigricans (SADDAN) (Bellus et al. 1999; Bonaventure et al. 1996).

REFERENCES

Bellus GA, Bamshad MJ, Przylepa KA, et al. Severe achondroplasia with developmental delay and acanthosis nigricans (SADDAN): phenotypic analysis of a new skeletal dysplasia caused by a Lys650Met mutation in fibroblast growth factor receptor 3. Am J Med Genet 1999;85:53–65.

Bellus GA, Escallon CS, Ortiz de Luna R, et al. First trimester prenatal diagnosis in couple at risk for homozygous achondroplasia. Lancet 1994;344:1511.

Bonaventure J, Rousseau F, Legeai-Mallet L, Le Merrer M, Munnich A, Maroteaux P. Common mutations in the fibroblast growth factor receptor 3 (*FGFR3*) gene account for achondroplasia, hypochondroplasia, and thanatophoric dwarfism. Am J Med Genet 1996;63:148–154.

Brust JS, Ford CV, Rimoin DL. Psychiatric aspects of dwarfism. Am J Psychiatry 1976;133:160–164.

Committee on Genetics, American Academy of Pediatrics. Health supervision for children with achondroplasia. Pediatrics 1995;95:443–451.

Cordone M, Lituania M, Bocchino G, Passamonti U, Toma P, Camera G. Ultrasonographic features in a case of heterozygous achondroplasia at 25 weeks' gestation. Prenat Diagn 1993;13:395–401.

Denny AD, Gingrass DJ, Ferguson DJ. Comprehensive correction of the craniofacial deformity in achondroplastic dwarfism. Ann Plast Surg 1992;29:550–558.

Elejalde R, de Elejalde MM, Hamilton PR, Lombardi JM. Prenatal diagnosis in two pregnancies of an achondroplastic woman. Am J Med Genet 1983;15:437–439.

Filly RA, Golbus MS, Carey JC, Hall JG. Short-limbed dwarfism: ultrasonographic diagnosis by mensuration of fetal femoral length. Radiology 1981;138:653–656.

Francomano CA. The genetic basis of dwarfism. N Engl J Med 1995;332:58–59.

Fryns JP, Kleczkowska A, Verresen H, Van den Berghe H. Germinal mosaicism in achondroplasia: a family with 3 affected siblings of normal parents. Clin Genet 1983;24:156–158.

Hecht F. Bes, Aesop, and Morgante: reflections of achondroplasia. Clin Genet 1990;37:279–282.

Hecht JT, Francomano CA, Horton WA, Annegers JF. Mortality in achondroplasia. Am J Hum Genet 1987;41:454–464.

Hecht JT, Hood OJ, Schwartz RJ, Hennessey JC, Bernhardt BA, Horton WA. Obesity in achondroplasia. Am J Med Genet 1988;31:597–602.

Hecht JT, Horton WA, Reid CS, Pyeritz RE, Chakraborty R. Growth of the foramen magnum in achondroplasia. Am J Med Genet 1989;32:528–535.

Horton WA, Hecht JT, Hood OJ, Marshall RN, Moore WV, Hollowell JG. Growth hormone therapy in achondroplasia. Am J Med Genet 1992;42:667–670.

Horton WA, Rotter JI, Rimoin DL, Scott CI, Hall JG. Standard growth curves for achondroplasia. J Pediatr 1978;93:435–438.

Hunter AG, Bankier A, Rogers JG, Sillence D, Scott CI Jr. Medical complications of achondroplasia: a multicentre patient review. J Med Genet 1998;35:705–712.

Kurtz AB, Filly RA, Wapner RJ, et al. In utero analysis of heterozygous achondroplasia: variable time of onset as detected by femur length measurements. J Ultrasound Med 1986;5:137–140.

Lattanzi DR, Harger JH. Achondroplasia and pregnancy. J Reprod Med 1982;27:363–366.

LeMerrer M, Rousseau F, Legai-Mallet L, et al. A gene for achondroplasia-hypochondroplasia maps to chromosome 4p. Nat Genet 1994;6:318–321.

Mahomed NN, Spellmann M, Goldberg, MJ. Functional health status of adults with achondroplasia. Am J Med Genet 1998;78:30–35.

Murdoch JL, Walker BA, Hall JG, et al. Achondroplasia—a genetic and statistical survey. Am J Hum Genet 1970;33:227–235.

Oberklaid F, Danks DM, Jensen F, Stace L, Rosshandler S. Achondroplasia and hypochondroplasia. J Med Genet 1979;16:140–146.

Pauli RM, Scott CI, Wassman ER Jr, et al. Apnea and sudden unexpected death in infants with achondroplasia. J Pediatr 1984;104:342–348.

Reid CS, Pyeritz RE, Kopits SE, et al. Cervicomedullary compression in young patients with achondroplasia: value of comprehensive neurologic and respiratory evaluation. J Pediatr 1987;110:522–530.

Rimoin DL, Silberberg R, Hollister DW. Chondro-osseous pathology in the chondrodystrophies. Clin Orthop 1976;114:137–152.

Rogers JG, Perry MA, Rosenberg LA. IQ measurement with skeletal dysplasia. Pediatrics 1979;63:894–897.

Roizen N, Ekwo E, Gosselink C. Comparison of education and occupation of adults with achondroplasia with same-sex sibs. Am J Med Genet 1990;35:257–260.

Rousseau F, Bonaventure J, Legeall-Mallet L, et al. Mutations in the gene encoding fibroblast growth factor receptor-3 in achondroplasia. Nature 1994;371:252–254.

Ryken TC, Menezes AH. Cervicomedullary compression in achondroplasia. J Neurosurg 1994;81:43–48.

Saleh M, Burton M. Leg lengthening: patient selection and management in achondroplasia. Orthop Clin North Am 1991;22:589–599.

Scott CI Jr. Achondroplastic and hypochondroplastic dwarfism. Clin Orthop Relat Res 1976;114:18–30.

Shiang R, Thompson LM, Zhu Y-Z, et al. Mutations in the transmembrane domain of *FGFR3* cause the most common genetic form of dwarfism, achondroplasia. Cell 1994;78:335–342.

Shohat M, Flaum E, Cobb SR, et al. Hearing loss and temporal bone structure in achondroplasia. Am J Med Genet 1993;45:548–551.

Stokes DC, Phillips JA, Leonard CO, et al. Respiratory complications of achondroplasia. J Pediatr 1983;102:534–541.

Thomas IT, Frias JL, Williams JL, Friedman WA. Magnetic resonance imaging in the assessment of medullary compression in achondroplasia. Am J Dis Child 1988;142:989–992.

Wilkin DJ, Szabo JK, Cameron R, et al. Mutations in fibroblast growth-factor receptor 3 in sporadic cases of achondroplasia occur exclusively on the paternally derived chromosome. Am J Hum Genet 1998;63:711–716.

and in approximately one third of cases, polydactyly (Tahernia and Stamps 1977; Tongsong et al. 1999). One report described the absence of fetal respiratory movements at 36 weeks of gestation in addition to a borderline low normal thoracic to abdominal circumference ratio (Chen et al. 1996).

▶ DIFFERENTIAL DIAGNOSIS

The major diagnostic criterion in Jeune syndrome is an abnormally small, narrow thorax, with short ribs. The chest configuration often leads to pulmonary hypoplasia and consequent respiratory insufficiency. On postnatal radiographs, typical skeletal changes in the thorax and pelvis of a patient who does not have polydactyly suggest a diagnosis of Jeune syndrome (Brueton et al. 1990). If the patient has polydactyly, it may be extremely difficult to distinguish between Jeune syndrome and Ellis–van Creveld syndrome (Giorgi et al. 1990). Ellis–van Creveld syndrome (see Chapter 94) may be differentiated from Jeune syndrome by the presence of congenital heart defects in 50% of affected patients (Schinzel et al. 1985), the presence of natal teeth and dental cysts (Oberklaid et al. 1977), and additional oral findings consisting of a frenulum binding to the upper lip or a partial cleft upper lip connected by multiple frenulae to the alveolar ridge. Polydactyly is a constant feature of Ellis–van Creveld syndrome, although it is present in only 30% of patients with Jeune syndrome. In addition, patients with Ellis–van Creveld syndrome have fingernail hypoplasia, a finding generally absent in Jeune syndrome.

On prenatal sonographic diagnosis, the presence of long-bone shortening with absence of other abnormalities may suggest achondroplasia (see Chapter 89). In fact, many of the patients described in the literature with Jeune syndrome were originally thought to have achondroplasia (Oberklaid et al. 1977). Renal and hepatic dysfunction will eventually develop in patients with Jeune syndrome. These findings are not present in achondroplasia.

An additional consideration in the differential diagnosis is Poland anomaly, but this condition is usually asymmetric. Patients with Poland anomaly have syndactyly as well as hypoplasia or aplasia of the thoracic muscles on the affected side. Metaphyseal chondrodysplasia can also be distinguished from Jeune syndrome by specific skeletal abnormalities, disproportionate short stature in the affected patient, the presence of thin and sparse hair, and fingernail hypoplasia.

▶ ANTENATAL NATURAL HISTORY

Very little is known about the antenatal natural history of Jeune syndrome. For example, it is not known whether the condition is associated with increased lethality in utero. In one report of a fetus studied after termination at 23 weeks of gestation, histologic examination of chondro-osseous tissue obtained at autopsy revealed normal resting cartilage and normal growth plate at the iliac crest (Lipson et al. 1984). The major abnormality seen was persistence of calcified cartilage cores within the bone trabeculae deep into the metaphysis. However, this finding is not unique to Jeune syndrome; it has also been documented in Ellis–van Creveld syndrome (Lipson et al. 1984).

▶ MANAGEMENT OF PREGNANCY

Definitive sonographic diagnosis of Jeune syndrome can probably be accomplished only in the setting of a known positive family history. For families who have had a previously affected child with Jeune syndrome, prenatal diagnosis is accomplished by serial measurements of long bones and careful assessment of the thoracic circumference. Without a positive family history, it is unlikely that a specific diagnosis of Jeune syndrome will be made antenatally. In Jeune syndrome, the chromosomes are normal. Thus, there is no specific indication for an amniocentesis to study the fetal karyotype. If the diagnosis of Jeune syndrome is made antenatally, we recommend that delivery should occur at a tertiary-care center because of the need for respiratory support in most of the infants affected with this condition. Cesarean section should be performed only for standard obstetric indications.

▶ FETAL INTERVENTION

There are no fetal interventions for Jeune syndrome.

▶ TREATMENT OF THE NEWBORN

Infants with Jeune syndrome are at high risk for respiratory distress syndrome. In one report, 7 of 10 patients described with Jeune syndrome had severe respiratory problems during the newborn period (Oberklaid et al. 1977). In this group of 7 infants, 2 died on the first day of life from very severe pulmonary abnormalities and 4 died between 5 weeks and 3 years of life. One patient survived and was a healthy 15-year-old with normal stature at the time of the report (Oberklaid et al. 1977). Patients with Jeune syndrome have pulmonary hypoplasia due to restriction of the chest circumference. In one study, the lungs of an affected patient weighed 31% of normal and demonstrated a disproportionate reduction of the alveoli, as compared with the bronchi and bronchioles (Tahernia and Stamps 1977).

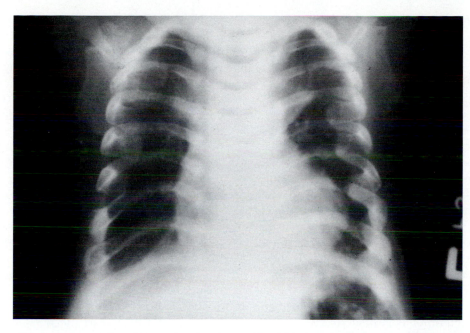

Figure 90-1. Postnatal radiograph of a 4-month-old infant with Jeune syndrome demonstrating narrow thorax and short ribs with expanded ends. *(Courtesy of Dr. Roy McCauley.)*

In addition to feeding problems, affected newborns with Jeune syndrome are also at risk for prolonged neonatal jaundice (Friedman et al. 1975; Hudgins et al. 1992). Definitive diagnosis is usually made radiographically. Chest x-ray films reveal short, horizontal ribs with a wide anterior portion and bulbous ends (Schinzel et al. 1985). The clavicles are described as having a "handle-bar" appearance (Fig. 90-1) (Rinaldi et al. 1990). The pelvis is small, with square-shaped iliac wings, a horizontal acetabular roof, and spur-shaped projections present on each side (Fig. 90-2). The pelvis has been described as having a "trident-like" appearance (Schmidt et al. 1972). The radiographic features in Jeune syndrome tend to be constant in the chest, although

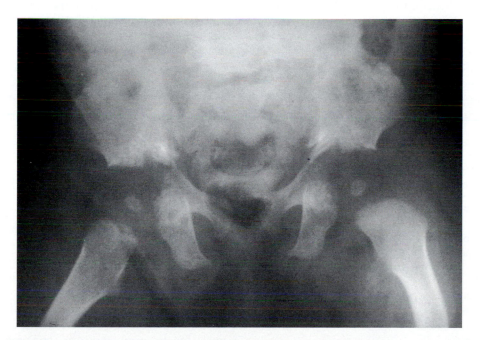

Figure 90-2. Postnatal radiograph of the same infant in Figure 90-1 demonstrating horizontal acetabular roof with spike of bone centrally, narrow sacrosciatic notches, and relatively mature ossification centers of the upper femora. *(Courtesy of Dr. Roy McCauley.)*

clinical severity may vary considerably (Oberklaid et al. 1977).

► SURGICAL TREATMENT

The alveolar hypoventilation seen in Jeune syndrome is due to impairment of expansion of the chest because of the short, horizontally positioned ribs, which results in pulmonary hypoplasia. In this condition, however, the lung alveolar growth potential is normal. Therefore, surgeons have postulated that expansion of the rib cage should allow further growth of the lungs. A surgical procedure has been described for thoracic expansion in Jeune syndrome (Davis et al. 1995). The chest wall is enlarged by lateral division of the ribs and underlying tissue in a staggered fashion so that either rib or periosteum covers the lung. The advantage of the lateral rib cage expansion is that it maintains anatomic protection of the anterior mediastinal structures. Subperiosteal rib osteotomies allow regrowth of the bone to stabilize rib expansion (Davis et al. 1995).

► LONG-TERM OUTCOME

A summary of the clinical findings in Jeune syndrome is listed in Table 90-1. Patients who survive infancy generally show improvement in pulmonary function but later die from progressive renal failure (Rinaldi et al. 1990). Progressive improvement also occurs in the appearance of the chest and the growth of the bony thorax in the patients who survive infancy (Gruskin and Fleischmann 1990).

The nature and extent of renal involvement depends on the age of the patient. In patients who died during infancy due to respiratory complications, autopsy studies revealed tubular dilatation, cortical cysts, cystic dysplasia, and diffuse cystic disease (Gruskin and Fleischmann 1990). In patients who survive infancy, renal

► TABLE 90-1. CLINICAL FINDINGS IN JEUNE SYNDROME

Short-limbed dwarfism
Long, narrow thorax, with short ribs
Respiratory problems
Brachydactyly with cone-shaped epiphyses
Short iliac wing with horizontal acetabulum
Polydactyly (+/−)
Progressive renal failure
Hepatic portal-tract fibrosis
Proliferation of bile ducts
Retinal abnormalities

Source: Wilson DJ, Weleber RG, Beals RK. Retinal dystrophy in Jeune's syndrome. Arch Ophthalmol 1987;105:651–657.

problems can present as polyuria, polydipsia, and hypertension manifesting as early as 2 or 3 years of age (Giorgi et al. 1990). Biopsy or autopsy studies have revealed tubular dilatation and atrophy, interstitial fibrosis, round lymphocytic cell infiltration of the kidney, glomerular sclerosis, and proteinuria (Gruskin and Fleischmann 1990). Patients in whom severe chronic renal failure develops but who are otherwise doing well have undergone successful renal transplantation (Giorgi et al. 1990; Gruskin and Fleischmann 1990). Some of the pathologic findings in this condition are considered to be indistinguishable from juvenile nephronophthisis (Shah 1980).

Another organ affected by this condition is the liver. Hepatic fibrosis, consisting of periportal fibrosis and bile-duct proliferation, is found consistently at autopsy and in liver-biopsy specimens. However, parenchymal changes are minimal (Hudgins et al. 1992; Oberklaid et al. 1977). Most patients with Jeune syndrome are free of symptoms related to the hepatic abnormalities, but occasionally patients do have persistent pruritus.

Other manifestations of Jeune syndrome include retinitis pigmentosa, optic atrophy, pigmentary retinopathy, polydactyly, hydrocephalus, pancreatic cysts, mitochondrial cytopathy, and cardiomyopathy (Gruskin and Fleischmann 1990). The retinal abnormalities occurring in this syndrome can include reduced visual acuity, photophobia, nystagmus, strabismus, and an abnormal electroretinogram (Wilson et al. 1987).

Mental and motor development in this syndrome is considered to be within normal limits (Friedman et al 1975; Giorgi et al. 1980).

In one case report, a 32-year-old male was described with Jeune syndrome. He was not dwarfed and had an adult height of 169 cm. He did, however, display the characteristic bony malformations of the thorax, pelvis, and extremities. The report stated that the thoracic malformations become less severe with age (Friedman et al. 1975). This adult individual had progressive renal disease due to cystic tubular dysplasia and glomerular sclerosis.

► GENETICS AND RECURRENCE RISK

Jeune syndrome is considered to be a single-gene disorder that is inherited as an autosomal recessive condition (Tahernia and Stamps 1977). Affected patients have been equally distributed between males and females. The disorder has been reported in individuals of both Caucasian and African-American ancestry. Parents who have previously had a pregnancy affected with Jeune syndrome have a 25% risk of recurrence. Prenatal diagnosis can be performed by serial measurement of the long bones. To date, the gene responsible for Jeune syndrome has not been identified.

REFERENCES

Brueton LA, Dillon MJ, Winter RM. Ellis-van Creveld syndrome, Jeune syndrome, and renal-hepatic-pancreatic dysplasia: separate entities or disease spectrum? J Med Genet 1990;27:252–255.

Chen CP, Lin SP, Liu FF, Jan SW, Lin SY, Lan CC. Prenatal diagnosis of asphyxiating thoracic dysplasia (Jeune Syndrome). Am J Perinatol 1996;13:495–498.

Davis JT, Ruberg RL, Leppink DM, McCoy KS, Wright CC. Lateral thoracic expansion for Jeune's asphyxiating dystrophy: a new approach. Ann Thorac Surg 1995;60:694–696.

de Elejalde BR, de Elejalde MM, Pansch D. Prenatal diagnosis of Jeune syndrome. Am J Med Genet 1985;21:433–438.

Friedman JM, Kaplan HG, Hall JG. The Jeune syndrome in an adult. Am J Med 1975;59:857–862.

Giorgi PL, Gabrielli O, Bonifazi V, Catassi C, Coppa GV. Mild form of Jeune syndrome in two sisters. Am J Med Genet 1990;35:280–282.

Gruskin AB, Fleischmann L. Clinical quiz. Pediatr Nephrol 1990;4:578–580.

Hudgins L, Rosengren S, Treem W, Hyams J. Early cirrhosis in survivors with Jeune thoracic dystrophy. J Pediatr 1992;120:754–756.

Lipson M, Waskey J, Rice J, et al. Prenatal diagnosis of asphyxiating thoracic dysplasia. Am J Med Genet 1984;18:273–277.

Oberklaid F, Danks DM, Mayne V, Campbell P. Asphyxiating thoracic dysplasia: clinical radiological, and pathological information on 10 patients. Arch Dis Child 1977;52:758–765.

Rinaldi S, Dionisi-Vici C, Goffredo B, Dallapiccola B, Rizzoni G. Jeune syndrome associated with cystinuria: report of two sisters. Am J Med Genet 1990;37:301–303.

Schinzel A, Savoldelli G, Briner J, Schubiger G. Prenatal sonographic diagnosis of Jeune syndrome. Radiology 1985;154:777–778.

Schmidt R, Pajewski M, Mundel G. Unusual features in familial asphyxiating thoracic dysplasia (Jeune's syndrome). Clin Genet 1972;3:90–98.

Shah KJ. Renal lesion in Jeune's syndrome. Br J Radiol 1980;53:432–436.

Tahernia AC, Stamps P. Jeune syndrome: report of a case, a review of the literature, and an editor's commentary. Clin Pediatr 1977;16:903–908.

Tongsong T, Chanprapaph P, Thongpadungroj T. Prenatal sonographic findings associated with asphyxiating thoracic dystrophy (Jeune syndrome). J Ultrasound Med 1999;18:573–576.

Wilson DJ, Weleber RG, Beals RK. Retinal dystrophy in Jeune's syndrome. Arch Ophthalmol 1987;105:651–657.

CHAPTER 91
Campomelic Dysplasia

► CONDITION

Campomelic dysplasia is a distinct clinical and radiologic entity characterized by symmetric bowing of the long bones of the lower extremity, sex reversal in some chromosomally male infants, and associated abnormalities, including cleft palate, flat facies, micrognathia, hydrocephalus, and renal abnormalities. The term campomelia comes from the Greek *camptos* meaning bent, and *melos,* meaning limbs. Despite the name of the condition, campomelia is not obligatory for a diagnosis of campomelic dysplasia (Ninomiya et al. 1995). MacPherson et al. (1989) described two newborn infants with respiratory distress who demonstrated all of the clinical and radiologic manifestations of campomelic dysplasia except the bent lower extremities. It is now known that the various skeletal and extraskeletal manifestations, including sex reversal, of campomelic dysplasia are part of a contiguous gene syndrome that maps to chromosome 17.

Classic campomelic dysplasia was first described by Maroteaux et al. (1971) and Bianchine et al. (1971) in independent reports. In a review of 43 affected patients, Hall and Spranger (1980) described four major radiologic features in patients with campomelic dysplasia: characteristic lower-limb bowing, absent or hypoplastic scapulas (which give rise to the "double clavicle" or "tomahawk" appearance on radiographs), nonmineralization of the thoracic pedicles, and narrow, vertical iliac bones (Fig. 91-1). They described other useful diagnostic features of the condition that included hypoplastic cervical vertebrae, widely spaced ischial bones, and absent ossification of the distal femoral and proximal tibial epiphyses. Khajavi et al. (1976) described campomelic dysplasia as a distinct entity consisting of short-limbed dwarfism with pretibial skin dimples, a

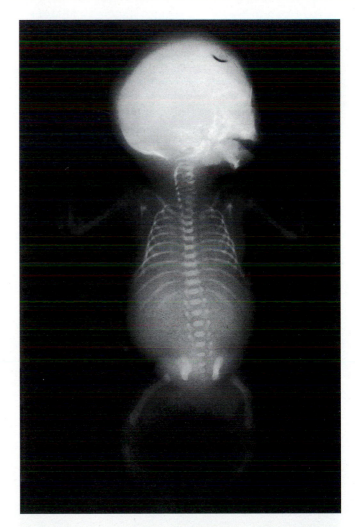

Figure 91-1. Postmortem radiograph obtained from a fetus with campomelic dsyplasia at 18 to 19 weeks of gestation. Note the bilateral sharp angulation of the femurs, hypoplastic scapulas and narrow, vertical ischial bones.

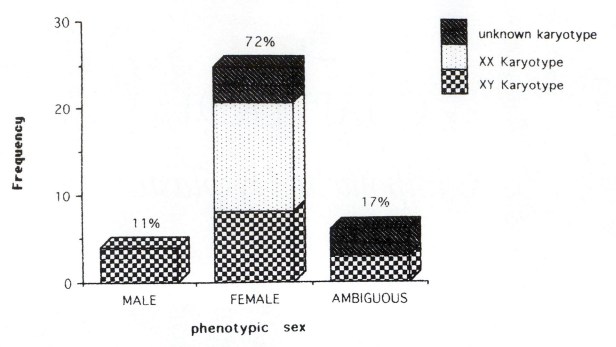

Figure 91-2. Association between phenotypic sex and karyotype in a population of individuals with campomelic dysplasia. *(Reprinted, with permission, from Mansour S, Hall CM, Pembrey ME, Young ID. A clinical and genetic study of campomelic dysplasia. J Med Genet 1995;32:415–420.)*

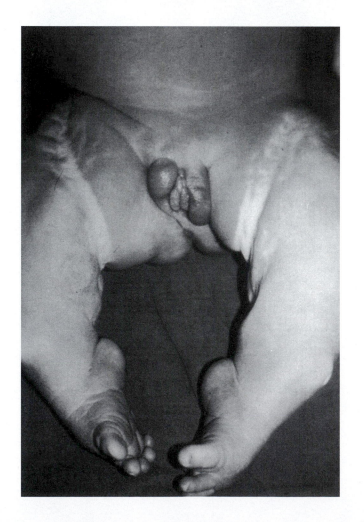

peculiar facies, cleft palate, hypotonia, absent olfactory bulbs, and respiratory distress ending in neonatal death. These authors suggested that the condition could be classified into three varieties: a long-limbed type, a short-limbed type with craniosynostosis, and a short-limbed type with normocephaly. The long-limbed variety is considered to be the most common (Khajavi et al. 1976).

A unique aspect of this condition is the sex reversal. Over half of the apparently female infants have a male, XY, karyotype (Fig. 91-2). In one study of 121 reported cases of campomelic dysplasia, 74 individuals had been karyotyped. Of these, 24 were 46,XX and phenotypically female. Of the remaining 50, who were 46,XY, 36 of them had normal female external genitalia, although a minority of them had some degree of ambiguity (Fig. 91-3) (Foster et al. 1994).

Over the past few years, much progress has been made with regard to understanding the underlying molecular mechanisms in campomelic dysplasia. The chromosomal location of the gene has been mapped,

Figure 91-3. An affected infant with campomelic dysplasia, demonstrating skin dimpling over angulation of the femurs, prominent labia majora suggesting ambiguous genitalia, and bilateral club feet. *(Reprinted, with permission, from Mansour S, Hall CM, Pembrey ME, Young ID. A clinical and genetic study of campomelic dysplasia. J Med Genet 1995;32:415–420.)*

the gene involved in the condition has been identified as *SOX9,* and the inheritance pattern has been clarified.

▶ INCIDENCE

The incidence of campomelic dysplasia is 0.05 in 10,000 to 1.6 in 10,000 live births (Mansour et al. 1995). There have been occasional case reports of infants affected with campomelic dysplasia in women who had taken oral contraceptives during the first trimester of pregnancy (Kim et al. 1995). This is probably incidental. There is no association between the incidence of campomelic dysplasia and advanced maternal or paternal age (Hall and Spranger 1980; Mansour et al. 1995).

▶ SONOGRAPHIC FINDINGS

Fetuses affected with campomelic dysplasia have a variety of anomalies. The most characteristic is the acute femoral angulation, which typically occurs at the junction of the upper third and lower third of both femora, with resulting symmetrical shortening (see Fig. 91-1). Other typical abnormalities include marked micrognathia, a small bell-shaped chest, mild bilateral hydronephrosis, hydrocephalus, cystic hygroma (Foster et al. 1994; Mansour et al. 1995), and club feet (Sanders et al. 1994) (Fig. 91-4). Polyhydramnios has been described in 25 to 48% of affected cases (Mansour et al. 1995; Slater et al. 1985). The associated hydrocephalus is thought to be due to atlanto-occipital occlusion (Deschamps et al. 1992). Approximately one fourth of patients may have associated cardiac malformations, which are always of the mild variety (Hall and Spranger 1980; Mansour et al. 1995). The associated genitourinary anomalies may include hydronephrosis, hydroureter, renal hypoplasia, or renal cysts (Argaman et al.1993; Slater et al. 1985). The femoral angulation is always anterior in the tibia and anterolateral in the femur (Pazzaglia and Beluffi 1987). Other bony abnormalities that have not been specifically described prenatally but are sufficiently unusual to warrant inspection include hypoplastic or absent scapulas and hypoplasia or absent fibulas.

The first successful prenatal diagnoses for this condition occurred in families with a previously affected child. In 1981, Fryns et al. described such a family and successfully diagnosed recurrence of the campomelic dysplasia in a fetus at 17 weeks of gestation with short, bowed limbs and hydrocephalus. Sonographic examination revealed poorly ossified long tubular bones that were not bowed and massive hydrocephaly. At autopsy the infant was also shown to have a high forehead and micrognathia (Fryns et al. 1981). Similarly, Winter et al. (1985) described a consanguineous couple who were

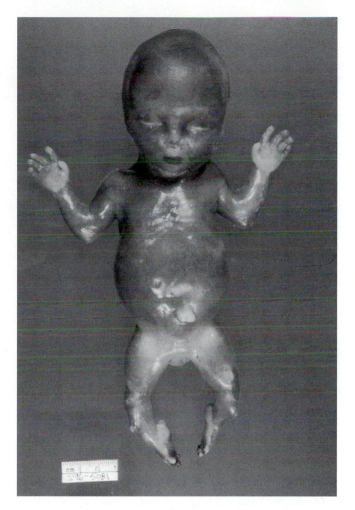

Figure 91-4. Postmortem appearance of the same fetus shown in Figure 91-1, showing characteristic hypoplastic midface, micrognathia, acute tibial angulation, and bilateral talipes equinovarus deformity.

second cousins and had previously delivered a term male with campomelic dysplasia. The diagnosis had previously been missed in the affected infant. Four sonographic examinations had been performed between 12 and 40 weeks of gestation, and normal growth had been observed. Postnatally, the affected infant had hypotelorism, micrognathia, campomelia, and talipes equinovarus. In the subsequent pregnancy, at 16 weeks of gestation, a discrepancy was noted between the length of upper and lower limbs. A repeat sonographic examination performed at 18 weeks demonstrated that the femurs were curved, the tibias were markedly curved, and the fibulas were not visible (Winter et al. 1985). In families not at risk for campomelic dysplasia, affected infants have been identified by a discrepancy between upper- and lower-limb lengths (Gillerot et al. 1989). Cordone et al. (1989) described a fetus at 26 weeks of gestation with a normal amniotic fluid volume who demonstrated symmetrical anterior bowing of the lower extremities with hypoplasia of the fibulas and talipes equinovarus, hypoplastic scapulas, a bell-shaped chest, and facial abnormalities including a flat nasal bridge and micrognathia.

▶ DIFFERENTIAL DIAGNOSIS

A prenatal diagnostic overlap occurs between campomelic dysplasia and osteogenesis imperfecta type II (see Chapter 98). This is due to the presence of bowing in the lower limbs, which can be a manifestation of osteogenesis imperfecta. The tibial bowing, however, is more pronounced in campomelic dysplasia (Sanders et al. 1994). Campomelic dysplasia is also accompanied by mild bowing of the femurs. In one report, the authors described three cases of osteogenesis imperfecta in which tibial bowing was present without apparent fractures. They also described two cases of campomelic dysplasia misdiagnosed as osteogenesis imperfecta because the femurs showed an acute angulation that was suggestive of a fracture (Sanders et al. 1994). The presence of additional fetal anomalies, including club feet, micrognathia, and hydronephrosis is more consistent with a diagnosis of campomelic dysplasia than osteogenesis imperfecta.

Other conditions that should be included in the differential diagnosis include diastrophic dysplasia (see Chapter 93). Both campomelic and diastrophic dysplasia share cervical vertebral anomalies, cleft palate, joint dislocations, bilateral talipes equinovarus, and laryngotracheal abnormalities, as well as abnormal ears, micrognathia, and brachydactyly (Hall and Spranger 1980). Individuals with Larsen syndrome also manifest many of these abnormalities as well as a flat nasal bridge and apparent hypertelorism. Hall and Spranger (1980) recommended comparison of the scapulas, thoracic pedicles, and iliac bones to allow a specific diagnosis of campomelic dysplasia. The following major features of campomelic dysplasia occur with greater than 50% frequency in affected individuals: hypoplastic scapulas, nonmineralized thoracic pedicles, and vertically narrow iliac bones. These are rare findings when seen individually, but pathognomonic for campomelic dysplasia when found in combination (Hall and Spranger 1980).

Other authors have indicated that in postnatal radiographs, scapular hypoplasia is the most consistent and unique feature. Potential overlap occurs between campomelic dysplasia and pelvis–shoulder dysplasia, which results in symmetric hypoplasia of the iliac wings and scapulas. In this condition, the iliac bones are small and square with flat acetabular roofs, which are different from the narrow iliac bones and steep acetabula of campomelic dysplasia. In pelvis–shoulder dysplasia, the lumbar vertebral bodies are rounded anteriorly, which gives them a bullet-like shape. Lordosis eventually de-

velops in these patients. In campomelic dysplasia, however, the cervical and thoracic vertebral bodies are dysplastic, small, and flattened, and eventually result in development of a thoracic scoliosis. In the chest, the lack of ossification of the thoracic pedicles is the major feature of campomelic dysplasia (MacPherson et al. 1989).

▶ ANTENATAL NATURAL HISTORY

The various manifestations of campomelic dysplasia are associated with an increased incidence of stillbirth. It is thought that up to 50% of cases are lost during gestation (Slater et al. 1985). It is currently unknown whether the initial factors responsible for the condition represent abnormalities of bone, nerves, or blood vessels. One investigator hypothesized that teratogenesis of the peripheral nerves results in adaptive shortening of the skeleton, and demonstrated that bone buckling occurred in duck embryos given neurotoxins (Roth 1991). Roth stated that bone buckling occurred because the growing bones accommodated the underdeveloped neurologic structures at the cost of a deformity. Other investigators have demonstrated that the main arterial axis of the lower limb is also abnormal in campomelic dysplasia (Rodriguez 1993). In careful postmortem vascular studies, Rodriguez demonstrated the absence or marked deficiency of the anterior tibial artery, which further proved the developmental association between vascular defects and limb anomalies (see Chapter 107). In addition, the profunda femoris and posterior tibial arteries were greater in diameter in fetuses affected with campomelic dysplasia than in age-matched controls.

Bone histology in infants affected with campomelic dysplasia suggests an ongoing repair process in the areas of angulation in the femur. New periosteal bone is laid down on the concave side, and remodeling of the mass of woven bone occurs. The process is similar to the healing of malaligned fractures. For most affected individuals, the growth plate cartilage and metaphyses appear normal (Pazzaglia and Beluffi 1987). Other investigators have identified identical changes occurring in the bend at the diaphysis. Parallel masses of periosteal bone have been demonstrated to extend into the medullary cavity at right angles to the axis of the bone. A triangular wedge of woven bone extends from the cortex into the medulla of the diaphysis (Khajavi et al. 1976). Type II collagen was measured in a 38-week, stillborn phenotypic female (karyotype 46,XY) affected with campomelic dysplasia. In this case, there was no suggestion of type II collagen abnormalities. These investigators showed that the nerves, muscles, and bones of the lower limbs were all affected. There were abnormalities seen in the cartilage, which suggested a disturbed structure of the extracellular matrix and possible abnormalities in the differentiation of the chondrocytes (Lazjuk et al. 1987). These investigators summarized previous work considering the cause of the bowing seen in the lower extremities in campomelic dysplasia. Previous theories included: (1) mechanical stress on the fetal lower extremities due to a faulty fetal position within the uterus; (2) a primary calf muscle imbalance resulting in shortening, providing traction on a weakened bone shaft; (3) intrauterine fracture occurring with subsequent healing; (4) an anomalous primary shaft ossification in the long bones developing early in embryogenesis; and (5) intrauterine hypotonia resulting in abnormal fetal positioning (Lazjuk et al. 1987). It is now appreciated that the *SOX9* mutation is the underlying basis for the disorder, although it is not known whether the *SOX9* mutation acts primarily on bone, nerves, or muscle.

▶ MANAGEMENT OF PREGNANCY

Fetuses in which campomelic dysplasia is suspected should be referred to a tertiary-care center capable of anatomic sonographic diagnosis of the fetus. Fetal karyotyping is indicated for two reasons: to determine the chromosomal gender and prepare the parents for the possibility of phenotypic sex reversal, and to specifically screen for chromosome 17 rearrangements, which can be associated with a milder phenotype (Foster et al. 1994). Once a definitive sonographic diagnosis has been made, the parents should meet with a medical geneticist and/or genetic counselor to discuss the implications of the diagnosis. The overwhelming majority of cases are lethal during the newborn period or during the first year of life. The poor prognosis should be discussed with the prospective parents, and termination of pregnancy can be offered at less than 24 weeks of gestation.

Rare survivors with campomelic dysplasia have been reported. All affected infants manifest respiratory distress. Delivery at a tertiary-care center is therefore indicated. The mean gestational age at delivery is 39.8 weeks (Mansour et al. 1995). There are no specific indications for delivery by cesarean section.

If the parents terminate the pregnancy or delivery results in a stillborn infant, placental material should be collected to establish a fibroblast culture, which can serve as a source of DNA for *SOX9* mutation analysis. Although the condition is now considered to be inherited as an autosomal dominant, with the majority of cases occurring as a new mutation, occasional cases of parental mosaicism warrant that prenatal diagnosis in subsequent pregnancies is indicated. The placental culture can serve as a source of the DNA mutation and will facilitate future DNA diagnosis.

▶ FETAL INTERVENTION

There are no fetal interventions for campomelic dysplasia.

▶ TREATMENT OF THE NEWBORN

A complete physical examination should be performed on all infants in whom campomelic dysplasia is suspected. The physical examination will typically include a low to normal birth weight, apparent macrocephaly (mean occipitofrontal circumference, 37 cm) (Argaman et al. 1993), extreme hypotonia, disproportionately short trunk and lower limbs, and flattened face, high forehead, and flattened nasal bridge. The palpebral fissures are narrow and give the appearance of hypertelorism. A cleft of the soft palate is present in two thirds of affected infants (Argaman et al. 1993). In the affected newborn the thighs are held in abduction (see Fig. 91-3). The hips are frequently dislocated. There are characteristic subcutaneous dimples present over the bend of the tibia. These dimples result from the loss of subcutaneous tissue secondary to in utero stretching at the point of curvature (Argaman et al. 1993; Gillerot et al. 1989).

A complete set of radiographs should be obtained during the newborn period, which will demonstrate the bladeless scapulas, the small bell-shaped chest, the frequent occurrence of only 11 pairs of ribs, and a poorly mineralized sternum. Radiographs may also demonstrate a short first metacarpal (Mansour et al. 1995). The characteristic clinical findings for infants affected with campomelic dysplasia are summarized in Table 91-1.

All affected infants manifest respiratory distress syndrome and generally require mechanical ventilation. Respiratory distress is due to a small thoracic cage with consequent pulmonary hypoplasia, a narrow larynx,

▶ TABLE 91-1. CHARACTERISTIC CLINICAL FINDINGS IN CAMPOMELIC DYSPLASIA

Bilateral bowing of the long bones of the legs, especially tibia	100%
Talipes equinovarus	100%
Skin dimpling overlying the tibial angulations	99%
Hypoplastic pelvis	97%
Hypoplastic scapulas	92%
Macrocephaly	90%
Cleft palate	50–80%
Scoliosis	70%
Cystic renal disease	33%
Hydrocephalus	23–25%
Polyhydramnios	25–48%

Source: Slater CP, Ross J, Nelson MM, Coetzee EJ. The campomelic syndrome: prenatal ultrasound investigations: a case report. S Afr Med J 1985;67:863–869.

and underlying abnormalities of the tracheobronchial cartilage (MacPherson et al. 1989). The majority of patients die during the neonatal period from the respiratory abnormalities.

▶ SURGICAL TREATMENT

Rare survivors with campomelic dysplasia have had severe orthopedic problems that can be treated surgically, including kyphoscoliosis, hip dislocation, and club feet (Gillerot et al. 1989). In one report, a 6.5-year-old girl was described who survived initial respiratory problems and was subsequently treated with a Pavlik harness for subluxation of the hips. She underwent two cervical and two thoracic spinal fusions, a release of complex foot deformities, and had an osteostomy of her right tibia (Ray and Bowen 1984). At 6.5 years of age, she had the height and weight of a 2.5-year-old child and the bone age of a 3.5-year-old child. She sat at 22 months of age. Despite the multiple orthopedic problems and apparent developmental delay, by age 6.5 years she was able to attend a normal first-grade class. In another report, an 18-year-old high school graduate with normal psychomotor development was described who required plastic surgery and orthodontic treatment to advance her hypoplastic midface (Mintz and Adibfar 1994).

▶ LONG-TERM OUTCOME

The outcome for most individuals with campomelic dysplasia is poor. Of 81 patients described with the more common long-limbed variety of campomelic dysplasia, 61 were stillborn or died during the first month of life. An additional 13 died between 35 days and 1 year of age. In this report, only 2 patients survived beyond the age of 2 years (Ray and Bowen 1984). Other authors emphasize that with few exceptions, the 50% of affected individuals who do not die during the perinatal period die within the first 10 months of life (Slater et al. 1985). Aspiration and severe feeding difficulties are common in affected infants, even while on mechanical ventilatory support. Infants who are on the respirator for prolonged periods tend to die of diffuse alveolar or massive tracheobronchial pulmonary hemorrhage (Argaman et al. 1993). Infants who come off the ventilator have complications of apnea, atalectasis, and pneumonia.

For individuals who survive beyond the first year of life, the outlook improves somewhat. Infants can still have stridor, retractions, and chronic pulmonary disease, as well as bronchitis and frequent otitis media. In one report, a 5-year-old girl with campomelic dysplasia was described whose condition was extremely unstable during her first year of life, but she eventually experienced a progressive decrease in the number of respiratory infections. Her early childhood years were characterized by marked hypotonia and mental retardation, but surprisingly, at 4 years of age she experienced a dramatic improvement in her development so that she could eventually speak and play and walk. At 5 years of age, however, her size was extremely small for her age (weight, 10.5 kg; height, 89 cm; normal head size of 53.5 cm). The original patient of Maroteaux was again reported on at 17 years of age, and was shown to have an IQ of 45, hearing loss, and severe kyphosis (Houston et al. 1983).

All patients who survive beyond the age of 6 months have been shown to have a profound hearing loss (Argaman et al. 1993; Takahasi et al. 1992). The deafness is now known to be due to histologic abnormalities in the temporal bone as well as deformities of the vestibular and semicircular canals. In this condition, the endochondral layer of the otic capsule contains no cartilage cells. In addition, the facial nerve follows an aberrant course. The size and position of the ossicles are abnormal (Takahasi et al. 1992; Tokita et al. 1979). Patients affected with campomelic dysplasia have a mixed type of hearing loss. Conductive hearing loss derives from anomalies of the ossicles and frequent otitis media. Sensorineural hearing loss derives from hypoplasia of the cochlea.

▶ GENETICS AND RECURRENCE RISK

Until recently, the inheritance pattern of campomelic dysplasia was thought to be autosomal recessive. This was on the basis of occasional cases recurring in families, especially consanguineous ones. In one report, 36 index cases of campomelic dysplasia were described with a total of 41 siblings. Analysis revealed a segregation ratio of 0.05, instead of the 0.25 expected for an autosomal recessive condition (Mansour et al. 1995). It is now known on the basis of molecular analysis that campomelic dysplasia is inherited as a autosomal dominant condition, with the majority of patients representing heterozygosity for a new mutation (Rimoin 1996). Recurrence in families is now thought to be due to rare cases of parental gonadal mosaicism. One case report described a mildly affected mother with a more severely affected daughter who died during the newborn period from respiratory distress (Lynch et al. 1993).

Cytogenetic studies performed in affected patients played a large role in gene mapping of this condition. In one patient with campomelic dysplasia, a de novo paracentric inversion of chromosome 17 was documented (Maraia et al. 1991). This report was followed by the description of a phenotypically female fetus with campomelic dysplasia whose karyotype was 46,XY,t(2;17)(q35;q23-24). These authors suggested that the long arm of chromosome 17 was likely to be the site of the gene mutation in campomelic dysplasia (Young et al. 1992). A total of 5 different patients with chromosomal rearrangements in campomelic dysplasia enabled the gene locus to be identified as 17q. Interestingly, the patients who have the translocation have, in general, survived longer (Foster et al. 1994). Ninomiya et al. (1995) suggested that campomelic dysplasia and sex reversal represented part of a contiguous-gene syndrome. They described a female patient with most manifestations of campomelic dysplasia except the bowed limbs, the so-called acampomelic campomelic syndrome. This female individual was noted to have a karyotype of 46,XY,t(12;17)(q21.32;q24.3 or q25.1) de novo. In 1993, these rare chromosomal rearrangements led the localization of the campomelic dysplasia gene to chromosome 17q24.1-25.2 (Tommerup et al. 1993). Among 33 cases of campomelic dysplasia with an XY karyotype, 21 were phenotypic females and 2 were ambiguous. These patients were studied for mutations in the testis-determining gene, *SRY,* but no mutations were demonstrated. It was therefore concluded that patients with campomelic dysplasia and an XY karyotype must have mutations in another autosomal locus that was important in sexual differentiation.

The gene *SOX9* encodes a putative transcription factor that is strongly conserved throughout mammalian evolution. *SOX9* is structurally related to the testis-determining factor *SRY,* and is expressed in many adult tissues, fetal testes, and fetal skeletal tissue (Wagner et al. 1994). It is now known that haploinsufficiency for the *SOX9* gene is the cause of campomelic dysplasia and autosomal XY sex reversal. This was proven by demonstration of inactivating mutations of one *SOX9* allele. In one of the cases reported by Wagner et al. (1994), one parent of an affected child was shown to have a low-grade mosaic mutation and had DNA that contained both the normal and mutant *SOX9* genes. Simultaneously, Foster et al. (1994) demonstrated that both campomelic dysplasia and sex reversal were caused by mutations in the *SOX9* gene. They described mutations in a single allele of *SOX9* on chromosome 17 in 6 of 9 patients affected with campomelic dysplasia. These mutations destroyed gene function by causing premature chain termination and loss of one-third of the protein gene product. DNA analysis of parents of affected children demonstrated the absence of similar mutations. Therefore, this conclusively proves that most cases of campomelic dysplasia are new mutations that are inherited as autosomal dominant conditions (Foster et al. 1994).

Subsequent research has shown that *SOX9* is a transcription factor that is essential for chondrocyte differentiation and cartilage formation (Bi et al. 1999). During embryogenesis, *SOX9* is expressed in all cartilage primordial tissue, coincident with the expression of the collagen alpha (II) gene *(COL2A1). SOX9* is also expressed in the central nervous and urogenital systems. Campomelic dysplasia arises by point mutations, truncations, and frameshift mutations that impede the ability of *SOX9* to activate target genes during organ development (McDowall et al. 1999).

Prenatal diagnosis is indicated for the rare survivors with mild manifestations of campomelic dysplasia, as their offspring will have a 50% likelihood of recurrence. Their offspring could be more severely affected, as demonstrated by the case of Lynch et al. (1993). For completely normal parents who have previously had an affected fetus or infant with campomelic dysplasia, prenatal diagnosis by sonography is indicated in subsequent pregnancies, although the recurrence risk is extremely low. Parental DNA can be studied to detect rare cases of mosaicism for *SOX9* mutations (Cameron et al. 1996).

REFERENCES

Argaman Z, Hammerman CA, Kaplan M, Schimmel M, Rabinovich R, Tunnessen WW Jr. Picture of the month: campomelic dysplasia. Am J Dis Child 1993;147:205–206.

Bi W, Deng JM, Zhang Z, Behringer RR, deCrombrugghe B. SOX9 is required for cartilage formation. Nat Genet 1999; 22:85–89.

Bianchine JW, Risenberg HM, Kanderian SS, Harrison HE. Campomelic dwarfism. Lancet 1971;1:1017.

Cameron FJ, Hageman RM, Cooke-Yarborough C, et al. A novel germ line mutation in SOX9 causes familial campomelic dysplasia and sex reversal. Hum Mol Genet 1996;5:1625–1630.

Cordone M, Lituania M, Zampatti C, Passamonti U, Magnano GM, Toma P. In utero ultrasonographic features of campomelic dysplasia. Prenat Diagn 1989;9:745–750.

Deschamps F, Teot L, Benningfield N, Humeau C. Ultrasonography of the normal and abnormal antenatal development of the upper limb. Ann Chir Main Memb Super 1992;11:389–400.

Foster JW, Dominguez-Steglich MA, Guioli S, et al. Campomelic dysplasia and autosomal sex reversal caused by mutations in an SRY-related gene. Nature 1994;372: 525–530.

Fryns JP, van den Berghe K, van Assche A, Van den Berghe H. Prenatal diagnosis of campomelic dwarfism. Clin Genet 1981;19:199–201.

Gillerot Y, Vanheck CA, Foulon M, Podevain A, Koulischer L. Campomelic syndrome: manifestations in a 20-week fetus and case history of a 5-year-old child. Am J Med Genet 1989;34:589–592.

Hall BD, Spranger JW. Campomelic dysplasia: further elucidation of a distinct entity. Am J Dis Child 1980;134: 285–289.

Houston CS, Opitz JM, Spranger JW, et al. The campomelic syndrome: review, report of 17 cases, and follow-up on the currently 17-year-old boy first reported by Maroteaux et al. in 1971. Am J Med Genet 1983;15:3–28.

Khajavi A, Lachman R, Rimoin D, et al. Heterogeneity in the campomelic syndromes: long and short bone varieties. Radiology 1976;120:641–647.

Kim MR, Qazi QH, Anderson VM, Valencia GB. A genetic male infant with female phenotype in campomelic syndrome: a possible relationship to exposure to oral contraceptives during pregnancy. Am J Obstet Gynecol 1995; 172:1042–1043.

Lazjuk GI, Shved IA, Cherstvoy ED, Feshchenko SP. Campomelic syndrome: concepts of the bowing and shortening in the lower limbs. Teratology 1987;35:1–8.

Lynch SA, Gaunt ML, Minford AM. Campomelic dysplasia: evidence of autosomal dominant inheritance. J Med Genet 1993;30:683–686.

MacPherson RE, Skinner SA, Donnenfeld AE. Acampomelic campomelic dysplasia. Pediatr Radiol 1989;20:90–93.

Mansour S, Hall CM, Pembrey ME, Young ID. A clinical and genetic study of campomelic dysplasia. J Med Genet 1995;32:415–420.

Maraia S, Saal HM, Wangsa D. A chromosome 17q de novo paracentric inversion in a patient with campomelic dysplasia: case report and etiologic hypothesis. Clin Genet 1991;39:401–408.

Maroteaux P, Spranger J, Opitz JM, et al. Le syndrome campomélique. Presse Med 1971;79:1157–1162.

McDowall S, Argentaro A, Ranganathan S, et al. Functional and structural studies of wild type SOX9 and mutations causing campomelic dysplasia. J Biol Chem 1999;274: 24023–24030.

Mintz SM, Adibfar A. Management of maxillofacial deformities in a patient with campomelic dysplasia. J Oral Maxillofac Surg 1994;52:618–623.

Ninomiya S, Narahara K, Tsuji K, Yokoyama Y, Ito S, Seino Y. Acampomelic campomelic syndrome and sex reversal associated with de novo t (12;17) translocation. Am J Med Genet 1995;56:31–34.

Pazzaglia UE, Beluffi G. Radiology and histopathology of the bent limbs in campomelic dysplasia: implications in the aetiology of the disease and review of theories. Pediatr Radiol 1987;17:50–55.

Ray S, Bowen JR. Orthopaedic problems associated with survival in campomelic dysplasia. Clin Orthop 1984;185: 77–82.

Rimoin DL. Molecular defects in the chondrodysplasias. Am J Med Genet 1996;63:106–110.

Rodriguez JI. Vascular anomalies in campomelic syndrome. Am J Med Genet 1993;46:185–192.

Roth M. Campomelic syndrome: experimental models and pathomechanisms. Pediatr Radiol 1991;21:220–225.

Sanders RC, Greyson-Fleg RT, Hogge WA, Blakemore KJ, McGowan DK, Isbister S. Osteogenesis imperfecta and campomelic dysplasia: difficulties in prenatal diagnosis. J Ultrasound Med 1994;13:691–700.

Slater CP, Ross J, Nelson MM, Coetzee EJ. The campomelic syndrome—prenatal ultrasound investigations: a case report. S Afr Med J 1985;67:863–869.

Takahasi H, Sando I, Masutani H. Temporal bone histopathological findings in campomelic dysplasia. J Laryngol Otol 1992;106:361–365.

Tokita N, Chandra-Sekhar HK, Daly JF, Becker MH, Aleksic S. The campomelic syndrome: temporal bone histopathologic features and otolaryngologic manifestations. Arch Otolaryngol 1979;105:449–454.

Tommerup N, Schempp W, Meinecke P, et al. Assignment of an autosomal sex reversal locus (SRA1) and campomelic dysplasia (CMPD1) to 17q24.3-q25.1. Nat Genet 1993;4:170–174.

Wagner T, Wirth J, Meyer J, et al. Autosomal sex reversal and campomelic dysplasia are caused by mutations in and around the SRY-related gene SOX9. Cell 1994;79:1111–1120.

Winter R, Rosenkranz W, Hofmann H, Zierler H, Becker H, Borkenstein M. Prenatal diagnosis of campomelic dysplasia by ultrasonography. Prenat Diagn 1985;5:1–8.

Young ID, Zuccollo JM, Maltby EL, Broderick NJ. Campomelic dysplasia associated with a de novo 2q;17q reciprocal translocation. J Med Genet 1992;29:251–252.

CHAPTER 92

Chondrodysplasia Punctata

▶ CONDITION

Chondrodysplasia punctata denotes a group of skeletal dysplasias characterized by locally disordered bone mineralization that results in bone stippling observed on radiographs obtained during the newborn period (Pryde et al. 1993). The areas of punctate calcification were first described by Conradi in 1914. In 1931, Hünermann designated the disorder "chondrodystrophia calcificans congenita." This term was defined as the x-ray finding of small calcific densities in the epiphyses (Hyndman et al. 1976). The disorder recognized by Hünermann also included micromelia, a saddle-nose deformity, flexion contractures, cataracts, and a dermopathy. As used today, the term chondrodysplasia punctata comprises a group of genetically heterogeneous disorders (Spranger et al. 1971). These include a nonrhizomelic type of skeletal dysplasia, known as Conradi–Hünermann syndrome. Rhizomelia refers to shortness of the proximal limb. At least four distinct genetic disorders are included under the umbrella term Conradi–Hünermann syndrome, including an autosomal dominantly inherited disorder, an X-linked dominantly inherited disorder that is lethal in males, an X-linked recessive disorder, and a disorder that is due to a deletion on the short arm of the X chromosome. In addition, a rarer disorder exists that is inherited as an autosomal recessive condition and is characterized by severe rhizomelic limb shortening. In rhizomelic chondrodysplasia punctata, additional findings include punctate calcifications of the epiphyses, facial abnormalities, mental retardation, skin changes, cataracts, joint contractures, calcification of the trachea and larynx, failure to thrive, and death within the first year of life.

It is now known that rhizomelic chondrodysplasia punctata is a disorder of the peroxisomes. Peroxisomes are intracellular organelles that catalyze a number of metabolic functions (Wanders et al. 1993). These include β oxidative chain shortening of fatty acids and their derivatives, synthesis of ether-phospholipids, and detoxification of glyoxalate (Hoefler et al. 1988; Schutgens et al. 1989; Wanders et al. 1993). Human peroxisomal disorders are subdivided into two categories: those in which the organelle is not normally formed, and those that involve a single peroxisomal enzyme (Moser 1999).

The peroxisomal disorders have been classified into three groups (A, B, and C) according to clinical presentation (Table 92-1). In patients with rhizomelic chondrodysplasia punctata, the peroxisomes are present, but they have lost many of their normal functions. Four distinct abnormalities have been found in patients with rhizomelic chondrodysplasia. These involve deficiency of enzymes important in phospholipid synthesis and phytanic acid oxidation (Hoefler et al. 1988; Schutgens et al. 1989; Wanders et al. 1993). A severe deficiency in plasmalogen synthesis is associated with deficient activities of the peroxisomal enzymes acyl-coenzyme A (acyl-CoA, dihydroxyacetone phosphate acyltransferase, and alkyl-dihydroxyacteone phosphate synthase. In addition, there is deficient activity of phytanic acid oxidase, and the enzyme peroxisomal 3-oxo acyl-CoA thiolase is present in an abnormal unprocessed form (Gendall et al. 1994; Suzuki et al. 1994). Because of these enzyme abnormalities, the characteristic biochemical abnormality in rhizomelic chondrodysplasia punctata is increased phytanic acid levels and decreased plasmalogens (Singh et al. 1988). In rhizomelic chondrodysplasia punctata, unlike in other peroxisomal conditions, the amount of very-long-chain fatty acids is normal. The method of choice to identify rhizomelic chondrodysplasia punctata prenatally is to analyze the plasmalogen levels in chorionic villi and erythrocytes (Wanders et al. 1993).

▶ **TABLE 92-1.** CLINICAL CLASSIFICATION OF PEROXISOMAL DISORDERS

Group A	Group B	Group C
Disease		
Zellweger syndrome	Rhizomelic	Conradi–Hünermann syndrome
Infantile Refsum disease	Chondrodysplasia punctata	(some cases)
Neonatal adrenoleukodystrophy	Nonrhizomelic	
Hyperpipecolic acidema	chondrodysplasia punctata	
	(Conradi–Hünermann)	
	syndrome [some cases])	
Symptoms		
Severe neurologic/hepatic	Growth defects	Milder symptoms
dysfunction	Epiphyseal calcifications	
Craniofacial abnormalities	Cataracts	
Hypotonia	Ichthyosis	
Early death	Midface hypoplasia	
Biochemical abnormalities		
Increased phytanic acid	Incresaed phytanic acid	
Increased VLCFAs	Normal VLCFAs	
Deficient in synthesis	Lack plasmalogens	
of plasmalogens		
Molecular abnormalities		
Mutations affect	Mutations affect	Mutations in
localization of	localization of	single genes
multiple peroxisomal	multiple peroxisomal	compromise activity
matrix proteins	matrix proteins	or localization of
		single enzymes

VLCFAs = very-long-chain fatty acids.

Source: Subrami S. PEX genes on the rise. Nat Genet 1997;15:331–333.

To date, 17 peroxisomal (peroxins, or *PEX*) genes have been identified. Most of them are also found in yeast, indicating their essential importance for cellular metabolism. Seven *PEX* genes are found in humans (Subramani 1997). Of these, five have been implicated in human disorders. Patients with rhizomelic chondrodysplasia punctata are deficient in a subset of peroxisomal enzymes whose transport depends on a peroxisome targeting signal 2 (PTS2) receptor, which is specified by the human *PEX7* gene. Mutations in *PEX7* cause rhizomelic chondrodysplasia punctata (Braverman et al. 1997; Motley et al. 1997; Purdue et al. 1997).

▶ INCIDENCE

The incidence of rhizomelic chondrodysplasia punctata varies between 0.9 in 100,000 live births (Stoll et al. 1989) and 1 in 84,442 live births in Western Scotland (Connor et al. 1985). Parental consanguinity has been noted in 8 to 10% of recessively inherited cases (Stoll et al. 1989). The incidence of dominantly inherited Conradi–Hünermann syndrome is presumably higher, as clinically the condition appears to be at least twice as common (Stoll et al. 1989). Precise incidence figures are unavailable because many mildly affected patients go unrecognized. The incidence of Zellweger syndrome,

another peroxisomal disorder that can be associated with punctate calcifications around the extremities is 1 in 50,000, with an estimated gene frequency of 1 in 110 individuals in the United States (Zellweger et al. 1988).

▶ SONOGRAPHIC FINDINGS

The major sonographic criteria for a diagnosis of chondrodysplasia punctata includes profound humeral shortening that is less marked than the femoral shortening, without shortening of other bones. In addition, expanded epiphyses are present, which contain multiple hyperechoic foci (the so-called puncta) (Fig. 92-1). In addition, nasal hypoplasia or midface depression with frontal bossing may be observed in the fetal profile. Approximately 10% of cases have associated congenital heart disease (Fourie 1995).

The first prenatal diagnosis of Conradi–Hünermann syndrome was made incidentally, when radiography was performed to assess fetal maturity in a woman who was post-term (Hyndman et al. 1976). The radiograph demonstrated stippling of the epiphyses at the fetal ankles, knees, pubic and ischial bones, and femur. At birth, the infant was noted to have a saddle-nose deformity, as well as coronal cleft vertebrae in the lumbar spine.

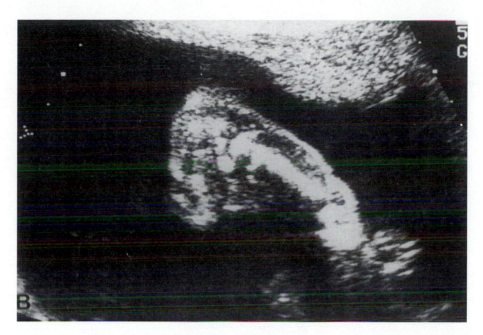

Figure 92-1. Prenatal sonographic image of a fetal femur at 22 weeks of gestation demonstrating proximal shortening and increased echogenicity due to punctate epiphyseal calcification. *(Reprinted, with permission, from Sastrowijoto SH, Vandenberghe K, Moerman P, Lauweryns JM, Fryns JP. Prenatal ultrasound diagnosis of rhizomelic chondrodyslasia punctata in a primigravida. Prenat Diagn 1994;14:770–776. Copyright 1994 John Wiley & Sons. Reprinted, by permission, of John Wiley & Sons, Ltd.)*

Prenatal sonographic diagnosis has been described more recently. In one report, Tuck et al. (1990) described a 21-year-old primigravida with a known diagnosis of Conradi–Hünermann syndrome. She had ichthyosis, sparse, dry hair, and asymmetrical limb shortening. She had surgery performed on her right hip at 6 years of age and subsequently had operations to lengthen her right femur at age 9. As an adult, she had short stature (144 cm) and a pronounced limp. When she became pregnant, she presented for prenatal diagnosis at 17 weeks of gestation, when a 3-mm asymmetry was noted between the right and left fetal femora and humeri. This asymmetry persisted on prenatal sonographic scans performed at 21, 24, 32, and 35 weeks of gestation. At birth, her infant was shown on radiographs to have epiphyseal stippling that was missed on prenatal sonogram. Physical examination also revealed a low nasal bridge, malar hypoplasia, and ichthyotic skin (Tuck et al. 1990). In another report, with no known family history, a fetus at 20 weeks of gestation was shown to have kyphoscoliosis, a shortened, bowed, left radius and ulnae, pelvic calcifications, and a prematurely calcified bifid sternum (Sherer et al. 1994). These observations prompted a retrospective analysis of sonography performed at 14 weeks of gestation, which revealed bilateral prematurely calcified epiphyses.

The diagnosis of Conradi–Hünermann syndrome is more straightforward when it is known that one of the parents is affected. In one report, Pryde et al. (1993) described a pregnant woman who herself had been diagnosed with Conradi–Hünermann syndrome at birth marked by scoliosis, punctate calcifications of the spine and femoral epiphyses, asymmetric limb shortening, postaxial polydactyly, cataracts, and irregular macular skin hyperpigmentation. In her first pregnancy, her fetus was noted to have asymmetrical short limbs, scoliosis, and mild fetal ventriculomegaly. In her second pregnancy, at 16 weeks of gestation a 5-mm difference was noted in the femoral lengths. At 32 weeks of gestation, severe polyhydramnios developed in her fetus. At birth, the diagnosis was confirmed by the presence of a saddle-nose, ichthyotic skin, and epiphyseal stipplings seen on radiographs. In this report, a fetus with a negative family history was also described. Prenatal sonograms were characterized by severe disorganization of the fetal spine observed at 18 weeks of gestation, represented by malsegmentation of the vertebrae along the entire length of the spine. No definitive scoliosis or shortness was observed. At 21 weeks of gestation, the fetal profile demonstrated and a flat nasal bridge. In addition, hyperechoic regions were observed at the femoral epiphyses that suggested premature calcification. In the same fetus, at 30 weeks of gestation, polyhydramnios was observed (Pryde et al. 1993).

The sonographer should look carefully at the fetal heart. Fourie (1995) reviewed 301 cases in the medical literature of nonrhizomelic chondrodysplasia punctata. Of these, 23 had confirmed congenital heart lesions

(7.6% of cases). There were numerous cases of pulmonic stenoses and pulmonary artery and aortic calcifications observed in this series.

The diagnosis of rhizomelic chondrodysplasia punctata is easier to make than Conradi–Hünermann syndrome due to the severe shortening of the extremities in combination with premature ossification and stippling of the ephiphyses (Hertzberg et al. 1999). Since the condition is inherited as an autosomal recessive gene, for most of these cases, there will be a negative family history. The prenatal sonographic findings reveal bilateral symmetric proximal shortening of the humeri and femora (less than the third percentile for gestational age) along with marked epiphyseal echogenicity that suggests the presence of the punctate epiphyseal calcifications (Sastrowijoto et al. 1994). Additional fetal findings may include brachycephaly, hydrocephalus, scalp edema, hypertelorism, hypoplastic nose, and coronal clefts of the vertebral bodies. Congenital heart disease has also been reported in the rhizomelic form of chondrodysplasia punctata (Sastrowijoto et al. 1994). Duff et al. (1990) described the diagnosis of rhizomelic chondrodysplasia punctata at 28 weeks of gestation in a woman whose previous infant was affected with this condition. She presented for prenatal sonography at 28 weeks of gestation. These investigators demonstrated stippling at the proximal end of the right humerus and both femurs over an 8-week period. The tibia consistently measured at the 20th percentile for gestational age, but both the femur and humerus were consistently at less than the 5th percentile. Over the period observed, a progressively more mottled appearance of the proximal end of the right humerus was demonstrated. The bone became more and more attenuated, irregular, and stippled in appearance, making it difficult to precisely define the end of it (Duff et al. 1990). In another report, a set of dichorionic twins was described, in which one was noted to have rhizomelic limb shortening at 25 weeks of gestation. In this fetus, the humeri were shaped like dumbbells and multiple hyperechoic foci were noted in the humeral epiphyses and the proximal femoral epiphyses. A 15-week sonogram was reanalyzed retrospectively; it revealed that the profound humeral shortening had previously been missed. Even at 15 weeks of gestation, flared humeral metaphyses and widened hyperechoic proximal ends of the humeri were visible (Gendall et al. 1994). Postmortem, the diagnosis of rhizomelic chondrodysplasia punctata was confirmed in this twin by demonstration of absent alkyldihydroxyacetone phosphate synthase activity in cultured skin fibroblasts.

▶ DIFFERENTIAL DIAGNOSIS

The differential diagnosis of conditions that result in limb shortening with punctate epiphyses is given in

▶ **TABLE 92-2.** DIFFERENTIAL DIAGNOSIS OF PUNCTATE EPIPHYSES

Skeletal dysplasias
  Chondrodysplasia punctata
  Conradi–Hünermann type
  Rhizomelic type
  Brachytelephalangic type
  Mesomelic metacarpal type
  Sheffield type
Other genetic disorders
  Zellweger syndrome
  Trisomy 21
  Trisomy 18
  Smith–Lemli–Opitz syndrome
  DeLange syndrome
  GM_1 gangliosidosis
  Child syndrome
Vitamin K disorders
  Warfarin embryopathy
  Vitamin K epoxide reductase deficiency
Teratogens
  Fetal alcohol effects
  Hydantoin exposure
  Phenacetin intoxication
  Maternal febrile illness

Source: Poznanski AK. Punctate epiphyses: a radiological sign, not a disease. Pediatr Radiol 1994;24:418–424.

Table 92-2. The conditions include skeletal dysplasias, other genetic or metabolic disorders, disorders of vitamin K metabolism, and teratogens. To distinguish among the conditions grouped under the term chondrodysplasia punctata, fetal-limb length must be measured. The humeri are the shortest in the rhizomelic form of chondrodysplasia punctata. The presence of polydactyly may suggest the more mildly X-linked dominant form of Conradi–Hünermann syndrome (Poznanski 1994). The major consideration in the differential diagnosis is to distinguish between the rhizomelic form of chondrodysplasia punctata and the milder, Conradi–Hünermann type. This is important in the determination of prognosis, as most infants with rhizomelic chondrodysplasia punctata die within the first year of life.

The other major condition that can present with punctate epiphyses is Zellweger (cerebrohepatorenal) syndrome, which is also characterized by lack of peroxisomes. In this condition, fetal-limb length should be appropriate for gestational age, but additional antenatal findings may include hepatomegaly, hypotonia, and cystic changes in the liver and kidney. The calcifications in Zellweger syndrome tend to be centered around the patella. A number of other metabolic conditions, such as Smith–Lemli–Opitz syndrome and GM_1 gangliosidosis can also present with punctate epiphyses (see Table 92-2).

Fetal exposure to warfarin, an anticoagulant, or the presence of a vitamin K epoxide reductase deficiency can result in stippled epiphyses. Warfarin exerts its effect on the developing fetus by inhibiting vitamin K–dependent posttranslational carboxylation of certain bone proteins. Vitamin K is normally converted to vitamin K epoxide. The enzyme vitamin K epoxide reductase then converts this metabolite back to vitamin K. Warfarin inhibits this reductase, so vitamin K–dependent carboxylases do not have their cofactor. The vitamin K disorders can result in fetal findings that are very similar to chondrodysplasia punctata, including nasal hypoplasia, calcification of the trachea, and brachytelephalangic changes of the digits (Poznanski 1994). The effects of warfarin and other coumarin derivatives are most significant when the fetus is exposed during the sixth to ninth week of gestation (Poznanski 1994). In both fetal alcohol exposure and the autosomal chromosome trisomies, the puncta are characteristically seen in the tarsal bones.

▶ ANTENATAL NATURAL HISTORY

The underlying bone abnormalities that result in the chondrodysplasia punctata phenotype are present in the early second trimester. In studies of fetuses from pregnancies that have been terminated, extensive characteristic calcifications have been noted in the sites of endochondral bone formation in the limbs and trunk. The calcifications are distinct from endochondral bone. Ossification appears delayed in areas where calcifications are most prominent (Silengo et al. 1980). In rhizomelic chondrodysplasia punctata, histopathologic studies reveal that the abnormal areas of calcification are characterized by irregular distribution of cartilage cells, mucoid degeneration, the presence of cystic spaces, increased vascularity, and proliferation of fibroblasts (Duff et al. 1990). The growth plates of the long bones are normal and the chondrocytes are arranged in normal columns (Sastrowijoto et al. 1994).

In fetuses with Zellweger syndrome, stippled calcifications of the patella, femur, and humerus are all observed by 20 weeks of gestation. In addition, the renal microcysts and macrocysts are also present. This condition is also characterized by neuronal migrational abnormalities. Cortical-plate defects and heterotopias that are apparent at the light microscope level are associated with lipid inclusions at the ultrastructural level (Powers 1995). These abnormalities are all due to the absence of peroxisomes.

▶ MANAGEMENT OF PREGNANCY

Fetuses who are suspected of having punctate calcifications or rhizomelic limb shortening should be referred to a center capable of detailed anatomic scanning. Once the suspected diagnosis of chondrodysplasia punctata has been confirmed, it is prudent to refer the parents to a medical geneticist, who could then examine both of them for mild signs of Conradi–Hünermann syndrome. This is extremely important, as the prognosis for the infant will differ depending on the cause of the puncta. If one of the parents is affected, as opposed to neither parent being affected, the prognosis will be considerably improved. It is critical that the person who examines the parents looks for nonskeletal manifestations of Conradi–Hünermann syndrome. As an example, Silengo et al. (1980) reported a 27-year-old woman who presented for genetic counseling because her 32-month-old daughter had Conradi–Hünermann syndrome. Despite the fact that the mother walked with a limp, was short, had patches of alopecia and had follicular atrophoderma, she herself had not been diagnosed as having Conradi–Hünermann syndrome. A slit-lamp examination revealed the presence of early lenticular cataracts in the mother. This woman had no abnormalities in her long bones or spine, but because of her hip dysplasia and eye and skin abnormalities, she was retrospectively diagnosed as affected. Therefore, for any fetus in which chondrodysplasia punctata is suspected, parents and close relatives should be specifically examined for the presence of a hypoplastic nose, cataracts, optic atrophy, alopecia, or pigmentary skin changes.

In addition, a chromosome analysis should be performed on the fetus. This is because one consideration in the differential diagnosis of chondrodysplasia punctata includes the X-linked recessive form, which may be due to a deletion of chromosome X at band p22.3 (Bick et al. 1992). Several investigators have described the existence of a contiguous-gene syndrome at Xp22.3 that consists of chondrodysplasia punctata, steroid sulfatase deficiency, and X-linked Kallman syndrome, which includes hypogonadism due to hypothalamic gonadotropin-releasing–hormone deficiency and anosmia secondary to absence of the olfactory bulbs and tracts (Bick et al. 1992).

For families who are known to be carriers of the rhizomelic form of chondrodysplasia punctata, prenatal diagnosis can be performed by biochemical analysis of either chorionic villi or amniocytes, although the recent identification of DNA mutations in the human *PEX7* gene should facilitate prenatal DNA diagnosis as well (Braverman et al. 1997). Prenatal sonography should be reserved for follow-up of fetuses who have been biochemically tested and are found to be normal.

No specific indication exists for cesarean delivery. Fetuses in which chondrodysplasia punctata is suspected should be delivered at a tertiary-care center because of the risk of respiratory distress.

▶ FETAL INTERVENTION

There are no fetal interventions for chondrodysplasia punctata.

► TREATMENT OF THE NEWBORN

Treatment of the newborn begins with an extensive and detailed physical examination. A list of the comparative clinical findings associated with nonrhizomelic chondrodysplasia punctata is given in Table 92-3. For many of the conditions associated with chondrodysplasia punctata, nasal hypoplasia is commonly seen (Fig. 92-2) (Seguin et al. 1993). This finding may be associated with a small and/or calcified airway. In one study, 29% of affected infants had respiratory distress syndrome during the newborn period that was attributed to the small airway (Seguin et al. 1993). The airway obstruction improves with age, as it is not typically found in older children (see Fig. 92-3).

Many of the typical radiographic findings that aid in obtaining the diagnosis are best observed during the newborn period, as they tend to disappear with age. These include the punctate epiphyses and vertebral clefts. A diagnosis of Conradi–Hünermann syndrome may be presumptively made by the characteristic facial appearance that consists of a flattened face due to malar hypoplasia, a small nose with a flat nasal bridge, a prominent forehead, wide-set eyes, and upslanting palpebral fissures. Cataracts are seen in 18% of affected infants (Poznanski 1994). Infants affected with Conradi–Hünermann syndrome may have ichthiosiform erythroderma or systemic atrophoderma. They may also have patches of alopecia and contractures of the extremities. The limb shortening is usually mild, but it can be asymmetric. Polydactyly may be observed in the X-linked dominant form.

Infants affected with rhizomelic chondrodysplasia punctata have much more marked shortening of the upper limbs. The metaphyses are generally flared. Radiographs demonstrate the puncta less commonly than in Conradi–Hünermann syndrome (see Fig. 92-4). The physical examination reveals the presence of full cheeks, giving the infant the appearance of a chipmunk (see Fig. 92-3). The skin changes are much less commonly observed in rhizomelic chondrodysplasia punctata. Cataracts are present in 75% of infants affected with this disorder (Poznanski 1994). Developmental abnormalities are typical of the rhizomelic form of chondrodysplasia punctata. Magnetic resonance imaging (MRI) may reveal the presence of migrational disturbances in the brain. An additional helpful radiographic finding is the presence of coronal clefts that can be seen on lateral films of the lumbar and thoracic vertebrae. There are several milder forms of chondrodysplasia punctata, characterized by abnormalities of the extremities. In the metacarpal type of chondrodysplasia punctata, short third and fourth metacarpals are observed. These children also have a hypoplastic midface and a flattened nasal bridge. In later life, they have a height that is 2 to 4 SD below normal. The brachytelphalangic type of chondrodysplasia punctata is characterized by an extremely small, anteverted, grooved nose that resembles the one in infants affected with Binder syndrome. On radiographs, the distal phalanges have a characteristic triangular appearance. This condition may be associated with a terminal deletion of the short arm of the X chromosome.

Another important consideration during the newborn period is the diagnosis of Zellweger syndrome,

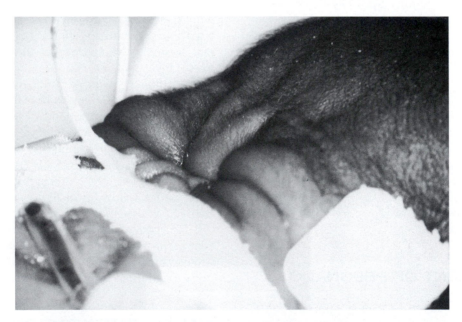

Figure 92-2. Newborn infant with rhizomelic chondrodysplasia punctata, demonstrating extreme nasal hypoplasia. The nasogastric feeding tube is seen taped to the nose. The infant is orally intubated. *(Courtesy of Dr. Marjorie C. Treadwell.)*

▶ **TABLE 92-3.** COMPARATIVE MANIFESTATIONS OF NONRHIZOMELIC CHONDRODYSPLASIA PUNCTATA SUBTYPES BY INHERITANCE PATTERNS

Inheritance	Synonyms	Punctate Calcifications	Limb Shortness	Saddle-Nose Deformity	Skin Changes (Ichthyosiform Erythroderma)	Cataracts	Mental Retardation	Other	Overall Prognosis
Autosomal dominant	Chondrodystrophia calcificans congenita	Variable severity asymmetric	Mild or none	Present	Present in 28% of cases	Symmetric, present in 17% of cases	None or minimal	Skeletal dysplasia	Good
X-linked recessive without chromosome deletion	Brachytelephalangic chondrodysplasia punctata	Mild severity, symmetric	Mild overall growth lag	Variable severity	No changes	None	None or mild	Uniform distal phalangeal hypoplasia	Good
X-linked recessive with Xp deletion	CPXR	Extensive bilateral symmetric	Shortness of stature	Typically severe with nasal hypoplasia	Marked skin changes	Occasional	IQ range, 50–70	Steroid sulfatase deficiency, and frequent distal phalangeal hypoplasia	Survival good, but neurodevelopmentally impaired
X-linked dominant	CPXD	Variable asymmetric	Proximal variable, asymmetric	Present	Marked cicatrical "patchy" changes	Asymmetric	Normal	Occasional scoliosis	Lethal in hemizygous males
Teratogenic phenocopy	Vitamin K–dependent coagulation defect, warfarin embryopathy	Irregular asymmetric pattern, variable severity	Moderate to severe	Moderate to severe with frequent nasal hypoplasia	None	None	Mild or none	Common mild distal phalangeal hypoplasia	Good

Source: Pryde PG, Bawle E, Brandt F, Romero R, Treadwell MC, Evans MI. Prenatal diagnosis of nonrhizomelic chondrodysplasia punctata. Am J Med Genet 1993;47:426–431.

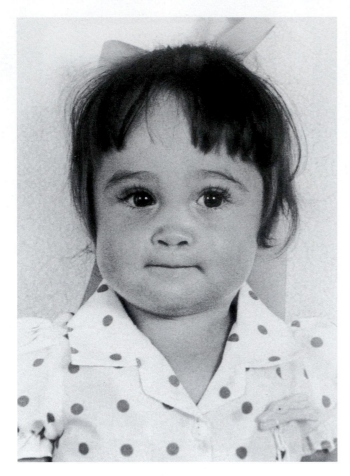

Figure 92-3. A child with chondrodysplasia punctata demonstrating severe nasal hypoplasia. *(Reprinted, with permission, from Fourie DT. Chondrodysplasia punctata: case report and literature review of patients with heart lesions. Pediatr Cardiol 1995;16:247–250.)*

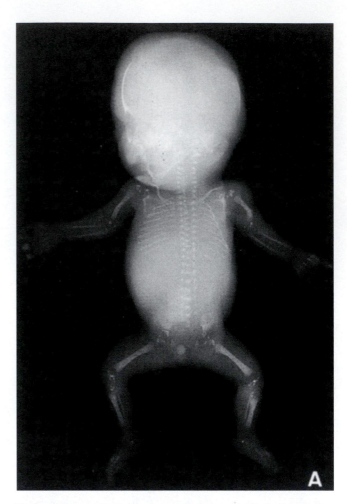

Figure 92-4. Postmortem radiograph demonstrating presence of epiphyseal calcifications in an infant with rhizomelic chondrodysplasia punctata. This is from the same individual shown in Figure 92-1. *(Reprinted, with permission, from Sastrowijoto SH, Vandenberghe K, Moerman P, Lauweryns JM, Fryns JP. Prenatal ultrasound diagnosis of rhizomelic chondrodypslasia punctata in a primigravida. Prenat Diagn 1994;14:770–776. Copyright 1994 John Wiley & Sons. Reprinted, by permission, of John Wiley & Sons, Ltd.)*

characterized by calcification of the patella. These infants are much more severely hypotonic than other infants. Renal sonography may also indicate the presence of cortical cystic changes. These infants also have progressive hepatic failure. The condition is generally lethal within the first year of life.

▶ SURGICAL TREATMENT

For more mildly affected patients with Conradi–Hünermann syndrome, orthopedic surgery may eventually be needed to correct limb-length asymmetry.

▶ LONG-TERM OUTCOME

The long-term outcome is related to the underlying condition. The rhizomelic form of chondrodysplasia punctata is the most severe, with a poor prognosis. Most

affected patients die during the first year of life (Sastrowijoto et al. 1994).

Patients affected with Conradi–Hünermann syndrome are shorter than normal at birth and remain so throughout life. The typical calcific stippling disappears by 3 to 4 years of age (Poznanski 1994). During infancy and early childhood, these infants may have cataracts, growth failure, or feeding problems. The presence of cataracts is considered by some investigators to carry a more worrisome prognosis. Affected infants are very susceptible to respiratory infections, generally because of the airway abnormalities. The laryngeal and tracheal calcifications usually resolve within the first 3 years of life (Seguin et al. 1993). Laryngoscopy and bronchoscopy can be considered electively during the first year of life to identify any lower-airway abnormalities (Seguin et al. 1993).

For infants who survive the first year of life, the skeletal deformities eventually become less pronounced and the contractures may disappear. The clinically unrecognized adults with Conradi–Hünermann syndrome described in the literature have had normal intelligence.

► GENETICS AND RECURRENCE RISK

To adequately calculate the recurrence risk, the definitive diagnosis must be known. For infants affected with rhizomelic chondrodysplasia punctata, the condition is inherited as an autosomal recessive and parents should be counseled that there is a 25% recurrence risk. Prenatal diagnosis is available as early 10 weeks of gestation by demonstration of decreased plasmalogen synthesis and decreased phytanic oxidation in chorionic villi. In addition, immunoblot studies of the peroxisomal 3-oxo-acyl-CoA thiolase can also definitively diagnose the presence of an affected fetus with rhizomelic chondrodysplasia punctata (Hoefler et al. 1988). If the biochemical studies of the chorionic villi or cultured amniocytes are normal, prenatal sonography can be used as additional confirmation of fetal status (Gray et al. 1990; Schutgens et al. 1989). Mutations in the human *PEX7* gene are now known to be the molecular cause for rhizomelic chondrodysplasia punctata. The *PEX7* gene maps to human chromosome 6q22-24 and consists of eight exons spanning more than 40 kilobases of DNA. In one study, 26 of 36 patients with rhizomelic chrondrodysplasia punctata had a single inactivating mutation known as L292 ter. This mutation was seen exclusively in patients of northern European descent (Braverman et al. 1997). Once a mutation is identified in a particular family, DNA diagnosis in subsequent pregnancies should be possible. Therefore, arrangements should be made to establish fibroblast-cell cultures from affected fetuses or infants who are electively terminated or die during the perinatal period.

Similarly, Zellweger syndrome is inherited as an autosomal recessive condition. This condition can be diagnosed definitively during the newborn period by measurement of plasma very-long-chain fatty acids. Prenatal diagnosis in subsequent pregnancies can demonstrate the very-long-chain fatty acid abnormalities and the absence of peroxisomes in cultured chorionic villus cells.

The definitive diagnosis of Conradi–Hünermann syndrome depends on a complete examination of both parents as well as taking a complete family history to rule out the autosomal dominant, X-linked dominant, and X-linked recessive forms. Parents who are retrospectively diagnosed as being affected with Conradi–Hünermann syndrome, such as in the case of Silengo et al. (1980), will be counseled that their fetuses have a 50% risk of recurrence. These patients should be followed prospectively with sonography.

Thus far, other gene-mapping studies have suggested that another form of chondrodysplasia maps to chromosome 4p16 (Dimmick et al. 1991), and that the X-linked dominant form maps to Xq28. The X-linked recessive and brachytelephalangic forms map to Xp22.3.

REFERENCES

Bick DP, Schorderet DF, Price PA, et al. Prenatal diagnosis and investigation of a fetus with chondrodysplasia punctata, ichthyosis, and Kallman syndrome due to an Xp deletion. Prenat Diagn 1992;12:19–29.

Braverman N, Steel G, Obie C, et al. Human PEX7 encodes the peroxisomal PTS2 receptor and is responsible for rhizomelic chondrodysplasia punctata. Nature Genet 1997;15:369–376.

Connor JM, Connor RAC, Sweet EM, et al. Lethal neonatal chondrodysplasias in the west of Scotland 1970–1983 with a description of a thanatophoric, dysplasialike, autosomal recessive disorder, Glasgow variant. Am J Med Genet 1985;22:243–253.

Conradi E. Vorzeitiges auftreten von konchen und eigenartigen verkalkunskernen vei condrodystrophia fotalis hypoplastica: histologische und ront neuntersuchungen. J Kinderheilkd 1914;80:86.

Dimmick J, Applegarth D, Chitayat D, Clarke L, Lau A, Moser H. Rhizomelic chondrodysplasia punctata in an infant with del (4) (p14p16). Am J Hum Genet 1991;49:155.

Duff P, Harlass FE, Milligan DA. Prenatal diagnosis of chondrodysplasia punctata by sonography. Obstet Gynecol 1990;76:497–500.

Fourie DT. Chondrodysplasia punctata: case report and literature review of patients with heart lesions. Pediatr Cardiol 1995;16:247–250.

Gendall PW, Baird CE, Becroft DM. Rhizomelic chondrodysplasia punctata: early recognition with antenatal ultrasonography. J Clin Ultrasound 1994;22:271–274.

Gray RG, Green A, Schutgens RB, Wanders RJ, Farndon PA, Kennedy CR. Antenatal diagnosis of rhizomelic chondrodysplasia punctata in the second trimester. J Inherit Metab Dis 1990;13:380–382.

Hertzberg BS, Kliewer MA, Decker M, Miller CR, Bowis JD. Antenatal ultrasonographic diagnosis of rhizomelic chondrodysplasia punctata. J Ultrasound Med 1999;18:715–718.

Hoefler S, Hoefler G, Moser AB, Watkins PA, Chen WW, Moser HW. Prenatal diagnosis of rhizomelic chondrodysplasia punctata. Prenat Diagn 1988;8:571–576.

Hyndman WB, Alexander DS, Mackie KW. Chondrodystrophia calcificans congenita: report of a case recognized antenatally. Clin Pediatr 1976;15:311–321.

Moser HW. Genotype-phenotype correlations in disorders of peroxisome biogenesis. Mol Genet Metab 1999;68:316–327.

Motley A, Hettema EH, Hogenhout EM, et al. Rhizomelic chondrodysplasia punctata is a peroxisomal protein targeting disease caused by non-functional *PTS2* receptor. Nat Genet 1997;15:377–380.

Powers JM. The pathology of peroxisomal disorders with pathogenetic considerations. J Neuropathol Exp Neurol 1995;54:710–719.

Poznanski AK. Punctate epiphyses: a radiological sign not a disease. Pediatr Radiol 1994;24:418–424.

Purdue PE, Zhang JW, Skoneczy M, Lazarow PW. Rhizomelic chondrodysplasia punctata is caused by deficiency of human *PEX7* a homologue of the yeast *PTS2* receptor. Nat Genet 1997;15:381–384.

Pryde PG, Bawle E, Brandt F, Romero R, Treadwell MC, Evans MI. Prenatal diagnosis of nonrhizomelic chondrodysplasia punctata. Am J Med Genet 1993;47:426–431.

Sastrowijoto SH, Vandenberghe K, Moerman P, Lauweryns JM, Fryns JP. Prenatal ultrasound diagnosis of rhizomelic chondrodypslasia punctata in a primagravida. Prenat Diagn 1994;14:770–776.

Schutgens RB, Schrakamp G, Wanders RH, Heymans HS, Tager JM, van den Bosch H. Prenatal and perinatal diagnosis of peroxisomal disorders. J Inherit Metab Dis 1989; 1:118–134.

Seguin JH, Baugh RF, McIntee RA. Airway manifestations of chondrodysplasia punctata. Int J Pediatr Otorhinolaryngol 1993;27:85–90.

Sherer DM, Glantz JC, Allen TA, Lonardo F, Metlay LA. Prenatal sonographic diagnosis of non-rhizomelic chondrodysplasia punctata. Obstet Gynecol 1994;83:858–860.

Silengo MC, Luzzatti L, Silverman FN. Clinical and genetics aspects of Conradi–Hunermann disease: a report of three familial cases and review of the literature. J Pediatr 1980; 97:911–917.

Singh I, Johnson GH, Brown FR. Peroxisomal disorders: biochemical and clinical diagnostic considerations. Am J Dis Child 1988;142:1297–1301.

Spranger JW, Opitz JM, Bidder U. Heterogenicity of chondrodysplasia punctata. Humangenetik 1971;11:190–212.

Stoll C, Dott B, Roth MP, Alembik Y. Birth prevalence rates of skeletal dysplasias. Clin Genet 1989;35:88–92.

Subramani S. PEX genes on the rise. Nat Genet 1997;15: 331–333.

Suzuki Y, Shimozawa N, Kawabata I, et al. Prenatal diagnosis of peroxisomal disorders: biochemical and immunocytochemical studies on peroxisomes in human amniocytes. Brain Dev 1994;16:27–31.

Tuck SM, Slack J, Buckland G. Prenatal diagnosis of Conradi's syndrome: case report. Prenat Diagn 1990;10: 195–198.

Wanders RJ, Schutgens RB, Barth PG, Tager JM, van den Bosch H. Postnatal diagnosis of peroxisomal disorders: a biochemical approach. Biochimie 1993;75:269–279.

Zellweger H, Maertens P, Superneau D, Wertelecki W. History of the cerebroheptaorenal syndrome of Zellweger and other peroxisomal disorders. South Med J 1988;81: 357–364.

CHAPTER 93

Diastrophic Dysplasia

► CONDITION

Diastrophic dysplasia is a distinct clinical entity characterized by disproportionate short stature, cleft palate, club foot, progressive scoliosis, limited joint mobility, proximally placed first metacarpals ("hitchhikers thumb"), and cystic degeneration of the pinnae of the ear ("cauliflower deformity") (Fig. 93-1) (Lachman et al. 1981). This condition was first described by Lamy and Maroteaux (1960) who used the Greek word *diastrophos,* meaning twisted, to describe the prominent involvement of the feet and spine in this type of dwarfism (Diab et al. 1994).

Diastrophic dysplasia exhibits distinctive histopathology, which consists of cytoplasmic accumulation of glycogen and fat in the chondrocytes, resulting in variability of chondrocyte size, shape, and viability (Diab et al. 1994). There is nonuniformity of the cartilage matrix with fibroblast and vascular ingrowth, resulting in fibrotic foci and areas of intracartilaginous calcification (Diab et al. 1994). The abnormalities of the cartilage matrix are considered pathognomonic and are visible with light microscopy. The underlying problem is an excessive amount of collagen deposition within the cartilage matrix rather than a lack of collagen. The excessive deposition of structurally abnormal collagen occurs in the growth cartilage rather than the resting cartilage (Shapiro 1992). This cartilage abnormality affects the entire epiphyseal area, which leads not only to shortening of the long bones, but to extreme malformation of the epiphyseal ends of the bones. This abnormality affects the articular surfaces, causing precocious osteoarthritis (Shapiro 1992). Furthermore, in one patient, a biochemical abnormality of type IX collagen has been described (Diab et al. 1994).

The underlying genetic basis of diastrophic dysplasia is now known (Hästbacka et al. 1994). The mutation involved in this condition is in a novel sulfate transporter gene, known as the diastrophic sysplasia sulfate transporter (*DTDST*) (Hästbacka et al. 1996). Impaired function of this gene product probably leads to undersulfation of proteoglycans in cartilage matrix, resulting in the disease phenotype (Hästbacka et al. 1994).

► INCIDENCE

Diastrophic dysplasia has been observed only in whites. To date, over 300 patients with diastrophic dysplasia have been described, and interestingly, at least 160 of them are in Finland (Ryöppy et al. 1992), where the gene for diastrophic dysplasia is unusually common due to an apparent founder effect in this relatively genetically isolated population (Hästbacka et al. 1994). The incidence of diastrophic dysplasia is 1 in 32,600 live births in Finland, where it is the most common skeletal dysplasia (Poussa et al. 1991).

► SONOGRAPHIC FINDINGS

Because of the rarity of this condition in the non-Finnish population, relatively few reports of the prenatal sonographic diagnosis of diastrophic dysplasia exist in the literature (Jung et al. 1998; Kaitila et al. 1983; Mantagos et al. 1981). To our knowledge, diastrophic dysplasia has not been diagnosed by sonography during the first trimester. The prenatal diagnosis of diastrophic dysplasia was first described in 1980, when O'Brien et al. (1980) reported the diagnosis in a family with a previous affected child. Prenatal sonography was performed at 13 weeks 5 days of menstrual age, and revealed a crown-to-rump length of 43 mm, which corresponded a gestational age of 11 weeks. The study was repeated

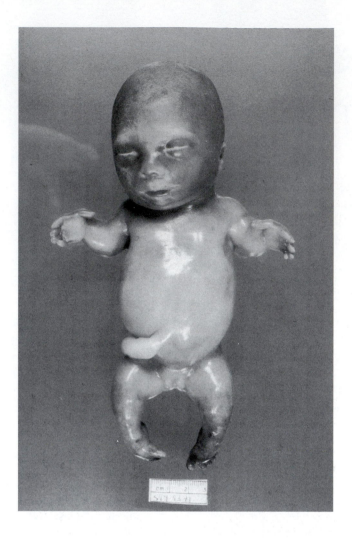

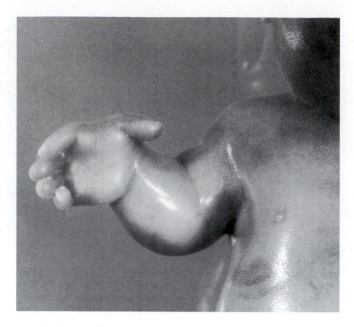

Figure 93-1. (Left) Postnatal photograph of a 19-week fetus with diastrophic dysplasia, illustrating severe micromelia, bilateral club feet, micrognathia, and bilateral hitchhiker thumbs. (Right) Close-up of extreme lateral displacement of thumbs. (*Courtesy of Dr. Joseph Semple.*)

at 16 weeks of gestation, when the femur length measured 13 mm (normal for gestational age: 19 to 26 mm). Thus, long-bone shortening was retrospectively demonstrated in this condition during the early second trimester (13 weeks 5 days). In this report, fetoscopy demonstrated extremely short and curved limbs in the affected fetus. Examination of the face and oral cavity also showed micrognathia and cleft palate, other findings that are typically seen in diastrophic dysplasia. In another case, also complicated by a positive family history, prenatal sonography performed at 16 weeks of gestation demonstrated abnormally short limbs (less than 3 SD below the mean for gestational age) and lateral projection of the thumbs (Fig. 93-2). These findings revealed an affected fetus. These authors recommended assessing fetuses at risk with serial examinations at 16, 20, 24, and 32 weeks of gestation because they were concerned that normal findings at 16 weeks might still be consistent with a diagnosis of an affected infant (Gollop and Eigier 1987). In another affected case with no family history of diastrophic dysplasia, ultrasound examination performed at 31 weeks revealed severe micromelia (all long bones less than 2 SD below

the mean for gestational age), normal amniotic fluid, ulnar deviation of the hands, abducted and proximally inserted thumbs and great toes, bilateral club feet, apparent elbow and knee joint contractures, cervical kyphosis (Fig. 93-3), and micrognathia. The diagnosis of diastrophic dysplasia was confirmed postnatally (Gembruch et al. 1988).

Other sonographic findings in diastrophic dysplasia include normal skull and vertebral-body ossification and occasional scoliosis. In a summary of 18 at-risk pregnancies in Finland, prenatal sonography performed during the second trimester was highly accurate for diagnosis of this condition (Hästbacka et al. 1993). Of the 18 fetuses at risk, 5 were predicted to be affected and 13 were predicted to be unaffected by long-bone measurements. All diagnoses were confirmed by postnatal or post-termination assessment.

▶ DIFFERENTIAL DIAGNOSIS

In the past, diastrophic dysplasia was considered to comprise two different clinical entities, the "classic"

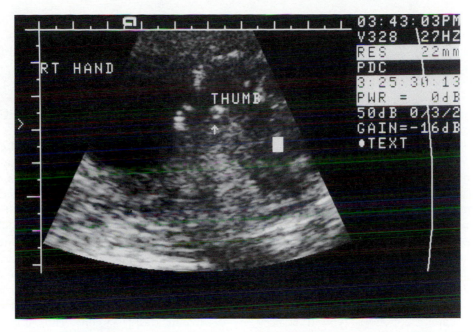

Figure 93-2. Prenatal sonogram of displaced ("hitchhiker") thumb in a fetus with diastrophic dysplasia.

diastrophic dysplasia and the "diastrophic variant." The term variant denoted a milder phenotype. Now all are considered to have one entity, diastrophic dysplasia, with variation in the phenotype (Horton et al. 1978). This was confirmed by Lachman et al. (1981), who studied 26 patients considered to have the variant form of diastrophic dysplasia, but in whom light and electron microscopic studies demonstrated the identical pathology present in the classic phenotype.

The differential diagnosis, therefore, includes the wide spectrum of clinical manifestations that occur in diastrophic dysplasia. Other conditions considered within the differential diagnosis include pseudodiastrophic dysplasia and atelosteogenesis type II. In pseudodiastrophic dysplasia, patients exhibit a large cranium with midface hypoplasia, long clavicles, short limbs, and platyspondyly (Eteson et al. 1986), but the cauliflower ear characteristic of diastrophic dysplasia does not occur in this

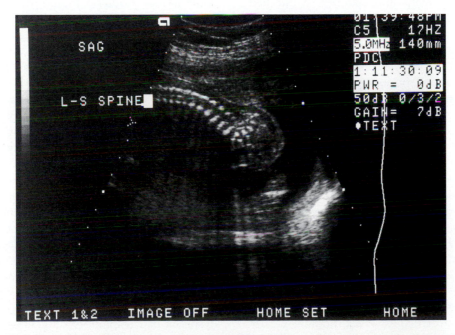

Figure 93-3. Prenatal sonogram demonstrating kyphosis in a fetus with diastrophic dysplasia.

condition. The distinguishing features of pseudodiastrophic dysplasia include elbow and proximal interphalangeal joint dislocation, and progressive scoliosis in infancy. Joint abnormalities seen in pseudodiastrophic dysplasia respond well to physical therapy. This is not true for diastrophic dysplasia. Pathologically, the two conditions are quite different. In pseudodiastrophic dysplasia, the resting cartilage is normal, with no areas of fibrous degeneration in the cartilage matrix of these patients.

In atelosteogenesis type II, patients exhibit marked shortness of limbs with metaphyseal widening, a characteristic bifid humerus, cervical scoliosis, and abnormalities of the digits. Radiographs reveal more severe abnormalities of the tubular bones of the hands and feet as compared with diastrophic dysplasia (Qureshi et al. 1995). On the other hand, the histologic abnormalities of the resting cartilage in atelosteogenesis type II are similar to those seen in diastrophic dysplasia. This is not surprising, as atelosteogenesis type II is now known to be caused by mutations in the same gene that causes diastrophic dysplasia, *DTDST* (Hästbacka et al. 1996).

▶ ANTENATAL NATURAL HISTORY

In one report, Qureshi et al. (1995) described characteristic histopathologic abnormalities seen in three cases of diastrophic dysplasia diagnosed by prenatal sonography. In all three cases, there was a negative family history, and routine second-trimester sonography diagnosed a nonspecific skeletal dysplasia. All pregnancies were terminated electively and extensively studied postmortem. Postmortem radiographs demonstrated moderately short long bones with a slight inward bowing. Broad metaphyses were demonstrated, especially in the femurs; mineralization of the bones was normal, and the vertebral bodies had normal widths. The ribs were normal, and there was no scoliosis demonstrated prenatally. On the postnatal radiographs, the characteristic hitchhiker thumb deformity was easily demonstrated.

Histopathologic studies demonstrated morphologic abnormalities that were very similar to those reported in postnatally diagnosed cases. The predominant changes were demonstrated in the resting cartilage, where chondrocytes were surrounded by a halo of dense-appearing cartilage matrix. The chondrocytic nuclei were larger than normal and some lacunae contained two or more nuclei. Degenerative changes were also seen in the vertebral bodies and tracheal cartilage. Cystic degeneration was demonstrated in the pinnae of the ears, the larynx, and the costal cartilages. These findings clearly demonstrate that the morphologic consequences of the abnormal sulfate transport gene occur relatively early in fetal life.

No evidence exists for increased in utero mortality due to diastrophic dysplasia.

▶ MANAGEMENT OF PREGNANCY

Pregnancy management will depend on whether there is a family history of a pregnancy previously affected with diastrophic dysplasia. If there is, and if DNA was obtained from the previously affected fetus or infant, DNA analysis should be performed. If DNA is available from a previously affected individual, family studies should be performed prior to planned pregnancy to identify the specific mutation that occurs in the family. It is likely that only one mutation exists for individuals of Finnish ancestry. For non-Finnish individuals, however, mutations can occur in several places within the diastrophic dysplasia gene. Thus, it is important to identify the mutation that occurs in a specific family. If the family previously had an affected child, and DNA was not obtained from the affected individual, prenatal diagnosis can be reliably performed by serial sonography, which is highly accurate in the detection of affected fetuses (Hästbacka et al. 1993).

The more likely scenario is a fetus that has no known family history of diastrophic dysplasia, but that has a skeletal dysplasia demonstrated on a sonogram performed for uterine size less than gestational date. If findings characteristic of diastrophic dysplasia are demonstrated by sonography, the potential diagnosis can be discussed with the family. Discussion of the outcome in this condition should include the facts that intelligence is normal and that wide variation in the phenotype of diastrophic dysplasia exists. Reported adult heights include a range of 100 to 159 cm (3 foot 9 inches to 6 feet) (Gembruch et al. 1988), although the mean height in a series of 72 American patients with diastrophic dysplasia was 118 cm (3 feet 11 inches) (Horton et al. 1982). Termination of pregnancy can be offered if the diagnosis is made prior to 24 weeks of gestation. If the family elects pregnancy termination, a complete perinatal autopsy should be performed, because the cartilage abnormalities demonstrated by light and electron microscopy are pathognomonic for this condition. At termination of pregnancy, DNA should be obtained from the fetus or placenta to store for future DNA analysis. There is no indication for cesarean delivery other than for standard obstetrical reasons. Consideration should be given, however, to delivery at a tertiary-care center for respiratory support of the newborn. In one report, 12% of patients with diastrophic dysplasia had respiratory difficulties at birth caused by glossoptosis (Rintala et al. 1986).

▶ FETAL INTERVENTION

There are no fetal inteventions for diastrophic dysplasia.

▶ TREATMENT OF THE NEWBORN

The characteristic postnatal clinical findings seen in patients with diastrophic dysplasia are summarized in Table 93-1. Because of the high incidence of cleft palate and micrognathia, a neonatologist should be present at the delivery to manage the airway. The lungs are normal and not hypoplastic. Postnatal radiographs can be obtained to confirm the diagnosis (Fig. 93-4). They may demonstrate calcification of the pinnae, precocious calcification of the larynx and costal cartilages, marked epiphyseal irregularities, delayed secondary ossification centers, and extreme shortening of the long bones (Diab et al. 1994). A clinical geneticist should be consulted for confirmation of the diagnosis and to provide genetic counseling for the family. The incidence of neonatal mortality is increased because of respiratory insufficiency related to tracheal cartilage weakness (Gustavson et al. 1985). After the newborn period, the lifespan is normal.

▶ LONG-TERM OUTCOME

Patients with diastrophic dysplasia exhibit normal intelligence and development. Long-term medical problems include short stature, cleft palate, scoliosis, and the need for osteotomies for hip, knee, and foot contractures (Shapiro 1992). Growth curves for height are available for patients with diastrophic dysplasia (Horton et al. 1982).

In one report, 95 Finnish patients with diastrophic dysplasia were studied until 79 years of age. Of these, 41 (43%) had an open cleft palate, and surgery was required in 37 of these patients. An additional 30 (32%) had submucous cleft palate or microforms of cleft palate. In these patients, no hypernasality of speech was noted. Only 16 (17%) of patients had a normal palate. Most patients had micrognathia (Rintala et al. 1986).

In another study of a large cohort (101 patients) with diastrophic dysplasia, one-third were noted to have cervical kyphosis. Three of these cases resolved spontaneously before 5 years of age. Scoliosis was demonstrated in 49% of females and only 22% of males with diastrophic dysplasia. Only 2 of these patients required operation. In addition, spina bifida occulta was demonstrated in 73% of females and 59% of males (Poussa et al. 1991). Spinal involvement may be severe in affected

▶ **TABLE 93-1.** CLINICAL FINDINGS IN DIASTROPHIC DYSPLASIA

Cleft palate
Cystic changes in pinnae ("cauliflower" ear)
Lordosis, scoliosis
Joint limitation
Rhizomelic and/or mesomelic shortening
Ulnar deviation of hand
Shortened ovoid first metacarpal ("Hitchhiker's" thumb)
Club foot deformity
Symphalangism

Modified from Lachman et al. 1981

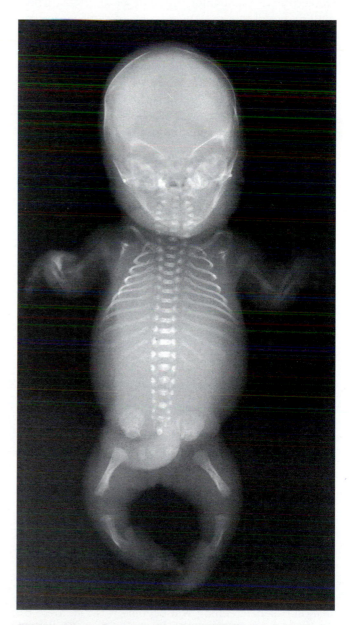

Figure 93-4. Post-mortem radiograph of the fetus shown in Figure 93-1.

patients, resulting in odontoid hypoplasia and C1-C2 subluxation. Atlanto-axial instability has also been reported (Diab et al. 1994; Richards 1991). Spinal stenosis with cord compression can lead to neurologic complications (Diab et al. 1994; Gembruch et al. 1988). Joint changes are progressive in nature and painful osteoarthroses and joint contractures can develop at an early age (Hästbacka et al. 1994).

A wide spectrum of foot deformities exists in patients with diastrophic dysplasia. In one study of 102 patients, 43% were demonstrated to have a foot with a tarsal valgus deformity and metatarsus adductus. An additional 29% of patients had equinovarus adductus and 8% had equinus deformity. Sixty-three percent of feet studied were plantigrade (Ryöppy et al. 1992). These authors noted that the abnormality of cartilage in diastrophic dysplasia results in cartilage that is softer than normal. Thus, the cartilaginous parts of the skeleton tend to become progressively deformed with weight bearing. This particularly involves the feet, hips, and knees of affected patients. Finally, sexual development is normal in patients with diastrophic dysplasia, and there is no indication that fertility is reduced.

▶ GENETICS AND RECURRENCE RISK

Diastrophic dysplasia is inherited as an autosomal recessive trait with a wide variability of expression, even among siblings. The gene for diastrophic dysplasia maps to the distal end of the long arm of chromosome 5 (Hästbacka et al. 1990, 1991). The Finnish population has been used to study this condition because the carrier frequency in Finland is 1 to 2%. Diastrophic dysplasia is one of the most common autosomal recessive disorders. The gene has been mapped based on linkage disequilibrium occurring in the Finnish population. A single ancestral mutation accounts for >95% of chromosomes bearing the mutation that causes diastrophic dysplasia (Hästbacka et al. 1994).

As noted earlier, the gene encodes a novel sulfate transporter now known as diastrophic dysplasia sulfate-transporter gene (DTDST). Impaired function of this gene product leads to undersulfation of proteoglycans in the cartilage matrix. It has been demonstrated that mRNA for this gene is minimally present in Finnish patients. Analysis of non-Finnish patients with diastrophic dysplasia has revealed two frame-shift mutations and one splice-acceptor change. In addition, evidence of deficient sulfate transport has been shown in skin fibroblasts from an affected patient (Hästbacka et al. 1994). Because of the founder effect occurring in Finland, population-based screening will become possible there because of the high carrier frequency for this condition.

Furthermore, the disorders atelosteogenesis type II and achondrogenesis type IB (see Chapter 88) are also caused by mutations in the DTDST gene (Hästbacka et al. 1993; Superti-Furga 1994; Superti-Furga et al. 1996). All three chrondrodysplasias appear to demonstrate a correlation between genotype and phenotype. The most severe disorder, achondrogenesis type IB, always shows mutations in the coding regions of both alleles, with most resulting in early termination codons. Patients with atelosteogenesis type II have mutations in the coding regions of both alleles of DTDST, but they involve less severe changes, such as frame-shift or missense mutations. No patient with diastrophic dysplasia has been demonstrated to have two mutations in the coding region of the gene (Hästbacka et al. 1993). This is presumably the reason that the phenotype associated with diastrophic dysplasia is the mildest of the groups of disorders now known to be due to sulfate-transporter-gene abnormalities.

First-trimester prenatal diagnosis has been performed successfully by DNA-based diagnosis for five fetuses at risk because of a positive family history. In fetal DNA obtained by chorionic villus sampling at 10 weeks, three fetuses were predicted to be unaffected and two were predicted to be affected with >95% probability. These diagnoses were considered to be concordant with the sonographic findings and were ultimately confirmed by analysis of DNA obtained at termination or after the birth of the infant (Hästbacka et al. 1993).

REFERENCES

Diab M, Wu JJ, Shapiro F, Eyre D. Abnormality of type IX collagen in a patient with diastrophic dysplasia. Am J Med Genet 1994;49:402–409.

Eteson DJ, Beluffi G, Burgio GR, Belloni C, Lachman RS, Rimoin DL. Pseudodiastrophic dysplasia: a distinct newborn skeletal dysplasia. J Pediatr 1986;109:635–641.

Gembruch U, Niesen M, Kehrberg H, Hansmann M. Diastrophic dysplasia: a specific prenatal diagnosis by ultrasound. Prenat Diagn 1988;8:539–545.

Gollop TR, Eigier A. Prenatal ultrasound diagnosis of diastrophic dysplasia at 16 weeks. Am J Med Genet 1987;27: 321–324.

Gustavson KH, Holmgren G, Jagell S, Jorulf H. Lethal and non-lethal diastrophic dysplasia: a study of 14 Swedish cases. Clin Genet 1985;28:321–324.

Hästbacka J, de la Chapelle A, Mahtani MM, et al. The diastrophic dysplasia gene encodes a novel sulfate transporter: positional cloning by fine-structure linkage disequilibrium mapping. Cell 1994;78:1073–1087.

Hästbacka J, Kaitila I, Sistonen P, de la Chapelle A. Diastrophic dysplasia gene maps to the distal long arm of chromosome 5. Proc Natl Acad Sci USA 1990;87:8056–8059.

Hästbacka J, Salonen R, Laurila P, de la Chapelle A, Kaitila I. Prenatal diagnosis of diastrophic dysplasia with polymorphic DNA markers. J Med Genet 1993;30: 265–268.

Hästbacka J, Sistonen P, Kaitila I, Weiffenbach B, Kidd KK, de la Chapelle A. A linkage map spanning the locus for diastrophic dysplasia (DTD). Genomics 1991;11:968–973.

Hästbacka J, Superti-Furga A, Wilcox WR, Rimoin DL, Cohn DH, Lander ES. Atelosteogenesis type II is caused by mutations in the diastrophic dysplasia sulfate-transporter gene (DTDST): evidence for a phenotypic series involving three chrondrodysplasias. Am J Hum Genet 1996; 58:255–262.

Horton WA, Hall JG, Scott CI, Pyeritz RE, Rimoin DL. Growth curves for height for diastrophic dysplasia, spondyloepiphyseal dysplasia congenita, and pseudo-achondroplasia. Am J Dis Child 1982;136:316–319.

Horton WA, Rimoin DL, Lachman RS, et al. The phenotypic variability of diastrophic dysplasia. J Pediatr 1978;93: 609–613.

Jung C, Sohn C, Sergi C. Care report: prenatal diagnosis of diastrophic dysplasia by ultrasound at 21 weeks of gestation in a mother with massive obesity. Prenat Diagn 18: 378–383.

Kaitila I, Ammala P, Karjalainen O, Liukkonen S, Rapola J. Early prenatal detection of diastrophic dysplasia. Prenat Diagn 1983;3:237–244.

Lachman R, Sillence D, Rimoin D, et al. Diastrophic dysplasia: the death of a variant. Radiology 1981;140:79–86.

Lamy M, Maroteaux P. Le nanisme diastrophique. Presse Med 1960;52:1977–1980.

Mantagos S, Weiss RR, Mahoney M, Hobbins JC. Prenatal diagnosis of diastrophic dwarfism. Am J Obstet Gynecol 1981;139:111–113.

O'Brien GD, Rodeck C, Queenan JT. Early prenatal diagnosis of diastrophic dwarfism by ultrasound. BMJ 1980;280:1300.

Poussa M, Merikanto J, Ryöppy S, Marttinen E, Kaitila I. The spine in diastrophic dysplasia. Spine 1991;16:881–887.

Qureshi F, Jacques SM, Johnson SF, et al. Histopathology of fetal diastrophic dysplasia. Am J Med Genet 1995;56: 300–303.

Richards BS. Atlanto-axial instability in diastrophic dysplasia: a case report. J Bone Joint Surg Am 1991;73:614–616.

Rintala A, Marttinen E, Rantala SL, Kaitila I. Cleft palate in diastrophic dysplasia: morphology, results of treatment and complications. Scand J Plast Reconstr Surg 1986;20: 45–49.

Ryöppy S, Poussa M, Merikanto J, Marttinen E, Kaitila I. Foot deformities in diastrophic dysplasia: an analysis of 102 patients. J Bone Joint Surg Br 1992;74:441–444.

Shapiro F. Light and electron microscopic abnormalities in diastrophic dysplasia growth cartilage. Calcif Tissue Int 1992;51:324–331.

Superti-Furga A. A defect in the metabolic activation of sulfate in a patient with achondrogenesis type IB. Am J Hum Genet 1994;55:1137–1145.

Superti-Furga A, Hästbacka J, Wilcox WR, Cohn DH, van der Harten HJ, Blau N. Achondrogenesis type IB is caused by mutations in the diastrophic dysplasia sulfate transporter gene. Nat Genet 1996;12:100–102.

CHAPTER 96

Hypophosphatasia

► CONDITION

The term hypophosphatasia was first used by Rathbun in 1948 to describe an infant with severe rickets and very low alkaline phosphatase activity in serum and tissues (Henthorn and Whyte 1992; Whyte et al. 1995). Hypophosphatasia is now considered to be a rare inherited metabolic bone disorder characterized by deficient activity of the liver/bone/kidney isoenzyme of alkaline phosphatase. This isoenzyme is also known as the tissue-nonspecific form of alkaline phosphatase (TNSALP).

Alkaline phosphatase was first discovered in 1923, when Robert Robinson noted a large amount of phosphatase activity within ossifying bone and cartilage in rats and rabbits. He was the first to suggest that this catalytic action was important for mineralization of the skeleton due to hydrolysis of a phosphate ester, which would result in the local increase of inorganic (free) phosphate (Whyte 1994). He subsequently showed that the enzyme functioned optimally at a distinctly alkaline pH, although he never specifically used the term *alkaline phosphatase*. Later, alkaline phosphatase was also demonstrated in tissues that normally do not mineralize, such as the liver, intestines, and placenta; thus, the role of alkaline phosphatase in skeletal mineralization was questioned. It is now known that at least four distinct genes encode four different human alkaline phosphatase isoenzymes. The TNSALP liver bone kidney form is especially rich in mineralizing bone. The location of this gene is on the short arm of chromosome 1, band p36.1-34 (Henthorn and Whyte 1992; Whyte et al. 1995). The other three genes are found in a cluster on the end of the long arm of chromosome 2. These include placental, intestinal, and placental-like isoenzymes of alkaline phosphatase. Each of the alkaline phosphatase genes have now been sequenced, and the TNSALP gene is the largest of the four (Whyte 1994).

Hypophosphatasia is a clinically variable condition. Mutations in the TNSALP gene are responsible for perinatal hypophosphatasia in which the severity of the disease generally correlates with the age of onset of symptoms. Fetuses detected in utero generally have the most severe form of hypophosphatasia, also known as the perinatal lethal form. Findings in this condition include profound undermineralization of the skeleton, lack of skull ossification resulting in a caput membraneceum, and shortened deformed limbs. Postnatal survival of affected infants is generally limited because of associated pulmonary hypoplasia and rachitic disease of the chest. Radiographic studies in the newborn are generally diagnostic. The infantile form of hypophosphatasia generally presents before the age of 6 months. The newborn can initially appear normal, but poor feeding subsequently develops, as do inadequate weight gain and symptoms of rickets. The initial problems include the development of craniosynostosis, increased intracranial pressure, hypercalcemia, renal failure, and seizures. Approximately 50% of affected infants die. The childhood form is variable in its clinical expression. It is characterized by premature loss of the deciduous teeth at an age of less than 5 years, resulting from abnormalities of the dental cementum, which is important for connection between the tooth roots and the periodontal ligament (Whyte 1994). Affected children also have short stature, rickets, deformation of the legs, knees, ankles, and wrists, although some of these improve with age. Affected patients have characteristic abnormalities on radiographs, which include focal bony defects near the ends of the major long bones. These manifest as a tongue-like shape of radiolucency that projects from the growth plate into the metaphysis (Whyte 1994). The adult form of hypophosphatasia generally presents during middle age. An additional childhood history of rickets or premature loss of deciduous teeth may or may not be elicited. In general, affected adults have enjoyed relatively good health as adolescents and young adults, but then recurrent metatarsal stress fractures develop and there is early loss of permanent teeth. The mildest form of hypophosphatasia is called "odontohypophosphatasia," which is reserved for patients whose only clinical manifestation is dental disease. No absolute diagnostic criteria exist for the separation of the various clinical presentations. A continuous spectrum of symptoms exists. It is anticipated that as the molecular basis for the disorders are increasingly identified, a more rational classification for the different clinical symptoms will be established. For the purposes of this book, however, the only condition that will be discussed subsequently is the perinatal form.

▶ INCIDENCE

The incidence of hypophosphatasia, based on 1957 data from Toronto, is 1 in 100,000 live births (Greenberg et al. 1990; Mulivor et al. 1978). Cases of hypophosphatasia have been described throughout the world, occurring in all races (Whyte 1994). During the years 1977 to 1986, six neonates affected with hypophosphatasia were born in southern Manitoba. After these infants were identified, it was appreciated that Mennonites in southern Canada have an unusually high carrier frequency for this disorder. Mennonites have a 1 in 25 chance of being a carrier for at least one mutation in the TNSALP gene. The birth incidence of affected infants with hypophosphatasia in Mennonites is 1 in 2500 (Chodirker et al. 1990). This unusually high incidence is presumably due to a founder effect with inbreeding.

▶ SONOGRAPHIC FINDINGS

The most striking abnormality described in cases of perinatal hypophosphatasia is the absence of a normally formed fetal skull (Kousseff and Mulivor 1981). The hallmarks for sonographic diagnosis of hypophosphatasia include a fetus who is small for gestational age with decreased echogenicity of the bones, a prominent falx cerebri due to undermineralization of the skull, various

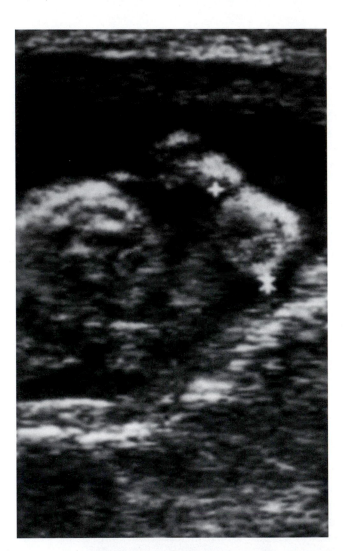

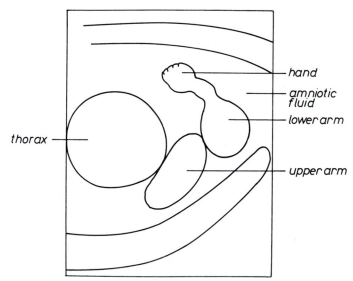

Figure 96-1. (Left) Sonographic image of a fetus at 24 weeks with hypophosphatasia, demonstrating severely shortened and bent forearm. (Right) Diagram of sonographic image in Panel A. *(Reprinted, with permission, from van Dongen PWJ, Hamel BCJ, Nijhuis JG, de Boer CN. Prenatal follow-up of hypophosphatasia by ultrasound: case report. Eur J Obstet Gynecol Reprod Biol 1990;34:283–288. Reprinted with the permission of Elsevier Science Ireland Ltd., Bay 15K, Shannon Industrial Estate, Co. Clare, Ireland.)*

skeletal deformities, and the presence of polyhydramnios occurring later in gestation (Wladimiroff et al. 1985). Also, pulmonary hypoplasia may be documented due to a severely reduced thoracic volume due to abnormal and short ribs. In one report, Van Dongen et al. (1990) described sonographic studies performed in a family with a previously affected child. Even as early as 8 weeks of gestation, the crown-to-rump length was indicative of a fetus 1.5 weeks younger than the actual gestational age. The family was lost to follow-up until 24 weeks of gestation, when severe polyhydramnios was noted. Other findings included an active fetus with shortened, bent, fixed limbs with markedly decreased echogenicity, which prevented separate visualization of the fingers and toes (Fig. 96-1). The falx cerebri and other central nervous system structures could be distinguished unusually clearly due to the low echogenicity

of the skull bones (Fig. 96-2A and B). This was described as being similar to the fetal appearance in hydrocephalus. In another report of prenatal diagnosis in a family at risk for recurrence of hypophosphatasia, the failure to outline a fetal head was noted at 16 weeks of gestation (Rudd et al. 1976). The skull was described as a very thin, faint circular outline. In addition, skip defects were noted in the cervical-spine vertebral bodies.

In another prenatal diagnostic report, with a negative family history, but a conception marked by consanguinity, underossification of the skull, facial bones, ribs, and limbs was noted at 27 weeks of gestation (DeLange and Rouse 1990). In addition, underossification of the metacarpals, neural arches of the spine, and vertebral bodies was noted. This group made a presumptive prenatal diagnosis of hypophosphatasia based on (1) the generalized underossification of the fetal bones, (2) shortening of the limbs, and (3) lack of ossification of groups of vertebral bodies, the neural arches, and the fetal hands.

More recently, a dominantly inherited form of mild hypophosphatasia has been described that presents in utero as severe bowing of the long bones (Moore et al. 1999; Pauli et al. 1999). Interestingly, in this condition, prenatal and postnatal improvement of the bone dysplasia occurs spontaneously. Some authors suggest that the condition should be called the benign prenatal form of hypophosphatasia.

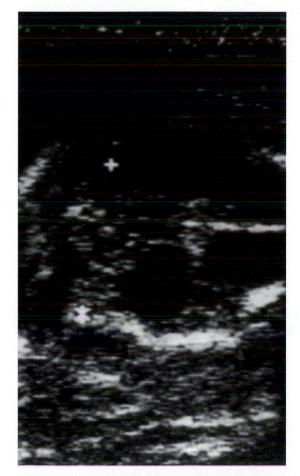

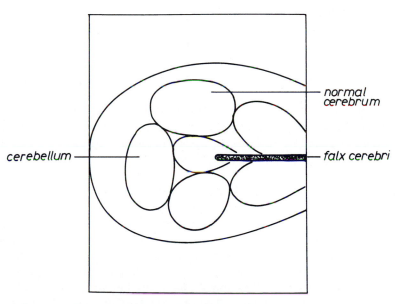

Figure 96-2. (Left) Sonographic image of the fetus seen in Figure 96-1A, demonstrating unusually clear visualization of the falx cerebri. (Right) Diagram of sonographic image in Panel A. *(Reprinted, with permission, from van Dongen PWJ, Hamel BCJ, Nijhuis JG, de Boer CN. Prenatal follow-up of hypophosphatasia by ultrasound: case report. Eur J Obstet Gynecol Reprod Biol 1990;34:283–288. Reprinted with the permission of Elsevier Science Ireland Ltd., Bay 15K, Shannon Industrial Estate, Co. Clare, Ireland.)*

▶ DIFFERENTIAL DIAGNOSIS

Failure to visualize the fetal skull leads to a presumptive differential diagnosis of hypophosphatasia versus anencephaly. An amniocentesis could be performed to measure amniotic fluid α-fetoprotein and acetylcholinesterase, although this is probably unnecessary, given the current state of sonographic imaging and the characteristic appearance of anencephaly. If these levels are normal, the diagnosis is likely to be hypophosphatasia. Other conditions associated with dwarfism that may result in malformation and undermineralization of the bones include type II osteogenesis imperfecta and achondrogenesis. Achondrogenesis (see Chapter 88) can be distinguished from hypophosphatasia by better ossification of the neural arches with nonossification of the vertebral bodies. To further distinguish between hypophosphatasia, osteogenesis imperfecta, and achondrogenesis, prenatal radiography may be considered to further define areas of calcification.

▶ ANTENATAL NATURAL HISTORY

Little is known about the antenatal natural history for fetuses affected with hypophosphatasia. There is an increased incidence of stillbirth for the severe perinatal form, although the cause for this is unknown.

▶ MANAGEMENT OF PREGNANCY

The strategies for the definitive prenatal diagnosis of hypophosphatasia have included fetal radiography (in the early 1980s), prenatal sonography, assay of alkaline phosphatase activity in cultured amniocytes, fibroblasts, or chorionic villus samples, measurement of alkaline phosphatase activity in fetal serum obtained by cordocentesis, or analysis of DNA linkage or mutation studies on fetal tissue (Henthorn and Whyte 1995). Management of pregnancy differs in the setting of a positive family history of hypophosphatasia versus a negative family history. If the family history is positive, ideally DNA has been previously obtained from the affected proband before death. This material, along with parental blood samples, should be sent to a reference laboratory with experience in the identification of mutations in the TNSALP gene. If the mutations in the family are previously known, prenatal diagnosis can best be performed by chorionic villus sampling (CVS) to identify the presence of both parental mutations in the fetus (Mornet et al. 1999). If parental mutations cannot be identified, one approach is to use the entire cDNA sequence for the TNSALP gene as a probe with restriction enzyme digest to perform restriction-fragment–length polymorphism (RFLP) linkage analysis. This approach has been successfully employed in a Japanese family with a previously affected child (Kishi et al. 1991). The disadvantage of this technique is that DNA from the prior affected child or fetus, the current fetus, and the parents are needed.

If mutation analysis has not been performed on a previously affected child, other approaches to prenatal diagnosis may include the use of monoclonal antibody to the TNSALP isoenzyme on fetal material obtained by CVS. In one report of 16 pregnancies at risk for hypophosphatasia, a normal range for the TNSALP levels was established (50 to 150 μmol per minute per gram of tissue; median = 130). In 11 of the 16 at-risk cases, the fetus had greater than 50 μmol per minute per gram of tissue. These values were considered to fall within the normal range. All pregnancies continued to term and all infants were normal. In 5 of the 16 at-risk pregnancies, the TNSALP values were <25 μmol per minute per gram of tissue and all fetuses were terminated. Four of the 5 affected fetuses were confirmed as abnormal either by documenting sonographic abnormalities, autopsy diagnosis of abnormally foreshortened limbs, or by subsequent biochemical confirmation on fibroblast or liver tissue. One family was lost to follow-up (Brock and Barron 1991). Muller and colleagues (1991) have cautioned that CVS material should be sampled at less than 12 weeks of gestation and that particular care should be taken to eliminate maternal decidual tissue from the sample. These authors have confirmed the very low activity of the TNSALP in early chorionic villus material in affected fetuses. Placental alkaline phosphatase was never detected by these authors before 9 weeks of gestation. Affected pregnancies have both low total alkaline phosphatase and 0% TNSALP (Muller et al. 1991). Thus, in families with a positive history of hypophosphatasia but with no knowledge of DNA mutation analysis, prenatal diagnosis may be performed in two different ways on chorionic villus material.

In the setting of a fetus with typical sonographic findings suggesting the presence of hypophosphatasia, but a negative or unknown family history, we suggest performing amniocentesis to measure amniotic fluid α-fetoprotein to rule out anencephaly and to confirm the fetal karyotype. The amniocytes may be placed into culture and may be used for both assay of alkaline phosphatase activity (Kousseff and Mulivor 1981; Mulivor et al. 1978) and DNA analysis (Mornet et al. 1999). Consultation with a clinical geneticist is indicated.

▶ FETAL INTERVENTION

There are no fetal interventions for hypophosphatasia.

► TREATMENT OF THE NEWBORN

No effective treatment is currently available for the perinatal form of hypophosphatasia. Vitamin D and mineral supplements normally used in the treatment of rickets should be avoided, since circulating levels of calcium, inorganic phosphorus, and the vitamin D metabolites are generally normal in affected patients with hypophosphatasia (Whyte 1994). Unsuccessful attempts have been made to infuse several types of alkaline phosphatase intravenously (Whyte 1994). Because perinatal hypophosphatasia is a lethal condition, treatment of the newborn should be directed toward confirming the diagnosis and ensuring that a mechanism is in place for follow-up genetic counseling.

Physical findings at birth include rhizomelic and asymmetric shortening of all four extremities, with very pliable skull bones and possible craniotabes (Fig. 96-3) (Kousseff and Mulivor 1981). The infant's thorax is extremely compliant and a respirator may be required for ventilation. This should be considered only for the time needed to confirm the diagnosis, as the abnormalities in the thorax will not improve. Confirmatory postnatal radiographs may be obtained, which should reveal the extreme hypomineralization that is considered diagnostic of this condition (Fig. 96-4). Serum may be obtained to demonstrate the decreased activity of TNSALP and increased urinary excretion of phosphoethanolamine. Serum calcium is typically normal except in infantile cases, in which hypercalcemia is a

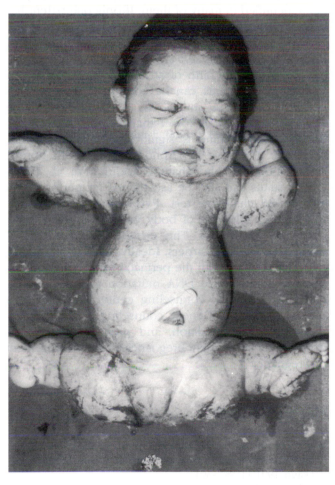

Figure 96-3. Postmortem photograph of a newborn infant with hypophosphatasia. Note the narrow chest and curved and shortened extremities. *(Reprinted, with permission, from van Dongen PWJ, Hamel BCJ, Nijhuis JG, de Boer CN. Prenatal follow-up of hypophosphatasia by ultrasound: case report. Eur J Obstet Gynecol Reprod Biol 1990;34:283–288. Reprinted with the permission of Elsevier Science Ireland Ltd., Bay 15K, Shannon Industrial Estate, Co. Clare, Ireland.)*

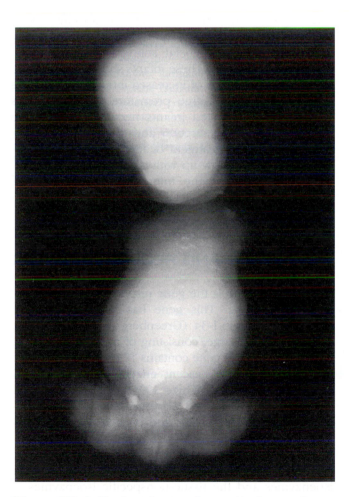

Figure 96-4. Postmortem radiograph of a newborn infant with hypophosphatasia. Note the severely hypomineralized bones. *(Reprinted, with permission, from van Dongen PWJ, Hamel BCJ, Nijhuis JG, de Boer CN. Prenatal follow-up of hypophosphatasia by ultrasound: case report. Eur J Obstet Gynecol Reprod Biol 1990;34:283–288. Reprinted with the permission of Elsevier Science Ireland Ltd., Bay 15K, Shannon Industrial Estate, Co. Clare, Ireland.)*

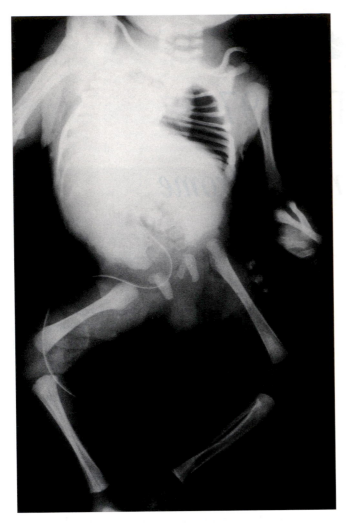

Figure 97-1. Anteroposterior radiograph of a newborn with Jarcho–Levin syndrome, demonstrating deformation of chest with characteristic "crab-claw" appearance.

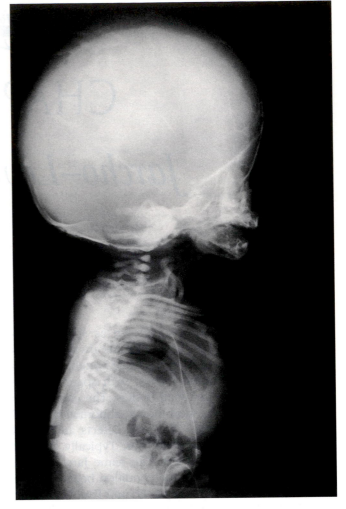

Figure 97-2. Lateral radiograph of the patient in Figure 97-1, showing the fan-like appearance of ribs.

glands. Simultaneously, another report at 22 weeks of gestation described the subtle spacing and widening of the fetal vertebrae seen in prenatal sonographic examination of a fetus with Jarcho–Levin syndrome (Apuzzio et al. 1987). At 22 weeks of gestation, a slightly smaller than normal chest diameter was appreciated but the diagnosis was unclear. In the same patient, by 28 weeks of gestation, an abnormally shaped chest was appreciated that included slight flattening of the ribs and irregularly spaced vertebrae (Apuzzio et al. 1987). In the third report, a fetus at 23 weeks of gestation was described with a shortened spine, disorganization of the vertebral bodies, posterior fusion of the ribs, with a short thorax but normal thoracic diameter. In a coronal view, narrowing of the lateral laminae in the lower thoracic and upper lumbar region was described. In the sagittal and coronal planes, grossly malaligned vertebrae, disorganization of vertebral bodies, and posteri-

orly fused ribs were appreciated (Romero et al. 1988). In 1989, Marks and colleagues reported two fetuses with sonographic findings of Jarcho–Levin syndrome. They described the following sonographic criteria for diagnosis of this condition (Marks et al. 1989):

1. Unpaired and poorly formed vertebral centers resulting in a "pebble-like" appearance of the spine
2. Multiple vertebral body fusion causing an irregular shortened spine
3. Indistinct or joined ribs posteriorly
4. A small or shortened thorax
5. A protuberant abdomen resulting from the shortened thorax
6. The presence of abdominal hernias
7. Normal amniotic fluid volume
8. Normal limb length and biparietal diameter measurements for gestational age

Subsequent reports have described the utility of prenatal sonographic diagnosis in families known to be at risk because of the prior birth of an affected infant (Lawson et al. 1997; Wong and Levine 1998). In one study, four fetuses were diagnosed as affected as early as 12 weeks of gestation (Eliyahu et al. 1997).

▶ DIFFERENTIAL DIAGNOSIS

The main consideration in the differential diagnosis is the determination of whether the findings are consistent with Jarcho–Levin syndrome or the related spondylocostal dysostoses, or whether the anomalies represent a more serious, lethal skeletal dysplasia. It is of great importance to rule out the most worrisome diagnoses of Jeune syndrome, campomelic dysplasia, and thanatophoric dysplasia (see Chapters 90, 91, and 100). These lethal conditions can be distinguished sonographically from Jarcho–Levin syndrome by the shortened limb measurements and narrowed chest deformity. In addition, in each of the other three conditions, there is no fusion of the ribs. Klippel–Feil syndrome can be distinguished from Jarcho–Levin syndrome because it affects the cervical rather than the thoracic ribs. The other conditions in the differential diagnosis include dyssegmental dysplasia and spondyloepiphyseal dysplasia congenita, but in this latter condition there is no rib fusion, and platyspondyly is present. In addition, any patient who presents with thoracic vertebral anomalies should be further investigated to rule out the VACTERL association, which consists of vertebral, anal, cardiac, tracheal and esophageal, renal, and radial limb anomalies.

The conditions most similar to Jarcho–Levin syndrome include COVESDEM (costovertebral-segmentation defects with mesomelia) syndrome (Wadia et al. 1978). In this condition, the thorax is not shortened, and mesomelia of the limbs is present, affecting the upper extremities more severely than the lower. It is sometimes difficult to distinguish Jarcho–Levin syndrome from spondylocostal dysostosis. This condition presents with less severe rib and vertebral anomalies, without the characteristic fan-like appearance of the rib fusion. This disorder is generally inherited as an autosomal dominant and it is consistent with survival into childhood.

▶ ANTENATAL NATURAL HISTORY

Morphologic studies of affected fetuses have shown that the vertebral bodies are malformed and consist of asymmetrically distributed ossification centers that vary greatly in size and shape and rarely cross the midline (Solomon et al. 1978). Microscopic examination of fetuses with Jarcho–Levin syndrome that were terminated during the second trimester has demonstrated disorganized vertebral endochondral bone formation with a lack of orderly column formation of mature chondrocytes. Although the ribs characteristically are fused, the endochondral bone formation within the ribs is normal (Marks et al. 1989). These defects undoubtedly occur extremely early in gestation, as the paraxial mesoderm undergoes segmentation between 21 and 28 days of gestation (Tolmie et al. 1987). Because certain homeobox genes important in formation of body structure are expressed uniquely in spinal cord, the question has been raised as to whether Jarcho–Levin syndrome could represent a mutation in one of the homeobox genes (Tolmie et al. 1987). Approximately one third of fetuses and infants with Jarcho–Levin syndrome have associated malformations that are outside of the thorax and vertebral bodies (Roberts et al. 1988). Some of the nonskeletal malformations that have been described in Jarcho–Levin syndrome include genitourinary anomalies, specifically uterus didelphys, bilobed bladder, hydronephrosis, undescended testes, urethral atresia, absent external genitalia, single umbilical artery, and cerebral polymicrogyria (Fig. 97-3) (Poor et al. 1983). Most reports do not emphasize central nervous system malformations, although in one report spina bifida and diastematomelia were described in a patient with Jarcho–Levin syndrome. Spina bifida occulta is reported to occur in 40.6% of patients with Jarcho–Levin syndrome (Giacoia and Say 1991).

▶ MANAGEMENT OF PREGNANCY

The main consideration in management of pregnancy is an accurate sonographic diagnosis. Prenatal sonograms should be reviewed by an expert in diagnosis of skeletal dysplasias. Both decreased and elevated maternal serum α-fetoprotein levels have been reported in this condition (Romero et al. 1988; Apuzzio et al. 1987). All reports of fetuses and infants affected with this condition have had normal chromosomes (Cantu et al. 1971; Karnes et al. 1991; Perez-Comas and Garcia-Castro 1974; Romero et al. 1988; Tolmie et al. 1987). Therefore, if the sonographic diagnosis is reasonably certain, there is no indication to obtain a fetal karyo-type. The route of delivery should be vaginal unless otherwise indicated for obstetric reasons. It is important for fetuses with Jarcho–Levin syndrome to be delivered in tertiary care centers because most of these infants will require neonatal resuscitation, mechanical ventilation, and postnatal genetic assessment.

▶ FETAL INTERVENTION

There are no fetal interventions for Jarcho–Levin syndrome.

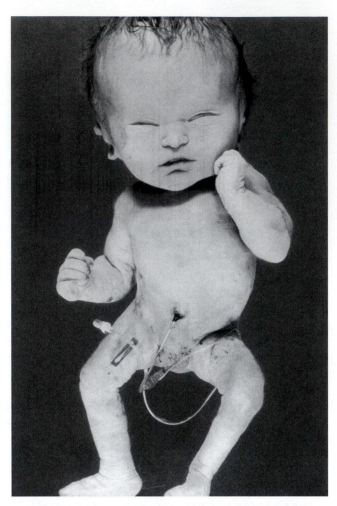

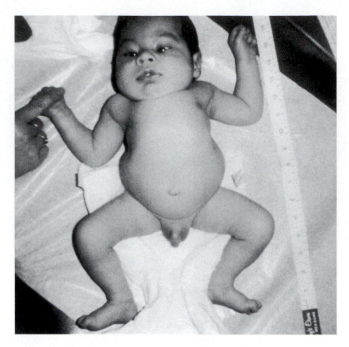

Figure 97-4. Infant with Jarcho–Levin syndrome who survived postnatally. *(Reprinted, with permission, from McCall CP, Hudgins L, Cloutier M, et al. Jarcho-Levin syndrome: unusual survival in a classical case. Am J Med Genet 1994;49:328–332.)*

Figure 97-3. Postmortem appearance of an infant with Jarcho–Levin syndrome. In addition to the bony abnormalities present, this infant had bilateral renal agenesis and a neural-tube defect. *(Courtesy of Dr. Mira Irons.)*

▶ TREATMENT OF THE NEWBORN

Because of the abnormally shaped chest, infants with Jarcho–Levin syndrome are likely to have pulmonary hypoplasia and to require resuscitation in the delivery room to begin adequate ventilation. Optimal treatment of the newborn with Jarcho–Levin syndrome should include delivery in a tertiary care center with a neonatologist prepared to provide immediate respiratory support and mechanical ventilation. A complete and detailed physical examination is indicated. Typical findings of the infant with Jarcho–Levin syndrome include a short neck, prominent occiput, low hairline, and a dysmorphic facial appearance that consists of a broad forehead, wide nasal bridge, prominent philtrum, anteverted nares, and a triangle-shaped mouth (Fig. 97-4). Additional physical findings include a protruberant abdomen,

poor muscle tone, abdominal hernias, long tapering fingers and toes, and soft-tissue syndactyly.

The major concern during the newborn period is the prevention of respiratory complications. The second most important consideration is an accurate diagnosis. Consultation with a clinical geneticist is indicated. In the newborn nursery, a complete postnatal skeletal survey should be performed. Radiographs should include the spine, which will demonstrate clefts, hemivertebrae, and abnormal vertebral-body fusion, and the chest, which may demonstrate hypoplasia and multiple rib fusion as well as a "scrambled" vertebral column (see Figs. 97-1 and 97-2) (Herold et al. 1988). Additional bony anomalies that may be diagnosed postnatally include an absent coccyx and a hypoplastic sacrum. The typical posteroanterior chest radiograph will show the rib anomalies in a distribution that appears similar to a crab. The lateral chest radiograph should show the rib fusion anomalies in a manner that appears like a fan (see Fig. 97-2). These findings are considered pathognomonic for this condition. In addition, long-bone films will be helpful to rule out another skeletal dysplasia.

▶ SURGICAL TREATMENT

The management of the orthopedic anomalies in Jarcho–Levin syndrome is difficult. The crab-like rib deformity and consequent pulmonary hypoplasia often require mechanical ventilatory support. This can be compounded by segments of the chest wall that are flail. In order to optimize respiratory mechanics and improve the affected infant's ability to be weaned from mechanical support, chest-wall reconstruction may be necessary. We successfully performed an extensive chest-wall reconstruction in an infant with Jarcho–Levin syndrome. In addition to a flail anterolateral right chest wall, he had diaphragmatic insertion at the 6th rib, further compromising ventilation. A prosthetic patch and rib graft were used to stent the flail-chest-wall segment, and the diaphragm was repositioned at the 12th rib posteriorly. The infant subsequently died from infection.

► LONG-TERM OUTCOME

All of the deaths reported in this condition have been due to respiratory insufficiency. This is presumably due to the severely deformed thoracic cage that results in pulmonary hypoplasia, followed by restrictive lung disease that predisposes the infants to severe pneumonia (Karnes et al. 1991). Patients with lethal cases generally die during the first 2 years of life. Although the restrictive effects of the thoracic cage have been considered to be responsible for these deaths, in one report, two infants with Jarcho–Levin syndrome underwent flexible fiberoptic bronchoscopy. In both of these patients, central airway abnormalities were visualized that were, according to the authors, not amenable to surgery. Specifically, the normal cartilaginous rings could not be seen bulging through the tracheal lining, and both mainstem bronchi were narrow with a shortened trachea

(Schulman et al. 1993). The patient who survived with this condition had chronic pulmonary disease due to chronic airflow obstruction. This patient wheezed and required supplemental oxygen and bronchodilators (Schulman et al. 1993). For a subset of Jarcho–Levin syndrome patients, the outcome appears to be less grim. Importantly, mental retardation is not a component of this condition. Herold et al. (1988) described 10 cases of Jarcho–Levin syndrome, 8 of whom survived well into childhood and adolescence. One of the patients described in this report included a 14-year-old who had no respiratory problems and had good compensatory movement in the hip joints despite marked restriction of the lumbar spine and rigidity of the cervical spine. This patient could bend and touch the floor without bending her knees. She was as active as other children with the exception of having back pain. In this report the 8 long-term survivors with the milder phenotype had a disease that was transmitted as an autosomal recessive disorder. Typically, the spinal abnormalities in these patients included a mild kyphosis and scoliosis for which no treatment was indicated because the curve of the scoliosis was not severe. The hemivertebrae in these patients appeared to compensate for each other. The opinion of the author of this report was that restriction of spinal mobility was inherent to the syndrome and not amenable to surgical treatment. The report of another long-term survivor, an 11-year-old Puerto Rican, was described in great detail in 1994 (McCall et al. 1994). This patient had the classic phenotype of Jarcho–Levin syndrome (Fig. 97-5). By 11 years of age his height was less than 3 SD below the mean. This equaled a height age of 8 years at a chronologic age of 11 years. His weight was between the 5th and 25th percentile for age

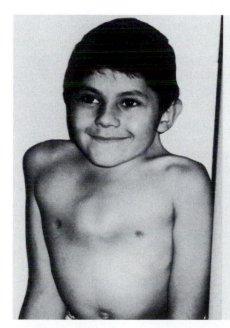 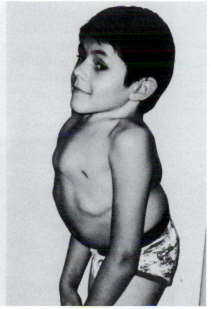

Figure 97-5. Same patient as in Figure 97-4, at age 7 years 8 months, demonstrating marked thoracic and neck shortness with severe pectus carinatum deformity. *(Reprinted, with permission, from McCall CP, Hudgins L, Cloutier M, et al. Jarcho-Levin syndrome: unusual survival in a classical case. Am J Med Genet 1994;49: 328–332.)*

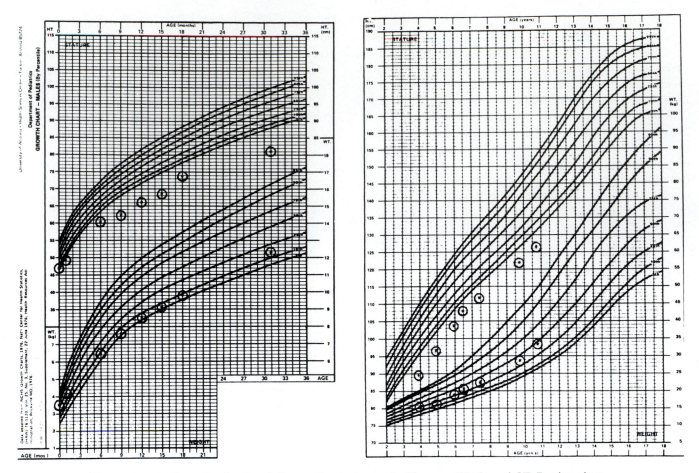

Figure 97-6. Growth charts of the patient shown in Figures 97-4 and 97-5, showing heights and weights from birth to age 10 years 9 months. *(Reprinted, with permission, from McCall CP, Hudgins L, Cloutier M, et al. Jarcho-Levin syndrome: unusual survival in a classical case. Am J Med Genet 1994;49:328–332.)*

(Fig. 97-6). His overall health was good, with the exception of recurrent otitis media in childhood and pneumonia at 5 months of age and then again at 3 years 6 months. This individual had normal development and hearing and was attending a regular fifth-grade class. He was extremely active in sports and was limited only by pulmonary function. His physical examination at age 11 showed an extremely short neck with low hairline and limited neck movement. His arms were long in relation to his body. He had a pectus carinatum deformity and an increased anteroposterior diameter of his chest (see Fig. 97-5). He had a dorsal kyphoscoliosis and a lumbar lordosis with a prominent abdomen. His face was normal and he had no other anomalies. Pulmonary function testing at age 11 years revealed a moderately severe restrictive pulmonary disease, with a decreased forced vital capacity and decreased forced expiratory volume. Although his pulmonary function tests are slightly worsening with time, these authors felt that for an individual diagnosed with Jarcho–Levin syndrome, the prognosis was less pessimistic than previously thought (McCall et al. 1994).

▶ GENETICS AND RECURRENCE RISK

The genetics of Jarcho–Levin syndrome are somewhat confused in the medical literature because of the different criteria used to establish the diagnosis. The clinical findings in 42 published patients were separated into three clusters based on their physical findings. The patients were grouped into the severely affected, recessively inherited patients with Jarcho–Levin syndrome, the more mildly affected patients with autosomal recessive or autosomal dominant disorders, and the patients who appeared to have the segmentation defects (Ayme and Preus 1986). In another study, 172 cases of spondylocostal dysostosis were reviewed for their patterns of inheritance. Of these, 78 appeared to be inherited as recessive disorders, 20 were dominantly inherited disorders, and 78 were new mutations in the family. The difficulty with this paper was that the spondylocostal dysostosis cases included cases of typical Jarcho–Levin syndrome with others.

There is good evidence for autosomal recessive inheritance of the classic phenotype of Jarcho–Levin syndrome. First of all, there is an increased incidence of consanguinity in affected cases (Herold et al. 1988). In a review of 21 patients with Jarcho–Levin syndrome of Puerto Rican or Hispanic ancestry, 43% had evidence of either consanguinity or more than one affected case in the family with normal parents.

Parents of a fetus or infant identified with features that are likely to represent Jarcho–Levin syndrome should meet with a genetic counselor to have a complete three generation family history taken. Once a clinical diagnosis is established for the fetus or infant, genetic counseling is indicated to discuss recurrence risk. If autosomal recessive inheritance appears likely, the recurrence risk is 25%. To date, the gene responsible for most classic cases of Jarcho–Levin syndrome has not been identified. Prenatal diagnosis in subsequent pregnancies is by second trimester sonographic examination.

REFERENCES

Apuzzio JJ, Diamond N, Ganesh V, et al. Difficulties in the prenatal diagnosis of Jarcho-Levin syndrome. Am J Obstet Gynecol 1987;156:916–918.

Ayme S, Preus M. Spondylocostal/spondylothoracic dysostosis: the clinical basis for prognosticating and genetic counseling. Am J Med Genet 1986;24:599–606.

Cantu JM, Urrusti J, Rosales G, et al. Evidence for autosomal recessive inheritance of costovertebral dysplasia. Clin Genet 1971;2:149–154.

Eliyahu S, Weiner E, Lahav D, Shalev E. Early sonographic diagnosis of Jarcho–Levin syndrome: a prospective screening program in one family. Ultrasound Obstet Gynecol 1997;9:314–318.

Giacoia GP, Say B. Spondylocostal dysplasia and neural tube defects. J Med Genet 1991;28:51–53.

Herold HZ, Edlitz M, Baruchin A. Spondylothoracic dysplasia. Spine 1988;13:478–481.

Jarcho S, Levin PM. Hereditary malformation of the vertebral bodies. Bull John Hopkins Hosp 1938;62:216–226.

Karnes PS, Day D, Berry SA, et al. Jarcho-Levin syndrome: four new cases and classification of subtypes. Am J Med Genet 1991;40:264–270.

Lawson ME, Share J, Benacerraf B, Krauss CM. Jarcho–Levin syndrome: prenatal diagnosis, prenatal care, and follow-up of siblings. J Perinatol 1997;17:407–409.

Marks F, Hernanz-Schulman M, Horii S, et al. Spondylothoracic dysplasia. J Ultrasound Med 1989;8:1–5.

McCall CP, Hudgins L, Cloutier M, et al. Jarcho-Levin syndrome: unusual survival in a classical case. Am J Med Genet 1994;49:328–332.

Miskin M, Baim RS, Allen LC, et al. Ultrasonic assessment of the fetal spine before 20 weeks' gestation. Radiology 1979;132:131–135.

Perez-Comas A, Garcia-Castro JM. Occipito-facial-cervico-thoracic-abdomino-digital dysplasia: Jarcho-Levin syndrome of vertebral anomalies: report of six cases and review of the literature. J Pediatr 1974;85:388–391.

Poor MA, Alberti O Jr, Griscom NT, et al. Nonskeletal malformations in one of three siblings with Jarcho-Levin syndrome of vertebral anomalies. J Pediatr 1983;103:270–272.

Roberts AP, Conner AN, Tolmie JL, et al. Spondylothoracic and spondylocostal dysostosis. J Bone Joint Surg Am 1988;70:123–126.

Romeo MG, Distenfano G, DiBella D, et al. Familial Jarcho-Levin syndrome. Clin Genet 1991;39:253–259.

Romero R, Ghidini A, Eswara MS, et al. Prenatal findings in a case of spondylocostal dysplasia type I (Jarcho-Levin syndrome). Obstet Gynecol 1988;71:988–991.

Schulman M, Gonzales MT, Bye MR. Airway abnormalities in Jarcho-Levin syndrome: a report of two cases. J Med Genet 1993;30:875–876.

Solomon L, Jimenez RB, Reiner L. Spondylothoracic dysostosis. Arch Pathol Lab Med 1978;102:201–205.

Tolmie JL, Whittle MJ, McNay MB, et al. Second trimester prenatal diagnosis of the Jarcho-Levin syndrome. Prenat Diagn 1987;7:129–134.

Wadia RS, Shirole DB, Dikshit MS. Recessively inherited costovertebral segmentation defect with mesomelia and peculiar facies (Covesdem syndrome). J Med Genet 1978;15:123–127.

CHAPTER 98
Osteogenesis Imperfecta

► CONDITION

Osteogenesis imperfecta is a clinically and genetically heterogeneous disorder of connective tissue, manifested by fragile, brittle, and osteoporotic bones. Affected patients have blue sclerae, hearing abnormalities, defective dentition, hyperlaxity of the joints, and normal intelligence (Brons et al. 1988). The majority of affected individuals are heterozygous for mutations of the *COL1A1* or *COL1A2* gene, which alters the structure of type I procollagen (Cole and Dalgleish 1995).

Osteogenesis imperfecta consists of at least four clinically distinct disorders that were first delineated by Sillence et al. (1979) (Table 98-1). Type I is the common mild form, type II is the perinatal lethal form, type III is the severe form, and type IV is the moderately clinically severe form (Cole and Dalgleish 1995).

Type I is a form of dominantly inherited osteoporosis that leads to fractures. Affected patients have distinctly blue sclerae and between 35 and 50% have presenile conductive hearing loss or deafness. The earliest age of onset of this hearing loss is 10 years, and 40% of affected adults eventually require hearing aids. Approximately one fifth of patients with type I osteogenesis imperfecta (OI) have kyphosis and scoliosis, although severe spinal curves are rarely seen. These patients also bruise easily. All patients with type I OI are able to walk independently. Type I is further subdivided into type IA, patients with normal teeth, and type IB, patients who have dentinogenesis imperfecta. Only 10% of patients with type I OI have fractures that are identifiable at birth (Sillence 1981). Patients affected with type I OI have a progressive loss of height due to platyspondyly and kyphosis. Birth weight and length are generally normal and short stature is of postnatal onset. These patients are also notable for a head size that appears large for height.

Patients with type II OI comprise the majority of cases prenatally detected and newborns with fractures. Most patients have blue sclerae that are noted at autopsy. Type II, the perinatal lethal form, has been further subdivided into types IIA, IIB, and IIC. In type IIA broad, crumpled femurs and continuous beading of the ribs are present. In addition, the patients are small for gestational age and have severe osteoporosis of the skull and face. In type IIB, there are minimal or no rib fractures present. Type IIB is the only form with potential postnatal survival. Because the ribs are less severely affected, the chest configuration is more normal and the resulting respiratory distress is less severe. In type IIC there are thin femurs and ribs with extensive fractures. In this form, the babies are very small for gestational age and severe osteopenia is present. However, many investigators state that distinction between the subgroups of type II is of limited value because all type II fetuses and infants die during the perinatal period.

Type III is a rare form of OI, characterized by marked bony fragility and fractures of the long bones and skull, which are sometimes present at birth (Sillence et al. 1986). In utero, the defect in ossification of the skull is not as marked as it is in Type II. Posnatally, there are spine and long bone fractures, which result in progressive short stature and kyphoscoliosis. Although blue sclerae are present at birth, they fade with time. Hearing impairment is rare in type III OI. Affected patients have a triangle-shaped face with a wide bitemporal diameter. These patients are among the smallest of adults with OI. They have considerable difficulty walking. They suffer from multiple pulmonary complications and die at an early age.

Type IV is a dominantly inherited form of osteoporosis that leads to fractures. Variable deformity of the long bones exists but affected patients have normal sclerae. There are no hearing abnormalites associated

▶ **TABLE 98-1.** OSTEOGENESIS IMPERFECTA: CLINICAL HETEROGENEITY AND BIOCHEMICAL DEFECTS

OI Type	Clinical Features	Inheritance Pattern	Biochemical Defects
I	Normal stature, little or no deformity; blue sclerae; hearing loss in about 50% of individuals; dentinogenesis imperfecta is rare and may distinguish a subset.	Autosomal dominant	Decreased production of type I procollagen
II	Lethal during the perinatal period, minimal calvarial mineralization, beaded ribs; compressed femurs; marked long bone deformity; platyspondyly.	Autosomal dominant (new)	Rearrangements in the *COLA1* and *COL1A2* genes Substitutions for glycine residues in the triple-helical domain of the $\alpha_1(I)$-chain
		Autosomal recessive (rare)	Small deletion in $\alpha_2(I)$-chain on the background of a null allele
III	Progressive deformation of bones, usually with moderate deformity at birth; sclerae variable in hue, but often lighten with age; dentinogenesis common, hearing loss common; very short stature.	Autosomal recessive	Frame-shift mutation that prevents incorporation of pro$\alpha_2(I)$ into molecules
		Autosomal dominant	Noncollagen defects Point mutations in the $\alpha_1(I)$- or $\alpha_2(I)$-chain
IV	Normal sclerae; mild to moderate bone deformity; variable short stature; dentinogenesis is common and hearing loss occurs in some.	Autosomal dominant	Point mutations in the $\alpha_2(I)$-chain Rarely, point mutations in the $\alpha_2(I)$-chain Small deletions in the $\alpha_2(I)$-chain

Source: Byers P.H. Osteogenesis imperfecta: an update. Growth Genet Horm 1988;14:1–5.

with type IV OI. Type IV has been further subdivided into IVA and IVB. In type IVA there is normal dentition and in IVB there is dentinogenesis imperfecta.

▶ INCIDENCE

The incidence of type I OI is 1 in 28,500 live births, of type II 1 in 62,000 live births; and of type III 1 in 68,800 live births (Sillence et al. 1979). In Sillence et al.'s original article, they did not quote an incidence for type IV OI. More recently, Rasmussen et al. (1996) identifed 16 cases of OI among 126,316 deliveries that occurred over a 15-year period in a single teaching hospital. These authors estimated a prevalence (with exclusion of high-risk patients) of 0.24 in 10,000 deliveries of type II OI and 0.4 in 10,000 of types II and III OI combined. OI has been described in all ethnic groups (Sykes et al. 1986).

In a review article, Sharony et al. (1993) described the accuracy of prenatal diagnosis in 226 fetuses and stillbirths referred for a suspected skeletal dysplasia. The most common final diagnosis in their series was OI, which was seen in 16% of cases.

▶ SONOGRAPHIC FINDINGS

The characteristic antenatal findings of OI include in utero fractures that occur with callus formation at the

site of healing. These result in prenatally acquired long-bone deformities and significant limb shortening (Fig. 98-1). Abnormalities of the fetal skull are the most striking findings in OI (Constantine et al. 1991). In addition, soft and fractured ribs contribute to a small thoracic subconference, which has been described as having a "champagne cork" appearance. The unusual clarity of intracranial structures is due to poor calvarial ossification (Fig. 98-2). This has led to the term *supervisualization* (Andrews and Amparo 1993). The compression of the fetal head by the ultrasound probe and the low echogenicity of the cranium should raise the suspicion of a skull dysplasia. However, this finding is not diagnostic for OI (Berge et al. 1995).

The following sonographic criteria have been proposed for type II OI: multiple fractures, demineralization of the calvarium, and a femoral length less than 3SD below the mean for gestational age, coupled with a wrinkled appearance of the long bones (Munoz et al. 1990).

In the absence of a known family history of OI, most fetuses detected prenatally will have type II. The major diagnostic criteria for this type of OI include shortened deformed long bones, underossification of the cranial vault, which results in easily seen intracranial structures, an abnormal and varying skull shape, a small chest circumference with broad and irregular ribs (Fig. 98-3), decreased fetal movements, and unusual fetal limb position (Constantine et al. 1991). In one case report, Morin et al. (1991) described a case of type IIA

with nor:
complete
develope
mileston
tion and
authors l
selves fr
pared the
a functio
ding. Th
tramedull
the age
ment in
considere
able to s
of achiev
ommend
ding shot
age to p
bert et al

▶ **LON**

Type I C
main pre:
patient at
may resu
predispos
who have
dentin. T
chips and
mal in ap
increased
may deve
OI. This i
being par
Patiei
incidence
ciuria is a
ity of the
renal son
et al. 199
Pater:
for 743 pa
natal leth
patient pc
77 with ty
and 70 wi
difference
Types IB,
pectancy a
patients w
life expect
19 occurre

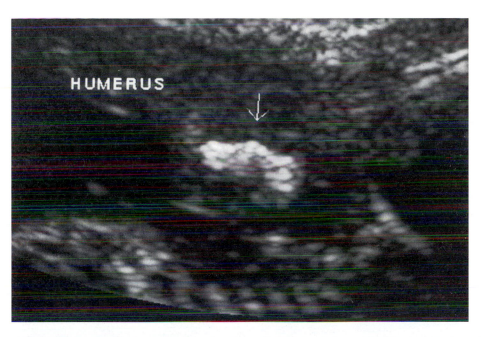

Figure 98-1. Sonographic image of a shortened and acutely angled humerus in a fetus with type II OI. Arrow indicates the site of fracture and callus formation.

OI in one of dizygotic twins diagnosed at 27 weeks of gestation. In this report, the affected fetus was so translucent that only one twin could be seen on a plain radiograph. In another case report, D'Ottavio et al. (1993) described a case of type II OI in the fetus of a woman at 14 weeks of gestation who underwent routine transvaginal ultrasonography. In this fetus, both femurs were short and severely angulated because of fractures. Even at this early point in gestation, the fetal skull was noted to be hypoechogenic, and an abnormal curvature of the right radius was present.

Prenatal diagnosis of OI types I and III is more difficult to make on a sonographic basis. Most of the cases described in the literature have been diagnosed in fetuses known to be at risk because of a positive family history. For example, Robinson et al. (1987) described a fetus at risk for type III OI who was followed with serial sonography. At 15 weeks of gestation, there was

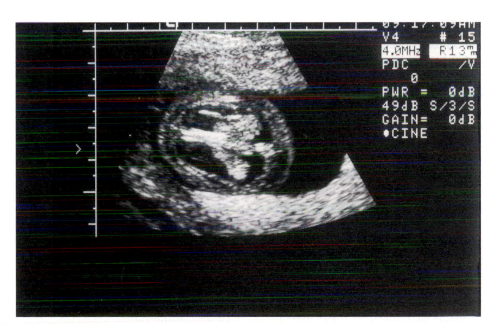

Figure 98-2. Cross-sectional view of a fetal head demonstrating significantly reduced skull ossification, resulting in unusually clear visualization of intracranial contents.

although heterozygous achondroplasia is clinically less severe than TD. It is of interest that patients with homozygous achondroplasia manifest a more severe clinical phenotype than patients with heterozygous achondroplasia. The features in homozygous achondroplasia clearly resemble TD and result in neonatal lethality (Tavormina et al. 1995).

▶ INCIDENCE

The incidence of thanatophoric dysplasia ranges from 0.27 in 10,000 to 0.4 in 10,000 live births (Martínez-Frías et al. 1988; Rasmussen et al. 1996). In a large series of 126,000 deliveries occurring at one institution, thanatophoric dysplasia was the most common osteochondrodysplasia observed (Rasmussen et al. 1996).

In individuals affected with thanatophoric dysplasia, the mean paternal age is elevated as compared with unaffected controls (Martínez-Frías et al. 1988; Orioli et al. 1995). In 50% of cases of thanatophoric dysplasia, the father is >35 years of age (Orioli et al. 1995). There is approximately a threefold increased risk for having a fetus with thanatophoric dysplasia when the father is between the ages of 35 and 39 (Martínez-Frías et al. 1988).

To date, most cases of thanatophoric dysplasia have occurred sporadically. The small number of familial cases reported reveal a paucity of well-documented sibling pairs, except in the case of monozygous twins. There is no evidence for parental consanguinity in affected fetuses (Martínez-Frías et al. 1988).

▶ SONOGRAPHIC FINDINGS

The sonographic findings in cases affected by thanatophoric dysplasia include severe micromelia with limited limb mobility. Although the femur is classically described as curved and resembling a telephone receiver (Fig. 100-2), affected fetuses can also have straight femurs. Additional sonographic findings include short, broad ribs, a narrowed chest circumference with consequent pulmonary hypoplasia, and hypoplastic vertebral bodies. The pelvic bones are characteristically small. Polyhydramnios is frequently present (Burrows et al. 1984; Stamm et al. 1987). In one report, an associated cardiac abnormality consisting of an atrioseptal defect and a bicuspid aortic valve was also described (Isaacson et al. 1983).

The *kleeblattschädel* (cloverleaf) deformity was first described in 1960 (Holtermüller and Wiedemann 1960). This cloverleaf shape of the skull is due to early fusion of the lambdoidal and coronal sutures. This results in a towering calvarium and lateral bulges of the temporal lobes, which form three leaves of the cloverleaf

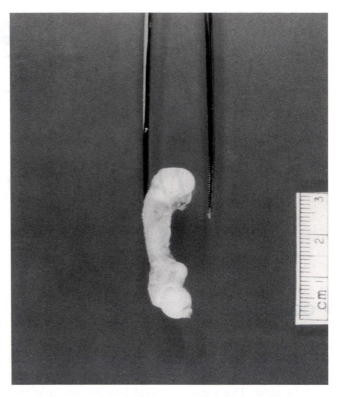

Figure 100-2. Postmortem photograph of an isolated femur from a fetus with thanatophoric dysplasia at 21 weeks of gestation, demonstrating its resemblance to a telephone receiver. *(Courtesy of Dr. Joseph Semple.)*

when the head is viewed from the face (Fig. 100-3). Because the lambdoidal and coronal sutures are fused, subsequent brain growth results in bulging in the regions of least resistance (Isaacson et al. 1983). The cloverleaf skull is present in only 14% of cases of thanatophoric dysplasia (Iannaccone and Gerlini 1974). Hydrocephalus is frequently associated with the cloverleaf skull (Issacson et al. 1983; Shaff et al. 1980). To diagnose the cloverleaf skull deformity, a coronal scan that shows the temporal lobes is recommended (Stamm et al. 1987).

In the literature, multiple reports exist of the second-trimester diagnosis of thanatophoric dysplasia on the basis of the severe micromelia (Camera et al. 1984; de Elejalde and de Elejalde 1985; Loong 1987; Meizner et al. 1990; Schild et al. 1996). These reports all describe fetuses with a long-bone length of less than the third percentile for gestational age, an extremely narrow chest, a protruberant abdomen, and vertebral bodies of reduced height. First-trimester diagnosis has also been reported (Benacerraf et al. 1988). Benacerraf and colleagues described a 13-week-old fetus with a narrow chest and foreshortened and bowed femurs. A repeat sonographic examination performed at 15 weeks again demonstrated the abnormalities. The pregnancy was

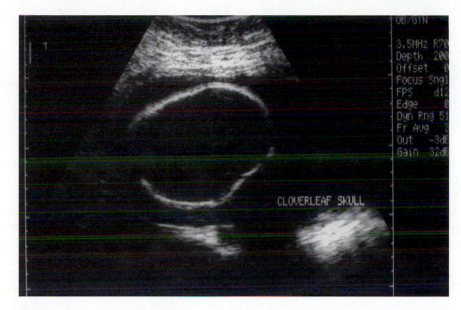

Figure 100-3. Antenatal sonogram demonstrating cloverleaf skull. (*Courtesy of Dr. Marjorie C. Treadwell.*)

electively terminated. In contrast, another group has described a fetus that appeared normal at 15 weeks of gestation and was subsequently diagnosed at 32 weeks of gestation with thanatophoric dysplasia (Macken et al. 1991).

▶ DIFFERENTIAL DIAGNOSIS

The differential diagnosis includes other skeletal dysplasias that manifest as severe micromelia, such as campomelic dysplasia (see Chapter 91), Ellis van–Creveld syndrome (see Chapter 94), and short-rib-polydactyly syndrome (see Chapter 99). Polydactyly is absent in thanatophoric dysplasia. In achondrogenesis, the bones are usually less mineralized than in thanatophoric dysplasia.

The cloverleaf skull is occasionally mistaken for an encephalocele (Chervenak et al. 1983; Mahony et al. 1985; Stamm et al. 1987; Weiner et al. 1986). Any soft-tissue bulge in the head or neck must be evaluated for its exact position. Encephalocele and cystic hygroma occur in the midline and most often are posterior. The cloverleaf skull is bilateral, with enlargement of the temporal lobes. The standard teaching that the skull is not intact in encephalocele is not helpful to distinguish between encephalocele and cloverleaf skull. This is because the bony calvarium may be expanded, thinned, or partially absent in the cloverleaf skull deformity, and conversely, in cases of encephalocele, the osseous defect in the skull may be very small (Stamm et al. 1987). A cloverleaf skull may also be noted in Apert, Carpenter, Crouzon, and Pfeiffer syndromes as well as in homozygous achondroplasia.

▶ ANTENATAL NATURAL HISTORY

The underlying defect in thanatophoric dysplasia is in the formation of bone from a cartilage model. There is generalized disruption and decrease in endochondral ossification, with membranous ossification being less affected (Lemyre et al. 1999). Fetuses affected with thanatophoric dysplasia show a progressive decrease in the growth rate of the long bones throughout gestation. While sometimes early in the second trimester the femur length can be in the normal range, the bones become progressively shortened and curved (Burrows et al. 1984).

The histologic abnormalities in thanatophoric dysplasia include the presence of abnormal mineralizing tissue at the growth plate. In the region normally occupied by growth-plate cartilage, cells and matrix have morphologic characteristics of epiphyseal cartilage, and the chondrocytes are not organized into columns or clusters. In addition, there are pyramidal areas of cartilage that resemble a shortened but normal growth plate, but the most characteristic finding is tufts of fibrous tissue scattered randomly along the growth plate. These have been termed "ossification tufts" (Horton et al. 1988). It is unclear whether these ossification tufts represent a primary phenomenon that disrupts endochondral bone growth or a secondary response to defective endochondral ossification. Marked abnormalities in endochondral and perichondral bone structures have been demonstrated by xeroradiography in a 20-week-old fetus (de Elejalde and de Elejalde 1985).

Increasing evidence exists that the brain is seriously involved in patients affected with thanatophoric dysplasia.

This is not surprising given that *FGFR3* expression is very high in the developing central nervous system (Tavormina et al. 1995). In a neuropathologic study of seven affected individuals, Wongmongkolrit and colleagues (1983) reported that all brains in thanatophoric dysplasia patients were larger than normal and demonstrated maldevelopment of the temporal lobes, characterized by extensive gyration and deep sulcation. The predominant findings were megencephaly, abnormal gyration, polymicrogyria in the temporal cortex, lateral displacement of the basal ganglia, reduced fiber tracts, and dysplasia of several nuclei. Ventricular dilation was present without evidence of obstruction. The most characteristic abnormality was the malformation of the temporal lobe with a pattern of disorganization that was distinctly different from any other condition. These investigators hypothesized that there was a relative vascular hypoperfusion of the developing temporal lobe, which resulted in polymicrogyria. In some cases, partial agenesis of the corpus callosum was also observed.

▶ MANAGEMENT OF PREGNANCY

If it is suspected that a pregnant woman is carrying a fetus with a severe skeletal dysplasia such as thanatophoric dysplasia, she should be evaluated at a center capable of performing a detailed fetal anatomic scan. Specific attention should be paid to measurement of the long bones and the chest circumference, as well as noting the presence or absence of polyhydramnios. There is no indication for a fetal karyotype, as in most cases the chromosomes are normal in thanatophoric dysplasia. However, an amniocentesis should be performed to obtain amniotic fluid cells for DNA analysis of *FGFR3*, which will provide a definitive diagnosis (Sawai et al. 1999). In addition, amniotic fluid α-fetoprotein and cholinesterase are also normal (de Elejalde and de Elejalde 1985). If the diagnosis is made prior to 24 weeks of gestation, the parents should be counseled regarding the extremely poor prognosis and be given the opportunity to terminate the pregnancy. Pregnancies with fetuses with thanatophoric dysplasia are frequently complicated by polyhydramnios, prematurity, malpresentation, and cephalopelvic disproportion. The presence of the cloverleaf deformity and hydrocephalus may necessitate cephalocentesis and assisted delivery. Vaginal breech deliveries are sometimes complicated by an extended short and rigid neck that may hinder the passage of the fetal head (Loong 1987). A cesarean section may sometimes be necessary to safely deliver the fetus, although it will not alter the otherwise grim prognosis for fetal survival (Wongmongkolrit et al. 1983).

▶ FETAL INTERVENTION

There are no fetal interventions for thanatophoric dysplasia.

▶ TREATMENT OF THE NEWBORN

Infants affected with thanatophoric dysplasia uniformly experience respiratory distress at birth. Potential explanations for the respiratory distress include the narrow chest with associated pulmonary hypoplasia, abnormalities of the bronchial cartilage, compression of brainstem respiratory centers, and altered pulmonary phospholipids (Issacson et al. 1983). If the diagnosis is known from antenatal studies, the parents may have the opportunity to request that no newborn resuscitation occurs.

Infants who are delivered with a severe skeletal dysplasia but without antenatal knowledge of the diagnosis may initially require resuscitation until a precise diagnosis can be made. A complete physical examination of the newborn is indicated, which will demonstrate the presence of a bulging forehead, prominent eyes, flattened nasal bridge, narrow chest, and severely shortened extremities (Fig. 100-4). Radiographs should be obtained, which will show the severe micromelia and femurs possibly shaped like telephone receivers (Fig. 100-5). The chest radiograph will also indicate the presence of short ribs, flat vertebral bodies that are H-shaped in the frontal projection, widened intervertebral disk spaces (Fig. 100-6), a short pelvis with a small sacroiliac notch, and a possible cloverleaf skull deformity (Fig. 100-7) (Andersen 1989). The most important differential radiologic features include the markedly flattened vertebral bodies with widened intervetebral spaces, the shortened bowed extremities, and the irregularly flared metaphyses (Campbell 1971).

Once the diagnosis of thanatophoric dysplasia has been confirmed, respiratory support may be electively withdrawn, given the nearly uniform neonatal lethality and poor outcome for the rare long-term survivors with this condition (MacDonald et al. 1989). Autopsy is indicated, and DNA mutation studies of the *FGFR3* gene should be performed to confirm the diagnosis.

▶ SURGICAL TREATMENT

Information exists on surgical treatment only for the extremely limited number of affected patients who survived past infancy. Affected infants eventually require tracheostomy for prolonged ventilatory support (see Fig. 100-4), ventriculoperitoneal shunt for hydrocephalus, and foramen magnum decompression (MacDonald et al. 1989).

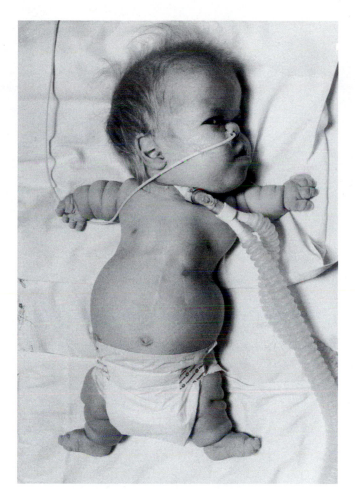

Figure 100-4. A long-term survivor with thanatophoric dysplasia. Note the placement of a tracheostomy tube. *(Reprinted, with permission, from MacDonald IM, Hunter AGW, MacLeod PM, MacMurray SB. Growth and development in thanatophoric dysplasia. Am J Med Genet 1989;33:508–512. Copyright 1989 Wiley-Liss. Reprinted, by permission, of Wiley-Liss, Inc., a subsidiary of John Wiley & Sons, Inc.)*

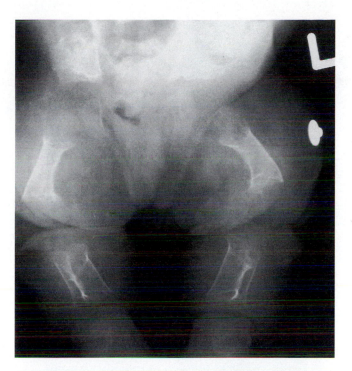

Figure 100-5. Postnatal radiograph of an affected infant demonstrating short tubular bones, metaphyseal widening, and spurs. *(Reprinted, with permission, from MacDonald IM, Hunter AGW, MacLeod PM, MacMurray SB. Growth and development in thanatophoric dysplasia. Am J Med Genet 1989;33:508–512. Copyright 1989 Wiley-Liss. Reprinted, by permission, of Wiley-Liss, Inc., a subsidiary of John Wiley & Sons, Inc.)*

▶ LONG-TERM OUTCOME

Several case reports discuss the longer survival of affected infants with thanatophoric dysplasia due to modern neonatal care (MacDonald et al. 1989; Stensvold and Hovland 1986; Tonoki 1987). In one report, a female with thanatophoric dysplasia who survived for 169 days was described. Her long-term course was complicated by hypotonic muscles and absent reflexes. Increasing hydrocephalus developed. Eventually she required supplemental oxygen but died from respiratory failure (Stensvold and Hovland 1986). In another case report, a male was described who survived for 212 days. His delivery was by cesarean section and complicated by severe birth asphyxia. He required oxygen supplementation but was discharged from the hospital at 35

days of age. At 4 months of age respiratory and cardiac failure developed and he required mechanical ventilation. His neurologic development was normal until 4 months of age, when frequent apnea and cyanosis developed, which was questionably due to cord compression and a small foramen magnum. He eventually died from respiratory failure secondary to pneumonia (Tonoki 1987).

The most informative reports come from two cases of prolonged survival with thanatophoric dysplasia. In both cases, ventilatory support was initiated due to respiratory distress of the newborn. Both patients eventually required ventriculoperitoneal shunts for hydrocephalus as well as decompression of the posterior fossa (MacDonald et al. 1989). The first patient survived to 5.2 years of age and was dependent on the ventilator. At age 4.75 years, development was estimated to be at the 2-week age level. At age 4.75 years, the patient weighed 8.82 kg (<3% for age), was 65 cm long (<3% for age), and had a head circumference of 47.5 cm (<3% for age) (Fig. 100-8). By 10 months of age, growth of the long bones ceased. The femurs maintained their telephone-receiver appearance. An electroencephalogram in this patient initially revealed epileptiform activity,

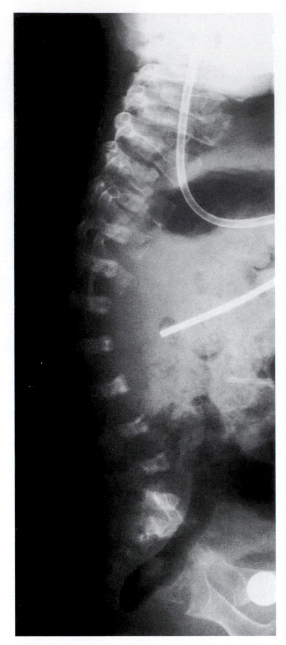

Figure 100-6. Spinal radiograph of an affected patient at 1.5 years of age, showing progressive lack of caudal ossification. *(Reprinted, with permission, from MacDonald IM, Hunter AGW, MacLeod PM, MacMurray SB. Growth and development in thanatophoric dysplasia. Am J Med Genet 1989;33:508–512. Copyright 1989 Wiley-Liss. Reprinted, by permission, of Wiley-Liss, Inc., a subsidiary of John Wiley & Sons, Inc.)*

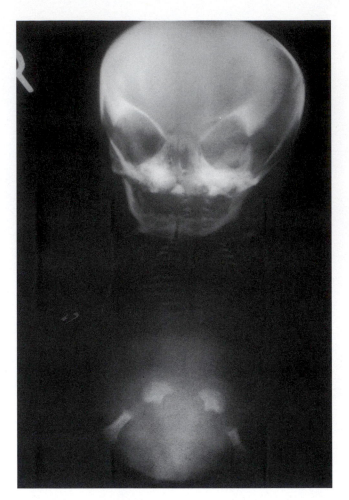

Figure 100-7. Postnatal skull radiograph of same fetus shown in Figure 100-3. *(Courtesy of Dr. Marjorie Treadwell.)*

There was a clinical question of brain-stem compression, so a posterior fossa decompression with laminectomy of the atlas and removal of the posterior third of bone around the foramen magnum occurred. At 4 months of age, the patient again required ventilatory support and a tracheostomy. Progressive hydrocephalus developed and a ventriculoperitoneal shunt was placed. At 3.7 years of age, the child could see and track objects, but had limited verbalization. After the placement of the ventriculoperitoneal shunt, the head circumference was <3% for age. This patient also manifested a prolonged period of nearly absent growth despite adequate nutrition.

On the basis of these two cases, these authors recommended that their long-term clinical experience with these two affected patients would "temper" their approach in the future (MacDonald et al. 1989).

followed later by background disturbance. The computed tomographic scan revealed abnormal differentiation of gray and white matter in both hemispheres.

The second affected patient initially required 40% inspired oxygen and did not need mechanical ventilation. At 2 months of age, however, a respiratory infection developed and intubation and ventilation were performed.

▶ GENETICS AND RECURRENCE RISK

Thanatophoric dysplasia is inherited as an autosomal dominant sporadic mutation with an extremely low risk

Growth and Development in Thanatophoric Dysplasia

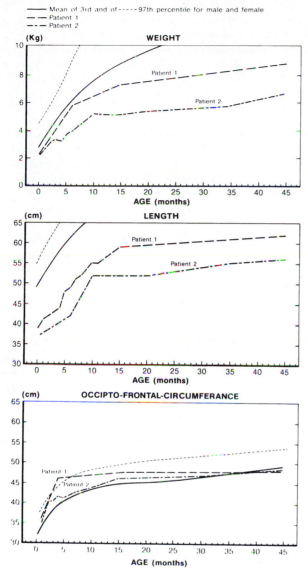

Figure 100-8. Growth curves of the two reported long-term survivors with thanatophoric dysplasia. *(Reprinted, with permission, from MacDonald IM, Hunter AGW, MacLeod PM, MacMurray SB. Growth and development in thanatophoric dysplasia. Am J Med Genet 1989;33:508–512. Copyright 1989 Wiley-Liss. Reprinted, by permission, of Wiley-Liss, Inc., a subsidiary of John Wiley & Sons, Inc.)*

gricans (SADDAN) (Bellus et al. 1999; Lemyre et al. 1999).

Several reports of thanatophoric dysplasia have been described in monozygous twins (Corsello et al. 1992; Young et al. 1989). Monozygous twins have been described who are discordant for the cloverleaf skull deformity (Corsello et al. 1992; Horton et al. 1983).

It is now known that a genotype–phenotype correlation exists in thanatophoric dysplasia. The subtype TD I consists of curved femurs with the variable presence of the skull deformity. In 22 of 39 patients affected with TD I there is an arginine-to-cysteine amino acid change at position 248. This mutation was not found in 50 control patients. In TD II, a lysine-to-glutamine amino acid change at position 650 was demonstrated in the intracellular tyrosine kinase domain of *FGFR3* in 16 of 16 affected individuals who presented with straight femurs and a severe cloverleaf skull deformity (Tavormina et al. 1995). Nested polymerase chain reaction primers have been designed for the rapid diagnosis of mutations in this condition. The mutations causing TD I and II are sporadic, as they were not seen in the parents who were tested (Tavormina et al. 1995). Of interest is that the manifestations of the disease are not simply due to heterozygous deletion of *FGFR3*, because a chromosomal abnormality syndrome, Wolf–Hirschhorn (4p−), does not result in a skeletal dysplasia. Thus, haploinsufficiency of the *FGFR3* gene is not the cause of thanatophoric dysplasia.

Additional mutations have been documented in TD I. Rousseau et al. (1995) found three different base substitutions in the chain termination (stop codon) of the *FGFR3* gene in 5 of 15 TD I patients without a cloverleaf skull deformity. These mutations cause protein elongation, resulting in a highly hydrophobic domain with an α-helix structure at its C-terminal end. This possibly impairs signal transduction. In another report, 7 different sporadic mutations in three different protein domains have now been identified in 25 of 26 patients with TD I. No correlation exists between the position of the mutation and phenotypic or radiologic abnormalities. *FGFR3* mutations in the extracellular receptor create new unpaired cysteine residues (Bonaventure et al. 1996). Review of 91 cases from the International Skeletal Dysplasia registry at Cedars-Sinai Hospital in Los Angeles revealed that every case of thanatophoric dysplasia had an identifiable *FGFR3* mutation (Wilcox et al. 1998). All cases with the Lys560Glu substitution had straight femora with craniosynostosis and frequently, a cloverleaf skull. Cases with this molecular phenotype had better preservation of the growth plate. In all other types of mutations in *FGFR3*, the femora were curved (Wilcox et al. 1998).

Prenatal diagnosis is characteristically performed by sonography with occasional supplementation by radiography. For families who have had a previously affected

of recurrence (Young et al. 1989). The chromosomes in affected patients have been normal, although one case has been described with a probably unrelated de novo 1:10 balanced translocation (Hersh et al. 1995). The disease is caused by missense mutations in the *FGFR3* gene, which maps to chromosome 4 band (McKusick et al. 1996). In addition to thanatophoric dysplasia, three other diseases are due to mutations in *FGFR3* gene: achondroplasia, hypochondroplasia, and severe achondroplasia with developmental delay and acanthosis ni-

infant in which the mutation was identified, definitive prenatal diagnosis can be performed as early as 10 weeks by chorionic villus sampling.

Parents who have an affected fetus with thanatophoric dysplasia may find comfort in an article written by a parent whose son was born with thanatophoric dysplasia and survived for 3 months in a newborn intensive care unit (Stabosz 1985).

REFERENCES

Andersen PE Jr. Prevalence of lethal osteochondrodysplasias in Denmark. Am J Med Genet 1989;32:484–489.

Bellus GA, Bamshad MJ, Pryzlepa KA, et al. Severe achondroplasia with developmental delay and acanthosis nigricans (SADDAN): mutation in fibroblast growth factor receptor 3. Am J Med Genet 1999;85:53–65.

Benacerraf BR, Lister JE, DuPonte BL. First trimester diagnosis of fetal abnormalities: a report of three cases. J Reprod Med 1988;33:777–780.

Bonaventure J, Rousseau F, Legeai-Mallet L, Le Merrer M, Munnich A, Maroteaux P. Common mutations in the fibroblast growth factor receptor 3 (FGFR3) gene account for achondroplasia, hypochondroplasia, and thanatophoric dwarfism. Am J Med Genet 1996;63:148–154.

Burrows PE, Stannard MW, Pearrow J, Sutterfield S, Baker ML. Early antenatal sonographic recognition of thanatophoric dysplasia with cloverleaf skull deformity. AJR Am J Roentgenol 1984;143:841–843.

Camera G, Dodero D, De Pascale S. Prenatal diagnosis of thanatophoric dysplasia at 24 weeks. Am J Med Genet 1984;18:39–43.

Campbell RE. Thanatophoric dwarfism in utero: a case report. Am J Roentgenol Radium Ther Nucl Med 1971;112:198–200.

Chervenak FA, Blakemore KJ, Isaacson G, Mayden K, Hobbins JC. Antenatal sonographic findings of thanatophoric dysplasia with cloverleaf skull. Am J Obstet Gynecol 1983;8:984–985.

Corsello G, Maresi E, Rossi C, Giuffre L, Cittadini E. Thanatophoric dysplasia in monozygotic twins discordant for cloverleaf skull: prenatal diagnosis, clinical and pathological findings. Am J Med Genet 1992;42:122–126.

de Elejalde BR, de Elejalde MM. Thanatophoric dysplasia: fetal manifestations and prenatal diagnosis. Am J Med Genet 1985;22:669–683.

Hersh JH, Yen FF, Peiper SC, et al. De novo 1:10 balanced translocation in an infant with thanatophoric dysplasia: a clue to the locus of the candidate gene. J Med Genet 1995;32:293–295.

Holtermüller K, Wiedemann HR. Kleblattschädel syndrome. Munch Med Wochenschr 1960;14:439–446.

Horton WA, Harris DJ, Collins DL. Discordance for the Kleeblattschadel anomaly in monozygotic twins with thanatophoric dysplasia. Am J Med Genet 1983;15:97–101.

Horton WA, Hood OJ, Machado MA, Ahmed S, Griffey ES. Abnormal ossification in thanatophoric dysplasia. Bone 1988;9:53–61.

Iannaccone G, Gerlini G. The so-called "cloverleaf skull syndrome." Pediatr Radiol 1974;2:175–184.

Isaacson G, Blakemore KJ, Chervenak FA. Thanatophoric dysplasia with cloverleaf skull. Am J Dis Child 1983;137:896–898.

Lemyre E, Azouz EM, Teebi AS, Glanc P, Chen MF. Bone dysplasia series. Achondroplasia, hypochondroplasia and thanatophoric dysplasia: review and update. Can Assoc Radiol J 1999;50:185–197.

Loong EPL. The importance of early prenatal diagnosis of thanatophoric dysplasia with respect to obstetric management. Eur J Obstet Gynecol Reprod Biol 1987;25:145–152.

MacDonald IM, Hunter AGW, MacLeod PM, MacMurray SB. Growth and development in thanatophoric dysplasia. Am J Med Genet 1989;33:508–512.

Macken MB, Grantmyre EB, Rimoin DL, Lachman RS. Normal sonographic appearance of a thanatophoric dwarf variant fetus at 13 weeks gestation. AJR Am J Roentgenol 1991;156:149–150.

Mahony BS, Filly RA, Callen PW, Golbus MS. Thanatophoric dwarfism with the cloverleaf skull: a specific antenatal sonographic diagnosis. J Ultrasound Med 1985;4:151–154.

Maroteaux P, Lamy M, Robert JM. Thanatophoric dwarfism. Presse Med 1967;75:2519–2524.

Martínez-Frías ML, Ramos-Arroyo MA, Salvador J. Thanatophoric dysplasia: an autosomal dominant condition? Am J Med Genet 1988;31:815–820.

McKusick VA, Amberger JS, Francomano CA. Progress in medical genetics: map-based gene discovery and the molecular pathology of skeletal dysplasias. Am J Med Genet 1996;63:98–105.

Meizner I, Carmi R, Levy A, Simhon T. Early prenatal ultrasonic diagnosis of thanatophoric dwarfism. Isr J Med Sci 1990;26:287–289.

Orioli IM, Castilla EE, Scarano G, Mastroiacovo P. Effect of paternal age in achondroplasia, thanatophoric dysplasia, and osteogenesis imperfecta. Am J Med Genet 1995;59:209–217.

Rasmussen SA, Bieber FR, Benacerraf BR, Lachman RS, Rimoin DL, Holmes LB. Epidemiology of osteochondrodysplasias: changing trends due to advances in prenatal diagnosis. Am J Med Genet 1996;61:49–58.

Rousseau F, Saugier P, Le Merrer M, et al. Stop codon FGFR3 mutations in thanatophoric dwarfism type 1. Nat Genet 1995;10:11–12.

Sawai H, Komori S, Ida A, Henmi T, Bessho T, Koyama K. Prenatal diagnosis of thanatophoric dysplasia by mutational analysis of the fibroblast growth factor receptor 3 gene and a proposed correction of previously published PCR results. Prenat Diagn 1999;19:21–24.

Schild RL, Hunt GW, Moore J, Davies H, Horwell DH. Antenatal sonographic diagnosis of thanatophoric dysplasia: a report of three cases and a review of the literature with special emphasis on the differential diagnosis. Ultrasound Obstet Gynecol 1996;8:62–67.

Shaff MI, Fleischer AC, Battino R, Herbert C, Boehm FH. Antenatal sonographic diagnosis of thanatophoric dysplasia. J Clin Ultrasound 1980;8:363–365.

Stabosz RD. Thanatophoric dwarfism: a parent's point of view. Delaware Med J 1985;57:221–225.

Stamm ER, Pretorius DH, Rumack CM, Manco-Johnson ML. Kleeblattschadel anomaly: in utero sonographic appearance. J Ultrasound Med 1987;6:319–324.

Stensvold K, Ek J, Hovland AR. An infant with thanatophoric dwarfism surviving 169 days. Clin Genet 1986;29:157–159.

Tavormina PL, Shiang R, Thompson LM, et al. Thanatophoric dysplasia (types I and II) caused by distinct mutations in fibroblast growth factor receptor 3. Nat Genet 1995;9:321–328.

Tonoki H. A boy with thanatophoric dysplasia surviving 212 days. Clin Genet 1987;30:415–416.

Weiner CP, Williamson RA, Bonsib SM. Sonographic diagnosis of cloverleaf skull and thanatophoric dysplasia in the second trimester. J Clin Ultrasound 1986;14:463–465.

Wilcox WR, Tavormina PL, Krakow D, et al. Molecular, radiologic, and histopathologic correlations in thanatophoric dysplasia. Am J Med Genet 1998;78:274–281.

Wongmongkolrit T, Bush M, Roessmann U. Neuropathological findings in thanatophoric dysplasia. Arch Pathol Lab Med 1983;107:132–135.

Young ID, Patel I, Lamont AC. Thanatophoric dysplasia in identical twins. J Med Genet 1989;26:276–279.

SECTION J

Extremities

CHAPTER 101

Amniotic Band Syndrome

► CONDITION

The amniotic band syndrome (ABS) is a group of spo-radic congenital anomalies that involve the limbs, cra-niofacial regions and trunk, ranging from constrictive bands, pseudosyndactyly to amputation, as well as multiple craniofacial, visceral, and body-wall defects (Higginbottom et al. 1979; Jones et al. 1974; Kulkarni et al. 1990; Lockwood et al. 1989; Ray et al. 1988; Seeds et al. 1982; Seidman et al. 1989; Torpin 1965). The term *amniotic band syndrome* encompasses many congeni-tal anomalies, including amniotic band disruption com-plex (Higginbottom et al. 1979), amniochorionic meso-blastic fibrous strings (Torpin 1965), aberrant tissue bands (Jones et al. 1974), amniotic deformity, adhe-sions, and mutilations (ADAM) complex (Keller et al. 1978), amniotic adhesion malformation syndrome (Herva et al. 1984), and the limb and/or body wall de-fect (Bamforth 1992).

Several theories have been advanced to explain the occurrence of these anomalies, but two are most com-monly held. In 1930 Streeter proposed that a disruption in embryogenesis at the time of formation of the germ disk and the amniotic cavity initiated a chain of events leading to the multiple defects. He suggested that am-niotic bands were the result, not the cause, of the patho-logic process. In 1992 Bamforth reviewed this theory in a series of 54 cases of ABS and concluded that it may be caused by a localized disturbance in establishment of basic embryonic organization. The most widely ac-cepted theory was proposed by Torpin in 1965. He ex-amined the placenta and fetal membranes in a number of affected individuals and concluded that the disorder was caused by primary rupture of the amnion early in gestation (Herva et al. 1984; Higginbottom et al. 1979; Keller et al. 1978; Seeds et al. 1982).

More recently, Moerman et al. (1992) proposed that the ABS is a collection of three distinct entities that can reconcile the adherents of Streeter's and Torpin's hy-potheses. They suggested that ABS consists of three dis-tinct lesions: (1) constrictive tissue bands; (2) amniotic adhesions; and (3) the more complex pattern of anom-alies designated the limb–body-wall complex (LBWC) (see Chapter 59). In this report of the fetopathologic evaluation of 18 cases of ABS, 4 had clearly constric-tive bands, which formed as a result of the amnion rupture sequence. The bands that resulted from amnion rupture encircled the limbs, resulting in annular constrictions, secondary syndactyly, and intrauterine amputations. In addition, constriction of the umbilical cord is a recognized cause of fetal death (Hong et al. 1963; Torpin 1965). These authors distinguish cases caused by constrictive bands from those caused by broad amniotic adhesions. Moerman et al. suggested that adhesive amniotic bands were morphologically and pathogenetically different from constrictive bands. Adhesive amniotic bands are usually associated with severe defects such as encephalocele and facial clefts. This group demonstrated pathologically that cranioplacental adhesions are broad adhesions, with the fetal skin fused to the amnion at the margins of the cranial defect. They speculated that the amnion covering the placenta or membranes seals the cranial defect separating the protruding brain from the chorion. Van Allen et al. (1987) proposed that the amnion becomes adherent to the embryo in areas of ischemic necrosis following vascular disruption. In short, the amniotic adhesions are secondary to fetal defects.

Moerman et al. (1992) considered the LBWC to be due to both band-related and non–band-related defects. The band-related defects include limb defects such as club foot. Non–band-related defects occur as a result of vascular disruptions or from compression (Miller et al. 1981). The thoracoabdominoschisis of LBWC is characterized by an anterolateral body-wall defect with evisceration of abdominal and/or thoracic organs. The eviscerated organs are in an extraamniotic sac bounded by the chorionic plate, a persistent extraembryonic coelom. The amnion is continuous with the skin. The umbilical cord is extremely short, with umbilical vessels running in the amniotic sac, often with an absent umbilical artery. The severe scoliosis is a postural deformity caused by abnormal fixation of the fetus to the placenta. They also cite the high incidence of internal structural defects such as cardiac anomalies, unilateral absence of a kidney, or intestinal atresia, which do not fit with simple amnion rupture.

The fetal malformations that can occur as a result of ABS can be categorized into neural-tube–like defects, craniofacial anomalies, limb anomalies, and constrictive bands (Ho and Liu 1987; Lubinsky et al. 1983; Seeds et al. 1982; Seidman et al. 1989). The neural-tube–like defects include cases of anencephaly and encephalocele, which may be asymmetric or multiple. The craniofacial anomalies include facial clefts, nasal deformity, asymmetric microphthalmia, and abnormal cranial calcification. Limb anomalies may be multiple and asymmetric, including limb or digital amputation, pseudosyndactyly, abnormal dermatoglyphics, and some cases of clubbed feet. Abdominal-wall and thoracic-wall defects can occur and some cases are mistaken for gastroschisis or omphalocele with rupture.

The most puzzling component of the ABS is its association with visceral anomalies, including bladder exstrophy, vertebral hypoplasia, and other renal, gonadal, cardiac, and pulmonary defects (Bamforth 1992). Constrictive bands involving the extremities are the most common defect associated with the ABS (Huang et al. 1995).

The variation in manifestations of the ABS are thought to be due to differences in timing of amniotic rupture and the degree to which the fetus becomes entangled by strands of amnion (Higginbottom et al. 1979; Seeds et al. 1982). The effect the amniotic bands have on the developing fetus have been classified into malformation, disruption, and deformation (Higginbottom et al. 1979). Amniotic bands that interrupt the normal sequence of embryologic development lead to malformations such as cleft lip and palate, and abdominal-wall defects. In contrast, bands may tear normally developed structures, leading to disruption such as central nervous system or calvarial defects, acrosyndactyly, amputations and nonanatomical facial clefts (Lockwood et al. 1989). The effects of fetal compression and tethering may lead to deformations such as clubbing of the feet and angulation of the spine.

The timing of amnion rupture has been suggested to occur between 28 days after conception to 18 weeks of gestation. If amnion rupture occurs prior to 45 days of gestation, the results are likely to be devastating, including severe skull defects and major visceral defects (Huang et al. 1995). Rupture occurring after 45 days of gestation is likely to result in more limited defects.

The cause of amnion rupture and band formation is not well understood, but it has been observed following amniocentesis (Rehder 1978). Late gestation bands, even in the absence of an amniocentesis, can also occur. Lage et al. (1988) reported ABS presenting at birth with multiple abnormalities of the extremities despite a normal sonographic appearance at 21 weeks of gestation. There have also been cases of ABS associated with underlying disease. Young et al. (1985) reported two cases in fetuses with Ehlers–Danlos syndrome type IV and one with osteogenesis imperfecta. They speculated that the premature amnion rupture may have been due to reduced or abnormal collagen in the amnion. There have been rare familial cases of ABS, and some teratogens, such as lysergic acid diethylamide and methadone, have been reported in association with the syndrome (Chemke et al. 1973; Daly et al. 1996; Lubinsky et al. 1983).

Chorioamniotic separation, occurring spontaneously or as a consequence of invasive procedures, is a potential cause of the amniotic band syndrome. The incidence of chorioamniotic separation diagnosed by ultrasound is reported to range from 1 in 187 to 1 in 4333 births (Borlum 1989; Kaufman et al. 1985). The natural history of chorioamniotic separation occurring in normal pregnancies was initially thought to be benign. However, Graf et al. (1997) reported a case of chorioamniotic separation that resulted in the formation of amniotic bands involving the umbilical cord, resulting in fetal death. The incidence of chorioamniotic separation may be even higher in cases of fetal surgery. In the same report Graf and colleagues described 5 cases of chorioamniotic separation occurring in a series of 40 patients undergoing open fetal surgery. Three of the 5 fetuses had amniotic bands involving the umbilical cord, leading to fetal death in 1. This report speculated that because the amnion is adherent and fixed to the umbilical cord, once formed amniotic bands may retract to the cord, causing strangulation. Heifetz (1984), in a review of amniotic band syndrome, reported that as many as 10% of cases had umbilical-cord strangulation.

ABS is often misdiagnosed, especially in cases of early amniotic band rupture. Infants affected by early amniotic rupture present with anencephaly, encephalocele, abdominal- or thoracic-wall defects, and severe limb abnormalities. The severity of the anomalies obscure the cause, especially if the amniotic bands are not evident at birth. It has been estimated that a correct neonatal diagnosis of ABS is made in only 24 to 50% of patients without specialized genetic consultation (Seeds et al. 1982).

▶ INCIDENCE

Due to difficulties in accurately diagnosing ABS, the estimates of its incidence vary widely. The reported incidence ranges from 1 in 1200 to 1 in 15,000 live births (Chemke et al. 1973; Ho and Liu 1987; Ray et al. 1988; Seeds et al. 1982). More recent estimates place the incidence of ABS at 1 in 1200 because of the more frequent recognition of an amniogenic cause for congenital anomalies (Moerman et al. 1992; Ossipoff and Hall 1977; Seeds et al. 1982).

▶ SONOGRAPHIC FINDINGS

ABS is associated with numerous antenatal sonographic features, as there are numerous forms of the syndrome and these features may occur as isolated problems or in combination. The earliest that amniotic bands have been seen is at 12 weeks of gestation, by endovaginal probe. The bands can be extremely difficult to detect sonographically and ABS is more often diagnosed by the effect that they have on fetal anatomy (Fig. 101-1). The effect of amniotic bands on the extremities may be manifested by absent digits or portions of limbs, or a swollen distal arm or leg resulting from constrictive amniotic bands (Fig. 101-2). ABS may affect the face with cleft lip or palate, asymmetric microphthalmia, or severe nasal deformity. Encephalocele may be a manifestation of ABS, especially when eccentrically placed (Fig. 101-3). Abdominal-wall defects can be the result of ABS, typically with large defects with free-floating intestine but large enough for the lines to herniate outside the abdomen. The characteristic appearance of an aberrant sheet or band of amnion attached to the fetus with resultant deformity and restriction of motion allows

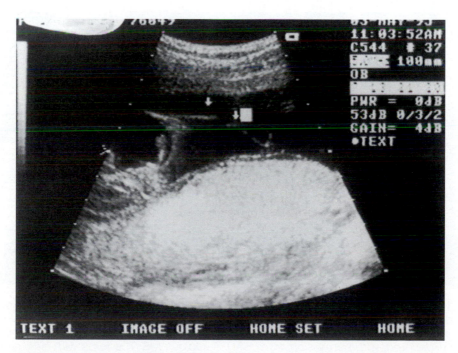

Figure 101-1. Sonographic image demonstating an amniotic band attached to the fetus and floating in the amniotic fluid.

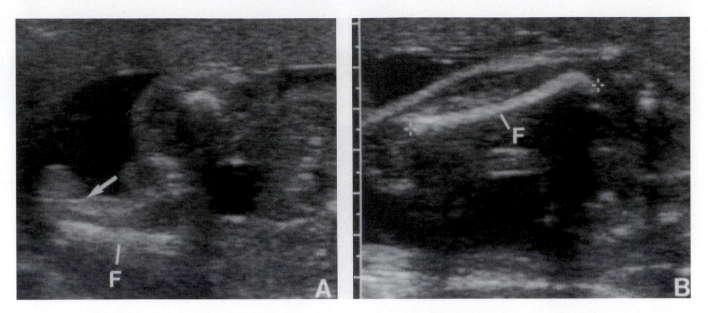

Figure 101-2. Sonographic image of a fetus with a constricting amniotic band of an extremity. (A) Amniotic bands result in amputation of the lower extremity immediately above the knee (arrow). (B) The normal contralateral femur (F) is shown for comparison. *(Reprinted, with permission, from Filly RA, Golbus MS. The fetus with amniotic band syndrome. In: Harrison MR, Golbus MS, Filly RA, ed. The unborn patient. 2nd ed. Philadelphia: Saunders, 1991:440–447.)*

a diagnosis of ABS to be made (Fig. 101-3). However, prenatal diagnosis is the exception rather than the rule.

The findings in ABS may be limited to isolated defects, including isolated facial cleft, digital amputation, or mild elephantiasis of an extremity beyond a con-

strictive band. These isolated features may be difficult to diagnose sonographically because the detailed fetal visualization required is beyond the scope of routine obstetrical ultrasound examinations. At the worst end of the spectrum, the fetus may be so severely deformed

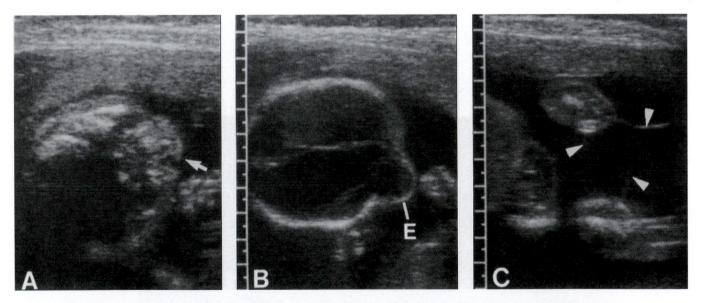

Figure 101-3. Sonographic image of a fetus with amniotic band syndrome manifesting as: (A) a "slash" defect in the maxillary region, and (B) an asymmetric encephalocele (E). (C) Amniotic bands were also noted to be attached to the extremities (arrowheads). *(Reprinted, with permission, from Filly RA, Golbus MS. The fetus with amniotic band syndrome. In: Harrison MR, Golbus MS, Filly RA, eds. The unborn patient. 2nd ed. Philadelphia: Saunders, 1991:440–447.)*

by the amniotic bands that the spine is contracted and organs are formed in perplexing and bizarre proportions. The head may be completely misshapen or absent. The bands responsible for these deformities are rarely seen and a presumptive diagnosis of ABS is made based on the commonly associated deformities.

The spinal deformities in ABS can be severe, manifesting as kyphotic lordosis or scoliosis as well as severe rotational abnormalities and even spinal amputation. While spinal deformity can be seen in other syndromes, severe spinal deformity should suggest ABS.

Spinal deformity associated with an abdominal-wall defect is particularly suggestive of ABS. While the typical appearance of an omphalocele is possible, the more common defect is a large slash-like defect of both the thoracic and abdominal cavities with evisceration. These defects are associated with exteriorized bowel, liver, and sometimes heart without an enveloping membrane. When associated with limb abnormalities this is characteristic of the limb–body-wall complex form of ABS (Fig. 101-4).

Deformation of the calvarium is another group of anomalies characteristic of ABS. If complete, the fetus may appear anencephalic. If partial, the fetus may appear to have an encephalocele. The distinguishing features that characterize these defects as ABS are their asymmetric nature and associated spinal deformity or abdominal-wall defects. In classic anencephaly the calvarial bones are symmetrically absent (see Chapter 5). In anencephaly caused by ABS there is some portion of calvarium present, usually near the base of the skull or near one other orbit. Similarly, classic encephaloceles occur near the midline, while ABS causes encephaloceles off the midline.

The presence of bands is unnecessary for the diagnosis of ABS in the presence of characteristic fetal anomalies. The sonographic detection of bands is helpful in confirming the diagnosis of ABS as the cause of fetal deformity. However, observation of these bands without fetal abnormality is not ABS. It is important for the sonographer to distinguish amniotic bands from other membranes and separations within the amnion. Separation of amnion and chorion is normal in early pregnancy until fusion occurs at approximately 16 weeks of gestation (Burrows et al. 1982; Patten et al. 1986; Sauerbrei et al. 1980).

Chorioamniotic separation may occur as a result of amniocentesis or fetal surgery, and extrachorionic hemorrhage may separate the chorioamniotic membrane from the uterine wall (Burrows et al. 1982; Graf et al. 1997; Spirit et al. 1979). In both of these instances a membrane may be observed sonographically. Other causes of membranes in the developing fetus include septate uterus, blighted twin, and circumvallate placenta (Filly et al. 1991).

Adhesions that form in the uterus as a result of curettage, cesarean section, or myomectomy may cause sheets of amnion that protrude into the lumen of the amniotic cavity (Asherman 1948; Comninos et al. 1969; Filly et al. 1991; Mahony et al. 1985; Randal et al. 1988). Randal et al. (1988) found that 76% of patients with amniotic sheets had undergone prior instrumentation. This results in an adhesion that becomes covered by chorion and amnion and has a thickness similar to the intertwin membrane of dichorionic diamniotic twins. These amniotic sheets do not adhere to the fetus because the amnion is intact. The uterine adhesion may rupture with growth of the fetus. Filly et al. (1991) have described

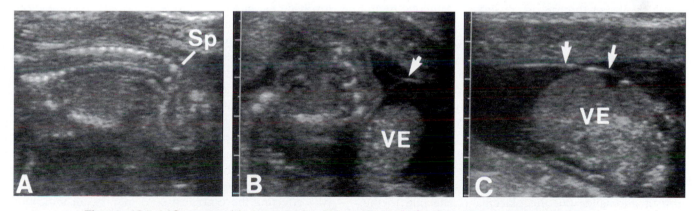

Figure 101-4. Sonographic image of a fetus with limb–body-wall complex showing severe twisting deformity of the spine associated with gastropleuroschisis and amniotic bands attached to the extremities. (A) The fetal spine (Sp) has a severe twisting deformity. (B) The twisting deformity is so severe that the viscera (VE) herniated through the gastropleuroschisis are found posterior to the fetus. (C) The amnion (arrows) encircles the exteriorized viscera. *(Reprinted, with permission, from Filly RA, Golbus MS. The fetus with amniotic band syndrome. In: Harrison MR, Golbus MS, Filly RA, eds. The unborn patient. 2nd ed. Philadelphia: Saunders, 1991:440–447.)*

the sonographic appearance of these synechiae as having a thickened base and a fine edge that undulates. There may be a bulbous edge, presumably due to the synechiae. There are no associated fetal abnormalities and there is free fetal movement around the sheet. The synechiae may not be seen in the third trimester, whether due to rupture or compression by the growing fetus.

In the limb–body-wall complex there is a constellation of abnormalities, including myelomeningoceles or caudal regression, thoracoabdominoschisis, or abdominoschisis and limb defects (see Fig. 101-4). At least two of the three abnormalities listed above are necessary to make a diagnosis of LBWC. The umbilical cord is usually short or absent, with the placenta attached to the fetus. If present, there may be only a two-vessel cord. The limbs may be missing or the feet clubbed. The spine is often short and curved and sacral regression is common. There may be Arnold–Chiari malformation and hydrocephalus associated with the meningomyelocele. There may be ectopia cordis as part of the thoracoabdominoschisis. Facial clefts may also be seen in LBWC.

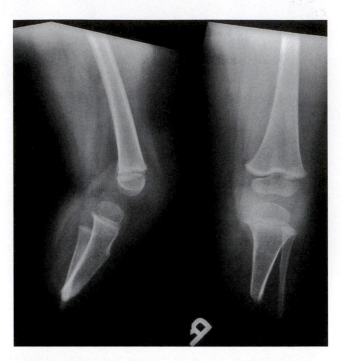

Figure 101-5. Plain radiograph of the right leg of a newborn who sustained amputation in utero of the right leg and foot from amniotic bands. *(Courtesy of Benjamin Alman, M.D.)*

▶ DIFFERENTIAL DIAGNOSIS

The differential diagnosis in ABS depends on the sonographic findings. In isolated constrictive amniotic bands associated with distal limb edema, possible lymphatic or vascular malformations should be considered. However, color Doppler studies should closely show the flow characteristics of a vascular malformation. Constrictive bands involving the upper extremity should suggest the possibility of the VACTERL association if the radius is affected, and Fanconi anemia if radial hypoplasia or absent thumbs are observed. Amniotic membranes within the amniotic cavity without associated fetal anomalies may be amniotic sheets secondary to intrauterine synechiae or remnant of a blighted twin, or secondary to amniocentesis or chorionic villus sampling.

A diagnosis of LBWC requires two of three of the following abnormalities: (1) myelomeningocele or caudal regression, (2) abdominal- or thoracoabdominal-wall defect, or (3) limb defects. The main differential diagnosis are cases of isolated neural-tube defects or ruptured omphalocele, which do not meet the criteria for LBWC. The body-stalk anomaly has a similar constellation of anomalies but the placenta is attached to the trunk of the fetus.

▶ ANTENATAL NATURAL HISTORY

There is great controversy about the pathogenesis of the various forms of ABS. Part of this controversy involves the timing in gestation of the development of amniotic bands. However, in constrictive amniotic bands of the extremities, the progression of constriction combined with fetal growth has resulted in extremity amputation (Fig. 101-5) (Hill et al. 1988). ABS can be associated with either polyhydramnios or oligohydramnios. Despite the severity of some forms of ABS, there are no adverse maternal consequences for this diagnosis. The incidence of intrauterine fetal death from ABS involving the umbilical cord is not known but numerous cases have been reported (Graf et al. 1997; Kanayama et al. 1995; Torpin 1965). However, the poorly characterized pathogenesis of this syndrome and limited sonographic surveillance limit our understanding of its prenatal natural history.

ABS is a relatively common, if underappreciated, cause of fetal and neonatal morbidity and mortality. The fetal-lamb model of ABS will be useful to better define the pathophysiology of ABS and to provide a tool to understand the unique fetal response to tissue injury, repair, and regeneration. Sonographic identification of ABS affecting the umbilical cord may be an indication for fetoscopic surgical intervention. In the future, intervention for nonlethal limb deformation may also be considered if maternal risk is sufficiently lowered. ABS is another in a growing list of conditions for which fetal surgery may be considered in the future.

Constrictive bands most commonly affect the extremities, but can also involve the umbilical cord, with resulting fetal death. Kanayama et al. (1995) described the reversal of diastolic flow observed in a fetus with umbilical-cord constriction due to amniotic bands. Graf et al. (1997) similarly reported a case of amniotic bands involving the umbilical cord following the development of chorioamniotic separation. Despite initially normal umbilical artery Doppler waveforms, this fetus died within 2 weeks from a constrictive amniotic band of the umbilical cord. Reports have described constrictive amniotic bands as a cause of fetal death (Moerman et al. 1992; Torpin 1965). However, until the reports by Kanayama and Graf and their colleagues, this was a diagnosis made pathologically after the fact. It is in cases like these that fetoscopic lysis of amniotic bands could be lifesaving.

▶ MANAGEMENT OF PREGNANCY

In managing a pregnancy with suspected ABS it is essential to have a detailed sonographic fetal survey to accurately assess any anomalies present. Fetal echocardiography is indicated in cases of abdominal-wall or abdominothoracic-wall defects because of the increased incidence of associated cardiac defects. Amniocentesis is not necessary in clear-cut cases of ABS as these are sporadic deformations with no association with chromosomal abnormalities. However, in instances in which the diagnosis is uncertain, genetic amniocentesis should be considered. For example, in cases of abdominal-wall defects in which a ruptured covered omphalocele cannot be excluded, genetic amniocentesis is indicated.

A fetus with ABS should pose no increased risk for the mother in the management of the pregnancy. There is no indication for cesarean section, except for obstetrical indications. In severe cases of ABS, such as LBWC, in which survival is not anticipated, conventional labor and vaginal delivery without intervention for fetal distress should be considered.

▶ FETAL INTERVENTION

The indications for fetal surgery are, with few exceptions, only for life-threatening conditions such as cystic adenomatoid malformation of the lung with hydrops, diaphragmatic hernia with a low lung:heart ratio, bladder-outlet obstruction with oligohydramnios, or sacrococcygeal teratoma with placentomegaly (see Chapters 3, 37, 38, 80, and 116). However, as experience with the techniques of fetal surgery has grown and the natural histories of certain non-life-threatening conditions have been better defined, the indications for fetal surgery have been extended. Two examples of this are in utero repair of meningomyelocele to prevent the devastating neurologic injury to the spinal cord

(Adzick et al. 1998) and fetoscopic cord ligation in monochorionic twins with imminent death of one twin to prevent neurologic injury in the surviving twin (Crombleholme et al. 1996). The indications for fetal surgery in the amniotic band syndrome may be either for a life-threatening condition if it involves constriction of the umbilical cord, or more commonly, threatened limb amputation due to amniotic band constriction (Ashkenazy et al. 1982; Kanayama et al. 1995; Tadmor et al. 1997; Torpin 1965).

Torpin (1965) reported 36 cases of fetal death due to cord constriction from amniotic bands. In each case the diagnosis was made retrospectively, however. Recognition of amniotic bands constricting the umbilical cord has been reported by Kanayama et al. (1995), who were able to document fetal compromise by reversal of diastolic flow in the umbilical artery by color Doppler. It is in cases like the one reported by Kanayama et al. that fetoscopic lysis of amniotic bands could be lifesaving.

Based on their experience with fetoscopy for cord ligation in TRAP sequence and the experimental work by Crombleholme et al. demonstrating the potential for functional recovery of banded extremities once released, Quintero et al. performed the first fetoscopic lysis of amniotic bands in human fetuses (Crombleholme et al. 1995; Quintero et al. 1997). Their first case was a fetus at 21 weeks of gestation with bilateral cleft lip and bands attached to the face and left upper extremity with distal limb edema. In order to avert limb amputation, fetoscopic lysis of bands was attempted at 22 weeks of gestation using a two-port technique. However, due to bleeding encountered on insertion of the second operating port, it was removed. The endoscissors were passed through the port used for the fetoscope, and the lysis was performed under ultrasound guidance. There was resolution of the distal edema within 6 days of the procedure. At 32 weeks, microphthalmia and anophthalmia of the right orbit were first noted at the site of the previously attached amniotic band. The infant was delivered at 39 weeks and was found to have a type IV Tessier craniofacial cleft and right microphthalmia. The extremity showed minimal residual scarring where the band had been attached and lysed. The infant's hand had radial paresis and mild hypoplasia.

The second case was a fetus at 23 weeks of gestation with a thick amniotic band constricting the left ankle of the fetus. There was marked edema distal to the band and minimal blood flow to the foot was observed by color and pulsed Doppler. Fetoscopy was performed using a 2.7-mm 5-degree endoscope and confirmed the sonographic findings. Again, bleeding was encountered on insertion of the operating port, necessitating its removal. Attempts at ultrasound-guided lysis using endoscissors were unsuccessful. A 2.4 mm 0-degree operating scope with a 400-μm contact YAG laser fiber was used to lyse approximately 85% of the band. Complete lysis of the band was not achieved for fear of injury to "important elements in the ankle." Postoperatively, the edema markedly improved, as did distal arterial blood flow, and there was return of flexion and extension on follow-up sonographic examination. The mother was hospitalized 8 weeks postoperatively at 31 weeks of gestation with premature rupture of membranes and delivered at 34.5 weeks of gestation. The infant underwent Z-plasties for residual effects of the amniotic band, and full functional recovery was anticipated.

The rationale for performing fetoscopic lysis of constricting extremity amniotic bands is based on the hypothesis that progressive compromise of fetal growth leads to amputation. However, this assumes that the procedure can be accomplished with no maternal morbidity and minimal fetal morbidity. This procedure would be hard to justify in the face of a serious maternal complication or a fetal death due to severely premature delivery at 21 or 23 weeks of gestation, even in the face of certain fetal limb amputation. While these two cases demonstrate the feasibility of fetoscopic lysis of amniotic bands, limiting application of these techniques to cases of umbilical-cord constriction would be on more solid ground given the potential risks to mother and fetus.

While extremity ABS may have devastating morphologic and functional effects on a limb, possibly resulting in amputation, it is not lethal. Extremity ABS is not an indication for fetoscopic surgery unless maternal risks and incidence of preterm labor can be markedly reduced from those that already exist. However, there are forms of ABS that are lethal or have devastating neurologic sequelae that may justify the current risks of intervention. Torpin (1965) has reported 36 cases of constrictive amniotic bands of the umbilical cord, which were uniformly fatal. Although rarer than other forms of ABS, umbilical-cord constriction, once diagnosed sonographically, may be amenable to fetoscopic release to avert fetal death.

▶ TREATMENT OF THE NEWBORN

A fetus known to have amniotic band syndrome should be delivered in a tertiary-care center with neonatologists, pediatric surgeons, and pediatric plastic and orthopedic surgeons available. Treatment depends on the nature of the amniotic band syndrome and the severity of the deformation. In cases of umbilical-cord involvement, early or even emergency delivery may be indicated if there are signs of fetal compromise (Kanayama et al. 1995). After delivery a careful physical examination should assess the severity of the amniotic band syndrome. Often there will be no evidence of the amniotic band at the time of delivery. In the case of extremity amniotic bands, treatment is dictated by the severity of the deformation. The severity of deformity can range from a mildly constrictive band, requiring release, to near amputation, requiring debridement. More often there is a band-like deformation that requires Z-plasties to surgically correct (Fig. 101-6).

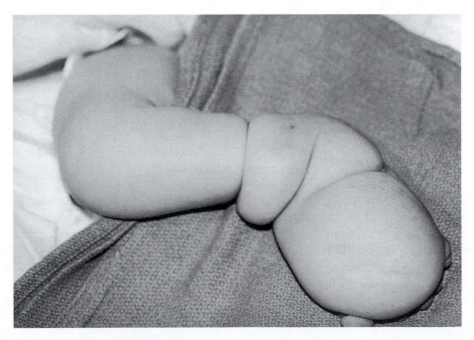

Figure 101-6. Postnatal appearance of the arm and hand of a newborn with extremity amniotic band syndrome.

In cases of amniotic bands involving the face and head, there may be severe facial clefts, anophthalmia, and encephalocele. These deformities may require many extensive reconstructive procedures to achieve an acceptable cosmetic result. Cases of the LBWC form of amniotic band syndrome are always fatal, and no reconstructive procedures are indicated.

▶ LONG-TERM OUTCOME

The outcome in amniotic band syndrome depends on the severity of the deformation. Cases of extremity amniotic band syndrome usually have an excellent long-term outcome. Even in cases of limb amputation, ambulation is possible with the aid of a prosthesis. The cosmetic results following extensive craniofacial reconstructive surgery are often acceptable, but the severity of these defects may leave these children permanently disfigured.

▶ GENETICS AND RECURRENCE RISK

Most cases of amniotic band syndrome are sporadic and there is no risk of recurrence in subsequent pregnancies. There have been cases of amniotic band syndrome associated with underlying disease, such as Ehlers–Danlos syndrome type III, or osteogenesis imperfecta. Similarly, amniotic band syndrome has been reported in association with teratogens such as methadone and lysergic acid diethylamide (Chemke et al. 1973; Daly et al. 1996). While associated maternal disease or teratogenic exposure may predispose to recurrence, these are rare causes of the amniotic band syndrome.

REFERENCES

Adzick NS, Sutton L, Crombleholme TM, et al. Successful fetal surgery for spina bifida. Lancet 1998;352:1675–1676.

Asherman JG. Amenorrhoea traumatic. Br J Obstet Gynaecol 1948;55:23–27.

Ashkenazy M, Borenstein R, Katz Z. Constriction of the umbilical cord by an amniotic band after midtrimester amniocentesis. Acta Obstet Gynecol Scand 1982;61:89–91.

Bamforth JS. Amniotic band sequence: Streeter's hypothesis reexamined. Am J Med Genet 1992;44:280–287.

Borlum KG. Second trimester chorioamniotic separation and amniocentesis. Eur J Obstet Gynecol Reprod Biol 1989;30:35–38.

Burrows PE, Lyons EA, Phillips HJ, et al. Intrauterine membranes: sonographic findings and clinical significance. J Ultrasound 1982;10:1–8.

Chemke J, Gaff G, Hurwitz N, et al. The ABS. Obstet Gynecol 1973;41:332–336.

Comninos AC, Zourlas PA. Treatment of intrauterine adhesions (Asherman's syndrome). Am J Obstet Gynecol 1969;105:862–867.

Crombleholme TM, Robertson FM, Marx G, et al. Fetoscopic cord ligation to prevent neurologic injury in monozygous twins. Lancet 1996;348:191.

Crombleholme TM, Dirkes K, Whitney TM, et al. Amniotic band syndrome in fetal lambs. I. Fetoscopic release and morphometric outcome. J Pediatr Surg 1995;30:974–978.

Daly CA, Freeman J, Weston W, et al. Prenatal diagnosis of ABS in a methadone user: review of the literature and a case report. Ultrasound Obstet Gynecol 1996;8:123–125.

Filly RA, Golbus MS. The fetus with amniotic band syndrome. In: Harrison MR, Golbus MS, Filly RA, eds. The unborn patient. 2nd ed. Philadelphia: Saunders, 1991:440–447.

Graf JL, Bealer JF, Gibbs DL, et al. Chorioamniotic membrane separation: a potentially lethal finding. Fetal Diagn Ther 1997;12:81–84.

Heifetz SA. Strangulation of the umbilical cord by amniotic bands. Pediatr Pathol 1984;2:285–304.

Herva R, Karkinen-Jaaskelainen M. Amniotic adhesion malformation syndrome: fetal and placental pathology. Teratology 1984;29:11–19.

Higginbottom MC, Jones KL. The amniotic band disruption complex: timing of amniotic rupture and variable spectra of consequent defects. J Pediatr 1979;96:544–549.

Hill L, Kislak S, Jones N. Prenatal ultrasound diagnosis of a forearm constrictive band. J Ultrasound Med 1988;7:293–295.

Ho DM, Liu HC. The ABS: report of two autopsy cases and review of the literature. Clin Med J 1987;39:429–436.

Hong CY, Simon MA. Amniotic bands knotted about umbilical cord: a rare cause of fetal death. Obstet Gynecol 1963;22:667–670.

Huang CC, Eng HL, Chen WJ. Amniotic band syndrome: report of two autopsy cases. Chang Gung Med J 1995;18:371–377.

Jones KL, Smith DW, Hall BD, et al. A pattern of craniofacial and limb defects secondary to aberrant tissue bands. J Pediatr 1974;84:90–95.

Kanayama MD, Gaffey TA, Ogburn PL Jr. Constriction of the umbilical cord by an amniotic band, with fetal compromise illustrated by reverse diastolic flow in the umbilical artery: a case report. J Reprod Med 1995;40:71–73.

Kaufman AJ, Fleischer AC, Thieme GA, et al. Separated chorioamnion and elevated chorion: sonographic features and clinical significance. J Ultrasound Med 1985;4:119–125.

Keller H, Neuhauser G, Durkin-Stamm MV, et al. "ADAM complex" (amniotic deformity, adhesions, mutilations): a pattern of craniofacial and limb defects. Am J Med Genet 1978;2:81–98.

Kulkarni ML, Gopal PV. Amniotic band syndrome. Indian Pediatr 1990;27:471–476.

Lage JM, VanMarter LJ, Bieber FR. Questionable role of amniocentesis in the etiology of amniotic band formation: a case report. J Reprod Med 1988;33:71–73.

Lockwood C, Ghidini A, Romero R, et al. ABS: reevaluation of its pathogenesis. Am J Obstet Gynecol 1989;160:1030–1033.

Lubinsky M, Sujansky E, Sanders W, et al. Familial amniotic bands. Am J Med Genet 1983;14:81–87.

Mahony BS, Filly RA, Callen PW, et al. The amniotic band syndrome: antenatal diagnosis and potential pitfalls. Am J Obstet Gynecol 1985;152:63–68.

Miller ME, Graham JM Jr, Higginbottom MC, et al. Compression-related defects from early amnion rupture: evidence for mechanical teratogenesis. J Pediatr 1981;98:292–297.

Moerman P, Fryns JP, Vandenberghe K, et al. Constrictive amniotic bands, amniotic adhesions, and limb-body wall complex: discrete disruption sequence with pathogenetic overlap. Am J Med Genet 1992;42:470–479.

Ossipoff V, Hall BD. Etiologic factors in the ABS: a study of twenty-four patients. Birth Defects 1977;13:117–121.

Patten RM, VanAllen MI, Mack LA, et al. Limb-body wall complex: in utero sonographic diagnosis of a complicated fetal malformation. AJR Am J Roentgenol 1986;146:1019–1024.

Quintero RA, Morales WJ, Phillips J, et al. In utero lysis of amniotic bands. Ultrasound Obstet Gynecol 1997;10:316–320.

Quintero RA, Reich H, Puder K, et al. Umbilical cord ligation of an acardiac twin by fetoscopy at 19 weeks of gestation. N Engl J Med 1994;330:469–471.

Randal SB, Filly RA, Callen PW, et al. Amniotic sheets. Radiology 1988;166:633–638.

Ray M, Hendrick SJ, Raimer SS, et al. ABS. Int J Dermatol 1988;27:312–314.

Rehder H. Fetal limb deformities due to amniotic constrictions (a possible consequence of preceding amniocentesis). Pathol Res Pract 1978;162:316–326.

Sauerbrei E, Cooperberg PL, Poland BJ: Ultrasound demonstration of the normal fetal yolk sac. J Clin Ultrasound 1980;8:217–220.

Seeds JW, Cefalo RC, Herbert WNP. Amniotic band syndrome. Am J Obstet Gynecol 1982;144:243–248.

Seidman JD, Abbondanzo SL, Watkin WG, et al. ABS: report of two cases and review of the literature. Arch Pathol Lab Med 1989;113:891–897.

Spirit BA, Kagan EH, Rozanski RM. Abruptio placenta: sonographic and pathologic correlation. AJR Am J Roentgenol 1979;133:877–881.

Streeter GL. Focal deficiencies in fetal tissues and their relation to intrauterine amputations. Contrib Embryol Carnegie Inst 1930;22:1–44.

Tadmor OP, Kreisberg GA, Achiron R, et al. Limb amputation in amniotic band syndrome: serial ultrasonographic and Doppler observations. Ultrasound Obstet Gynecol 1997;10:312–315.

Torpin R. Amniochorionic mesoblastic fibrous strings and amniotic bands. Am J Obstet Gynecol 1965;91:65–75.

Van Allen MI, Curry C, Gallagher L. Limb body wall complex. I. Pathogenesis. Am J Med Genet 1987;28:529–548.

Ville Y, Hyett J, Hecher K, et al. Preliminary experience with endoscopic laser surgery for severe twin–twin transfusion syndrome. N Engl J Med 1995;332:224–227.

Young ID, Lindenbaum RH, Thompson EM, et al. Amniotic bands in connective tissue disorders. Arch Dis Child 1985;60:1061–1063.

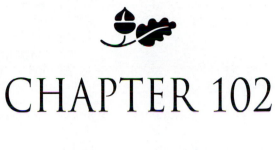

CHAPTER 102

Arthrogryposis

► CONDITION

The term arthrogryposis, a mixture of Latin and Greek words, means curved or crooked joint (Hageman et al. 1988). This term was first used in 1923 by Stern. The first medical description of arthrogryposis occurred in 1841, when Otto described an infant with multiple congenital contractures and referred to the condition as "congenital myodystrophy" (Swinyard and Bleck 1985).

Arthrogryposis refers to a symptom complex characterized by multiple joint contractures that are present at birth. The muscles in the affected area or areas are replaced by fat and fibrous tissue (Shapiro and Specht 1993). Although the term arthrogryposis is in wide use, the preferred descriptive term is multiple congenital contractures. Multiple congenital contractures do not represent a syndrome but a compensatory connective tissue response (Swinyard and Bleck 1985).

According to Hall (1981), the term arthrogryposis multiplex congenita was coined to describe infants with multiple congenital contractures. Confusion has arisen because the term was used as a diagnosis. The term is descriptive, and the presence of congenital contractures only indicates a clinical sign with multiple underlying causes. In general, anything that decreases intrauterine movement may lead to limitation of joint movement and the subsequent formation of contractures. The earlier in development it occurs and the longer the duration of limitation of movement will result in more severe contractures at birth.

There are four major causes of congenital contractures (Hall 1981). The first is an abnormality of muscle tissue. Examples of this are muscular dystrophy, congenital myopathies, and congenital absence of muscle. The second cause is abnormal nerve function or innervation. This includes central nervous system malformations, a congenital neuropathy, and failure of the nerves to form or myelinate, or exposure to toxins that affect nerve function. A third cause of congenital contractures is an abnormality of connective tissue. This interferes with the normal development of tendons, bone, cartilage, or joint tissue. The fourth cause is mechanical limitation to movement in utero. This includes the presence of uterine fibroids, oligohydramnios, amniotic bands, or the presence of a multiple gestation.

Clinical features of arthrogryposis include rigidity of several joints, resulting from short, tight muscles and capsular contractures, dislocation of joints, "featureless" extremities (normal skin creases are absent and there is an increase in the amount of subcutaneous fat), presence of deep skin dimples in the vicinity of affected joints, absence or fibrosis of muscles, and normal intellectual development (Williams 1978).

► INCIDENCE

The incidence of multiple congenital contractures is approximately 1 in 3000 live births (Hall 1985). In one study of 66 cases of arthrogryposis multiplex congenita, the mothers were significantly older than average (Wynne-Davies and Lloyd-Roberts 1976). Davis and Kalousek (1988) identified 16 cases of fetal akinesia deformation sequence in 948 not yet viable fetuses at 9 to 20 weeks of gestation. The fetal akinesia deformation sequence was defined as joint contractures with or without formation of webs, with intrauterine growth restriction, pulmonary hypoplasia, micrognathia, short umbilical cord, and a short gut (Davis and Kalousek 1988). In addition, arthrogryposis multiplex congenita has been described in association with cases of failed termination of pregnancy (Hall et al. 1996). These authors hypothesized that the contractures were due to vascular compromise during attempted termination with a secondary loss of functional neurons leading to fetal akinesia and subsequent contractures. A rupture of membranes with continuous leakage of amniotic fluid after attempted termination may have worsened the existing contractures.

▶ SONOGRAPHIC FINDINGS

Examination of the fetal extremities is not listed in the American Institute of Ultrasound and Medicine (AIUM) guidelines, but it is a critical adjunct to fetal imaging and is needed to diagnose many syndromes (Bromley and Benacerraf 1995). The sonographic diagnosis of arthrogryposis is made by observation of the malposition of the limbs (Fig. 102-1). The morphologic aspects of the bones are normal but the range of movements is limited (Deschamps et al. 1992). Increased nuchal edema and polyhydramnios are commonly observed in association with arthrogryposis.

Baty et al. (1988) reported the prenatal diagnosis of distal arthrogryposis type I by sonographic examination at 18 weeks of gestation in a family with two other affected members. Real-time sonographic evaluation demonstrated a flexed position of the fingers and extension of the right wrist, which did not change despite active motion of the shoulders and elbows. The fetal hands were in a fist and the fingers did not extend (Fig. 102-2). These authors described the following important variables in the sonographic diagnosis of fetal joint contractures (Baty et al. 1988):

1. The gestational age of the fetus
2. The timing of the development of the joint contractures

3. The severity of the joint contractures
4. The index of suspicion of the ultrasonographer
5. The skill, patience, and previous experience of the sonographer
6. The divergence of the affected joints from the neutral position
7. The amount of joint movement
8. The presence of other sonographically detectable anomalies
9. The persistence of findings over time

Amyoplasia is the most common cause of joint contractures. Sepulveda et al. (1995) diagnosed a case of fetal amyoplasia at 19 weeks of gestation with absent fetal movements, severe multiple congenital contractures, hydrops fetalis, and polyhydramnios. No spontaneous fetal movements were seen over a 40-minute period of observation. Autopsy of this affected fetus revealed small groups of poorly developed muscle fibers within areas of fat. These authors noted that fetal movements were absent during intrahepatic venous sampling in the fetus with amyoplasia. This was in contrast to their previous observations that second-trimester fetuses normally react with vigorous movements during venipuncture.

A unique type of arthrogryposis has been observed in Scandinavia. This condition, which is lethal, presents with progressive subcutaneous edema from the 13th week of gestation onward and decreased fetal-limb movements. In this Scandinavian type of lethal congenital contracture syndrome, abnormal findings uniformly develop between 13 and 16 weeks of gestation (Kirkinen et al. 1987).

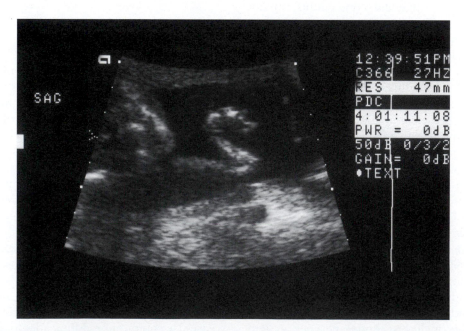

Figure 102-1. Sagittal sonographic image of a fetal lower extremity with contractures at the knee and ankle.

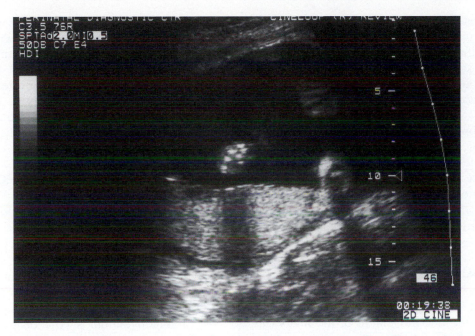

Figure 102-2. Sonographic image of a fetal hand demonstrating fixed flexion of all digits.

Stoll and colleagues (1991) studied two children born to a mother with myasthenia gravis. Her first pregnancy was a 33-week-old fetus with multiple flexion contractures, who died 1 hour after birth from respiratory insufficiency. Her second pregnancy was remarkable for an abnormal ultrasound examination at 20 weeks, which showed decreased fetal movements and multiple flexion contractures. In myasthenia gravis, a maternal factor is transferred to the fetus, which affects the fetal joints.

Goldberg et al. (1986) described a case of fetal arthrogryposis at 30 weeks of gestation in a fetus with scalp edema but no ascites. Moderate polyhydramnios was present. In this fetus, the lower extremities were tightly flexed and crossed in a squatting position. No normal limb activity was noted. These authors stated that late identification of arthrogryposis was valuable in minimizing the birth trauma associated with the vaginal delivery of an infant with fixed joints.

► DIFFERENTIAL DIAGNOSIS

Over 150 conditions are known in which multiple congenital contractures are a predominant sign (Hall 1986). In a review of 155 patients with arthrogryposis, Sarwark et al. (1990) noted that 43% of patients had amyoplasia, 35% had other contracture syndromes, 7% had the dominantly inherited form of distal arthrogryposis, 6% had multiple congenital anomalies, and 2% had chromosomal abnormalities.

Amyoplasia is the single most common cause of multiple congenital contractures. A very specific limb positioning exists in this condition. There is a marked decrease in muscle mass. Contractures are symmetric, with all four limbs affected. The patients have a round face with a mild micrognathia and a midline hemangioma. Intelligence is normal in this condition.

Distal arthrogryposis is a dominantly inherited disorder. There is a lesser degree of involvement of the extremities and preservation of good muscle tone and bulk. Affected patients have a clenched-fist deformity of the hand, occasional congenital dislocation of the hip, and mild to severe positional deformities of the foot (Baty et al. 1988). In distal arthrogryposis, the function of the hands improves with time, use, and physical therapy. There is intrafamilial and interfamilial variability in expression; however, the manifestations of this condition are limited to the joints.

Another consideration in the differential diagnosis is Pena–Shokeir syndrome, which manifests as severe intrauterine growth restriction, a short umbilical cord, pulmonary hypoplasia, micrognathia, and facial anomalies. The overall appearance, however, is somewhat nonspecific.

Only a small percentage of patients with arthrogryposis will have a chromosomal abnormality. The most common abnormalities associated with this condition are trisomy 18 and mosaic trisomy 8. Maternal myasthenia gravis is in the differential diagnosis, as neonatal myasthenia develops in 12% of babies born to mothers with this condition.

In Scandinavia, a lethal congenital contracture syndrome is inherited as an autosomal recessive condition. This condition is lethal in utero at a mean gestational age of 29 weeks. Affected fetuses present with hydrops fetalis and malpositioning of the hips and knees with webbing of the neck and elbows. The muscles are hypoplastic, and there is severe thinning of the ventral half of the spinal cord (Herva et al. 1988).

In the subgroup of patients with contractures due to neurogenic abnormalities, spinal muscular atrophy is a consideration. DNA analysis of 12 unrelated patients with congenital contractures, generalized muscle weakness, evidence of denervation on electromyographic studies, and muscle-biopsy evidence of denervation, revealed that 50% of affected patients lacked the survival motor neuron gene (Börglen et al. 1996). The survival motor neuron (*SMN*) gene is absent or interrupted in 90 to 100% of patients with spinal muscular atrophy.

▶ ANTENATAL NATURAL HISTORY

Joint development starts at 5.5 weeks of gestation, and by the 8th week, the first movement of the limbs can be observed (Ajayi et al. 1995). Absence of motion leads to stiff joints, pterygium formation, pulmonary hypoplasia, and a short umbilical cord. The primary underlying problem in arthrogryposis is due to degeneration of the anterior horn cells, occurring during the early months of gestation (Williams 1978). Early destruction of muscle fibers in utero will result in certain muscles being affected earlier or more severely. Affected muscles tend to lose tone and to fail to counterbalance the tone of the normally developed antagonist muscles. This further restricts the normal movements of the muscles and joints during periods of rapid fetal growth (Williams 1978). According to Hall (1996), an ischemic event occurring during a critical period of anterior horn development may result in contractures. Handling of the pregnant uterus disturbs uterine blood flow, which may result in temporary hypoxia and bradycardia of the embryo. Disruption or decreased flow in the anterior spinal arteries or decreased uterine vessel blood flow will lead to damage or loss of neurons or muscles. The anterior horn cells are particularly susceptible to hypoxic damage or loss at 8 to 14 weeks of gestation (Hall 1996). The subsequent lack of normal anterior-horn-cell function leads to fetal akinesia and secondarily to multiple joint contractures.

Moessinger (1983) developed an animal model of fetal akinesia deformation sequence by paralyzing rat fetuses with injections of curare. The anomalies noted at the time of delivery included multiple joint contractures, pulmonary hypoplasia, micrognathia, intrauterine growth restriction, short umbilical cord, and polyhydramnios. The polyhydramnios in association with fetal akinesia is mediated by lack of swallowing activity.

Clarren and Hall (1983) studied the neuropathologic findings in the spinal cords of 10 infants with neurogenic arthrogryposis and compared them to 8 infants with spinal muscular atrophy type I and 11 age matched controls. The numbers of α-motor neurons were reduced in affected patients with arthrogryposis and spinal muscular atrophy. Abnormal histology was seen in patients with arthrogryposis. In 5 patients, the pathologic pattern was consistent throughout the entire spinal cord. In 5 patients there was an unequal distribution across the spinal cord, and this correlated with the muscle groups involved clinically.

▶ MANAGEMENT OF PREGNANCY

The pregnant patient should be asked whether there is a history of decreased fetal movement. This may be difficult to ascertain in a first pregnancy. She should also be asked whether there is a history of infection, fever or hypothermia, or exposure to teratogens. Additional considerations include the exclusion of uterine masses, the presence of a twin gestation, placental abnormalities, or oligohydramnios. The diagnoses of myotonic dystrophy or myasthenia gravis should be ruled out in the pregnant patient. The pregnant woman should be specifically asked whether she has any history of use of phenytoin, insulin, ethanol, or angel dust (Thompson and Bilenker 1985). A prenatal karyotype should be obtained to rule out an associated chromosomal abnormality. Prenatal factors that potentially predict severe respiratory insufficiency at birth include decreased fetal movements, presence of polyhydramnios, micrognathia, and thin ribs (Bianchi and Van Marter 1994). If the fetus appears to have arthrogryposis and has a strong likelihood of respiratory insufficiency at birth, the prospective parents can be offered termination of pregnancy. If the diagnosis is made later than 24 weeks of gestation, or if the parents do not desire termination, the fetal position should be checked close to term. There is an increased incidence of breech positioning associated with arthrogryposis. Delivery can be complicated by abnormal fetal position and lack of flexibility of the limbs (see Fig. 102-1) (Hall 1981). Therefore, an elective cesarean section may be necessary for safe delivery. We recommend delivery in a tertiary-care center because of the potential for respiratory difficulties at birth and the potential need for mechanical ventilation.

▶ FETAL INTERVENTION

There are no fetal interventions for arthrogryposis.

▶ TREATMENT OF THE NEWBORN

The primary consideration in the treatment of the newborn is to determine if only the limbs are affected, if there is evidence of central nervous system dysfunction, or if there is evidence of additional organs being affected

(Hall 1981). A complete and detailed physical examination should be performed, including specific notation of the appearance and position of the joints and the passive range of motion of the joints. The physical examination should specifically rule out the presence of micrognathia, cleft palate (including the submucous isoform), scoliosis, muscular imbalance, hemivertebrae, or a covered neural-tube defect. Common skin defects associated with arthrogryposis include scalp defects, amniotic bands, and dimples over the joints with limitation of movement. Midline hemangiomas are particularly common in amyoplasia.

Laboratory tests that are recommended for diagnosis include cranial imaging by computed tomographic or magnetic resonance imaging scan (Hageman et al. 1988), chromosome analysis if not performed antenatally, electroencephalography, electromyography with nerve-conduction-velocity studies (Thompson and Bilenker 1985), and radiography. Thin ribs are associated with congenital muscular disease (Chassevent et al. 1978). Creatine kinase levels are nonspecifically elevated and are not useful in obtaining a diagnosis (Bianchi and Van Marter 1994). A muscle biopsy can be performed as early as days 6 to 15 of postnatal life (Bianchi and Van Marter 1994). Physical examination findings consistent with a diagnosis of amyoplasia include a round face with a midline hemangioma (Fig. 102-3), the presence of bilateral club feet, hands that are always flexed at the wrists, and shoulders that are internally rotated. The elbows are usually straight and the hand is rotated posteriorly in what is known as the "policeman's-tip" or "waiter's tip" position. Affected children with amyoplasia have decreased muscle mass. It is important to mobilize the joints as soon as possible after birth. Physical therapy for children with amyoplasia should be initiated during the newborn period. Treatment includes a mixture of application of plaster casts with periods of vigorous therapy (Fig. 102-4).

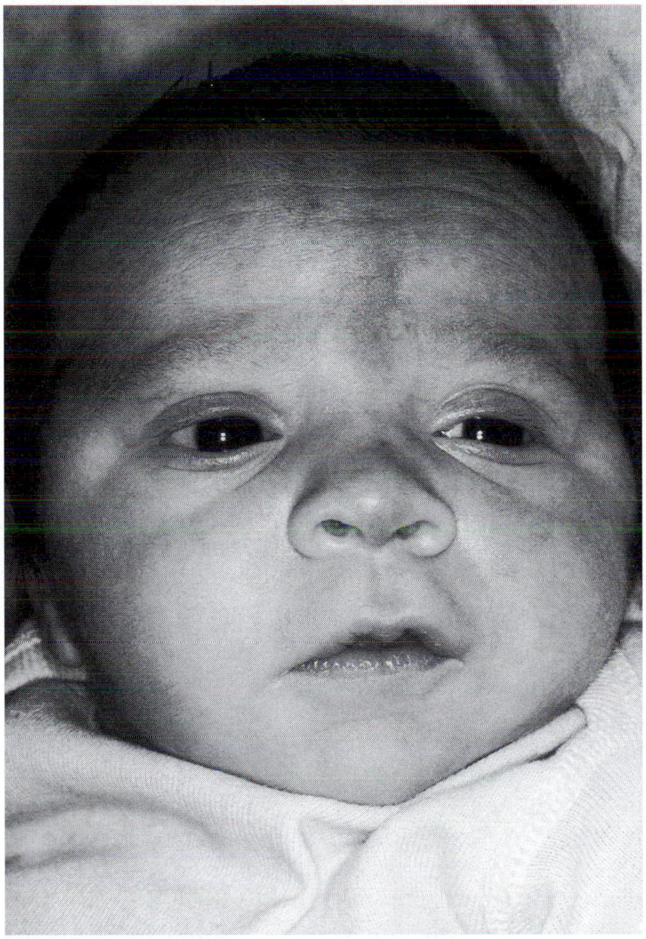

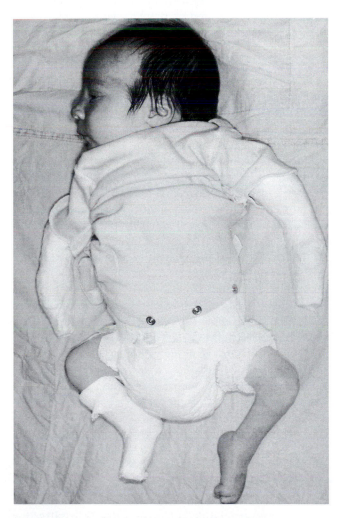

Figure 102-4. Postnatal appearance of same infant in Figure 102-3, demonstrating early treatment with plaster casts. At the time the photograph was taken, the left club foot was receiving a new cast. Symmetric contractures of all 4 extremities are found in amyoplasia.

Figure 102-3. Postnatal photograph of a newborn infant with amyoplasia, demonstrating typical round face and a midline hemangioma on forehead and tip of nose.

A neuromuscular workup may be warranted in cases of arthrogryposis. Patients should be closely examined for the occurrence of perinatal fractures. This can be suspected if a localized deformity, soft-tissue swelling, or irritability occurs. Rigid joints and hypotonia contribute to the occurrence of fractures at delivery (Shapiro and Specht 1993).

▶ SURGICAL TREATMENT

The goal of surgical treatment is to achieve the maximum function possible for each involved joint. Club foot is the common abnormality in arthrogryposis. Ninety percent of children with arthrogryposis have severe bilateral club feet (Solund et al. 1991). Treatment of the foot is the dominant orthopedic problem throughout the first year of life. Solund et al. (1991) treated 10 children with 17 affected feet for a mean follow-up period of 13 years. Fourteen of the 17 feet were satisfactorily treated, defined as painless and plantigrade at the time of examination. These authors recommended performing a talectomy (removal of the talus) before the expected age of walking.

Knee contractures are generally treated with physical therapy to extend the range of motion. If operative correction is necessary, this is performed with lengthening of the hamstrings with a posterior capsulotomy. Thomas et al. (1985) reported on 104 patients treated between 1952 and 1982. Seventy-four of the 104 had significant knee contractures, and they were followed for a period of 2 to 20 years. Of the 74, 43 had nonoperative treatment, which included physical therapy, bracing, or serial casting. Thirty-one patients had operative procedures, and these authors stated that the most useful procedure in the growing child was a posterior capsule release with hamstring tenotomy.

Affected patients can also have hip dislocation. The characteristic deformity is flexion abduction–external rotation contractures, accompanied by unilateral or bilateral hip dislocation (Shapiro and Specht 1993).

Scoliosis often occurs in patients with arthrogryposis due to contractures of the muscles of the trunk. This almost invariably responds to stretching and orthopedic management. Most patients have a history of uterine malposition. Surgical correction is recommended for curves of greater than 15 degrees (Sarwark at al 1990).

▶ LONG-TERM OUTCOME

Bianchi and Van Marter (1994) performed a retrospective medical review and identified 15 newborns over a 10-year period who had arthrogryposis multiplex congenita and required ventilatory support at birth. Fourteen of the 15 patients died; 13 were electively extubated after a variable time course (2 hours to 64 days). All were totally apneic without respiratory support. Autopsies were performed on all 14 nonsurvivors and revealed an approximately equal distribution of central nervous system malformations, peripheral neuropathies, and peripheral myopathies. The single patient who survived had a different clinical course from the other infants. She weaned spontaneously from the ventilator at age 7 days and was ultimately diagnosed with myasthenia gravis. These authors recommended performing an edrophonium challenge test prior to elective extubation of any infant with arthrogryposis multiplex congenita and inability to breathe. However, most infants with arthrogryposis do not have respiratory problems, and their prognoses are considerably better.

Sarwark et al. (1990) described a better than expected prognosis in amyoplasia. The size of the limbs at birth and presence or absence of pterygia (webs) can be used to predict response to therapy. Amyoplasia is an example of a severe birth defect that can improve with appropriate intervention. Sells et al. (1996) reviewed the outcome of 38 children with amyoplasia, diagnosed by a medical geneticist. Eighty-four percent of the 38 had symmetrical four-limb involvement. Affected patients had an average of 5.7 orthopedic procedures performed. By age 5 years, 85% of affected children were ambulatory, although mobility aids were used by a large proportion of them. Most of the children were relatively or completely independent in their activities of daily living. Most were in regular classrooms at the appropriate grade level. Although infants with amyoplasia have pronounced musculoskeletal involvement at birth and require orthopedic and rehabilitative interventions during childhood, the authors concluded that functional outcome in physical and education areas is excellent (Sells et al. 1996). Of note, 11.6% of the children with amyoplasia had anomalies suggesting a vascular compromise in utero, including gastroschisis, bowel atresia, or abdominal-wall defects.

Carlson et al. (1985) identified a different population of 52 patients who were at least 16 years old with arthrogryposis. The mean age was 27.3 years (range, 17 to 42 years). Although these patients had limitation in shoulder motion they had no significant functional handicaps despite the presence of elbow deformities. Fifty-two percent had wrist deformities, and approximately half of them were not treated. Fifteen of 27 patients with wrist deformities had serial casts and splints, and 7 required subsequent surgical correction. Following carpectomy or wrist fusions patients had no pain and had satisfactory wrist function. Seventy-one percent of the 52 patients had knee involvement and 85% had foot involvement, mainly club foot. Twenty-six patients required surgery and an average of 4.9 procedures on each foot. Fifty-six percent of patients had hip problems but functioned well as adults. The majority of patients had normal intelligence and 50% of adults were married. In this mixed population of patients with arthrogryposis, half walked independently, 9 walked with crutches or other mobility aids and only 8 were nonambulatory. Most of the patients had no limitations in their activities of daily living.

▶ GENETICS AND RECURRENCE RISK

The recurrence risk for arthrogryposis depends on the underlying cause for the condition. Amyoplasia is sporadic with little or no recurrence risk. Distal arthrogryposis type I is an autosomal dominant condition with a 50% risk of recurrence. The gene for distal arthrogryposis type I has been mapped to the pericentromeric region of chromosome 9 (Bamshad et al. 1994). The Scandinavian form of lethal congenital contracture syndrome is an autosomal recessive condition with a 25% risk of recurrence (Vuopala and Herva 1994).

There is an increased incidence of club feet, dislocated hips, and hyperextensibility in children with multiple contractures (Hall 1981). Hall (1986) personally studied a group of over 350 children with congenital contractures. Twenty-eight percent of these cases had a known recognizable genetic disorder caused by a single-gene, chromosomal, or multifactorial condition. Six percent were the result of an environmental insult or exposure to a teratogen. Forty-six percent of cases had known diagnoses (such as amyoplasia) with no risk of recurrence. In only 20% of cases there was no diagnosis made. In situations where there was no diagnosis or cause for the arthrogryposis, Hall stratified the recurrence risk. If the limbs are primarily affected, there is a recurrence risk of 4.7%. If the limbs are affected in addition to other malformations, there is a recurrence risk of 1.4%. If the limbs and the central nervous system are both affected, there is a recurrence risk of 7%. However, Hall cautioned that these numbers should be used only if a specific diagnosis has not been made for the index case with arthrogryposis.

REFERENCES

Ajayi RA, Keen CE, Knott PD. Ultrasound diagnosis of the Pena Shokeir phenotype at 14 weeks of pregnancy. Prenat Diagn 1995;15:762–764.

Bamshad M, Watkins WS, Zenger RK, et al. A gene for distal arthrogryposis type I maps to the pericentromeric region of chromosome 9. Am J Hum Genet 1994;55:1153–1158.

Baty BJ, Cubberley D, Morris C, Carey J. Prenatal diagnosis of distal arthrogryposis. Am J Med Genet 1988;29:501–510.

Bianchi DW, Van Marter LJ. An approach to ventilator dependent neonates with arthrogryposis. Pediatrics 1994;94:682–686.

Börglen L, Amiel J, Viollet L, et al. Survival motor neuron gene deletion in the arthrogryposis multiplex congenita-spinal muscular atrophy association. J Clin Invest 1996;98:1130–1132.

Bromley B, Benacerraf B. Abnormalities of the hands and feet in the fetus: sonographic findings. AJR Am J Roentgenol 1995;165:1239–1243.

Carlson WO, Speck GJ, Vicari V, Wenger DR. Arthrogryposis multiplex congenita. Clin Orthop Relat Res 1985;194:115–123.

Chassevent J, Sauvegrain J, Besson-Leaud M, Kalifa G. Myotonic dystrophy (Steinert's disease) in the neonate. Radiology 1978;127:747–749.

Clarren SK, Hall JG. Neuropathologic findings in the spinal cords of 10 infants with arthrogryposis. J. Neurol Sci 1983;58:89–102.

Davis JE, Kalousek DK. Fetal akinesia deformation sequence in previable fetuses. Am J Med Genet 1988;29:77–87.

Deschamps F, Teot L, Benninfield N, Humeau C. Ultrasonography of the normal and abnormal antenatal development of the upper limb. Ann Hand Surg 1992;11:389–400.

Goldberg JD, Chervenak A, Lipman RA, Berkowitz RL. Antenatal sonographic diagnosis of arthrogryposis multiplex congenita. Prenat Diagn 1986;6:45–49.

Hageman G, Ippel EPF, Beemer FA, dePater JM, Lindhout D, Willemse J. The diagnostic management of newborns with congenital contractures: a nosologic study of 75 cases. Am J Med Genet 1988;30:883–904.

Hall JG. An approach to congenital contractures (arthrogryposis). Pediatr Ann 1981;10:15–26.

Hall JG. Arthrogryposis associated with unsuccessful attempts at termination of pregnancy. Am J Med Genet 1996;63:293–300.

Hall JG. Genetics aspects of arthrogryposis. Clin Orthop Relat Res 1985;194:44–53.

Herva R, Conradi NG, Kalimo H, Leisti J, Sourander P. A syndrome of multiple congenital contractures: neuropathological analysis on five fatal cases. Am J Med Genet 1988;29:67–76.

Kirkinen P, Herva R, Leisti J. Early prenatal diagnosis of a lethal syndrome of multiple congenital contractures. Prenat Diagn 1987;7:189–196.

Moessinger AC. Fetal akinesia deformation sequence in an animal model. Pediatrics 1983;72:857–863.

Sarwark JF, MacEwen GD, Scott CI. Current concepts review: amyoplasia (a common form of arthrogryposis). J Bone Joint Surg Am 1990;72:465–469.

Sells JM, Jaffe KM, Hall JG. Amyoplasia, the most common type of arthrogryposis: the potential for good outcome. Pediatrics 1996;97:225–231.

Sepulveda W, Stagiannis KD, Cox PM, Wigglesworth JS, Fisk NM. Prenatal findings in generalized amyoplasia. Prenat Diagn 1995;15:660–664.

Shapiro F, Specht L. The diagnosis and orthopaedic treatment of childhood spinal muscular atrophy, peripheral neuropathy, Friedreich ataxia, and arthrogryposis. J Bone Joint Surg Am 1993;75:1699–1714.

Solund K, Sonne-Holm S, Kjolbye JE. Talectomy for equinovarus and deformity in arthrogryposis: a 12 (2-20) year review of 17 feet. Acta Orthop Scand 1991;62:372–374.

Stern WG. Arthrogryposis multiplex congenita. J Am Med Assn 1923;81:1507.

Stoll C, Ehret-Mentre MC, Treisser A, Tranchant C. Prenatal diagnosis of congenital myasthenia with arthrogryposis in a myasthenic mother. Prenat Diagn 1991;11:17–22.

Swinyard CA, Bleck EE. The etiology of arthrogryposis (multiple congenital contractures). Clin Orthop Relat Res 1985;194:15–29.

Thomas B, Schopler S, Wood W, Oppenheim WL. The knee in arthrogryposis. Clin Orthop Relat Res 1985;194:87–92.

Thompson GH, Bilenker RM. Comprehensive management of arthrogryposis multiplex congenita. Clin Orthop Relat Res 1985;194:6–14.

Vuopala K, Herva R. Lethal congenital contracture syndrome: further delineation and genetic aspects. J Med Genet 1994;31:521–527.

Williams P. The management of arthrogryposis. Orthop Clin North Am 1978;9:67–89.

Wynne-Davies R, Lloyd-Roberts GC. Arthrogryposis multiplex congenita: search for prenatal factors in 66 sporadic cases. Arch Dis Child 1976;51:618–623.

CHAPTER 103
Clinodactyly

► **CONDITION**

The term clinodactyly derives from the two Greek words—*kleinin,* meaning "to bend," and *dactylos,* which means "finger." Clinodactyly is a descriptive term that refers to incurving or medial deviation of the finger at the distal interphalangeal joint (Fig. 103-1). The fifth finger is most frequently affected. Usually, this is due to wedging of the middle phalanx so that the planes of the proximal and distal ends are not parallel but converge toward the radial side (Birkbeck 1975). There have been several attempts to provide an objective definition of clinodactyly. In one approach, clinodactyly is defined as the relationship between the length of the

fifth middle phalanx to the length of the fourth middle phalanx (Birkbeck 1975). Other authors have used an angle of greater than 8 degrees between the long axis of the distal phalanx and the middle phalanx (Birkbeck 1975). Yet other groups use a more stringent definition and use a distal phalanx deviation of at least 15 degrees (Skvarilova and Smahel 1984).

Clinodactyly is frequently accompanied by brachymesophalangy, which means that the middle phalanx of the fifth finger is short and has increased breadth.

Clinodactyly may be isolated or part of a syndrome. It may be a sporadic developmental event or it may be familial (Poznanski et al. 1969). Approximately 60% of newborns with Down syndrome have bilateral fifth

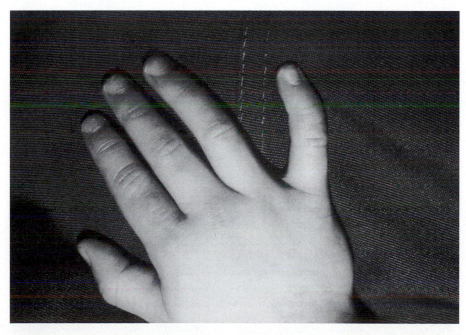

Figure 103-1. Photograph of a child's hand demonstrating medial incurving of the fifth finger consistent with a clinical diagnosis of clinodactyly.

finger clinodactyly (Hall 1970). The association between clinodactyly and Down syndrome has been known for over 100 years. In 1896 Smith published the first roentgenogram illustrating fifth finger clinodactyly in a patient with Down syndrome (Smith 1896).

► INCIDENCE

Several large population studies have addressed the incidence of clinodactyly in healthy infants and children. In Czechoslovakia, Skvarilova and Smahel (1984) studied 911 healthy children from Prague, age 6 to 18 years. They defined clinodactyly as the presence of any distal phalanx axis deviation of greater than 15 degrees on clinical examination. Affected children underwent radiography and the hands of their immediate family members were examined. Clinodactyly of the fifth finger was seen in 10 individuals (1.1%). Of these, 6 individuals also had brachymesophalangy. In 9 of the 10 affected cases at least one parent was confirmed as being similarly affected. In the remaining case, the father was unavailable for examination. Affected children had considerable bilateral symmetry. The ratio of boys to girls affected was 6:4. The incidence of clinodactyly in approximately 1% of the normal population was confirmed in a study of healthy white newborns, in which clinodactyly of the fifth finger was seen in 0.99% of cases (Marden et al. 1964). Poznanski and colleagues (1969) have noted significant racial and ethnic differences in fifth finger clinodactyly. For example, they cite an incidence of 3.4% in a Guatemalan population and an incidence of 5% in a population from Hong Kong. Clinodactyly is not an anomaly, per se, but rather a developmental delay or arrest. Mehes (1973) reported that 0.5% of normal full-term Hungarian newborns had

clinodactyly, but that this percentage increased to 0.9% in full-term small-for-gestational-age infants. This study also noted an increased incidence of clinodactyly in preterm infants at less than 25 weeks of gestation, in which the incidence was 2.56%.

► SONOGRAPHIC FINDINGS

Although ossification of the middle phalanx of the fifth finger occurs normally early during the second trimester of pregnancy, the major concern when fifth-finger clinodactyly is detected on a prenatal sonogram is its potential association with trisomy 21 (Deren et al. 1998). In one study of ultrasound markers of chromosomal disease, 3 of 21 cases of Down syndrome had postmortem or postnatal findings of fifth-finger clinodactyly (Twining and Zuccollo 1993).

In 1988, Benacerraf et al. demonstrated hypoplasia of the middle phalanx of the fifth digit in four of five fetuses with Down syndrome examined at 17 to 20 weeks of gestation. They described a radial curve to the fifth digit. One of the 5 affected fetuses had no visible ossification of the middle phalanx of the fifth digit (Fig. 103-2). These authors suggested that fifth-finger clinodactyly could be used in addition to other sonographic signs in screening for trisomy 21. This observation was followed by a prospective study examining the middle phalanx of the fourth and fifth digits in 1032 fetuses between 15 and 20 weeks of gestation prior to routine genetic amniocentesis (Benacerraf et al. 1990). These authors constructed a ratio of the middle phalanx of the fifth digit divided by the middle phalanx of the fourth digit and obtained a median value for normal fetuses of 0.85. In eight fetuses with trisomy 21, the median ratio was 0.59. These authors suggested a cut-

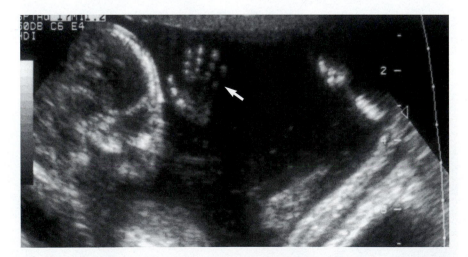

Figure 103-2. Prenatal sonographic image demonstrating absent ossification of the middle phalanx of the fifth finger (arrow) with radial incurving, suggesting a diagnosis of clinodactyly.

off value of 0.70, which would identify 75% of the Down syndrome fetuses and 18% of normal fetuses at the same gestational age. This gave a positive predictive value of this finding of 3.2%. These authors noted that the ratio appeared to rise slightly between 15 and 16 weeks of gestation and at greater than 17.5 weeks of gestation in normal fetuses, implying that the ratios would be affected by normal developmental maturation of this bone. Ossification of the middle phalanx was completely absent in 65 (6.3%) of normal fetuses, although 50% of these fetuses were between 15 and 16 weeks of gestation. Thus, ossification of the middle phalanx of the fifth finger is a gradual process that is not normally complete at 15 weeks of gestation. This has also been confirmed by other investigators (Birkbeck 1975). The conclusion of this report was that measurement of the middle phalanx of the fourth and fifth digits may be useful as an adjunct to sonographic screening for Down syndrome (Benacerraf et al. 1990).

More recently, Deren et al. (1998) examined whether the detection of subtle sonographic abnormalities, including clinodactyly, improved screening efficiency for fetal trisomy 21. Clinodactyly alone had a 28.6% detection rate. Clinodactyly, when seen in association with increased nuchal thickness or short humerus, increased the detection rate of trisomy 21 from 53.3% to 63.2%.

▶ DIFFERENTIAL DIAGNOSIS

Clinodactyly has been observed in 1% of normal individuals. Therefore, the most likely diagnosis is a normal fetus. However, the finding should elicit some concern, as clinodactyly is a component of many genetic syndromes, including Down syndrome (clinodactyly observed in 60% of cases), Russell–Silver dwarfism (76% of cases), Cornelia de Lange syndrome (88% of cases), Klinefelter syndrome (84% of cases), oto-palatal-digital syndrome, oro-facial-digital syndrome, oculo-dento-digital syndrome, Holt–Oram syndrome, Prader–Willi syndrome, and Turner syndrome, (Poznanski et al. 1969). Many of these syndromes will be characterized by the presence of additional anomalies or a chromosomal abnormality.

▶ ANTENATAL NATURAL HISTORY

Birkbeck (1975) examined radiographs of the silver-stained hand bones of 210 human fetuses obtained between 8 and 20 weeks of gestation. In 179 (85%) of fetuses studied, clinodactyly of the fifth finger was demonstrated. He suggested that clinodactyly and brachymesophalangy of the fifth finger were both normal developmental stages that diminished with advancing age and bone development. He demonstrated that

a normal transition occurs from the characteristic wedge shape of the middle phalanx of the fifth finger to the more typical postnatal form with a series of radiographs taken at different gestational age intervals.

Thus, demonstration of clinodactyly and brachymesophalangy in the fetus after 16 weeks of gestation should be considered examples of subtle developmental delays and not malformations.

▶ MANAGEMENT OF PREGNANCY

The documentation of fifth-finger clinodactyly mandates that a targeted fetal sonographic scan should be performed to screen for additional anomalies typical of Down syndrome, including increased nuchal membrane, cystic hygroma, atrioventricular canal defect of the heart, duodenal atresia, polyhydramnios, and an increased gap between the first and second toes (see Chapter 134). We do not advocate karyotyping for isolated fifth-finger clinodactyly, especially if both parents have been examined and at least one has fifth-finger clinodactyly. In the setting of the fifth-finger clinodactyly and an additional fetal anomaly, we would recommend obtaining a prenatal chromosome analysis, as there are many reports in the literature of abnormal karyotypes associated with these findings.

▶ FETAL INTERVENTION

There are no fetal interventions for clinodactyly.

▶ TREATMENT OF THE NEWBORN

No treatment is required for isolated fifth-finger clinodactyly. However, a thorough physical examination of the newborn is indicated to elicit subtle anomalies that may have been missed on the prenatal sonographic examination. If not examined prior to their infant's birth, an attempt should be made to examine the hands of both parents. If a hand of one of the parents demonstrates clinodactyly on physical examination, radiographic studies are not necessary. Parental hand films might be helpful to detect subtle abnormalities of the phalanges.

▶ SURGICAL TREATMENT

For most cases of fifth-finger clinodactyly, there is no indication for surgical treatment. However, rare case reports exist in which the clinodactyly has been treated surgically (Godunova 1982). In most of these case reports, additional hand anomalies, such as the absence

of th
a m

▶ L

For i
pect
seld

▶ G

For a
ter 1
gene
varia
Skva
featu
agno
synd
of cl
fifth-
and

REF

Benac
   mic
   9:3
Benac
   den

CHAPTER 105

Ectrodactyly

► CONDITION

The term ectrodactyly derives from the Greek *ektroma,* meaning "abortion," and *daktylos,* meaning "finger." Ectrodactyly is a human developmental malformation that consists of missing digits, a deep median cleft, and fusion of remaining digits, all of which result in claw-like extremities (Scherer et al. 1994). A central ray defect is the hallmark of the split-hand and split-foot malformation. This deformity was first reported in the medical literature in 1575, when Ambroise Paré described a 9-year-old boy with a right split hand and an absence deformity of the long bones of the legs (cited in Temtamy and McKusick 1978) (Fig. 105-1). The split hand/split

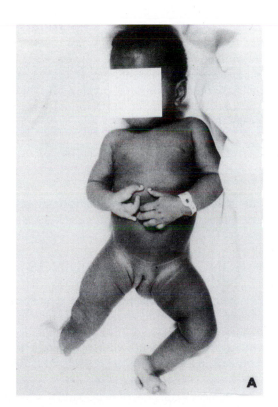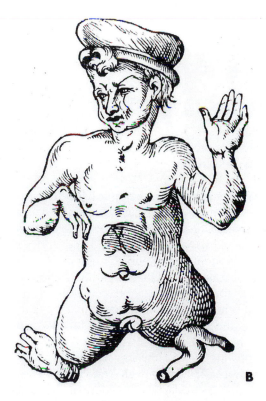

Figure 105-1. Similarities occurring between two cases of split hand/split foot malformation in cases separated by four centuries. (A) Affected infant with ectrodactyly of the right hand. (B) Nine-year-old affected boy described by Ambroise Paré in 1575. *(Reprinted, with permission, from Temtamy S, McKusick V. The genetics of hand malformations. New York: Liss, 1978. Copyright 1978 Alan R. Liss. Reprinted, by permission, of John Wiley and Sons, Inc.)*

▶ **TABLE 105-1.** CLINICAL FEATURES OF THE ECTRODACTYLY SYNDROMES

Condition	Mode of Inheritance	Ectrodactyly	Ecto-dermal Dysplasia	Cleft Lip/ Palate	Tear-Duct Abnormality	Genito-urinary Abnormality	Hearing Loss	Dysmor-phic Facies
EEC	autosomal dominant	+	+	+	+	+	+	+
EE	autosomal dominant	+	+		+			
ECP	autosomal dominant	+		+				
E-HL	autosomal dominant	+					+	
LADD	autosomal dominant	+	+		+			
ADULT	autosomal dominant	+	+		+			
Goltz–Gorlin	X-linked dominant			+	+	+	+	

For definitions of abbreviations, see text

Source: Scherer SW, Poorkaj P, Massa H, et al. Physical mapping of the split hand/split foot locus on chromosome 7 and implication in syndromic ectrodactyly. Hum Mol Genet 1994;3:1345–1354.

foot malformation has been classified into two subtypes. In type I, there is an absence of the central ray of either the hand or the foot, with syndactyly occurring between fingers or toes on each side of the cleft. These abnormalities result in an appearance that is similar to a lobster's claw. In type II ectrodactyly, only one digit, usually the fifth, is present. This is known as the monodactyly subtype of ectrodactyly (Temtamy and McKusick 1978). Although these subclassifications are helpful because they are descriptive, they do not reflect distinct genetic entities.

Although the common usage of the term ectrodactyly is as a descriptive term for the split hand or foot malformation, the term was actually first used in 1832 by St. Hilaire to denote "absence of fingers." According to Temtamy and McKusick (1978), ectrodactyly refers to a specific hand deformity with a partial or total absence of the distal segments of the hand, and normal proximal segments. In this broader definition, ectrodactyly may involve certain phalanges (aphalangia), only the digits (adactylia), or the full hand (acheiria). More recently, it has become clear that ectrodactyly occurs in two clinical settings: the split hand/foot malformation, a single-gene defect that is transmitted as an autosomal dominant disorder in families; and the syndromic ectrodactylies that include split hand and split foot as one component of a group of anomalies. It has therefore been recommended that the nomenclature for split hand/split foot syndromes be changed to split hand/foot malformation to emphasize the fact that a malformation is the developmental cause for the disorder (Nunes et al. 1995).

The syndromic ectrodactylies encompass many different conditions. The most well known of these is the EEC syndrome (ectrodactyly, ectodermal dysplasia, cleft lip and palate). In the EEC syndrome, the ectodermal dysplasia is manifested by lightly pigmented, sparse and wiry hair, a decreased number of hairs in the eyelashes and eyebrows, hypopigmented skin with numerous pigmented nevi in the head and neck

region, abnormalities of the primary and permanent teeth, including hypoplasia of the enamel, severe caries, brittle or dystrophic nails, atretic lacrimal puncta, a decrease or absence of the orifices of the meibomian glands, and corneal vascularization and scarring, which results in limitation of visual acuity or functional blindness (Bystrom et al. 1975). A conductive sensorineural hearing loss may be a complication of the cleft palate seen in EEC syndrome (Anneren et al. 1991). In one large study of 123 affected patients, 100% had ectodermal dysplasia, 84% had tear-duct anomalies, 83.7% had ectrodactyly, 72.4% had cleft lip and/or palate, 33.3% had genitourinary anomalies, and 14% had deafness (Rodini and Richieri-Costa, 1990). EEC syndrome is characterized by variability in clinical expression. A variety of other disorders overlap the EEC syndrome. These are listed under "Differential Diagnosis" and in Table 105-1.

▶ INCIDENCE

The incidence of split hand malformation is 1 in 90,000 live births (Temtamy and McKusick 1978).

▶ SONOGRAPHIC FINDINGS

Relatively few reports exist in the prenatal diagnosis literature that describe the sonographic findings for fetuses with ectrodactyly. The characteristic sonographic findings are the absence of the central digits of the hand with normal or enlarged digits at the lateral aspects (Fig. 105-2) (Leung et al. 1995).

Prenatal diagnosis of ectrodactyly was first reported in 1980, when a fetus was studied at 16 and 19 weeks of gestation and was noted to have one hand with syndactyly and both feet with lobster-claw deformities. This diagnosis occurred in the setting of a father known to be affected with ectrodactyly. These parents elected to

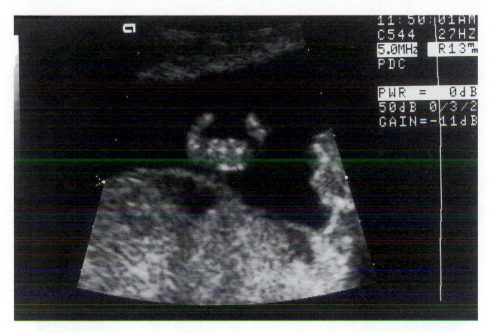

Figure 105-2. Prenatal sonographic image of a fetal hand with ectrodactyly. Note the absence of central digits.

terminate the pregnancy. Examination following termination confirmed bilateral syndactyly of the third and fourth fingers and bilateral lobster-claw deformities of the feet (Henrion et al. 1980). Kohler and colleagues (1989) described the detection of a 30-week appropriate-for-gestational-age male fetus with cleft palate, syndactyly, and lobster-claw deformity and no family history of ectrodactyly. More recently, transvaginal sonography has also been used to diagnose bilateral cleft lip with lobster-claw deformities of the hands and feet in a fetus with an apparently negative family history at 14 weeks of gestation (Fig. 105-3). Posttermination studies confirmed the diagnosis of EEC syndrome. The mother was a 24-year-old, healthy woman who had sonography performed as an anatomic screen without a specific clinical indication. After diagnosis of EEC syndrome in this fetus, the mother was more closely examined and was found to have microdontia of two lateral upper incisors. This was not apparent initially because cosmetic dental work had been preformed. The authors suggested that the dental anomalies could represent an extremely mild form of EEC syndrome. She was advised to have her next pregnancy followed by transvaginal sonography from the 10th week of gestation onward, when fetal fingers and toes can be visualized (Bronshtein and Gershoni-Baruch 1993).

▶ DIFFERENTIAL DIAGNOSIS

The main consideration in the prenatal diagnosis of ectrodactyly is the distinction between the split hand and foot malformation, inherited as a single-gene autosomal dominant disorder, versus the syndromic ectrodactylies. Some of the clinical features of the various ectrodactyly syndromes are described in Table 105-1. As stated earlier, EEC syndrome is characterized by ectrodactyly, ectodermal dysplasia, cleft lip and palate, nasolacrimal-duct abnormalities, genitourinary abnormalities, hearing loss, and a mildly dysmorphic facies. The EE syndrome (Wallis 1988) is a distinct autosomal dominant disorder that manifests as ectrodactyly and ectodermal dysplasia. Wallis (1988) described six members of a four-generation Mauritian family with ectrodactyly and ectodermal dysplasia but no evidence of cleft lip and/or palate, no abnormalities in the nasolacrimal ducts or sac, and no abnormalities of the scalp. Similarly, families have been described with ectrodactyly and cleft lip (ECP syndrome) but no evidence of ectodermal dysplasia. To further confuse matters, there is another autosomal dominant disorder that presents as ectrodactyly and absent or hypoplastic long bones of the extremities (Genuardi et al. 1990; Hoyme et al. 1987). In this latter condition, approximately 68% of patients have hand malformations and 64% have foot malformations. The associated defects observed in affected kindreds include craniosynostosis, a bifid xiphoid process, and kidney stones. The other abnormalities characteristic of EEC syndrome are not observed in this unique disorder. Patients have also been described with ectrodactyly and hearing loss (E-HL syndrome). The lacrimo-auriculo-dental-digital syndrome (LADD) is characterized by tear-duct abnormalities, nasolacrimal-duct obstruction, ear anomalies, deafness, small and peg-shaped teeth

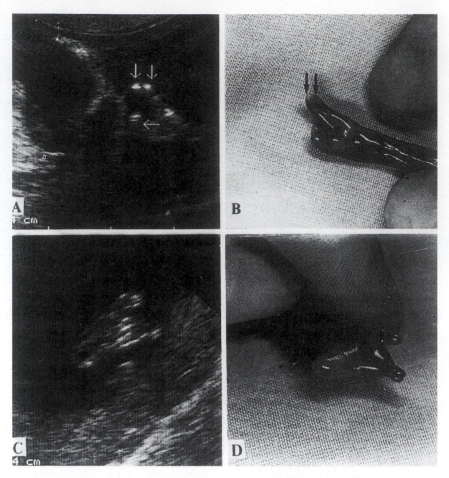

Figure 105-3. Corresponding transvaginal sonographic and pathologic views at 14 weeks of gestation of the fetal hand, demonstrating absent digits and synphalangism (panels A and B) and the fetal foot, showing absent digits and split foot malformation (panels C and D). *(Reprinted, with permission, from Bronshtein M, Gershoni-Baruch R. Prenatal transvaginal diagnosis of the ectrodactyly, ectodermal dysplasia, cleft palate (EEC) syndrome. Prenat Diagn 1993;13:519–522. Copyright 1993 John Wiley and Sons. Reprinted, by permission, of John Wiley and Sons, Inc.)*

with hypoplastic enamel, and renal anomalies. These patients are distinguished from patients with EEC by the lack of characteristic lobster-claw deformities (Rodini and Richieri-Costa, 1990). The acro-dermato-ungual-lacrimal-tooth (ADULT) syndrome is another dominantly inherited disorder characterized by hypodontia, early loss of permanent teeth due to weak fixation, ectrodactyly, obstruction of the tear ducts, onychodysplasia, and excessive freckling (Propping and Zerres 1993). In this unique disorder, intelligence is normal and skin pigmentation with sun exposure is normal. Patients have some overlap with EEC syndrome. In Goltz–Gorlin syndrome, affected patients are female. This disorder is inherited as an X-linked dominant condition with lethality in males. Affected patients have ectodermal dysplasia, facial clefts, limb abnormalities, (but not typically ectrodactyly), tear-duct and genitourinary abnormalities,

and hearing loss. These patient also typically exhibit growth and neuropsychomotor delay, which is not a characteristic of EEC syndrome or the split hand and foot malformation. In patients with Goltz–Gorlin syndrome, the presence of characteristic focal dermal hypoplasia facilitates the diagnosis (Rodini et al. 1992).

A newly appreciated genetic disorder, limb mammary syndrome, consists of mammary hypoplasia, ectrodactyly, and other anomalies (van Bokhoven et al. 1999).

▶ ANTENATAL NATURAL HISTORY

Little is known about the antenatal natural history of the ectrodactyly syndromes. Pregnancy loss is not a characteristic feature of these syndromes.

▶ MANAGEMENT OF PREGNANCY

Fetuses ascertained to have ectrodactyly on a prenatal sonographic examination should be referred to a perinatal center capable of performing a complete anatomic study. Particular attention should be paid to the diagnosis of cleft lip and/or palate, genitourinary abnormalities, and other anatomic defects. Once ectrodactyly has been diagnosed, it is important to examine both parents and to obtain a complete family history. The ectrodactyly syndromes are characterized by extreme variation in clinical expression. Thus, it is important to be aware of extremely mild manifestations of these disorders. A number of ectrodactyly conditions have been associated with chromosomal abnormalities, particularly involving chromosome 7q22 (McElveen 1995; Naritomi et al. 1993; Scherer et al. 1994). Therefore, prenatal karyotyping is recommended when ectrodactyly is observed in the fetus.

Patients with EEC syndrome have been described with low birth weight and a slightly increased incidence of prematurity (Anneren et al. 1991).

There is no indication for delivery by cesarean section solely for the diagnosis of ectrodactyly. Decisions regarding route of delivery should proceed according to standard obstetrical management. There is no indication for delivery in a tertiary-care center, as many of the malformations characteristic of the ectrodactyly syndromes generally present with symptoms later in life. However, arrangements should be made for postnatal referral to a clinical genetics unit and a plastic surgeon. Infants with severe cleft lip and cleft palate may need to have a feeding team evaluation.

▶ FETAL INTERVENTION

There are no fetal interventions for ectrodactyly.

▶ TREATMENT OF THE NEWBORN

Infants affected with split hand/foot malformation or one of the ectrodactyly syndromes generally do not have difficulty with their cardiopulmonary systems and do not require neonatal resuscitation. A thorough postnatal physical examination is mandatory. Infants diagnosed prenatally with ectrodactyly should have a complete examination of the palate, including the soft palate and the uvula. Given that these infants are at a reasonably high risk for underlying genitourinary abnormalities, we recommend administration of prophylactic antibiotics until renal anatomy can be studied postnatally. In addition, an early audiologic investigation should be performed, as there is also a significant risk of associated hearing loss. For further management of cleft lip and cleft palate, see Chapter 24. If evidence of decreased lacrimal secretion is present, consideration can be given to administration of artificial tears.

▶ SURGICAL TREATMENT

Surgical treatment for affected patients with EEC syndrome includes functional improvement of the hands, repair of cleft lip and/or cleft palate, and removal of lacrimal duct blockage. None of these surgical procedures are performed during the newborn period. Although the hands will never appear normal, the main surgical consideration is the successful establishment of opposition between two digits.

▶ LONG-TERM OUTCOME

Functional impairment of the hands of affected patients with ectrodactyly is not usually a problem, provided that opposition of two digits can be obtained (Buss et al. 1995). Surgical procedures are directed mainly toward closing an exceptionally wide cleft of the hands and separating syndactylous digits. Patients with ectrodactyly also have difficulty finding proper-fitting shoes. For patients with split hand/foot malformation or EEC syndrome, there is little evidence that intelligence is affected. In one study of 24 cases of patients with EEC syndrome, there was no evidence of mental retardation or developmental delay (Buss et al. 1995). In this study, every affected patient attended a normal school and each patient had normal language milestones despite some of them having problems with hearing loss.

The major difficulties associated with EEC syndrome with regard to long-term outcome include visual difficulties resulting from corneal scarring due to meibomian-gland dysfunction and recurrent blepharitis. This latter condition has been ameliorated by operations that improve lacrimal drainage. Orofacial clefting, seen in 14 of 24 patients described with EEC syndrome, may also affect hearing (Buss et al. 1995).

Since the major complications of EEC syndrome are related to repeated infections of the eyes, upper respiratory tract, teeth, and urogenital system, the question has been raised as to whether these patients have an underlying immunodeficiency. In one report, four patients with EEC syndrome were studied and shown to have normal immunoglobulin production, complement activity, and lymphocyte and granulocyte function. These authors concluded that the recurrent infections in EEC syndrome were due to the predisposing anatomic abnormalities and recommended surgical repair of the nasolacrimal duct and extraction of hypoplastic teeth to reduce the frequency of infections (Obel et al. 1993). They also recommended prophylactic use of antibiotics to prevent deafness and ophthalmic sequelae.

▶ GENETICS AND RECURRENCE RISK

The split hand/foot malformation and the ectrodactyly syndromes are characterized by wide variability of clinical expression with occasional nonpenetrance. Autosomal dominant inheritance of ectrodactyly was first suggested in 1908 (Temtamy and McKusick 1978). Families with pedigree evidence of autosomal dominant inheritance have a 50% risk of recurrence.

The autosomal dominant form of split hand/foot malformation was mapped to chromosome 7q21.3-q22.1 by studying multiple patients with cytogenetic rearrangements (Scherer et al. 1994). Naritomi et al. (1993) reported an inverted insertion of 7q22-q34 into chromosome 3q21. These authors suggested that 7q22 was the location for at least one gene associated with ectrodactyly. This report was validated by McElveen et al. (1995), who described a patient with cleft feet, a cleft right hand, seizures, mental retardation, scoliosis and a dysmorphic facies. This patient was shown to have an interstitial deletion of 7q11.23q22 (McElveen et al. 1995). Ectrodactyly is present in 41% of patients who have a deletion of 7q21.2-7q22.1. Based on cytogenetic information, molecular mapping has identified a critical interval of 1.5 megabases of DNA for a locus designated as *SHFM1* (split hand/foot malformation number 1). In six patients with cytogenetic translocations or inversions, breakpoints have been mapped within 700 kilobases of DNA of each other to identify a critical region for the gene (Scherer et al. 1994). Of note, a potential candidate gene for ectrodactyly, *DLX5*, has also been mapped within this region. This gene is called the "distal-less gene," which is critical for limb development in drosophila. It may possibly act through disruption of *cis*-acting regulatory signals or position affects (Scherer et al. 1994).

It is now known that there are at least three separate genetic loci for the split hand/foot malformation. As mentioned above, 7q21.22 is the location of *SHFM1*. On the basis of a single large Pakistani pedigree there is also an X-linked gene that maps to Xq26.1, known as *SHFM2*. Most recently, an additional locus, *SHFM3*, has been identified at chromosome 10q25, on the basis of gene mapping in a stillborn infant with ectrodactyly and other malformations (Nunes et al. 1995). This infant was the product of a father with a known balanced translocation that involved chromosomes 4 and 10, and had monosomy for 4p15.1-4pter and trisomy for 10q25.2-qter. The fact that SHFM is genetically heterogeneous was verified in an additional large fam-

ily transmitting an autosomal dominant form of SHFM and did not show linkage to 7q22 (Nunes et al. 1995).

Families with clear cut evidence of a dominantly inherited form of SHFM should be encouraged to submit blood samples to one of the laboratories investigating the various ectrodactyly genes. If linkage is documented within an individual family, prenatal DNA diagnosis is possible. When the case is isolated or there is no evidence of DNA linkage to one of the previously identified SHFM loci, prenatal diagnosis of ectrodactyly can be performed by sonography starting at 10 weeks using a transvaginal probe.

EEC syndrome is an autosomal dominant disorder that has been mapped to chromosome 3q27. In 9 unrelated families affected with EEC, mutations have been demonstrated in the p63 gene (Celli et al. 1999).

REFERENCES

Anneren G, Andersson T, Lingren PG, Kjartansson S. Ectrodactyly-ectodermal dysplasia-clefting syndrome (EEC): the clinical variation and prenatal diagnosis. Clin Genet 1991; 40:257–262.

Buss PW, Hughes HE, Clarke A. Twenty-four cases of the EEC syndrome: clinical presentation and management. J Med Genet 1995;32:716–723.

Bronshtein M, Gershoni-Baruch R. Prenatal transvaginal diagnosis of the ectrodactyly, ectodermal dysplasia, cleft palate (EEC) syndrome. Prenat Diagn 1993;13: 519–522.

Bystrom EB, Sanger RG, Stewart R. The syndrome of ectrodactyly, ectodermal dysplasia and clefting. J Oral Surg 1975;33:192–198.

Celli J, Duijf P, Hamel BC, et al. Heterozygous germlike mutations in the p53 homolog p63 are the cause of EEC syndrome. Cell 1999;99:143–153.

Genuardi M, Zollino M, Bellussi A, Fuhrmann W, Neri G. Brachy/ectrodactyly and absence or hypoplasia of the fibula: an autosomal dominant condition with low penetrance and variable expressivity. Clin Genet 1990;38: 321–326.

Henrion R, Oury JF, Aubry JP, Aubry MC. Prenatal diagnosis of ectrodactyly. Lancet 1980;2:319.

Hoyme HE, Lyons-Jones K, Nyhan WL, Pauli RM, Robinow M. Autosomal dominant ectrodactyly and absence of long bones of upper or lower limbs: further clinical delineation. J Pediatr 1987;111:538–543.

Kohler R, Sousa P, Santos-Jorge C. Prenatal diagnosis of the ectrodactyly, ectodermal dysplasia, cleft palate (EEC) syndrome. J Ultrasound Med 1989;8:337–339.

Leung KY, MacLauchlan NA, Sepulveda W. Prenatal diagnosis of ectrodactyly: the "lobster-claw" anomaly. Ultrasound Obstet Gynecol 1995;6:443–446.

McElveen C, Carvajal MV, Moscatello D, Towner J, Lacassie Y. Ectrodactyly and proximal/intermediate interstitial deletion 7q. Am J Med Genet 1995;56:1–5.

Naritomi K, Izumikawa Y, Tohma T, Hirayama K. Inverted

insertion of chromosome 7q and ectrodactyly. Am J Med Genet 1993;46:492–493.

Nunes ME, Schutt G, Kapur RP, et al. A second autosomal split hand/split foot locus maps to chromosome 10q24-q25. Hum Mol Genet 1995;4:2165–2170.

Obel N, Hansen B, Black FT. Normal immunological status in four patients with ectrodactyly-ectodermal dysplasia-clefting syndrome (EEC-syndrome). Clin Genet 1993;43:146–149.

Propping P, Zerres K. Adult syndrome: an autosomal dominant disorder with pigment anomalies, ectrodactyly, nail dysplasia, and hypodontia. Am J Med Genet 1993;45:642–648.

Rodini ESO, Nardi A, Guion-Almedia ML, Richieri-Costa A. Ectodermal dyplasia, ectrodactyly, clefting, anophthalmia/microphthalmia, and genitourinary anomalies: nosology of Goltz-Gorlin syndrome versus EEC syndrome. Am J Med Genet 1992;42:276–280.

Rodini ESO, Richieri-Costa A. EEC Syndrome: report on 20 new patients, clinical and genetic considerations. Am J Med Genet 1990;37:42–53.

Scherer SW, Poorkaj P, Massa H, et al. Physical mapping of the split hand/split foot locus on chromosome 7 and implication in syndromic ectrodactyly. Hum Mol Genet 1994;3:1345–1354.

Temtamy S, McKusick V. The genetics of hand malformations. New York: Liss, 1978.

van Bokhoven H, Jung M, et al. Limb mammary syndrome: a new genetic disorder with mammary hypoplasia, ectrodactyly, and other hand/foot anomalies maps to human chromosome 3q27. Am J Hum Genet 1999;64:538–546.

Wallis CE. Ectrodactyly (split-hand/split-foot) and ectodermal dysplasia with normal lip and palate in four generation kindred. Clin Genet 1988;34:252–257.

Weissenbach J, Boncinelli E, Trask B, Tsui L-C, Evans JP. Physical mapping of the split hand/split foot focus on chromosome 7 and implication in syndromic ectrodactyly. Hum Mol Genet 1994;3:1345–1354.

CHAPTER 106

Polydactyly

► CONDITION

Polydactyly is the presence of a hand or a foot with more than five fingers or toes. Although the medical term polydactyly was first ascribed to the Amersterdam physician Theordor Kerckring (Blauth and Olason 1988), the presence of polydactyly was mentioned in the Bible (Nicolai and Schoch 1986). Polydactyly is the most frequent congenital anomaly of the human hand (Tsukurov et al. 1994). Polydactyly is classified as "preaxial," which refers to a duplication of digits on the radial side of the hand and the tibial side of the foot, and "postaxial," in which the extra digits occur on the ulnar and fibular sides of the hand and foot, respectively. The boundary between the preaxial and postaxial segments is somewhat controversial. It has variously been placed between the first and second ray, the middle of the second ray, and the second and third ray (Blauth and Olason 1988). The term preaxial has also been used for polydactyly involving the first ray; axial for rays II, III, and IV; and postaxial for the fifth ray. In general, postaxial polydactyly is more common than preaxial polydactyly (Temtamy and McKusick 1978). Polydactyly has been further subclassified on a descriptive basis. In postaxial polydactyly, type A denotes fully developed extra digits. Type B describes rudimentary extra digits or a pedunculated skin tag that is usually found on the hands and only rarely on the feet. This type is very common among blacks. In preaxial polydactyly, when the thumb is polydactylous it is known as type I, when a triphalangeal thumb is present it is known as type II, when the index finger is polydactylous it is type III, and when polysyndactyly occurs it is known as type IV.

Morphogenetically, the hand and foot malformations can be considered as a process of bifurcation of one or several finger or toe rays in the longitudinal axis progressing from peripheral to central. Segment polar-

ity genes initially identified in Drosophila, such as sonic hedgehog (*SHH*), may eventually be shown to play a critical role in this process.

► INCIDENCE

Notable differences exist in the incidence of polydactyly according to race and gender. In a 1963 study performed in New York City, the incidence of postaxial polydactyly in blacks was 10.7 in 1000 live births, whereas in a comparable white population, the incidence was 1.6 in 1000 live births. In this study, polydactyly was noted to be twice as common in males as in females (Mellin 1963). In general, there is a 1% incidence of postaxial polydactyly of the hand in black individuals. This is inherited as an autosomal dominant trait. There is also a high frequency of postaxial polydactyly in some Latino populations (Orioli 1995). In one Japanese study, preaxial polydactyly has been demonstrated in the hand and postaxial polydactyly in the foot (Masada et al. 1986). Affected females predominated when the foot was involved and males predominated when the hand was involved. In this study of 523 cases, associated anomalies were seen in 5% of patients (Masada et al. 1986). In another Japanese study of 330 feet in 265 patients affected with foot polydactyly, a 10% incidence of positive family history was noted (Watanabe et al. 1992).

► SONOGRAPHIC FINDINGS

The phalanges are identifiable as early as the 13th week of gestation by transabdominal sonographic examination (Figs. 106-1 and 106-2) (Deschamps et al. 1992), and by 11 weeks of gestation by transvaginal scan (Hobbins et al. 1994). The major consideration in the

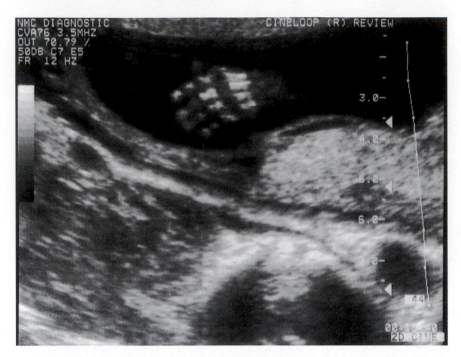

Figure 106-1. Prenatal sonographic image of a fetus with five normal digits. In this image two phalangeal bones are demonstrated in the thumb, whereas the other digits each have three clearly visualized phalangeal bones.

prenatal sonographic examination is to determine whether the polydactyly is isolated. As polydactyly is a component of many genetic syndromes, it especially important to a perform a thorough anatomic survey to look for associated anomalies. Specific associations that should be ruled out include skeletal dysplasia, poly-cystic kidneys, and encephalocele. Once polydactyly is identified it is especially important to note the length of the long bones (Bromley and Benacerraf 1995). Poly-dactyly of the hand is easier to diagnose than that of the foot (Figs. 106-3 and 106-4). A postaxial skin tag can be easily overlooked, whereas a normally formed

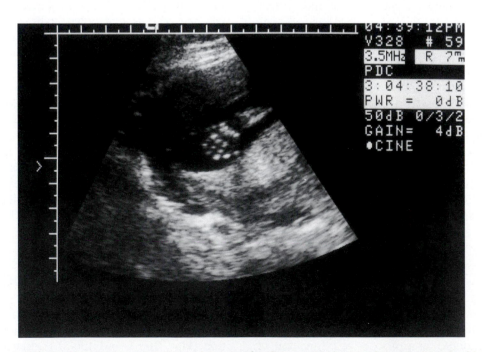

Figure 106-2. Prenatal sonographic image of a fetus with postaxial polydactyly. Note the presence of a single phalanx that appears to be on the ulnar side of the fifth digit.

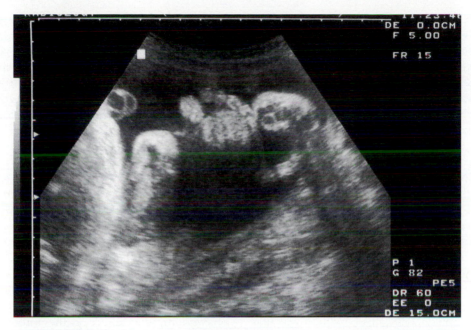

Figure 106-3. Sonographic image of the base of a normal fetal foot indicating the great toe and four additional smaller toes.

extra digit will be more easily visualized. Triphalangeal thumbs are also considered within the diagnostic spectrum of polydactyly.

▶ DIFFERENTIAL DIAGNOSIS

The majority of antenatally diagnosed cases of polydactyly will be isolated and consistent with a normal prognosis in families of African-American descent. The major consideration in the differential diagnosis is to determine whether the condition is isolated and familial or due to a syndrome. Isolated polydactyly is also considered to be a manifestation of the heterozygote (carrier) state for Ellis–van Creveld and Meckel–Gruber syndromes (Goldblatt et al. 1992; Nelson et al. 1994; Wright et al. 1994). Trisomy 13, which manifests as polydactyly in 75% of affected patients (Tsukurov et al. 1994) should

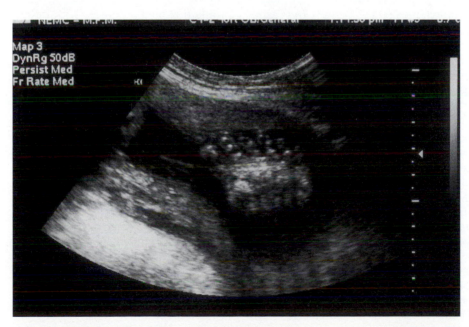

Figure 106-4. Sonographic view of a fetus with polydactyly of the foot, indicating the presence of six well-formed toes.

be ruled out by prenatal karyotyping if additional sonographic abnormalities are present (see Chapter 132). Patients with trisomy 13 have polydactyly, cardiac defects, central nervous system defects including holoprosencephaly, and other major organ abnormalities. If the chromosomes are normal but the fetus is noted to have polydactyly and holoprosencephaly, a possible diagnosis is pseudotrisomy 13, which is inherited as an autosomal recessive condition (Verloes et al. 1991). For patients to receive this diagnosis, the karyotype must be normal and holoprosencephaly must be present with polydactyly or other anomalies. Alternatively, polydactyly with other serious central nervous system defects can be present (Lurie and Wulfsberg 1993). The constellation of brain abnormalities in polydactyly can suggest Meckel–Gruber syndrome, which is also inherited as an autosomal recessive trait (Gershoni-Baruch et al. 1992). Patients with Meckel–Gruber syndrome characteristically have an occipital encephalocele, polycystic kidneys, and polydactyly. This condition was first described in 1822 (Ueda et al. 1987). Isolated polydactyly has been questioned in carriers of the Meckel–Gruber syndrome. Nelson et al. (1994) described a family in which three boys were affected. Their father and paternal first cousin had bilateral postaxial polydactyly, which raised the question of whether they were manifesting heterozygotes. One hundred percent of patients affected with Meckel–Gruber syndrome have cystic renal dysplasia, and 55% of these patients have polydactyly. The constellation of polydactyly, mental retardation, obesity, retinal dystrophy, and hypogonadism suggests the diagnosis of Bardet–Biedel syndrome, which is also inherited as a recessive trait. Bardet–Biedel syndrome is now known to be caused by four independent loci on chromosomes 3, 11, 15, and 16 (Carmi et al. 1995; Leppert et al. 1994). The combination of short-limb dysplasia, thoracic hypoplasia, multiple visceral abnormalities, and polydactyly suggest a diagnosis of short-rib polydactyly syndrome (see Chapter 99). Ellis–van Creveld syndrome (see Chapter 94) presents with polydactyly and a skeletal dysplasia, along with cardiac malformations. If a midline abdominal cyst is seen in association with the polydactyly, the underlying diagnosis could be McKusick–Kaufman syndrome (Chitayat et al. 1987). The findings of preaxial polydactyly and club hands with hypoplastic first metacarpal have been described in DiGeorge syndrome and 22q11 deletion (Fryer 1996; Cormier-Daire et al. 1995). Additional considerations in the differential diagnosis are given in Table 106-1.

▶ ANTENATAL NATURAL HISTORY

The antenatal natural history depends entirely on the underlying associated diagnosis. Isolated polydactyly has no apparent effect on the antenatal natural history. Conditions such as trisomy 13 have a profound effect on the antenatal natural history and may result in miscarriage.

▶ MANAGEMENT OF PREGNANCY

Fetuses in which polydactyly is suspected should be referred to a tertiary-care center capable of detailed fetal anatomic diagnosis. A complete family history should be obtained regarding the occurrence of polydactyly in other family members. Occasionally, parents are unaware of the fact of they have had small digits removed during their own infancy. Both parents should be examined for the presence of scars near both of their little fingers. For fetuses with isolated polydactyly, there is no indication for delivery at a tertiary-care center, especially in light of a positive family history. However,

▶ **TABLE 106-1.** DIFFERENTIAL DIAGNOSIS OF POLYDACTYLY

Condition	Major Associated Findings
Isolated (familial)	None
Trisomy 13	Central nervous system, cardiac, renal anomalies
Pseudotrisomy 13	Holoprosencephaly
Meckel–Gruber syndrome	Encephalocele, renal dysplasia, liver cysts
Bardet–Biedl syndrome	Obesity, mental retardation, hypogenitalism
Short-rib polydactyly syndromes	Skeletal dysplasia
Ellis–van Creveld syndrome	Skeletal dysplasias, cardiac anomalies
Smith–Lemli–Opitz syndrome	Intrauterine growth retardation, holoprosencephaly, ambiguous genitalia
Pallister–Hall syndrome	Midline central nervous system anomalies
McKusick–Kaufman syndrome	Cystic abdominal mass (hydrometrocolpos)
Cephalopolysyndactyly (Greig syndrome)	Craniosynostosis, syndactyly
Holt–Oram syndrome	Cardiac anomalies
DiGeorge syndrome	Cardiac, renal anomalies
Chondrodysplasia punctata (X-linked)	Skeletal, midface anomalies

if the fetus is shown to have associated abnormalities, consideration should be given to delivery in a tertiary-care center, where clinical geneticists are available for syndromic diagnosis. Consideration should be given to performing antenatal karyotyping to specifically rule out trisomy 13. As stated earlier, attention should be paid to length of the long bones, the central nervous system, the heart, and the kidneys, as these are the organs that are abnormal in the major conditions that are associated with polydactyly. For families known to be at risk for a single-gene disorder associated with polydactyly, embryofetoscopy has been performed successfully to diagnose polydactyly (Quintero et al. 1993). In one report, in a family at risk for recurrence for Meckel–Gruber syndrome, postaxial polydactyly was observed on both the hands and feet of a fetus at 10 menstrual weeks (Dumez et al. 1994). In addition, bilateral cystic lesions in the mesonephros and metanephros were visualized. The fingers and toes can be observed as early as 9 weeks of gestation by embryoscopy in fetuses at high risk for an inherited abnormality (Dumez et al. 1994).

▶ FETAL INTERVENTION

There is no fetal intervention for polydactyly.

▶ TREATMENT OF THE NEWBORN

Newborns who are delivered with polydactyly should have a thorough physical examination by a clinical geneticist to rule out associated findings (Figs. 106-5 and 106-6A). If karyotyping has not been performed prenatally, it should be considered at the time of birth to rule out trisomy 13. A case of 22q11 deletion has been associated with polydactyly (Fryer 1996). If evidence of polysyndactyly is present, radiographs may be obtained to document the underlying bony anatomy (see Fig. 106-6). A pediatric orthopedic surgeon should be consulted.

In cases of postaxial polydactyly that consist of a small skin tag, consideration can be given to their removal. Pediatricians are commonly taught to ligate the base of these lesions with suture material as a simple, inexpensive form of removal (Frieden et al. 1995). However, because these supernumerary digits may vary in size and internal contents, consultation with a pediatric orthopedic surgeon may be advisable. Extra digits with a wide pedicle at the base are at increased risk for infection, scarring, or incomplete removal. Frieden et al. (1995) suggest infiltrating the base of the extra digit with a local anesthetic and removing the lesion with sterile iris scissors. They suggest that hemostasis will occur with firm, direct pressure for several minutes, or with

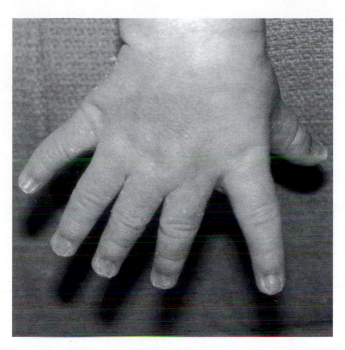

Figure 106-5. Postnatal photograph of a newborn infant at term with six well-formed fingers. This patient has preaxial polydactyly of the index finger (type III). At 3 months of age this infant was diagnosed with Pallister–Hall syndrome.

20% ammonium chloride or ferric subsulfate solution or a silver nitrate stick.

▶ SURGICAL TREATMENT

For well-formed digits that interfere with hand function, consultation with a hand surgeon is advisable. The goal of surgical treatment is to achieve optimal function and as normal an appearance as possible. In one report, Ganley and Lubhan (1995) performed a follow-up study of 21 patients with preaxial polydactyly who were treated between 1979 and 1994. There were 26 thumbs affected. Of their patients, 9 were boys and 12 were girls. Of the 26 thumbs, 6 were treated with ablation alone, 10 were treated with ablation and radial collateral ligament reconstruction and shaving of the metacarpal, 5 thumbs were treated with the Bihaut–Cloquet procedure (see below), and 5 thumbs were treated conservatively with only observation. Of the 6 thumbs treated with ablation alone, 5 required subsequent radial collateral ligament reconstruction. Patients who underwent ablation with ligament reconstruction showed improvement in clinical alignment and stability of the thumbs, but they did not have normal joint motion. The Bilhaut–Cloquet procedure involves removing the middle portions of the two adjoining thumbs; the remaining thumbs are sewn together, resulting in a narrower single digit. Patients who underwent this procedure had

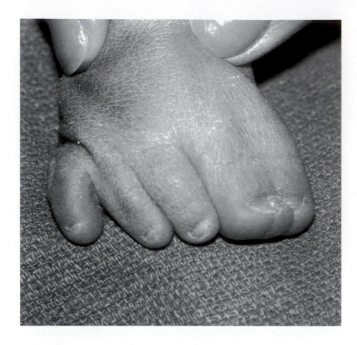

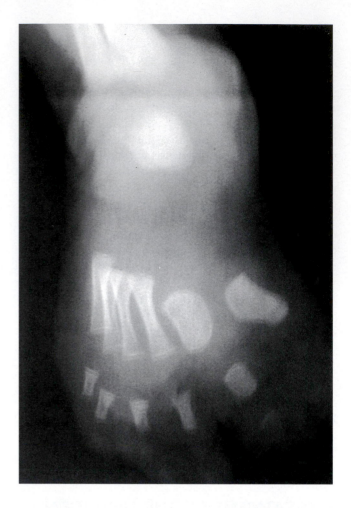

Figure 106-6. (Left) Postnatal photograph of the same infant in Figure 106-5 with polysyndactyly of the toes. (Right) Radiograph of the foot shown in panel A.

improved cosmetic appearance and function, however, they did not have normal joint motion. These authors recommended that ablation be performed only in the context of reconstruction of the radial collateral ligament. They also cautioned that no surgical techniques guarantee ultimately normal joint motion. However, all of their patients were satisfied that the postoperative thumb was significantly improved as compared with their preoperative condition (Ganley and Lubahn 1995).

▶ LONG-TERM OUTCOME

See under "Surgical Treatment."

▶ GENETICS AND RECURRENCE RISK

Patients with isolated postaxial polydactyly generally inherit this trait as an autosomal dominant condition. In one report, Radhakrishna et al. (1993) described a five-generational pedigree of 71 affected members of an Indian family in Gujarat. All affected family members had preaxial polydactyly manifesting as a well-formed, articulated digit of the hand or foot. An addi-

tional 20 family members had triphalageal thumbs or duplication of the great toe. The digital anomalies were isolated. Patients had no other abnormalities, and the polydactyly did not interfere with their work as agricultural laborers. There was no effect of this gene on reproductive fitness. This autosomal dominant gene was manifested by three different phenotypes: preaxial polydactyly, duplication of the thumbs or great toes, and the presence of triphalangeal thumbs.

Several genes responsible for polysyndactyly have been mapped to chromosome 7q36 (Roberts and Tabin 1994; Zguricas et al. 1999). Hing et al. (1995) described a six-generation North American white kindred with preaxial polydactyly; they showed linkage to chromosome 7q36. In addition, genes responsible for polysyndactyly and preaxial polydactyly types II and III have also been mapped to the same region (Tsukurov et al. 1994; Zguricas et al. 1999). Interestingly, both *EN2*, the human homologue of the engrailed gene of Drosophila, which is important for axial patterning, and *SHH*, sonic hedgehog, have been mapped to the same region of the human genome.

Greig cephalopolysyndactyly syndrome is a rare autosomal dominant disorder characterized by craniofacial abnormalities, pre- and post-axial polydactyly, as well as syndactyly of the hands and feet. Point mutations in the human *GLI3* gene, as well as cytogenetic rearrangements of chromosome 7p13 that disrupt the *GLI3* gene, are the underlying basis of this condition (Wild et al. 1997).

The recurrence risk for isolated familial polysyndactyly is 50%. The recurrence risk for many of the associated conditions depends on the specific condition. Many of these conditions are inherited as autosomal recessive genes, which carry a 25% recurrence risk. Trisomy 13 has a 1% recurrence that is independent of maternal age. Prenatal diagnosis is possible as early as 11 weeks of gestation by transvaginal sonography.

REFERENCES

Blauth W, Olason AT. Classification of polydactyly of the hands and feet. Arch Orthop Trauma Surg 1988;107:334–344.

Bromley B, Benacerraf B. Abnormalities of the hands and feet in the fetus: sonographic findings. AJR Am J Roentgenol 1995;165:1239–1243.

Carmi R, Elbedour K, Stone EM, Sheffield VC. Phenotypic differences among patients with Bardet-Biedl syndrome linked to three different chromosome loci. Am J Med Genet 1995;59:199–203.

Chitayat D, Hahm SYE, Marion RW, et al. Further delineation of the McKusick-Kaufman hydrometrocolpos-polydactyly syndrome. Am J Dis Child 1987;141:1133–1136.

Cormier-Daire V, Iserim L, Theophile D, et al. Upper limb malformations in DiGeorge syndrome. Am J Med Genet 1995;56:39–41.

Deschamps F, Teot L, Benningfield N, Humeau C. Ultrasonography of the normal and abnormal antenatal development of the upper limb. Ann Hand Surg 1992;11:389–400.

Dumez Y, Dommergues M, Gubler M-C, et al. Meckel-Gruber syndrome: prenatal diagnosis at 10 menstrual weeks using embryoscopy. Prenat Diagn 1994;14:141–144.

Frieden IJ. Suture ligation of supernumerary digits and 'tags': an outmoded practice? Arch Pediatr Adolesc Med 1995;149:1284.

Fryer A. Monozygotic twins with 22q 11 deletion and discordant phenotype. J Med Genet 1996;33:173.

Ganley TJ, Lubahn JD. Radial polydactyly: an outcome study. Ann Plast Surg 1995;35:86–89.

Gershoni-Baruch R, Nachlieli T, Leibo R, Degani S, Weissman I. Cystic kidney dysplasia and polydactyly in 3 sibs with Bardet-Biedl syndrome. Am J Med Genet 1992;44:269–273.

Goldblatt J, Minutillo C, Pemberton PJ, Hurst J. Ellis-van Creveld syndrome in a Western Australian Aboriginal community. Med J Aust 1992;157:271–272.

Hing AV, Helms C, Slaugh R, et al. Linkage of preaxial polydactyly type 2 to 7q36. Am J Med Genet 1995;58:128–135.

Hobbins JC, Jones OW, Gottesfeld S, Persutte W. Transvaginal ultrasonography and transabdominal embryoscopy in the first-trimester diagnosis of Smith-Lemli-Opitz syndrome, type II. Am J Obstet Gynecol 1994;171:546–549.

Leppert M, Baird L, Anderson KL, Otterud B, Lupski JR, Lewis RA. Bardet-Biedl syndrome is linked to DNA markers on chromosome 11q and is genetically heterogeneous. Nat Genet 1994;7:108–112.

Lurie IW, Wulfsberg EA. "Holoprosencephaly-polydactyly" (pseudotrisomy 13) syndrome: expansion of the phenotypic spectrum. Am J Med Genet 1993;47:405–409.

Masada K, Tsuyuguchi Y, Kawabata H, Kawai H, Tada K, Ono K. Terminal limb congenital malformations: analysis of 523 cases. J Pediatr Orthop 1986;6:340–345.

Mellin GW. The frequency of birth defects. In: Fishbein M, ed. Birth defects. Philadelphia: Lippincott, 1963.

Nelson J, Nevin NC, Hanna EJ. Polydactyly in a carrier of the gene for the Meckel syndrome. Am J Med Genet 1994;53:207–209.

Nicolai J-PA, Schoch SL. Polydactyly in the Bible. J Hand Surg 1986;11A:293.

Orioli IM. Segregation distortion in the offspring of Afro-American fathers with postaxial polydactyly. Am J Hum Genet 1995;56:1207–1211.

Quintero RA, Abuhamad A, Hobbins JC, Mahoney MJ. Transabdominal thin-gauge embryofetoscopy: a technique for early prenatal diagnosis and its use in a case of Meckel-Gruber syndrome. Am J Obstet Gynecol 1993;168:1552–1557.

Radhakrishna U, Multani AS, Solanki JV, Shah VC, Chinoy NJ. Polydactyly: a study of a five-generation Indian family. J Med Genet 1993;30:296–299.

Roberts DJ, Tabin C. The genetics of human limb development. Am J Hum Genet 1994;55:1–6.

Temtamy SA, McKusick VA. Part V: Polydactyly. In: The genetics of hand malformations. New York: Liss, 1978:364–437.

Tsukurov O, Boehmer A, Flynn J, et al. A complex bilateral polysyndactyly disease locus maps to chromosome 7q36. Nat Genet 1994;6:282–286.

Ueda N, Sasaki N, Sugita A, et al. Encephalocele, polycystic kidneys, and polydactyly with other defects: a necropsy case of Meckel syndrome and a review of literature. Acta Pathol Jpn 1987;37:323–330.

Verloes A, Ayme S, Gambarelli D, et al. Holoprosencephaly-polydactyly ('pseudotrisomy 13') syndrome: a syndrome with features of hydrolethalus and Smith-Lemli-Opitz syndromes: a collaborative multicentre study. J Med Genet 1991;28:297–303.

Watanabe H, Fujita S, Oka I. Polydactyly of the foot: an analysis of 265 cases and a morphological classification. Plast Reconstr Surg 1992;89:856–877.

Wild A, Kalff-Suske M, Vortkamp A, Bornholdt D, Konig R, Grzeschik KH. Point mutations in human *GLI3* cause Greig syndrome. Hum Mol Genet 1997;6:1979–1984.

Wright C, Healicon R, English C, Burn J. Meckel syndrome: what are the minimum diagnostic criteria? J Med Genet 1994;31:482–485.

Zguricas J, Heus H, Morales-Peralta E, et al. Clinical and genetic studies on 12 preaxial polydactyly families and refinement of the localization of the gene responsible to a 1.9 cM region on chromosome 7q36. J Med Genet 1999;6:32–40.

CHAPTER 107

Radial Aplasia

► CONDITION

Radial aplasia is one manifestation of a spectrum of anomalies known as radial ray malformations. These may occur unilaterally or bilaterally, and either as isolated malformations or in association with other birth defects (Fig. 107-1). In radial aplasia, the defect occurs on the preaxial side of the forearm. Skeletal findings in radial ray malformations may include absence or hypoplasia of the radius, with associated absence or hypoplasia of the scaphoid and trapezium bones of the wrist, with or without first metacarpal and thumb abnormalities (Brons et al. 1990; Lamb 1972).

Radial aplasia results from arrest of radial longitudinal development, which may be secondary to damage at the apical ectoderm of the limb bud occurring between 6 and 12 weeks of gestation. One hypothesis regarding its cause is that radial aplasia may result from abnormal blood-vessel development, which causes an abnormal gradient of nutrients important for the differentiation of mesenchyme into bone or muscle (Van Allen et al. 1982). In radial aplasia, bones as well as associated muscles, nerves, and joints may be affected. Other causes for the developmental arrest of the radius include maternal infectious agents and local biochemical abnormalities secondary to maternal diabetes or medication.

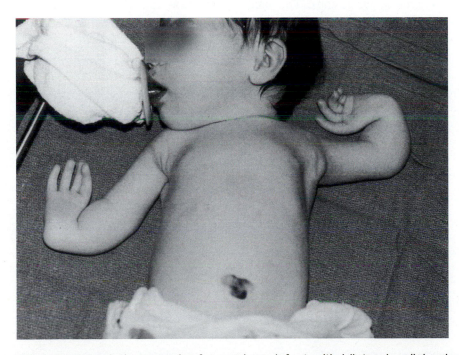

Figure 107-1. Postnatal photograph of a newborn infant with bilateral radial aplasia and absent thumbs.

In many cases, a correlation exists between the specific type of radial deformity and associated hematologic abnormalities (Bay and Levine 1988). For example, absence of the radius with presence of the thumb affects the platelets and is a characteristic finding in the thrombocytopenia–absent radius (TAR) syndrome. If both the radius and thumb are absent, the hematologic findings are more severe; aplastic anemia generally results (Bay and Levine 1988).

▶ INCIDENCE

The incidence of radial aplasia is approximately 1 in 30,000 live births (Brons et al. 1990; Sofer et al. 1983). The condition is bilateral in approximately 50% of cases (Bay and Levine 1988).

▶ SONOGRAPHIC FINDINGS

In radial aplasia, a single fetal forearm bone is identified, with acute radial deviation of the hand (Fig. 107-2). The single forearm bone can be identified as an ulna by comparison with standard tables of ulnar lengths (Ylagan and Budorick 1994). Published standards exist for normal humeral, radial, and ulnar bone lengths at different points in gestation (Jeanty et al. 1985). The examination of the fetal extremities is not listed in the American Institute of Ultrasound in Medicine (AIUM) guidelines for standard obstetric sonography. However, examination of the extremities is critically important in the diagnosis of many genetic syndromes. The fetal

limb buds may be seen sonographically as early as 8 weeks of gestation, with the limb articulations and digits becoming visible by 11 to 12 weeks of gestation (Bromley and Benacerraf 1995).

The diagnosis of radial aplasia may be made as early as 14 to 15 weeks of gestation by noting the absence of the radius and the hand in varus position. Prolonged observation of the fetus will reveal that malposition of the hand persists during the entire sonographic examination. When the fetus moves its arms, the hand remains flexed but not rigid (Deschamps et al. 1992).

In one report, Meizner et al. (1986) described the prenatal diagnosis of an affected fetus with absence of the radius and thumb at 18 weeks of gestation. They noted shortening and bowing of the ulna. The fetal hands were clubbed and deviated laterally. An additional finding included crossed renal ectopy of the right kidney. The family history was notable for an affected father and sibling (Meizner et al. 1986; Sofer et al. 1983). In a retrospective study of seven affected fetuses and infants with radial aplasia diagnosed during the perinatal period at the University Hospitals of Amsterdam and Rotterdam, six affected patients were noted to have associated abnormalities of the central nervous system, gastrointestinal tract, kidneys, or heart (Brons et al. 1990). Three of these affected fetuses had trisomy 18. A high degree of perinatal lethality was noted in this report; however, there may have been bias of ascertainment. These authors recommended both longitudinal visualization and transverse scanning of the bones of the extremities to clearly delineate the ulna from the radius. They recommended that the best time for visualization and separate measurements of the radius and

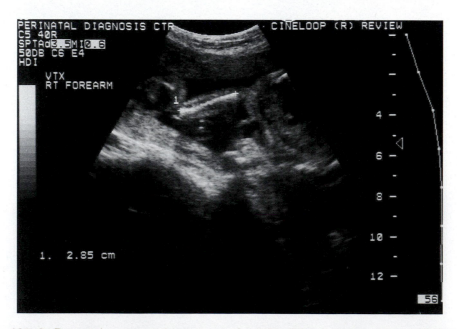

Figure 107-2. Prenatal sonographic image of a fetal right forearm, demonstrating the presence of a single bone, the ulna.

ulna was approximately 13 to 16 weeks of gestation. Many of the cases in this report were complicated by abnormalities in amniotic fluid, including both oligohydramnios and polyhydramnios. These authors emphasized, however, that special attention should be paid to the central nervous system, heart, kidneys, vertebral column, and monitoring of fetal growth.

▶ DIFFERENTIAL DIAGNOSIS

The differential diagnosis for conditions associated with radial aplasia is listed in Table 107-1. The conditions comprise four different categories: single-gene disorders,

multiple congenital anomaly syndromes of unknown or sporadic cause, chromosomal abnormalities, and teratogen exposures. The most common chromosomal abnormality associated with radial aplasia is trisomy 18, although radial abnormalities are generally uncommon in trisomy 18 (Sepulveda et al. 1995). More commonly, a shortened radial ray is present. Although many authors list trisomy 13 as potentially being associated with radial aplasia, this is not the most commonly observed skeletal abnormality in trisomy 13. Trisomy 13 is much more commonly characterized by polydactyly (see Chapters 106 and 132). In one report, a case of mosaic trisomy 22 was associated with radial aplasia (Dulitzky et al. 1981). In another case report, a translocation

▶ **TABLE 107-1.** DIFFERENTIAL DIAGNOSIS OF RADIAL APLASIA

Condition	Associated Findings in Addition to Radial Aplasia	Mode of Inheritance
Single-gene disorders		
Holt–Oram syndrome	Cardiac abnormalities	Autosomal Dominant
Acrorenal syndrome	Crossed renal ectopy, single kidney, ear malformations	Autosomal Dominant
Acrofacial dysostosis (Nager type)	Malar and mandibular hypoplasia, deafness, coloboma of lower eyelids	Autosomal Dominant
IVIC (oculo-oto-radial syndrome)	Hearing impairment, external ophthalmoplegia, thrombocytopenia, urogenital anomalies	Autosomal Recessive
Fanconi anemia	Pancytopenia, microcephaly, hyperpigmentation, increased chromosome breakage	Autosomal Recessive
Thrombocytopenia–absent radius (TAR)	Thrombocytopenia	Autosomal Recessive
Aase syndrome	Cleft lip and/or palate, hypoplastic anemia	Autosomal Recessive
Baller–Gerold syndrome	Carniosynostosis, short stature	Autosomal Recessive
RAPADILINO syndrome	Absent patellae, dislocated joints, diarrhea, short stature, long nose	Autosomal Recessive
Roberts syndrome	Cardiac anomalies, cleft lip and/or palate, tetraphocomelia	Autosomal Recessive
Seckel syndrome	Dwarfism, microcephaly, mental retardation, prominent nose	Autosomal Recessive
Multiple anomalies, unknown cause		
VACTERL association	Vertebral, anal, cardiac, tracheo-esophageal, renal, and limb defects	Sporadic
Cornelia de Lange syndrome	Dwarfism, microcephaly, synophrys	Unknown
Poland anomaly	Breast and chest wall deformities on affected side	Vascular accident
Lacrimo-auriculo-dental-digital syndrome (LADD)	Lacrimal duct stenosis, cupped external ear, dental anomalies	Unknown
Chromosomal abnormalities		
Trisomy 18	Intrauterine growth restriction, micrognathia, cardiac anomalies, clenched hand	Chromosomal
Trisomy 13	Polydactyly, central nervous system abnormalites, cardiac and renal abnormalities	Chromosomal
Mosaic trisomy 22	Ectopic kidney, mental retardation	Post-meiosis nondisjunction
46,XY,t(1 : 7)(q42;p15)	Wilms' tumor	Chromosomal (familial)
Teratogen exposure		
Valproic acid	Neural-tube defects, vertebral and cardiac abnormalities	Environmental
Thalidomide	Tetraphocomelia	Environmental

occurring between chromosomes 1 and 7 was associated with the presence of Wilms tumor and bilateral radial aplasia (Hewitt et al. 1991).

With regard to maternal teratogen exposure, valproic acid is of the most concern (Verloes et al. 1990). Valproic acid is the most effective antiepileptic drug for simple petit mal seizures, which is the most commonly occurring type of epilepsy in women of childbearing age. Unfortunately, valproic acid is associated with a higher prevalence of fetal anomalies than other antiepileptic agents (Ylagan and Budorick 1993). The risk of neural-tube defects with valproic acid exposure during pregnancy is on the order of 1 to 2%. Valproic acid crosses the placenta, and the fetal serum concentration is greater than the maternal serum concentration. Limb anomalies have been reported in 47 to 65% of mothers exposed to valproic acid. These figures, however, include even minor abnormalities of the nails such as hypoplasia (Ylagan and Budorick 1994).

Several disorders characterized by autosomal dominant patterns of inheritance are associated with radial ray malformations. These include Holt–Oram syndrome, the acrorenal syndrome, and acrofacial dysostosis (Nager type) (see Table 107-1). A complete family history is essential for any fetus diagnosed with radial ray aplasia. Many of the autosomal recessive conditions associated with radial aplasia are also associated with hematologic disturbances. The major disorders in this category include Fanconi anemia, thrombocytopenia–absent radius (TAR) syndrome, and Aase syndrome. In the TAR syndrome, thrombocytopenia results in symptomatic bleeding in more than 90% of affected cases during the first 6 months of life (Adeyokunnu 1984; Bhargava et al. 1972; O'Flanagan et al. 1989). Cordocentesis results documenting a thrombocytopenia will diagnose this condition (Boute et al. 1996; Shelton et al. 1999). The Baller–Gerold syndrome is distinguishable by the hallmark findings of craniosynostosis, short stature, and radial aplasia. In this condition, cases are divisible into two groups: those who do not have additional malformations and those who have a broad range of additional abnormalities. In Baller–Gerold syndrome, the chromosomes are normal and most patients are intellectually normal (Anyane-Yeboa et al. 1980; Boudreaux et al. 1990; Feingold et al. 1979; Galea and Tolmie 1990; Greitzer et al. 1974). The acronym RAPADILINO stands for radial aplasia, patella absent, diarrhea, dislocated joints, little size/limb malformations, nose long, normal intelligence. To date, affected patients have been of Finnish ancestry (Kaariainen et al. 1989).

The finding of associated vertebral, cardiac, renal, or tracheoesophageal abnormalities may also lead to a presumed diagnosis of VACTERL association (Tongsong et al. 1999).

▶ ANTENATAL NATURAL HISTORY

At 6 weeks of gestation, the upper limb buds are recognized by small bumps on the lateral side of the embryo's body. Embryonic mesenchyme induces a thickening of the covering ectoderm. This ectoderm secondarily induces mesenchymal differentiation. The proximal segment of the limb bud develops first (Deschamps et al. 1992). At 7 weeks the limb buds first become visible sonographically (Bromley and Benacerraf 1995). At 8 weeks, the distal limb buds flatten to become the hand and foot plates. The limbs subsequently develop and flex. Development of the upper limb occurs approximately 2 days ahead of the lower limbs (Bromley and Benacerraf 1995). By 9 weeks the fetal forearms can raise progressively above the shoulder level. The hands are often observed to cover the mouth and nose. At this point, however, sonographic differentiation of the digits is still not possible (Deschamps et al. 1992). At 10 weeks of gestation, posterior rotation of the upper limb occurs, and for the first time, individual digits can be identified. At 12 weeks, primary ossification centers of the long bones are present. By 14 weeks of gestation, the whole hand is fully formed and one can observe full movements of the fetal arm, including abduction, flexion, scratching, and movements toward the mouth. By 15 weeks of gestation, differentiation of the carpal bones is possible and individual phalanges are identifiable (Deschamps et al. 1992).

Any disruption in the process of limb development occurring between 6 and 12 weeks of gestation will result in a limb defect (Bay and Levine 1988). Vascular differentiation may have a role in this process. The radial artery is the last major vessel of the arm to appear, at 39 days of embryonic life. The radial bone develops later than the ulna. The difference in timing may contribute to the increased frequency of radial versus ulnar defects observed in humans (Van Allen et al. 1982). Vasculogenesis precedes differentiation of the mesenchyme into muscle and bone. The formation of arteries does not require the presence of bone. Van Allen and colleagues (1982) described three different patterns of vascular abnormalities in spontaneously miscarried fetuses with radial aplasia. In type 1 cases, a single midline superficial vessel was observed, with no radial or ulnar artery. This pattern of malformation was characteristic of fetuses with acardia (see Chapter 118). In type 2 cases, absence of the radial artery was seen with or without persistence of the median artery. Other vessels were within normal limits. This pattern was observed in fetuses with multiple malformations of unknown cause. In type 3 cases, the radial artery was present but had an abnormal course. All other vessels were normal. This pattern was characteristic of TAR syndrome. These authors hypothesized that the morphogenesis of the entire limb was determined by a previously established pattern of blood vessels. They hypothesized that radial aplasia may be the result of abnormal vessel development. The early capillaries form a three-dimensional network that gives the appearance of a humerus, radius, and ulna even before chondrogenesis ensues. The existing vasculature establishes gradients that are important in the determination of mesenchymal differentiation into bone or muscle. Therefore, it is not unreasonable to imply that abnormalities in vessel development will have important consequences for subsequent bone and muscle development.

In one case, a fetus with radial ray aplasia was described in a mother with a petit mal seizure disorder who took valproic acid from 2 to 8 menstrual weeks. After 8 weeks, when it was determined that she was pregnant, her therapy was changed to carbamazepine for the remainder of the pregnancy (Ylagan and Budorick 1994). Multidrug therapy has been noted to be a primary factor associated with an increased incidence of malformations in offspring of women with epilepsy (Delgado-Escueta and Janz 1992).

▶ FETAL INTERVENTION

There are no fetal interventions for radial aplasia.

▶ MANAGEMENT OF PREGNANCY

Fetuses in which radial aplasia is ascertained need to have a detailed anatomic survey to specifically delineate the presence of other anatomic abnormalities. Areas of concern include the central nervous system, heart, vertebral column, gastrointestinal system, and kidneys. A complete family history should be obtained, ideally by a genetic counselor, to specifically rule out consanguinity, which may predispose the fetus to an autosomal recessive disorder. The parents should be examined for subtle malformations such as ear abnormalities (present in the acrorenal syndrome) or minor, clinically subtle hand abnormalities that may occur in the Holt–Oram syndrome. A history of teratogen exposure should be obtained from the mother, specifically with regard to valproic acid treatment during the pregnancy. Maternal diabetes should be ruled out. An amniocentesis should be performed to study the fetal karyotype. The most likely underlying chromosomal abnormality is trisomy 18. If Fanconi anemia is a consideration, karyotyping should be performed, with specific documentation of the presence of chromosomal breaks and the formation of quadriradial figures. To rule out Fanconi anemia, the chromosomes must also be studied after exposure to the clastogenic agent diepoxybutane. This is best per-

formed by a specialty laboratory with experience in the prenatal diagnosis of Fanconi anemia.

In the setting of a positive family history for TAR syndrome, or to rule out associated hematologic abnormalities, consideration should be given to cordocentesis. Cordocentesis can provide both chromosome analysis and diagnosis of hematologic abnormalities. It is potentially useful in ruling out thrombocytopenia or early signs of aplastic anemia, such as an increased mean corpuscular volume for gestational age.

Consideration should be given to delivery of the infant by cesarean section because of the presence of bilateral flexion contractures at the elbow, which might result in dystocia. Delivery is recommended at a tertiary-care center to permit early consultation with experts in clinical genetics, orthopedic surgery, and pediatric radiology.

▶ TREATMENT OF THE NEWBORN

A complete physical examination is essential at birth. The newborn should be evaluated by individuals with experience in clinical genetics, pediatric orthopedic surgery, pediatric hematology, and pediatric radiology. Confirmatory skeletal radiography of the extremities

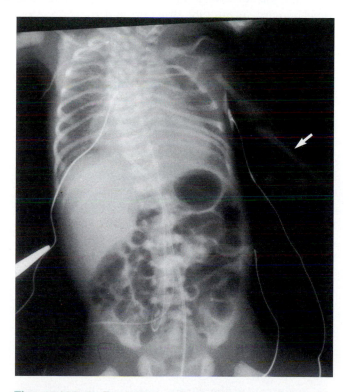

Figure 107-3. Postnatal radiograph of an infant with VATER association. Note the presence of vertebral malformations. The arrow indicates a single left forearm bone with clubbed hand.

should be performed (Fig. 107-3). If a chromosome analysis was not performed prenatally, full-scale banded karyotyping with observation for chromosome breaks and a diepoxybutane study should be performed. A complete blood count with a differential and platelet counts should also be obtained to rule out Fanconi anemia and TAR and Aase syndromes. A subtle manifestation of aplastic anemia during the newborn period is an increased elevation in the mean cellular volume as compared with normal neonates.

▶ SURGICAL TREATMENT

The child with radial aplasia will have displacement of the wrists and hand to the radial side of the ulna, producing a characteristic deformity (see Fig. 107-1). This is initially correctable with manipulation by casts or by splinting. The soft tissues of the wrists can be tight and contracted on the radial side. This is generally due to the presence of a strong, fibrous band that replaces the absent radius. With subsequent long-bone growth, bowing of the ulna increases. Therefore, splinting is an essential part of the early treatment of radial aplasia (Lamb 1972). The two digits on the ulnar side of the hand are almost always normal in appearance and function. The two digits on the radial side of the hand usually have some impairment in joint structure and function. Most affected children prefer to use the ulnar two digits for prehension (Lamb 1972).

Surgical treatment depends on whether the affected patient has unilateral or bilateral radial aplasia. If the case is unilateral, the normal arm will be the functional one and the affected arm will serve only as an aid. In this case, the major goal is to improve the appearance of the affected arm. Functional outcome is a secondary consideration. In bilateral cases, the goal is to improve function to permit independent living. In general, treatment begins during the newborn period and operative intervention occurs within the first year of life. All therapies are designed to improve mobility, strength, and stability of the forearm and wrist, and to improve the dexterity of the hand and fingers (Bay and Levine 1988). The four basic principles of treatment are (Lamb 1972):

1. Prevent soft-tissue contractures by short casts or by creating splints for the patient to wear at night
2. Excise the fibrous band that causes radial contractures
3. Centralize the carpus over the ulna. This produces wrist stability with a limited range of wrist movement
4. Pollicize the index finger

▶ LONG-TERM OUTCOME

In one report, 10 patients were described with congenital anomalies of the radius diagnosed at birth. None of the cases were isolated . Two of the patients had TAR syndrome, 1 had VACTERL association, 1 had Holt–Oram syndrome, and 1 had Poland anomaly. All patients had concomitant abnormalities of the ulna. Four patients had associated congenital cardiac disease. Three patients had vertebral defects and 2 had abnormalities of the sacrum. Seven of the 10 cases were bilateral. Three patients had a positive family history and 2 were infants of diabetic mothers. Of the 10 patients, 5 required surgery: 3 had centralization of the carpus over the ulna, 1 had pollicization of the index finger, and 1 had local reconstructive hand surgery. In all 5 cases, the limb function improved to some degree (Bay and Levine 1988).

▶ GENETICS AND RECURRENCE RISK

The genetics and recurrence risk of radial aplasia depends on the underlying condition responsible for this bony abnormality. If a chromosomal abnormality was diagnosed, the recurrence risk for a condition such as trisomy 18 will be the maternal age-related risk or 1%, whichever is greater. If an unbalanced chromosomal abnormality was diagnosed, both parents need to be studied to determine whether a parental translocation was responsible for the unbalanced situation in the offspring. If a single-gene disorder was diagnosed, the recurrence risk will be 25 or 50%, depending on whether the condition is inherited as an autosomal recessive or autosomal dominant condition, respectively (see Table 107-1). The VACTERL association is considered to be sporadic, with a negligible recurrence risk. If maternal valproic acid exposure has been determined to be the underlying cause for the radial aplasia, consideration should be given to stopping the antiepileptic medication prior to conception after consultation with a neurologist. If necessary, medication can be restarted during the second trimester.

In the event that the fetus or infant dies from associated malformations, a perinatal autopsy is strongly recommended to determine the underlying diagnosis.

REFERENCES

Adeyokunnu AA. Radial aplasia and amegakaryocytic thrombocytopenia (TAR syndrome) among Nigerian children. Am J Dis Child 1984;138:346–348.

Anyane-Yeboa K, Gunning L, Bloom AD. Baller-Gerold syndrome craniosynostosis—radial aplasia syndrome. Clin Genet 1980;17:161–166.

Bay K, Levine C. Congenital radial aplasia. Mo Med 1988; 85:87–92.

Bhargava SK, Pal V, Gupta R. Congenital aplasia and hypoplasia of radius. Indian Pediatr 1972;15:599–600.

Boudreaux JM, Colon MA, Lorusso GD, Parro EA, Pelias MZ. Baller-Gerold syndrome: an 11th case of craniosynostosis and radial aplasia. Am J Med Genet 1990;37:447–450.

Boute O, Depret-Mossser S, Vinatier D, et al. Prenatal diagnosis of thrombocytopenia-absent radius syndrome. Fetal Diagn Ther 1996;11:224–230.

Bromley B, Benacerraf B. Abnormalities of the hands and feet in the fetus: sonographic findings. AJR Am J Roentgenol 1995;165:1239–1243.

Brons JTJ, van der Harten HJ, Van Geijn HP, et al. Prenatal ultrasonographic diagnosis of radial-ray reduction malformations. Prenat Diagn 1990;10:279–288.

Delgado-Escueta AV, Janz D. Consensus guidelines: preconception counseling, management, and care of the pregnant woman with epilepsy. Neurology 1992;42:149–160.

Deschamps F, Teot L, Benningfield N, Humeau C. Ultrasonography of the normal and abnormal antenatal development of the upper limb. Ann Hand Surg 1992;11:389–400.

Dulitzky F, Shabtai F, Zlotogora J, Halbrecht I, Elian E. Unilateral radial aplasia and trisomy 22 mosaicism. J Med Genet 1981;18:473–476.

Feingold M, Sklower SL, Willner JP, Desnick RH. Craniosynostosis-radial aplasia: Baller-Gerold syndrome. Am J Dis Child 1979;133:1279–1280.

Galea P, Tolmie JL. Normal growth and development in a child with Baller-Gerold syndrome (craniosynostosis and radial aplasia). J Med Genet 1990;27:784–787.

Greitzer LJ, Jones KL, Schnall BS, Smith DW. Craniosynostosis—radial aplasia syndrome. J Pediatr 1974;84:723–724.

Hewitt M, Lunt PW, Oakhill A. Wilms' tumour and a de novo (1;7) translocation in a child with bilateral radial aplasia. J Med Genet 1991;28:411–412.

Jeanty P, Romero R, D'Alton M, Venus I, Hobbins JC. In utero sonographic detection of hand and foot deformities. J Ultrasound Med 1985;4:595–599.

Kaariainen H, Ryoppy S, Norio R. RAPADILINO syndrome with radial and patellar aplasia/hypoplasia as main manifestations. Am J Med Genet 1989;33:346–351.

Lamb DW. The treatment of radial club hand. Hand 1972; 4:22–30.

Meizner I, Bar-Ziv J, Barki Y, Abeliovich D. Prenatal ultrasonic diagnosis of radial-ray aplasia and renal anomalies. Prenat Diagn 1986;6:223–225.

O'Flanagan SJ, Cunningham JM, McManus S, Otridge BW, McManus F. Thrombocytopenia—radial aplasia (TAR) syndrome with associated immune thrombocytopenia. Postgrad Med J 1989;65:485–487.

Sepulveda W, Treadwell MC, Fisk NM. Prenatal detection of preaxial upper limb reduction in trisomy 18. Obstet Gynecol 1995;85:847–850.

Shelton SD, Paulyson K, Kay HH. Prenatal diagnosis of thrombocytopenia absent radius (TAR) syndrome and vaginal delivery. Prenat Diagn 1999;19:54–57.

Sofer S, Bar-Ziv J, Abeliovich D. Radial ray aplasia and renal anomalies in a father and son: a new syndrome. Am J Med Genet 1983;14:151–157.

Tongsong T, Wanapirak C, Piyamongkol W, Sudasana J. Prenatal sonographic diagnosis of VATER association. J Clin Ultrasound 1999;27:378–384.

Van Allen MI, Hoyme HE, Jones KL. Vascular pathogenesis of limb defects. I. Radial artery anatomy in radial aplasia. J Pediatr 1982;101:832–838.

Verloes A, Frikiche A, Gremillet C, et al. Proximal phocomelia and radial ray aplasia in fetal valproic syndrome. Eur J Pediatr 1990;149:266–267.

Ylagan LR, Budorick NE. Radial ray aplasia in utero: a prenatal finding associated with valproic acid exposure. J Ultrasound Med 1994;13:408–411.

CHAPTER 108

Syndactyly

► CONDITION

The term syndactyly comes from the Greek *syn,* meaning together and *daktylos,* meaning finger. It describes an apparent fusion of the digits. Syndactyly can be osseous, which refers to fusion of the bones, or cutaneous, defined as webbing of the skin between two digits. In fetal life, the limb buds may be recognized sonographically as early as 8 weeks of gestation, but the digits become visible only at 11 to 12 weeks (Bromley and Benacerraf 1995). After the 12th week, the hand is fully formed, but separate movements of the digits are not easily observed until 15 weeks of gestation (Deschamps et al. 1992). Absence of digital dissociation implies a diagnosis of syndactyly.

Although mild cutaneous syndactyly, or webbing, of the toes is a common familial trait, it is generally too subtle to be appreciated on a prenatal sonogram. Syndactyly severe enough to interfere with digital movement suggests a more serious pathology, such as one of the acrocephalosyndactyly syndromes. These syndromes are generally associated with abnormalities of the skull shape due to craniosynostosis (Chapter 9).

► INCIDENCE

Mild syndactyly is relatively common. It has an incidence of 1 in 1650 to 1 in 3000 live births (Temtamy and McKusick 1978). Syndactyly severe enough to interfere with fetal digital movement is rare. Triploidy, which is associated with syndactyly, has a incidence of 1 in 10,000 live births. The incidence of Apert syndrome, which includes syndactyly as one component, is 1 in 160,000 live births, but a high neonatal mortality rate results in a 1 in 2 million incidence in the general population (Boog et al. 1999; Finkels et al. 1997; Hill et al. 1987).

► SONOGRAPHIC FINDINGS

Syndactyly is suggested by the inability to distinguish separate digits of the fingers and toes or to demonstrate independent movement of the fingers. Syndactyly is excluded if the fetus splays or interdigitates the fingers (Ginsberg et al. 1994).

Syndactyly may be one component of a syndrome. To make a syndromic diagnosis, the sonographer needs to decide if all four limbs are involved and what associated anomalies are present. Many of the syndromes associated with syndactyly also have synostosis of the cranial sutures. This may appear as acrocephaly, a tall, peaked skull shape with a high forehead, frontal bossing, and a prominent metopic suture.

One of the better known acrocephalosyndactyly syndromes is Apert syndrome. In Apert syndrome, complete syndactyly of the second through fourth digits is present, which leads to the characteristic "mitten-like" hands and feet (Figs. 108-1 and 108-2). This condition also frequently involves the fifth finger. Multiple case reports have appeared in the literature regarding the prenatal sonographic diagnosis of Apert syndrome (Boog et al. 1999; Filkins et al. 1997; Hill et al. 1987; Kim et al. 1986; Narayan and Scott 1991; Parent et al. 1994). The hallmark of the sonographic diagnosis of this condition is that despite prolonged observation, the fetus is never noted to have distinct or separate finger movements. The hands are never seen to open in this condition (Fig. 108-3). In addition, the toes appear fused (Fig. 108-4). Additional abnormalities characteristic of Apert syndrome include polyhydramnios and an acrocephalic calvarium (Hill et al. 1987), ventriculomegaly, partial agenesis of the corpus callosum (Parent et al. 1994), hydrocephalus (Kim et al. 1986), and dysmorphic features, including a high forehead, hypertelorism, and a depressed nasal bridge (Parent et al. 1994). Prenatal sonographic diagnosis of Apert syndrome has been made in both the setting of

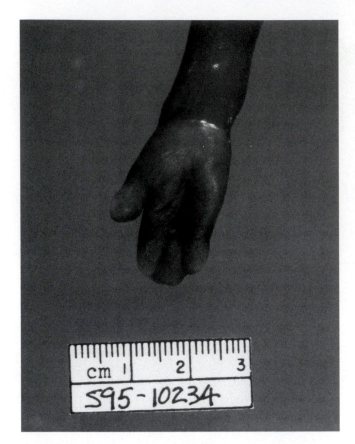

Figure 108-1. Postmortem photograph of a hand from a fetus at 21 weeks of gestation demonstrating the "mitten-like" appearance due to syndactyly of the second, third, and fourth digits. *(Courtesy of Dr. Joseph Semple.)*

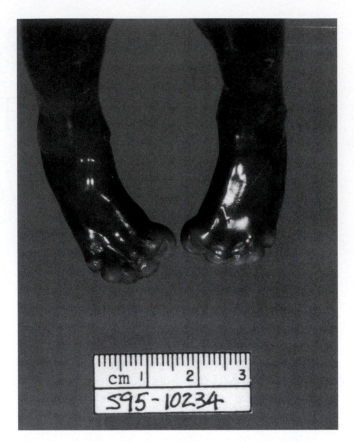

Figure 108-2. Postmortem photograph of the fetus in Figure 108-1 demonstrating syndactyly of all of the toes. The pregnancy was terminated due to a diagnosis of Apert syndrome. *(Courtesy of Dr. Joseph Semple.)*

an affected mother with a fetus at 50% risk for inheriting the condition (Narayan and Scott 1991), as well as in the setting of a negative family history with the disorder presumably due to a spontaneous mutation (Filkins et al. 1997; Hill et al. 1994; Parent et al. 1994).

Prenatal sonographic diagnosis of Carpenter syndrome has been reported in a twin gestation first studied at 17 weeks (Ashby et al. 1994). In this case report, one twin was noted to have club-like fetal hands, with the fingers maintained permanently in a flexed position. At 20 weeks of gestation, an abnormal, diamond-shaped head was noted in the axial plane along with preaxial polydactyly of the feet and duplication of the great toe. The fingers were described as being "pulled together," and they never spread normally, which was noticed easily because the other twin had normal digital movements (Ashby et al. 1994).

▶ DIFFERENTIAL DIAGNOSIS

The differential diagnosis of syndactyly is listed in Table 108-1. Fetuses with triploidy (see Chapter 131) have char-

acteristic, pathognomonic cutaneous syndactyly of the third and fourth digits. Fetuses with triploidy also have second-trimester growth restriction, cystic and/or small placentae, ventriculomegaly, and congenital heart defects (Mittal et al. 1998). The differential diagnosis also includes Apert syndrome (acrocephalosyndactyly type II). Patients with Carpenter syndrome have acrocephaly, with variable synostosis of the sagittal lambdoid, and coronal sutures (see Chapter 9). They also have syndactyly, preaxial polydactyly of the toes, and brachydactyly of the hands and feet with short or absent middle phalanges. One of the difficulties in the prenatal diagnosis of Carpenter syndrome is that marked variability exists even within a family. Pfeiffer syndrome, another acrocephalosyndactyly syndrome, is characterized by craniosynostosis, hydrocephalus, large thumb, and partial cutaneous soft-tissue syndactyly of the hands and feet (Hill and Grzybek 1994). Syndactyly that occurs between the second and third digits is a major manifestation of Smith–Lemli–Opitz syndrome, a recessively inherited disorder of cholesterol metabolism. Fraser syndrome (see Chapter 30) is characterized by cryptophthalmos and syndactyly (Fryns et al. 1997). Patients with Fraser syndrome

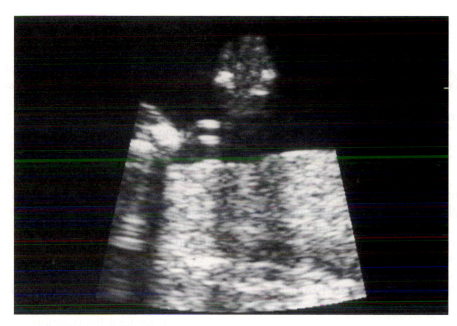

Figure 108-3. Corresponding prenatal sonographic image obtained from the fetus shown in Figures 108-1, showing syndactyly.

also have renal agenesis, laryngeal stenosis or atresia, abnormalities of the ears and external genitalia, and other minor anomalies. Syndactyly is a major feature of Fraser syndrome. It occurs in 77% of patients with this condition (Ramsing et al. 1990). The syndactyly in Fraser syndrome is always cutaneous and most often involves fingers and toes. Its severity may vary from slight interdigital webbing to complete syndactyly. Another consideration in the differential diagnosis of syndactyly is short-rib poly-

dactyly syndrome (SRPS) type II, Majewski (see Chapter 99). In type II SRPS, patients have polysyndactyly, short ribs, cleft lip, and short tibiae (Thomson et al. 1982).

▶ ANTENATAL NATURAL HISTORY

Syndactyly is due to deficiency in the normal pattern of preprogrammed cell death that occurs with the radial

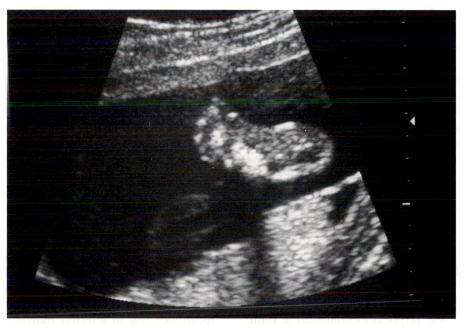

Figure 108-4. Corresponding prenatal sonographic image obtained from the fetus shown in Figure 108-2, showing fusion of the toes.

▶ **TABLE 109-1.** ABNORMALITIES OF THE UMBILICAL CORD

Umbilical cord
 Abnormal length and diameter
 Neoplasms
  Thrombosis
  Hemangioma
  Hematoma
  Teratoma
 Edema
 Distortional abnormalities
  Loops
  Knots
  Torsions
  Twists
Vascular malformations
 Abnormal vessel number
 Abnormal vascular spiraling
 Umbilical-cord varix
 Umbilical-artery aneurysm
 Persistent right umbilical vein
Wharton jelly
 Aberrations in amount
 Mucinous degeneration
Other
 Allantoic-duct cysts
 Omphalomesenteric-duct cysts
 Varix of the umbilical cord
 Urachal cyst
 Omphalocele
 Gastroschisis

Source: Persutte WH, Hobbins J. Single umbilical artery: A clinical enigma in modern prenatal diagnosis. Ultrasound Obstet Gynecol 1995;6:216–229.

include umbilical-artery aneurysm (Siddiqui et al. 1992), umbilical-vein varix (Estroff and Benacerraf 1992; Mahony et al. 1992), and persistent right umbilical vein (Hill et al. 1994; Jeanty 1989). The distance between spirals (helixes) in the umbilical cord can be measured. Normally, this distance is 2 to 2.5 cm. If the distance decreases to less than 2 cm between helixes, acute torsion of the cord is possible (Collins et al. 1993). Umbilical-cord knots are difficult to identify prospectively; as many as 72% of cases are missed on third-trimester color Doppler studies (Sepulveda et al. 1995).

▶ DIFFERENTIAL DIAGNOSIS

The major consideration in the differential diagnosis is to determine if the umbilical-cord abnormality is a false positive finding. Most umbilical-cord abnormalities are descriptive. Sensitivity and specificity of diagnosis can be improved by the use of Doppler studies.

▶ ANTENATAL NATURAL HISTORY

The umbilical cord grows by tension generated by fetal movement; Naeye (1985) has measured umbilical-cord lengths of 35,779 singletons and determined that a length of at least 32 cm is necessary to prevent traction on the cord during a vaginal delivery. The majority of umbilical-cord growth occurs during the first and second trimesters. Walker and Pye (1960) demonstrated that the cord length of premature babies is similar to that

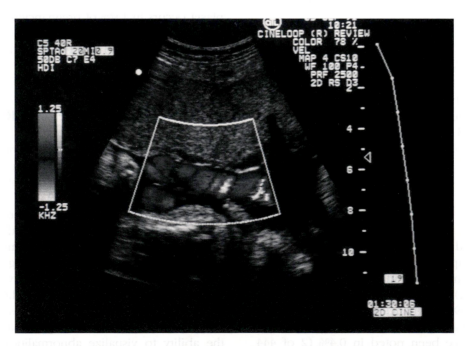

Figure 109-1. Color Doppler velocimetry studies showing the normal coiling of the umbilical cord. See color plate.

of full-term babies. The mean length of a full-term newborn's umbilical cord is 60 cm. There is no correlation between umbilical-cord length and parity, maternal age, maternal weight or height, presence of preeclampsia, or fetal gender, weight, length, or presenting part (Walker and Pye 1960).

Short umbilical cords are significantly associated with low IQ values and neuromuscular abnormalities, such as the fetal akinesia deformation sequence or severe infantile spinal muscular atrophy (Naeye 1985). In infants with trisomy 21, the average cord length is 45 cm; this is almost certainly due to in utero hypotonia, which causes decreased tension to be placed on the cord (Moessinger et al. 1982). Miller et al. (1981) studied infants with a variety of pathologic conditions. They found the most dramatically shortened cords in patients with early evidence of amnion rupture. Restriction of fetal movement was thought to be the effect of tethering by amniotic bands. The lesser degree of cord shortening seen in renal agenesis is presumably due to a later decrease in intrauterine space resulting from oligohydramnios.

Experiments on rat fetuses have confirmed that early oligohydramnios affects the cord length by limiting the intrauterine environment. Conversely, rat fetuses allowed to develop in the maternal abdomen have a cord length that is 147% greater than controls. In addition, rat fetuses whose movements are paralyzed by curare have cord lengths that are 85% of control values (Moessinger et al. 1986; Skupski et al. 1992).

Umbilical vascular coiling is established by the end of the first trimester. A sinistral (counterclockwise) rotation is present in most pregnancies (Fletcher 1993; Strong et al. 1993). The absence of the normal coiling of the umbilical cord has been identified as an antenatal risk factor for perinatal morbidity and mortality. This so-called straight cord may be structurally weaker and more susceptible to external tension (Fig. 109-2) (Strong et al. 1993). Lacro et al. (1987) noted a 10% stillbirth rate in newborns with absent umbilical coiling. In a prospective study, 38 fetuses with noncoiled umbilical vessels were identified. As compared with normal control fetuses, the noncoiled group had a significantly increased incidence of intrauterine death, preterm delivery, repetitive intrapartum fetal heart rate decelerations, operative delivery for fetal distress, meconium staining, and anatomical–karyotypic abnormalities (Strong et al. 1993). Other investigators have calculated an umbilical coiling index by dividing the total number of coils observed by the length of the cord. Subjects with below the 10th percentile and above the 90th are defined as hypocoiled and hypercoiled, respectively. In one study of 635 placentas from deliveries of at least 24 weeks of gestation, Rana et al. (1995) found that subjects with hypocoiled cords had increased rates of fetal heart rate disturbances and interventional delivery.

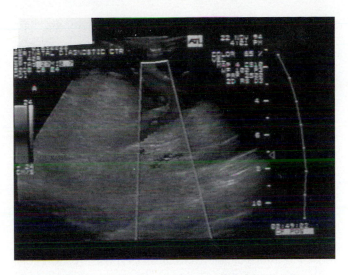

Figure 109-2. Color Doppler velocimetry studies demonstrating a straight umbilical cord. Note the lack of coiling as compared with Figure 109-1. See color plate.

Fetuses with hypercoiled cords had a higher rate of premature delivery as compared with fetuses with normally coiled cords.

To our knowledge, prospective outcome studies related to a sonographic finding of umbilical-cord ulceration have not yet been performed. The finding is described here because of the reported association of umbilical-cord ulceration noted at birth with intestinal atresia in two infants and one stillborn fetus (Bendon et al. 1991). In two of three cases, severe in utero hemorrhage occurred from the ulcers. The intestinal atresia is the primary problem, with umbilical-cord ulceration occurring as a secondary phenomenon. The following hypotheses have been proposed to account for this association: vascular reactivity, gastric reflux, and epithelial abnormalities (Bendon et al. 1991).

In one case report, an infant with four umbilical arteries and one vein was described (Beck and Naulty 1985). The infant had multiple medical problems due to *Escherichia coli* sepsis, but ultimately survived with age-appropriate growth and development. There were no associated anomalies. The patient was shown to have triplication of the right umbilical artery.

Umbilical-artery hypoplasia has been defined as a difference in the diameter between both umbilical arteries of >2 mm (Sepulveda et al. 1992). The umbilical arteries have discordant blood flow velocity waveforms in the absence of associated placental pathology. In one series, two of six affected fetuses with this finding had an adverse perinatal outcome (Dolkart et al. 1992). In another case report with pathologic follow-up of the umbilical cord after birth, no adverse effect was seen (Sepulveda et al. 1992).

Vascular malformations of the umbilical cord, such as umbilical-vein varix and umbilical-artery aneurysm, are extremely rare. Umbilical-artery aneurysm is potentially lethal in utero, due to umbilical venous compression (Siddiqui et al. 1992). Cystic dilatation of the umbilical vein has been variously associated with an increased incidence of in utero death (Mahony et al. 1992) and a normal outcome (Estroff and Benacerraf 1992).

▶ MANAGEMENT OF PREGNANCY

When a short cord is diagnosed, detailed level II sonography is indicated to look for evidence of oligohydramnios, amniotic bands, body-wall defects, neuromuscular abnormalities, and arthrogryposis. A short cord in the setting of abnormalities such as increased nuchal translucency measurement and a decreased femur:foot length ratio may suggest trisomy 21. Fetuses with noncoiled umbilical cords may be at increased risk for aneuploidy. In one study of 48 consecutive live-born neonates with noncoiled umbilical vessels, four cases of trisomy (8.3%) and one case of mosaic trisomy (2.1%) were identified (Strong 1995). However, all of these fetuses had additional anomalies detected with sonography. It is therefore unclear at present whether amniocentesis is indicated for an isolated noncoiled cord. Fetuses with noncoiled umbilical cords are at increased risk for perinatal mortality; antepartum testing and early documentation of fetal lung maturity should be considered. Fetuses with evidence of bowel atresia should be monitored for sonographic findings consistent with umbilical-cord ulceration and resulting hemorrhage. Fetuses with vascular malformations such as umbilical-artery aneurysm may need to be delivered as soon as lung maturity is ensured (Siddiqui et al. 1992). Fetuses with true knots of the umbilical cord ascertained prenatally may need to be delivered by cesarean section.

▶ FETAL INTERVENTION

There are no fetal interventions for umbilical-cord abnormalities.

▶ TREATMENT OF THE NEWBORN

For all of the conditions discussed here, a thorough physical examination of the newborn is indicated. In the setting of the short cord, observation of newborn movements, with particular emphasis on the neurologic examination, is important. Tables of normal values exist for the measurement of periumbilical skin length in the newborn. These standards are useful in the neonatal diagnosis of syndromes that include umbilical dysmorphology (O'Marcaigh et al. 1992).

▶ SURGICAL TREATMENT

There is no surgical treatment indicated for umbilical-cord abnormalities.

▶ LONG-TERM OUTCOME

Follow-up is indicated for associated abnormalities. The isolated umbilical-cord findings do not need follow-up.

▶ GENETICS AND RECURRENCE RISK

None of the conditions discussed, when present as an isolated finding, have implications for familial recurrence.

REFERENCES

Aokio S, Hata T, Ariyuki Y, Makirara K, Hata K, Kitao M. Antenatal diagnosis of aberrant umbilical vessels. Gynecol Obstet Invest 1997;43:232–235.

Beck R, Naulty CM. A human umbilical cord with four arteries. Clin Pediatr 1985;24:118–119.

Bendon RW, Tyson FW, Baldwin VJ, Cashner KA, Mimouni F, Miodovnik M. Umbilical cord ulceration and intestinal atresia: a new association? Am J Obstet Gynecol 1991;164:582–586.

Collins JC, Muller RJ, Collins CL. Prenatal observation of umbilical cord abnormalities: a triple knot and torsion of the umbilical cord. Am J Obstet Gynecol 1993;169:102–104.

Dolkart LA, Reimers FT, Kuonen CA. Discordant umbilical arteries: ultrasonographic and Doppler analysis. Obstet Gynecol 1992;79:59–63.

Estroff JA, Benacerraf BR. Umbilical vein varix: sonographic appearance and postnatal outcome. J Ultrasound Med 1992;11:69–73.

Fletcher S. Chirality in the umbilical cord. Br J Obstet Gynaecol 1993;100:234–236.

Hill LM, Mills A, Peterson C, Boyles D. Persistent right umbilical vein: sonographic detection and subsequent neonatal outcome. Obstet Gynecol 1994;84:923–925.

Jauniaux E, Campbell S, Vyas S. The use of color Doppler imaging for prenatal diagnosis of umbilical cord anomalies: report of three cases. Am J Obstet Gynecol 1989;161:1195–1197.

Jeanty P. Fetal and funicular vascular anomalies: identification with prenatal US. Radiology 1989;173: 367–370.

Lacro RV, Jones KL, Benirschke K. The umbilical cord twist: origin, direction, and relevance. Am J Obstet Gynecol 1987;157:833–838.

Mahony BS, McGahan JP, Nyberg DA, Reisner DP. Varix of the fetal intra-abdominal umbilical vein: comparison with normal. J Ultrasound Med 1992;11:73–76.

Miller ME, Higginbottom M, Smith DW. Short umbilical cord: Its origin and relevance. Pediatrics 1981;67: 618–621.

Moessinger AC, Blanc WA, Marone PA, Polsen DC. Umbilical cord length as an index of fetal activity: experimental study and clinical implications. Pediatr Res 1982;16: 109–112.

Moessinger AC, Mills JL, Harley EE, et al. Umbilical cord length in Down syndrome. Am J Dis Child 1986;140: 1276–1277.

Naeye RL. Umbilical cord length: clinical significance. J Pediatr 1985;107:278–281.

O'Marcaigh AS, Folz LB, Michels VV. Umbilical morphology: normal values for neonatal periumbilical skin length. Pediatrics 1992;90:47–49.

Persutte WH, Hobbins J. Single umbilical artery: a clinical enigma in modern prenatal diagnosis. Ultrasound Obstet Gynecol 1995;6:216–229.

Rana J, Ebert GA, Kappy KA. Adverse perinatal outcome in patients with an abnormal umbilical coiling index. Obstet Gynecol 1995;85:573–577.

Sepulveda W, Addis JR. Romero R, Greb AE, Jacques SM, Qureshi F. Umbilical artery hypoplasia. Fetus 1992;3:9–12.

Sepulveda W, Shennan AH, Bower S, Nicolaidis P, Fisk NM. True knot of the umbilical cord: a difficult prenatal ultrasonographic diagnosis. Ultrasound Obstet Gynecol 1995; 5:106–108.

Siddiqui TA, Bendon R, Schultz DM, Miodovnik M. Umbilical artery aneurysm: prenatal diagnosis and management. Obstet Gynecol 1992;80:530–533.

Skupski D, Bond A, Kogut E, Chervenak F. Umbilical cord, short. Fetus 1992;2:1–2.

Strong TH. Trisomy among fetuses with noncoiled umbilical blood vessels. J Reprod Med 1995;40:789–790.

Strong TH Jr, Elliott SP, Radin TG. Non-coiled umbilical blood vessels: a new marker for the fetus at risk. Obstet Gynecol 1993;81:409–411.

Walker CW, Pye BG. The length of the human umbilical cord: a statistical report. BMJ 1960;1:546.

CHAPTER 110

Single Umbilical Artery (SUA)

► CONDITION

The normal umbilical cord consists of three vessels—two arteries and one vein (Fig. 110-1). Single umbilical artery (SUA) refers to the congenital absence of one of the arteries. The condition was originally described by Vesalius in 1543, Fallopio in 1561, and by Bauhin in 1621 (Persutte and Hobbins 1995). The first prenatal diagnosis of SUA was made in 1980 (Jassani et al. 1980). SUA is one of the most common malformations found in humans.

► INCIDENCE

In prospective studies of live-born infants, the incidence of SUA varied from 344 in 39,773 (0.9%) to 782 in 372,066 (0.48%) births in the United States National Collaborative Perinatal Project and a Swedish registry, respectively (Froelich and Fujikura 1973; Lilja 1991). The incidence was twofold to threefold higher in a survey of spontaneous abortuses (Byrne and Blanc 1985). In most studies, the gender distribution is equal. In the National Collaborative Perinatal Project, SUA was noted in 1.2% of white infants and 0.5% of black infants (Froelich and Fujikura 1973). SUA occurs three to four times more frequently among twins than among singletons (Heifetz 1984). Other conditions associated with SUA include maternal diabetes, epilepsy, hypertension, antepartum hemorrhage, polyhydramnios, and oligohydramnios (Persutte and Hobbins 1995).

► SONOGRAPHIC FINDINGS

The normal umbilical cord contains two arteries and one vein (see Fig. 110-1). SUA is easiest to demonstrate

in cross-sectional images (Fig. 110-2) but may also be visualized longitudinally (Fig. 110-3). Diagnosis prior to 20 weeks of gestation may be difficult because of the small size of the cord. Fetuses with SUA have an increased diameter of the umbilical artery with no changes of the umbilical vein (Sepulveda et al. 1996b). Color flow Doppler techniques have greatly enhanced the ability to both visualize the umbilical cord (Catanzarite et al. 1995; Jauniaux et al. 1989); and measure its flow velocity waveforms (Sepulveda et al. 1996a; Ulm et al. 1997). Fetal umbilical arteries should be examined near the bifurcation of the aorta with color Doppler if available (see Fig. 110-3). The intrafetal portion of the umbilical arteries may be easier to visualize than the free-floating cord. A single umbilical artery may have a diameter that approaches that of the umbilical vein. Diagnosis of SUA by sonography has a sensitivity of 64.9%, a specificity of 99.9%, and a positive predictive value of 64.9% (Jones et al. 1993).

► DIFFERENTIAL DIAGNOSIS

Nonvisualized second umbilical artery should be ruled out. False positive diagnoses are more likely to occur before 22 weeks of gestation.

► ANTENATAL NATURAL HISTORY

The umbilical arteries develop from the allantois, a diverticulum of the yolk sac. Between 3 and 5 weeks of gestation, a transient common umbilical artery is normally present in all embryos, replacing a plexus of arteries around the allantois. Subsequently, the common umbilical artery becomes shorter, and right and left umbilical arteries advance within the body stalk

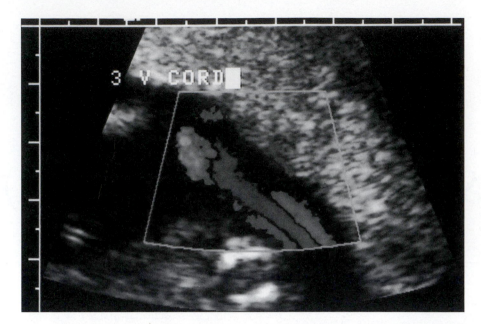

Figure 110-1. Color Doppler study demonstrating the presence of two umbilical arteries and one umbilical vein. See color plate.

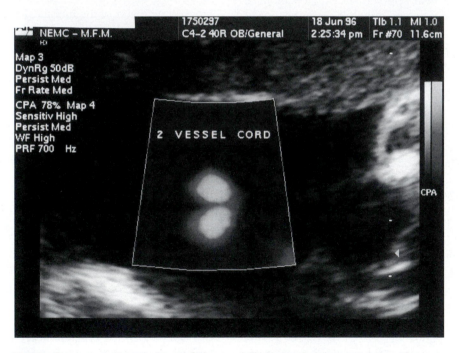

Figure 110-2. Cross-sectional view of the umbilical cord demonstrating the presence of two umbilical vessels. See color plate.

(Monie 1970). SUA can result from one of three mechanisms: primary agenesis of one of the definitive umbilical arteries, a secondary atrophy or atresia of a previously normal umbilical artery, or persistence of the common allantoic/umbilical artery. In one prospective study of 77 cases of antenatally diagnosed SUA, the left artery was absent 73% of the time. In addition, the presence of multiple anomalies and/or abnormal karyotype were seen more commonly with absence of the left artery (Abuhamad et al. 1995). However, another study did not demonstrate an association between the side of the single artery and presence of malformations (Blazer et al. 1997). An increased risk of perinatal mortality exists when SUA is diagnosed. Much of this is due to the associated

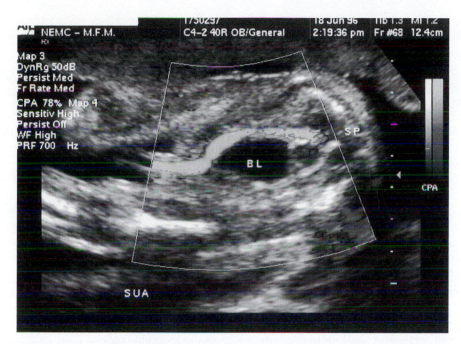

Figure 110-3. Longitudinal view of the umbilical arteries at the bifurcation of the aorta, demonstrating the presence of a single umbilical artery. BL = bladder. See color plate.

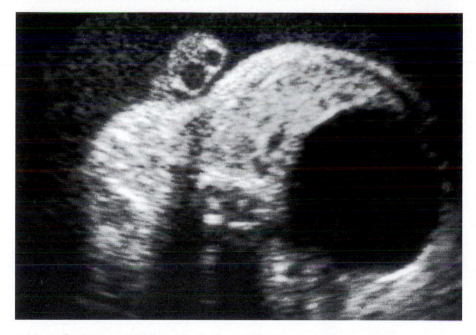

Figure 110-4. Cross-sectional view of an umbilical cord with two vessels, in association with a large simple ovarian cyst. *(Courtesy of Dr. Wolfgang Holzgreve.)*

congenital malformations (see above). Independent of the presence of malformations, several studies have documented an increased chance of intrauterine growth restriction (with an average birth weight of less than 2.5 kg) and preterm delivery (with an average gestation of 35.9 weeks) for infants with SUA (Heifetz 1984; Jones et al. 1993; Leung and Robson 1989; Lilja 1991).

▶ MANAGEMENT OF PREGNANCY

The key determinant of prognosis for a fetus with SUA is to detect the presence of associated anomalies (Fig. 110-4). For this reason, detailed level II sonography is recommended for all cases of SUA. Some groups advocate fetal echocardiographic studies as well (Abuhamad et al. 1995; Persutte and Hobbins 1995). The incidence of major malformations in newborns ranges from 17.5 to 44% (Leung and Robson 1989). These malformations affect a wide variety of organ systems, including heart, brain, skeletal, gastrointestinal, and renal. Prospective studies of fetuses with SUA indicate a 26–31% chance of associated structural anomalies (Abuhamad et al. 1995; Chow et al. 1998). The distribution of anomalies differs somewhat in fetuses (Table 110-1). The documentation of anomalies in addition to the SUA puts the fetus at a significant risk for a chromosomal abnormality (Byrne and Blanc 1985; Nyberg et al. 1991, 1988); prenatal karyotyping is recommended. Retrospective studies of cytogenetically abnormal pregnancies, however, reveal a relatively low incidence of SUA (10 to 11%) (Khong and George 1992; Saller et al. 1990). Trisomies 13, 18, and 21 and Turner syndrome have been reported in association with SUA (Saller et al. 1990). If the karyotype is normal but there are associated anomalies, the fetus should be considered high risk and delivered in a tertiary-care center capable of newborn resuscitation and sophisticated syndrome diagnosis. If the karyotype reveals a diagnosis incompatible with prolonged extrauterine survival, the infant can be delivered in a community hospital with pediatric consultation and an antenatal agreement to not perform heroic resuscitative efforts.

Many questions arise regarding the appropriate subsequent management of a fetus with an isolated SUA. Based on our experience and review of the literature, prenatal karyotype is not indicated (Nyberg et al. 1991). However, in one study of 167 cases of SUA, among 85 cases that were apparently isolated prenatally, 6 (7%) had anomalies that were detected at birth (Chow et al. 1998). Careful attention to fetal growth during the third trimester with serial ultrasound examinations and eval-

uation for symptoms of preterm labor is warranted. (Catanzarite et al. 1995; Khong and George 1992; Nyberg et al. 1991).

▶ FETAL INTERVENTION

There are no fetal interventions indicated for SUA.

▶ TREATMENT OF THE NEWBORN

As discussed above, the newborn with associated malformations needs treatment and diagnostic evaluation in a tertiary-care center. The newborn with isolated SUA needs no immediate treatment other than a thorough physical examination.

A somewhat controversial area has been the need for a renal workup following the demonstration of SUA. This originated from a study by Feingold (1964), who performed intravenous pyelography on 24 children with isolated SUA at birth and found genitourinary tract abnormalities in one third of cases. These findings have been more recently confirmed by an Irish study of 112 infants who were found to have isolated SUA at delivery. In this study 19 infants were documented with abnormal postnatal renal sonography. Eight of 112 (7.1%) had significant persisting abnormalities, with vesicoureteric reflux found in five infants (Bourke et al. 1993). The morphologic abnormalities found in three patients included megaureter, pelvic kidney, and dilation of the collecting system. Although the authors recommend postnatal renal ultrasonography for all infants with SUA, their maternal population did not have detailed level II antenatal sonograms. If a level II sonogram is normal, we do not advocate confirmatory postnatal renal screening in the absence of clinical symptoms.

A more recent meta-analysis of 37 postnatal studies on SUA published over a 40 year period confirms this approach (Thummala et al. 1998). The mean incidence of associated anomalies in liveborn infants with SUA was 27% (range 22–32%). Additional urologic studies were performed on 204 infants with apparently isolated SUA. Of these, 33 (16.2%) had some form of renal anomaly, but over half of these anomalies were minor or self-limiting. Thummala et al. concluded that current data do not justify extensive urologic radiographic investigations for asymptomatic newborns with isolated SUA.

▶ SURGICAL TREATMENT

There is no surgical treatment for isolated SUA. If a genitourinary abnormality is detected, consultation with a

▶ **TABLE 110-1.** ANOMALIES ASSOCIATED WITH A SINGLE UMBILICAL ARTERY

Fetuses*	Newborn malformations†
Multiple congenital anomalies	Skeletal system
ADAM sequence	Cardiovascular
Urogenital malformation	Urogenital
Craniospinal malformations	Gastrointestinal
Meckel syndrome	Central nervous system
Nonimmune hydrops	Respiratory tract
	Integumentary (skin)

*Data from Csécsei K, Kovacs T, Hinchliffe SA, Papp Z. Incidence and associations of single umbilical artery in prenatally diagnosed, malformed, midtrimester fetuses: a review of 62 cases. Am J Med Genet 1992;43:524–530.

†Data from Froehlich LA, Fujikura T. Follow-up of infants with single umbilical artery. Pediatrics 1973;52:6–13; and Leung AK, Robson WL. Single umbilical artery: a report of 159 cases. Am J Dis Child 1989;143:108–111.

pediatric urologist is warranted. Postnatal follow-up may include renal sonography and voiding cystourethrography.

► LONG-TERM OUTCOME

For surviving infants, the prognosis is excellent. The National Collaborative Perinatal Project noted that growth-retarded infants caught up with their peers (Froelich and Fujikura 1973). Intelligence was in the normal range. The one surprising finding was the increased incidence of inguinal hernias in survivors.

► GENETICS AND RECURRENCE RISK

Isolated SUA is thought to be a developmental anomaly, with no risk for familial recurrence. In the setting of associated anomalies, it is important to make an accurate diagnosis to permit proper genetic counseling.

REFERENCES

Abuhamad AZ, Shaffer W, Mari G, Copel JA, Hobbins JC, Evans AT. Single umbilical artery: does it matter which artery is missing? Am J Obstet Gynecol 1995;173:728–732.

Blazer S, Sujov P, Escholi Z, Itai B-H, Bronshtein M. Single umbilical artery—right or left? Does it matter? Prenat Diag 1997;17:5–8.

Bourke WG, Clarke TA, Mathews TG, et al. Isolated single umbilical artery—the case for routine renal screening. Arch Dis Child 1993;68:600–601.

Byrne J, Blanc WA. Malformations and chromosome anomalies in spontaneously aborted fetuses with single umbilical artery. Am J Obstet Gynecol 1985;151:340–342.

Catanzarite VA, Hendricks SK, Maida C, Westbrook C, Cousins L, Schrimmer D. Prenatal diagnosis of the two-vessel cord: implications for patient counseling and obstetric management. Ultrasound Obstet Gynecol 1995;5:98–105.

Chow JS, Benson CB, Doubilet PM. Frequency and nature of structural anomalies in fetuses with single umbilical arteries. J Ultrasound Med 1998;17:765–768.

Csécsei K, Kovacs T, Hinchliffe SA, Papp Z. Incidence and associations of single umbilical artery in prenatally diagnosed, malformed, midtrimester fetuses: a review of 62 cases. Am J Med Genet 1992;43:524–530.

Feingold M. Intravenous pyelograms in infants with single umbilical artery. N Engl J Med 1964;270:1178–1180.

Froehlich LA, Fujikura T. Follow-up of infants with single umbilical artery. Pediatrics 1973;52:6–13.

Heifetz SA. Single umbilical artery: a statistical analysis of 237 autopsy cases and review of the literature. Perspect Pediatr Pathol 1984;8:345–378.

Jassani MN, Brennan JN, Merkatz IR. Prenatal diagnosis of a single umbilical artery by ultrasound. J Clin Ultrasound 1980;8:447–448.

Jauniaux E, Campbell S, Vyas S. The use of color Doppler imaging for prenatal diagnosis of umbilical cord anomalies: report of three cases. Am J Obstet Gynecol 1989;161:1195–1197.

Jones TB, Sorokin Y, Bhatia R, et al. Single umbilical artery: accurate diagnosis? Am J Obstet Gynecol 1993;169:538–540.

Khong TY, George K. Chromosomal abnormalities associated with a single umbilical artery. Prenat Diagn 1992;12:965–968.

Leung AK, Robson WL. Single umbilical artery: a report of 159 cases. Am J Dis Child 1989;143:108–111.

Lilja M. Infants with single umbilical artery studied in a national registry. Paediatr Perinat Epidemiol 1991;5:27–36.

Monie IW. Genesis of single umbilical artery. Am J Obstet Gynecol 1970;108:400–405.

Nyberg DA, Mahony BS, Luthy D, et al. Single umbilical artery: prenatal detection of concurrent anomalies. J Ultrasound Med 1991;10:247–253.

Nyberg DA, Shepard T, Mack LA, et al. Significance of a single umbilical artery in fetuses with central nervous system malformations. J Ultrasound Med 1988;7:265–273.

Persutte WH, Hobbins JC. Single umbilical artery: a clinical enigma in modern prenatal diagnosis. Ultrasound Obstet. Gynecol 1995;6:216–229.

Saller DN Jr, Keene CL, Sun CC, et al. The association of single umbilical artery with cytogenetically abnormal pregnancies. Am J Obstet Gynecol 1990;163:922–925.

Sepulveda W, Nicolaidis P, Bower S, Ridout DA, Fisk NM. Common iliac artery flow velocity waveforms in fetuses with a single umbilical artery: a longitudinal study. Br J Obstet Gynaecol 1996a;103:660–663.

Sepulveda W, Peek MJ, Hassan J, Hollingsworth J. Umbilical vein to artery ratio in fetuses with single umbilical artery. Ultrasound Obstet Gynecol 1996b;8:23–26.

Thummala MR, Raju TN, Langenberg P. Isolated single umbilical artery anomaly and the risk for congenital malformations: a meta-analysis. J Pediatr Surg 1998;33:580–585.

Ulm B, Ulm MR, Deutinger J, Bernaschek G. Umbilical artery Doppler velocimetry in fetuses with a single umbilical artery. Obstet Gynecol 1997;90:205–209.

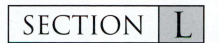

CHAPTER 111

Cervical Teratoma

► CONDITION

Cervical teratoma is a rare tumor. Only 150 congenital cases have been described. Since the first prenatal diagnosis of fetal cervical teratoma in 1978, there have been only 18 published reports of cervical masses detected in utero (Baumann et al. 1993; Cunningham et al. 1987; Hitchcock et al. 1987; Holinger et al. 1987; Jordan et al. 1988; Kagan et al. 1983; Kelly et al. 1990; Liechty et al. 1997; O'Callaghan et al. 1997; Patel et al. 1982; Pearl et al. 1986; Roodhooft et al. 1987; Schoenfeld et al. 1978; Suita et al. 1982; Thurkow et al. 1983; Trecet et al. 1984; Zerella et al. 1990).

As in other teratomas, cervical teratomas are composed of tissues foreign to their normal anatomic sites. All three germ layers are represented within the tumor. Neural tissue is the most common histologic component, with cartilage and respiratory epithelium also observed (Schoenfeld et al. 1982). Thyroid tissue occurs in 30 to 40% but it is uncertain whether this represents actual involvement of the gland or ectopic thyroid tissue (Jordan et al. 1988). Theories regarding the origin

of cervical teratoma include derivation from totipotential germ cells or abnormal development of a conjoined twin (Ashley 1973; Hitchcock et al. 1987).

► INCIDENCE

As stated above, these tumors are extremely rare. There is no apparent relationship to maternal age or parity (Hitchcock et al. 1987). Unlike other teratomas, males and females are equally affected (Batsakis et al. 1964; Tapper and Lack 1983) and there is no racial predilection (Suita et al. 1982).

► SONOGRAPHIC FINDINGS

On ultrasound examination, cervical teratomas are typically asymmetric, unilateral, mobile and well demarcated (Fig. 111-1). Most are multiloculated, irregular masses with solid and cystic components. As many as 50% have calcifications present (Gundry et al. 1983;

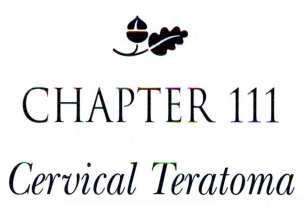

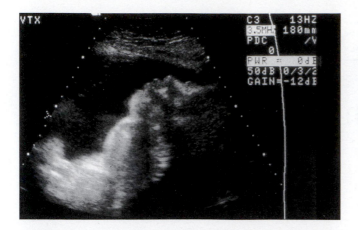

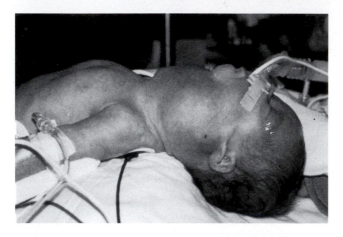

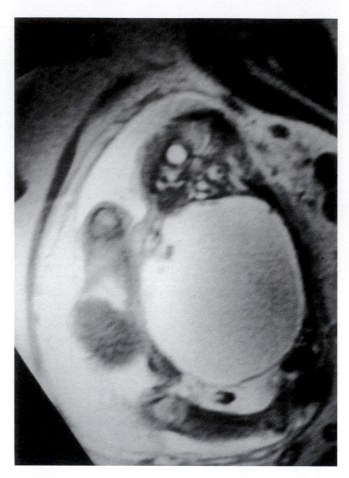

Figure 111-1. (Top) Prenatal sonographic image of a fetus in sagittal section demonstrating a complex cervical mass resulting in hyperextension of the neck due to a cervical teratoma. This has been referred to as the "flying fetus" sign, as the head extension is similar to that observed in ski jumpers when they fly off the ski jump. (Bottom) Postnatal appearance of the same patient.

Figure 111-2. Fetal magnetic resonance image (MRI) showing a giant cervical teratoma with a huge cystic component. The cervical teratoma was larger than the fetus. (Reprinted, with permission, from Liechty KW, Crombleholme TM, Flake AW, et al. Intrapartum airway management for giant fetal neck masses: the EXIT procedure (ex-utero intrapartum treatment). Am J Obstet Gynecol 1997;177:870–874.)

Kelly et al. 1990). Calcifications may be difficult to appreciate on ultrasound examination and are more easily seen on plain radiographs (Goodwin et al. 1965; Hajdu et al. 1966; Suita et al 1982). Calcifications, when present in a partially cystic and solid neck mass, are virtually diagnostic of cervical teratoma (Gundry et al. 1983).

Cervical teratomas are usually large and bulky, typically measuring 5 to 12 cm in diameter (Batsakis 1964; Silberman and Mendelson 1960). Tumor masses greater than the size of the fetal head have also been reported (Fig. 111-2) (Batsakis et al. 1964; Jordan et al. 1988; Owor and Master 1974). These tumors usually extend to the mastoid process and body of the mandible, superiorly displacing the ear. Inferiorly they can extend to the clavicle and suprasternal notch or extend into the mediastinum. Posteriorly, they can extend to the anterior border of the trapezius. Involvement of the oral

floor, protrusion into the oral cavity (epignathus) and extension into the superior mediastinum have also been noted in cervical teratomas (Jordan et al. 1988).

Polyhydramnios will complicate 20 to 40% of the prenatally diagnosed cases and is more commonly observed in large tumors (Bale 1949; Hajdu et al. 1966; Lloyd and Clatworthy 1958; Trecet et al. 1984). Polyhydramnios is thought to be due to esophageal obstruction, as has been demonstrated by contrast amniography (Mochizuki et al. 1986; Rosenfeld et al. 1979). An empty stomach may be the first sonographic clue to esophageal obstruction from cervical teratoma (Rosenfeld et al. 1979; Suita et al. 1982). Other anomalies have been reported in association with cervical teratomas, including one case each of chondrodystrophia fetalis and imperforate anus (McGoon 1952). Hypoplastic left ventricle and trisomy 13 have also been reported in association with cervical teratoma (Dische and Gardner 1987; Gundry et al. 1983). Mandibular hypoplasia may also be seen as a direct result of mass effect on the developing mandible (Liechty et al. 1997).

▶ DIFFERENTIAL DIAGNOSIS

Cystic hygroma is the most likely entity to be mistaken for cervical teratoma in cases detected prenatally (see Chapter 32). The similarities in size, sonographic findings, clinical characteristics, location, and gestational age at presentation make this distinction difficult (Batsakis et al. 1964). Cystic hygromas are typically multi-loculated cystic masses with poorly defined borders that infiltrate the normal structures of the neck. This contrasts with the usually well-defined borders of cervical teratomas. Furthermore, cystic hygromas tend to be smaller than cervical teratomas, unilateral, and more frequently involve the posterior triangle (Pearl et al. 1986).

Many other entities may resemble cervical teratoma on sonographic imaging (Table 111-1). Amniotic fluid α-fetoprotein (AFP) has been suggested as an aid in the differential diagnosis of a cervical mass. AFP levels may be either elevated or normal in cervical teratomas. Because fewer than 30% of cervical teratomas have an elevated AFP (Schoenfeld et al. 1982; Trecet et al. 1984), this assay is not particularly helpful in the differential diagnosis of fetal cervical masses. An elevated serum AFP level in the newborn, however, may be helpful in following the patient for signs of teratoma recurrence after successful resection.

Fetal MRI has proven particularly useful in distinguishing the complex septic and solid teratoma from lymphangioma (see Figure 111-2) (Liechty et al. 1997).

▶ ANTENATAL NATURAL HISTORY

The antenatal natural history of fetal cervical teratomas is not well defined. Although they are most often malignant in adults, the vast majority of cervical teratomas in fetuses and infants are benign (Mochizuki et al. 1986). However, rare cases of malignancies in this age group have been described (Azizkhan et al. 1995; Baumann et al. 1993; Heys et al. 1967; Schoenfeld et al. 1982; Thurkow et al. 1983; Touran et al. 1989). The true malignant potential of cervical teratoma is uncertain (Batsakis et al. 1964; Cunningham et al. 1987; Gundry et al. 1983; Owor and Master 1974; Pupovac 1986; Watanatittan et al. 1981). Despite the existence of primitive tissue types in the tumor and metastases to regional lymph nodes, many infants have remained free from recurrence following complete resection of a cervical teratoma. These cases suggest that malignant biologic behavior is uncommon in this population (Batsakis et al. 1964; Dunn et al. 1992; Gundry et al. 1983). Imma-

▶ **TABLE 111-1.** DIFFERENTIAL DIAGNOSIS OF CERVICAL TERATOMA

Congenital goiter
Solid thyroid tumors
Thyroid cyst or thyroglossal duct cyst
Branchial cleft cyst
Neuroblastoma
Hamartoma
Hemangioma
Lipoma
Laryngocele
Lymphangioma
Parotid tumor
Neural-tube defects, such as occipital encephalocele or cervical myelomeningocele

ture tissue seen on histologic examination may merely represent the immaturity of the host; thus pathologic studies are not completely reliable in predicting prognosis (Batsakis et al. 1964; Tapper and Lack 1983).

▶ MANAGEMENT OF PREGNANCY

Fetal cervical teratoma can profoundly affect the course of pregnancy. Repeated ultrasound examinations are indicated to monitor amniotic fluid volume, tumor size, and fetal well-being. In cases followed by serial sonography, rapid tumor growth has been noted (Baumann et al. 1993; Hitchcock et al. 1987). Stillbirth rates of 10 to 50% have been reported (Hajdu et al. 1966; Hawkins and Park 1972; Roodhooft et al. 1987; Silberman and Mendelson 1960; Trecet et al. 1984). There is a high incidence of preterm labor and preterm delivery, thought to be secondary to the increase in uterine size due to polyhydramnios and/or tumor. Because of the hyperextension of the neck, the so-called flying fetus sign (see Fig. 111-1), and the often large tumor size, there is an increased incidence of malpresentation and dystocia (Gonzalez-Crussi 1982; Owor and Master 1974). Cesarean section is often recommended because of the abnormal fetal position (Chervenak et al. 1985; Kagan et al. 1983; Levine et al. 1990; Rempen et al. 1985). Stabilization of the newborn's airway at delivery is facilitated by the assembly of a team qualified to obtain a bronchoscopic or surgical airway if orotracheal intubation is unsuccessful (Zerella et al. 1990). Currently, a fetus with cervical teratoma is best managed by the EXIT (ex utero intrapartum treatment) procedure, which provides time for laryngoscopy, bronchoscopy, and even tracheostomy, if necessary, to secure the airway (Liechty et al. 1997).

Airway obstruction and respiratory compromise at birth can be life-threatening and accounts for up to 45% of the mortality seen with this abnormality. Consequently, delivery should occur at a tertiary-care center. There have been anecdotal reports of intrapartum laryngoscopy or bronchoscopy in cases of fetal neck masses in which the fetus is delivered but the cord is not clamped (Kelly et al. 1990). Unfortunately, this procedure offers no advantage over standard cesarean section, as the removal of the fetus from the womb results in uterine contraction and cessation of uteroplacental gas exchange (Liechty et al. 1997; McNamara and Johnson 1995).

▶ FETAL INTERVENTION

The ex utero partum treatment, or EXIT, procedure was specifically designed to provide time to secure an airway while preserving uteroplacental gas exchange (Fig. 111-3). While Langer and Schwartz and their colleagues had each reported a case using this approach, the technique was not fully developed until it was applied in diaphragmatic hernia (Langer et al. 1992; Mychalishka et al. 1997; Schwartz et al. 1993). When tracheal-clip application was applied in human fetuses with diaphragmatic hernia, it was necessary to develop a technique to allow time for neck dissection, clip removal, bronchoscopy, and intubation. Several individual case reports have described operating on placental support for fetal airway management, but none presented a systematic approach and correlated cord blood gases with time or placental support (Catalano et al. 1992; Langer et al. 1992; Schwartz et al. 1993; Skarsgard et al. 1996;

Tanaka et al. 1994). Recently Crombleholme et al. (1997) applied the lessons learned from use of the EXIT procedure in diaphragmatic hernia to the management of giant fetal neck masses in a small series of five patients, three with cervical teratomas and two with lymphangioma (Crombleholme et al. 1997; Liechty et al. 1997). The mean duration of the EXIT procedure was 28 minutes, with a range of 8 to 54 minutes. Direct laryngoscopy was performed in all five cases. Although orotracheal intubation was possible in two of the five, in one of the two intubation was possible only after drainage of 1800 ml of cyst fluid. In one case, massive involvement of the chest, neck, and face by the lymphangioma precluded orotracheal intubation, and, in accordance with the family's wishes, a surgical airway was not attempted. In the remaining two patients, who had teratomas, there was severe distortion of the airway, rendering intubation by direct laryngoscopy impossible. In each of these cases bronchoscopy and tracheostomy were required to secure the airway. In both cases the mass effect of the tumor had pulled the thoracic trachea into the neck. In the first case this resulted in a tracheostomy 1.5 cm above the carina and in the second case the tracheostomy was performed between the 8th and 10th tracheal rings, as this was the only available site due to mass effect of the tumor (Fig. 111-4). This infant subsequently underwent resection of the mass closure of this distal tracheostomy and creation of a new tracheostomy between the 2nd and 3rd tracheal rings.

Unlike a conventional cesarean section, the EXIT procedure maintains uteroplacental blood flow and

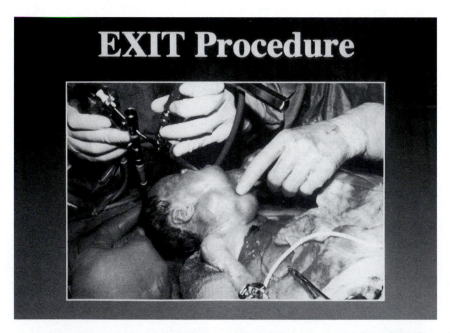

Figure 111-3. EXIT procedure being performed on a fetus with a cervical teratoma. Only the head and the upper chest are removed from the uterus to maintain uterine volume. A pulse oximetry probe is on the right hand and a bronchoscope is inserted into the fetus's airway.

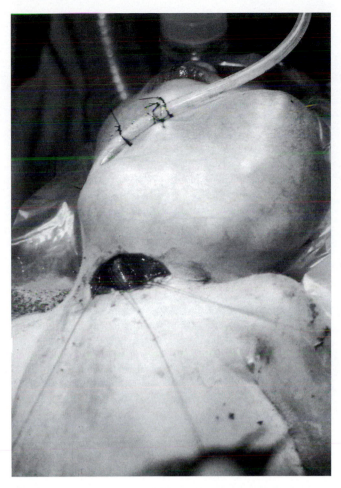

Figure 111-4. The same patient in Figure 111-3 during the EXIT procedure. The cervical teratoma had so distorted the airway that an endotracheal tube had to be tunneled through the soft tissue of the neck and entered the trachea between the 8th and 10th tracheal rings.

fetal gas exchange by keeping the uterus relaxed through the use of inhalational agents and the maintenance of uterine volume by only partially exposing the fetus. This is apparent in the relatively normal venous cord blood gases seen after up to 54 minutes of uteroplacental support (Liechty et al. 1997). By preserving uteroplacental blood flow, the EXIT procedure allows time to perform multiple procedures such as direct laryngoscopy, bronchoscopy, tracheostomy, surfactant administration, and cyst decompression, some or all of which may be required to secure the airway.

There are a number of potential risks to the mother who undergoes an EXIT procedure. Because inhalational agents keep the uterus very relaxed, there is a risk of increased hemorrhage because of uterine atony. The risk of uterine atony and hemorrhage can be minimized through coordination between the surgeon and the anesthesiologist to decrease the concentration of inhalational anesthetic and administer oxytocin at the time of umbilical-cord ligation. The use of the uterine stapling device and coordination with the anesthesiologist kept the average intraoperative blood loss at 950 ml, well within the accepted range for traditional cesarean section (Hood and Holubec 1990).

Lower-uterine-segment hysterotomy is preferred for the EXIT procedure, as it allows the possibility of future vaginal delivery. However, a low anterior placenta or extremely large neck mass may make lower uterine section impossible. In such cases, a classical hysterotomy is necessary. This approach necessitates cesarean delivery for all future deliveries because of the risk of uterine rupture during labor. Prior to an EXIT procedure, mothers should be counseled about the possibility that future pregnancies would require cesarean delivery.

▶ TREATMENT OF THE NEWBORN

Airway obstruction at birth is life-threatening and associated with a high mortality rate (Azizkhan et al. 1995). In giant fetal neck masses this mortality is usually associated with a delay in obtaining an airway and an inability to ventilate the infant effectively. This delay can result in hypoxia and acidosis and, if the delay is greater than 5 minutes, anoxic injury may occur (Dawes 1968). This complication is all the more tragic as most of these children have an isolated benign tumor and do well after postnatal resection.

Mortality can be as high as 80 to 100% in untreated infants, regardless of the tumor size (Garmel and Crombleholme 1994; Batsakis et al. 1964; Goodwin et al. 1965; Gundry et al. 1983; Hurlbut et al. 1967; Silberman and Mendelson 1960). Delaying surgery can result in retention of secretions, atelectasis, and/or pneumonia due to interference with swallowing (Batsakis et al. 1964; Gonzalez-Crussi 1982). In addition, precipitous airway obstruction may occur due to hemorrhage into the tumor (Batsakis et al. 1964; Gundry et al. 1983; Hurlbut et al. 1967; Silberman and Mendelson 1960) even in minimally symptomatic newborns. For this reason, orotracheal intubation is indicated in all patients regardless of the presence or absence of symptoms. Mortality decreases to between 9 and 17% in infants treated surgically (Batsakis et al. 1964; Goodwin et al. 1965; Gundry et al. 1983; Hajdu et al. 1966; Hurlbut et al. 1967; Silberman and Mendelson 1960).

▶ SURGICAL TREATMENT

These tumors tend to be large, disfiguring masses that envelop vital structures in the neck. Extensive neck dissection and multiple procedures are often necessary to achieve the goals of complete extirpation of the tumor with acceptable functional and cosmetic results.

In a review of 18 cases of cervical and oral facial teratomas, Azizkhan and colleagues reported that life-threatening airway obstruction occurred in 7 infants (39%), 2 of whom died without ever having a secure airway (Azizkhan et al. 1995). Two neonates with prenatally diagnosed tumors survived because tracheostomies were performed in the delivery room by an attending pediatric surgeon. Survival was observed in 15 of the 18 cases (83%). One neonate required multiple surgeries to achieve complete tumor extirpation. Morbidity included two cases with recurrent laryngeal-nerve injury, two with hypothyroidism, and two with developmental delay and mental retardation secondary to airway obstruction and asphyxia at birth.

▶ LONG-TERM OUTCOME

Infants with cervical teratoma are at risk for transient or permanent hypoparathyroidism and hypothyroidism. Cervical teratoma may completely replace the thyroid gland, and tumor resection may result in permanent hypothyroidism. More commonly, thyroid tissue may be preserved but may not be adequately functioning and an interval of thyroxine supplementation may be necessary. Because of the massive nature of these tumors and the difficulty in identifying parathyroid glands, transient or permanent hypoparathyroidism may be observed. Calcium and vitamin D supplementation may be needed postoperatively. A pediatric endocrinologist should be consulted if these complications are encountered. In approximately two-thirds of the cases, cervical teratomas produce markedly elevated levels of AFP. However, an elevated AFP level obtained immediately postoperatively must be interpreted with caution. AFP levels in normal newborns have an enormous range, with some as high as 20,000 units during the first month of life. The AFP values progressively fall during infancy until levels of less than 4 units are obtained at 1 year of age. While an elevated AFP level may not necessarily be abnormal, the levels should decrease during infancy. A rising AFP should alert the clinician to the possibility of teratoma recurrence. While cervical teratoma is generally a benign tumor, there is the possibility of malignant transformation, and close surveillance for tumor recurrence is essential. We recommend following AFP levels at three month intervals in infancy and yearly thereafter, with CT or MRI scanning twice a year for the first three years of life.

▶ GENETICS AND RECURRENCE RISK

There has been one report of congenital cervical teratoma occurring in siblings, but no other familial cases have been described (Hurlbut et al. 1967).

REFERENCES

Ashley DJB. Origin of teratomas. Cancer 1973;32:390–394.

Azizkhan RG, Haase GM, Applebaum H, et al. Diagnosis, management and outcome of cervicofacial teratomas in neonates: a children's cancer group study. J Pediatr Surg 1995;30:312–316.

Bale GF. Teratoma of the neck in the region of the thyroid gland. Am J Pathol 1949;26:565–579.

Batsakis JG, Littler ER, Oberman HA. Teratomas of the neck. Arch Otolaryngol 1964;79:619–624.

Baumann FR, Nerlich A. Metastasizing cervical teratoma of the fetus. Pediatr Pathol 1993;13:21–27.

Catalano PJ, Urken ML, Alvarez M, et al. New approach to the management of airway obstruction in "high risk" neonates. Arch Otolaryngol Head Neck Surg 1992;118:306–309.

Chervenak FA, Isaacson G, Touloukian R, Tortora M, Berkowitz RL, Hobbins JC. Diagnosis and management of fetal teratomas. Obstet Gynecol 1985;66:666–671.

Crombleholme TM, Hubbard A, Howell L, et al. EXIT procedure (ex utero intrapartum treatment) for giant fetal neck masses. Am J Obstet Gynecol 1997;176:S84.

Cunningham MJ, Myers EN, Bluestone CD. Malignant tumors of the head and neck in children: a twenty-year review. Int J Pediatr Otorhinolaryngol 1987;13:279–292.

Dawes G. Fetal and neonatal physiology. Chicago: Year Book, 1968.

Dische MR, Gardner HA. Mixed teratoid tumors of the liver and neck in trisomy 13. Am Soc Clin Pathol 1987;69:631–637.

Dunn CJ, Nguyen DL, Leonard JC. Ultrasound diagnosis of immature cervical teratoma: a case report. Am J Perinatol 1992;9:445–447.

Garmel S, Crombleholme TM. The ultrasound diagnosis and management of fetal tumors. Postgrad Obstet Gynecol 1985;15:1–8.

Gonzalez-Crussi F. Extragonadal teratomas. In: Atlas of tumor pathology. Series 2. Fascicle 18. Bethesda, MD: Armed Forces Institute of Pathology, 1982:118–127.

Goodwin BD, Gay BB. The roentgen diagnosis of teratoma of the thyroid region. AJR Am J Roentgenol 1965;95:25–31.

Gundry SR, Wesley JR, Klein MD, Barr M, Coran AG. Cervical teratomas in the newborn. J Pediatr Surg 1983;18:382–386.

Hajdu SI, Faruque AA, Hajdu E, Morgan WS. Teratoma of the neck in infants. Am J Dis Child 1966;3:412–416.

Hawkins DB, Park R. Teratoma of the pharynx and neck. Ann Otol Rhinol Laryngol 1972;81:848–853.

Heys RF, Murray CP, Kohler HG. Obstructed labour due to fetal tumours: cervical and coccygeal teratoma. Gynaecologia 1967;164:43–54.

Hitchcock A, Sears RT, O'Neill T. Immature cervical teratoma arising in one fetus of a twin pregnancy. Acta Obstet Gynecol Scand 1987;66:377–379.

Holinger LD, Birnholz JC. Management of infants with prenatal ultrasound diagnosis of airway obstruction by teratoma. Ann Otol Rhinol Laryngol 1987;96:61–64.

Hood DD, Holubec DM. Elective repeat cesarean section. Effect of anesthesia type on blood loss. J Reprod Med 1990;35:368–372.

Hurlbut HJ, Webb HW, Moseley T. Cervical teratoma in infant siblings. J Pediatr Surg 1967;2:424–426.

Jordan RB, Gauderer MWL. Cervical teratomas: an analysis, literature review and proposed classification. J Pediatr Surg 1988;23:583–591.

Kagan AR. Cervical mass in a fetus associated with maternal hydramnios. AJR Am J Roentgenol 1983;140:507–509.

Kelly MF, Berenholz L, Rizzo KA, et al. Approach for oxygenation of the newborn with airway obstruction due to a cervical mass. Ann Otol Rhinol Laryngol 1990;99:179–182.

Langer JC, Tabb T, Thompson P, Paes BA, Caco CC. Management of prenatally diagnosed tracheal obstruction: access to the airway in utero prior to delivery. Fetal Diagn Ther 1992;7:12–16.

Levine AB, Alvarez M, Wedgewood J, Berkowitz RL, Holzman I. Contemporary management of a potentially lethal fetal anomaly: a successful perinatal approach to epignathus. Obstet Gynecol 1990;76:962–966.

Liechty KW, Crombleholme TM, Flake AW, et al. Intrapartum airway management for giant fetal masses: the EXIT procedure (ex-utero intrapartum treatment). Am J Obstet Gynecol 1997;177:870–874.

Lloyd JR, Clatworthy HW. Hydramnios as an aid to the early diagnosis of congenital obstruction of the alimentary tract: a study of the maternal and fetal factors. Pediatrics 1958;21:903–909.

McGoon DC. Teratomas of the neck. Surg Clin North Am 1952;32:1389–1395.

McNamara H, Johnson N. The effect of uterine contractions on fetal oxygen saturation. Br J Obstet Gynecol 1995;102:644–647.

Mochizuki Y, Noguchi S, Yokoyama S, et al. Cervical teratoma in a fetus and an adult. Acta Pathol Jpn 1986;36:935–943.

Mychalishka GB, Bealor JF, Graf JL, Adzick NS, Harrison MR. Operating on placental support: the ex utero intrapartum treatment (EXIT) procedure. J Pediatr Surg 1997;32:227–230.

O'Callaghan SP, Walker P, Wohle C, et al. Perinatal care of a woman with the prenatal diagnosis of a massive fetal neck tumor (cervical teratoma). Br J Obstet Gynecol 1997;104:261–263.

Owor R, Master SP. Cervical teratomas in the newborn. East Afr Med J 1974;51:376–381.

Patel RB, Gibson YU, D'Cruz CA, Burkhalter JL. Sonographic diagnosis of cervical teratoma in utero. AJR Am J Roentgenol 1982;139:1220–1222.

Pearl RM, Wisnicki J, Sinclair G. Metastatic cervical teratoma of infancy. Plast Reconstr Surg 1986;77:469–473.

Pupovac D. Ein fall von teratoma colli mit veranderungen in den regionaren lymphdrusen. Arch Klin Chir 1986;53:59–67.

Rempen A, Feige A. Differential diagnosis of sonographically detected tumours in the fetal cervical region. Eur J Obstet Gynecol Reprod Biol 1985;20:89–105.

Roodhooft AM, Delbeke L, Vaneerdeweg W. Cervical teratoma: prenatal detection and management in the neonate. Pediatr Surg Int 1987;2:181–184.

Rosenfeld CR, Coln CD, Duenhoelter JH. Fetal cervical teratomas as a cause of polyhydramnios. Pediatrics 1979;64:174–179.

Schoenfeld A, Edelstein T, Joel-Cohen SJ. Prenatal ultrasonic diagnosis of fetal teratoma of the neck. Br J Radiol 1978;51:742–744.

Schoenfeld A, Ovadia J, Edelstein T, Liban E. Malignant cervical teratoma of the fetus. Acta Obstet Gynecol Scand 1982;61:7–12.

Schwartz MZ, Silver H, Schulman S. Maintenance of the placental circulation to evaluate and treat an infant with massive head and neck hemangioma. J Pediatr Surg 1993;28:52–62.

Silberman R, Mendelson IR. Teratoma of the neck. Arch Dis Child 1960;35:159–170.

Skarsgard ED, Chitkara U, Krane EJ, Riley ET, Halamek LP, Dedo HH. The OOPS procedure (operation on placental support): in utero airway management of the fetus with prenatally diagnosed tracheal obstruction. J Pediatr Surg 1996;31:826–828.

Suita S, Ikeda K, Nakano H, et al. Teratoma of the neck in a newborn infant—a case report. Z Kinderchir 1982;35:9–11.

Tanaka M, Sato S, Naito H, Nakayama H. Anesthetic management of a neonate with prenatally diagnosed cervical tumour and upper airway obstruction. Can J Anaesth 1994;41:236–240.

Tapper D, Lack EE. Teratomas in infancy and childhood. Ann Surg 1983;198:398–410.

Thurkow AL, Visser GHA, Oosterhuis JW, de Vries JA. Ultrasound observations of a malignant cervical teratoma of the fetus in a case of polyhydramnios: case history and review. Eur J Obstet Gynecol Reprod Biol 1983;14:375–384.

Touran T, Applebaum H, Frost DB, Richardson R, Taber P, Rowland J. Congenital metastatic cervical teratoma: diagnostic and management considerations. J Pediatr Surg 1989;24:21–23.

Trecet JC, Claramunt V, Larraz J, Ruiz F, Zusyarregui M, Ugalde FJ. Prenatal ultrasound diagnosis of fetal teratoma of the neck. J Clin Ultrasound 1984;12:509–511.

Watanatittan S, Othersen HB, Hughson MD. Cervical teratoma in children. Prog Pediatr Surg 1981;14:225–239.

Zerella JT, Finberg FJ. Obstruction of the neonatal airway from teratomas. Surg Gynecol Obstet 1990;170:126–131.

CHAPTER 112

Liver Tumors

► CONDITION

Tumors of the liver are rare during the perinatal period. They account for only 5% of all neoplasms that occur in the fetus and the newborn (Borch et al. 1992; Broadbent 1992; Campbell et al. 1987; Isaacs 1997; Werbe et al. 1992). The most common primary hepatic tumor is hemangioma, followed by mesenchymal hamartoma, and hepatoblastoma (Davenport et al. 1995; Davis et al. 1988; Isaacs 1985). Each has been detected prenatally by ultrasound examination and can be detected postnatally by palpation of an abdominal mass (Garmel et al. 1994; Isaacs 1997; Romero et al. 1988). However, metastatic lesions are more common than primary liver tumors (Coffin and Dehner 1992; Dehner 1978). The most common tumor that metastasizes to the liver in the fetus and newborn is neuroblastoma, followed by leukemia, yolk-sac tumor from sacrococcygeal teratoma, and rhabdoid tumor of the kidney (Dehner 1978; Isaacs 1985, 1997). The majority of hepatic hemangiomas are diagnosed before 6 months of age and almost 50% appear within the first week of life (Davis et al. 1988; Dehner 1978, 1981, 1987; Dehner et al. 1975; Drut et al. 1992; Ehren et al. 1983; Golitz et al. 1986; Laird et al. 1976; Luks et al. 1991; Miller and Greenspan 1985a and b; Stanley et al. 1977, 1989; Werbe et al. 1992). There are at least five reports in the literature of hepatic hemangiomas diagnosed by prenatal sonographic examination (Horgan et al. 1984; Nakamoto et al. 1983; Petrovic et al. 1992; Platt et al. 1983; Sepulveda et al. 1993). It is likely that more hemangiomas occur in the liver than are actually recognized, because many are asymptomatic or silent conditions that regress or are discovered as only an incidental finding on clinical imaging or postmortem examination (Dehner 1978). Some hemangiomas, in contrast, present with hepatomegaly or a mass lesion and high-output cardiac failure, while others may be life-threatening during the

perinatal period due to rupture of the hemangioma and hemoperitoneum during delivery (Berry 1993; Davenport et al. 1995; Dehner 1981, 1987; Larcher et al. 1981; Miller and Greenspan 1985a and b; Romero et al. 1988; Stanley et al. 1989; Weinberg and Finegold 1986). Hemangiomas have been associated with consumptive coagulopathy resulting from disseminated intravascular coagulation (DIC), sequestration of platelets causing a bleeding diathesis (Kasabach–Merritt syndrome), and anemia (Berry 1993; Dehner 1987; Isaacs et al. 1991; Slopeck and Lakatau 1989; Tur et al. 1981). High-output cardiac failure leading to in utero demise at 33 weeks of gestation as a result of hepatic hemangioma has been described by Nakamoto et al. (1983). In a report from Stanley et al. (1989) a palpable abdominal mass and cardiac failure were the most frequent presenting findings in 20 infants diagnosed with hepatic hemangiomas. In about 50% of newborns, hepatic hemangiomas are associated with hemangiomas of the skin and other organs (Berry 1993; Davenport et al. 1995; Dehner 1978, 1987; Golitz et al. 1986; Isaacs 1985; Larcher et al. 1981; Leonidas et al. 1993; Shturman-Ellstein et al. 1978; Stanley et al. 1989). The fatal combination of cutaneous and hepatic hemangiomas, hydrops fetalis, hydramnios, and premature delivery has been reported by Shturman-Ellstein et al. (1978). This case was also notable for associated placental edema and chorioangioma, with a terminal clinical course complicated by thrombocytopenia and DIC in the Kasabach–Merritt syndrome that was further compromised by respiratory distress syndrome (Shturman-Ellstein et al. 1978).

Congenital malformations may also be observed in association with hepatic hemangiomas. Werbe et al. (1992) described two such cases in stillborn infants. One infant had a 4-cm hemangioma and an encephalocele, while the other had two liver lesions in addition to encephalomyelitis, partial gut malrotation, and single umbilical artery. In another report, congenital heart disease and prune belly syndrome, respectively, occurred with hepatic hemangiomas in two other neonates (Ehren et al. 1983). Shah et al. (1987) reported a 6-hour-old full-term female infant who died during surgery for repair of a left congenital diaphragmatic hernia who was found to have hemangioma rising from the lobe of the liver in the left thorax. Hepatic hemangiomas have also been described in association with the Beckwith–Wiedmann syndrome, placental chorioangioma, and dysmorphic kidneys (Drut et al. 1992).

The second most common benign hepatic tumor that occurs during the perinatal period is mesenchymal hamartoma (Davis et al. 1988; Dehner 1978, 1981; De-Maioribus et al. 1990; Isaacs 1983, 1991, Stocker et al. 1983; Weinberg and Finegold 1986). Over 50% of cases of mesenchymal hamartoma are diagnosed in infants and about 25% are in newborns. In a report by Keeling (1971), five of seven patients with this condition were 2 months of age or younger. The lesion was an incidental postmortem finding in three newborns, including one stillborn infant.

The pathogenesis of mesenchymal hamartoma is incompletely understood and, as the name *hamartoma* implies, it is of a developmental rather than a neoplastic origin (Dehner 1978, Weinberg and Finegold 1986). Lennington et al. (1993) have suggested that mesenchymal hamartomas result from anomalous blood supply to a liver lobule, leading to ischemia and subsequent cystic change and fibrosis. Consistent with this premise is the observation that some hamartomas have necrotic centers and are attached to the liver by a pedi-

cle (Lennington et al. 1993). In addition, neither recurrence following complete resection nor malignant transformation have been reported in mesenchymal hamartomas (Dehner 1978, Isaacs 1983; Stanley et al. 1986; Stocker et al. 1983). Mesenchymal hamartoma can readily be detected by prenatal sonographic examination (Foucar et al. 1983; Garmel et al. 1994; Hirata et al. 1990; Mason et al. 1992; Wienk et al. 1990). In general, mesenchymal hamartomas are not associated with other congenital malformations (Weinberg and Finegold 1986), but occasional exceptions have been noted, including Keeling's (1971), report of excessive oral mucus secretions and an abdominal mass. This infant was found to have a tracheoesophageal fistula with an annular pancreas in addition to the hamartoma. Stocker et al. reported that 5 of their 30 patients with mesenchymal hamartoma had various anomalies and associated conditions (Stocker et al. 1983). Most mesenchymal hamartomas occur in the right lobe of the liver but up to 10% can be bilateral (Dehner 1978, 1987; Weinberg and Finegold 1986).

Hepatoblastoma is the leading primary hepatic malignant tumor occurring during the first year of life (Isaacs et al. 1997). Over half of all hepatoblastomas are diagnosed in infants, but less than 10% are found in newborns (Campbell et al. 1987; Exelby et al. 1975; Gonzalez-Crussi et al. 1982; Isaacs et al. 1991; Keeling 1971; Weinberg and Finegold 1983, 1986).

Typically, hepatoblastoma presents as an upper abdominal mass arising from a single area, more often from the right lobe of the liver than the left (Fig. 112-1).

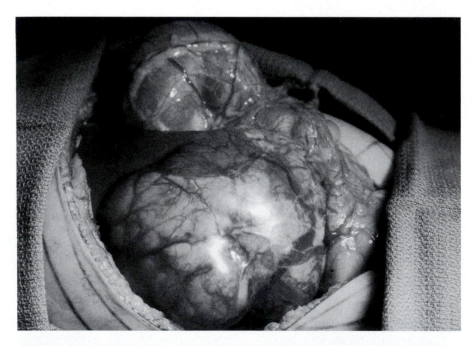

Figure 112-1. Intraoperative view of a newborn with congenital hepatoblastoma arising from the right lobe of the liver.

Hepatoblastoma can be detected by antenatal sonography (Garmel et al. 1994; Orozco-Florian et al. 1991; van de Bor et al. 1985). In one prenatally detected case, hepatoblastoma was responsible for compression of the inferior vena cava leading to fetal hydrops and intrauterine death at 36 weeks of gestation (Benjamin et al. 1981). Kazzi et al. (1989) described a similar case in a newborn with hepatoblastoma that was diagnosed antenatally. Hydrops fetalis, consumptive coagulopathy associated with massive hemorrhage into the tumor, and anemia were present at birth in this fetus. Orozco-Florian et al. (1991) reported a fetus with hepatoblastoma detected antenatally that had associated nephromegaly and pancreatic nesidioblastosis consistent with the diagnosis of Beckwith–Wiedemann syndrome; however, the affected neonate did not have either macroglossia or omphalocele. In addition to neuroblastoma and leukemia, hepatoblastoma is one of the rare perinatal malignancies that can metastasize to the placenta and cause fetal death (Bond 1976; Dinmick 1991; Robinson and Bolande 1985). A broad range of congenital anomalies and malformation syndromes have been reported to occur in association with hepatoblastoma. Hemihypertrophy can occur in as many as 2 to 3% of affected patients. Beckwith–Wiedemann syndrome and intestinal adenomatous polyposis are the most common associated syndromes (Dehner 1981; Fraumeni et al. 1978; Geiser et al. 1970; Giardiello et al. 1991; Greenberg et al. 1993; Hartley et al. 1990; Kazzi et al. 1989; Landing et al. 1976; Li et al. 1987; Orozco-Florian et al. 1991; Rubie et al. 1993; Weinberg and Finegold 1986). In the combination of hepatoblastoma and familial adenomatous polyposis, which is an autosomal dominant disorder, often ophthalmoscopic examination of the affected individual reveals hypertrophy of the retinal pigment epithelium, which appears to be a sensitive and a specific marker for the polyposis gene (Giardiello et al. 1991). Hepatoblastoma, in addition, has been described in siblings in a variety of clinical settings, including in the fetal alcohol syndrome, in association with the maternal use of contraceptives, in trisomy 18, in patients with Wilms tumor, and in newborns with adenomatoid malformation of the renal epithelium (Greenberg et al. 1993; Khan et al. 1979; Knowlson and Cameron 1979; Landing et al. 1976; Mamlok et al. 1989; Riikonen et al. 1990). Aicardi syndrome (infantile spasms, agenesis of the corpus callosum, and multiple ocular malformations) has been described in a 2-month-old female infant with hepatoblastoma (Tanaka et al. 1985).

No clearly defined factors have been implicated in the development of these tumors and the causes of these entities are unknown. Because of the rarity of these lesions, much remains to be learned about the prenatal sonographic findings, natural history, and optimal pregnancy management for these unusual cases.

▶ INCIDENCE

Tumors of the liver presenting during the perinatal period are rare. Primary hepatic neoplasms account for only 0.5 to 2% of pediatric tumors (Alagille and Odievre 1979). Hemangiomas are relatively common, occurring in as many as 1 in 100 newborns and in 1 in 5 premature infants with a birth weight less than 1000 g (Enjorlas et al. 1990; Folkman 1984). The specific incidence of hepatic hemangioma is not known. The annual incidence of hepatoblastoma in the United States is estimated to be 0.9 in 1 million children, with a 2:1 male predominance (Fraumeni et al. 1978, Young et al. 1975). The incidence of mesenchymal hemartoma is uncertain, but there appears to be a male predominance. The prenatal incidence of each of these hepatic tumors is unknown.

▶ SONOGRAPHIC FINDINGS

There have been at least five reported cases of hepatic hemangiomas diagnosed prenatally by ultrasound examination (Horgan et al. 1984; Nakamoto et al. 1983; Petrovic et al. 1992; Platt et al. 1983; Sepulveda et al. 1993;). These lesions can be single or multiple and can appear hypoechogenic, hyperechogenic, or mixed in appearance depending on the degree of fibrosis and the stage of evolution (Gonen et al. 1989; Horgan et al. 1984; Nakamoto et al. 1983). The reported sizes of hemangiomas have ranged from 1.1 by 0.9 cm to 7.8 by 6.4 cm (Petrovic et al. 1992; Sepulveda et al. 1993). Hepatomegaly may also be seen. Polyhydramnios has been noted occasionally, which is thought to be due to either a hyperdynamic state induced by this vascular tumor or gastrointestinal-tract compression secondary to mass effect (Nakamoto et al. 1983; Petrovic et al. 1992). In addition, fetal hydrops has been reported in one case by Shturman-Ellstein et al. (1978).

Mesenchymal hamartomas have also been described prenatally (Foucar et al. 1983; Hirata et al. 1990; Mason et al. 1992). Hamartomas typically appear as an irregular cyst on ultrasound examination (Nyberg et al. 1990). Both oligohydramnios and polyhydramnios have been reported in association with mesenchymal hamartomas (Mason et al. 1992).

Hepatoblastoma develops in fetal life and is the most common primary liver malignancy in infancy and childhood, yet only rare cases have been detected prenatally (Garmel et al. 1994; Isaacs 1997; van de Bor et al. 1985). Neonatal hepatoblastomas are typically solid and echogenic and calcifications may be present. Two-thirds involve only one lobe (Exelby et al. 1975). Associated anomalies have been reported in the neonate, including hemihypertrophy, Down syndrome, cardiovascular defects, and genitourinary anomalies (Gonzalez-Crussi et al. 1982). Whether most of these are chance associations is not clear. In van de Bor et al.'s (1985) case report of hepatoblastoma, polyhydramnios was noted in association with hepatomegaly; this was due to a gastrointestinal obstruction.

▶ DIFFERENTIAL DIAGNOSIS

The differential diagnosis of fetal hepatomegaly, usually involving splenomegaly as well, includes hydrops, fetal infection, anemia, metabolic abnormalities (e.g., hypothyroidism) and, certain syndromes such as Beckwith–Wiedemann and Zellweger (Nyberg et al. 1990; Schutgens et al. 1985). The differential diagnosis of prenatally diagnosed hepatic masses should include isolated nonparasitic cysts (Chung 1986), cysts associated with polycystic kidney disease, and metastatic neuroblastoma. Gonen et al. (1989) prenatally confirmed the vascular nature of hemangioma with pulse Doppler studies showing drainage into an enlarged hepatic vein. This technique may prove useful in a differential diagnosis of prenatally detected hepatic lesions. In addition to hemangioma, hepatoblastoma, and mesenchymal hamartomas, one should also consider the possibility of hepatic adenoma. There has been one reported case of prenatally diagnosed hepatic adenoma. Marks et al. (1990) noted a 4-by-4-cm hypoechoic liver mass with no associated anomalies. An autopsy confirmed the diagnosis of hepatic adenoma. Hepatic hemangioendothelioma has also been diagnosed prenatally as a cystic and solid lesion with Doppler imaging, confirming the vascular nature of the tumor (Gonen et al. 1989). While this fetus progressed to nonimmune hydrops, another case was noted to spontaneously regress (Horgan et al. 1984).

α-Fetoprotein (AFP) levels are markedly elevated in neonatal cases of hepatoblastoma and mesenchymal hamartoma (Exelby et al. 1975; Ito et al. 1984; Pollice et al. 1992). This has not yet been reported with prenatal lesions, and the usefulness of maternal serum AFP levels in the diagnosis and management of prenatally detected hepatic tumors is unknown.

▶ ANTENATAL NATURAL HISTORY

Because of the rarity of these lesions, little is known about the antenatal natural history of hepatic tumors. Hemangiomas are histologically benign, and postnatally the natural history tends toward spontaneous regression after infancy. However, there is great variability in severity and complications (Larcher et al. 1981). Occasionally, hemangiomas are associated with arteriovenous shunting and subsequent congestive heart failure. Heart failure in hydrops, with resultant intrauterine neonatal

death, has been reported (Berdon and Baker 1969; Gonen et al. 1989; Nakamoto et al. 1983). These cases may represent the prenatal correlate of infants with hemangiomas and arteriovenous shunting, resulting in congestive heart failure. Others have reported either no change or spontaneous resolution (Horgan et al. 1984; Platt et al. 1983; Sepulveda et al. 1993). Once the diagnosis of hemangioma is confirmed postnatally, by computed tomographic (CT) or magnetic resonance imaging (MRI) scans, the asymptomatic neonate can be treated conservatively with counseling to alert the family of potential complications (Horgan et al. 1984; Platt et al. 1983). In the absence of complications, such as heart failure, the prognosis is good (Slovis et al. 1975).

van de Bor et al.'s (1985) report of prenatally detected hepatomegaly, later found to be hepatoblastoma, ended in neonatal death from liver rupture. Benjamin et al. (1981) reported hepatoblastoma as a cause of intrauterine fetal death. Similarly, Robinson and Bolande (1985) reported a stillborn infant with metastases to the lungs, placenta, and cord from hepatoblastoma. Experience with infants and children is slightly more encouraging. In patients in whom complete resection is possible, the long-term survival rate is 60% (Exelby et al. 1975). However, local extension and recurrence occurs in more than 40% of patients with hepatoblastoma. Hepatoblastoma is usually fatal if it cannot be completely resected, despite preoperative chemotherapy (Gonzalez-Cruzzi et al. 1982).

There is one reported case of stillbirth associated with mesenchymal hamartoma, and no other fetal abnormalities potentially responsible for fetal death were noted at autopsy (Foucar et al. 1983). Two other fetuses with prenatally diagnosed hamartomas did well after surgical resection. This last scenario is more consistent with neonatal mesenchymal hamartoma, in which the prognosis is favorable following tumor resection (Hirata et al. 1990)

▶ MANAGEMENT OF PREGNANCY

A pregnant woman carrying a fetus in which a hepatic tumor is suspected should undergo an extensive prenatal evaluation. This should include a detailed sonographic examination to define the nature of the mass, location, blood supply, and any associated anomalies. Color Doppler studies may be helpful in distinguishing hemangioma from hepatoblastoma, mesenchymal hamartoma, or adenoma. Evidence of other hemangiomas should be sought. While mesenchymal hamartoma is usually an isolated finding, associated anomalies such as tracheoesophageal fistula and annular pancreas have been reported (Keeling 1971; Stocker et al. 1983). Hepatoblastoma has been reported in Beckwith–Wiedemann syndrome and a fetus with a hepatic tumor should be examined for evidence of organomegaly or macroglossia. Hepatoblastoma also occurs in the Aicardi syndrome, and care should be taken to rule out agenesis of the corpus callosum (Jones 1997). Every fetus with a hepatic mass should undergo echocardiography to obtain base-line values and be followed for development of high-output cardiac physiology. Serial scans in fetuses with hepatic tumors are indicated because of the potential for the development of oligohydramnios, polyhydramnios, nonimmune hydrops, and intrauterine fetal death. Fetal MRI scanning may be helpful in establishing a diagnosis of a liver tumor.

Pregnancies complicated by hepatic tumors should be delivered in a tertiary-care center, with neonatologists, pediatric surgeons, and pediatric oncologists available. Depending on the size of the lesion, cesarean section may be necessary. Because of the vascular nature of these lesions, any chance of tumor rupture should be minimized.

▶ FETAL INTERVENTION

There are no fetal interventions for liver tumors.

▶ TREATMENT OF THE NEWBORN

Once an infant with a hepatic tumor is born, attention should focus on establishing a definitive diagnosis. In the cases of hepatic hemangiomas, more than 50% will have associated cutaneous hemangiomas. The infant's platelet count, fibrinogen, and fibrin split products should be checked to exclude DIC and platelet trapping. Follow-up echocardiography should be performed to exclude high-output cardiac physiology. An initial bedside ultrasound examination may be helpful in establishing the diagnosis, however, CT or MRI scans are usually indicated to more fully define these lesions.

In the newborn with a hepatic mass suspected of being a hepatoblastoma, the serum AFP level should be measured. However, values in normal term infants may be between 20,000 and 120,000 ng per milliliter, which may make interpretation difficult in the newborn, but markedly elevated AFP levels are usually seen in hepatoblastoma. Ultrasound examination is helpful in differentiating solid from cystic masses. Hepatoblastoma usually shows a large hyperechoic mass. Color Doppler imaging is also helpful in evaluating the involvement of the portal vein, hepatic veins, and the inferior vena cava.

CT scanning of the liver is helpful in defining the extent of the tumor and assessing resectability of the tumor (Fig. 112-2). MRI scans give detailed information not only on segmental anatomy of a hepatic tumor but also on vascular anatomy of the liver, making angiography unnecessary.

The distinction between hepatic hemangioma and arteriovenous malformations is an important one.

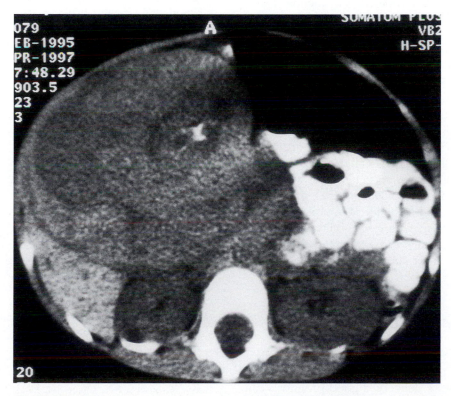

Figure 112-2. CT scan of a patient with a hepatoblastoma largely replacing the right lobe of the liver.

Hepatic arteriovenous malformations require embolization or surgical resection and do not respond to corticosteroids or interferon-α.

▶ SURGICAL TREATMENT

In the experience with 34 hepatic hemangiomas causing congestive heart failure, surgical resection of solitary lesions mortality was 25%, and 45% when embolization was used for solitary and multiple lesions (Folkman 1984). The mortality rate was only 20% when corticosteroids were used. Eleven patients who did not respond to corticosteroids received interferon-α, resulting in a mortality rate of only 9%. Currently, interferon-α is restricted to treatment of serious or life-threatening hemangioma that fails to respond to corticosteroids or develops complications of corticosteroid administration or has a contraindication to long-term corticosteroids (gastrointestinal bleeding, vomiting, infection), or parental refusal of corticosteroids. An initial 2-week course of oral corticosteroids at 2 to 3 mg per kilogram of body weight per day is tried. If the hemangioma responds, as evidenced by shrinkage, decreased turgor, pallor, or arrest of growth then it is continued for 4 weeks before beginning a slow taper over 8 to 10 months (Folkman et al. 1997).

Interferon-α is not without potential complications; its recognized toxicities include fever, elevated liver function tests, transient neutropenia, and anemia. These toxicities are reversible. One worrisome complication associated with interferon-α is the development of long-tract signs and increased motor tone in the lower limbs.

In cases of mesenchymal hamartoma, definitive treatment consists of a frozen section to confirm the diagnosis and exclude the possibility of malignancy and then complete resection of the mass.

Surgical resection is the primary mode of treatment in hepatoblastoma. However, in tumors that are found to be unresectable at operative staging, biopsy is performed to make a diagnosis, and chemotherapy is begun, with reexploration for resection after several cycles of chemotherapy and evidence of tumor regression. In some centers a decision on resectability is made on the basis of imaging studies and a percutaneous biopsy is obtained to make a tissue diagnosis before starting chemotherapy.

▶ LONG-TERM OUTCOME

In hepatic hemangiomas in the absence of complications such as congestive heart failure, platelet trapping, or rupture at the time of delivery, a good prognosis can be anticipated. Most hepatic hemangiomas are asymptomatic and go unrecognized and do not develop complications. Even in the face of complications there has been significant improvement in survival with the treatment of hepatic hemangiomas with corticosteroids and interferon-α (Folkman et al. 1997). The natural history of hemangiomas is to progress during infancy and then to steadily regress thereafter (Folkman et al. 1997).

There has also been steady progress in the outcome of patients treated for hepatoblastoma. The combination of surgery and chemotherapy has achieved disease-free survival rates of 100% for stage I, 75% for stage II, and 67% for stage III disease (Tagge et al. 1997). Unfortunately, no disease-free survival has been achieved with stage IV disease.

The long-term prognosis in mesenchymal hamartoma is excellent following complete resection. These tumors are not associated with malignant transformation and do not recur following complete resection.

▶ GENETICS AND RECURRENCE RISK

Most of the hepatic lesions discussed in this chapter are sporadic in nature, without an associated risk for recurrence in subsequent pregnancies. There are however, two notable exceptions associated with hepatoblastoma. Hepatoblastoma occurs in up to 10% of children with Beckwith–Wiedemann syndrome, which is inherited as an autosomal dominant condition (see chapter 28). There is also an increased risk of hepatoblastoma in kindreds of familial adenomatous polyposis. This is inherited as an autosomal dominant gene predisposing to colonic adenomas and carcinomas. It is estimated that the risk of hepatoblastoma in children of patients with familial adenomatous polyposis is 0.42% (Li et al. 1987, Tagge et al. 1997).

REFERENCES

Alagille D, Odievre M. Liver and biliary tract disease in children. New York: Wiley, 1979:311.

Benjamin E, Lendon M, Marsden HB. Hepatoblastoma as a cause of intrauterine fetal death: case report. Br J Obstet Gynaecol 1981;88:329.

Berdon WE, Baker DH. Giant hepatic hemangioma with cardiac failure in the newborn infant: value of high-dosage intravenous urography and umbilical angiography. Radiology 1969;92:1523–1528.

Berry PJ. Congenital tumors. In: Keeling JW, ed. Fetal and neonatal pathology. 2nd ed. Berlin: Springer-Verlag, 1993:273.

Bond JV. Neuroblastoma metastatic to the liver in infants. Arch Dis Child 1976;51:879–881.

Borch K, Jacobsen T, Olsen JH, et al. Neonatal cancer in Denmark 1943–1985. Pediatr Hematol Oncol 1992;9:209–216.

Broadbent VA. Malignant disease in the neonate. In: Robertson NRC, ed. Textbook of neonatology. 2nd ed. Edinburgh: Churchill Livingstone, 1992:879.

Campbell AN, Chen HSL, O'Brien A, et al. Malignant tumors in the neonate. Arch Dis Child 1987;62:19–24.

Chung W-M. Antenatal detection of hepatic cyst. J Ultrasound Med 1986;14:217–219.

Coffin CM, Dehner LP. Congenital tumors. In: Stocker JT, Dehner LP, eds. Pediatric pathology. Vol. 1. Philadelphia: Lippincott 1992:325.

Davenport M, Hansen L, Heaton ND, et al. Hemangioendothelioma of the liver in infants. J Pediatr Surg 1995;30:44–48.

Davis CF, Carachi R, Young DG. Neonatal tumors: Glasgow 1966–1986. Arch Dis Child 1988;63:1075–1081.

Dehner LP, Ewing SL, Sumner HW. Infantile mesenchymal hamartoma of the liver: histologic and ultrastructural observations. Arch Pathol 1975;99:379–384.

Dehner LP. Hepatic tumors in the pediatric age group: a distinctive clinico-pathologic spectrum. Perspect Pediatr Pathol 1978;4:217–232.

Dehner LP. Neoplasm of the fetus and neonate. In: Naeye RL, Kissone JM, Kauffman N, eds. Perinatal diseases: International Academy of Pathology monograph no. 22, Baltimore: Williams & Wilkins, 1981:286.

Dehner LP. Pediatric surgical pathology. 2nd ed. Baltimore: Williams & Wilkins, 1987.

DeMaioribus CA, Lally KP, Sim K, et al. Mesenchymal hamartoma: a 35 year review. Arch Surg 1990;125:598–605.

Dinmick JE. Liver disease in the perinatal infant. In: Wigglesworth JS, Singer DB, eds. Textbook of fetal and perinatal pathology. Vol. 2. London: Blackwell, 1991:981.

Drut R, Drut RM, Toulause JC. Hepatic hemangioendotheliomas, placental chorangiomas and dysmorphic kidneys in Beckwith–Wiedmann syndrome. Pediatr Pathol 1992;12:197–203.

Ehren H, Mahour GH, Isaacs H Jr. Benign liver tumors in infancy and childhood: report of 48 cases. Am J Surg 1983;145:325–331.

Enjorlas O, Riche MC, Merland JJ, et al. Management of alarming hemangiomas in infancy: a review of 25 cases. Pediatrics 1990;5:491–496.

Exelby PR, Filler RM, Grosfeld JL: Liver tumors in children, the particular reference to hepatoblastoma and hepatocellular carcinomas: American Academy of Pediatrics Surgical Section Survey 1974. J Pediatr Surg 1975;10:329–337.

Folkman J. Towards a new understanding of vascular proliferative disease in children. Pediatrics 1984;74:850–855.

Folkman J, Mulliken JB, Ezekowitz AB. Angiogenesis and hemangiomas. In: Oldham KT, Colombani PM, Foglia RP. eds. Surgery of infants and children: scientific principles and practice. Philadelphia: Lippincott-Raven, 1997:569–580.

Foucar E, Williamson R, Yiu-Chiu V, et al. Mesenchymal hamartoma of the liver identified by fetal sonography. AJR Am J Roentgenol 1983;140:970–972.

Fraumeni JF Jr, Miller RW, Hill JA. Primary carcinoma of the liver in childhood: an epidemiological study. J Natl Cancer Inst 1978;40:1087–1095.

Garmel S, Crombleholme TM, Semple J, et al. Prenatal diagnosis and management of fetal tumors. Semin Perinatol 1994;18:350–365.

Geiser CF, Balz A, Schindler AM. Epithelial hepatoblastoma associated with congenital hemihypertrophy and cystathioninuria. Pediatrics 1970;46:66–70.

Giardiello FM, Offerhaus GJA, Krush AJ, et al. Risk of hepatoblastoma in familial adenomatosis polyposis. J Pediatr 1991;118:766–771.

Golitz LE, Rudikoff J, O'Meara OP. Diffuse neonatal hemangiomatosis. Pediatr Dermatol 1986;3:145–151.

Gonen R, Fong K, Chiasson DA. Prenatal sonographic diagnosis of hepatic hemangioendothelioma with secondary non-immune hydrops fetalis. Obstet Gynecol 1989;73:485–487.

Gonzalez-Crussi F, Upton MP, Maurer HS: Hepatoblastoma: "attempt at characterization of histologic subtypes." Am J Surg Pathol 1982;6:599–612.

Greenberg M, Filler RM: Hepatic tumors. In: Rizzo PA, Poplock DG, eds. Principles and practice of pediatric oncology. 2nd ed. Philadelphia: Lippincott, 1993:697.

Hartley AL, Birch JM, Kelsey AM, et al. Epidemiological and familial aspects of hepatoblastoma. Med Pediatr Oncol 1990;18:103–109.

Hirata G, Matsunaga M, Medcaris A, et al. Ultrasonographic diagnosis of a fetal abdominal mass: a case of a mesenchymal liver hamartoma and a review of the literature. Prenat Diagn 1990;10:507–512.

Horgan JG, King DL, Taylor KJW. Sonographic detection of prenatal liver mass. J Clin Gastroenterol 1984;6:277–282.

Isaacs H Jr. Liver Tumors. In: Isaacs H Jr. Tumors of the fetus and newborn, Philadelphia, WB Saunders, 1991:275–297.

Isaacs H Jr. Neoplasms in infants: report of 265 cases. Pathol Ann 1983;18:165–177.

Isaacs H Jr. Perinatal (congenital and neonatal) neoplasms: a report of 110 cases. Pediatr Pathol 1985;3:165–172.

Isaacs H Jr. Liver tumors in tumors of the fetus and newborn. Philadelphia: Saunders, 1997:278–297.

Ito H, Kishikawa T, Toda T, et al. Hepatic mesenchymal hamartoma of an infant. J Pediatr Surg 1984;19:315–317.

Jones KL. Aicardi syndrome in Smith's recognizable patterns of human malformation. Philadelphia: Saunders, 1997:534–535.

Kazzi NJ, Chang CH, Robertts EC, et al. Fetal hepatoblastoma presenting as non-immune hydrops. Am J Perinatol 1989;6:278–280.

Keeling JW. Liver tumors in infancy and childhood. J Pathol 1971;103:69–76.

Khan A, Boder JL, Hoy GR, et al. Hepatoblastoma in a child with fetal alcohol syndrome. Lancet 1979;1:1403–1405.

Knowlson GRG, Cameron AH. Hepatoblastoma with adenomatoid renal epithelium. Histopathology 1979;3:201–204.

Laird WB, Friedman S, Koop CE, et al. Hepatic hemangiomatosis. Am J Dis Child 1976;130:657–662.

Landing BH. Tumors of the liver in childhood. In: Okuda K, Peters RL, eds. Hepatocellular carcinoma. New York: Wiley, 1976:59–75.

Larcher VF, Howard ER, Mowat AP. Hepatic haemangiomata: diagnosis and management. Arch Dis Child 1981;56:4–14.

Li FP, Thurber WA, Seddon J, et al. Hepatoblastoma in families with polyposis coli. JAMA 1987;257:2475–2479.

Leonidas JC, Strauss L, Beck AR. Vascular tumors of the liver in newborns. Am J Dis Child 1993;147:193–198.

Lennington WJ, Gray JF Jr, Page DL. Mesenchymal hamartoma of the liver: a regional ischemic lesion of a sequestered lobe. Am J Dis Child 1993;147:193–197.

Luks FI, Yazheck S, Brandt ML, et al. Benign liver tumors in children: a 25 year experience. J Pediatr Surg 1991;26:1326–1331.

Mamlok V, Nichols M, Lockhart L, et al. Trisomy 18 and hepatoblastoma. Am J Med Genet 1989;33:125–128.

Marks F, Thomas P, Lustig I, et al. In utero sonographic description of a fetal liver adenoma. J Ultrasound Med 1990;9:119–122.

Mason BA, Hodges W, Ricci-Goodman J. Antenatal sonographic detection of a rare solid hepatic mesenchymal hamartoma. J Matern Fetal Med 1992;1:134–136.

Miller JH, Greenspan BS. Integrated imaging of hepatic tumors in childhood. Part I. Malignant lesions (primary and metastatic). Radiology 1985a;154:83–90.

Miller JH, Greenspan BS. Integrated imaging of hepatic tumors in childhood. Part II. Benign lesions (congenital reparative, and inflammatory). Radiology 1985b;154:91–98.

Nakamoto SK, Dreilinger A, Dattel B, et al. The sonographic appearance of hepatic hemangioma in utero. J Ultrasound Med 1983;2:239–241.

Nyberg DA, Mahoney BS, Pretorius DH, eds. Diagnostic ultrasound of fetal anomalies: text and atlas. Chicago: Year Book, 1990:382–387.

Orozco-Florian R, McBride JA, Favara BE, et al. Congenital hepatoblastoma and Beckwith-Wiedemann syndrome: a case study including DNA ploidy profiles of tumor and adrenal cytomegaly. Pediatr Pathol 1991;11:131–137.

Petrovic O, Haller H, Rukavina B, et al. Prenatal diagnosis of a large liver cavernous hemangioma associated with polyhydramnios. Prenat Diagn 1992;12:70–71.

Platt LD, Devore GR, Benner P, et al. Antenatal diagnosis of a fetal liver mass. J Ultrasound Med 1983;2:521–524.

Pollice L, Zito FA, Troia M. Hepatoblastoma: a clinicopathologic review. Pathologica 1992;84:25–32.

Riikonen P, Toumineul, Seppa A, et al. Simultaneous hepatoblastomas in identical twins. Cancer 1985;66:2429–2432.

Robinson HB Jr, Bolande RP. Case 3: fetal hepatoblastoma with placental metastases. Pediatr Pathol 1985;4:163–165.

Romero R, Pilu G, Jeanty P, et al. Prenatal diagnosis of fetal anomalies. Norwalk, CT: Appleton & Lange, 1988:249–251.

Rubie H, Baunin C, Guitard J, et al. Tiemeurs neonatales malignes. Rev Prat (Paris) 1993;43:2203–2204.

Schutgens RBH, Schrakamp G, Wanders RJA, et al. The cerebro-hepatorenal syndrome (Zellweger) syndrome: prenatal detection based on impaired biosynthesis of plasmologens. Prenat Diagn 1985;5:337–341.

Sepulveda WH, Donetch G, Giuliano A. Prenatal sonographic diagnosis of fetal hepatic hemangioma. Eur J Obstet Gynecol Reprod Biol 1993;48:73–76.

Shah KD, Beck AR, Jhaveri MK, et al. Infantile hemangioendothelioma of heterotopic intrathoracic liver associated with diaphragmatic hernia. Hum Pathol 1987;18:754–759.

Shturman-Ellstein R, Greco MA, Myrie C, et al. Hydrops fetalis and hepatic vascular malformation associated with cutaneous hemangioma and chorioangioma. Acta Paediatr Scand 1978;67:239–243.

Slovis TL, Berdon WE, Haller JO, et al. Hemangiomas of the liver in infants: review of diagnosis, treatment, and course. AJR Am J Roentgenol 1975;123:791.

Slopeck LL, Lakatau DJ. Non-immune fetal hydrops with hepatic hemangioepithelioma and Kasabach-Merritt syndrome: a case report. Pediatr Pathol 1989;9:987–990.

Stanley P, Gates GF, Eto RT, et al. Hepatic cancerous hemangiomas and hemangioendotheliomas in infancy. AJR Am J Roentgenol 1977;129:317–323.

Stanley P, Geer GD, Miller JH, et al. Infantile hepatic hemangiomas clinical features, radiologic investigations, and treatment of two patients. Cancer 1989;64:936–941.

Stocker JT, Ishak KG. Mesenchymal hamartoma of the liver: report of 30 cases and review of the literature. Pediatr Pathol 1983;1:245–251.

Tagge EP, Tagge DU. Hepatoblastoma and hepatocellular carcinoma. In: Oldham KT, Colombani PM Foglia RP, eds. Surgery of infants and children: scientific principles and practice. Philadelphia: Lippincott-Raven, 1997:633–643.

Tanaka T, Takakura H, Takeshima S, et al. A rare case of Aicardi syndrome with severe brain malformation and hepatoblastoma. Brain Dev 1985;7:507–511.

van de Bor M, Verwey RA, Van Pel R. Acute polyhydramnios associated with fetal hepatoblastoma. Eur J Obstet Gynecol Reprod Biol 1985;20:60–69.

Weinberg AG, Finegold MJ. Primary hepatic tumors of childhood. Hum Pathol 1983;14:512–528.

Weinberg AG, Finegold MJ. Primary hepatic tumors in childhood. In: Finegold M, ed. Pathology of neoplasia in children and adolescents. Major Problems in Pathology, vol 18. Philadelphia: Saunders, 1986:353.

Werbe P, Scurry J, Ostor A, et al. Survey of congenital tumors in perinatal necropsies. Pathology 1992;24:247–253.

Wienk M, Van Geijn H, Copray F, et al. Prenatal diagnosis of fetal tumors by ultrasonography. Obstet Gynecol Survey 1990;45:639–653.

Young JL Jr Miller RW: Incidence of malignant tumors in U.S. children. J Pediatr 1975;86:254–258.

CHAPTER 113
Mesoblastic Nephroma

► CONDITION

Although in general, congenital renal tumors are rare, mesoblastic nephroma is among the most common to present during the first few months of postnatal life. Mesoblastic nephroma is also known as fetal renal hamartoma, lyomyomatous hamartoma, and mesenchymal hamartoma (Slasky et al. 1982; Wigger 1975). These tumors are composed of mesenchymal tissue, in the form of interlacing bundles of ovoid or spindle-shaped cells. Since this "classical" form of mesoblastic nephroma was reported, a cellular variant has been described that may account for a large proportion of cases (Pettinato et al. 1989). The cause of mesoblastic nephroma is unknown, but it has been suggested that mesoblastic nephroma is a differentiated form of Wilms tumor (Bolande 1974) or a derivative of secondary mesenchyme (Wigger 1975). Current opinion favors classification of mesoblastic nephroma as a distinct, usually benign neoplasm arising from renal mesenchyme.

► INCIDENCE

A mesoblastic nephroma is a rare tumor, with only 120 cases reported during the neonatal period. Only 13 cases have been described in utero. The rarity of this tumor makes estimates of the incidence of this lesion difficult.

► SONOGRAPHIC FINDINGS

Ehman et al. (1983) described the first case of mesoblastic nephroma detected prenatally by ultrasound examination—a 4-cm solid mass in the left upper quadrant of a twin fetus at 35 weeks of gestation. They also noted mild to moderate polyhydramnios. A nephrectomy performed after birth confirmed the diagnosis of mesoblastic nephroma. Since then, other authors have described the detection of these tumors prenatally with ultrasound imaging during the third trimester (Appuzio et al. 1986; Boulot et al. 1989; Burtner and Willard 1988; Geirsson et al. 1985; Giulian 1984; Howey et al. 1985; Kuo et al. 1989; Ohmichi et al. 1989; Rempen et al. 1992; Romano 1984; Walter and McGahan 1985; Yamboa et al. 1986). However, most of these authors did not consider the diagnosis of mesoblastic nephroma prenatally. Mesoblastic nephroma can present as a large (4 to 8 cm), unilateral renal mass with nodular densities or as diffuse renal enlargement (Figure 113-1). These tumors are predominantly solid, but cystic areas are occasionally seen (Slasky et al. 1982). Unlike Wilms tumor, there is no well-defined capsule, most likely due to hemorrhage with subsequent cystic degeneration.

Many fetal mesoblastic nephromas are initially detected by ultrasound examination because of a discrepancy between uterine size and gestational dates due to associated polyhydramnios. Polyhydramnios has been detected in most of the published cases of mesoblastic nephroma (Appuzio et al. 1986; Boulot et al. 1989; Burtner and Willard 1988; Geirsson et al. 1985; Giulian 1984; Howey et al. 1985; Ohmichi et al. 1989; Rempen et al. 1992; Romano 1984; Walter and McGahan 1985; Yamboa et al. 1986). The mechanism of polyhydramnios is unclear (Favara et al. 1968; Howey et al. 1985; Walter and McGahan 1985). Theories regarding cause include impaired gastrointestinal function due to mass effect of the tumor (Geirsson et al. 1985; Howey et al. 1985) and increased renal blood flow or impaired renal concentrating ability (Geirsson et al. 1985; Perlman et al. 1976), with subsequent increase in fetal urine production (Ohmichi et al. 1989).

Associated anomalies have been reported with congenital mesoblastic nephroma; these include neuroblastoma (Blank et al. 1978) and central nervous system

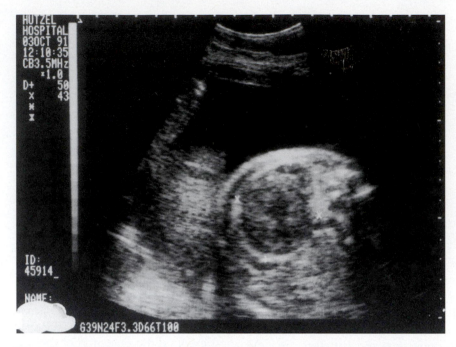

Figure 113-1. Transverse sonographic image of a fetal abdomen revealing a complex renal mass, consistent with mesoblastic nephroma. *(Courtesy of Dr. Marjorie Treadwell.)*

(Howell et al. 1982; Werb et al. 1992), genitourinary, gastrointestinal, and limb abnormalities (Howell et al. 1982).

▶ DIFFERENTIAL DIAGNOSIS

The differential diagnosis of mesoblastic nephroma includes hydronephrosis and multicystic dysplastic kidney, which are both more common than mesoblastic nephroma and appear typically cystic on ultrasound examination. The more malignant nephroblastoma, or Wilms tumor (see Chapter 117), may be indistinguishable from mesoblastic nephroma antenatally (Giulian 1984; Walter and McGahan 1985). Wilms tumor usually has a well-defined capsule and, although an embryonic tumor, is more likely to be seen in the infant or young child. Focal renal dysplasia should also be considered in the differential diagnosis (Gordillo et al. 1987; Sanders et al. 1988). In addition, diffuse nephroblastomatosis should be considered, in which case both kidneys are involved and can be seen as acoustic shadowing due to calcifications (Ambrosino et al. 1990). Infantile polycystic kidney disease can be recognized by nonvisualization of the bladder, oligohydramnios, and bilaterally enlarged echogenic kidneys (Rempen et al. 1992). Adult polycystic kidney disease can be presumed in the presence of a positive family history of this condition (see Chapter 85). Kidney enlargement in other inherited disorders, such as Meckel–Gruber syndrome, is usually bilateral.

In the differential diagnosis, one must also rule out masses extending from adjacent organs such as the adrenal gland or the liver. Solid tumors, such as neuroblastoma of the adrenal or extra-adrenal neuroblastoma and extrathoracic bronchopulmonary sequestration, may be mistaken for mesoblastic nephroma. Careful sonography can usually distinguish the normal-appearing kidney adjacent to these external tumors.

▶ ANTENATAL NATURAL HISTORY

Mesoblastic nephromas are usually benign. In the vast majority of cases, total nephrectomy is curative. However, infiltration of adjacent structures, local recurrence, and metastases have been reported (Bolande 1974; Fu and Kay 1973; Gonzalez-Crussi et al. 1980; Howell et al. 1982; Joshi et al. 1973, 1986; Shen and Yunis 1980; Steinfeld et al. 1984; Walker and Richard 1973). These unusual cases may be due to incomplete excision (Beckwith and Weeks 1986; Slasky et al. 1982). However, mesenchymal tumors are a heterogeneous group, with malignant tumors comprising one end of the spectrum and the majority (the benign tumors) at the other end (Beckwith and Weeks 1986; Gonzalez-Crussi et al. 1981; Joshi et al. 1986). At this time there is no way to predict which tumors will recur or metastasize, based on clinical pathologic features, and close postnatal follow-up is warranted (Joshi et al. 1986). There have been no cases of recurrence or metastases in any of the prenatally diagnosed tumors with follow-up to 12 months of age.

► MANAGEMENT OF PREGNANCY

Because of the benign nature of most mesoblastic nephromas, if ultrasound examination convincingly shows a renal lesion, it is recommended to allow the pregnancy to go to term (Giulian 1984). There appears to be a higher incidence of preterm labor and/or preterm rupture of membranes in pregnancies complicated by mesoblastic nephroma, as a result of associated polyhydramnios (Haddad et al. 1996; Walter and McGahan 1985). In a review of prenatally diagnosed mesoblastic nephroma, 9 of 13 (69%) cases were complicated by preterm labor and/or preterm rupture of membranes as early as 26 weeks of gestation (Appuzio et al. 1986; Rempen et al. 1992). When prematurity is likely, it is recommended to deliver these patients in tertiary care centers to optimize care of the neonate.

Dystocia may complicate these deliveries due to the large size of these renal tumors (Yamboa et al. 1986). There has also been one report of hydrops in association with a large mesoblastic nephroma. Possible mechanisms include obstruction of the portal vein or inferior vena cava circulations, increased vascularity with subsequent arteriovenous shunting, massive hemorrhage into the tumor with resultant anemia, or some combination of these factors (Gray 1989). Serial ultrasound examinations should be performed to monitor tumor size, amniotic fluid volume, and fetal well-being. The prospective parents should be advised that the prognosis for cases of fetal mesoblastic nephroma is excellent with current surgical techniques and close postoperative surveillance for possible recurrence.

► FETAL INTERVENTION

There is no fetal treatment for mesoblastic nephroma.

► TREATMENT OF THE NEWBORN

The main differential diagnosis in an infant with a large heterogeneous renal mass is between mesoblastic nephroma and malignant neoplasms, such as Wilms tumor, clear tumor, clear-cell sarcoma of the kidney, and malignant rhabdoid tumor. The infant should be delivered in a tertiary care setting with consideration given to cesarean section delivery to obviate the potential for dystocia or hemorrhage into the tumor. Once the infant has been stabilized, further preoperative evaluation should include an ultrasound examination with color flow Doppler to evaluate the presence of tumor thrombus within the renal veins or inferior vena cava, as is commonly seen with Wilms tumor, but is uncommonly associated with mesoblastic nephroma. Computed tomographic scanning of the abdomen is useful to best define the extent of the tumor and plan the surgical resection.

► SURGICAL TREATMENT

Radical resection of the tumor is the therapy of choice, and it is usually curative (Bolande 1974; Wigger 1975). Although resection alone is usually curative for mesoblastic nephroma, a small percentage may have local recurrence or present later with metastases. It is thought that these local recurrences are due to inadequate resection during the primary procedure. It was observed by Beckwith and Weeks (1986) that many of the specimens of patients in whom metastases subsequently developed showed either focal or diffuse increases in cellularity, with high mitotic rates. Some have suggested that the so-called cellular or atypical congenital mesoblastic nephroma should be treated as a potentially malignant tumor (Joshi et al. 1986). However, a review of all cases of recurrent or metastatic mesoblastic nephroma demonstrated that the cellular variant is not associated with adverse outcome in infants younger than 3 months, with the exception of one instance in which incomplete removal of the tumor was documented (Beckwith and Weeks 1986).

Because of the tendency to extend into perirenal tissues and subsequently recur, appropriate treatment of mesoblastic nephroma includes a radical surgical approach with efforts to secure wide margins of uninvolved tissue on all aspects of the specimen. In addition, the cellular variant of mesoblastic nephroma carries no adverse prognostic significance in infants younger than 3 months of age. However, in older infants the demonstration of increased cellularity and high mitotic rate is of some concern because a few patients with such lesions will experience local recurrence or distant metastases. Infants older than 3 months of age with the cellular variant of congenital mesoblastic nephroma should probably receive adjuvant chemotherapy, whereas in infants younger than 3 months of age, resection alone is adequate therapy (Beckwith and Weeks 1986; Berry 1987).

► LONG-TERM OUTCOME

Because of the potential in a small percentage of patients with these tumors for local recurrence or distant metastases, these patients need to be followed closely for evidence of recurrence so that they can be treated aggressively.

▶ GENETICS AND RECURRENCE RISK

Mesoblastic nephroma is not known to be familial and there is no known risk of recurrence in subsequent siblings.

REFERENCES

Ambrosino MM, Hernanz-Schulman M, Horii SC, et al. Prenatal diagnosis of nephroblastomatosis in two siblings. J Ultrasound 1990;9:49–51.

Appuzio JJ, Unwin W, Adhate A, Nichols R. Prenatal diagnosis of fetal renal mesoblastic nephroma. Am J Obstet Gynecol 1986;154:636–637.

Beckwith JB, Weeks DA. Congenital mesoblastic nephroma: when should we worry? Arch Pathol Lab Med 1986; 110:98–99.

Berry PJ. Congenital tumors in fetal and neonatal pathology. In: Keeling JW, ed. Fetal and neonatal pathology. London: Springer-Verlag 1987:229.

Blank E, Neerhout RC, Burry KA. Congenital mesoblastic nephroma and polyhydramnios. JAMA 1978;240:1504–1505.

Bolande RP. Congenital and infantile neoplasia of the kidney. Lancet 1974;2:1497–1499.

Boulot P, Pages A, Deschamps F, et al. Nephrome mesoblastique congenital (tumeur de Bolande). J Gynecol Obstet Biol Reprod 1989;18:1037–1040. (English summary.)

Burtner CD, Willard O. Prenatal diagnosis of congenital mesoblastic nephroma in association with polyhydramnios. W V Med J 1988;84:393–394.

Ehman RL, Nicholson SF, Machin GA. Prenatal sonographic detection of congenital mesoblastic nephroma in a monozygotic twin pregnancy. J Ultrasound Med 1983;2: 555–557.

Favara BE, Johnson W, Ito J. Renal tumors in the neonatal period. Cancer 1968;22:845–855.

Fu Y, Kay S. Congenital mesoblastic nephroma and its recurrence. Arch Pathol 1973;96:66–70.

Geirsson RT, Ricketts NEM, Taylor DJ, Coghill S. Prenatal appearance of a mesoblastic nephroma associated with polyhydramnios. J Clin Ultrasound 1985;13:488–490.

Gonzalez-Crussi F, Sotelo-Avila C, Kidd JM. Malignant mesenchymal nephroma of infancy. Am J Surg Pathol 1980;4:185–190.

Gonzalez-Crussi F, Sotelo-Avila C, Kidd JM. Mesenchymal renal tumors in infancy: a reappraisal. Hum Pathol 1981;12:78–85.

Gordillo R, Vilaro M, Sherman NH, et al. Circumscribed renal mass in dysplastic kidney. J Ultrasound Med 1987; 6:613–617.

Gray ES. Mesoblastic nephroma and non-immunological hy-drops fetalis (letter to the editor). Pediatr Pathol 1989; 9:607–609.

Giulian BB. Prenatal ultrasonographic diagnosis of fetal renal tumors. Radiology 1984;152:69–70.

Haddad B, Haziza J, Touboul C, et al. The congenital mesoblastic nephroma: a case report of prenatal diagnosis. Fetal Diagn Ther 1996;11:61–66.

Howell CG, Othersen HB, Kiviat NE, et al. Therapy and outcome in 51 children with mesoblastic nephroma: a report of the National Wilms Tumor Study. J Pediatr Surg 1982;17:826–831.

Howey DD, Farrell EE, Shyoff J, et al. Congenital mesoblastic nephroma: prenatal ultrasonic findings and surgical excision in a very-low-birth-weight infant. J Clin Ultrasound 1985;13:506–508.

Joshi VV, Kasznicka J, Walters TR. Atypical mesoblastic nephroma. Arch Pathol Lab Med 1986;110:100–106.

Kuo C, Tsau Y, Yau KT, Chuang S. Congenital mesoblastic nephroma: report of a case. J Formos Med Assoc 1989; 88:836–838.

Ohmichi M, Tasaka K, Sugita N, et al. Hydramnios associated with congenital mesoblastic nephroma: a case report. Obstet Gynecol 1989;74:469–471.

Perlman M, Potashnik G, Wise S. Hydramnion and fetal anomalies. Am J Obstet Gynecol 1976;24:966–968.

Pettinato G, Manivel JC, Wick MR, Dehner LP. Classical and cellular (atypical) congenital mesoblastoma nephroma: a clinicopathologic, ultrastructural, immunohistochemical and flow cytometric study. Hum Pathol 1989;20:682–690.

Rempen A, Kirchner T, Frauendienst-Egger G, Hocht B. Congenital mesoblastic nephroma. Fetus 1992;2:1–5.

Romano WL. Neonatal renal tumor with polyhydramnios. J Ultrasound Med 1984;3:475–476.

Sanders RC, Nussbaum AR, Solez K. Renal dysplasia: sonographic findings. Radiology 1988;167:623–626.

Shen SC, Yunis EJ. A study of the cellularity and ultrastructure of congenital mesoblastic nephroma. Cancer 1980; 45:306–314.

Slasky BS, Penkrot RJ, Bron KM. Cystic mesoblastic nephroma. Urology 1982;19:220–223.

Steinfeld AD, Crowley CA, O'Shea PA, Tefft M. Recurrent and metastatic mesoblastic nephroma in infancy. J Clin Oncol 1984;2:956–960.

Walker D, Richard GA. Fetal hamartoma of the kidney: recurrence and death of a patient. J Urol 1973;110:352–353.

Walter JP, McGahan JP. Mesoblastic nephroma: prenatal sonographic detection. J Clin Ultrasound 1985;13:686–689.

Werb P, Scurry J, Ostor A, et al. Survey of congenital tumors in perinatal necropsies. Pathology 1992;24:247–253.

Wigger HJ. Fetal mesenchymal hamartoma of kidney. Cancer 1975;36:1002–1008.

Yamboa TJ, Schwartz D, Henderson R, et al. Prenatal diagnosis of a congenital mesoblastic nephroma. J Reprod Med 1986;31:257–259.

CHAPTER 114

Neuroblastoma

▶ CONDITION

Neuroblastomas arise from undifferentiated neural tissue of the adrenal medulla (40 to 70%) or extraadrenal sympathetic ganglia (30 to 60%) in the abdomen, thorax, pelvis, or head and neck (Beckwith and Perrin 1963; Birner 1961; Ferraro et al. 1988; Janetschek et al. 1984; Schneider et al. 1965). Neuroblastic nodules appear to be normal fetal structures within the adrenal gland that regress or differentiate throughout gestation. Greater numbers of these nodules are present early in gestation than at birth or during early infancy (Grosfeld et al. 1993; Turkel and Habashi 1974). Neuroblastic nodules were found in 100% of the adrenal glands studied in second-trimester abortuses (Ikeda et al. 1981; Turkel and Habashi 1974) (Fig. 114-1). Postnatal autopsy studies of newborn and young infants who died of unrelated causes reveal nodules to be present in 0.5 to 2.5% of carefully sectioned specimens (Beckwith and Perrin 1963; Grosfeld et al. 1993; Guin et al. 1969). These figures contrast with the incidence of symptomatic neuroblastoma of 1 in 10,000 to 1 in 30,000 children. This calls into question the clinical significance of these early lesions and the need for treatment. It is also of interest that adrenal cysts are more commonly seen in fetal neuroblastoma, but are relatively uncommon in postnatal life (Turkel and Habashi 1974). Cystic change may also represent a phase of normal adrenal development,

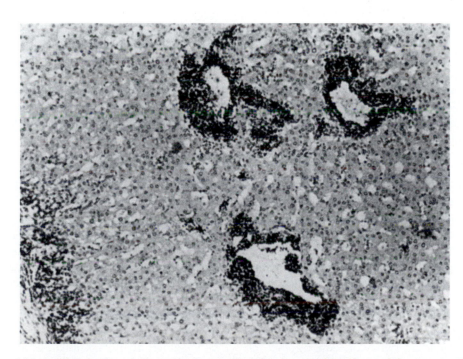

Figure 114-1. Histologic section demonstrating fetal neuroblastic nodules, or rests.

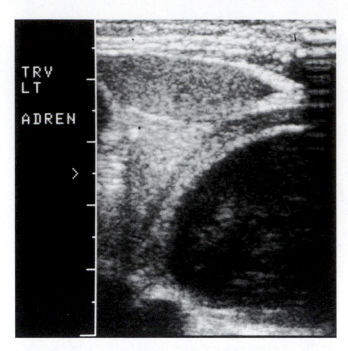

Figure 114-2. Prenatal sonographic image of an adrenal cyst from a fetal neuroblastoma. *(Reprinted, with permission, from Garmel SH, Crombleholme TM, Semple JP et al. Prenatal diagnosis and management of fetal tumors. Semin Perinatol 1994b;18:350–365.)*

thus accounting for prenatal detection of sonographically apparent but possibly clinically insignificant tumors (Tubergen and Heyn 1970) (Fig. 114-2). Although these tumors may represent rests of neural tissue with persistence into neonatal life, the potential for malignant transformation due to defective regression or differentiation must be considered (Grosfeld et al. 1993; Turkel and Habashi 1974).

The results of mass infant screening programs in Japan using urinary vanillylmandelic acid (VMA) and homovanillic acid (HVA) support the view that neuroblastoma in situ may not represent clinically significant disease (Bessho et al. 1991; Grosfeld et al. 1993). Screening infants at 6 months of age has resulted in a doubling of the incidence of neuroblastoma detected in infants. However, the expected fall in the incidence of neuroblastoma detected in older age groups has not been shown. Furthermore, survival in the screened groups has approached 100%. The asymptomatic cases detected by screening may represent a subset of tumors destined to regress or differentiate without posing any clinical risk. This would explain both the high incidence in infants detected by screening programs and their excellent survival. The group detected by newborn screening may be the same subset of tumors detected prenatally with ultrasound examination. In contrast, there is a subset of neuroblastoma diagnosed in utero or in newborns which displays aggressive biologic behavior. Among the 39 cases of fetal neuroblastoma reported, the vast majority

were stage I or II, but there were also one each with stage III and IV disease (Atkinson et al. 1986; Crombleholme et al. 1994; deFilippi et al. 1986; Fenart et al. 1983; Forman et al. 1990; Gadwood and Reynes 1983; Giulian et al. 1986; Goldstein et al. 1994; Gormel et al. 1994; Hosoda et al. 1992; Kurtz and Hilberg 1989; Newton et al. 1985; Pley et al. 1989; Sones 1983; Suresh et al. 1993; Tovar et al. 1988) and five with stage IVS disease (Ho et al. 1993; Hainaut et al. 1987). All children affected with stage IV disease died. In a review of congenital neuroblastoma reported between 1985 and 1991, Jennings et al. (1993) found 14 stillbirths, 44 neonatal deaths, and 2 late deaths, with only 10 known survivors. Eight cases were associated with metastases to the placenta, and 1 had umbilical-cord metastases. This subset of aggressive tumors associated with such poor outcomes may be quite different from the subset detected by the Japanese screening programs (Grosfeld et al. 1993) or prenatal ultrasound examination. The cause of neuroblastoma is unclear, although most cases appear sporadic (Behrman 1992). At least one hypothesis is that antenatal factors play a role, with some adverse stimulus or stimuli occurring in late pregnancy. Preterm delivery is protective, while growth-restricted term infants are at risk (Johnson and Spitz 1985). There have been reports of congenital neuroblastoma in association with maternal phenytoin and phenobarbital use (Allen et al. 1980; Sherman and Roizen 1976). The causative effect of phenytoin in neuroblastoma has been questioned and this is most likely a coincidental finding.

► INCIDENCE

Neuroblastoma is one of the most common tumors of infancy and childhood, with a clinical incidence of between 1 in 10,000 and 1 in 30,000 individuals (Fowlie et al. 1986; Janetschek et al. 1984). Neuroblastoma may be more common in white children than in other ethnic groups and more common in male than in female children (Askin and Geschickter 1985; Behrman 1992; Miller et al. 1968; Turkel and Habashi 1974).

► SONOGRAPHIC FINDINGS

Since the first case of prenatally detected neuroblastoma was reported, 38 cases of neuroblastoma have been suspected or diagnosed by prenatal ultrasound examination. All have been visualized during the third trimester of pregnancy (Atkinson et al. 1986; Crombleholme et al. 1994; deFilippi et al. 1986; Fenart et al. 1983; Ferraro et al. 1988; Forman et al. 1990; Fowlie et al. 1986; Gadwood and Reynes 1983; Gormel et al. 1994; Goldstein et al. 1994; Giulian et al. 1986; Hainaut et al. 1987; Ho et al. 1993; Hosoda et al. 1992; Jaffa et al.

1993; Janetschek et al. 1984; Jennings et al. 1993; Kurtz and Hilberg 1989; Liyanage and Katoch 1992; Newton et al. 1985; Pley et al. 1989; Sones 1983; Suresh et al. 1993; Tovar et al. 1988). The sonographic findings described by these studies were quite variable. The primary tumor is often small (only a few millimeters or centimeters in greatest diameter). Ninety percent of cases involve the adrenal gland, creating difficulties in distinction between the mass itself and the upper pole of the ipsilateral kidney. Cystic and solid areas within the mass are typically seen, which may be related to hemorrhage and necrosis of the tumor (Atkinson et al. 1986). Purely cystic lesions have also been reported in fetal neuroblastoma and may indicate a more favorable prognosis (Atkinson et al. 1986; Crombleholme et al. 1994; Gormel et al. 1994; Kurtz and Hilberg 1989). Occasionally, calcifications can be seen within the tumor (Fowlie et al. 1986; Giulian et al. 1986; Potter and Parrish 1961). The tumor is usually well encapsulated and may displace the kidney inferiorly and laterally but preserves the renal outline. If arising in the sympathetic ganglia, the mass may be seen in the chest, cervical region, or intraabdominal paravertebral locations.

Occult neuroblastomas are rarely metastatic, but prenatal detection of liver metastases has been reported (Jaffa et al. 1993; Liyanage and Katoch 1992). A suprarenal mass associated with hepatomegaly is highly suggestive of the diagnosis of neuroblastoma. Likewise, if a liver mass is seen on prenatal ultrasound examination, one needs to carefully examine all neural-crest regions, especially in the renal and suprarenal areas, to rule out a primary tumor locus (Jaffa et al. 1993). Several cases have been reported with neuroblastoma metastatic to the placenta and umbilical cord. Careful imaging of the placenta and umbilical cord is also indicated because of reports of metastases to these areas.

Occasionally, ultrasound examination may also reveal polyhydramnios and/or hydrops (Falkinburg and Kay 1953; Forman et al. 1990). Although the underlying mechanism is unknown, numerous hypotheses have been proposed, including hepatomegaly with subsequent mechanical obstruction of the umbilical vein or vena cava (Moss and Kaplan 1978; Van der Slikke and Balk 1980), compromised liver function with resultant hypoproteinemia (Adzick and Harrison 1994); metastatic involvement of the placenta with placentomegaly and hydrops (Janacek et al. 1984), tumor infiltration of bone marrow with subsequent anemia and heart failure (Moss and Kaplan 1978), or arrhythmia and heart failure due to catecholamine release (Moss and Kaplan 1978).

Malformations have occasionally been noted in association with neuroblastoma in children, including microcephaly, hydrocephaly, absence of the corpus callosum, cleft lip and palate, tracheoesophageal fistula, heart defects, skeletal abnormalities, genitourinary abnormalities, polydactyly, and single umbilical artery

(Andersen and Hariri 1983; Berry et al. 1970; Bodian 1963; Kouyoumdjian and McDonald 1951; Potter and Parrish 1942). A consistent pattern of associated anomalies has not been demonstrated however, and the majority have been isolated cases of fetal neuroblastomas (Berry et al. 1970; Miller 1966; Sy et al. 1968).

▶ DIFFERENTIAL DIAGNOSIS

The differential diagnosis in neuroblastoma is extensive, as these tumors can be found in the adrenal gland and elsewhere along the sympathetic ganglia. The involvement of the adrenals can be mistaken for hydronephrosis, multicystic kidney, or upper-pole cystic dysplasia seen in obstructive duplex collecting systems, unless a clear distinction from the adjacent kidney is made. Less common entities are outlined in Table 114-1. Demonstration of low-impedance waveforms by color Doppler studies and flow mapping may be helpful in differentiating neuroblastoma from adrenal hemorrhage (Goldstein et al. 1994). If the liver is involved, hamartoma, hepatoblastoma, and hemangioma must be considered. A case report of a solid neck mass seen prenatally on ultrasound examination was found postmortem to be consistent with either primary or metastatic cervical neuroblastoma (Gadwood and Reynes 1983). In this case, the differential diagnosis included cystic hygroma, neural-tube defect, cervical teratoma, and goiter. In one case report of cerebral neuroblastoma, the differential diagnosis included teratoma, glioblastoma, and craniopharyngioma. Prenatal tumor biopsy confirmed the diagnosis of neuroblastoma (Suresh et al. 1993).

▶ ANTENATAL NATURAL HISTORY

Our understanding of the antenatal natural history of prenatally diagnosed neuroblastoma is still evolving, and much remains uncertain. The incidence of adrenal neuroblastoma in situ at neonatal autopsy has been reported to occur in 1 of 40 patients dying from unrelated causes

▶ TABLE 114-1. DIFFERENTIAL DIAGNOSIS OF FETAL SUPRARENAL MASS OR CYST

Adrenal hematoma
Duplex collecting system with dysplastic changes
Neuroblastoma
Extralobar bronchopulmonary sequestration
Liver cyst
Hepatoblastoma
Lymphangioma
Mesenteric cyst
Meconium cyst
Splenic cyst

(Grosfeld et al. 1993). The majority of occult neuroblastomas are most likely developmental variants, which regress spontaneously before becoming clinically evident, or differentiate into benign ganglioneuromas (Beckwith and Perrin 1963; Miller et al. 1968; Pley et al. 1989; Turkel and Habashi 1976).

Among the 39 reported cases of fetal neuroblastoma, 33 developed in the adrenal glands, 4 were intrathoracic tumors, 1 was an intracranial tumor, and 1 developed from an unknown primary site (deFilippi et al. 1986; Jaffa et al. 1993; Ho et al. 1993; Gadwood and Reynes 1983; Suresh et al. 1993). Thirty of these patients had neuroblastoma in situ or were Evans stage I or II, 2 were stage IV, 5 were stage IVS, and 2 were not staged (Gadwood and Reynes 1983; Hainaut et al. 1987; Ho et al. 1993; Jaffa et al. 1993; Kurtz and Hilberg 1989; Liyanage and Katoch 1992; Newton et al. 1985; Suresh et al. 1993). It is interesting that in two patients initially diagnosed and treated as stage I postnatally, hepatic metastases developed and later evolved to stage IV (Fenart et al. 1983; Ferraro et al. 1988). One patient with neuroblastoma initially diagnosed and treated as stage II later had hepatic and bone marrow metastases, which evolved into stage IVS (Ho et al. 1993). These cases underscore the need for close postoperative surveillance even in patients with stage I disease. Hydrops developed in three fetuses with stage IV or IVS and liver metastases (Gadwood and Reynes 1983; Hainaut et al. 1987; Newton et al. 1985). In addition, hypertension and preeclampsia reportedly developed in three mothers, thought to be induced by catecholamines secreted from functional tumors (Jennings et al. 1993; Newton et al. 1985; Pley et al. 1989).

The two most important factors in the prognosis of clinical neuroblastoma are the age of the patient at diagnosis and the stage of the disease. Patients presenting at less than 1 year of age have a favorable prognosis. The overall survival is only 10 to 20% in children presenting after 1 year of age, but is greater than 90% in patients younger than 1 year of age at the time of diagnosis (Estroff et al. 1991; Grosfeld et al. 1993). Patients with disease at an earlier stage and well-differentiated tumors have a better prognosis than those with disease at a more advanced stage and poorly differentiated tumors. Early diagnosis is important in identifying patients prior to 1 year of age and at an early stage of disease. The increasing use of prenatal ultrasound imaging may allow diagnosis at a younger age and earlier stage with the hope of improved survival. The caveat is that the clinical significance of fetal neuroblastoma remains unknown. It is not clear that the natural history of fetal neuroblastoma parallels that of clinical neuroblastoma presenting later in life. The true prenatal history of fetal neuroblastoma may never be determined because potentially malignant tumor will not be managed expectantly. Because of this we may be subjecting neonates, many of whom have biologically benign lesions, to unnecessary risks of surgery and chemotherapy.

▶ MANAGEMENT OF PREGNANCY

Serial ultrasound examinations to assess tumor size, amniotic fluid volume, and fetal well-being play an important role in pregnancy management. A search should also be made for evidence of metastatic spread. An attempt should be made to stage the disease prenatally by sonographic examination. The presence of extensive hepatic metastases places the fetus at markedly increased risk for the development of hydrops. Significant and rapid tumor growth has been noted in at least two reports and may not be predictable (Fowlie et al. 1986; Janetschek et al. 1984). Others have reported an association with placentomegaly and hydrops, with subsequent death in utero or early during neonatal life (Anders et al. 1973; Birner 1961; Gadwood and Reynes 1983; Hainaut et al. 1987; Jaffa et al. 1993; Newton et al. 1985; Potter and Parrish 1942; Van der Slikke and Balk 1980). Because of the poor prognosis, delivery is recommended if hydrops develops.

Dystocia at delivery has been reported due to liver enlargement with capsule rupture and subsequent hemoperitoneum (Askin and Geschickter 1985; Birner 1961; Hagstrom 1929; Potter 1961). Cesarean section should be considered to avoid tumor hemorrhage during labor, as has been reported by Murthy, Weinberg, and others (Jaffa et al. 1993; Murthy et al. 1978; Weinberg and Radman 1943). However, Ho et al. (1993) reported no peripartum delivery complications in their series. We recommend an ultrasound examination late in gestation to evaluate the likelihood of dystocia and the need for cesarean section.

Maternal symptoms related to fetal catecholamine production, including sweating, flushing, palpitations and hypertension, have been reported during the third trimester of pregnancy (Newton et al. 1985; Voute et al. 1970). Development of hypertension is a potential complication in pregnancies associated with either a functioning fetal adrenal tumor or a hydropic fetus (Newton et al. 1985; Nicolay and Gainey 1964; Voute et al. 1970). Early delivery may be indicated if maternal health is jeopardized. Delivery should take place at a tertiary-care center, with neonatologists, pediatric surgeons and oncologists available.

It has been suggested that a 24-hour maternal urine assay or amniocentesis for fetal urinary catecholamine metabolites (VMA, HVA) may be helpful when the prenatal diagnosis of neuroblastoma is unclear or the cause of maternal hypertension is suspected (Crombleholme et al. 1994; Gormel et al. 1994; Newton et al. 1985, Zambotti et al. 1975). However, most neuroblastomas are nonfunctional, and thus far, amniotic fluid catecholamine studies have not been helpful in establishing the prenatal diagnosis of neuroblastoma (Hosoda et al. 1992). Therefore, in the absence of maternal or fetal complications, no invasive diagnostic testing is warranted, but serial examinations of the mother and fetus are recommended (Crombleholme et al. 1994; Gormel et al. 1994).

▶ FETAL INTERVENTION

There is currently no indication for fetal intervention in fetal neuroblastoma. However, if fetal or maternal complications arise, early delivery should be considered in cases of catecholamine-induced hypertension or fetal hydrops.

▶ TREATMENT OF THE NEWBORN

An infant with a prenatal diagnosis of suspected fetal neuroblastoma should undergo a detailed physical examination. In cases of stage IVS disease, bluish subcutaneous nodules (the so-called blueberry muffin) from metastatic neuroblastoma may be seen all over the infant's body. The blood pressure should be noted prior to and during palpation of the suspected tumor mass. Among postnatal neuroblastomas, approximately 20% may release vasoactive peptides on palpation. The abdomen should be gently palpated to discern an abdominal mass and its relationship to other viscera. The liver should be assessed for size and evidence of metastases. Simi-

larly, gentle palpation of a cervical mass will offer clues to histology and relationship to adjacent structures.

The newborn with suspected congenital neuroblastoma should have plain radiography of the abdomen, chest, or neck region (depending on tumor location). Neuroblastoma has characteristic finely stippled calcifications. A postnatal ultrasound examination may be useful to correlate with prenatal findings. Chest radiography should be performed to exclude pulmonary metastases. In most instances a computed tomographic (CT) scan is indicated to more accurately stage the disease and define the extent of the primary tumor (Fig. 114-3).

Urine should be collected for spot measurement of catecholamines and tumor metabolites, including epinephrine, norepinephrine, dopamine, VMA, and HVA. Baseline liver-function tests should be determined in all patients even without evidence of hepatic metastases. Serum ferritin and neuron-specific enolase should be assayed, as they have prognostic significance in patients under 1 year of age. As part of the preoperative staging, a technetium-99m bone scan, and bone marrow aspiration and biopsy should be performed.

The child should undergo surgery for biopsy, staging, and resection of the primary tumor, if possible without jeopardizing adjacent structures. Similarly, in stage IVS disease, resection of the primary tumor is indicated. This will provide tissue for determination of N-*myc* amplification and DNA ploidy. In stage IVS disease, with the presence of diploid DNA complement and N-*myc* amplification, chemotherapy is indicated. In the absence of these findings, observation alone is indicated. The treatment of neuroblastoma depends on the clinical

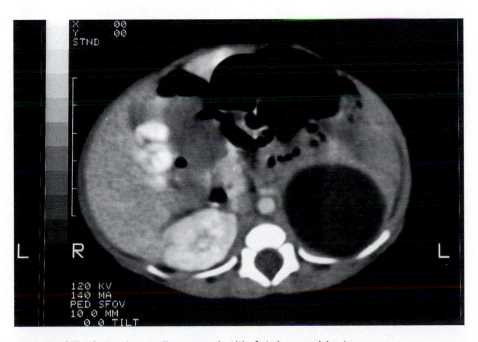

Figure 114-3. CT of newborn diagnosed with fetal neuroblastoma.

staging. In stage I (primary with regional or distant metastases) or stage II (regional lymph node metastases but no distant metastases), surgery alone is sufficient. But in stage III (tumor extends beyond midline and bilateral lymph nodes may be involved) or stage IV (distant metastases) postoperative chemotherapy is indicated.

▶ LONG-TERM OUTCOME

The newborn with congenital neuroblastoma may initially present with stage I disease that subsequently progresses. This does not represent disease recurrence but rather a delayed presentation of metastases, which results in restaging to stage IVS or IV, which requires chemotherapy. As with all pediatric oncology patients, close long-term follow-up is essential even after completion of therapy to ensure early detection of recurrence.

▶ GENETICS AND RECURRENCE RISK

Several cytogenetic abnormalities can be seen in neuroblastoma, including deletion of the short arm of chromosome 1, abnormal chromosome fragments known as "double minutes" (DMs, N-*myc* amplification), and integrated homogeneously staining regions (HSRs) (Brodeur et al. 1981; Brodeur and Fong 1989). The chromosome 1p deletion may represent loss of a tumor suppressor gene involved in neuroblastoma, while the DMs and the HSRs may represent gene amplification. Neuroblastomas can be familial, but no characteristic genetic syndrome or congenital anomaly is associated with a predisposition for this tumor. The proto-oncogene N-*myc* was found initially because it was amplified in neuroblastoma cell lines (Schwab et al. 1983). N-*myc* amplification (3- to 300-fold) is found in primary neuroblastoma and is associated with advanced stages of disease, rapid progression, and poor outcome (Brodeur 1990; Brodeur et al. 1984; Seeger et al. 1985). Neuroblastomas with favorable prognoses are diagnosed early in life, at an early stage, with hyperdiploid karyotypes, and without abnormalities of chromosome 1p or N-*myc* amplification (Jennings et al. 1993). To date, only eight fetal neuroblastomas have had their tumors analyzed for N-*myc* amplification (Crombleholme et al. 1994; Gormel et al. 1994; Ho et al. 1993; Hosoda et al. 1992; Jennings et al. 1993) and all showed a normal copy number of N-*myc* oncogenes. This correlated with disease-free survival after surgery without chemotherapy at 3 to 16 months of age at follow-up.

Familial cases of neuroblastoma have been observed in siblings, identical twins, and one case in which mother and child were both affected (Emery et al. 1983; Pendergrass and Hanson 1976; Grotting et al. 1983). Neu-

roblastoma has also been reported in patients with the Beckwith–Wiedemann syndrome, pancreatic islet-cell dysplasia, and infants born to mothers taking phenytoin. There have also been occasional reports of familial neuroblastoma. One report involved four or five siblings, which suggests that some neuroblastomas may be inherited as an autosomal dominant trait (Dodge and Benner 1945; Chatten and Voorhees 1967). There is also an increased incidence of neuroblastoma in infants with the fetal alcohol syndrome (Kinney et al. 1980; Seeler et al. 1979). Neuroblastoma has also been reported in infants with Hirschsprung's disease, with both rectosigmoid and total colonic Hirschsprung's disease (Corochi et al. 1982; Michna et al. 1988) usually a mediastinal primary.

REFERENCES

Adzick NS, Harrison MR. The unborn surgical patient. Curr Prob Surg 1994;31:33–35.

Allen RW, Ogden B, Bentley FL, Jung AL. Fetal hydantoin syndrome, neuroblastoma, and hemorrhagic disease in a neonate. JAMA 1980;244:1464–1465.

Anders D, Kindermann G, Pfeifer U. Metastasizing fetal neuroblastoma with involvement of the placenta simulating fetal erythroblastosis. J Pediatr 1973;82:50–53.

Andersen JH, Hariri J. Congenital neuroblastoma in a fetus with multiple malformations. Virchows Arch A Pathol Anat 1983;400:219–222.

Askin JA, Geschickter CF. Neuroblastoma of the adrenal in children. J Pediatr 1985;935:157–178.

Atkinson GO, Zaatari GS, Lorenzo RL, Gay BB, Garvin AJ. Cystic neuroblastoma in infants: radiographic and pathologic features. AJR Am J Roentgenol 1986;146:113–117.

Beckwith JB, Perrin EV. In situ neuroblastomas: a contribution to the natural history of neural crest tumor. Am J Pathol 1963;43:1089–1104.

Behrman RE. Neoplasms and neoplasm-like structures. In: Behrman RE, Kliegman RM, Aruin AM, ed. Nelson textbook of pediatrics. Philadelphia: Saunders 1992:1304–1307.

Berry CL, Keeling J, Hilton C. Coincidence of congenital malformation and embryonic tumors of childhood. Arch Dis Child 1970;45:229–231.

Bessho F, Hashizume K, Nakajo T, Kamoshita S. Mass screening in Japan increased the detection of infants with neuroblastoma without a decrease in older children. J Pediatr 1991;119:237–241.

Birner WF. Neuroblastoma as a cause of antenatal death. Am J Obstet Gynecol 1961;82:1388–1391.

Bodian M. Neuroblastoma: an evaluation of its natural history and the effects of therapy. Arch Dis Child 1963;38:606–609.

Brodeur GM. Neuroblastoma: clinical significance of genetic abnormalities. Cancer Surv 1990;9:673–688.

Brodeur GM, Fong CT. Molecular biology and genetics of human neuroblastoma. Cancer Genet Cytogenet 1989;41:153–174.

Brodeur GM, Green AA, Hayes FA, et al. Cytogenetic features of human neuroblastomas and cell lines. Cancer Res 1981;41:4678–4686.

Brodeur GM, Seeger RC, Schwab M, Varmus HE, Bishop JM. Amplification of N-*myc* in untreated human neuroblastomas correlates with advanced disease stage. Science 1984;224:1121–1124.

Chatten J, Voorhees ML. Familial neuroblastoma. N Engl J Med 1967;277:1230–1236.

Crombleholme TC, Murray TA, Harris BH. Diagnosis and management of fetal neuroblastoma. Curr Opin Obstet Gynecol 1994a;6:199–202.

DeFilippi G, Canestri G, Bosio U, Derchi LE, Coppi M. Thoracic neuroblastoma: antenatal demonstration in a case with unusual postnatal radiographic findings. Br J Radiol 1986;59:704–706.

Dodge HJ, Benner MC. Neuroblastoma of the adrenal medulla in siblings. Rocky Mt Med J 1945;42:35–38.

Emery LG, Shields M, Shah NR, et al. Neuroblastoma associated with Beckwith–Wiedemann syndrome. Cancer 1983; 52:176–179.

Estroff JA, Shamberger RC, Diller L, Benacerraf BR. Neuroblastoma. Fetus 1991;1:1–4.

Falkinburg LW, Kay MN. A case of congenital sympathogonioma (neuroblastoma) of the right adrenal simulating erythroblastosis fetalis. J Pediatr 1953;42:462–465.

Fenart D, Deville A, Donzeau M, Bruneton JN. Neuroblastome retroperitoneal diagnostique in utero. J Radiol 1983; 64:359–361.

Ferraro EM, Fakhry J, Aruny JE, Bracero LA. Prenatal adrenal neuroblastoma. J Ultrasound Med 1988;7: 275–278.

Forman HP, Leonidas JC, Berdon WE, et al. Congenital neuroblastoma: evaluation with multimodality imaging. Radiology 1990;175:365–368.

Fowlie F, Giacomantonio M, McKenzie E, Baird D, Covert A. Antenatal sonographic diagnosis of adrenal neuroblastoma. J Can Assoc Radiol 1986;37:50–51.

Gadwood KA, Reynes CJ. Prenatal sonography of metastatic neuroblastoma. J Clin Ultrasound 1983;11:512–551.

Garmel SH, Crombleholme TM, Semple JP, et al. Prenatal diagnosis and management of fetal tumors.Semin Perinatol 1994b;18:350–365.

Giulian BB, Chang CCN, Yoss BS. Prenatal ultrasonographic diagnosis of fetal adrenal neuroblastoma. J Clin Ultrasound 1986;14:225–227.

Goldstein I, Gomez K, Copel JA. The real-time and color doppler appearance of adrenal neuroblastoma in a third-trimester fetus. Obstet Gynecol 1994;83:854–856.

Grosfeld JL, Rescoria FJ, West KW, Goldman J. Neuroblastoma in the first year of life: clinical and biologic factors influencing outcome. Semin Pediatr Surg 1993;2:37–46.

Grotting JC, Kossel C, Demner L. Nesidioblastosis and congenital neuroblastoma. Arch Pathol Lab Med 1983;103: 642–646.

Guin GH, Gilbert EF, Jones B. Incidental neuroblastoma in infants. Am J Clin Pathol 1969;51:126–136.

Hagstrom HT. Fetal dystocia due to metastatic neuroblastoma of the liver. Am J Obstet Gynecol 1929;19:673–676.

Hainaut F, Bouton JM, Plot C, Denhez M. Anasarque foeto-placentaire secondaire a un neuroblastome. J Gynecol Obstet Biol Reprod 1987;16:367–372.

Ho PTC, Estroff JA, Kozakewich H, et al. Prenatal detection of neuroblastoma: a ten-year experience from the Dana

Farber Cancer Institute and Children's Hospital. Pediatrics 1993;92:258–264.

Hosoda Y, Miyano T, Kimura K, et al. Characteristics and management of patients with fetal neuroblastoma. J Pediatr Surg 1992;27:623–625.

Ikeda Y, Lister J, Bouton JM, Buyukpamukcu M. Congenital neuroblastoma in situ, and the normal fetal development of the adrenal. J Pediatr Surg 1981;16:636–644.

Jaffa AJ, Many A, Hartoov J, Kupfermic MJ, Peyser MR. Prenatal sonographic diagnosis of metastic neuroblastoma: report of a case and review of the literature. Prenat Diagn 1993;13:73–77.

Janetschek G, Weitzel D, Stein W, Munterfering H, Alken P. Prenatal diagnosis of neuroblastoma by sonography. Urology 1984;24:397–402.

Jennings RW, LaQuaglia MP, Leong K, Hendren WH, Adzick NS. Fetal neuroblastoma: prenatal diagnosis and natural history. J Pediatr Surg 1993;28:1168–1174.

Johnson CC, Spitz MR. Neuroblastoma: case-control analysis of birth characteristics. J Natl Cancer Inst 1985;74:789–792.

Kinney H, Faix R, Brazy J. The fetal alcohol syndrome and neuroblastoma. Pediatrics 1980;66:130–132.

Kouyoumdjian AO, McDonald JJ. Association of congenital adrenal neuroblastoma with multiple anomalies, including an unusual oropharyngeal cavity (imperforate buccopharyngeal membrane). Cancer 1951;4:784–788.

Kurtz AB, Hilbert P. Ultrasound case of the day. Radiographics 1989;9:361–364.

Liyanage IS, Katoch D. Ultrasonic prenatal diagnosis of liver metastases from adrenal neuroblastoma. J Clin Ultrasound 1992;20:401–403.

Michna BA, McWilliams NB, Kuemmel TM, et al. Multifocal ganglioneuroblastoma coexistent with total colonic aganglionosis. J Pediatr Surg 1988;23:57–59.

Miller RW. Relation between cancer and congenital defects in man. N Engl J Med 1966;275:87–93.

Miller RW, Fraumeni JF, Hill JA. Neuroblastoma: epidemiologic approach to its origin. Am J Dis Child 1968;115: 253–261.

Moss TJ, Kaplan L. Association of hydrops fetalis with congenital neuroblastoma. Am J Obstet Gynecol 1987;132: 905–906.

Murthy TVM, Irving IM, Lister J. Massive adrenal hemorrhage in neonatal neuroblastoma. J Pediatr Surg 1978;13: 31–34.

Newton ER, Louis F, D'Alton ME, Feingold M. Fetal neuroblastoma and catacholamine-induced maternal hypertension. Obstet Gynecol 1985;65:49S–52S.

Nicolay KS, Gainey HL. Pseudotoxemic state associated with severe Rh isoimmunization. Am J Obstet Gynecol 1964;89:41–45.

Pendergrass TW, Hanson JW. Fetal hydantoin syndrome and neuroblastoma. Lancet 1976;2:250.

Pley EAP, Wouters EJM, de Jong PA, Tielens AGWM, Clemonts GJF. The sonographic imaging of fetal adrenal neuroblastoma: a case report. Eur J Obstet Gynecol Reprod Biol 1989;31:95–99.

Potter EL. Tumors. In: Gilbert-Barnes E, ed. Potter's pathology of the fetus and infant. 3rd ed. Chicago: Year Book, 1961:195–198.

Potter EL, Parrish JM. Neuroblastoma, ganglioneuroma, and

of cases are diagnosed before the age of 3 to 4 years, with a mean time of presentation at 2 years of age. Bilateral retinoblastoma typically becomes clinically apparent earlier, with the average age at diagnosis being 12 months (Shields and Shields 1990). In rare cases, multiple congenital anomalies may be seen in association with retinoblastoma. However, these cases represent only 0.05% of cases of retinoblastoma reported in the United States (Jensen and Miller 1971). The reported anomalies include congenital heart disease, cleft palate, Bloch–Sulzberger syndrome, infantile corital hyperasthosis, dentinogenesis imperfecta, incontinentia pigmenti, and familial congenital cataracts (Green 1985).

▶ SONOGRAPHIC FINDINGS

In the case reported by Maat-Kievit et al. (1993), a fetus at 21 weeks of gestation had an oval-shaped mass protruding from the right side of the face (Fig. 115-1). The tumor was an irregular echogenic mass measuring 8 by 6 by 3 cm. The tumor was covered by a thin membrane with an echolucent rim between the membrane and the tumor. The majority of the face was obscured by the tumor. The tumor deformed the normal anatomy of the facial bones, and the contralateral orbit could not be seen. The differential diagnosis of a facial tumor detected by prenatal ultrasound examination and the features that distinguish them are listed in Table 115-1. It

▶ **TABLE 115-1.** DIFFERENTIAL DIAGNOSIS OF FACIAL/ORBITAL TUMORS DETECTED BY PRENATAL SONOGRAPHIC STUDIES

Epignathus
  Sonolucent and (highly) echogenic areas
  Irregular shape
  Localization: nasopharyngeal area
Cephalocele
  Intracranial abnormalities, hydrocephaly, skull defect
  Smooth, rounded shape
  Localization: skull
Hemangioma
  Echogenic or sonolucent areas
  Pulsations, flow (Doppler)
  Localization: oral cavity
Myoblastoma
  Echogenic with small sonolucent areas
  Multilobular shape
  Localization: oral cavity
Dacryocystocele
  Sonolucent
  Small cyst
  Localization: inferomedial to the orbit
Retinoblastoma
  Irregular, echogenic, surrounded by sonolucent area
  Oval shape, covered by membrane
  Localization: eye

Source: Matt-Kievet JA, Oepkes D, Hartwig NG, et al. A large retinoblastoma detected in a fetus at 21 weeks of gestation. Prenat Diagn 1993;13:377–384.

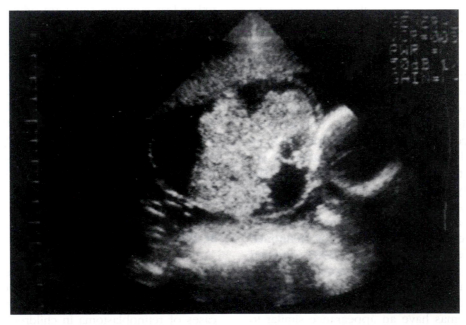

Figure 115-1. Fetus at 22 weeks of gestation with a large tumor originating from the right eye. *(Reprinted from Maat-Kievit JA, Oepkes D, Hartwig NG, et al. A large retinoblastoma detected in a fetus at 21 weeks of gestation. Prenat Diagn 1993;13:377–384. Copyright John Wiley & Sons Limited. Reproduced with permission.)*

should be noted that ultrasound examination is an extremely insensitive screening technique for heritable retinoblastoma in families at risk for recurrence. In these instances, percutaneous umbilical blood sampling or amniocentesis to obtain fetal tissue should be considered, as DNA-based prenatal diagnosis is now available.

▶ DIFFERENTIAL DIAGNOSIS

The case of retinoblastoma diagnosed at 21 weeks of gestation was found to have a very large oval-shaped mass protruding from the right side of the fetal face (Maat-Kievit et al. 1993). Histologic studies confirmed the diagnosis of retinoblastoma with extension beyond the orbit with an 8-by-6-by-3-cm mass rounded by a transonic area covered by a thin membrane. Because of the location and the size of this tumor the differential diagnosis included most causes of facial tumors (see Table 115-1). Epignathus is a tumor that grows through the floor of the mouth, is usually quite irregular in shape, and is localized primarily in the nasopharyngeal area. Although it has a heterogeneous appearance, with sonolucent and highly echogenic areas, its location usually distinguishes it from retinoblastoma. Cephalocele (see Chapter 11) is usually associated with intracranial abnormalities, such as hydrocephalus and calvarial defects. It is usually smooth, contoured, round in shape, and localized to the skull. In contrast, hemangiomas are usually readily identified by color flow Doppler studies, which show significant blood flow within the tumor mass. Myoblastomas are ordinarily localized to the oral cavity and tend to be echogenic, with other sonolucent areas within it. Dacryocystocele may be more difficult to distinguish from retinoblastoma because of its proximity to the eye. It is usually localized in the inframedial aspect of the orbit. Retinoblastoma is an irregular echogenic mass that may be surrounded by the sonolucent area that arises specifically from the eye (see Fig. 115-1).

▶ ANTENATAL NATURAL HISTORY

Retinoblastoma is a congenital tumor that arises from embryonic neural-crest cells. In most newborns, as well as fetuses, retinoblastomas remain undetected until ophthalmologic symptoms arise during childhood (Abramson et al. 1983; Gallie and Phillips 1982; Liebman and Gellis 1966). It is thought that the onset of retinoblastoma must be after the transformation and first differentiation of the nervous layer of the pars optica of the retina in the fifth to eighth weeks of embryogenesis (England 1983). In the case reported by Maat-Kievit et al. (1993), the fetus presented at 21 weeks with a large

mass extending beyond the orbit. This suggests that the tumor cells must have undergone enormous mitotic activity to create such a large tumor in a brief time. This is not the usual presentation of retinoblastoma, which may not be detected for the first several years of life. Whether the natural history of retinoblastoma presenting prenatally is distinct from more typical cases that present in early childhood is unknown.

▶ MANAGEMENT OF PREGNANCY

Fetuses in which retinoblastoma is suspected should be referred to a tertiary-care center capable of anatomic sonographic diagnosis of the fetus. Level 2 sonograms should be obtained to exclude the possibility of associated congenital anomalies, including cleft palate and congenital heart disease. Because of the potential for associated congenital heart disease, if any abnormalities are detected on four-chamber view of the heart, or the outflow tracts or abnormalities in cardiac axis are detected, formal echocardiography is indicated.

If retinoblastoma is detected prior to 24 weeks of gestation, the parents should be counseled about the option of terminating the pregnancy. No treatment options are currently available in utero, and the parents should be informed that a retinoblastoma of a sufficient size to be detected sonographically places the fetus in a very poor prognostic category. Postnatal survival with tumors of this nature are poor, with only a third of the eyes being salvageable, and the cure rate is less than 25%.

Although data regarding the management of the pregnancy are scarce, as few cases have been diagnosed prenatally, consideration should be given to delivery at lung maturity for immediate postnatal therapy. It is unclear if cesarean section is warranted and should be based on an assessment of the size of the tumor close to the time of delivery. Delivery should be planned in a tertiary-care setting, with pediatric ophthalmologists, oncologists, and radiation therapists available to plan the treatment of the newborn.

▶ FETAL INTERVENTION

There is no fetal treatment for retinoblastoma.

▶ TREATMENT OF THE NEWBORN

The neonate should be carefully examined for the presence of associated anomalies. An ophthalmologic consultation should be obtained to assess the extent of the tumor, as well as the contralateral eye.

► SURGICAL TREATMENT

Coordinated follow-up between the ocular oncologist and the primary care specialist is essential because of the likelihood of retinoblastoma recurrence, treatment-associated morbidity, and development of a second tumor that is not retinoblastoma.

The critical objective of retinoblastoma treatment is the survival of the patient, and retinoblastoma cure rates now exceed 90% with current treatment methods (Shields and Shields 1990). Specific treatment approaches vary from center to center, and increasing attention is now focused on preservation of visual function. Enucleation of the eye is considered when there is no hope for useful vision, even if the tumor is thought to be eradicated. A cosmetic disadvantage of this approach is that in children under 3 years of age the orbit ceases to grow normally after the eye is removed, and as the face of the infant grows the orbit looks increasingly sunken (see Chapters 23 and 30). External-beam radiation therapy produces the same appearance due to inhibition of bone growth. The indication for cryotherapy and photocoagulation are similar; however, both techniques can successfully treat only small lesions, less than 3 mm in diameter and 2 mm thick. Episcleral-plaque radiotherapy may be superior to external-beam irradiation in delivering a higher local tumor radiation dose with considerably lower orbital and facial radiation and may be used in solitary tumors less than 8 mm in thickness.

Retinoblastomas are considered radiosensitive. The purpose of radiation therapy for retinoblastomas is control of local disease while preserving vision. Because the majority of patients will have multiple tumors in one or both eyes and these tumors may be multifocal in origin, radiation fields must include the entire geographic extent of the retina, the anterior border of which is the ora serrata. In an attempt to preserve vision, external-beam or episcleral-plaque radiotherapy has become the treatment of choice for the majority of children with retinoblastoma. Any eye that has a chance for useful vision should be considered for radiation therapy rather than enucleation. The results of chemotherapy treatment for intraocular retinoblastoma have been disappointing because intraocular penetration of systemic drugs is poor and tumors often express the membrane glycoprotein p170 and become drug-resistant (Chan et al. 1989). Adjuvant chemotherapy has been tested in children with group V disease (tumors involving more than half the retina or with vitreous seeding) after enucleation, with no survival advantage over enucleation alone (Abramson 1985). Chemotherapy is best restricted to patients with extraocular disease or regional or distant metastases (Pizzo et al. 1985).

After initial treatment, patients must be examined closely for tumor regrowth, extraocular extension, and/or vitreous seeding, and additional radiation, laser, cryotherapy, or adjuvant chemotherapy may be indicated in these cases.

► LONG-TERM OUTCOME

Patients with heritable retinoblastoma have an increased risk for other malignancies developing (Abramson et al. 1984; Roarty et al. 1988; Wilson et al. 1996). In one study, 13% of patients with retinoblastoma, treated by radiation therapy, had second malignancies. Seventy percent of these tumors were in and 30% outside the irradiation field (Abramson et al. 1984). In the same study there were 23 patients who did not receive radiation therapy and 5 of these had second malignant tumors. These tumors were predominately sarcomas, with osteosarcoma being the tumor most frequently reported. The incidence of second malignant tumors appears to increase with time, with a 20% incidence after 10 years. This rises to 50% at 20 years, and at 30 years it approaches 90% (Abramson et al. 1984).

There is considerable controversy regarding the true rate of second malignancy in retinoblastoma survivors. Long-term follow-up studies vary widely with respect to long-term incidence, with reported rates of second malignancy between 25 and 90% at 30-year follow-up. Because of the increasing risk of the development of a second tumor, patients should be examined periodically by the primary care physician. In particular, patients with bilateral retinoblastoma are always at risk for the development of second tumor; the longest reported interval is 57 years between primary retinoblastoma diagnosis and second tumor presentation (Wilson et al. 1996).

► GENETICS AND RECURRENCE RISK

The retinoblastoma locus has been assigned to chromosome 13q14 (Sparkes et al. 1980). Cytogenetic analysis has revealed that there is a deletion of band 13q14 in 5 to 10% of patients with retinoblastoma (Howard 1982; Lemieux and Richer 1990). Genetic and physical mapping indicates that the retinoblastoma gene is closely linked to the genetic locus for esterase D, which maps exactly to this region (Lee and Lee 1986; Sparkes et al. 1983; Squire et al. 1986). The loss of one retinoblastoma allele is insufficient for tumor development, whereas the loss of both alleles is associated with tumor formation. The retinoblastoma gene *(Rb)* is 200,000 base pairs in size and it encodes a protein of 928 amino acids. The *Rb* gene product is a nuclear phosphoprotein with DNA-binding activity that is expressed in many different types of cells (Lee et al. 1987). Rb protein forms complexes with viral oncoproteins of several DNA tumor viruses (DeCaprio et al. 1988; Whyte et al. 1988). Many studies have suggested that the Rb protein plays a role in the regulation of cell growth (Chan et al. 1989)

Retinoblastoma may be either nonheritable or of the heritable type that shows an autosominal dominant inheritance pattern with a high degree of penetrance (Nussbaum and Puck 1976; Vogel 1979). If there is a positive family history, genetic counseling becomes more straightforward because this is clearly a heritable case of retinoblastoma (Cavenee et al. 1986; Draper et al. 1992; Yandell et al. 1989). In sporadic cases, which includes the majority of patients, this may be either heritable or nonheritable. Bilateral sporadic cases are always heritable, and each child of the affected patients who survive will have a 50% risk of having retinoblastoma. Unilateral sporadic cases may be either heritable or nonheritable, with empiric risk studies revealing a 10 to 12% risk of having heritable type and that the first child of a survivor has a 5 to 6% chance of having the disease (Vogel 1979). If normal parents have one affected child, the risk of their next child having a retinoblastoma is about 1% if the first child has a unilateral tumor and 6% if the child has bilateral tumors. To rule out the possibility that one parent is silently clinically affected with an unsuspected retinoblastoma, both parents should have ophthalmologic examinations to facilitate accurate genetic counseling.

Because the *Rb* gene has been cloned, DNA-based prenatal diagnosis is available for families in which one parent is affected, and a 50% recurrence risk exists. DNA analysis is much more accurate than prenatal sonography (Dryja et al. 1989; Gollie et al. 1991; Naumova et al. 1994).

REFERENCES

Abramson DH, Notterman RB, Ellsworth RM. Retinoblastoma treated in infants in the first six months of life. Arch Ophtholmol 1983;101:1362–1366.

Abramson DH, Ellsworth RM, Kitchin FD, Tung G. Second nonocular tumors in retinoblastoma survivors: are they radiation induced? Ophthalmology 1984;91:1351–1355.

Abramson DH. Treatment of retinoblastoma. In: Blandi FC, ed. Contemporary issues in ophthalmology. Vol. 2. Retinoblastoma. New York: Churchill Livingstone, 1985:63–93.

Cavenee WK, Murphree L, Shull MM, et al. Prediction of familial predisposition to retinoblastoma. N Engl J Med 1986;314:1201–1206.

Chan SL, Canton MD, Gallie BL. Chemosensitivity and multi-drug resistance to antineoplastic drugs in retinoblastoma cell lines. Anticancer Res 1989;9:469–474.

DeCaprio JA, Ludlow JW, Figge J, et al. SV40 large tumor antigen forms a specific complex with the product of the retinoblastoma susceptibility gene. Cell 1988;54:275–283.

Devesa SS. The incidence of retinoblastoma. Am J Ophthalmol 1975;80:263–265.

Donaldson SS, Egbert PR, Lee WH. Retinoblastoma. In: Pizzo PA, Poplack DG, eds. Principles and practice of pediatric oncology. Philadelphia: Lippincott, 1993:683–696.

Dryja TP, Mukai S, Petersen R, et al. Parental origin of mutations of the retinoblastoma gene. Nature 1989;339:556–558.

England MA. A color atlas of life before birth: normal fetal development. Chicago: Year Book Medical Publisher 1983:66–68.

Gallie BL, Dunn JM, Chan HSL, et al. The genetics of retinoblastoma: relevance to the patient. Pediatr Clin North Am 1991;38:299–315.

Gallie BL, Ellsworth RM, Abramson DH, et al. Retinoma: spontaneous regression of retinoblastoma or benign manifestation of the mutation? Br J Cancer 1982;45:513–521.

Gallie BL, Phillips RA. Multiple manifestations of the retinoblastoma gene. Birth Defects Original Article Series 1982;18:689–701.

Green DM. Retinoblastoma. In: Green DM, ed. Diagnosis and management of malignant solid tumors in infants and children. Boston: Martinus Nijhoff, 1985:90–128.

Howard RO. Chromosome errors in retinoblastoma. Birth Defects Original Article Series 1982;18:705–715.

Jensen RD, Miller RW. Retinoblastoma: epidemiologic characteristics. N Engl J Med 1971;285:307–311.

Lee EY-HP, Lee W-H. Molecular cloning of the human esterase D gene, a genetic marker of retinoblastoma. Proc Natl Acad Sci USA 1986;88:6337–6341.

Lee W-H, Shew JY, Hong FD, et al. The retinoblastoma susceptibility gene encodes a nuclear phosphoprotein associated with DNA binding activity. Nature 1987;329:642–645.

Lemieux N, Richer CL. Chromosome evolution and high-resolution analysis of leukocytes, bone marrow and tumor cells of retinoblastoma patients. Am J Med Genet 1990;36:456–462.

Liebman SD, Gellis SS. The pediatrician's ophthalmology, St. Louis: Mosby, 1966:257–260.

Maat-Kievit JA, Oepkes D, Hartwig NG, et al. A large retinoblastoma detected in a fetus at 21 weeks of gestation. Prenat Diagn 1993;13:377–384.

Marga CE, Hidayat A, Kopelman J, et al. Retinocytoma: a benign variant of retinoblastoma. Arch Ophthal 1983;101:1519–1531.

Murphree AL, Benedict WF. Retinoblastoma: clues to human oncogenesis. Science 1984;223:1028–1033.

Naumova A, Sapienza C. The genetics of retinoblastoma, revisited. Am J Hum Genet 1994;54:264–273.

Nussbaum R, Puck J. Recurrence risks for retinoblastoma: a model for autosomal dominant disorders with complex inheritance. J Pediatr Ophthalmol 1976;13:89–98.

Pizzo PA, Mises JS, Cassody JR, et al. Solid tumors of childhood. In: Devita UT, Hellman S, Rosenberg SA, eds. Cancer: principles and practice of oncology. 2nd ed. Philadelphia: Lippincott, 1985:1536–1540.

Roarty JD, McLean IW, Zimmerman LE. Incidence of second neoplasms in patients with bilateral retinoblastoma. Ophthalmology 1988;95:1583–1587.

Shields JA, Shields CL. Update on retinoblastoma. Semin Ophthalmol 1990;5:183–192.

Sparkes RS, Murphree AL, Lingua RW, et al. Gene for hereditary retinoblastoma assigned to human chromosome 13 by linkage to esterase D. Science 1983;219:971–973.

Sparkes RS, Sparkes MC, Wilson MG, et al. Regional assignment of genes for human esterase D and retinoblastoma to chromosome band 13q14. Science 1980;208:1042–1044.

Squire J, Dryja TP, Dunn J, et al. Cloning of the esterase D gene: a polymorphic gene probe closely linked to the retinoblastoma on chromosome 13. Proc Natl Acad Sci USA 1986;83:6573–6577.

Vogel F. Genetics of retinoblastoma. Hum Genet 1979;52: 1–54.

Whyte P, Buchkovich KJ, Horowitz JM, et al. Association between an oncogene and an anti-oncogene: the adenovirus E1A proteins bind to the retinoblastoma gene product. Nature 1988;334:124–129.

Wiggs J, Nordenskjold M, Yandell D, et al. Prediction of the risk of hereditary retinoblastoma, using DNA polymorpisms within the retinoblastoma gene. N Engl J Med 1988;318:151–157.

Wilson MG, Ebbin AJ, Towner JW, et al. Chromosomal anomalies in patients with retinoblastoma. Clin Genet 1977;12:1–8.

Wilson MC, Shields JA, Shields CL, et al. Orbital rhabdomyosarcoma fifty-seven years after radiotherapy for retinoblastoma. Orbit 1996;15(2):97–100.

Yandell DW, Campbell TA, Dayton SH, et al. Oncogenic point mutations in the human retinoblastoma gene: their application to genetic counseling. N Engl J Med 1989; 321:1689–1694.

Zimmerman LE. Retinoblastoma and retinocytoma. In: Spencer WH. ed. Ophthalmic pathology: an atlas and textbook. 3rd ed. vol. 2. Philadelphia: Saunders, 1985: 1292–1351.

CHAPTER 116

Sacrococcygeal Teratoma

▶ CONDITION

Sacrococcygeal teratoma (SCT) is defined as a neoplasm composed of tissues from either all three germ layers or multiple foreign tissues lacking an organ specificity (Gross et al. 1951; Mahour et al. 1975). Because of the multiple cell lineages that characterize these tumors, it was previously suggested that SCT was of germ-cell origin or a form of fetus in fetu (Linder et al. 1975; Theiss et al. 1960). However, more recently, SCT has been thought to arise from a totipotent somatic cell originating in Hensen's node. This node is a caudal-cell mass in the embryo that appears to escape normal inductive influences (Bale et al. 1984)

SCT has been classified by the relative amounts of presacral and external tumor present (American Academy of Pediatrics Surgery Section [AAPSS] Classification [Table 116-1, Fig. 116-1) (Altman et al. 1974). The utility of this classification scheme lies in the relationship between stage and timing of diagnosis, ease of resection, and malignant potential. Type I SCT is evident at birth, is usually easily resected, and has a low malignant potential. Similarly, types II and III SCT are recognized at birth, but resection may be difficult, requiring both an anterior and a posterior approach. In type IV SCT, the diagnosis may be delayed until it becomes symptomatic at a later age. Malignant transformation has frequently occurred by the time a type IV SCT is diagnosed. Although the cause is unknown, one hypothesis suggests that SCT is derived from totipotent cells in Hensen's node (Gross et al. 1987) or in reproductive-gland anlage (Abbott et al. 1966). Others have suggested a "twinning accident," with incomplete separation during embryogenesis and abnormal development of one fetus (Ashley 1973; Cousins et al. 1980; Waldhausen et al. 1963). In support of this latter theory, several authors have noted a family history of twinning in many of these patients (Gross et al. 1987; Grosfeld et al. 1976; Hickey and Layton 1954).

▶ INCIDENCE

SCT is one of the most common tumors in newborns; however, it is still rare, occurring in 1 in 35,000 to 1 in 40,000 live births (Schiffer and Greenberg 1956). Females are four times more likely to be affected as males, however, malignant change is more frequently observed in males (Abbott et al. 1966; Altman et al. 1974; Carney et al. 1972; Conklin and Abell 1967; Fraumeni et al. 1973).

▶ SONOGRAPHIC FINDINGS

Retrospective prenatal diagnosis of SCT was first made in the mid-1970s, and the first prospective prenatal diagnosis was reported by Horger and McCarter in 1979. They described a 13-cm complex mass at the fetus's caudal end, with solid and cystic areas and bizarre internal echoes associated with polyhydramnios. This

▶ **TABLE 116-1.** AAPSS STAGING CLASSIFICATION OF SACROCOCCYGEAL TERATOMAS

Type	Description
I	Completely external; no presacral component
II	External component and internal pelvic component
III	External component and internal component extending into abdomen
IV	Completely internal and no external component

Adapted from Altman RP, Randolph JG, Lilly JR. Sacrococcygeal teratoma: American Academy of Pediatrics Surgical Section survey 1993. J Pediatr Surg 1974;9:389–398.

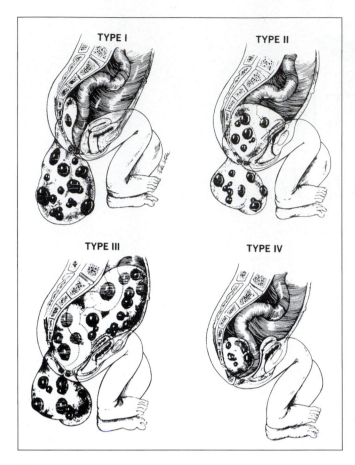

Figure 116-1. AAPSS classification of the different types of sacrococcygeal teratoma, based on the location of the tumor. *(Reprinted, with permission, from Holzgreve W, Flake AW, Langer JC. The fetus with sacrococcygeal teratoma. In: Harrison MR, Golbus MS, Filly RA (eds). The unborn patient. Philadelphia: WB Saunders 1991;461.)*

typical prenatal appearance has been confirmed by other authors (Fig. 116-2) (Seeds et al. 1982). Approximately 60 cases of SCT diagnosed prenatally with ultrasound imaging have been reported (Bond et al. 1990; Grisoni et al. 1988). The most common clinical presentation is uterine size greater than gestational dates, initiating an ultrasound examination (Seeds et al. 1982). To date, the earliest diagnosis of SCT has been made at 13.5 weeks of gestation (Kuhlmann et al. 1987).

SCTs can grow at an unpredictable rate to tremendous dimensions. Several case reports note fetal tumors as large as 25 by 20 cm (Heys et al. 1967; Weiss et al. 1976). These tumors are generally exophytic (AAPSS type I), but may extend retroperitoneally displacing pelvic (type II) or abdominal structures (type III) (Litwiller 1967).

Most SCTs are solid or mixed solid and cystic, consisting of randomly arranged irregularly shaped cysts (Chervenak et al. 1985; Seeds et al. 1982). Purely cystic SCT has also been described prenatally (Hogge et al. 1987; Seeds et al. 1982). Calcifications can be seen microscopically, although the majority are not visible on prenatal ultrasound examination. Most prenatally diagnosed SCTs are extremely vascular, which is easily demonstrated with the use of color flow Doppler studies (Fig. 116-3). Polyhydramnios has been noted in most cases of prenatally diagnosed SCT, although the mechanisms for this are not known (Chervenak et al. 1985).

Hepatomegaly, placentomegaly, and nonimmune hydrops have also been seen in association with SCT and appear to be secondary to high-output cardiac failure (Bond et al. 1990; Cousins et al. 1980; Flake 1993; Gergely et al. 1980; Heys et al. 1967; Kapoor and Saha 1989). High-output failure may be due to tumor hem-

Figure 116-2. Prenatal sonographic image demonstrating large type II sacrococcygeal tumor in a 23-week-old fetus. In this view the intrapelvic extent of the tumor cannot be seen.

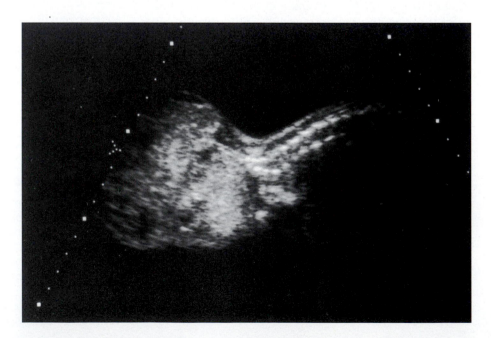

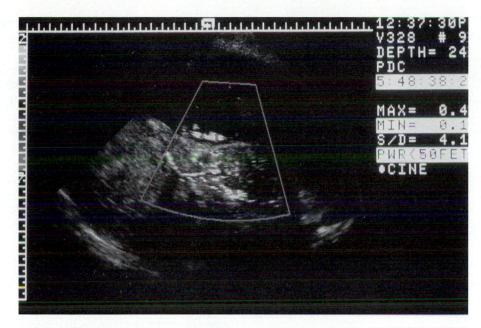

Figure 116-3. Color flow Doppler study of the same fetus shown in Figure 116-1 demonstrating the vascularity of the tumor. See color plate.

orrhage or arteriovenous shunting within the tumor (Alter et al. 1988; Bond et al. 1990; Cousins et al. 1980; Flake et al. 1986; Schmidt et al. 1989). Some authors have attributed heart failure with subsequent hydrops to severe fetal anemia secondary to tumor hemorrhage (Alter et al. 1988). However, normal fetal hematocrits have also been reported, suggesting that congestive heart failure is more often due to high-output cardiac failure from arteriovenous shunting within the tumor (Schmidt et al. 1989). The demonstration of heart failure or hydrops on ultrasound examination is usually a preterminal event (Bond et al. 1990; Flake et al. 1986; Kuhlmann et al. 1987).

Controversy exists regarding the presence of associated anomalies and the need for chromosome analysis. The incidence of coexisting anomalies is 11 to 38%, primarily involving the nervous, cardiac, gastrointestinal, genitourinary, and musculoskeletal systems (Altman et al. 1974; Carney et al. 1972; Ein et al. 1980; Fraumeni et al. 1973; Gonzalez-Crussi et al. 1978; Hickey and Layton 1954; Holzgreve et al. 1985; Izant and Filston 1975; Kuhlmann et al. 1987; Schiffer and Greenberg 1956; Werb et al. 1992). Several authors postulate that at least some of these anomalies are related to tumor development. Others have reported an increased incidence of spinal deformities (Alexander and Stevenson 1946; Bentley and Smith 1960; Carney et al. 1972; Ewing 1940; Gruenwald 1941; Wilson et al. 1963). Most authors agree with Berry et al.'s (1970) observation of an increased incidence of local abnormalities only, such as rectovaginal fistula and imperforate anus, which are thought to be directly related to tumor growth during

fetal development. Aneuploidy has not been reported with SCT and we do not recommend amniocentesis for karyotype analysis unless fetal surgery is contemplated.

▶ DIFFERENTIAL DIAGNOSIS

The differential diagnosis of SCT includes lumbosacral myelomeningocele, which invariably demonstrates a spinal defect. Myelomeningoceles have a cystic or semicystic rather than a solid appearance and do not contain calcifications. Examination of the fetal brain is helpful in establishing the diagnosis, as most fetuses with lumbosacral myelomeningocele will have cranial signs. Rarer entities that mimic SCT include neuroblastoma, glioma, hemangioma, neurofibroma, cordoma, leiomyoma, lipoma, melanoma, and any of the 50 tumors or malformations of the sacrococcygeal region that may be seen (Table 116-2) (Lemire and Beckwith 1982)

Biochemical markers such as α-fetoprotein (AFP) and acetylcholinesterase are not reliable in distinguishing SCTs from other abnormalities (Holzgreve et al. 1987). It has been suggested, however, that AFP can be used to differentiate benign from malignant tumors, as marked elevations of AFP may reflect the presence of a malignant endodermal sinus component to the tumor (Gonzalez-Crussi 1978, 1982; Grosfeld et al. 1976; Tsuchilda et al. 1975). AFP levels can be extremely high in normal newborns, limiting the utility of this marker to distinguish benign from malignant lesions (Ohama et al. 1997).

▶ **TABLE 116-2.** TUMORS AND MALFORMATIONS OF THE SACROCOCCYGEAL REGION*

Subcutaneous lipoma
Teratoma
Endodermal sinus tumor
Neuroblastoma
Ganglioneuroma
Myxopapillary ependymoma
Fibromatosis
Neurofibroma
Ependymoma
Giant cell tumor of sacrum
Leiomyoma
Lymphoma
Rhabdomyosarcoma
Mesenchymoma
Wilms' tumor in teratoma
Paraganglioma
Glomus tumor
Lumbosacral lipoma
Tail appendage
Hamartoma
Hemangioma
Hemangioendothelioma
Teratoma in meningomyelocele
Myelocystocele
Meningocele

*This table lists reported tumors and malformations of the sacro-coccygeal region in postnatal patients. Not all have been diagnosed prenatally.
Source: Lemire RJ, Beckwith JB. Pathogenesis of congenital tumors and malformations in the sacrococcygeal region. Teratology 1982;25:201–213.

▶ ANTENATAL NATURAL HISTORY

The antenatal natural history of prenatally detected SCT is not as favorable as that of SCT presenting at birth. Well-defined prognostic factors for SCT diagnosed postnatally, as outlined in the AAPSS classification system, do not necessarily apply to fetal cases (Altman et al. 1974; Bond et al. 1990) (see Table 116-1). While the mortality rate for SCT diagnosed in the newborn is at most 5%, the mortality rate for fetal SCT approaches 50% (Bond et al. 1990; Flake et al. 1986; Flake 1993).

Most SCTs are histologically benign. Malignancy appears to be more common in males, especially with solid versus complex or cystic tumors (Schey et al. 1977). The presence of histologically immature tissue does not necessarily signify malignancy (Carney et al. 1972; Gonzalez-Crussi 1982). Calcifications occur more often in benign tumors but may also be seen in malignant tumors and are unreliable indicators of malignant potential (Grosfeld et al. 1976; Hickey et al. 1954; Horger and McCarter 1979; Schey et al. 1977; Waldhausen et al. 1963). Although there is one reported case of malignant yolk sac differentiation in a fetal SCT, there

has not been a case of metastatic teratoma in a neonate with a prenatally diagnosed SCT (Flake 1993; Holzgreve et al. 1985).

The prenatal history of SCT is quite different from the postnatal natural history. Flake et al. (1986) reviewed 27 cases of prenatally diagnosed SCT. Five cases were electively terminated and 15 of the remaining 22 died, either in utero or shortly after delivery. The majority of these patients presented between 22 and 34 weeks of gestation with a uterus large for gestational age secondary to severe polyhydramnios. The presence of hydrops and/or polyhydramnios was associated with intrauterine fetal death in 7 of 7 cases. Bond et al. reported survey data from the International Fetal Medicine and Surgery Society on prenatally diagnosed SCT, confirming the high mortality, with a rate of 52% (Bond et al. 1990). When SCT was seen in association with placentomegaly or hydrops all 15 fetuses died precipitously in utero. The indication for ultrasound examination was also found to be a predictive factor. If SCT was an incidental finding, the prognosis was favorable at any gestational age. However, if the ultrasound examination was performed for maternal indications, 22 of 32 fetuses died. In addition, diagnosis prior to 30 weeks was associated with a poor outcome.

Sheth et al. (1988) also reported significant perinatal mortality associated with SCT, with only 6 survivors of 15 cases diagnosed prenatally. Three of 4 cases associated with hydrops were rapidly fatal. The sole survivor was salvaged by emergency cesarean section at 35 weeks. This series was unusual because 3 cases had severe obstructive uropathy and secondary renal dysplasia. A more favorable outcome was reported by Gross et al. (1987) in which 8 of 10 fetuses with prenatally diagnosed SCT survived. However, no fetus had hydrops or placentomegaly, and the 2 nonsurvivors were electively terminated.

Hydrops in SCT is usually, but not always, fatal. Nakayama et al. (1991) reported survival in two fetuses with SCT presenting with hydrops at 27 and 30 weeks of gestation. In addition, Robertson et al. (1995) were able to salvage a hydropic fetus at 26 weeks of gestation by staged resection of the SCT (Fig. 116-4). Acute rapid growth of the SCT with polyhydramnios and preterm labor had developed in this fetus. The newborn was in a high-output state from shunting through the tumor. In a staged resection, the tumor was initially devascularized by ligation of both internal iliac arteries. Twenty-four hours later the external portion of the mass was resected. The infant underwent resection of the intrapelvic portion of the tumor at 3 months of age, and did well.

Sonographic features of SCT including size, AAPSS classification, solid or cystic composition, or presence or absence of calcifications have not been predictive of either fetal survival or future malignant potential

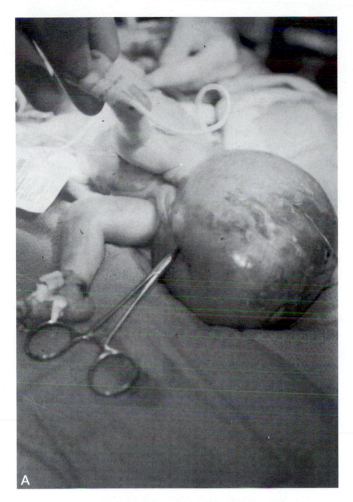
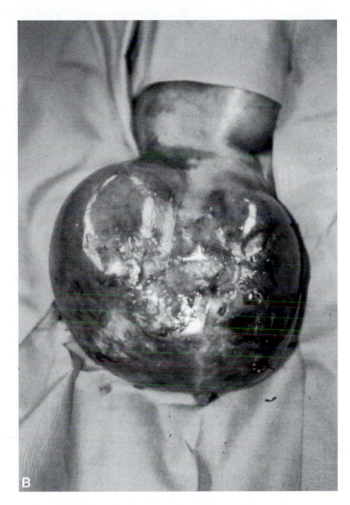

Figure 116-4. Postnatal photograph of a 26-week-gestation premature newborn with a large SCT. (A) The SCT has distorted the perineum so that the anus is in a plane anterior to the genitalia. The tip of the clamp is in the anal orifice. (B) The same tumor following devascularization. *(Reprinted, with permission, from Robertson FR, Crombleholme TM, Frantz ID III, Shepard BA, D'Alton ME, Bianchi DW. Devascularization and staged resection of giant SCT in the preterm infant. J Pediatr Surg 1995;30:309–311.)*

(Altman et al. 1974; Flake 1993). One exception to this may be the unilocular cystic form of SCT, which has a relatively favorable prognosis because of benign histology and limited vascular and metabolic demand (Horger and McCarter 1979; Mintz et al. 1983). The growth of the SCT in relation to the size of the fetus is unpredictable and may increase, decrease, or stabilize as gestation proceeds. However, a rapid phase of tumor growth usually precedes the development of placentomegaly and hydrops. One sonographic feature that appears to be associated with rapid tumor growth and the development of placentomegaly and hydrops is the color Doppler appearance of the tumor itself, with highly vascular lesions more likely to develop complications.

The prenatal mortality, unlike postnatal mortality, is not due to malignant degeneration, but to complications of tumor mass or tumor physiology (Flake et al. 1983). The tumor mass may result in malpresentation or dystocia, which in turn may result in tumor rupture and hemorrhage during delivery. Dystocia has been reported as an obstetric problem in 6 to 13% of cases in postnatal series (Giugiaro et al. 1977; Gross et al. 1987; Musci et al. 1983). The most important benefit of prenatal diagnosis is prevention of dystocia by elective or emergency cesarean section. Tumor mass effect may also result in uterine instability and preterm delivery because of uterine distention (Bond et al. 1990; Flake et al. 1986). Massive polyhydramnios is frequently seen in large fetal SCT, which also predisposes to uterine irritability and preterm delivery and resulting perinatal morbidity and mortality. The cause of polyhydramnios in fetal SCT is uncertain, but may be hyperfiltration of the fetal kidney due to the high-output cardiac state.

The physiologic consequence of fetal SCT depends on the metabolic demands of the tumor, blood flow to the tumor, and the presence and degree of anemia. The nature of the SCT—whether cystic or solid, size, and rate of growth—all affect the metabolic demands of fetal SCT. While classically thought to derive its blood supply from the middle sacral artery (Smith et al. 1961) these large tumors often parasitize blood supply from the internal and external iliac systems. This may result in vascular "steal" from the umbilical-artery blood flow to the placenta. A confounding factor is the development of fetal anemia either from external tumor rupture or hemorrhage into the tumor. The latter may occur as a result of necrosis caused by the tumor outgrowing its blood supply. Either anemia or vascular steal, or both, may contribute to the high-output physiology seen in fetal SCT.

The high-output cardiac failure in fetal SCT can be diagnosed by fetal echocardiography and Doppler study (Flake et al. 1986; Langer et al. 1989; Schmidt et al. 1989). When hydrops develops in fetuses with SCT, all have dilated ventricles and dilated inferior venae cavae due to increased venous return from the lower body (Flake 1993). Serial sonographic examinations in fetal SCT often show progressive increases in combined ventricular output and descending aortic flow velocity. In general, placental blood flow is decreased by the vascular steal by the SCT (Flake 1993; Schmidt et al. 1989). Postnatal measurements of umbilical arterial blood gases before and after removal of a large SCT demonstrate that the tumor acts as a large arteriovenous shunt.

▶ MANAGEMENT OF PREGNANCY

Although the primary cause of death in neonatal SCT is malignant invasion, in prenatal SCT the complications of prematurity or exsanguinating tumor hemorrhage at delivery predominate (Adzick and Harrison 1994; Bond et al. 1990; Flake et al. 1986). Weekly sonographic examinations should be performed during pregnancy to assess amniotic fluid index, tumor growth, fetal well-being, and early evidence of hydrops (Chervenak et al. 1985; Langer et al. 1989). Serial Doppler echocardiographic evaluations should be performed in all patients to detect early signs of high-output state, as evaluated by an increased diameter of the inferior vena cava, increased descending aortic flow velocity, or increased combined ventricular output (Alter et al. 1988; Flake 1993). Evidence of heart failure, placentomegaly, and/or hydrops should be sought, as these may progress rapidly and are harbingers of preterminal events (Langer et al. 1989). Bond et al. (1990) reported a uniformly fatal outcome when SCT was associated with placentomegaly and/or hydrops. Only 2 of 17 deaths occurred when neither placentomegaly nor hydrops was present. Flake et al. (1986) reported seven of seven fetal deaths in pregnancies complicated by placentomegaly and hydrops. Weekly amniocenteses to determine pulmonary maturity are recommended by some physicians after 36

weeks of gestation, with delivery once fetal lung maturity is established (Adzick and Harrison 1994). Warning signs and symptoms of preterm labor should be stressed at prenatal visits, and limitation of activity, treatment, and cervical checks may be indicated (Garmel et al. 1994). The recommended mode of delivery is determined by the size of the tumor. Vaginal delivery may be possible with some small tumors (Flake 1993; Grisoni et al. 1988). Complications of vaginal delivery have included fetal death after rupture, avulsion, or asphyxia (Chervenak et al. 1985; Giugiaro et al. 1977; Grosfeld et al. 1976; Heys et al. 1967; Holzgreve et al. 1987; Schiffer and Greenberg 1956; Werb et al. 1992). Cesarean delivery is recommended to avoid trauma-induced hemorrhage or dystocia, especially in large (>5 to 10 cm) tumors (Chervenak et al. 1985; El-Qarmalaui et al. 1990; Flake 1993; Gross et al. 1987; Hoag et al. 1987). The size of the tumor may also influence the type of uterine incision. A large tumor may warrant a classical uterine incision, especially in a preterm infant (Chervenak et al. 1985).

Dystocia has been reported when the diagnosis of SCT was unsuspected in as many as 6 to 13% of cases (Abbott et al. 1966; Desai et al. 1968; Edwards 1983; El-Shafie et al. 1988; Heys et al. 1967; Hickey and Layton 1954; Hickey and Martin 1964; Johnson et al. 1988; Kowalski et al. 1968; Litwiller 1969; Lowenstein et al. 1963; Lu and Lee 1966; Mintz et al. 1983; Musci et al. 1983; Schiffer and Greenberg 1956; Seeds et al. 1982; Seidenberg and Hurwitt 1958; Tanaree 1982; Varga et al. 1987; Weiss et al. 1976; Werner and Swiecicka 1968). Transabdominal and transvaginal aspirations of large cysts have been attempted with variable results to facilitate delivery in the face of significant dystocia (Abbott et al. 1966; Desai et al. 1968; Edwards 1983; El-Shafie et al. 1988; Johnson et al. 1988; Litwiller 1969; Mintz et al. 1983; Musci et al. 1983; Tanaree 1982; Weiss et al. 1976). It is hoped that prenatal detection of SCT will prevent such unforeseen emergencies (Musci et al. 1983).

Fetal SCT is sometimes associated with maternal complications. The mother should be observed for signs and symptoms of preeclampsia, such as the "mirror syndrome" described by Nicolay et al. in association with SCT and hydrops (Bond et al. 1990; Coleman et al. 1987; Cousins et al. 1980; Flake et al. 1986; Langer et al. 1989; Nicolay and Gainey 1964). Delivery should be performed in a tertiary-care center, with neonatologists and pediatric surgeons available.

▶ FETAL INTERVENTION

The uniformly dismal outcome in fetuses with SCT complicated by placentomegaly and hydrops has been the impetus for resection of this tumor in utero. Harrison was the first to attempt antenatal resection of an SCT (Langer et al. 1989). The first case, at 24 weeks of gestation, was markedly hydropic (Flake 1993; Langer et al. 1989) with a significantly elevated combined ventricular output of 972 ml per kilogram of body weight per minute documented by echocardiography. In addition, the mother had mild hypertension, edema, and proteinuria. Preterm labor developed, which was controlled with tocolytic agents. At surgery, the exophytic portion of the tumor was dissected free of the anus and rectum and amputated at its base with a stapling device. Despite the resection, the fetus remained hydropic, with an elevated combined ventricular output of 869 ml per kilogram of body weight per minute. Percutaneous umbilical-cord blood sampling showed the fetal hematocrit to be only 16%. This was increased to 27% by blood transfusion. The fetus subsequently improved significantly, with sonographic resolution of hydrops, and a decrease in descending aortic flow to 524 ml per kilogram of body weight per minute. However, the maternal mirror syndrome progressed to pulmonary edema and on postoperative day 12, a 26-week-gestation fetus was delivered by cesarean section and died of pulmonary immaturity at 6 hours of age. The mother's illness resolved within 2 days. Autopsy showed no evidence of hydrops and no residual tumor.

A second case was attempted at 26 weeks of gestation, when dramatic enlargement of the tumor resulted in early hydrops, elevated combined ventricular output, and severe polyhydramnios (Flake 1993). The surgery went uneventfully, and the base of the tumor was stapled to excise the exophytic portion and reverse the hyperdynamic state. The fetus did well until postoper-

ative day 8, when irreversible preterm labor developed and the fetus was delivered by emergency cesarean section. Because the histology of the resected specimen was interpreted as an immature teratoma grade III/III, with predominance of neuroepithelial elements and foci of yolk sac differentiation, resection of residual tumor was attempted on the 13th day of life. During dissection of the presacral space the baby experienced complete cardiovascular collapse due to a paradoxical air embolism. The histology of the tumor revealed grade III/III immature teratoma, but the residual tumor was more mature than the previous tumor specimen and contained no foci of yolk sac differentiation.

The first successful resection of fetal SCT with long-term survival was reported by Adzick et al. (1997). At 25 weeks of gestation a type II SCT had rapid enlargement and development of polyhydramnios and placentomegaly, with associated maternal tachycardia and proteinuria suggesting impending maternal mirror syndrome (Fig. 116-5). At surgery, the exophytic portion of the tumor was dissected free of the anus and rectum and the base of the tumor excised with a thick-tissue stapling device (Fig. 116-6). The mother and fetus did well postoperatively, with resolution of hydrops and placentomegaly within 10 days. Pathology of the tumor showed grade III/III immature teratoma without evidence of yolk sac differentiation. At 29 weeks of gestation preterm labor prompted cesarean delivery. Postnatally, the female infant underwent resection of the coccyx and surrounding tissue at 2 months of age, but no residual tumor was found. She did well until 1 year of age when

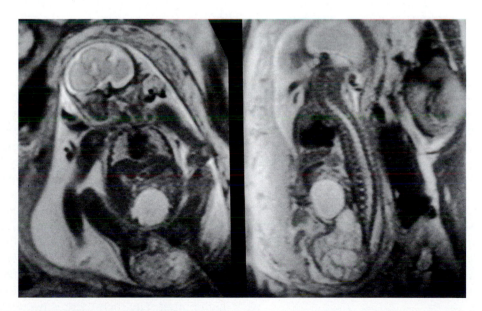

Figure 116-5. Fetal magnetic resonance imaging scan demonstrating in coronal (left) and sagittal (right) sections a fetus at 25 weeks of gestation with type II SCT. The large intrapelvic portion of tumor has completely blocked the bladder outlet, causing megacystis. The fetal urine is detectable by the presence of contrast dye. *(Reprinted, with permission, from Quinn TM, Hubbard AM, Adzick NS. Prenatal magnetic resonance imaging enhances fetal diagnosis. J Pediatr Surg 1998;33:553–558.)*

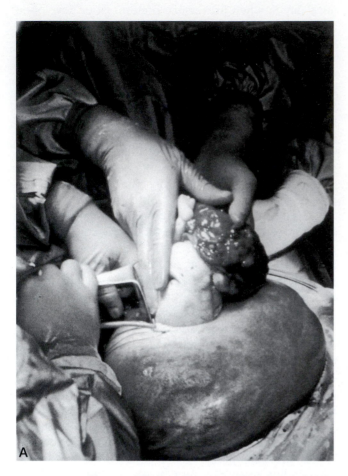
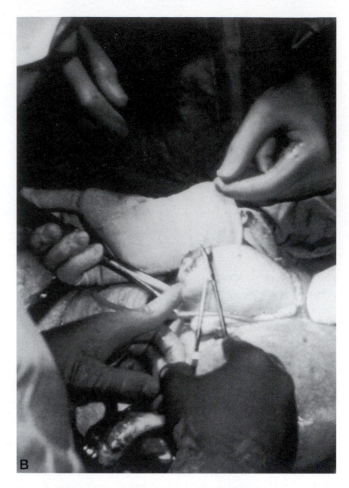

Figure 116-6. Intraoperative view of a 25-week-gestation fetus undergoing resection in utero. (A) The ruptured tumor and lower extremities of the fetus are delivered from the wound. (B) The fetal buttock wound is closed immediately following resection. *(Reprinted, with permission, from Adzick NS, Crombleholme TM, Morgan MA, Quinn TM. A rapidly growing fetal teratoma. Lancet 1997;349:538.)*

AFP levels became elevated to 22,000ng/ml and she presented with pleural effusions, lung nodules, and a recurrent buttock mass from a metastatic yolk sac tumor. She has had an excellent response to chemotherapy.

While clinical experience remains limited, there have been two other cases of SCT successfully resected in utero, at Children's Hospital of Philadelphia and at the University of California, San Francisco. For the fetus with a large SCT associated with early signs of hydrops or placentomegaly, resection in utero remains a viable option. Primary resection of the external portion of the tumor was performed with interval resection of the pelvic extension of SCT. This approach may be useful in managing the common association of prematurity, large tumor, and hyperdynamic state.

▶ TREATMENT OF THE NEWBORN

A neonatologist should attend the delivery and be prepared to provide respiratory support. Careful handling of the infant is important to prevent exsanguinating hemorrhage into the tumor. Umbilical-artery and venous catheters should be placed. Excellent venous access is paramount should hemorrhage in the tumor occur. The infant should be started on pressor agents such as dopamine or dobutamine to support the heart in its hyperdynamic state. Transfusion may be necessary immediately postnatally because hemorrhage into the tumor may have occurred during the delivery.

Severely premature infants should be intubated and treated for respiratory distress with surfactant-replacement therapy. Echocardiography should be obtained to assess the cardiac status of the newborn. Abdominal ultrasound examination can be performed at the bedside to assess the intrapelvic extent of tumor. If there is no high-output state then there is no urgency to resect the tumor, and attention should focus on the treatment of respiratory distress and correction of anemia. If a hyperdynamic state exists with an elevated cardiac output, attention should focus on supporting the newborn heart with inotropic agents and urgent resection of the SCT.

▶ SURGICAL TREATMENT

The goal of this resection is reversal of the high-output state, and this can usually be accomplished by resection of the exophytic portion of the tumor. We have used aortic occlusion by vessel loop to minimize hemorrhage when resecting a SCT in a severely premature infant. If residual pelvic tumor remains, the urgency of resection can be guided by the pathology. The presence of yolk sac differentiation would necessitate earlier resection. In the absence of yolk sac differentiation, however, several months of growth of the infant can facilitate subsequent resection of the coccyx and the intrapelvic portion of the tumor. Usually an abdominoperitoneal approach is required for resection of the pelvic tumor. The operating table should be kept in a slight reverse Trendelenburg position to prevent air embolism (Seeds et al. 1982).

Large SCTs often result in polyhydramnios and in twin preterm labor. Complications of prematurity are a leading cause of mortality in fetal SCT. In one report, a fetus had been followed closely but preterm labor developed that could not be controlled (Robertson et al. 1995). The newborn had significant respiratory distress syndrome and was in a high-output state from a tumor 1.5 times its size. Because the primary physiologic derangement was the high-output state, the baby underwent an initial devascularization by ligating the internal iliac arteries and colostomy for fecal diversion. Initial ligation of the middle sacral and internal iliac arteries eliminated the hyperdynamic high-output state. This returned cardiac output to normal and allowed time to respond to surfactant-replacement therapy. Thirty-six hours later primary resection of the residual tumor was performed. The infant underwent subsequent resection of the intrapelvic portion of the tumor at 2 months of age. She has done well and is now 4 years of age and free of disease.

▶ LONG-TERM OUTCOME

The most important prognostic factor for SCT appears to be the age at diagnosis (Conklin and Abell 1967). When the diagnosis is made prior to 2 months of postnatal age, or excision is performed prior to 4 months of age, the malignant potential is only 5 to 10% (Donnellan and Swenson 1988; Gross et al. 1951; Hickey and Layton 1954; Waldhausen et al. 1963). This increases from 50% to 90% if the diagnosis is delayed until after 2 to 4 months of age (Hickey and Layton 1954; Altman et al. 1974). The mortality in a newborn with SCT is not primarily due to malignant potential, but rather from difficulty in resection, and possibility of tumor hemorrhage (Alter et al. 1988; Altman et al. 1974; Grissoni et al. 1988; Schey et al. 1977). Gestational age at diagnosis

may also affect prognosis, as fetuses diagnosed with SCT after 30 weeks of gestation tend to fare better than those diagnosed earlier (Flake et al. 1986; Kuhlmann et al. 1987; Schey et al. 1977). Cystic tumors may carry a better prognosis, most likely because of the lower incidence of tumor hemorrhage or vascular steal (Hogge et al. 1987).

Prompt excision of both the tumor and the coccyx is thought to be essential to prevent recurrence (Gross et al. 1987). Delay may result in infection, hemorrhage, pressure necrosis, and malignant degeneration (Holzgreve et al. 1985). Fortunately, with benign SCT there is usually no serious bowel or bladder dysfunction after surgery and most neonates do well following resection (Gross et al. 1987; Litwiller 1969; Tapper and Lack 1983).

The long-term outcome in newborns with SCT is generally excellent. These tumors are benign but do have premalignant potential, and close follow-up is important. Most SCTs that undergo malignant transformation are type IV, with no external component to indicate the diagnosis. We currently recommend that all newborns with SCT have serum AFP levels measured and physical examinations performed, including digital rectal examinations every 3 months. If the SCT was nonfunctional, postnatal pelvic sonographic examinations should be obtained at similar intervals. Although SCTs are usually benign, they are prone to recurrence. Surveillance for tumor recurrence is essential postoperatively. In SCTs that are functional, AFP levels may be a useful marker for possible recurrence. If the initial serum AFP level is not elevated, then pelvic ultrasound examinations should be obtained on a yearly basis. Recurrence of the tumor does not necessarily indicate recurrence of malignancy. It should be treated as a premalignant lesion and excised. Even with malignant transformation of SCT, results with current chemotherapeutic regimens have achieved excellent survival rates. Misra et al. (1997) reported survival rates of 88% with local disease and 75% even in the face of distant metastases.

▶ GENETICS AND RECURRENCE RISK

Some cases of SCT appear to be familial, with a suggestion of an autosomal dominant inheritance (Gonzalez-Crussi 1982; Hunt et al. 1977).

REFERENCES

Abbott PD, Bowman A, Kantor HI: Dystocia caused by sacrococcygeal teratoma. Obstet Gynecol 1966;27:571–579.

Adzick NS, Harrison MR. The unborn surgical patient. Curr Probl Surg 1994;35:1.

Adzick NS, Crombleholme TM, Morgan MA, Quinn TM. A rapidly growing fetal teratoma. Lancet 1997;349:538.

Alexander CM, Stevenson LD. Sacral spina bifida, intrapelvic meningocele, and sacrococcygeal teratoma. Am J Clin Pathol 1946;16:466–471.

Alter DN, Reed KL, Marx GR, Anderson CF, Shenker L. Prenatal diagnosis of congestive heart failure in a fetus with a sacrococcygeal teratoma. Obstet Gynecol 1988;71:978–981.

Altman RP, Randolph JG, Lilly JR. Sacrococcygeal teratoma. American Academy of Pediatrics Surgical Section Survey—1973. J Pediatr Surg 1974;9:389–398.

Ashley DJB. Origin of teratomas. Cancer 1973;32:390–394.

Bale PM: Sacrococcygeal developmental abnormalities and tumors in children. Perspect Pediatr Pathol 1984;1:9–56.

Bentley JFR, Smith JR. Developmental posterior enteric remnants and spinal malformations. Arch Dis Child 1960; 35:76–86.

Berry CL, Keeling J, Hilton C. Coincidence of congenital malformation and embryonic tumours of childhood. Arch Dis Child 1970;45:229–231.

Bond SJ, Harrison MR, Schmidt KG, et al. Death due to high-output cardiac failure in fetal sacrococcygeal teratoma. J Pediatr Surg 1990;25:1287–1291.

Carney JA, Thompson DP, Johnson CL, Lynn HB. Teratomas in children: clinical and pathologic aspects. J Pediatr Surg 1972;7:271–282.

Chervenak FA, Isaacson G, Touloukian R, et al. Diagnosis and management of fetal teratomas. Obstet Gynecol 1985;66:666–671.

Conklin J, Abell MR. Germ cell neoplasms of sacrococcygeal region. Cancer 1967;12:2105–2117.

Cousins L, Benirschke K, Porreco R, Resnik R. Placentomegaly due to fetal congestive failure in a pregnancy with a sacrococcygeal teratoma. J Reprod Med 1980;25: 142–144.

Desai V. Dystocia due to fetal sacrococcygeal teratoma. J Obstet Gynaecol Br Commw 1968;75:1074–1075.

Donnellan WA, Swenson O. Benign and malignant sacrococcygeal teratomas. Pediatr Surg 1988;64:834–846.

Edwards WR. A fetal sacrococcygeal tumor obstructing labor after attempted home confinement. Obstet Gynecol 1983;61:19S–21S.

Ein SH, Adeyemei SD, Mancer K. Benign sacrococcygeal teratomas in infants and children. Ann Surg 1980;191: 382–384.

El-Qarmalaui MA, Saddik M, El Abdel Hadi F, Muwaffi R, Nageeb K. Diagnosis and management of fetal sacrococcygeal teratoma. Int J Gynecol Obstet 1990;31:275–281.

El-Shafie M, Naylor D, Schaff E, Conrad M, Miller D. Unexpected dystocia secondary to a fetal sacrococcygeal teratoma: a successful outcome. Int J Gynecol Obstet 1988;27:431–438.

Flake AW. Fetal sacrococcygeal teratoma. Semin Pediatr Surg 1993;2:113–120.

Flake AW, Harrison MR, Adzick NS, Laberge J, Warsof SL. Fetal sacrococcygeal teratoma. J Pediatr Surg 1986;21: 563–566.

Fraumeni JR, Li FP, Dalager N. Teratomas in children: Epidemiologic features. J Natl Cancer Inst 1973;1425–1430.

Garmel SH, Crombleholme TM, Semple J et al. Prenatal diagnosis and management of fetal tumors. Semin Perinatol 1994;18:350–365.

Gergely RZ, Eden R, Schifrin BS, Wade ME. Antenatal diagnosis of congenital sacral teratoma. J Reprod Med 1980;24:229–231.

Giugiaro A, Boario U, DiFrancesco G, Freni G. Considerazioni su tre casi di rottura intraparto di teratoma sacro-coccigeo. Minerva Pediatr 1977;29:1517–1524. (English summary.)

Gonzalez-Crussi F. Extragonadal teratomas. Atlas of tumor pathology. 2nd series, fascicle 18. Bethesda, MD: Armed Forces Institute of Pathology, 1982:50–76.

Gonzalez-Crussi F, Winkler RF, Mirkin DL. Sacrococcygeal teratomas in infants and children. Arch Pathol Lab Med 1978;102:420–425.

Grisoni ER, Gauderer MWL, Wolfson RN, Jassani MN, Olsen MM. Antenatal diagnosis of sacrococcygeal teratomas: prognostic features. Pediatr Surg Int 1988;3:173–175.

Grosfeld JL, Ballantine TVN, Lowe D, Baehner RL. Benign and malignant teratomas in children: analysis of 85 patients. Surgery 1976;80:297–305.

Gross RE, Clatworthy HW, Meeker IA. Sacrococcygeal teratomas in infants and children. Surg Gynecol Obstet 1951;92:341–354.

Gross SJ, Benzie RJ, Sermer M, Skidmore MB, Wilson SR. Sacrococcygeal teratoma: prenatal diagnosis and management. Am J Obstet Gynecol 1987;156:393–396.

Gruenwald P. Tissue anomalies of probable neural crest origin in a twenty millimeter human embryo with myeloschysis. Arch Pathol 1941;31:489–500.

Heys RF, Murray CP, Kohler HG. Obstructed labour due to foetal tumours: cervical and cocygeal teratoma. Gynaecologia 1967;164:43–54.

Hickey RC, Layton JM. Sacrococcygeal teratoma: emphasis on the biological history and early therapy. Cancer 1954; 7:103l–1043.

Hickey RC, Martin RG. Sacrococcygeal teratomas. Ann NY Acad Sci 1964;114:951–957.

Hogge WA, Thiagarajah S, Barber VG, Rodgers BM, Newman BM. Cystic sacrococcygeal teratoma: ultrasound diagnosis and perinatal management. J Ultrasound Med 1987;6:707–710.

Holzgreve W, Mahony BS, Glick PL, et al. Sonographic demonstration of fetal sacrococcygeal teratoma. Prenat Diagn 1985;5:245–257.

Holzgreve W, Miny P, Anderson R, Golbus MS. Experience with 8 cases of prenatally diagnosed sacrococcygeal teratomas. Fetal Ther 1987;2:88–94.

Horger E, McCarter LM. Prenatal diagnosis of sacrococcygeal teratoma. Am J Obstet Gynecol 1979;134:228–229.

Hunt PT, Kendrick CD, Ashcraft KW, et al. Radiography of hereditary presacral teratoma. Radiology 1977;122:187–191.

Izant RJ Jr, Filston HC. Sacrococcygeal teratomas: analysis of forty-three cases. Am J Surg 1975;130:617–621.

Johnson JWC, Porter J, Kellner KR, et al. Abdominal rescue after incomplete delivery secondary to large fetal sacrococcygeal teratoma. Obstet Gynecol 1988;71:981–983.

Kapoor R, Saha MM. Antenatal sonographic diagnosis of fetal sacrococcygeal teratoma with hydrops. Australas Radiol 1989;33:285–287.

Kowalski E, Sokolowska-Pituchowa J. Teratoma of the fetal sacral as a delivery obstacle. Gin Pol 1968;39:123–124. (English summary.)

Kuhlmann RS, Warsof SL, Levy DL, Flake AJ, Harrison MR. Fetal sacrococcygeal teratoma. Fetal Ther 1987;1:95–100.

Langer JC, Harrison MR, Schmidt KG, et al. Fetal hydrops and death from sacrococcygeal teratoma: rationale for fetal surgery. Am J Obstet Gynecol 1989;160:1145–1150.

Lemire RJ, Beckwith JB. Pathogenesis of congenital tumors and malformations in the sacrococcygeal region. Teratology 1982;25:201–213.

Linder D, Hecht F, McCaw BK, et al. Origin of extragonadal teratoma and endodumal sinus tumors. Nature 1975;254:597–600.

Litwiller MR. Dystocia caused by sacrococcygeal teratomas. Obstet Gynecol 1969;34:783–786.

Lowenstein A, Schwartz H, Simon SR, Roth E, Scheininger LM. Delivery of a fetus with a large sacrococcygeal tumor, an unusual case. J Newark Beth Israel Hosp 1963;14:78–84.

Lu T, Lee KH. Two cases of congenital sacral teratoma obstructing labour. J Obstet Gynaecol Br Commonw 1966;73:852–854.

Mahour GH, Woolley MM, Trinedi SN, et al. Sacrococcygeal teratoma: a 33-year experience. J Pediatr Surg 1975;10:183–188.

Mintz MC, Mennuti M, Fishman J. Prenatal aspiration of sacrococcygeal teratoma. AJR Am J Roentgenol 1983;141:367–368.

Misra D, Pritchard J, Drake DP, et al. Markedly improved survival in malignant sacrococcygeal teratomas—16 years' experience. Eur J Pediatr Surg 1997;7:152–155.

Musci MN, Clark MJ, Ayres RE, Finkel MA. Management of dystocia caused by a large sacrococcygeal teratoma. Obstet Gynecol 1983;62:10S–12S.

Nakoyama DK, Killion A, Hill LM, et al. The newborn with hydrops and sacrococcygeal teratoma. J Pediatr Surg 1991;26:1435–1438.

Nicolay KS, Gainey HL. Pseudotoxemic state associated with severe Rh isoimmunization. Am J Obstet Gynecol 1964;89:41–45.

Ohama K, Nagase H, Ogina K, et al. Alpha-fetoprotein levels in normal children. Eur J Pediatr Surg 1997;7:267–269.

Robertson FR, Crombleholme TM, Frantz ID III, et al. Devascularization and staged resection of giant SCT in the preterm infant. J Pediatr Surg 1995;30:309–311.

Schcy WL, Shkolnik A, White H. Clinical and radiographic considerations of sacrococcygeal teratomas: an analysis of 26 new cases and review of the literature. Radiology 1977;125:189–195.

Schiffer MA, Greenberg E. Sacrococcygeal teratoma in labor and the newborn. Am J Obstet Gynecol 1956;72:1054–1062.

Schmidt KG, Silverman NH, Harrison MR, Callen PW. High-output cardiac failure in fetuses with large SCT: diagnosis by echocardiography and Doppler ultrasound. J Pediatr 1989;114:1023–1028.

Seeds JW, Mittelstaedt CA, Cefalo RC, Parker TF. Prenatal diagnosis of sacrococcyge alteratoma: an anechoic caudal mass. J Clin Ultrasound 1982;10:193–195.

Seidenberg B, Hurwitt ES. Clinical aspects and management of sacrococcygeal teratoma. Arch Surg 76:429–436 1958.

Sheth S, Nussbaum AR, Sanders RC, et al. Prenatal diagnosis of sacrococcygeal teratomas: sonographic-pathologic correlation. Radiology 1988;169:131–136.

Smith B, Passaro E, Clatworthy HW. The vascular anatomy of sacrococcygeal teratomas: its significance in surgical management. Surgery 1961;49:534–539.

Tanaree P. Delivery obstructed by sacrococcygeal teratoma. Am J Obstet Gynecol 1982;142:239.

Tapper D, Lack EE. Teratomas in infancy and childhood. Ann Surg 1983;198:398–410.

Theiss EA, Ashley DJB, Mostofi FK. Nuclear sex of testicular tumors and some related ovarian and extragonadal neoplasms. Cancer 1960;13:323–330.

Tsuchilda Y, Urano Y, Endo Y, et al. A study on alpha-fetoprotein and endodermal sinus tumor. J Pediatr Surg 1975;10:501–506.

Varga DA, Kaplan RF, Kellner KR, Johnson JW, Miller D. Vaginal delivery impeded by a large sacrococcygeal teratoma: anesthetic considerations. Anesth Analg 1987;66:1325–1327.

Waldhausen JA, Kilman JW, Vellios F, Battersby JS. Sacrococcygeal teratoma. Pediatr Surg 1963;54:933–949.

Weiss DB, Wajntraub G, Abulafia Y, Schiller M. Vaginal surgical intervention for a sacrococcygeal teratoma obstructing labor. Acta Obstet Gynecol Scand 1976;55:183–185.

Werb P, Scurry J, Ostor A, Fortune D, Attwood H. Surgey of congenital tumors in perinatal necropsies. Pathology 1992;24:247–253.

Werner B, Swiecicka K. Teratoma of the sacro-coccygeal region of the fetus resulting as a delivery obstacle. Gin Pol 1968;39:925–927. (English summary.)

Wilson CA, Litton C, Capinpin A. Sacrococcygeal teratoma associated with congenital spinal deformity. Plast Reconstr Surg 1963;31:289–293.

CHAPTER 117

Wilms' Tumor

► CONDITION

Renal neoplasms account for approximately 10% of all malignant tumors in children (Breslow and Beckwith 1982). Nephroblastoma (Wilms' tumor) accounts for 80% of renal neoplasms in children, while other tumor types, such as anaplastic sarcoma, clear-cell sarcoma, rhabdoid tumor, and renal-cell carcinoma account for the rest. Wilms' tumor has a peak incidence at 2 to 3 years of age, but it can be present from infancy to adulthood (Breslow et al. 1988a and b). Five cases have been diagnosed in utero (Guillian 1984; Ritchey et al. 1995).

Nephroblastoma is a tumor that arises within the kidney and consists of a variety of embryonic tissues such as glomeruli and tubules, spindle cells, smooth and skeletal muscle fibers, cartilage, and bone. Wilms' tumor is associated with many genetic conditions, including Beckwith–Wiedemann, Drash, and Klippel–Trenaunay syndromes and neurofibromatosis (King 1993). However, the most common presentation of Wilms' tumor is an asymptomatic abdominal mass. Abdominal pain, hematuria or malaise, weakness, anorexia, and weight loss may also be presenting symptoms.

Fetal Wilms' tumor may present as part of Perlman syndrome, which is characterized by familial nephroblastomatosis, fetal ascites, polyhydramnios, hepatomegaly, macrosomia, and Wilms' tumor (Greenberg et al. 1986; Perlman 1986). Wilms' tumor in Perlman syndrome occurs in the absence of chromosomal abnormalities, enzymatic defects, or somatic conditions known to be associated with Wilms' tumor. Nephroblastomatosis may present as either diffuse or discrete rests of abnormally persistent embryonic renal blastema. In some instances, this condition is believed to be a premalignant precursor of Wilms' tumor (Kulkarni et al. 1980; Stone et al. 1990). Nephroblastomatosis has been defined by Ambrosino et al. (1990) as either persistent metanephric blastema in infants over 36 weeks of gestation or the presence of persistent metanephric blastema in an abnormal location and/or quantity in younger fetuses. Nephrogenic rests occur as two main types, perilobar and intralobar (Beckwith et al. 1990). Nephroblastomatosis occurs in four patterns: perilobar only, intralobar only, combined, and universal or panlobar (Beckwith et al. 1990). The diffuse, panlobar type is characterized by diffuse superficial blastemal tissue that surrounds and compresses the normal parenchyma. In contrast, in the multifocal, perilobar, or intralobar types, nodular renal blastoma is found in the subcapsular cortex and in the deep cortex above the columns of Bertin. Nephroblastomatosis is considered a precursor of Wilms' tumor, especially when it is of the multifocal type (Ambrosino et al. 1990, Kulkarni et al. 1980; Stone et al. 1990).

► INCIDENCE

Only rarely have cases of Wilms' tumor been diagnosed prenatally. However, our current understanding of the disease suggests that at least the predisposition to developing Wilms' tumor is present before birth. The incidence of Wilms' tumor is thought to be 1 in 10,000 live births, with an estimated 8 cases in 1 million children under the age of 15 years (Kramer 1985). The fetal and neonatal incidence of the disease is unknown. In 50% of cases the left kidney is affected, in 45% of the cases the right is affected, and in 5% the tumor is bilateral. The tumor can be seen in association with specific anomalies, including aniridia (8.5 in 1000 cases), hemihypertrophy (25 in 1000 cases), cryptorchidism (28 in 1000 cases), and hypospadias (18 in 1000) (Breslow et al. 1988a and b).

▶ SONOGRAPHIC FINDINGS

The sonographic features of Wilms' tumor are indistinguishable from those of mesoblastic nephroma. Both present as complex masses that arise from or may completely replace the normal kidney. These tumors are predominantly solid, but cystic areas also can be seen. There may be a well-defined pseudocapsule in Wilms' tumor as opposed to mesoblastic nephromas (Fig. 117-1A) (Guillian et al. 1984; Walter and McGahan 1985). In mesoblastic nephroma, polyhydramnios is a feature of most cases that have been reported (Yambao et al. 1986). Few antenatally detected cases of Wilms' tumor have been described thus far, so it is uncertain if polyhydramnios may occur in association with Wilms' tumor. Magnetic resonance imaging (MRI) may be used to enhance anatomic delineation of a renal mass (Fig. 117-1B) (Tomá et al. 1990). Three cases of prenatally diagnosed nephroblastomatosis have been reported (Ambrosino et al. 1990; Gaulier et al. 1993). One was the stillborn product of a 28-weeks gestation complicated by polyhydramnios, ascites, pleural effusion, nephromegaly, and calcific foci in one kidney. The second case similarly showed polyhydramnios, homogeneous nephromegaly, and calcific foci within the kidney. The lungs of both fetuses were hypoplastic. The kidneys at autopsy showed diffuse nephroblastomastosis and were thought to represent Perlman syndrome. The third case occurred within a multicystic dysplastic kidney.

▶ DIFFERENTIAL DIAGNOSIS

The differential diagnosis of a fetal renal mass includes hydronephrosis (see Chapters 78, 79, and 80) and multicystic dysplastic kidney (see Chapter 82). While far more common, the typical cystic appearance of hydronephrosis and multicystic dysplastic kidney distinguishes them from Wilms' tumor. However, mesoblastic nephroma (see Chapter 113) may be indistinguishable from Wilms' tumor (Garmel et al. 1994; Guillian et al. 1984; Walter and McGahan 1985). Focal renal dysplasia should also be considered in the differential diagnosis (Gordillo et al. 1987; Sanders et al. 1988) as well as masses extending from adjacent organs such as the adrenal gland or liver. In addition, nephroblastomatosis occuring in multicystic dysplastic kidney was detected by prenatal ultrasound examination as a renal mass indistinguishable from a Wilms' tumor (Gaulier et al. 1993).

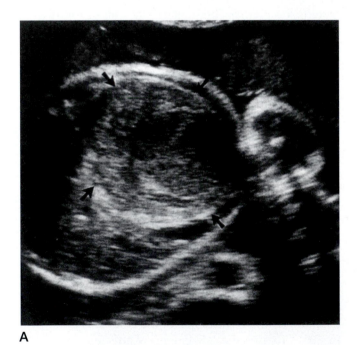

A

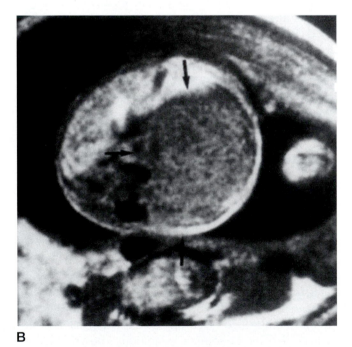

B

Figure 117-1. (A) Fetal transverse sonographic image at 37 weeks of gestation demonstrating an echogenic mass with well-defined borders arising from the left renal fossa (arrows). (B) Transverse T$_1$-weighted image of the same fetus, showing the mass to be hypointense relative to the liver (arrows). *(Reprinted, with permission, from Tomá P, Lucigrai G, Dodero P, et al. Prenatal detection of an abdominal mass by MR imaging performed while the fetus is immobilized with pancuronium bromide. AJR Am J Roentgenol 1990;154:1049–1050.)*

▶ ANTENATAL NATURAL HISTORY

The antenatal natural history of Wilms' tumor remains undefined because of the infrequent prenatal ascertainment of these tumors.

▶ MANAGEMENT OF PREGNANCY

The fetus with a suspected renal tumor should undergo a detailed sonographic evaluation to detect associated anomalies and clues to the cause of the mass. The features of Perlman syndrome, including fetal ascites, hepatomegaly, macrosomia, and polyhydramnios should be sought. A family history of Wilms' tumor should also be excluded. The contralateral kidney should be closely examined for anomalies or masses.

Because of the possibility of polyhydramnios in mesoblastic nephroma (the main consideration in the differential diagnosis) as well as in Perlman syndrome, these pregnancies should be followed closely, as polyhydramnios may precipitate preterm labor and premature birth. These tumors seldom achieve a size that might preclude vaginal delivery; however, an ultrasound examination should be done close to term to assess this possibility. Fetal MRI may be helpful in defining the anatomy and potentially in assisting in the differential diagnosis (Fig. 117-1B).

▶ FETAL INTERVENTION

No fetal intervention is necessary in Wilms' tumors.

▶ TREATMENT OF THE NEWBORN

Physical examination of the newborn should confirm the presence of an abdominal mass. The affected newborn's blood pressure should be monitored, as 50% of Wilms' tumors may have associated hypertension. Associated anomalies (aniridia, cryptorchidism, and hypospadias) or physical signs of Beckwith–Wiedemann syndrome (macrosomia and macroglossia) should be excluded. A diagnostic workup for the presence of metastases should include chest radiography and abdominal computed tomographic (CT) scanning.

A newborn with suspected Wilms' tumor should undergo an exploratory laparotomy for nephroureterectomy and exploration of the contralateral kidney to exclude synchronous bilateral lesions. If a complete resection is achieved and the histology reveals mesoblastic nephroma, no further treatment is indicated. In the National Wilms' Tumor Study-5 protocol, in cases of stage I Wilms' tumors that weigh less than 550 g in a patient under 2 years of age, a complete surgical resection is all that is necessary (Green et al. 1994; Ritchey 1998). In other tumors, adjuvant treatment with chemotherapy and radiation therapy is planned according to stage of disease and histology as defined by the National Wilms' Tumor Study.

▶ LONG-TERM OUTCOME

The long-term outcome for infants with Wilms' tumor depends on histology and stage of the tumor. In general, the 4-year survival of all patients with favorable histology approaches 90% (Haase and Ritchey 1997). Unfavorable histology include Wilms' tumors with anaplasia, and two other distinct renal tumors—clear-cell sarcoma of the kidney and malignant rhabdoid tumor of the kidney. Anaplasia is present in approximately 4.5% of tumors and is more common in older children, with a peak incidence of 5 years. Stage I anaplastic tumors have a biologic behavior similar to stage I patients with a favorable histology with similar survival and relapse rates (Shochat 1997). The survival rates in patients with focal anaplasia, stages II to IV, was 100%. However, this is a small percentage of patients with anaplasia. The 4-year survival of patients with diffuse anaplasia was only 52% (Shochat 1997). The 4-year survival is 75% for patients with clear-cell sarcoma of the kidney, and 25% for malignant rhabdoid tumors (D'Angio et al. 1989).

One concern for patients undergoing treatment for Wilms' tumor is the potential for the development of second malignant neoplasms. Li et al. (1983) reported that in 11 (2%) of 487 children treated at the Dana–Farber Cancer Institute second primary malignancies developed 7 to 34 years after treatment. The National Wilms' Tumor Study has reported similar findings, with 1% of survivors having a second malignancy at 10 years (Breslow et al. 1988). These malignancies ranged from leukemia or lymphoma to hepatocellular carcinoma and soft-tissue sarcomas. Children with Wilms' tumor who are long-term survivors require ongoing surveillance for the development of a second malignant neoplasm during their adult life.

Other late effects in Wilms' tumor survivors are problems with fertility and pregnancy and low-birth-weight infants. Green et al. (1982) reviewed the reproductive histories of 36 Wilms' tumor survivors and found a significant increase (6.7%) in the perinatal mortality of their offspring. This was thought to be primarily the result of prematurity and the low birth weight of infants born to mothers who had previously undergone abdominal radiation. The risk of low-birth-weight infants in this group of patients was 30%. Li et al. (1987) observed similar problems in 34 of 114 pregnancies in female Wilms' tumor survivors who underwent radiation.

Because of the increased risk in mothers who are Wilms' tumor survivors, prenatal counseling and referral to a maternal and fetal medicine specialist is recommended when pregnancy is contemplated (Byrne et al. 1988).

▶ GENETICS AND RECURRENCE RISK

Recent advances suggest that there are hereditary and nonhereditary forms of Wilms' tumor, depending on whether the initial mutational event occurred in a germ cell or a somatic cell (Knudson and Strong 1978). Younger patients; those with aniridia, genitourinary anomalies, and bilateral disease; and familial cases have been considered to be in the hereditary group. It has been estimated that this group accounts for 20% of cases of Wilms' tumors. Of the patients registered with the National Wilms' Tumor Study, 1% of the cases have at least one family member similarly affected (Breslow et al. 1982).

Patients with Wilms' tumor and aniridia, genitourinary anomalies, and mental retardation (WAGR) syndrome frequently demonstrate a deletion of band 11p13 (Francke et al. 1979; Kofous et al. 1984). The loss of function of a recessive tumor-suppressor gene located in the 11p13 region may be responsible for the development of Wilms' tumor. Call et al. (1990) have identified a *WT1* (Wilms' tumor) gene from the 11p13 region. *WT1* acts by binding to other DNA sequences that control the expression of renal genes. *WT1* appears to be essential for normal development of the kidney and genitourinary tract. However, *WT1* mutations occur in fewer than 10% of cases. A second gene, *WT2*, has been identified at the end of chromosome 11p in association with the Beckwith–Wiedemann syndrome locus. In addition, a third Wilms' tumor locus has been suggested by lack of linkage to either *WT1* or *WT2* in the rare families affected with Wilms' tumor (Grundy et al. 1988; Strong et al. 1988). Other genes and chromosomal abnormalities have been identified at the 11p15 locus and on chromosome 16q (Maw et al. 1992; Waley et al. 1990). The sporadic form of Wilms' tumor is not associated with recurrence in subsequent pregnancies. However, about 20% of patients with Wilms' tumor are at risk for recurrence in a sibling. These pregnancies should be closely observed by ultrasound examination and amniocentesis should be considered for genetic testing. Most Wilms' tumors diagnosed in the newborn or infant are stage I or II and the long-term prognosis appears to be excellent, with a survival rate of 95% (Ritchey et al. 1995). Not only is survival influenced by the early stage of neonatal Wilms' tumor, but unfavorable histology is rare in patients under 2 years of age (Isaacs 1997). It is important to emphasize, however, that the rarity of neonatal Wilms' tumor precludes definitive statements regarding survival.

REFERENCES

Ambrosino MM, Hernanz-Schulman M, Horrii SC, et al. Prenatal diagnosis of nephroblastomatosis in two siblings. J Ultrasound Med 1990;9:49–51.

Beckwith J, Kiviat NB, Bonadio JF, Nephrogenic rests, nephroblastomatosis, and the pathogenesis of Wilms' tumor. Pediatr Pathol 1990;10:1–6.

Breslow N, Beckwith JB. Epidemiologic features of Wilms' tumor: results of the National Wilms' Tumor Study. J. Natl Cancer Inst 1982;68:429–436.

Breslow N, Beckwith JB, Ciol M, et al. Age distribution of Wilms' tumor: report from the National Wilms' Tumor Study. Cancer Res 1988a;48:1653–1657.

Breslow N, Norkool PA, Olshan A, et al. Second malignant neoplasms in survivors of Wilms' tumor: a report from the National Wilms' Tumor Study. J Natl Cancer Inst 1988b;80:592–595.

Byrne J, Mulvihill JJ, Connelly RR, et al. Reproductive problems and birth defects in survivors of Wilms' tumor and their relatives. Med Pediatr Oncol 1988;16:1233–1240.

Call KM, Glaser T, Ito CY, et al. Isolation and characterization of a zinc finger polypeptide gene at the human chromosome 11: Wilms' tumor locus. Cell 1990;60:509–520.

D'Angio GJ, Breslow N, Beckwith JB. Treatment of Wilms' tumor: results of the third National Wilms' Tumor Study. Cancer 1989;64:349–356.

Francke U, Holmes LB, Atkins L, et al. Aniridia-Wilms' tumor association: evidence for specific deletion of 11p13. Cytogenet Cell Genet 1979;24:184–192.

Garmel SH, Crombleholme TM, Semple JP, et al. Prenatal diagnosis and management of fetal tumors. Semin Perinatol 1994;18:350–358.

Gaulier A, Bascon-Gibad L, Sobatier P, et al. Panlobar nephroblastomastosis with cystic dysplasia: an unusual case with diffuse renal involvement studied by immunohistochemistry. Pediatr Pathol 1993;15: 741–747.

Gordillo R, Vilaro M, Shuman NH, et al. Circumscribed renal mass in dysplastic kidney. J Ultrasound Med 1987;6: 613–617.

Green DM, Beckwith JB, Weeks DA, et al. The relationship between microsubstaging variables, tumor weight and age at diagnosis of children with stage I favorable histology Wilms' tumor: a report from the National Wilms' Tumor Study. Cancer 1994;74:1817–1820.

Green DM, Fine WE, Li FP. Offspring of patients treated for unilateral Wilms' tumor in childhood. Cancer 1982; 49:2285–2288.

Greenberg F, Stein F, Greisch MV, et al. The Perlman familial nephroblastomatosis syndrome. Am J Med Genet 1986; 24:101–110.

Grundy P, Kaufos A, Morgan K, et al. Familial predisposition to Wilms' tumor does not map to the short arm of chromosome 11. Nature 1988;336:374–376.

Guillian BB. Prenatal ultrasonographic diagnosis of fetal renal tumors. Radiology 1984;152:69–70.

Haase GM, Ritchey ML. Nephroblastoma. Semin Pediatr Surg 1997;6(1):11–16.

Isaacs H Jr. Renal tumors. In: Tumors of the fetus and newborn. Philadelphia: WB Saunders, 1997:244–277.

King DR. Renal neoplasms in pediatric surgery. In: Ashkraft KW, Holder TM, eds. Philadelphia: Saunders 1993:784–797.

Knudson AG, Strong LC. Mutation and cancer: a model for Wilms' tumor of the kidney. J Natl Cancer Inst 1978;48: 313–324.

Kofous A, Hansen MF, Lampkin BC, et al. Loss of alleles at loci on human chromosome 11 during genesis of Wilms' tumor. Nature 1984;309:170–172.

Kramer SA. Pediatric urological oncology. Urol Clin North Am 1985;12:31–39.

Kulkarni R, Bailie MD, Bernstein J. Progression of nephroblastomatosis to Wilms' tumor. J Pediatr Surg 1980;96: 178–181.

Li FP, Ginbrere K, Gelber RD, et al. Outcome of pregnancy in survivors of Wilms' tumor. JAMA 1987;257:216–219.

Li FP, Yan JC, Sallon S, et al. Second neoplasms after Wilms' tumor in childhood. J Natl Cancer Inst 1983;71: 1205–1209.

Maw MA, Grundy PE, Millow LJ, et al. A third Wilms' tumor locus on chromosome 16q. Cancer Res 1992;53: 3094–3098.

Perlman M. Perlman syndrome: familial renal dysplasia with Wilms' tumor, fetal gigantism, and multiple congenital anomalies. Am J Med Genet 1986;25:793–795.

Ritchey ML, Azizkhan RG, Beckwith JB, et al. Neonatal Wilms' tumor. J Pediatr Surg 1995;30:856–863.

Ritchey ML. Wilms' tumor in pediatric surgical oncology. In: Andressy RJ, ed. Pediatric Surgical Oncology. Philadelphia: Saunders, 1998:155–174.

Sanders RC, Nussbaum AR, Solez K. Renal dysplasia: sonographic findings. Radiology 1988;167:623–626.

Shochat SJ. Renal tumors in surgery of infants and children: scientific principles and practice. In: Oldham KT, Columbani PM, Foglia RP, eds. Surgery of infants and children: scientific principles and practice. Philadelphia: Lippincott-Raven, 1997:581–592.

Stone MM, Beaver BL, Sun C-CJ, et al. The nephroblastomatosis complex and its relation to Wilms' tumor. J Pediatr Surg 1990;25:933–937.

Strong LC, Coruptan DA, Chao L, et al. Task of linkage of familial Wilms' tumor to chromosome band 11p13. Nature 1988;336:377–378.

Tomá P, Lucigrai G, Dodero P, et al. Prenatal detection of an abdominal mass by MR imaging performed while the fetus is immobilized with pancuronium bromide. AJR Am J Roentgenol 1990;154:1049–1050.

Waley RB, Pol N, Bucke B, et al. Loss of heterozygosity in Wilms' tumor involves two distinct regions of chromosome 11. Oncogene 1990;5:901–907.

Walter JP, McGahan JP. Mesoblastic nephroma: prenatal sonographic detection. J Clin Ultrasound 1985;13:686–689.

Yambao TJ, Schwartz D, Henderson R, et al. Prenatal diagnosis of a congenital mesoblastic neophroma: a case report. J Reprod Med 1986;31:257–259.

▶ **TABLE 118-1.** CLASSIFICATION OF THE CONDITIONS OF ACARDIA

Acardius acephalus: This is the most frequent variety, responsible for 60% to 75% of cases (Lachman et al. 1980). The head is absent but the trunk and limbs are more or less well developed (Das 1902; Robie et al. 1989; Simonds and Gowen 1925).

Acardius acormus: This is a very rare type of acardia in which there is development of the fetal head only (Robie et al. 1989). The head is usually directly attached to the placenta via a cord arising in the cervical region (Das 1902; Kappelman 1944; Simonds and Gowen 1925).

Acardius amorphus, or anideus: This type of acardia occurs in about 20% of cases (Lachman et al. 1980). The defect consists of an irregular, skin-covered mass of bone, muscle, fat, and connective tissue without the external form of a fetus (Das 1902; Kappelman 1944). The umbilical cord is inserted anywhere on the surface.

Acardius anceps or paracephalus: The head is poorly formed, but trunk and limbs are fairly well developed (Das 1902; Simonds and Gowen 1925). This form is sometimes included with the acephalus group.

Acardius myelacephalus: This form consists of an amorphous mass, with some development of one or more limbs (Kappelman 1944; Simonds and Gowen 1925).

1994). The karyotypic abnormalities included monosomy, trisomy, deletions, mosaicism, and polyploidy.

The members of a TRAP sequence are known as the perfused twin and the pump twin. The perfused twin in a TRAP sequence is an example of the impact of vascular disruption on morphogenesis. Multisystem malformations, as well as unusual body form, are found in the perfused twin. Figure 118-1 illustrates the gradation of loss of normal body form ranging from an amorphous appearance to an individual with more severe abnormalities found in the upper part of the body. The malformations found in cases of acardia include growth abnormalities, partial or complete absence of the cranial vault, anencephaly, holoprosencephaly, absent or rudimentary facial features, absent or rudimentary upper and/or lower limbs, absent lungs and heart, gastrointestinal atresias, omphalocele, gastroschisis, and absent liver, pancreas, spleen, and kidneys (Van Allen et al. 1983). The pattern of structural abnormalities found in the perfused twins with abnormal karyotypes is not appreciably different from those with normal karyotypes (Van Allen et al. 1983). Van Allen et al. suggested that the abnormal karyotype per se is not responsible for the malformation complex, but rather that it contributes to the discordant development between

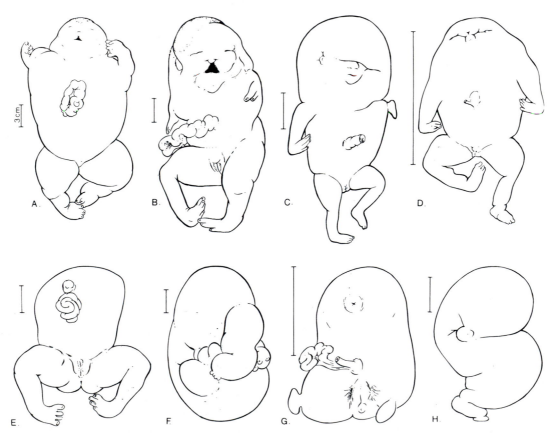

Figure 118-1. Gradation of loss of normal body form in acardia. *(Reprinted, with permission, from Van Allen MI, Smith SW, Shepard TH. Twin reversed arterial perfusion (TRAP) sequence: a study of 14 twin pregnancies with acardius. Semin Perinatol 1983;7:288.)*

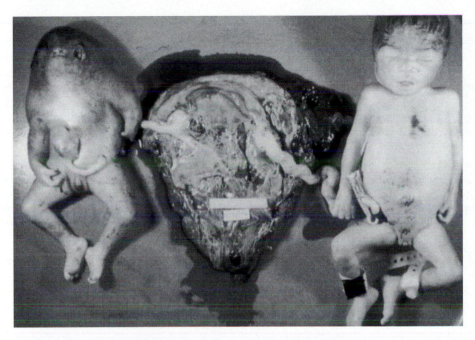

Figure 118-2. An acardiac fetus and its pump twin delivered at 26 weeks of gestation following spontaneous premature labor.

twins, increasing the likelihood of reversal of arterial blood flow if an anastomosis occurs.

The presence of an acardiac twin requires one normal or "pump" twin to provide circulation for itself as well as its acardiac sibling. In many cases the acardiac twin is almost equal in size to the normal twin (Fig. 118-2). The pump twin is usually morphologically normal. In a review of 34 pump fetuses with a known karyotype, 3 (8.8%) were abnormal as a result of trisomy. The pump twin may show evidence of the physiologic consequence of fetal cardiac overload and congestive heart failure with hepatosplenomegaly. The principal perinatal problems associated with acardiac twinning are pump twin congestive heart failure, maternal hydramnios, and preterm delivery (Moore et al. 1990).

Prematurity is the most important factor in determining the prognosis for the pump twin (see Fig. 118-2) (Healey 1994; Moore et al. 1990; Van Allen et al. 1983;). Fifty percent of acardiac pregnancies will result in fetal or neonatal death. Only a quarter can be expected to be delivered after 36 weeks. Preterm delivery and the attendant long-term morbidities can be expected for the remaining quarter (Moore et al. 1990).

▶ INCIDENCE

The frequency of acardia has been estimated from birth records in New York City to be 1 in 35,000 (Napolitani and Schreiber 1960). A virtually identical estimate of 1 in 34,000 births was suggested by Gillim and Hendricks (1953) using data from Johns Hopkins University Hos-

pital. Acardia was observed in 1 of 606 twin pregnancies, and the rate of twins was calculated at 1 in 86.5 births in the United States (Gillim and Hendricks 1953). Such an estimate must be very approximate. Van Allen et al. (1983) have suggested these figures to be a gross underestimate of the true frequency of the TRAP sequence because most cases go unrecognized and unreported as a result of early pregnancy loss. In contrast, an analysis of data from the Eurocat Network (European Registration of Congenital Anomalies and Twins) gave a prevalence of acardia of 0.064 in 10,000 births, which is much lower than were previous estimates in the literature (Haring et al. 1993). Acardia is unique to multiple pregnancies, and of those occurs almost exclusively in monochorionic pregnancies. The incidence of acardia is higher in monoamniotic than in diamniotic monochorionic twin pairs. The TRAP sequence is more common in monozygotic triplets than in monozygotic twins (James 1977; Healey 1994). Acardia is more common in multiparous women (Healey 1994). Some authors have suggested a slight female preponderance in acardiac twins (James 1977); however, in the most recent review, the sex ratio of acardiac twins was not significantly different from the sex ratio of all infants born in Victoria, Australia in 1988 and 1989 (Healey 1994).

▶ SONOGRAPHIC FINDINGS

Antenatal diagnoses of acardia have been reported in the literature only since 1980. From 1980 to 1991 antenatal diagnosis was made in 59% of the 74 cases in which the time of diagnosis was reported (Healey 1994). The gestational age at the time of sonographic diagnosis of acardia had a range of 12 to 34 weeks, with a mean of 23.

Ultrasonographic features useful in the diagnosis of acardia include absence of normal cardiac structure and cardiac movement, the presence of limb movements, and variable structural abnormalities. Common structural abnormalities identified in the acardiac fetus include anencephaly, omphalocele, and absence of upper limbs. Most cases have edematous soft tissue, and large cystic hygroma–like spaces are commonly identified in the skin (Fig. 118-3) (Mack et al. 1982).

The placentation is most commonly monochorionic diamniotic (74%), in which a thin membrane will be seen dividing the sac of the acardiac fetus from the pump fetus (Healey 1994). Monoamnionicity is present in approximately 24% of cases (Healey 1994), and in such pregnancies there is failure to visualize a dividing membrane. In exceptional cases, dichorionicity may be diagnosed (Healey 1994). The umbilical cord will demonstrate a single umbilical artery in approximately two thirds of cases, and in one third the number of cord vessels will be normal (Healey 1994). Polyhydramnios is a common feature. Color flow Doppler velocimetry may demonstrate a velamentous insertion of the cord in the acardiac fetus.

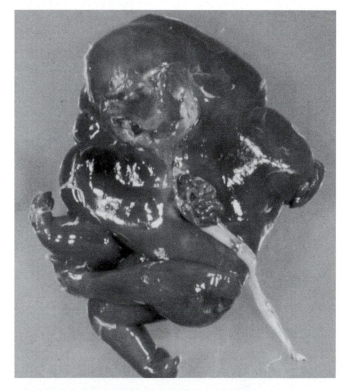

Figure 118-3. An acardiac chorangiopagus parasiticus fetus with a more marked degree of malformation that seen in Figure 118-2. *(Courtesy of Dr. Joseph Semple.)*

Measurement of the acardiac twin should be performed, because the ratio of the weight of the acardiac twin to that of the pump twin is useful for prediction of pregnancy outcome. Because of the nature of the structural abnormality the biometric parameters of biparietal diameter, abdominal circumference, and femur length are usually not available or reliable in an acardiac fetus. This problem of the antenatal determination of the acardiac twin's weight has been addressed by Moore et al. (1990). The dimensions and weights of 23 acardiac twins were used for the analysis. A second-order regression equation (weight [g] = $-1.66 \times$ length $+ 1.21 \times$ length^2) was computed and was predictive of acardiac weight with the use of its longest linear measurement ($r = .79$; $P < 0.001$; SEE = 326 g). When the actual and equation-predicted weights were compared, the mean error ($\pm$SE) in prediction was 240 $\pm$ 156 g.

The pump twin should have a detailed structural survey performed because trisomy has been reported in up to 9% of cases (Healey 1994) and sonographic features typical of a trisomic fetus may be identified. A detailed examination of the heart is helpful in detecting early signs of in utero congestive heart failure in the normal twin. Atrial and ventricular enlargement can be an initial feature of impending cardiac decompensation and can be measured using M-mode echocardiography by obtaining a transverse view through the cardiac chambers (Allan 1986; DeVore 1987). The ventricular fractional shortening capacity can also be calculated using M-mode echocardiography with the formula (D $-$ S)D $\times$ 100, where D is the diastolic and S is the systolic ventricular size. A low value is indicative of poor cardiac contractility. A pericardial effusion may be demonstrated either by real-time or M-mode echocardiography and is a sign of congestive heart failure. Tricuspid regurgitation may be identified by Doppler studies of the tricuspid valve and is an early sign of congestive heart failure (Shenker et al. 1988; Silverman et al. 1985).

Verification of circulatory reversal by pulsed Doppler sonography of an acardiac twin has been reported with reversed direction of flow in the umbilical artery and vein (Benson et al. 1989; Donnenfeld et al. 1991; Langlotz et al. 1991; Pretorius et al. 1988; Sherer et al. 1989).

▶ DIFFERENTIAL DIAGNOSIS

Acardia has been mistaken for intrauterine fetal death. Evidence of growth in the "dead" fetus and a "twitching" noted on repeat ultrasound examination has allowed the diagnosis of an acardiac twin to be made (Cardwell 1988). In a severely macerated fetus, the skeletal and visceral forms are more differentiated, and the soft-tissue edema is less advanced than in a case of acardia (Mack et al. 1982).

The acardiac fetus may also be mistaken for an anencephalic fetus. The sonographic features of absent trunk region in addition to increased soft tissue in the body aid in the correct diagnosis (Billah et al. 1984). Pulsed Doppler examination has been used to demonstrate reversed flow through the umbilical artery of the acardiac twin (Pretorius et al. 1988).

▶ ANTENATAL HISTORY

The principal perinatal problems associated with acardiac twinning are pump twin congestive heart failure, maternal hydramnios, and preterm delivery. The antenatal diagnosis of acardia can be made only through sonographic examination and has been reported in the literature only since 1980. Two large series of acardiac twins have attempted to identify factors prognostic of favorable outcome for the pump twin (Healey 1994; Moore et al. 1990).

In the series of 49 cases reported by Moore et al. (1990), one third of fetuses were delivered before they were viable. Viability was defined as delivery at or beyond 25 weeks of gestation. Of the potentially viable 33 cases, 4 (12%) ended in death of the pump twin in utero. The overall perinatal mortality was 55% and was primarily associated with prematurity (Table 118-2).

Hydramnios was a major maternal complication, occurring in 46% of all acardiac pregnancies, and it was strongly associated with preterm labor and congestive heart failure in the pump twin. Eighty-two percent of patients with hydramnios experienced preterm labor requiring hospital admission and treatment, as compared with 22% of pregnancies with normal amniotic fluid (P < 0.01). Hydramnios was observed in 78% of pump twins with congestive heart failure as compared with 13% of those in whom congestive heart failure was not confirmed (P < 0.001). The perinatal outcome was strongly related to the ratio of the weight of the acardiac twin to that of the pump twin. The mean overall ratio of the twin weights was 52 ± 42%. The twin weight ratio was more than 70% in 25% of cases. When this characteristic was present, the incidence of preterm delivery was 90%, hydramnios 40%, and congestive cardiac failure in the pump twin 30%, as compared with 75%, 30%, and 10%, respectively, when the ratio was less than 70% (Moore et al. 1990).

In the series by Healey (1994), of 5 cases at Monash Medical Centre and a review of 184 case reports in the literature from 1960 to 1991, the overall perinatal mortality for the pump fetus was 35% in twins and 45% in triplets. Factors associated with a significant increase in perinatal mortality for the pump fetus included delivery before 32 weeks of gestation, the acardius anceps form of acardia, and the presence of arms, ears, larynx, trachea, pancreas, kidney, or small intestine in the acardiac fetus.

▶ MANAGEMENT OF PREGNANCY

When the diagnosis of multiple pregnancy with an acardiac fetus is made, the high and low risk factors for perinatal mortality in the pump fetus must be evaluated through sonographic examination. The presence of polyhydramnios, a ratio of the weight of the acardiac twin to that of the pump twin of greater than 70%, and congestive heart failure are all poor prognostic signs. Evaluation of the structure of the acardiac fetus may also be helpful. Factors that place the pregnancy at high risk for perinatal mortality include features of acardius anceps demonstrating the presence of arms, ears, larynx, trachea, pancreas, renal tissue, and small intestine. Features that indicate a lower risk include features of acardius amorphous with absence of arms, legs, brain, esophagus, trachea, and omphalocele (Healey 1994). The gestational age should be documented by maternal history and standard biometric measurements of the pump fetus. Karyotyping of the pump twin should be offered because as many as 9% of pump twins have an abnormal karyotype (Healey 1994). The treatment options for acardia are listed in Table 118-3 (Ash et al. 1990; Holzgreve et al. 1994; Porreco et al. 1991; Quintero et al. 1994; Robie et al. 1989; Simpson et al. 1983; Van Allen et al. 1983). It is our opinion that observation with serial sonographic measurements is the management of choice when the twin weight ratios are less than 70% (D'Alton

▶ TABLE 118-2. PERINATAL COMPLICATIONS OF 49 PREGNANCIES WITH ACARDIAC TWINNING

Delivery mode	
Spontaneous abortion	18%
Elective	14%
Cesarean section, all cases	38%
Cesarean section, potentially viable cases	58%
Pump twin	
Male/female	57%/43%
Malpresentation	29%
Major structural anomaly	9%
Hydramnios	46%
Congestive heart failure	53%
Previable	32%
Live-born	59%
Premature (<37 wk)	35%
Gestational age at delivery (wk)	29 ± 7
Birth weight (g)*	
Acardiac	651 ± 571
Pump twin	1378 ± 1047

*Mean ±SD.
Source: Moore TR, Gale S, Benirschke K. Perinatal outcome of 49 pregnancies complicated by acardiac twinning. Am J Obstet Gynecol. 1990;163:907–912.

▶ **TABLE 118-3.** TREATMENT OPTIONS FOR ACARDIA

	Reference
Observation	
Medical therapy	
Digoxin	Simpson et al. 1983
Indomethacin	Ash et al. 1990
Selective delivery	Robie et al. 1989
Umbilical cord blockade	
Platinum coil	Porreco et al. 1991
Silk suture in alcohol	Holzgreve et al. 1994
Fetoscopic cord ligation	Quintero et al. 1994

Source: D'Alton ME, Simpson LL. Syndromes in twins. Semin Perinatol 1995;19:375–386.

and Simpson 1995). Steroids should be given if delivery is expected between 24 and 34 weeks of gestation (NIH Consensus Development Panel 1995). Preterm labor should be suppressed with tocolytic agents.

The use of maternal digitalization to treat cardiac failure in the pump twin was reported by Simpson et al. in 1983. Marked edema of the trunk in the normal twin was present. Fetal ascites, pleural effusion, or cardiomegaly was not demonstrated. Serial ultrasound examinations demonstrated resolution of the edema and continued normal growth of the viable fetus. Delivered at 34 weeks, the normal twin weighed 1860 g. The acardiac twin weighed 1810 g. No subsequent reports of this digoxin therapy for acardia have been reported.

Ash et al. (1990) reported the use of indomethacin in an acardiac pregnancy complicated by polyhydramnios at 21 weeks. No evidence of cardiac failure was visualized in the pump twin. Indomethacin, 50 mg daily, was given to treat the symptomatic hydramnios because of the high risk of premature labor. The indomethacin was continued for 8.5 weeks. Oligohydramnios at 34 weeks prompted induction of labor, and spontaneous vaginal delivery occurred. The normal twin weighed 1865 g at birth, and the acardiac twin weighed 785 g (Ash et al. 1990).

Delivery should occur in a tertiary-care hospital because of the risk of preterm delivery and congestive cardiac failure in the pump twin. The vaginal route is the preferred mode of delivery. The indications for cesarean section include the standard obstetric reasons. In Moore et al.'s series, abnormal presentation and fetal distress necessitated cesarean delivery in more than half of the potentially viable pregnancies.

▶ FETAL INTERVENTION

Robie et al. (1989) reported a case of selective delivery by hysterotomy of an acardiac acephalic twin fetus at 22.5 weeks of gestation with the subsequent delivery of the normal twin at 33 weeks of gestation. Fries et al. (1992) subsequently reported 5 cases of selective delivery in 1992. In one case, placental abruption occurred shortly after the procedure, leading to fetal death. Two cases delivered at 35 weeks of gestation, and the remaining 2 delivered at 27 and 28 weeks.

Porreco et al. (1991) described the insertion of a helical metal coil under sonographic guidance to induce thrombosis in the umbilical artery of the acardiac twin at 24 weeks. The co-twin delivered at 39 weeks and had a normal course.

Quintero et al. (1994) described a percutaneous fetoscopic procedure that treated this condition at 19 weeks of gestation and was followed by the birth of a normal twin at 36 weeks of gestation. A further case was reported by McCurdy et al. (1993). A trial of maternal digoxin administration failed and was followed by a fetoscopic ligation of the acardiac twin's cord at 19 weeks. Ultrasound examination on the first postoperative day indicated death of the pump twin.

Holzgreve et al. (1994) injected multiple pieces of silk suture soaked in 96% alcohol into the umbilical cord of an acardiac twin at 21 weeks of gestation. This resulted in immediate interruption of flow in the cord and the ultimate delivery at term of a 2780-g healthy newborn. The advantage of this approach in comparison to umbilical-cord ligation is the use of a much thinner needle. Less operative time is required, and there is no need for general anesthesia (Holzgreve et al. 1994).

Other methods of interrupting the circulation in the acardiac twin involve direct coagulation of the umbilical vessels or the aorta, using either laser photocoagulation or diathermy themocoaglulation. Laser photocoagulation of umbilical vessels using a neodymium yttrium aluminum garnet laser has been successfully reported, although this approach appears less likely to be successful when performed after 24 weeks gestation (Arias et al. 1998). This may be because umbilical vessels are too large to adequately photocoagulate when the gestational age is greater than 24 weeks. Thermocoagulation of the aorta of the acardiac fetus using diathermy via a wire passed through an 18-gauge needle has been successfully reported in four cases at 24 weeks gestation or less (Rodeck et al. 1998). The advantages of this latter approach include avoiding the need for microendoscopic instruments or skills, and avoiding the difficulties in identifying the target umbilical cord. Successful interruption of the acardiac circulation after 24 weeks gestation may require a more invasive approach, such as fetoscopic ligation of the umbilical cord (Arias et al. 1998; NcCurdy et al. 1993; Quintero et al. 1994).

All of the invasive procedures described have the goal of interrupting the umbilical circulation. It has been recommended that invasive procedures be performed only after heart failure has developed (Platt et al. 1983). Some have recommended surgical intervention only after medical therapy has failed (Ash et al. 1990). Others have suggested intervening before heart failure is present in the pump twin (Platt et al. 1983).

▶ TREATMENT OF THE NEWBORN

A neonatologist should attend the delivery. In Moore et al.'s (1990) series, admission to a newborn intensive care unit was required in 41% of the pregnancies and 59% of those reaching viability. Five of 29 live-born pump twins died during the newborn period. There is little information in the literature on the neonatal course of the pump twin. The main problems for the pump twin include complications of prematurity and congestive heart failure (Moore et al. 1990; Van Allen et al. 1983).

Other frequent neonatal findings include massive hepatosplenomegaly, ascites with hypoplasia of abdominal musculature, edema, and hypoalbuminemia due to inadequate liver synthesis of albumin (Van Allen et al. 1983).

Respiratory assistance as well as support of myocardial function with inotropic medication may be required. Early administration of surfactant therapy is indicated when premature delivery at less than 30 weeks of gestation is anticipated. Postnatal consultation with a pediatric cardiologist and echocardiography are recommended.

▶ LONG-TERM OUTCOME

There is no information in the literature concerning long-term outcome for the pump twin. Considerations for the long-term prognosis must include the degree of prematurity, the severity of the neonatal course, and the degree of congestive heart failure.

▶ GENETICS AND RECURRENCE RISK

Estimates of the recurrence risk of acardiac twin pregnancy are on the order of 1 in 10,000 (Van Allen et al. 1983). This recurrence risk is calculated from the recurrence risk for monoamniotic twinning, which is 1% (Myrianthopoulos 1970), multiplied by the frequency of the occurrence of the TRAP sequence, which is approximately 1% of all monozygous twins (Napolitani and Schreiber 1960; Gillim and Hendricks 1953).

REFERENCES

Ahlfeld F. Die Entstehung der Acardiaci. Arch Gynakol 1879;14:321.

Allan LD. Manual of fetal echocardiography. Boston: MTP 1986.

Arias F, Sunderji S, Gimpleson R, et al. Treatment of acardiac twinning. Obstet Gynecol 1998;91:818–821.

Ash K, Harman CR, Gritter H. TRAP sequence—successful outcome with indomethacin treatment. Obstet Gynecol 1990;76:960.

Bieber FP, Nance WE, Morton CC, et al. Genetic studies of an acardiac monster: evidence of polar body twinning in man. Science 1981;213:755.

Benirschke K, Kim CK. Multiple pregnancy. Part I. N Engl J Med 1973;288:1276–1284.

Benson CB, Bieber FR, Genest DR, et al. Doppler demonstration of reversed umbilical blood flow in an acardiac twin. J Clin Ultrasound 1989;17:291–295.

Billah KL, Shah K, Odwin C. Ultrasonic diagnosis and management of acardius acephalus twin pregnancy. Med Ultrasound 1984;8:108

Cardwell MS. The acardiac twin, a case report. J Reprod Med 1988;33:320–322.

D'Alton ME, Simpson LL. Syndromes in twins. In: Chervenak FA, D'Alton ME, eds. Multiple gestation. Semin Perinatol 1995;19:375–386.

Das K. Acardius anceps. Br J Obstet Gynaecol 1902;2:341.

DeVore GR. Cardiac imaging. In: Sabbagha RE, ed. Diagnostic ultrasound. 2nd ed. Philadelphia: Lippincott 1987: 324–362.

Donnenfeld AE, van de Woestijne J, Craparo F, et al. The normal fetus of an acardiac twin pregnancy: perinatal management based on echocardiographic and sonographic evaluation. Prenat Diagn 1991;11: 235–244.

Fisk NM, Ware M, Stanier P, et al. Molecular genetic etiology of twin reversed arterial perfusion sequence. Am J Obstet Gynecol 1996;174:891–894.

Fries MH, Goldberg JD, Golbus MS. Treatment of acardiac-acephalus twin gestations by hysterotomy and selective delivery. Obstet Gynecol 1992;79:601–604.

Gillim DL, Hendricks CH. Holocardius: review of the literature and case report. Obstet Gynecol 1953;2:647.

Haring DAJP, Cornel MC, Van der Linden JC, et al. Acardius acephalus after induced ovulation: a case report. Teratology 1993;47:257–262.

Healey MG. Acardia: predictive risk factors for the co-twin's survival. Teratology 1994;50:205–213.

Holzgreve W, Tercanli S, Krings W, et al. A simpler technique for umbilical-cord blockade of an acardiac twin. N Engl J Med 1994;331:56–57.

James WH. A note on the epidemiology of acardiac monsters. Teratology 1977;16:211–216.

Kappelman MD. Acardius amorphus. Am J Obstet Gynecol 1944;47:412.

Lachman R, McNabb M, Furmanski M, et al. The acardiac monster. Eur J Pediatr 1980;134:195.

Langlotz H, Sauerbrei E, Murray S. Transvaginal Doppler sonographic diagnosis of an acardiac twin at 12 weeks gestation. J Ultrasound Med 1991;10:175–179.

Mack LA, Gravett MG, Rumack CM, et al. Antenatal ultrasonic evaluation of acardiac monsters. J Ultrasound Med 1982;1:13–18.

McCurdy CM Jr, Childers JM, Seeds JW. Ligation of the umbilical cord of an acardiac-acephalus twin with an endoscopic intrauterine technique. Obstet Gynecol 1993; 82:708–711.

Moore TR, Gale S, Benirschke K. Perinatal outcome of forty-nine pregnancies complicated by acardiac twinning. Am J Obstet Gynecol 1990;163:907–912.

Myrianthopoulos NC. An epidemiologic survey of twins in a large, prospectively studied population. Am J Hum Genet 1970;22:662.

Napolitani FD, Schreiber I. The acardiac monster: a review of the world literature and presentation of 2 cases. Am J Obstet Gynecol 1960;80:582.

NIH Consensus Development Panel on the Effect of Corticosteroids for Fetal Maturation on Perinatal Outcomes. JAMA 1995;273:413–418.

Platt LD, DeVore GR, Bieniarz A, et al. Antenatal diagnosis of acephalus acardia: a proposed management scheme. Am J Obstet Gynecol 1983;146:857.

Porreco RP, Barton SM, Haverkamp AD. Occlusion of umbilical artery in acardiac, acephalic twin. Lancet 1991; 337:326–328.

Pretorius DH, Leopold GR, Moore TR, et al. Acardiac twin: report of Doppler sonography. J Ultrasound Med 1988; 7:413.

Quintero RA, Rich H, Puder K, et al. Umbilical-cord ligation of an acardiac twin by fetoscopy at 19 weeks gestation. N Engl J Med 1994;330:469–471.

Robie GJ, Payne GG, Morgan MA. Selective delivery of an acardiac, acephalic twin. N Engl J Med 1989;320:512.

Rodeck C, Deans A, Jauniaux E. Thermocoagulation for the early treatment of pregnancy with an acardiac twin. N Engl J Med 1998;339:1293–1295. ,

Schatz CF. Die Acardii und ihre Verwandten. Berlin: A. Hirschwald, 1898.

Shenker L, Reed KL, Marx GR, et al. Fetal cardiac Doppler flow studies in prenatal diagnosis of heart disease. Am J Obstet Gynecol 1988;158:1267–1273.

Sherer DM, Armstrong B, Shah YG, et al. Prenatal sonographic diagnosis, Doppler velocimetric umbilical cord study, and subsequent management of an acardiac twin pregnancy. Obstet Gynecol 1989;74:472–475.

Silverman NH, Kleinman CS, Rudolph AM, et al. Fetal atrioventricular valve insufficiency associated with nonimmune hydrops: a two dimensional echocardiographic and pulse Doppler ultrasound study. Circulation 1985;72:825–831.

Simonds JP, Gowen GA. Fetus amorphus: report of a case. Surg Gynecol Obstet 1925;41:171.

Simpson PC, Trudinger BJ, Walker A, et al. The intrauterine treatment of fetal cardiac failure in a twin pregnancy with an acardiac, acephalic monster. Am J Obstet Gynecol 1983;147:842–844.

Van Allen MI, Smith SW, Shepard TH. Twin reversed arterial perfusion (TRAP) sequence: a study of 14 twin pregnancies with acardius. Semin Perinatol 1983;7:285.

CHAPTER 119

Conjoined Twins

► CONDITION

Although a rare event, the birth of conjoined twins has always fascinated both the physician and the layperson. The first well-documented case was reported in A.D. 1100 and described the Biddenden maids, who were joined at the hips and shoulders. In 1134, when the maids had lived together for 34 years, Mary was suddenly taken ill and died. Eliza, her sister, died 6 hours later (Bondeson 1992). The most famous conjoined twins were Eng and Chang Bunker, born in Siam in 1811. The inappropriate term "Siamese twins" was coined by P.T. Barnum, who promoted the exhibition of Chang and Eng Bunker. An early medical description of these most famous conjoined twins, who lived unseparated until they died at age 63, can be found in the works of Warren (1829). Many conjoined twins are stillborn. In one series 40% of conjoined twins were stillborn and an additional 35% survived only 1 day (Edmonds and Layde 1982). Konig recorded the first successful separation of conjoined twins in 1689. These twins were joined at the umbilicus, and the division was accomplished by necrosing the band of tissue between the two children with a constricting ligature. Kiesewetter (1966) reviewed 24 surgical attempts at separation that appeared in the literature from 1689 to 1962. There are now over 100 reports of successful separations in the medical literature or lay press (Filler 1986). Conjoined twins may be joined at a variety of anatomic sites, and classifications have been developed to describe all the possibilities (Guttmacher and Nichols 1967). The nomenclature in use clinically is derived from the most prominent site of conjunction. The common twin types include thoracopagus, xiphopagus or omphalopagus, pygopagus, ischiopagus, and craniopagus.

Thoracopagus is the most common type of conjoined twin and with omphalopagus (or xiphopagus) represents about 75% of cases reported. The two individuals lie face to face and share a common sternum, diaphragm, and upper abdominal wall from xiphoid to umbilicus. An extensive review of the anatomy of thoracopagus twins has been published by Nichols et al. (1967). In data from 32 cases, 75% have conjoined hearts. Because of the abnormal ventricular arrangements and associated anomalies of the great arteries and veins, successful surgical division is usually not possible. In about half of these cases, the intestinal tracts are also joined. Occasionally, the esophagus and stomach are single, but usually the union starts in the distal duodenum and ends in a pouch at the site of a Meckel diverticulum. The biliary tree is joined in 25% of cases.

Xiphopagus or omphalopagus twins, usually considered a subgroup of thoracopagus, also face one another and usually have the least-complicated union of all conjoined twins. They are joined at the anterior abdominal wall from xiphoid to umbilicus. The peritoneal cavity of one communicates with that of the other, but the upper intestinal tracts are usually separate. A bridge of liver connects the infants in the majority of cases. Evaluation of the single umbilical cord in twins joined at the umbilicus has revealed the presence of two to seven umbilical vessels. An omphalocele is often present at the umbilical-cord insertion.

Pygopagus twins represent about 20% of cases, are joined at the buttocks and perineum, and face away from each other. A significant length of sacrum may be fused, and as a result, the twins often share the sacral spinal canal. A single lower rectum and anus is common, and often the lower genital tract and external genitalia are fused.

Ischiopagus accounts for 5% of cases. These twins are united at a single bony pelvis. Four normal lower extremities (ischiopagus tetrapus) may be attached to the pelvis, but often two of the four lower extremities are fused into one malformed limb (ischiopagus tripus). The intestinal tracts usually join at the terminal ileum, which empties into a single colon.

Craniopagus is the least common type of conjoined twins and accounts for 2% of cases. There is always fusion of the skull, and often the twins share large dural sinuses and vascular structures. A classification into partial or total forms, having a junction at either brow, vertex, or parietal bone, has been devised by O'Connell (1976). In the partial forms, the brains are separated by bone or dura and each brain has separate leptomeninges. In the total form, the brains of each twin are connected, or they are separated only by arachnoid. Separation of the total type is extremely difficult, and feasibility is often determined by the presence of a superior sagittal sinus for each brain that will provide adequate venous drainage.

▶ INCIDENCE

The exact incidence of conjoined twins is not known, but estimates have varied from 1 in 80,000 to 1 in 25,000 births (Freedman, et al. 1962; Siegel 1950). In Africa, reports indicate that this anomaly occurs as often as 1 in 14,000 births, suggesting an increased incidence among African Americans (Bhettay et al. 1975; Bland and Hammar 1962). Other reports on the frequency of conjoined twinning show the incidence to be between 1 in 2800 to 1 in 200,000 (Hanson 1975). Three conjoined twins over a 10-month period among residents of South Glamorgan with approximately 5400 deliveries a year is the highest reported incidence of conjoined twinning so far described (Rees et al. 1993). In Rudolph et al.'s (1967) review, about 70% of conjoined twins were female. Maternal age and parity do not appear to be factors that influence the occurrence of this type of twinning.

▶ SONOGRAPHIC FINDINGS

The first report of conjoined twins diagnosed ultrasonographically was in 1977 (Fagan 1977). Since then prenatal diagnosis has been reported many times and can be made in the first trimester (Hill, 1997; Hubinot et al, 1997; Lam et al, 1998; Maymon et al, 1998). Suspicion of conjoined twins should arise when a dividing membrane cannot be visualized. van den Brand et al. (1994) have suggested nine sonographic findings to diagnose conjoined twins (Table 119-1). Polyhydramnios is present in 75% of thoracopagus twins (Harper et al. 1980). Congenital anomalies are common in conjoined twins, even in the organs that are not shared. Congenital heart disease, renal and genitourinary abnormalities,

▶ **TABLE 119-1.** SONOGRAPHIC FINDINGS USED TO DIAGNOSE CONJOINED TWINS

Bifid appearance of the first-trimester fetal pole
Lack of a separating membrane between the twins
Inability to separate the fetal bodies
Detection of fetal anomalies
More than three vessels in the umbilical cord
Heads at same level and body plane
Spines unusually extended
Extremities in unusual proximity
Fetuses do not change position relative to one another after movement or manipulation, or with passage of time

Source: van den Brand SFJJ, Nijhuis JG, van Dongen PWJ. Prenatal ultrasound diagnosis of conjoined twins. Obstet Gynecol Surv 1994;49:656–662

intestinal duplication, and omphalocele have all been reported. Ultrasound examination has been found useful in describing the extent of joining of the cardiovascular system in thoracoabdominally joined twins (Fig. 119-1 and 2). Sanders et al. (1985) have reviewed their experience in four pairs of thoracoabdominally joined twins and demonstrated that prenatal echocardiography correctly diagnosed major cardiac anomalies, although they missed certain important features because of their inability to detect abnormal pulmonary venous connections. In addition, the investigators concluded that conjoined twins were more easily and thoroughly examined in utero because more views could be obtained as compared with the postnatal examination, which is hampered by the conjunction and the associated omphalocele. With the use of ultrasound equipment it is always possible to detect whether bone tissue is interposed between the two brains (Fig. 119-3). However, it is impossible to detect if the two cerebral hemispheres are joined or separated by either the dura or pia mater. Color flow mapping may be useful in craniopagus twins to determine vascular connections (Loverro et al. 1991).

▶ DIFFERENTIAL DIAGNOSIS

In a retrospective review of 14 cases of conjoined twinning diagnosed prenatally between 1984 and 1989, no false positive or false negative diagnoses of conjoined twins were made. Transvaginal sonographic studies significantly improved the delineation of conjunction in two patients, and computed tomography permitted the diagnosis to be confirmed in two patients (Barth et al. 1990). There are several pitfalls for the sonographic diagnosis of conjoined twins. Inseparable fetal skin contours must be a persistent finding at the same anatomic level to avoid the false positive diagnosis of conjoined twins (Barth et al. 1990). Even discordant presentation does not exclude the diagnosis, particularly in

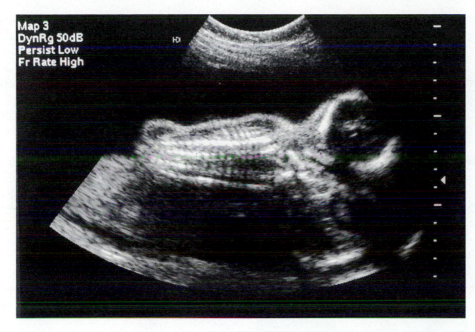

Figure 119-1. Prenatal sonographic image of thoracopagus twins, demonstrating duplication of vertebral column.

omphalopagus twins. The joining bridge may be sufficiently small to allow for rotation of the twins. Finally, with severe conjoining, twins may be melded into a conglomerative tissue mimicking a single pregnancy (Weingast et al. 1984). The diagnosis of conjoined twins does not however exclude the presence of other problems unique to twinning. One case has been reported of an acardiac set of conjoined twins, coexisting in a triplet pregnancy (Sanjaghsaz et al, 1998).

► ANTENATAL NATURAL HISTORY

Little is known about the antenatal natural history of conjoined twins. Polyhydramnios has been reported in 75% of thoracopagus twins (Harper et al. 1980). In the older obstetric literature on the subject, stillbirth occurred in approximately 20 to 40% of cases (Harper et al. 1980). More recently, many prenatally diagnosed patients elect termination, leaving single case reports and small series

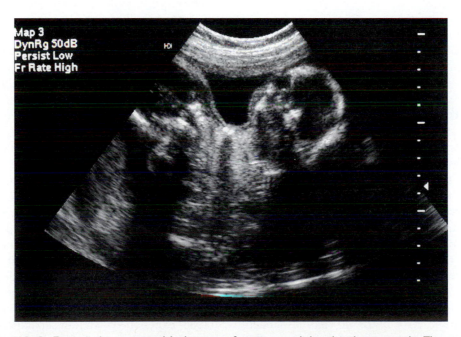

Figure 119-2. Prenatal sonographic image of same conjoined twins seen in Figure 119-1, demonstrating the presence of two separate heads on a joined thorax.

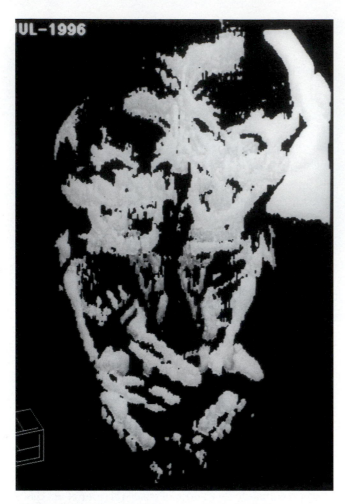

Figure 119-3. Prenatal CT scan seen with three-dimensional reconstruction of dicephalic tribrachii dipus conjoined twins.

in the literature. Most of the literature regarding recent case reports has concentrated on the subject of surgical separation.

▶ MANAGEMENT OF PREGNANCY

When the diagnosis of conjoined twins is made before viability, the option of pregnancy termination should be discussed with the parents. Since mortality and the ability to separate thoracopagus twins is directly related to the union of two hearts and associated cardiac abnormalities, echocardiography is recommended in all cases and may be of significant value to parents faced with the decision of whether to terminate the pregnancy. Although sonography is a standard technique for evaluation of fetal anatomy, its ability to characterize certain tissues is limited. Additional testing, including computed tomographic (CT) scanning, has also been used in utero to delineate the extent of the conjunction (see Fig. 119-2).

Magnetic resonance imaging (MRI) improves soft-tissue definition and has been reported to be of additional use in the antenatal evaluation of conjoined twins. Zoppini et al. (1993) used MRI following fetal paralysis with pancuronium and identified bowel-to-bowel anastomosis. Prior to the MRI, a solution of gadolinium DTPA was also inected into the stomach of one twin to aid in the diagnosis of bowel-to-bowel anastomosis. Early prenatal diagnosis and precise character relation of conjoined twins are essential for optimal obstetric and postnatal management. Vaginal delivery may be possible for preterm conjoined twins for which postnatal survival is impossible. Near-term cesarean section is the delivery method of choice for conjoined twins to maximize survival and prevent birth trauma. Dystocia occurs frequently (Nichols et al. 1967), and in omphalopagus twins it has been reported in 36% of cases (Harper et al. 1980). Delivery at a tertiary-care center is recommended for optimal neonatal intensive care and pediatric surgical support.

▶ FETAL INTERVENTION

There are no fetal interventions for conjoined twins.

▶ TREATMENT OF NEWBORN

Except for life-threatening emergencies that must be treated by immediate separation of the twins, surgery should be delayed until an accurate assessment of shared structures is completed (Filler 1986). Table 119-2 lists the important diagnostic studies, the structures that each study will best evaluate, and the type of twin that requires such a study. Comprehensive evaluation of the cardiovascular system is necessary in all thoracopagus twins (Fig. 119-4). These studies should begin immediately after birth because of the high likelihood of an abnormality in one or both twins. The most important factor in prognosis is the degree of separation of the two hearts. Of the conjoined twins who are born alive, the potential long-term survivors fall into two groups. The first group involves children who thrive despite being joined. Pygopagus, ischiopagus, and xiphopagus twins usually fall into this category. In this group there is sufficient time to evaluate organ sharing and to plan operative separation. Separation in these children should probably be delayed several months until the infants are larger. The advantages of waiting are that the infants will be larger, important congenital anomalies not obvious at birth will have become apparent, and the risks of surgery and anesthesia should be less. In Filler's (1986) experience with four separations, delay was clearly beneficial. The second group involves twins whose lives are threatened because of the conjunction or coexistent

▶ **TABLE 119-2.** MOST USEFUL DIAGNOSTIC STUDIES FOR EVALUATING DIFFERENT TYPES OF TWINS

Test	Evaluation of	Type of Union in Twin
MRI	Nervous system	Cranial and thoracoabdominal
CT scan	Bony unions, kidneys, urinary tract, central nervous system	All types
Ultrasound	Liver, biliary system, pancreas	Thoracoabdominal
Plain films	Extremities	Ischiopagus
Radionuclide scans	Liver, spleen, biliary tract	Thoracoabdominal
Cystography, urethrography	Bladder, urethra	Abdominal and pelvic
Barium studies of gastrointestinal tract	Small bowel, colon	Abdominal and pelvic
Angiography	Heart and major blood vessels	Thoracoabdominal and cranial
Echocardiography*	Heart and great vessels	Thoracoabdominal
Electrocardiography		
Cardiac catheterization		

*Prenatal test appears to be especially useful.
Source: Filler RM. Conjoined twins and their separation. Semin Perinatol 1986;10(1):82–91.

congenital abnormalities. Emergency surgery with or without separation may be required before appropriate diagnostic studies can be completed. Urgent surgery is indicated in three clinical situations: (1) when the existence of one twin threatens the life of the other (Graivier and Jacoby 1980); (2) when a potentially correctable life-threatening anomaly is present (e.g., severe congenital heart disease or intestinal obstruction); and (3) when surgical intervention is necessary for a traumatic injury to the bridge of tissue and underlying viscera joining the twins.

▶ SURGICAL TREATMENT

Many descriptions of surgical procedures to separate different types of conjoined twins appear in the literature (DeVries 1967; Gans et al. 1968; James et al. 1985; Kiesewetter 1966; Kling et al. 1975; Koop 1961). It is beyond the scope of this review to describe the individual operations in detail. However, the surgeon is faced with two general considerations. First, the surgical team must try to separate the shared structures, leaving each child with functional residual organs and limbs whenever possible. Second, the skin, muscle, and bony defect at the site of conjunction must be closed after separation is completed. Closure of defects can be relatively simple when the defect is small, as in the case of omphalopagus twins. When the defect is large, closure can be extremely difficult. In cases of large defects, a flap of skin and muscle may be available for coverage. Silastic tissue expanders have been used to provide additional skin and muscle to aid closure in several cases (Filler 1986). Teflon mesh and acrylic prostheses have also been described (DeVries 1967; Wilson 1957). It is essential to have a coordinated approach of the operating team, consisting of duplicate anesthesiologists, surgeons, and nursing personnel. The anesthesia team should be responsible for setting up methods of physiologic monitoring (James et al. 1985; Simpson et al. 1967). Existing operating tables may need to be modified as the standard tables are not properly designed for the separation of conjoined twins. The modifications

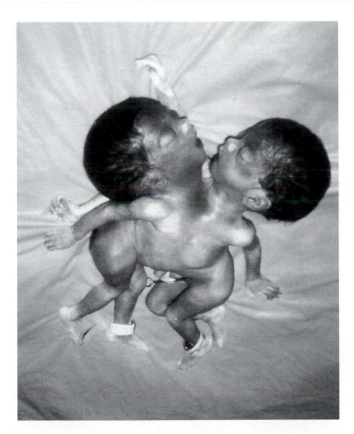

Figure 119-4. Postnatal appearance of thoracopagus twins.

required will depend on the type of separation (Savickis 1984).

Significant ethical considerations arise in cases in which it is not possible to achieve separation without sacrificing the life or the quality of the life of one of the two twins. These issues have been the subject of a review by Pepper (1967) and Raffensperger (1997).

► LONG-TERM OUTCOME

The prognosis for surgery depends on the type of conjunction. The results for omphalopagus and xiphopagus twins are particularly good. Even 30 years ago, in a review of 11 sets of omphalopagus twins, 19 of the 22 children survived (Nichols et al. 1967). When omphalocele is present in this type of twinning, the prognosis appears to be somewhat worse. Votteler (1986) reviewed the results of separation in seven sets of omphalopagus twins with an associated omphalocele treated between 1963 and 1981. The omphalocele had ruptured in four sets. One twin in three of the four sets died, and one twin from two of the three sets with an intact omphalocele also died.

With the exception of a single case of a successful separation of a set of twins who shared a right atrium (Synhorst et al. 1979), thoracopagus twins sharing hearts have not survived. Survival is more frequent in those sharing a single pericardium (Edmonds and Layde 1982). The most common causes of death in thoracopagus twins include cardiac abnormalities, infections, and respiratory failure. In many failures, closure of the chest wall has contributed to the poor outcome, either because of tight closure that restricts chest motion or a defect in the sternum that allows paradoxical respiratory motion (Filler 1986). The outcome for craniopagus twins relates to whether the union is total or partial (Bucholz et al. 1987; Votteler 1986). In a review of 21 cases of craniopagus, temporoparietal and occipital junctions had a worse outcome than frontal and parietal junctions (Bucholz et al. 1987). In the Votteler series, 50% had residual neurologic abnormalities, whereas in the Bucholz series only one of nine had severe neurologic deficit. The prognosis appears better when surgery is performed during the neonatal period and when craniopagus twins are separated in stages rather than in one procedure (Bucholz et al. 1987).

Successful separations of pygopagus twins have been reported by Koop (1961), Votteler (1982), Cloutier et al. (1979) and Fowler et al (1999). The prognosis is usually good for pygopagus twins mainly because the joined structures are not essential for life. In most reported cases, both twins have survived (Filler 1986).

The separation of ischiopagus twins is usually difficult because most of the abdominal viscera are joined. There is only one pelvis and often only three lower extremities. Votteler compiled a list of 12 ischiopagus separations from 1955 to 1981 in which one or both ischiopagus twins survived. Filler (1986), Ross et al. (1985), and Grantzow et al. (1985) have successfully separated four other sets. Albert et al. (1992) further reported on the orthopedic management of four cases treated at Children's Hospital in Philadelphia. Six of the eight infants survived. Significant postseparation orthopedic problems persisted in all of the successful separations. These included but were not limited to hip flexures, club foot, recurrent dislocated hip, one functional deformed foot, and quadriceps contractures. In addition to orthopedic problems, successfully separated ischiopagus twins require long-term rehabilitation because of gynecologic, urologic, and intestinal disabilities. In Filler's (1986) series of three cases of ischiopagus twins, one set at age 17 used a prosthesis for an absent lower extremity, and each had a colostomy. In a second set, at age 4 each child had a colostomy and an artificial limb. Because they shared a single set of male genitalia, one child is being raised as a boy and the other as a girl. In a further set reported at age 1.5 years, each had a colostomy, a suprapubic bladder catheter, and normal lower extremities (Filler 1986).

► GENETICS AND RECURRENCE RISK

To our knowledge, the recurrence risk is not increased above background for conjoined twins.

REFERENCES

Albert MC, Drummond DS, O'Neill J, et al. The orthopedic management of conjoined twins: a review of 13 cases and report of 4 cases. J Pediatr Orthop 1992;2:300–307.

Barth RA, Filly RA, Goldberg JD, et al. Conjoined twins: prenatal diagnosis and assessment of associated malformations. Radiology 1990;177:201–207.

van den Brand et al. SFJJ, Nijhuis JG, van Dongen PWJ. Prenatal ultrasound diagnosis of conjoined twins. Obstet Gynecol Surv 1994;49:656–662.

Bhettay E, Nelson MS, Beighton P. Epidemic of conjoined twins in southern Africa. Lancet 1975;2:741–743.

Bland KG, Hammar B. Xiphopagus twins. Cent Afr J Med 1962;8:371.

Bondeson J. The Biddenden maids: a curious chapter in the history of conjoined twins. J R Soc Med 1992;85:216–221.

Bucholz RD, Yoon KW, Shively RE. Temporoparietal craniopagus: case report and review of the literature. J Neurosurg 1987;66:72–79.

Cloutier R, Levassiur L, Copty M, et al. The surgical separation of pygopagus twins. J Pediatr Surg 1979;14:554–556.

DeVries PA. Separation of the San Francisco twins. Birth Defects 1967;3:75.

Edmonds LD, Layde PM. Conjoined twins in the United States 1970–1977. Teratology 1982;25:301–308.

Fagan CJ. Antepartum diagnosis of conjoined twins by ultrasonography. AJR Am J Roentgenol 1977;129:921–922.

Filler RM. Conjoined twins and their separation. Semin Perinatol 1986;10:82–91.

Fowler CL, Pulito AR, Warf BC, et al. Separation of complex pygopagus conjoined twins. J Pediatr Surg 1999;34:619–622.

Freedman HL, Tafeen CH, Harris H. Conjoined thoracopagus twins. Am J Obstet Gynecol 1962;84:1904.

Gans SL, Morgenstern L, Gettelman E, et al. Separation of conjoined twins in the newborn period. J Pediatr Surg 1968;3:565–574.

Graivier L, Jacoby MD. Emergency separation of newborn conjoined (Siamese) twins. Tex Med 1980;76:60–62.

Grantzow R, Heckler WC, Holschneider AM, et al. Separation of an asymmetric xipho-omphalo-ischiopagus tripus. Langenbecks Arch Chir 1985;363:195–206.

Guttmacher AF, Nichols BL. Teratology of conjoined twins. Birth Defects 1967;3:3.

Hanson JW. Incidence of conjoined twinning. Lancet 1975;2:1257.

Harper RG, Kenigsberg K, Sia CG, et al. Xiphopagus conjoined twins: a 300-year review of the obstetric, morphopathologic, neonatal, and surgical parameters. Am J Obstet Gynecol 1980;137:617.

Hill LM. The sonographic detection of early first-trimester diagnosis of conjoined twins. Prenat Diagn 1997;17:961–963.

Hubinot C, Kollman P, Malvaux V, et al. First-trimester diagnosis of conjoined twins. Fetal Diagn Ther 1997;12:185–187.

James RD, McLeod ME, Relton JES, et al. Anesthetic considerations for separation of omphalo-ischopagus tripus twins. Can Anaesth Soc J 1985;33:402–411.

Kiesewetter WB. Surgery on conjoined (Siamese) twins. Surgery 1966;59:860–871.

Kling S, Johnston RJ, Michalyshyn B, et al. Successful separation of xiphopagus-conjoined twins. J Pediatr Surg 1975;10:267–271.

Koop CE. The successful separation of pygopagus twins. Surgery 1961;49:271.

Konig G. Sibi invicem adnati feliciter separati. Ephemerid Natur Curios Dec II, Ann VIII Obs 145, 1689.

Lam YH, Sin SY, Lam C, et al. Prenatal sonographic diagnosis of conjoined twins in the first trimester: two case reports. Ultrasound Obstet Gynecol 1998;1:289–291.

Loverro G, Occhiogrosso M, Caruso G, et al. Prenatal diagnosis of craniopagus (case report). Acta Obstet Gynecol Scand 1991;70:237–239.

Maymon R, Halperin R, Weinraub Z, et al. Three-dimensional transvaginal sonography of conjoined twins at 10 weeks: a case report. Ultrasound Obstet Gynecol 1998;11:292–294.

Nichols BL, Blattner RJ, Rudolph AJ. General clinical management of thoracopagus twins. Birth Defects 1967;3:38.

O'Connell JEA. Craniopagus twins: surgical anatomy and embryology and their implications. J Neurol Neurosurg Psychiatry 1976;39:1–22.

Pepper CK. Ethical and moral considerations in the separation of conjoined twins. Birth Defects 1967;3:128.

Raffensperger J. A philosophical approach to conjoined twins. Pediatr Surg Int 1997;12:249–255.

Rees AEJ, Vujanic GM, Williams WM. Epidemic of conjoined twins in Cardiff. Br J Obstet Gynaecol 1993;100:388–391.

Ross AJ, O'Neill JA, Silverman DG, et al. A new technique for evaluating cutaneous vascularity in complicated conjoined twins. J Pediatr Surg 1985;20:743–746.

Rudolph AJ, Michaels JP, Nichols BL. Obstetric management of conjoined twins. Birth Defects 1967;3:28.

Sanders SP, Chin AJ, Parness IA, et al. Prenatal diagnosis of congenital heart defects in thoracoabdominally conjoined twins. N Engl J Med 1985;313:370–374.

Sanjaghsaz H, Bayram MO, Qureshi F. Twin reversed arterial perufsion sequence in conjoined, acardiac, acephalic twins associated with a normal triplet. A case report. J Reprod Med 1998;43L1046-1050.

Savickis J. The separation of conjoined twins—an OR nursing perspective. Can Nurse 1984;80:21–23.

Siegel I. Thoracopagus: vaginal delivery without destructive operation. Ill Med J 1950;97:40.

Simpson JS, Pelton DA, Swyer PR. The importance of monitoring during operations of conjoined twins. Can Med Assoc J 1967;96:1463.

Synhorst D, Matlak M, Roan Y, et al. Separation of conjoined thoracopagus twins joined at the right atria. Am J Cardiol 1979;43:662–665.

Votteler TP. Necrotizing enterocolitis in a pygopagus conjoined twin. J Pediatr Surg 1982;17:555–557.

Votteler TP. Conjoined twins. In: Welch KJ, Randolph JG, Ravitch MM, et al., eds. Pediatric surgery. Vol 2. Chicago: Year Book, 1986:771–779.

Warren JC. An account of the siamese twin brothers united together from their birth. Am J Med Sci 1829;52:255.

Weingast GR, Johnson ML, Pretorius DH, et al. Difficulty in sonographic diagnosis of cephalothoracopagus. J Ultrasound Med 1984;3:421–423.

Wilson H. Surgery in Siamese twins: a report of three sets of conjoined twins treated surgically. Ann Surg 1957;145:718.

Zoppini C, Vanzulli A, Kustermann A, et al. Prenatal diagnosis of anatomical connections in conjoined twins by use of contrast magnetic resonance imaging. Prenat Diagn 1993;13:995–999.

occurred in multiple gestations (Landy and Weingold 1989). However, only a few cases of biochemical rather than clinical coagulopathy have been reported under these circumstances, and the 25% incidence may be an overestimation (Anderson et al. 1990; Carlson and Towers 1989). In one series of 16 pregnancies complicated by intrauterine fetal death of one twin, no cases of maternal disseminated intravascular coagulation were found (Fusi and Gordon 1990). In another series, transient fibrin-split products and hypofibrinogenemia was found in 2 of 20 cases of single IUFD in twins, neither of which was clinically apparent or required medical therapy (Eglowstein and D'Alton 1993). It is also reassuring to note that no cases of clinical coagulopathy have been reported in the extensive literature on selective termination and multifetal pregnancy reduction (Malone and D'Alton 1999).

▶ INCIDENCE

Single IUFD in the first trimester may occur in up to 50% of cases of twin pregnancies (Varma 1979). The reported frequency of a single IUFD in multiple gestations in the second or third trimester is much less, and varies from 0.5 to 6.8% (Litschgi and Stucki 1980). It is estimated that there is a threefold to fourfold increase in intrauterine death with monochorionic twins as compared with dichorionic twins (Burke 1990; Kilby et al. 1994). A single fetal death is also more common among twins with a structural abnormality (Kilby et al. 1994). Death of a single fetus has also been observed in higher-order pregnancies, complicating 14 to 17% of triplet gestations (Borlum 1991; Gonen et al. 1990).

▶ SONOGRAPHIC FINDINGS

The sonographic findings in single IUFD in twin pregnancy vary, depending on whether there is an identifiable cause for the death and on the interval between the death and performance of the ultrasound examination. Sonographic assessment should include complete biometric and anatomic assessments of the dead and surviving twins, an assessment of fluid volumes in both sacs, evaluation of the cord insertion sites, and determination of chorionicity. If the fetal death is due to placental insufficiency associated with maternal medical disease, there may be evidence of intrauterine growth restriction in the surviving twin. Sonographic examination may reveal a fetal abnormality or a placental abruption as a causative factor. Sonographic features of twin-to-twin transfusion syndrome should also be searched for, as described in Chapter 123.

The determination of chorionicity is important in the counseling and treatment of patients with single IUFD in twin pregnancy. If two separate placentas are visualized or the fetuses are of unlike gender the pregnancy is dichorionic. If only one placenta is identified and the fetuses are of the same sex, the separating membrane should then be examined. If two layers are present the placentation is monochorionic. If three or four layers are visualized the placentation is dichorionic (D'Alton and Dudley 1989). Membrane thickness has been used to assess chorionicity, with a thin membrane indicating monochorionicity and a thick membrane indicating dichorionicity (Barss et al. 1985). However, there is some concern that a membrane may appear both thin and thick at different times during the same ultrasound examination and at different gestational ages (D'Alton and Dudley 1989; Hertzberg et al. 1987; Samuels 1988). The "twin peak" sign, identified on ultrasound examination by the presence of a triangular projection of placental tissue between the layers of the separating membrane, has been suggested to provide reliable evidence of dichorionicity (Malone and D'Alton 1999) (Fig. 120-1). However, the absence of the twin peak sign does not help to determine chorionicity, which limits its usefulness as a clinical marker (Malone and D'Alton 1999).

Sonographic examination can only establish the diagnosis of chorionicity with absolute certainty when there are clearly two separate placentas or there are fetuses of opposite gender. None of the methods of examining the membrane are completely reliable. Furthermore, assessment of chorionicity may be difficult with single IUFD in a twin gestation if there is a single placenta. Oligohydramnios in the sac of the dead fetus may make the diagnosis of fetal gender difficult. Sonographic examination of the dividing membrane may also be difficult because the membrane may be tightly adherent to the dead fetus (D'Alton and Dudley 1989). Therefore, if a certain diagnosis of chorionicity is needed, in the presence of a single placenta and same-sex fetuses, DNA studies on amniocytes may be required (Malone and D'Alton 1999).

▶ DIFFERENTIAL DIAGNOSIS

There is no differential diagnosis for this condition.

▶ ANTENATAL HISTORY

An accurate assessment of the antenatal history of multiple pregnancies complicated by single IUFD is hampered by the lack of a single large study (Landy and

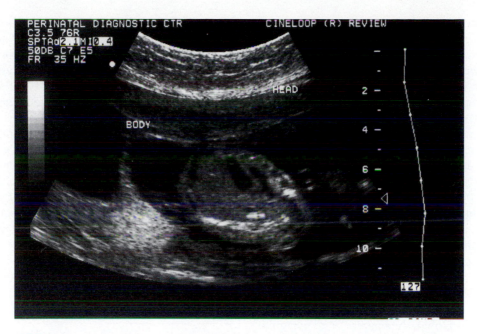

Figure 120-1. Sonographic image demonstrating the "twin peak" sign, a triangular projection of placental tissue. This sign has been suggested as evidence of a dichorionic gestation.

Weingold 1989). Most of the available data consist of case reports and small retrospective series dealing with unfavorable outcomes (Enbom 1985). Many cases will not represent a management problem because labor will already have begun by the time the diagnosis of single IUFD is made. However, some patients with single IUFD in a multiple gestation will remain pregnant with one or more surviving fetuses, which creates a management dilemma. Elective delivery after confirmation of pulmonary maturity does not necessarily prevent the development of multicystic encephalomalacia in the surviving fetus or fetuses (Malone and D'Alton 1999). Therefore, elective delivery is not recommended before 37 weeks of gestation for the surviving co-twin of a stillbirth in utero unless antenatal surveillance is suggestive of fetal compromise. Similarly, close fetal surveillance after the diagnosis of single IUFD cannot necessarily guarantee a good outcome for the surviving fetus or fetuses. This is most likely because the insult causing multicystic encephalomalacia probably occurs at the moment of the single fetal death (Malone and D'Alton 1999).

In 14 cases in Landy and Weingold's (1989) series, expectant management was instituted in an attempt to delay delivery in order to benefit the surviving co-twin. The interval between diagnosis of fetal death and delivery ranged between 2 and 12 weeks. One of the survivors had neurologic deficits, and 11 of the 14 pregnancies delivered before 37 weeks of gestation. In addition to the 14 cases identified by Landy, Santema et al. (1995) have identified from 8 reports 123 cases

that were managed expectantly. The overall incidence of neurologic morbidity was 12%; the mortality rate for the surviving twin was 4.3%.

► MANAGEMENT OF PREGNANCY

Maternal referral to a tertiary-care perinatal unit is advised when a single IUFD in a multiple gestation is diagnosed. However, in many cases labor will already have started and in others coexisting maternal illness or placental abruption may make it necessary to deliver the surviving fetus or fetuses (D'Alton et al. 1984). Sonographic evaluation of the surviving fetus or fetuses for fetal growth and surveillance, such as a nonstress test or biophysical profile, should be performed on admission. Delivery is indicated if fetal monitoring in the surviving twin demonstrates fetal compromise. Delivery is also appropriate when the gestational age is known to be 37 weeks or greater. When the gestational age is less than 37 weeks, it is advisable to determine the chorionicity. If the chorionicity is determined to be dichorionic, the main risk to the surviving twin is to be born prematurely. If the chorionicity is determined to be monochorionic, the risk to the surviving twin is premature birth with the added neurologic risk of multicystic encephalomalacia, which occurs in 12% of cases (D'Alton and Simpson 1995). It is important to realize that immediate delivery may not prevent neurologic handicap (D'Alton et al. 1984). Therefore, in preterm gestation, the risk of prematurity outweighs the potential risk of neurologic handicap in the surviving twin.

Serial ultrasound examinations are performed to monitor fetal growth and to visualize the fetal brain in order to look for evidence of multicystic encephalomalacia or other reported neurologic sequelae (D'Alton and Simpson 1995). In cases in which sonography of the fetal brain appears normal 2 weeks after the death of the co-twin there have been no case reports of multicystic encephalomalacia occurring at a later time interval; therefore, a patient can be reassured at this time (Carlson and Towers 1989). Base-line maternal coagulation studies should be performed. It is not necessary to obtain further coagulation studies unless there is a clinical indication (Malone and D'Alton 1999). The mode of delivery will depend on the presentation of the surviving twin and on the indication for delivery. Cesarean delivery is recommended only for standard obstetric indications. At the time of delivery umbilical-cord gas measurements, hemoglobin, hematocrit, and coagulation profile should be obtained on the surviving infant.

In known monochorionic pregnancies with impending death of one twin, preterm delivery may be indicated in order to prevent neurologic injury to the survivor or potentially to salvage both twins. DNA zygosity studies on amniocytes can be used for rapid and certain confirmation of the chorionicity (Norton et al. 1997). In a monochorionic twin pregnancy with a gestational age of greater than 28 weeks, the risk of neurologic handicap to the surviving twin in the case of death of the co-twin seems to be higher than the risk of prematurity. Neurologic injury to the surviving co-twin does not seem to be preventable by prompt delivery following death of one twin (D'Alton et al. 1984). Therefore, delivery should be considered if it appears likely that one fetus is about to die in utero. If chorionicity is unclear and the death of one twin seems imminent, it is necessary to weigh the risks and benefits to each twin of expectant management versus early delivery. If dichorionicity can be clearly demonstrated there is no benefit to the healthy, appropriately grown co-twin of elective preterm delivery in cases in which the smaller twin is likely to die.

▶ FETAL INTERVENTION

No fetal intervention is recommended before 37 weeks in cases in which a single IUFD has already been documented. As described above, in cases of the impending death of one fetus in a multiple gestation, DNA studies on amniocytes should be performed when ultrasound examination cannot clearly demonstrate chorionicity (Norton et al. 1997).

In addition, selective termination of a fetus that is about to die in a monochorionic gestation may be con-

sidered, in an effort to protect the healthy co-fetus or fetuses. We have reported a case of fetoscopic cord ligation in one member of a monochorionic twin pregnancy with a cardiac defect incompatible with life and hydrops, which was thought to be at significant risk of IUFD. The normal co-twin was delivered 6 weeks after the cord-ligation procedure and had a normal neonatal course (Crombleholme et al. 1996). Indications for considering a fetoscopic cord-ligation procedure to prevent neurologic handicap in twins would include anomalies incompatible with life in monochorionic pregnancies at a gestational age less than 28 weeks or significant growth discordance in monochorionic gestations with fetal testing suggestive of impending fetal death at extremes of prematurity. Because of the inaccuracy inherent in ultrasonic determination of monochorionicity, zygosity testing with DNA studies is important in these clinical situations.

▶ TREATMENT OF THE NEWBORN

All surviving infants of a multiple gestation following single IUFD should be evaluated postnatally for neurologic damage, and a thorough neurological assessment should be performed. Pediatric follow-up to assess growth and development is advisable. Otherwise no additional special precautions or investigations are required for such surviving infants.

▶ SURGICAL TREATMENT

There is no requirement for neonatal surgical evaluation for surviving infants of multiple gestations following single IUFD, unless additional anomalies are present in the survivors.

▶ LONG-TERM OUTCOME

The literature regarding the clinical significance of single IUFD in twins spans 34 years and includes more than 150 cases, most of which do not address long-term outcome for the survivor (Eglowstein and D'Alton 1993). In one series of 188 confirmed monozygous twin pairs, there were 7 in utero deaths (Melnick 1977). Five of the seven co-twin survivors had normal head circumference and psychomotor development. Head circumferences ranged between the 35th and 97th percentiles, and the IQs were all within 1 SD of the mean for sex, race, and zygosity. One co-twin died at 2 months, and postmortem studies revealed necrosis of the white matter of the cerebellum. A different co-twin had a head circumference at the 3rd percentile from 1 to 7 years of age, but psychomotor development at 1, 4, and 7 years was normal (Melnick 1977).

In another series of 206 pregnancies with death of at least one twin before delivery, follow-up 8 years or more after birth revealed that three twins (5%) had cerebral palsy or mental retardation (Rydhstrom and Ingemarsson 1993). All three were second twins and of the same sex as their co-twins.

▶ GENETICS AND RECURRENCE RISK

There is unlikely to be an increased risk of single IUFD if future pregnancies involve multiple gestations, although there are no data to confirm this assessment.

REFERENCES

Anderson RL, Golbus MS, Curry CJR, et al. Central nervous system damage and other anomalies in surviving fetus following second trimester antenatal death of co-twin. Prenat Diagn 1990;10:513–8.

Barss VA, Benacerraf BR, Frigoletto FD Jr. Ultrasonographic determination of chorion type in twin gestation. Obstet Gynecol 1985;66:779–783.

Benirschke K, Kim CK. Multiple pregnancy. N Engl J Med 1973;288:1276–1284.

Benirschke K. Multiple gestation: incidence, etiology and inheritance. In: Creasy RK, Resnik R, eds. Maternal-fetal medicine. 4th ed. Philadelphia: Saunders, 1999:585–597.

Borlum KG. Third-trimester fetal death in triplet pregnancies. Obstet Gynecol 1991;77:6–9.

Burke MS. Single fetal demise in twin gestation. Clin Obstet Gynecol 1990;33:69–78.

Carlson NJ, Towers CV. Multiple gestation complicated by the death of one fetus. Obstet Gynecol 1989;73:685–689.

Colburn DW, Pasquale SA. Monoamnionic twin pregnancy. J Reprod Med 1982;27:165–168.

Crombleholme TM, Robertson F, Marx G, et al. Fetoscopic cord ligation to prevent neurological injury in monozygous twins. Lancet 1996;348:191.

D'Alton ME, Dudley DK. The ultrasonographic prediction of chorionicity in twin gestation. Am J Obstet Gynecol 1989;160:557–561.

D'Alton ME, Newton ER, Cetrulo CL. Intrauterine fetal demise in multiple gestation. Acta Genet Med Gemellol 1984;33:43–49.

D'Alton ME, Simpson LL. Syndromes in twins. Semin Perinatol 1995;19:375–386.

Dudley DK, D'Alton ME. Single fetal death in twin gestation. Semin Perinatol 1986;10:65–72.

Eglowstein M, D'Alton ME. Intrauterine demise in multiple gestation: theory and management. J Matern Fetal Med 1993;2:272–275.

Enbom JA. Twin pregnancy with intrauterine death of one twin. Am J Obstet Gynecol 1985;152:424–429.

Fusi L, Gordon H. Multiple pregnancy complicated by single intrauterine death: problems and outcome with conservative management. Br J Obstet Gynaecol 1990;97:511–516.

Gonen R, Heyman E, Asztalos E, et al. The outcome of triplet gestations complicated by fetal death. Obstet Gynecol 1990;75:175–178.

Hertzberg BS, Kurtz AB, Choi HY, et al. Significance of membrane thickness in the sonographic evaluation of twin gestations. AJR Am J Roentgenol 1987;148:151–153.

Kilby MD, Govind A, O'Brien PM. Outcome of twin pregnancies complicated by a single intrauterine death: a comparison with viable twin pregnancies. Obstet Gynecol 1994;84:107–109.

Landy HJ, Weiner S, Corson SL, et al. The "vanishing twin": ultrasonographic assessment of fetal disappearance in the first trimester. Am J Obstet Gynecol 1986;155:14–19.

Landy HJ, Weingold AB. Management of a multiple gestation complicated by an antepartum fetal demise. Obstet Gynecol Surv 1989;44:171–176.

Litschgi M, Stucki D. Course of twin pregnancies after fetal death in utero. Z Geburtshilfe Perinatol 1980;184:227–230.

Malone FD, D'Alton ME. Multiple gestation: clinical characteristics and management. In: Creasy RK, Resnik R, eds. Maternal-fetal medicine. 4th ed. Philadelphia: Saunders, 1999:598–615.

Melnick M. Brain damage in survivor after in-utero death of a monozygous co-twin. Lancet 1977;2:1287.

Naeye RL. Placental infarction leading to fetal or neonatal death. Obstet Gynecol 1977;50:583–588.

Norton ME, D'Alton ME, Bianchi DW. Molecular zygosity studies aid in the management of discordant multiple gestations. J Perinatol 1997;17:202–207.

Prompeler HJ, Madjar H, Klosa W, et al. Twin pregnancies with single fetal death. Acta Obstet Gynecol Scand 1994;73:205–208.

Rydhstrom H, Ingemarsson I. Prognosis and long-term follow-up of a twin after antenatal death of the co-twin. J Reprod Med 1993;38:142–146.

Samuels P. Ultrasound in the management of the twin gestation. Clin Obstet Gynecol 1988;31:110–122.

Santema JG, Swaak AM, Wallenburg HCS. Expectant management of twin pregnancy with single fetal death. Br J Obstet Gynaecol 1995;102:26–30.

Varma TR. Ultrasound evidence of early pregnancy failure in patients with multiple conceptions. Br J Obstet Gynecol 1979;86:290–292.

CHAPTER 121

Malformations in Twins

► CONDITION

When congenital malformations occur in a multiple gestation, management decisions can be difficult for both parents and physicians because the fates of such sibling fetuses are necessarily linked. Given that the incidence of multiple gestations is increasing in industrialized countries, primarily because of assisted reproductive technologies (Jewell and Yip 1995), the management dilemma for twins with malformations will also inevitably increase. Congenital malformations occur more commonly in twin as compared with singleton gestations and are an important contributor to the increased perinatal mortality associated with twin gestation. Some malformations in twins are inherent to the monozygotic twinning process, such as acardiac twinning, conjoined twins, and twin-to-twin-transfusion syndrome. These malformations are discussed separately (see Chapters 118, 119, and 123). Other malformations in twins are deformation abnormalities, such as club foot, which result from the crowding of the intrauterine environment.

► INCIDENCE

The incidence of congenital malformations in twins from the British Columbia Health Surveillance Registry up to 1975 was estimated at 6% of twin pairs (Schinzel et al. 1979). In this series, the incidence of congenital anomalies was found to be 2.5 times more common in monozygotic twins than in dizygotic twins or singletons. The incidence of chromosomal abnormalities is increased twofold in dizygotic twins as compared with age-matched singleton pregnancies, but the incidence of nonchromosomal abnormalities does not seem to be increased (Drugan et al. 1996).

In one series of 1424 twin pairs, 445 pairs were monozygotic, 26 of which (6%) had congenital malformations (Cameron et al. 1983). Even among monozygotic twin pairs with malformations, however, the majority of fetuses will be discordant for the abnormality, with only 6 of the 26 twin pairs (23%) in Cameron et al.'s study showing concordance for the abnormality. In another registry of 4490 twins, there was a 50% increase in incidence of congenital malformations among twins as compared with singletons, 4.9 versus 3.3%, respectively, with this increase being almost entirely limited to same sex—and therefore presumably monozygotic—twin pairs (Layde et al. 1980).

The incidence of open neural-tube defects in twins is controversial. In one study from California and Norway, anencephaly and encephalocele, but not meningomyelocele, were found more commonly in twins as compared with singletons (Windham et al. 1982). In a national survey from England and Wales, there was a threefold increased incidence of anencephaly in twins as compared with singletons, while the incidence of encephalocele and meningomyelocele was similar in twins and singletons (Doyle et al. 1991). In a further study from Spain, the incidence of anencephaly was 0.1% for twins as compared with 0.03% for singletons, and this increase was almost entirely in same-sex twin pairs (Ramos-Arroyo 1991). However, in a study from Northern Ireland, the incidence of anencephaly was decreased in twins, while the incidence of meningomyelocele was similar to that of singletons (Little and Nevin 1989a). The incidence of congenital cardiovascular malformations was also found to be modestly increased in twins as compared with singletons, 0.9 versus 0.7%, with the increase again being confined to same-sex twin pairs (Little and Nevin 1989b).

▶ SONOGRAPHIC FINDINGS

The ability of sonographic examination to detect congenital malformations in twin pregnancies has not been adequately evaluated, with no large patient series available for review. In one series of 33 fetuses from twin pregnancies with anomalies, none of 8 cardiac anomalies were diagnosed prenatally, while 11 of 20 (55%) other major anomalies and none of 12 minor anomalies were diagnosed prenatally (Allen et al. 1991). In another series of 24 fetuses with anomalies, it was considered that by using serial ultrasonography in a tertiary-care center it may be possible to achieve an 88% detection rate, with 100% specificity, in the prenatal diagnosis of anomalies in twin pregnancies (Edwards et al. 1995). However, almost 40% of fetuses with anomalies in this series were not diagnosed until 24 weeks gestation or later, when options for management are more limited. More recently, it has been suggested that up to 88% of cases of Down syndrome in twin pregnancies could be detected by combining risks derived from maternal age and sonographic nuchal translucency thickness measurement at 10 to 14 weeks of gestation (Sebire et al. 1996).

▶ DIFFERENTIAL DIAGNOSIS

The differential diagnosis following the prenatal diagnosis of a congenital malformation in a twin pregnancy is extensive and is dependent on the particular abnormality that is suspected. For differential diagnoses for individual malformations, the corresponding chapters in this textbook should be consulted. Judging from the few published series of sonographic diagnosis of congenital malformations in twins, there seems to be a high degree of specificity involved in the correct prenatal identification of anomalies (Allen et al. 1991; Edwards et al. 1995).

▶ ANTENATAL NATURAL HISTORY

Specific information on the antenatal natural history of individual malformations is available in the corresponding chapters in this textbook. The history of such pregnancies becomes even more complicated when, as in the majority of cases, there is discordance for the malformation in question. While a range of interventions has been available for patients diagnosed with congenital malformations in twins, only recently has information become available on the outcome of twin gestations complicated by fetal anomalies that are expectantly managed. In a series of 14 expectantly managed twin gestations in which only one fetus had a con-genital malformation, Malone et al. (1996) found a significantly increased risk of preterm delivery in such pregnancies, in addition to the base-line risk of prematurity already seen with normal twin gestations. There was a 20% additional risk of preterm delivery, attributable to the presence of an anomalous fetus. Birth weight was significantly lower, and both cesarean delivery rate and perinatal mortality rate were increased in anomalous twin pregnancies as compared with control twins. These data were subsequently confirmed by Alexander et al. (1997), who found both lower gestational age at delivery and lower birth weight in a group of 18 expectantly managed anomalous twin pregnancies as compared with control twins.

▶ MANAGEMENT OF PREGNANCY

When both fetuses in a twin pregnancy are concordant for malformations, subsequent management of that pregnancy is straightforward and should involve both the usual obstetric management of twin gestations and any required interventions for the particular malformation. However, pregnancy management becomes considerably more complex when one twin has a congenital malformation but the co-twin is normal. Counseling of parents depends on the type of abnormality and the prognosis for the anomalous twin as well as on the likely outcome for the normal co-twin. Three management options are available in this situation: expectant management, selective termination of the anomalous fetus, and termination of the entire pregnancy (Malone and D'Alton 1997). Selective termination of an anomalous twin is described in detail under "Fetal Intervention."

For pregnancy management, we recommend karyotyping for twins with malformations. As already described, parents should be counseled that expectant management of an anomalous twin pregnancy is associated with an increased risk of preterm delivery. In addition to the risk of prematurity, expectant management can also be complicated by intrauterine death of the anomalous fetus, which can have profound implications for the well-being of the normal co-twin, especially in a monochorionic twin gestation (see Chapter 120). If one fetus in a monochorionic twin pair dies, there is a 12% risk in the remaining co-twin of multicystic encephalomalacia, leading to profound neurologic handicap (Malone and D'Alton 1997). This risk is present from the moment of the death of the first twin, and may not be predictable, even by intensive surveillance with sonographic examination or fetal heart rate monitoring. Therefore, serious consideration should be given to delivering the twins if an anomalous fetus in a monochorionic gestation appears to be in a premorbid condition. This decision will depend on the gestational age, so that the risks of neurologic morbidity associated with expectant management are balanced against the iatrogenic risk of prematurity associated with delivery. If an anomalous twin in a monochorionic twin pair has already died in utero, close fetal surveillance for the surviving co-twin is recommended, although it must be realized that this may not prevent neurologic morbidity, which may already have occurred. Similarly, delivery immediately after diagnosis of the intrauterine death of one twin may not protect against neurologic morbidity in the surviving co-twin. Delivery at 37 weeks, or after measuring lung indexes consistent with maturity, is reasonable in such situations.

Antenatal surveillance of twin gestations complicated by congenital malformations should at least involve the usual fetal surveillance given to normal twin pregnancies. This includes serial sonographic examinations every 3 to 4 weeks from approximately 18 weeks for fetal growth, or every 2 weeks if growth restriction or growth discordance greater than 20% is present. Further intensive fetal surveillance with nonstress tests and Doppler velocimetry is also reserved for cases of growth restriction or significant growth discordance. Additional fetal testing may also be indicated depending on the particular type of congenital malformation present.

The decision on location of delivery will depend entirely on the nature of the congenital malformation, presence of associated anomalies, and availability of postnatal therapies. With regard to mode of delivery, the choice between vaginal and cesarean delivery will also be dictated by the individual malformation and fetal prognosis. This is described in detail in the appropriate section in the chapters describing each abnormality. In addition, the usual obstetric indications for determining mode of delivery of normal twin gestations may also apply. Typically, all vertex:vertex twins are candidates for vaginal delivery, while most obstetricians perform a cesarean delivery if the presenting twin is nonvertex. When the presenting twin is vertex and the second twin is nonvertex, a vaginal breech delivery of the second twin is generally acceptable if the estimated fetal weight is greater than 1500 g. There are insufficient data to confirm the optimal mode of delivery when a nonvertex second twin weighs less than 1500 g.

▶ FETAL INTERVENTION

The main fetal intervention available for twin gestations in which one fetus has a congenital malformation is selective termination. Whether selective termination is considered a reasonable option will depend on the severity of the anomaly, the chorionicity of the pregnancy, and the moral and ethical beliefs of the parents. Selective termination may appear unreasonable in the case of minor congenital malformations. It has also been argued that selective termination should not be performed in cases of lethal anomalies because it is difficult to justify the additional risk to the normal fetus of an invasive procedure designed to terminate a co-twin that is already nonviable (Stone and Berkowitz 1995). An exception may be the presence of polyhydramnios in a twin gestation discordant for anencephaly because such pregnancies are at much higher risk of preterm delivery than are normal twin pregnancies (Sebire et al. 1997). Another option in the case of twins discordant for anencephaly is to perform serial amnioreduction if polyhydramnios develops, with a view toward reducing the risk of preterm delivery (Sebire et al. 1997).

Determining chorionicity is vital prior to considering selective termination of an anomalous fetus in a twin pregnancy. This can be determined sonographically by identifying fetal gender, observing the thickness of the dividing membranes, or observing separate placentae. Alternatively, at the time karyotyping is performed, the amniocyte culture can also be used as a source of fetal DNA for zygosity testing (Norton et al. 1997). Monozygous twins will have identical DNA polymorphisms at all loci analyzed, whereas dizygous twins will differ.

Selective termination by potassium chloride injection is contraindicated with monochorionic gestations because death of the unaffected twin occurs in 80 to 100% of cases within several days of termination of the anomalous fetus (Evans et al. 1994; Golbus et al. 1988). Other methods of performing selective termination of an anomalous fetus in a monochorionic twin pair have been described, but all are considered experimental at this time. Each of these experimental techniques must ensure rapid occlusion of the umbilical vessels of the anomalous fetus to prevent acute hypotension and subsequent mortality or neurologic morbidity in the normal fetus (Malone and D'Alton 1997). Successful techniques that have been described to date include hysterotomy (Robie et al. 1989), fetoscopic cord ligation (Fig. 121-1) (Crombleholme et al. 1996; Quintero et al. 1996), fetoscopic laser ablation of umbilical vessels (Hecher et al. 1996), and percutaneous injection of absolute alcohol (Denbow et al. 1997) into the intra-abdominal umbilical vessels.

Selective termination in dichorionic pregnancies is now most commonly performed by ultrasound-guided intracardiac potassium chloride injection, and is almost always performed during the second trimester. Before performing the termination procedure it is essential to confirm that the targeted fetus has the abnormality in question. This identification is fairly straightforward if a structural abnormality is present. However, in cases of chromosomal abnormality without obvious structural malformation, there may be some doubt about correct identification of the anomalous fetus, especially if some time has passed since karyotyping or if careful intrauterine mapping was not performed initially. In cases

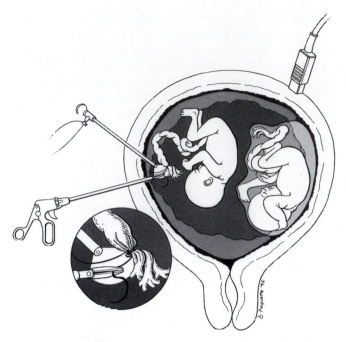

Figure 121-1. Diagram of fetoscopic cord ligation technique used in the selective termination of a twin fetus with a malformation.

in which there is some doubt regarding fetal identification it is recommended to perform repeat chromosomal analysis using rapid techniques (such as fluorescence in situ hybridization or fetal blood sampling) immediately before selective termination.

The loss rate prior to 24 weeks of gestation following selective termination with potassium chloride injection is 8%, with a further 4% of patients delivering between 25 and 28 weeks, 10% between 29 and 32 weeks, and 22% between 33 and 36 weeks (Evans et al. 1994). The largest series of selective terminations from a single center, consisting of 69 twin pregnancies, demonstrated increased risks of preterm delivery if the presenting twin is terminated, as well as increased risks of preterm delivery and membrane rupture following selective termination at greater than 20 weeks of gestation (Lynch et al. 1996).

▶ TREATMENT OF THE NEWBORN

The treatment of neonatal twins with malformations is entirely dependent on the type of abnormality and is described for each abnormality under the appropriate "Treatment of the Newborn" section in this textbook.

▶ SURGICAL TREATMENT

The only surgical treatment that has been described antenatally in the management of twins with malformations is various surgical forms of selective termination, such as hysterotomy and fetoscopy (Crombleholme et al. 1996; Robie et al. 1989). As with treatment of the newborn, neonatal surgery is also entirely dependent on the type of abnormality and is described for that abnormality under the appropriate "Surgical Treatment" section in this textbook.

▶ LONG-TERM OUTCOME

No data are available on the long-term outcome of normal co-twins following selective termination of an anomalous twin. The long-term outcome of anomalous fetuses that are managed expectantly is also entirely dependent on the type of abnormality and is described for each abnormality under the appropriate "Long-Term Outcome" section in this textbook.

▶ GENETICS AND RECURRENCE RISK

The recurrence risk for malformations seen in twin pregnancies varies greatly depending on the particular abnormality. For deformations such as club foot that probably occur as a result of crowding of the intrauterine environment, the risk of recurrence is relatively small. For malformations such as acardiac twinning and twin-to-twin-transfusion syndrome that occur secondary to vascular communications across a monochorionic placenta, the recurrence risk is also relatively small. Recurrence risks for other abnormalities are described under the "Genetics and Recurrence Risk" sections in the relevant chapters in this textbook.

REFERENCES

Alexander JM, Ramus R, Cox SM, et al. Outcome of twin gestations with a single anomalous fetus. Am J Obstet Gynecol 1997;177:849–852.

Allen SR, Gray LJ, Frentzen BH, et al. Ultrasonographic diagnosis of congenital anomalies in twins. Am J Obstet Gynecol 1991;165:1056–1060.

Cameron AH, Edwards JH, Derom R, et al. The value of twin surveys in the study of malformations. Eur J Obstet Gynecol Reprod Biol 1983;14:347–356.

Crombleholme TM, Robertson F, Marx G, et al. Fetoscopic cord ligation to prevent neurologic injury in monozygous twins. Lancet 1996;348:191.

Denbow ML, Battin MR, Kyle PM, et al. Selective termination by intrahepatic vein alcohol injection of a monochorionic twin pregnancy discordant for fetal abnormality. Br J Obstet Gynaecol 1997;104:626–627.

Drugan A, Johnson MP, Krivchenia EL, et al. Genetics and genetic counseling. In: Gall SA, ed. Multiple pregnancy and delivery. St. Louis: Mosby, 1996:85–97.

Doyle PE, Beral V, Botting B, et al. Congenital malformations in twins in England and Wales. J Epidemiol Community Health 1991;45:43–38.

Edwards MS, Ellings JM, Newman RB, et al. Predictive value of antepartum ultrasound examination for anomalies in twin gestations. Ultrasound Obstet Gynecol 1995;6:43–49.

Evans MI, Goldberg JD, Dommergues M, et al. Efficacy of second-trimester selective termination for fetal abnormalities: international collaborative experience among the world's largest centers. Am J Obstet Gynecol 1994;171:90–94.

Golbus MS, Cunningham N, Goldberg JD, et al. Selective termination of multiple gestations. Am J Med Genet 1988;31:339–348.

Hecher K, Reinhold U, Gbur K, et al. Interruption of umbilical blood flow in an acardiac twin by endoscopic laser coagulation. Geburt Frauenheilkd 1996;56:97–100.

Jewell SE, Yip R. Increasing trends in plural births in the United States. Obstet Gynecol 1995;85:229–232.

Layde PM, Erickson JD, Falek A, et al. Congenital malformations in twins. Am J Hum Genet 1980;32:69–78.

Little J, Nevin NC. Congenital anomalies in twins in Northern Ireland II: Neural tube defects 1974–1979. Acta Genet Med Gemellol (Roma) 1989a;38:17–25.

Little J, Nevin NC: Congenital anomalies in twins in Northern Ireland III: Anomalies of the cardiovascular system 1974–1979. Acta Genet Med Gemellol (Roma) 1989b;38:27–35.

Lynch L, Berkowitz RL, Stone J, et al. Preterm delivery after selective termination in twin pregnancies. Obstet Gynecol 1996;87:366–369.

Malone FD, Craigo SD, Chelmow D, et al. Outcome of twin gestations complicated by a single anomalous fetus. Obstet Gynecol 1996;88:1–5.

Malone FD, D'Alton ME. Management of multiple gestations complicated by a single anomalous fetus. Curr Opin Obstet Gynecol 1997;9:213–216.

Norton ME, D'Alton ME, Bianchi DW. Molecular zygosity studies aid in the management of disocordant multiple gestations. J Perinatol 1997;17:202–207.

Quintero RA, Romero R, Reich H, et al. In utero percutaneous umbilical cord ligation in the management of complicated monochorionic multiple gestations. Ultrasound Obstet Gynecol 1996;8:16–22.

Ramos-Arroyo MA. Birth defects in twins: study in a Spanish population. Acta Genet Med Gemellol (Roma) 1991;40:337–344.

Robie GF, Payne GG, Morgan MA. Selective delivery of an acardiac acephalic twin. N Engl J Med 1989;320:512–513.

Schinzel AAGL, Smith DW, Miller JR. Monozygotic twinning and structural defects. J Pediatr 1979;95:921–930.

Sebire NJ, Snijders RJM, Hughes K, et al. Screening for trisomy 21 in twin pregnancies by maternal age and fetal nuchal translucency thickness at 10–14 weeks of gestation. Br J Obstet Gynaecol 1996;103:999–1003.

Sebire NJ, Sepulveda W, Hughes KS, et al. Management of twin pregnancies discordant for anencephaly. Br J Obstet Gynaecol 1997;104:216–219.

Stone J, Berkowitz RL. Multifetal pregnancy reduction and selective termination. Semin Perinatol 1995;19:363–374.

Windham GC, Bjerkedal T, Sever LE. The association of twinning and neural tube defects: studies in Los Angeles, California, and Norway. Acta Genet Med Gemellol (Roma) 1982;31:165–172.

CHAPTER 122

Monoamniotic Twins

▶ CONDITION

Monoamniotic twinning is an unusual form of twinning in which both twins occupy a single amniotic sac. Monoamniotic twins account for 1% of all monozygotic twin pregnancies (D'Alton and Simpson 1995). This form of monozygotic twinning typically occurs when a single embryo splits during postovulation days 8 to 10. Splitting before this time gives rise to either dichorionic diamniotic twins, or more commonly, monochorionic diamniotic twins. Splitting later in embryogenesis gives rise to conjoined twins.

Although a rare event, monoamniotic twinning is important because of the high perinatal mortality rate associated with these pregnancies. The first comprehensive review of the world literature was performed in 1935 by Quigley, who found an overall mortality rate of 68% in 94 pregnancies. His opinion was that the poor prognosis was due mainly to twisting and knotting of the umbilical cords with subsequent occlusion of the blood supply to one or both twins. A subsequent review in 1959 added 35 new cases to the world literature and reported a high fetal mortality rate of 30% (Salerno 1959). More recent data have suggested a 54% perinatal mortality rate, which may be due to premature delivery, growth restriction, congenital anomalies, vascular anastomoses between twins, and umbilical-cord entanglement or cord accidents (Carr et al. 1990; Malone and D'Alton 1999).

▶ INCIDENCE

It is difficult to ascertain the exact incidence of monoamniotic twins, but they account for 1% of all monozygotic twin pregnancies (D'Alton and Simpson 1995). The incidence has ranged in various studies from 1 in 1650 to 1 in 93,734 live births (Colburn and Pasquale 1982; Simonsen 1966). There seems to be a preponderance of female twins among monoamniotic twin pairs (Derom and Vlietinck 1988). In a study of 26 sets of monoamniotic twins, 20 (77%) were female pairs. However, this difference was not as evident in Carr et al.'s (1990) series of 24 sets, which included 11 (46%) sets of females and 13 (54%) sets of males.

▶ SONOGRAPHIC FINDINGS

Ultrasound examination has been demonstrated to be helpful in determining the chorionicity of twin pregnancy. The most common way of diagnosing monoamniotic twins has been failure to identify a dividing membrane in the presence of a single placental mass and like-gender twins. However, failure to visualize a dividing membrane does not ensure that the pregnancy is monoamniotic because such a membrane may be missed even with well-performed sonography (Blane et al. 1987). Color flow Doppler has also been described in the diagnosis of umbilical-cord entanglement in three monoamniotic twin gestations (Belfort et al. 1993) (Fig. 122-1). In another series, ultrasound diagnosis of cord entanglement was used to predict abnormalities in fetal heart rate tracings (Aisenbrey et al. 1995). Ultrasound-guided injection of indigocarmine dye mixed with air into the amniotic sac during genetic amniocentesis has been said to enhance the diagnosis of monoamniotic twins (Tabsh 1990). If microbubbles are seen around both fetuses, the diagnosis of monoamniotic twinning is made with accuracy.

If monoamniotic twinning is suspected, amniography may increase the accuracy of diagnosis (Lavery and Gadwood 1990). In this report, 30 ml of 61% iopamidol (Isovue-M 300, Squibb) was injected into the amniotic

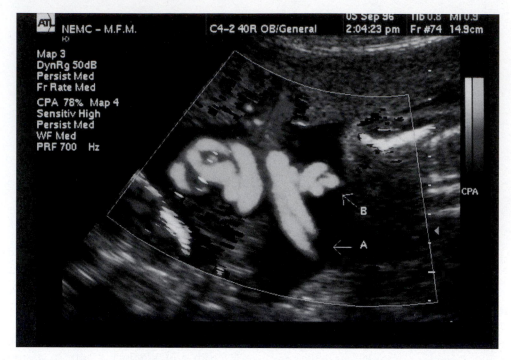

Figure 122-1. Power Doppler imaging of entangled umbilical cords in a case of monoamniotic twins. See color plate.

fluid. Maternal abdominal x-ray films taken 24 hours after the injection revealed that both fetuses had swallowed contrast medium injected into a shared single amniotic sac. Computed tomography following intraamniotic injection of Renografin has also been suggested to confirm the diagnosis of monoamniotic twinning (Carlan et al. 1990; Perkins and Terry 1992).

▶ DIFFERENTIAL DIAGNOSIS

The main difficulty in differential diagnosis of monoamniotic versus monochorionic diamniotic pregnancies is that ultrasound examination may not always allow visualization of the dividing membrane. In cases in which visualization is limited because the mother is obese, the use of color flow Doppler and amniocentesis techniques with Renografin or air may help to confirm the diagnosis. We have not found it necessary to use any of these additional techniques in nine cases prenatally diagnosed (Harney et al. 1995). In this study, all cases of monoamnionicity were confirmed by pathologic examination of the placenta.

A major consideration in differential diagnosis is the intrauterine rupture of a diamniotic twin membrane, which can then mimic the sonographic appearance of true monoamniotic twins. Actual differential diagnosis between these two conditions is probably not necessary, as intrauterine membrane rupture has a perinatal mortality rate consistent with that of true monoamniotic

gestations (Gilbert et al. 1991). This clinical scenario should be suspected when there is failure to visualize a dividing membrane following previous sonographic confirmation of a membrane. Possible causes for this intrauterine rupture include trauma during amniocentesis, infection, and developmental disturbances of the membranes (Gilbert et al. 1991).

▶ ANTENATAL NATURAL HISTORY

Both monozygotic and dizygotic twins have a higher morbidity and mortality rate than single fetuses (Malone and D'Alton 1999). Particularly high intrauterine morbidity and mortality rates are seen in monoamniotic twins (Carr et al. 1990; Quigley 1935; Raphael 1961; Salerno 1959; Simonsen 1966). This has been attributed to premature delivery, growth restriction, congenital anomalies, vascular anastomoses between twins, and umbilical-cord entanglement or cord accidents (Fig. 122-2). Cord accidents seem to contribute the most to these high intrauterine mortality rates. In one of the earliest series of monoamniotic twins it was stated that double survival of such twins is a rare event (Quigley 1935). In the most recent series, however, the reported double perinatal survival rate has been 100% (Harney et al. 1995).

Most of the reports on monoamniotic twins are not helpful for antenatal counseling because in almost all cases the diagnosis of monoamnionicity was made postnatally. In one report of three consecutive cases of

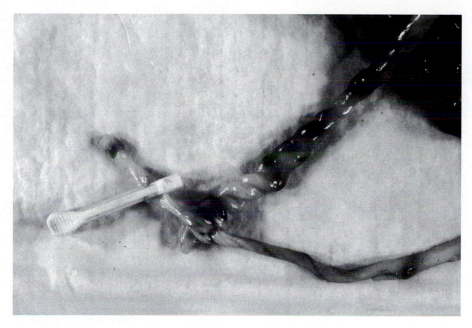

Figure 122-2. Postnatal photograph of a true knot in a case of double fetal death in a monoamniotic twin pregnancy. *(Courtesy of Dr. Michael Paidas.)*

prenatally diagnosed monoamniotic twins, one pregnancy was delivered because of preterm labor, one for persistent variable decelerations at 34 weeks, and one electively at 34 weeks after confirmation of pulmonary maturity (Rodis et al. 1987). Double survival occurred in all three cases. In our series of nine cases of antenatally diagnosed monoamniotic twins, delivery occurred between 26 and 34 weeks of gestation (Harney et al. 1995). In seven of the nine cases, delivery was performed because of fetal decelerations noted during nonstress testing. It is our hypothesis that increasing frequency of decelerations noted on nonstress testing may be a warning sign of more serious cord compression yet to occur. For example, we have noted that mild decelerations become much more serious and frequent, leading to profound bradycardia over a period of 2 hours. In addition, there seems to be a higher incidence of twin-to-twin transfusion syndrome and intrauterine growth restriction in monoamniotic twins (Harney et al. 1995).

▶ MANAGEMENT OF PREGNANCY

Because of the paucity of published data concerning antenatally diagnosed monoamniotic twins there is little information from which to draw conclusions concerning the proper management of these very-high-risk pregnancies. There are two studies that attempt to address issues concerning the antepartum and intrapartum management of monoamniotic twins. One study was a retrospective evaluation of 24 sets of histologically con-

firmed monoamniotic twin pregnancies, with particular attention paid to the optimal timing of delivery (Carr et al. 1990). There were no perinatal deaths after 30 weeks of gestation, and therefore the authors saw no advantage to elective premature delivery. In their series, however, the diagnosis of monoamniotic twins was made prenatally in only 21% of cases, and the diagnosis of twins was known prenatally in only 29% of cases. In a second study the cases of 20 monoamniotic twin pregnancies at the University of Iowa from 1961 to 1989 were reviewed (Tessen and Zlatnik 1991). In their retrospective series no perinatal death occurred after 32 weeks of gestation, and the authors therefore suggested that prophylactic premature delivery might not be indicated. However, in an addendum to the original paper the authors report a double fetal death of 35-week monoamniotic twins just after completion of their study, again demonstrating that the safety of expectant management of monoamniotic twin pregnancies is unproven beyond 34 weeks.

Antenatal testing in the form of nonstress tests and biophysical profile scores is recommended in the case of monoamniotic twins. Nonstress testing should occur at least daily from 26 weeks of gestation (Malone and D'Alton 1999). The objective of antenatal testing is to determine the presence and frequency of variable decelerations, as these changes may precede intrauterine fetal death. Continuous fetal heart rate monitoring of both twins is recommended if variable decelerations increase in frequency or severity. Biophysical testing is performed only for evaluation of nonreactive nonstress tests and cannot predict variable decelerations. Serial ultrasound examinations are performed every month to evaluate fetal growth and to rule out the development of polyhydramnios and the twin-to-twin transfusion syndrome. Antenatal corticosteroid therapy is used to enhance fetal pulmonary maturity because of the high incidence of premature delivery in monoamniotic twins. In general the delivery of monoamniotic twins requires the setting of a tertiary-care center. However, after 32 weeks of gestation delivery may be accomplished in a community hospital with level-two nursery capabilities.

In regard to the timing of delivery, some authors have advocated delivery of all monoamniotic twin pregnancies immediately on demonstration of fetal pulmonary maturity (Kassam and Tompkins 1980). Others have recommended elective delivery at 32 weeks of gestation because of a presumed increased risk of cord accidents as the pregnancy progresses (Rodis et al. 1987). The optimal timing of delivery is still unknown. It is our practice to perform elective delivery following antenatal corticosteroid therapy at 34 weeks. Delivery at this time carries with it a low risk of neonatal morbidity when weighed against the uncertain risk of continuing the pregnancy. Although some series have questioned the need for early delivery, the double death referred to in the addendum to Tessen's report is particularly troubling (Carr et al. 1990; Tessen and Zlatnik 1991). In addition, at present we do not have the technology to continuously trace both fetal hearts for a prolonged time. Consequently, it is our preference to perform elective delivery at 34 weeks of gestation. However, it is not unreasonable to manage selected cases of monoamniotic twins expectantly beyond 34 weeks of gestation, with careful fetal surveillance, and to decide on timing of delivery based on fetal lung maturity (Malone and D'Alton 1999).

The optimal mode of delivery of monoamniotic twins also remains undefined. Cesarean section has been recommended by some authors to eliminate the risk of intrapartum cord accidents (Rodis et al. 1987). However, there are data to support vaginal delivery of monoamniotic twins. In one series, no fetal deaths and only one case of nonreassuring fetal testing requiring emergency cesarean delivery occurred during labor in 15 monoamniotic twin pregnancies delivered vaginally (Tessen and Zlatnik 1991). In another series of 24 cases, vaginal delivery was accomplished in 75% of individual neonates and in 48% of liveborn infants, although the antenatal diagnosis of monoamniotic twins was unknown in most cases and so could not have influenced management (Carr et al. 1990). Cesarean section was performed in our series because of abnormal fetal testing in seven of nine cases (Harney et al. 1995). In one case there was severe preeclampsia with growth discordance requiring delivery, and elective induction was attempted in one case, followed by cesarean delivery because of failure to progress in the second stage of labor (Harney et al. 1995). There are also data suggesting potential difficulties with vaginal delivery of monoamniotic twins. In one case, a nuchal cord affecting the first twin was cut to facilitate delivery, and on delivery of this twin's body it was noted that the cut cord was actually that of the second twin (McLeod and McCoy 1981). Given these issues and the high incidence of nonreassuring fetal testing, we have generally delivered all monoamniotic twin pregnancies by cesarean section (Malone and D'Alton 1999).

▶ FETAL INTERVENTION

Because of the limited published experience on antenatal management of monoamniotic twins it is unclear how often fetal intervention is necessary. Daily nonstress testing only tests fetal heart patterns for a short period, which is the main limitation of this method of antenatal surveillance. Continuous recording of the fetal heart rate would be optimal for a monoamniotic twin. This is not practical with current monitoring equipment. It is theoretically possible to insert subcutaneously in the fetus a monitor that will continuously record the fetal heart rate (Crombleholme et al. 1996). As fetoscopic methods of in utero diagnosis and therapy become more refined, continuous monitoring may become an option when monoamniotic twins are diagnosed prenatally.

The only intervention described to reduce the incidence of cord accidents in monoamniotic twins is medical amnioreduction. In one small series, the prostaglandin inhibitor sulindac, 200 mg orally twice daily, was administered to three patients carrying monoamniotic twins, beginning at 24 to 29 weeks of gestation (Peek et al. 1997). In two of the three cases, dose-related reduction in amniotic fluid volume was noted, and in all three cases fetal lie was stabilized. All fetal heart rate tracings remained normal, and all six infants survived. Although this is a very limited study, the authors also pointed out the difficulty of performing a randomized controlled trial given the rarity of the condition. Another possible, but unproven, side effect of this approach is the potential benefit of maintenance tocolysis with sulindac.

▶ TREATMENT OF THE NEWBORN

It is recommended that cord hematocrits be obtained in monoamniotic twins because of the higher incidence of twin-to-twin transfusion syndrome. Prematurity is the most important concern, together with growth restriction. Detailed examination should also be performed because of the higher incidence of congenital anomalies in monoamniotic twins. No other specific neonatal intervention is required. Placental pathologic tests should be performed in all cases to confirm the prenatal diagnosis. It is possible that the incidence of true monoamniotic placentas may be less than that reported because many suspected monoamniotic placentas may represent disrupted diamniotic-monochorionic placentas (Gilbert et al. 1991).

▶ SURGICAL TREATMENT

No surgical treatments have been described.

▶ LONG-TERM OUTCOME

There are no data available for long-term outcome.

▶ GENETICS AND RECURRENCE RISK

There are no genetics and recurrence risks described in the literature.

REFERENCES

Aisenbrey GA, Catanzarite VA, Hurley TJ, et al. Monoamniotic and pseudomonoamniotic twins: sonographic diagnosis, detection of cord entanglement, and obstetric management. Obstet Gynecol 1995;86:218–22.

Belfort MA, Moise KJ, Kirshon B, et al. The use of color flow Doppler ultrasonography to diagnose umbilical cord entanglement in monoamniotic twin gestations. Am J Obstet Gynecol 1993;168:601–604.

Blane CE, DiPietro MA, Johnson MZ, et al. Sonographic detection of monoamniotic twins. J Clin Ultrasound 1987; 15:394–396.

Carlan SJ, Angel JL, Sawai SK, et al. Late diagnosis of non-conjoined monoamniotic twins using computed tomographic imaging: a case report. Obstet Gynecol 1990;76: 504–506.

Carr SR, Aronson MP, Coustan DR. Survival rates of monoamniotic twins do not decrease after 30 weeks' gestation. Am J Obstet Gynecol 1990;163:719–722.

Colburn DW, Pasquale SA. Monoamniotic twin pregnancy. J Reprod Med 1982;27:165–168.

Crombleholme TM, D'Alton MD, Cendron M, et al. Prenatal diagnosis and the pediatric surgeon: the impact of prenatal consultation on perinatal management. J Pediatric Surg 1996;31:156–163.

D'Alton ME, Simpson LL. Syndromes in twins. Semin Perinatol 1995;19:375–386.

Derom C, Vlietinck R. Population-based study of sex proportion in monoamniotic twins. N Engl J Med 1988;319: 119.

Gilbert WM, Davis SE, Kaplan C, et al. Morbidity associated with prenatal disruption of the dividing membrane in twin gestations. Obstet Gynecol 1991;78:623–630.

Harney K, Craigo S, Chelmow D, D'Alton M. The management of monoamniotic twin pregnancies. Presented to the British Congress of Obstetrics and Gynecology, Dublin, Ireland, July 5, 1995.

Kassam SH, Tompkins MG, Monoamniotic twin pregnancy and modern obstetrics: report of a case with a peculiar cord complication. Diagn Gynecol Obstet 1980;2:213–220.

Lavery J, Gadwood KA. Amniography for confirming the diagnosis of monoamniotic twinning: a case report. J Reprod Med 1990;35:911–914.

Malone FD, D'Alton ME. Multiple gestation: clinical characteristics and management. In: Creasy RK, Resnik R, eds. Maternal-fetal medicine. 4th ed. Philadelphia: Saunders, 1999:598–615.

Peek MJ, McCarthy A, Kyle P, et al. Medical amnioreduction with sulindac to reduce cord complications in monoamniotic twins. Am J Obstet Gynecol 1997;176:334–336.

Perkins RP, Terry JD. Exclusion of monoamniotic twinning by contrast-enhanced computed tomography. Obstet Gynecol 1992;79:876–878.

Quigley JK. Monoamniotic twin pregnancy: a case record with review of the literature. Am J Obstet Gynecol 1935; 29:354–362.

Raphael SI. Monoamniotic twin pregnancy—a review of the literature and a report of 5 new cases. Am J Obstet Gynecol 1961;81:323–330.

Rodis JF, Vintzileos AM, Campbell WA, et al. Antenatal diagnosis and management of monoamniotic twins. Am J Obstet Gynecol 1987;157:1255–1257.

Salerno LJ. Monoamniotic twinning—a survey of the American literature since 1935 with a report of four new cases. Obstet Gynecol 1959;14:205–213.

Simonsen M. Monoamniotic twins. Acta Obstet Gynecol Scand 1966;45:43–52.

Tabsh K. Genetic amniocentesis in multiple gestation: a new technique to diagnose monoamniotic twins. Obstet Gynecol 1990;75:296–298.

Tessen JA, Zlatnik FJ. Monoamniotic twins: a retrospective controlled study. Obstet Gynecol 1991;77:832–834.

CHAPTER 123

Twin-to-Twin Transfusion Syndrome

▶ CONDITION

The twin-to-twin transfusion syndrome (TTS) is a complication of multiple gestation resulting from imbalanced blood flow through vascular communications in the placenta (chorioangiopagus), such that one twin is compromised and the other is favored. The prognosis is poor, with a perinatal mortality rate ranging from 60 to 100% for both twins (Cheschier and Seeds 1988; Gonsoulin et al. 1990; Rausen et al. 1965).

The earliest description of TTS may have been in the book of Genesis. At the birth of Esau and Jacob it was recorded that "the first one came out red," possibly describing the birth of a polycythemic twin. In 1752 William Smellie reported the injection of the umbilical artery of one twin with the injection material flowing out the vessel of the co-twin.

Research in the area of vascular anastomoses in twin placenta in the late 1800s was dominated by the German obstetrician Friedreich Schatz, who described four types of vascular connections within monochorionic placentas:

1. Superficial connections between capillaries
2. Superficial arterial connections between large vessels
3. Superficial venous connections between large vessels
4. Vascular communications between capillaries in the villi

He described three circulatory systems in monochorionic twins. The first two were the circulations in either twin. The third circulation consisted of the arteriovenous communications bridging the two fetal circulations below the placental surface (Schatz 1882).

Schatz proposed that when superficial artery-to-artery and vein-to-vein anastomoses are absent or insufficient, imbalances may occur in the common circulation of the twins. Such imbalances favor the transfer of blood from one twin to the other and result in TTS. A study demonstrating fewer anastomoses from placentas complicated by TTS (Bajoria et al. 1995) confirms Schatz's observations from the late 1800s. Ten placentas from pregnancies with evidence of midtrimester TTS diagnosed using ultrasound criteria were compared with 10 placentas from pregnancies without TTS. Placentas from pregnancies with TTS had significantly fewer anastomoses than did those without TTS, both overall and for each of the different types (arterioarterial, venovenous, and arteriovenous). Whereas multiple anastomoses were present in all controls, only one TTS placenta had more than a single communication. Anastomoses in the TTS group were more likely to be of the deep than the superficial type.

▶ INCIDENCE

Vascular communications occur in all monochorionic but rarely in dichorionic placentas. TTS is therefore almost exclusively found in monochorionic twins. TTS is estimated to occur in 5 to 15% of monochorionic twin pregnancies (Benirschke and Kim 1973; Rausen et al. 1965). Lage (1989) described a case of TTS resulting from vascular anastomoses within a fused dichorionic twin placenta. Robertson and Neer (1983) reported 2 cases of TTS in dichorionic pregnancies.

The true incidence of TTS is difficult to ascertain. TTS may occur very early during the second trimester, with loss of both fetuses; in mid-gestation or at term. It is of most concern to the perinatologist when it occurs in mid-second trimester, when the syndrome results in polyhydramnios, often with spontaneous rupture of membranes, or in spontaneous labor that leads to premature delivery. Because TTS can have such a wide spectrum of clinical presentation, in many cases the diagnosis may go undocumented.

▶ SONOGRAPHIC FINDINGS

Wittmann et al. (1981) and Brennan et al. (1982) have suggested the sonographic criteria for the diagnosis of TTS, including: (1) significant size disparity in fetuses of the same sex, (2) disparity in size between two amniotic sacs, (3) disparity in size of the umbilical cords, (4) single placenta, and (5) evidence of hydrops in either fetus or findings of congestive cardiac failure in the recipient. However, discordant growth is a common complication of twin pregnancies, and causes other than TTS exist for discordant amniotic fluid volumes. The criterion of a birth-weight difference of greater than 20% for the diagnosis of TTS is based on the belief that the donor twin becomes growth-restricted as a result of anemia and hypoalbuminemia. However, Sherer et al. (1994) reported a case of acute intrapartum TTS so severe as to cause the death of both twins. In this report, the birth weights of the infants differed by only 2%.

In some cases, the discordance in amniotic fluid volume is so great that the amnion adheres to the smaller baby, so that it appears "stuck" to the wall of the uterus (Fig. 123-1). In this situation it may be extremely difficult to visualize the dividing membrane between the twins. The "stuck twin" phenomenon is not pathognomonic for TTS; it may also result from structural fetal anomalies, congenital infection, chromosomal abnormalities, or ruptured membranes (Patten et al. 1989). In contrast, the co-twin moves freely in a normal or increased amniotic fluid volume (see Fig. 123-1). On ultrasound examination, signs of hydrops fetalis are occasionally found in the recipient (Brennan et al. 1982), rarely in the donor (Rausen et al. 1965), and exceptionally in both (McCafee et al. 1970).

▶ DIFFERENTIAL DIAGNOSIS

Because all of the above sonographic features described for the diagnosis of TTS are nonspecific, the use of Doppler ultrasound and fetal blood sampling has been suggested to improve the accuracy of diagnosis (Fig. 123-2). Giles et al. (1990) described 11 cases of TTS diagnosed on the basis of like-gender twins with monochorionic placentation and umbilical venous blood hemoglobin differences exceeding 5 g per deciliter at delivery. The umbilical-artery systolic:diastolic ratios were concordant, even in the presence of differences in fetal size. The authors suggested that Doppler velocimetry of the umbilical artery is important in differentiating TTS from fetal growth discordance and hypothesized that

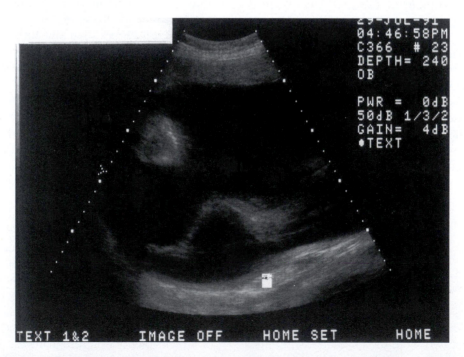

Figure 123-1. Prenatal sonographic image demonstrating a "stuck" twin in the upper left section of the image and the co-twin in a sac with polyhydramnios. See color plate.

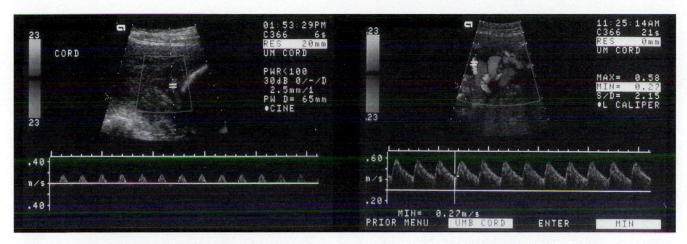

Figure 123-2. Composite ultrasound images demonstrating absent end diastolic flow in the umbilical artery of the donor stuck twin and normal flow velocity waveforms in the recipient fetus. See color plate.

the concordance in waveforms was due to the absence of an underlying placental vascular pathologic lesion. However, Pretorius et al. (1988) reported abnormal Doppler findings in eight cases of TTS. Five of eight twins demonstrated umbilical-artery waveforms with absent or reversed diastolic flow. Our data agree with those of Pretorius et al. In Table 123-1, data on 14 cases of TTS at our institution (Castaner et al. 1992) are presented and compared with Giles et al.'s (1990) data. Different diagnostic criteria were used in both studies. We used the classic sonographic findings to make the diagnosis, whereas Giles et al. made the diagnosis based on a discordant hemoglobin at birth. All of our cases had a "stuck" twin. There was a very high perinatal death rate in our series, which is consistent with most other series of severe TTS. There were no perinatal deaths in Giles et al. series. It is our opinion that Giles et al. observed a much less severe expression of TTS that presented during the third trimester. The differences in outcome found between Giles et al.'s series and ours may represent variation in diagnostic criteria for TTS.

Fisk et al. (1990) described fetal blood sampling in six cases compromised by TTS. Difference in hemoglobin concentration of 5 g per deciliter was found in only one pregnancy. Confirmation of a shared circula-

tion was achieved in two pregnancies by transfusing adult Rh-negative red cells into the smaller fetus and then detecting them by Kleihauer–Betke testing in blood aspirated from the larger fetus. Bruner and Rosemond (1993) further reported successful fetal blood sampling in six of nine cases with the ultrasonographic diagnosis of TTS. Hemoglobin difference was present in only one case. Shared circulation was demonstrated and confirmed in four (44%) of those initially identified by ultrasonographic criteria through the transfusion of O-negative red cells into the small twin and the performance of Kleihauer–Betke analysis on blood obtained from the larger twin. The author concluded that the currently accepted prenatal criteria are insufficient for the diagnosis of TTS and suggested that the sonographic findings of marked growth discordance with oligohydramnios, polyhydramnios, monochorionic placenta, and like gender should more accurately be described as the twin oligohydramnios/polyhydramnios sequence.

The injection of intravascular pancuronium bromide has been suggested as an alternative to the injection of adult red cells to confirm TTS (Tanaka et al. 1992). Paralysis of both fetuses can be detected through the examination of fetal heart rate tracings. There is an absence of accelerations noted with a reduction in fetal

▶ **TABLE 123-1.** DOPPLER ULTRASOUND STUDIES IN TWIN-TO-TWIN TRANSFUSION

Diagnostic criteria	Castaner et al. 1992 *Ultrasound Examination*	Giles et al. 1990 *Hemoglobin Difference at Birth*
Presentation <20 weeks	11	2
Mean gestational age at delivery	29.7 weeks	34 weeks
Weight difference >20%	11 of 14	5 of 11
Absent end-diastolic flow	6	0
Neonatal deaths	8	0
Intrauterine deaths	3	0

heart rate variability and a persistent tachycardia seen following pancuronium injection.

TTS is generally diagnosed during the neonatal period by demonstration of a hemoglobin difference of greater than 5 g per deciliter (Rausen et al. 1965; Tan et al. 1979) and a difference in birth weight between twins of greater than 20% (Tan et al. 1979). Untimely umbilical-cord clamping of either donor or recipient, erythropoietic changes, and reversed intrapartum shunting may result in false positive and false negative diagnosis when the determination is based on hemoglobin disparity alone. The cutoff value between normal and abnormal intertwin birth-weight differences also remains controversial (Blickstein 1990). In fact, all the classically accepted neonatal criteria of discordant hemoglobin, hematocrit, and weight have been challenged.

Danskin and Neilson (1989) found that hemoglobin differences of greater than 5 g per deciliter occur at similar rates in twins with dichorionic and monochorionic placentation. They reported birth-weight differences greater than 20% equally in monochorionic and dichorionic pregnancies. Wenstrom et al. (1992) reviewed 97 cases of pathologically proven monochorionic twin pregnancies and observed all combinations of weight and hemoglobin/hematocrit discordance. Of 97 twin pairs, 34 were discordant for weight, and in half of these the hemoglobin and hematocrit were concordant. In 18% of cases the smaller twin had the higher hematocrit, and in 32% the smaller twin had the lower hematocrit. The authors concluded that weight and hemoglobin/hematocrit discordance is common in monochorionic twins and in itself is not sufficient for a diagnosis of TTS. Conflicting information regarding both the fetal and neonatal hematologic criteria for the diagnosis of TTS, together with the potential risk inherent in fetal blood sampling, has led us to avoid this procedure at our institution for the definitive diagnosis of TTS.

▶ ANTENATAL NATURAL HISTORY

TTS was first characterized by Herlitz in 1941, who reported anemia in one twin and polycythemia in the other. TTS occurs in acute and chronic forms. In early pregnancy an acute transfusion may result in an early fetal death, resulting in the so-called vanishing twin syndrome. Later in pregnancy, TTS may cause death of one or both twins (Fig. 123-3). Sometimes, a rapid transfer of blood from one twin to the other occurs during delivery. In such cases the twins are similar in weight and length, but one is polycythemic and hypervolemic and the other is anemic and hypovolemic.

In the chronic form of the transfusion syndrome, the transfusion of blood from one twin to the other occurs over an extended period during the pregnancy.

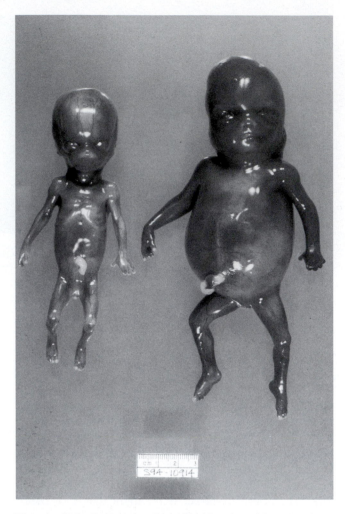

Figure 123-3. Death of both twins in mid-gestation as a result of twin-to-twin transfusion syndrome. The smaller, growth-restricted donor twin is on the left and the larger recipient twin on the right. *(Courtesy of Dr. Joseph Semple.)*

In chronic TTS, the donor twin is generally hypovolemic and anemic and shows varying degrees of growth restriction. In severe cases the donor may die in utero and present at delivery as a fetus papyraceous. The recipient twin is hypervolemic, often larger than the donor, and may develop cardiac hypertrophy and congestive heart failure. Because of increased urine output, severe polyhydramnios frequently develops in the recipient twin and leads to premature delivery. Oligohydramnios is generally associated with the donor twin. The organ changes seen in donor twins in chronic TTS resemble abnormalities observed in malnourished singletons. Weights of the heart, liver, spleen, thymus, and fetal adrenal cortex are proportionately smaller in the donor than in the recipient twin and suggest antenatal malnutrition (Naeye 1965) (Fig. 123-4). A much higher concentration of atriopeptin (atrionatriuretic peptide) has been reported in the serum from the recipient twin

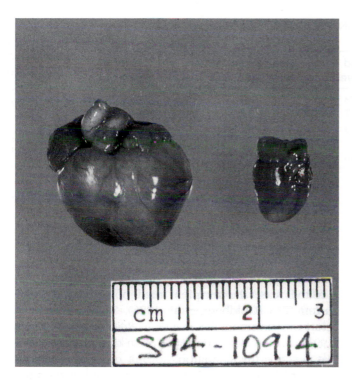

Figure 123-4. At the right is the paler, smaller heart of the donor fetus. At the left is the plethoric, larger heart of the recipient fetus.

as compared with the donor twin in two cases of severe transfusion syndrome. One may infer from this that atriopeptin plays a role in the pathophysiology of the syndrome (Nageotte et al. 1989). Atriopeptin, produced by mammalian atria, is a peptide that promotes diuresis and vascular changes. In TTS, atriopeptin released from the atria of the recipient may lead to increased urine output that results in polyhydramnios and vascular changes that in turn lead to hydrops (Nageotte et al. 1989). Untreated, the natural history of TTS is associated with a 60 to 100% mortality rate for both twins in severe or chronic cases (Benirschke and Kim 1973; Cheschier and Seeds 1988).

▶ MANAGEMENT OF PREGNANCY

In the assessment of discordant growth in twins in utero it is important to differentiate TTS from isolated growth failure of one twin. The cause of stuck twin syndrome includes twin-to-twin transfusion, fetal anomalies, placental insufficiency, and possibly abnormal cord insertion. A detailed anatomic survey is recommended to rule out any associated congenital abnormalities. Such a survey may be difficult if the fetus is stuck because of substantial oligohydramnios, which impairs ultrasonic visualization. Color Doppler studies are useful to visualize where the cord inserts into the placenta. It is our

practice to perform amniocentesis on both sacs to exclude a chromosomal abnormality. Amniotic fluid is also sent for cytomegalovirus culture because of the reported association of stuck twin syndrome with viral infections. The definitive antenatal diagnosis is difficult, and therapy is usually based on a presumptive diagnosis. It is our practice to inform patients of the various available treatment options, summarized in Table 123-2.

In general, the type of treatment selected will depend on the gestational age at presentation. Expectant management has been associated with 100% perinatal mortality in one review (Weir et al. 1979) and with a 90% mortality in a further review by Elliott (1992). In some cases, one of the twins may die in utero. As discussed in the chapter on intrauterine fetal death in twins, this is associated with increased neurologic morbidity of the surviving twin. When intrauterine death occurs, the polyhydramnios resolves, and hydrops fetalis may also resolve (Kirshon et al. 1990). In our experience, however, it may take as long as 6 weeks for the polyhydramnios to resolve.

Reported medical therapies include digoxin and indomethacin. In one case report, digoxin was administered to the mother at 27 weeks of gestation when edema, ascites, and hydramnios were noted in the recipient twin. The heart failure resolved, and the twins were delivered by elective cesarean section at 34 weeks and had a normal outcome (De Lia et al. 1985). Successful use of indomethacin has been reported in twins with polyhydramnios (Lange et al. 1989). The chorionicity was not described, and discordant birth weights were seen in only two of six cases. Therefore, it is unlikely that the polyhydramnios was due to TTS. We have reported two cases of TTS complicated by single intrauterine fetal death within 72 hours of initiating indomethacin therapy (Jones et al. 1993). In one case, the smaller (donor) fetus died. In the second case, the larger (recipient) fetus died. Because of this experience, indomethacin is no longer offered for treatment of TTS at our institution.

Decompression amniocentesis was initially used to reduce maternal discomfort owing to associated

▶ TABLE 123-2. REPORTED TREATMENT OPTIONS FOR TTS*

Conservative
Medical therapy
   Indomethacin
   Digoxin
Repetitive amniocentesis
Amniotic septostomy
Selective feticide
Hysterotomy with removal of one fetus
Laser obliteration of placental anastomoses

*Gestational age is the most important factor in deciding the options.

this opinion still needs to be confirmed by a randomized trial.

In a study of TTS from Germany, 73 patients at a single center were treated with fetoscopic laser ablation, while 43 patients at a separate center were treated with serial reduction amniocentesis (Hecher et al. 1999). Patients in the fetoscopic laser group had a higher proportion of pregnancies with at least one survivor, fewer fetal deaths, higher gestational age at delivery, and fewer cases of abnormal sonographic findings in the brain of survivors. It was therefore concluded that fetoscopic laser ablation is a more effective treatment for TTS than serial reduction amniocentesis.

A reasonable approach to fetal intervention for TTS may be to incorporate several of these possible interventions. At initial presentation, amniocentesis of both sacs should be performed to obtain karyotype information and to perform amnioreduction. Amniotic septostomy may also be performed at this time. If the sonographic findings fail to resolve, or if they deteriorate, and there is evidence of fetal cardiac compromise, then laser ablation of placental vessels may be reasonable. Another option in severe cases at less than 24 weeks of gestation may be to perform fetoscopic laser coagulation of the cord of the compromised twin (see Chapter 121). The sonographic features of TTS affecting the surviving twin would then be expected to resolve.

▶ TREATMENT OF THE NEWBORN

Both acute and chronic cases of TTS must be managed expeditiously by trained neonatologists. Two neonatal resuscitation teams are required. Because the incidence of prematurity is so high, many complications of prematurity are present, including the need for respiratory support, transfusion, and supplemental glucose. Specific problems unique to newborn cases of TTS include severe anemia in the donor and severe polycythemia and hypervolemia in the recipient newborn. Either one or both twins may have hydrops. Exchange transfusions may be necessary to correct the anemia and polycythemia.

▶ SURGICAL TREATMENT

No surgical treatment has been described for newborns with TTS.

▶ LONG-TERM OUTCOME

One of the concerns associated with in utero treatment for TTS is that prolongation of pregnancy might produce survivors with excessive neonatal or infant complications (Mahony et al. 1990). There are few data available on the long-term follow-up of infants diagnosed prenatally with TTS. In the older literature thrombocytopenia has been suggested as a cause of cataracts, impaired hearing, and growth restriction of the donor twin (Corney and Aherne 1965). Intrauterine growth deficiency of the brain (Naeye 1963) and profound neonatal hypoglycemia (Reisner et al. 1965) have been implicated as a cause for cerebral impairment of the donor, resulting in subsequent lower intelligence as compared with the recipient twin. Cardiomyopathy and associated cardiac dysfunction has been reported (Elliott 1992; Mahony et al. 1990). In one study, five of five recipient twins were found to have cardiomegaly and tricuspid regurgitation prenatally; four had cardiac dysfunction after birth (Zosmer et al. 1994). In Elliott's (1992) experience there were two cardiac abnormalities in 12 fetuses (one critical aortic stenosis, one cardiopathy). Renal cortical necrosis (Dimmick et al. 1971; Feingold et al. 1986) and brain infarction have been reported in the donor twin (Mahony et al. 1990). These complications have also been described in the surviving co-twin of intrauterine fetal death in utero. The mechanism may be hypovolemia and ischemic injury in the smaller donor twin (Elliott 1992). In Reisner et al.'s series, the 15% incidence of confirmed cerebral palsy was similar to the background incidence in reports from their institution when corrected for gestational age (Reisner et al. 1993; Shy et al. 1990). Other significant long-term complications such as blindness, deafness, chronic cardiac disease, severe chronic lung disease, or renal insufficiency were described as "minimal." No late infant deaths occurred in the series.

▶ GENETICS AND RECURRENCE RISK

There are no reports of recurrence of TTS in the literature.

REFERENCES

Bajoria R, Wigglesworth J, Fisk NM. Angioarchitecture of monochorionic placentas in relation to the twin-twin transfusion syndrome. Am J Obstet Gynecol 1995;172: 856–863.

Benirschke K, Kim CK. Multiple pregnancy. N Engl J Med 1973;288:1276–1284, 1329–1336.

Blickstein I. The twin-twin transfusion syndrome. Obstet Gynecol 1990;76:714–721.

Brennan JN, Diwan RJ, Rosen MG, et al. Fetofetal transfusion syndrome: prenatal ultrasonographic diagnosis. Radiology 1982;143:535–536.

Bruner JP, Rosemond RL. Twin-to-twin transfusion syndrome: a subset of the twin oligohydramnios-polyhydramnios sequence. Am J Obstet Gynecol 1993;169:925–930.

Castaner J, Baker E, Cetrulo CL, et al. Umbilical artery Dopplers in twin to twin transfusion syndrome. J Ultrasound Med 1992;11:S51.

Cheschier NC, Seeds JW. Polyhydramnios and oligohydramnios in twin gestations. Obstet Gynecol 1988;71:882–884.

Corney G, Aherne W. The placental transfusion syndrome in monozygous twins. Arch Dis Child 1965;40:264–270.

Danskin FH, Neilson JP. Twin-to-twin transfusion syndrome: what are appropriate diagnostic criteria? Am J Obstet Gynecol 1989;161:365–368.

De Lia JE, Emery MG, Sheafor SA, et al. Twin transfusion syndrome: successful in utero treatment with digoxin. Int J Gynaecol Obstet 1985;23:197–201.

De Lia JE, Cruikshank DP, Keye WR Jr. Fetoscopic neodymium: YAG laser occlusion of placental vessels in severe twin-twin transfusion syndrome. Obstet Gynecol 1990;75:1046–1053.

De Lia JE, Kuhlmann RS, Harstad TW, et al. Fetoscopic laser ablation of placental vessels in severe previable twin-twin transfusion syndrome. Am J Obstet Gynecol 1995;172:1202–1211.

Dimmick JE, Hardwick DF, Yuen BH. A case of renal necrosis and fibrosis in the immediate newborn period: association with the twin-twin-transfusion syndrome. Am J Dis Child 1971;122:345–347.

Donnenfeld AE, Glazerman LR, Cutillo DM, et al. Fetal exsanguination following intrauterine angiographic assessment and selective termination of a hydrocephalic, monozygotic co-twin (case report). Prenat Diagn 1989;9:301–308.

Elliott JP, Urig MA, Clewell WH. Aggressive therapeutic amniocentesis for treatment of twin-twin transfusion syndrome. Obstet Gynecol 1991;77:537–540.

Elliott JP. Amniocentesis for twin-twin transfusion syndrome. Contemp Obstet Gynecol 1992;August:30–47.

Feingold M, Cetrulo CL, Newton ER, et al. Serial amniocenteses in the treatment of twin to twin transfusion complicated with acute polyhydramnios. Acta Genet Med Gemellol 1986;35:107–113.

Fisk NM, Borrell A, Hubinont C, et al. Fetofetal transfusion syndrome: do the neonatal criteria apply in utero? Arch Dis Child 1990;65:657–661.

Giles WB, Trudinger BJ, Cook CM, et al. Doppler umbilical artery studies in the twin-twin transfusion syndrome. Obstet Gynecol 1990;76:1097–1099.

Golbus MS, Cunningham N, Goldberg JD, et al. Selective termination of multiple gestations. Am J Med Genet 1988;31:339–348.

Goldberg HJ, Oats JN, Ratten V, et al. Timely diagnosis by cardiotocography of critical fetal reserve due to fetofetal transfusion syndrome. Aust NZ J Obstet Gynaecol 1986;26:182–184.

Gonsoulin W, Moise KJ Jr, Kirshon B, et al. Outcome of twin-twin transfusion diagnosed before 28 weeks of gestation. Obstet Gynecol 1990;73:214–216.

Hecher K, Plath H, Bregenzer T, et al. Endoscopic laser surgery versus serial amniocenteses in the treatment of severe twin-twin transfusion syndrome. Am J Obstet Gynecol 1999;180:717–724.

Herlitz G. Zur kenntnis der anämischen und polyzytämischen Zustände bei Neugeborenen sowie des Icterus gravis neonatorum. Acta Pediatr 1941;29:211.

Jones JM, Sbarra AJ, Dilillo L, et al. Indomethacin in severe twin-to-twin transfusion syndrome. Am J Perinatol 1993;10:24–26.

Kirshon B, Moise KJ, Mari G, et al. In utero resolution of hydrops fetalis following the death of one twin in twin-twin transfusion. Am J Perinatol 1990;7:107–109.

Lage JM, Van Marter LJ, Mikhail E. Vascular anastomoses in fused, dichorionic twin placentas resulting in twin transfusion syndrome. Placenta 1989;10:55.

Lange IR, Harman CR, Ash KM, et al. Twin with hydramnios: treating premature labor at source. Am J Obstet Gynecol 1989;160:552–557.

Mahony BS, Petty CN, Nyberg DA, et al. The "stuck twin" phenomenon: ultrasonographic findings, pregnancy outcome, and management with serial amniocenteses. Am J Obstet Gynecol 1990;163:1513–1521.

McCafee CA, Fortune DW, Beischer NA. Non-immunological hydrops fetalis. J Obstet Gynaecol Br Commonw 1970;77:226–237.

Nageotte MP, Hurwitz SR, Kaupke CJ, et al. Atriopeptin in the twin transfusion syndrome. Obstet Gynecol 1989;73:867.

Naeye RL. Human intrauterine parabiotic syndrome and its complications. N Engl J Med 1963;268:804–809.

Naeye RL. Organ abnormalities in a human parabiotic syndrome. Am J Pathol 1965;46:8–29.

Patten RM, Mack LA, Harvey D, et al. Disparity of amniotic fluid volume and fetal size: Problem of the stuck twin—US studies. Radiology 1989;172:153–157.

Pinette MG, Yuqun P, Pinette SG, et al. Treatment of twin-twin transfusion syndrome. Obstet Gynecol 1993;82:841–846.

Pretorius DH, Manchester D, Barkin S, et al. Doppler ultrasound of twin transfusion syndrome. J Ultrasound Med 1988;7:117–124.

Rausen AR, Seki M, Strauss L. Twin transfusion syndrome. J Pediatr 1965;66:613–628.

Reisner SH, Forbes AE, Cornblath M. The smaller of twins and hypoglycemia. Lancet 1965;1:524–526.

Reisner DP, Mahony BS, Petty CH, et al. Stuck twin syndrome: outcome in thirty-seven consecutive cases. Am J Obstet Gynecol 1993;169:991–995.

Robertson EG, Neer KJ. Placental injection studies in twin gestation. Am J Obstet Gynecol 1983;147:170.

Saade GR, Olson G, Belfort MA, et al. Amniotomy: a new approach to the "stuck twin" syndrome. Am J Obstet Gynecol 1995;172:429.

Saunders NJ, Snijders RJM, Nicolaides KH. Therapeutic amniocentesis in twin-twin transfusion syndrome appearing in the second trimester of pregnancy. Am J Obstet Gynecol 1992;166:820–824.

Schatz F. Eine besondere Art von einseitiger Polyhydramnie mit anderseitiger Oligohydramnie bei eineiigen Zwillingen. Arch Gynaekol 1882;19:329.

Sherer DM, Glantz JC, Metlay LA, et al. Marked twin-twin transfusion in the absence of nonimmune hydrops. Am J Perinatol 1994;11:317–319.

Shy K, Luthy DA, Bennett FC, et al. Effects of electronic fetal-heart-rate monitoring, as compared with periodic auscultation, on the neurologic development of premature infants. N Engl J Med 1990;322:588–593.

▶ **TABLE 124-1.** TENTH PERCENTILE BIRTH WEIGHT CUTOFFS, IN GRAMS, BY GESTATIONAL AGE AND FETAL GENDER, FROM 1991 NATIONAL UNITED STATES POPULATION DATA

Gestational age (weeks)	Male	Female
20	270	256
21	328	310
22	388	368
23	446	426
24	504	480
25	570	535
26	644	592
27	728	662
28	828	760
29	956	889
30	1117	1047
31	1308	1234
32	1521	1447
33	1751	1675
34	1985	1901
35	2205	2109
36	2407	2300
37	2596	2484
38	2769	2657
39	2908	2796
40	2986	2872
41	3007	2891
42	2998	2884
43	2977	2868
44	2963	2853

Reproduced from Alexander GR, Himes JH, Kaufman RB, Mor J, Kogan M: A United States national reference for fetal growth. Obstet Gynecol 87:163–8 1996. Reprinted, with permission, from the American College of Obstetricians and Gynecologists.

et al. 1996; Williams et al. 1982). Commonly used cutoffs for defining IUGR in male and female fetuses at various gestational ages are shown in Table 124-1. A further problem with the use of such cutoff values for diagnosing IUGR is that they cannot identify a fetus that has failed to reach its own growth potential, but whose weight is not yet below the usual cutoff value. Such a fetus may be identified through serial sonography, in which sequential weight estimates are associated with decreasing percentile values for gestational age.

The term intrauterine growth restriction is frequently and erroneously used as a substitute for the original term small for gestational age. SGA describes a population of fetuses with a weight below the 10th percentile without reference to the cause. Most SGA fetuses are normal but small fetuses that simply reflect the normal weight distribution within a population. The use of a particular cutoff value such as the 10th percentile is clearly arbitrary, and will inevitably include a large number of fetuses that are constitutionally small, without any evidence of pathology. Up to 70% of SGA infants are small because of such constitutional reasons

as maternal ethnicity, parity, or body-mass index (Lin and Santolaya-Forgas 1998). IUGR describes a subset of these SGA fetuses whose weight is below the 10th percentile as a result of a pathologic process that is due to a diverse group of disorders. The term intrauterine growth restriction is preferred to intrauterine growth retardation, as the word retardation has a tremendously negative influence on patients.

IUGR has classically been subdivided into two patterns: asymmetric and symmetric IUGR. This provides further information on fetal body size and length, rather than a simple reliance on fetal weight. With symmetric IUGR, both head and abdomen are decreased proportionately, while asymmetric IUGR refers to a greater decrease in abdominal size, which is also referred to as the head-sparing effect (Lin and Santolaya-Forgas 1998). Approximately 70 to 80% of cases of IUGR are asymmetric, with the remaining 20 to 30% being symmetric. It was commonly believed that asymmetric IUGR represented placental insufficiency, while symmetric IUGR was more likely to be associated with constitutional problems, such as aneuploidy. However, it is now recognized that the timing of the pathologic insult is of more importance than the actual nature of the underlying pathology in determining the pattern of IUGR, thereby calling into question the clinical utility of subdividing IUGR into such patterns (Lin and Santolaya-Forgas 1998). Symmetric IUGR can be caused by placental insufficiency occurring early in gestation, so that by the time the fetus is examined it has evolved from an initial asymmetric pattern to a pattern of symmetric IUGR. Overall infant body proportions can be described also using the ponderal index, which is the birth weight in grams divided by the crown-to-heel length in cubic centimeters.

The list of possible causes of IUGR is extensive and is summarized in Table 124-2. These causes can be conveniently divided into fetal, placental, and maternal factors (Lin and Santolaya-Forgas 1998). The most common fetal factors associated with IUGR include fetal chromosomal abnormalities, structural fetal malformations, fetal infections, and complications related to multiple gestations (Figure 124-1). Approximately 2 to 5% of all IUGR fetuses can be expected to have a chromosomal abnormality (Creasy and Resnik 1999). Up to one-fourth of all infants with congenital structural malformations will have IUGR, and the incidence of growth restriction increases significantly as the number of different malformations per infant increases (Khoury et al. 1988). The number of infectious agents proven to cause IUGR is limited; they include rubella and cytomegalovirus, although no known bacterial infections have been linked to IUGR (Creasy and Resnik 1999).

The importance of defining a subpopulation of fetuses with IUGR lies in the association with adverse pregnancy outcome. The likelihood of perinatal morbidity

▶ **TABLE 124-2.** RISK FACTORS FOR INTRAUTERINE GROWTH RESTRICTION

Fetal factors	Placental factors	Maternal factors

Chromosomal abnormalities:
  Trisomies 21, 18, 13
  Turner syndrome
  Chromosomal deletions
  Uniparental disomy
  Confined placental mosaicism
Structural malformations:
  Anencephaly
  Omphalocele/gastroschisis
  Diaphragmatic hernia
  Renal agenesis/dysplasia
  Cardiac malformations
  Multiple malformations
Multiple pregnancies:
  Monochorionic gestation
  Single anomalous fetus
  Twin-to-twin transfusion
Fetal infections:
  Rubella
  Cytomegalovirus
  Varicella-zoster
	Abnormal trophoblast invasion
	Placental infarction
	Abruption
	Vascular malformations
	Velamentous cord insertion
	Placenta previa
	Circumvallate placenta
	Chorioangioma
		Constitutional factors:
		  Race
		  Height/weight
		Nutritional factors:
		  Poor pregnancy weight gain
		  Low prepregnancy weight
		  Inflammatory bowel disease
		  Chronic pancreatitis
		  Gastrointestinal surgeries
		Hypoxic conditions:
		  Severe lung disease
		  Cyanotic heart disease
		  Sickle cell anemia
		Vascular problems:
		  Chronic hypertension
		  Preeclampsia
		  Collagen vascular disease
		  Insulin-dependent diabetes
		  Antiphospholipid antibodies
		Renal disease:
		  Glomerulonephritis
		  Renal transplantation
		  Chronic renal failure
		Environmental factors:
		  High altitude
		  Cigarette smoking
		  Substance abuse
		  Medications
		Past obstetric history:
		  Previous stillbirth
		  Previous IUGR
		  Previous preterm birth

Adapted from Lin CC, Santolaya-Forgas J: Current concepts of fetal growth restriction: part I. Causes, classification, and pathophysiology. Obstet Gynecol 92:1044–55 1998. Reprinted, with permission, from the American College of Obstetricians and Gynecologists.

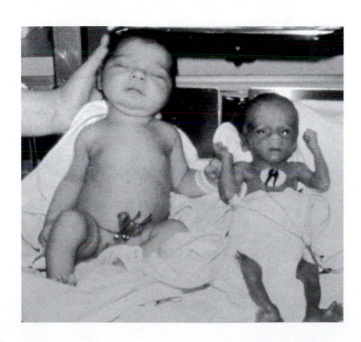

and perinatal mortality increases significantly as the birth-weight percentile decreases, so that once below the third to fifth percentiles, the chances of fetal death increase by as much as 20-fold (Scott and Usher 1966). For infants weighing less than 1500 g at term, the perinatal mortality rate is increased at least 70-fold as compared with appropriately grown term infants (Williams et al. 1982). Much of the increased perinatal morbidity and mortality in IUGR fetuses is due to the strong association between aneuploidy and structural fetal malformations with IUGR (Scott and Usher 1966).

Figure 124-1. Monozygotic twins in which the twin on the right is severely growth restricted compared to its co-twin.

▶ INCIDENCE

The incidence of IUGR varies depending on the population examined and the standard growth curves used to make the diagnosis (Goldenberg et al. 1989). Using the commonly quoted cutoff of the 10th percentile for defining pregnancies at risk for IUGR implies that at least 10% of the entire obstetric population will be labeled as being IUGR. In Europe, the commonly used cutoff for defining IUGR of 2 SD below the mean will include 5% of the total population. Approximately one third of all infants weighing less than 2500 g at birth are not just small for gestational age, but have sustained IUGR (Lin and Santolaya-Forgas 1998). Approximately 4 to 7% of all infants born in developed countries and 6 to 30% in developing countries are classified as growth-restricted (Galbraith et al. 1979; Lugo and Cassady 1971; Scott and Usher 1966).

▶ SONOGRAPHIC FINDINGS

Prenatal ultrasonography is the imaging method of choice for diagnosing and evaluating possible cases of IUGR. The typical finding is a significant discrepancy in some or all of the fetal biometric parameters as compared with measurements expected based on gestational age alone. The most common biometric parameters evaluated are the biparietal diameter, head circumference, abdominal circumference, and femur length. These measurements can then be used in a variety of formulas to provide an estimate of fetal weight (Hadlock et al. 1984; Shepard et al. 1982). However, it should be noted that sonographic prediction of fetal weight using such formulas may vary by up to 20% from actual fetal weight, thereby calling into question the accuracy of prenatal sonographic diagnosis of IUGR. For this reason, diagnosis and management of IUGR is generally guided by serial sonographic assessments of the fetus.

In cases of symmetric IUGR, measurements of the fetal head, abdomen, and femur should all be below the expected values for a given gestational age. By contrast, with asymmetric IUGR, measurements of the fetal abdomen will be less than expected, while fetal head and femur measurements will be appropriate for gestational age. While it is generally considered that symmetric IUGR represents an intrinsic insult to the fetus (chromosomal abnormality, fetal infection) and asymmetric IUGR represents an extrinsic insult (placental insufficiency), sonographic differentiation of these patterns may not be clinically relevant (Creasy and Resnik 1999). Mixed patterns of fetal growth restriction are also possible, which further limits the clinical utility of subdividing IUGR into symmetric and asymmetric types.

Improvements in the accuracy of prenatal diagnosis of IUGR may occur with the advent of three-dimensional ultrasonography. Three-dimensional measurements of the fetal thigh to predict birth weight have been shown in one study to be more accurate than weight prediction using standard biometric formulas and conventional two-dimensional sonography (Chang et al. 1997). In that study, the error in birth-weight prediction was 0.7% using three-dimensional assessment of the fetal thigh volume, as compared with 6 to 20% using standard biometric formulas.

Following the diagnosis of IUGR, a careful sonographic survey should be performed to search for some of the possible causes listed in Table 124-2. In cases of severe IUGR associated with placental problems, oligohydramnios is a frequent finding. In cases of severe IUGR but normal or increased amniotic fluid volume, fetal aneuploidy or structural malformation is likely. Pulsed Doppler sonographic assessment of the umbilical artery may reveal abnormalities of flow in true cases of IUGR. As placental resistance increases, umbilical arterial flow toward the placenta during diastole will decrease, leading to an increase in the ratio of systolic to diastolic flow (S:D ratio). Eventually, umbilical arterial diastolic flow disappears and may even reverse direction toward the fetus, (absent end-diastolic flow and reversed end-diastolic flow). These sonographic findings, in the presence of severe IUGR, are ominous for continued in utero fetal well-being (Reed et al. 1987).

▶ DIFFERENTIAL DIAGNOSIS

A very likely alternative cause of apparent IUGR following prenatal ultrasonography is incorrect pregnancy dating. Also, because of the inherent inaccuracy of all forms of prenatal estimation of fetal weight, the differential diagnosis of IUGR should always include a normally grown fetus. In addition, at least 70% of all cases of SGA infants are constitutionally small, and do not reflect a pathologic impairment of fetal growth (Lin and Santolaya-Forgas 1998). Once a diagnosis of pathologic IUGR is considered likely, the differential diagnosis for the underlying cause is extensive and is listed in Table 124-2.

▶ ANTENATAL NATURAL HISTORY

The antenatal natural history of IUGR is difficult to predict in individual cases. Overall, perinatal mortality increases significantly as the birth-weight percentile decreases, from 20 in 1000 births at the fifth percentile to 150 in 1000 births at the first percentile (Creasy and Resnik 1999).

In cases of IUGR secondary to placental insufficiency, the typical in utero progression involves redistribution of fetal blood flow away from noncritical organs and maintaining cerebral blood flow. This leads to reduced fetal renal blood flow, which manifests as worsening oligohydramnios. In addition, further growth of the fetal abdominal dimensions is decreased and subcutaneous fat is no longer deposited. Doppler studies demonstrate decreased umbilical arterial diastolic flow, which may become absent or reversed as the IUGR worsens. In contrast, cerebral end-diastolic blood flow increases and, as fetal death nears, central cerebral vasodilation is lost (Arias 1994).

Because of this apparent sequence in fetal deterioration with IUGR, many investigators have used intensive fetal surveillance in an effort to predict when a fetus with IUGR is sufficiently compromised that in utero death is likely. Unfortunately, the predictive value of such antenatal surveillance is imperfect. It has been suggested that, in fetuses with IUGR, the development of absent or reversed end-diastolic umbilical arterial flow heralds imminent fetal death, and therefore may warrant elective delivery (Reed et al. 1987). However, the time interval between development of such Doppler abnormalities and fetal death may be up to 2 weeks, and therefore abnormal Doppler findings alone cannot be relied on to dictate elective premature delivery of a fetus with IUGR (Lin and Santolaya-Forgas 1999).

The antenatal history of fetuses with IUGR secondary to aneuploidy, structural malformation, or infection will be dictated in large part by the nature of the particular abnormality.

▶ MANAGEMENT OF PREGNANCY

When the prenatal diagnosis of IUGR is suspected, the patient should be referred to a maternal–fetal medicine physician for targeted ultrasound examination and counseling regarding further pregnancy management. The ultrasound examination should be repeated, with particular attention paid to all biometric parameters, amniotic fluid status, umbilical arterial Doppler indexes, and the presence of any structural fetal malformations or stigmata of aneuploidy. Invasive testing for fetal karyotype should be offered, as 2 to 5% of all fetuses with IUGR will have a chromosomal abnormality (Creasy and Resnik 1999). Maternal evaluation should include careful obstetric, medical, family, and genetic histories to evaluate for possible causes of IUGR, as listed in Table 124-2. Maternal serum should be sent for rubella titers, and maternal urine should be evaluated with cytomegalovirus culture. Antiphospholipid antibody testing should be considered in a patient with a history suspicious for this syndrome.

Further pregnancy management will depend on the gestational age and on the presence of additional malformations. If the pregnancy has already reached 37 weeks of gestation, delivery should be arranged promptly, as the extremely low risk of pulmonary immaturity cannot justify the ongoing risk of intrauterine fetal death. If the pregnancy is at less than 34 weeks of gestation and fetal testing is reassuring, expectant management is generally favored. Expectant management includes modified bed rest, smoking cessation, and treating maternal hypertension (Lin and Santolaya-Forgas 1999). The extent of antenatal testing depends on the degree of IUGR, the amniotic fluid status, and umbilical-artery Doppler indexes. In general, we recommend twice-weekly testing with a fetal nonstress test, together with a biophysical profile, and such expectant management can continue as long as these tests remain reassuring. These tests should be supplemented by daily counting of fetal movements by the mother. If umbilical-artery Doppler indexes are abnormal, especially in the presence of absent or reversed end-diastolic flow, daily fetal testing with nonstress tests and at least twice-weekly biophysical profiles are recommended. Pregnancies may continue for a further 2 weeks with reassuring fetal testing despite the presence of absent or reversed end-diastolic umbilical arterial flow, so this finding alone is not an indication to deliver the fetus (Lin and Santolaya-Forgas 1999).

For pregnancies between 34 and 37 weeks of gestation, further pregnancy management should be individualized, and may be guided by fetal lung maturity indexes. It is not unreasonable to manage all pregnancies with IUGR and reassuring fetal testing expectantly until 37 weeks of gestation, at which time elective delivery is arranged (Craigo et al. 1996). Using this management scheme, delivery before 37 weeks occurs only with nonreassuring fetal testing. The presence of oligohydramnios or abnormal umbilical-artery Doppler indexes are not used to decide on timing of delivery. If amniocentesis has documented fetal lung maturity during this 34-to-37-week gestational age range, there is no further role for expectant management, and delivery should be arranged promptly.

The mode of delivery for fetuses with IUGR should be based entirely on standard obstetric practices. There is no evidence to support a policy of routine cesarean delivery for all fetuses with IUGR. However, because many of these fetuses will have decreased placental reserve and therefore may not tolerate a prolonged labor, serious consideration should be given to elective cesarean delivery for a fetus with nonreassuring antenatal testing with an unfavorable cervix (Creasy and Resnik 1999). If induction of labor and vaginal delivery are deemed appropriate for an individual fetus with IUGR, continuous electronic monitoring of the fetal heart rate should be conducted. Such fetuses are at increased risk of having heart-rate decelerations and decreased heart-rate variability (Lin and Santolaya-Forgas 1999). The

Disorders of Amniotic Fluid Volume

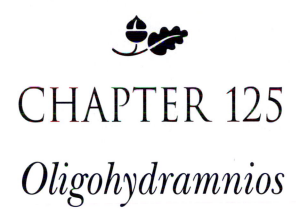

CHAPTER 125

Oligohydramnios

► CONDITION

Oligohydramnios is a decrease in the volume of amniotic fluid. The diagnosis of oligohydramnios is most frequently made by ultrasound examination. Oligohydramnios was initially defined as a subjective decrease in amniotic fluid volume resulting in fetal crowding as compared with normal values (Crowley et al. 1984). Objective sonographic estimation of amniotic fluid volume involves measuring different dimensions of amniotic fluid pockets. Various definitions of oligohydramnios exist. Oligohydramnios has been defined as a maximal vertical pocket (MVP) of less than 1 cm, but has also been defined as a MVP of less than 2 cm (Chamberlain et al. 1984; Manning et al. 1981). A semiquantitative four-quadrant technique, known as the amniotic fluid index (AFI) is also widely used. Oligohydramnios can be defined as an AFI of less than 5 cm, but has also been defined as an AFI of less than 8 cm (Moore 1993; Phelan et al. 1987).

Amniotic fluid volume is the result of a balance between inflow and outflow to and from the amniotic cavity. In the first half of pregnancy, the majority of amniotic fluid is a result of active transport of sodium and chloride across the amniotic membrane and fetal skin, with water moving passively in response (Brace and Resnik 1999). In the second half of pregnancy, the majority of amniotic fluid is a result of fetal micturition. Another major source of amniotic fluid is secretion from the respiratory tract. The average amniotic fluid volume is 30 ml at 10 weeks of gestation, rising to 780 ml at 32 to 35 weeks, after which time a natural decrease in volume occurs (Brace and Resnik 1999). The amniotic fluid volume is not stagnant, but is completely turned over at least once daily. Fetal urine first appears at 8 to 10 weeks of gestation, and reaches a production rate of 700 to 900 ml per day near term (Brace and Resnik 1999).

Oligohydramnios can occur as a result of decreased urinary production or excretion, or can be a result of fluid loss, such as with premature rupture of membranes. Causes of oligohydramnios include ruptured membranes, placental insufficiency, fetal anomalies, medication use by the mother, abnormalities of multiple gestations, chromosomal abnormalities, and idiopathic causes (Garmel et al. 1997). In the second trimester, premature rupture of membranes accounts for 50% of all cases of oligohydramnios; fetal anomalies, 15%; abruption, 7%; abnormal twinning, 5%; intrauterine growth restriction, 18%; and idiopathic causes, 5% (Shenker et al. 1991). The presence of oligohydramnios in a twin gestation may be due to twin-to-twin transfusion syndrome, intrauterine growth restriction of one twin, or intrauterine fetal death.

Premature rupture of membranes may be suggested with the sonographic appearance of oligohydramnios and an appropriately grown, structurally normal fetus. A sterile speculum examination demonstrating the absence of pooling following a negative phenaphthazine (Nitrazine) test will usually rule out rupture of membranes. Occult rupture of membranes may occur, and amniocentesis with indigocarmine-dye infusion may be necessary in some cases to rule out membrane rupture as an causative factor of oligohydramnios. Significant oligohydramnios occurring prior to 22 weeks of gestation is associated with a poor prognosis, most likely because of a high likelihood of pulmonary hypoplasia, and also because of a high incidence of congenital malformations.

Medication use by the mother, such as prostaglandin synthetase inhibitors and angiotensin-converting–enzyme inhibitors, has been reported to cause oligohydramnios. Indomethacin is used to treat preterm labor and can result in oligohydramnios, although this is usually reversible following discontinuation of the drug (Kirshon et al. 1991). Oligohydramnios, prolonged neonatal anuria, and ossification defects in the neonatal skull have been reported with in utero exposure to angiotensin-converting–enzyme inhibitors (Cunniff et al. 1990; Barr and Cohen 1991). The use of angiotensin-converting–enzyme inhibitors is absolutely contraindicated during pregnancy.

▶ INCIDENCE

Because of differing definitions, the reported incidence of oligohydramnios varies from 0.5 to 8% of all pregnancies (McCurdy and Seeds 1993; Phelan et al. 1987). When an MVP of less than 2 cm is used as a cutoff, the incidence of oligohydramnios is 3% of all pregnancies (Chamberlain et al. 1984). When an AFI of less than 5 cm is used, the incidence of oligohydramnios is 8% (Phelan et al. 1987). Norms for amniotic fluid volume across gestation were established in one report of sonographic amniotic fluid measurements in 791 patients (Moore and Cayle 1990). The fifth percentile for amniotic fluid index at term was approximately 7 cm. Interobserver variability may account for some of the variations in quoted incidences of oligohydramnios;

however, interobserver and intraobserver variability have been reported as reliable and reproducible (Halperin et al. 1985; Moore and Cayle 1990).

▶ SONOGRAPHIC FINDINGS

A diagnosis of oligohydramnios is almost always made on the basis of sonographic findings. Several methods of sonographic amniotic fluid assessment have been described. The subjective assessment of amniotic fluid volume with ultrasound examination was the earliest technique described (Crowley et al. 1984). This method involved the assessment of the relative amount of amniotic fluid present by comparing the amount of echo-free fluid areas in the uterus with the space occupied by the fetus. Disadvantages of this method include the requirement of a trained observer and the lack of a numerical result that can be used to follow a trend in amniotic fluid volume. Studies of interobserver variability for subjective sonographic assessment of amniotic fluid volume found that among experienced observers subjective estimates had good agreement rates and that this was not improved by the use of an arbitrary amniotic fluid volume classification such as vertical pocket depth (Goldstein and Filly 1988; Halperin et al. 1985).

However, most clinicians today use some form of objective semiquantitative estimate of amniotic fluid volume, based on the MVP or the AFI. The MVP involves surveying the entire uterus and measuring the depth of the deepest pocket of amniotic fluid in centimeters. Only amniotic fluid pockets free of fetal parts and umbilical cord are measured. The criteria for defining oligohydramnios vary, with some suggesting an MVP of less than 1 cm as an appropriate cutoff for oligohydramnios, while others use a cutoff of less than 2 cm to diagnose oligohydramnios (Chamberlain et al. 1984; Manning et al. 1981).

The AFI involves summing the maximum vertical pockets from each of the four quadrants of the uterus. In a report of sonographic AFI measurements in 197 patients, the mean AFI rose from 7 cm at 12 weeks of gestation to 20 cm at 26 weeks gestation, and then plateaued for the remainder of gestation at approximately 16 cm (Phelan et al. 1987). In a cross-sectional study of 791 pregnancies with AFI measurements, an AFI of 7 cm was at the fifth percentile at term, and only 1% of all pregnancies had an AFI of less than 5 cm at term (Moore and Cayle 1990).

It is important to measure the AFI with the patient supine, to orient the transducer in the maternal sagittal plane, to measure the sonographic planes perpendicular to the floor, to measure fluid pockets free from umbilical cord or fetal extremities, and to use the umbilicus and linea nigra as landmarks for dividing the uterus into four quadrants (Phelan et al. 1987).

There is no agreement in the obstetric literature as to which method of sonographic measurement of amniotic fluid volume is best. In one study comparing MVP with AFI, the correlation coefficient was 0.51, and the MVP was associated with a lower sensitivity (Moore 1990). Others have found good correlation between the MVP and AFI methods, with the MVP being better (Magann et al. 1994). Both MVP and AFI should therefore be considered reasonable methods for quantifying the amniotic fluid volume.

Whenever a diagnosis of oligohydramnios is made, a careful sonographic fetal anatomy survey should be performed to evaluate for fetal abnormalities, such as features of urinary tract obstruction or malformation. Absence of bladder filling following a 1-hour period of observation suggests a urinary-tract abnormality. Fetal renal anomalies including renal agenesis (see Chapter 86), urethral obstruction (see Chapter 80), and multicystic kidneys (see Chapter 82) account for 11% of cases of oligohydramnios discovered during the second trimester (Shenker et al. 1991).

If severe oligohydramnios is present at less than 24 weeks of gestation, the possibility of pulmonary hypoplasia should be considered. Numerous sonographic criteria to predict pulmonary hypoplasia have been described. Measurements of chest circumference are highly predictive of pulmonary hypoplasia in patients with either severe oligohydramnios or prolonged premature rupture of membranes (D'Alton et al. 1992). Normal values for fetal thoracic circumference and for the ratio of thoracic circumference to abdominal circumference have been established, and this ratio has been found to remain constant throughout pregnancy (D'Alton et al. 1992). A thoracic:abdominal circumference ratio of less than 0.80 in the setting of severe oligohydramnios in the second trimester is suspicious for pulmonary hypoplasia.

▶ DIFFERENTIAL DIAGNOSIS

The differential diagnosis for oligohydramnios includes normal pregnancy during the late third trimester, postmaturity, intrauterine growth restriction, premature rupture of membranes, fetal death, fetal renal anomalies (bilateral multicystic dysplastic kidneys, bilateral renal agenesis, bilateral ureteral obstruction, posterior urethral valves, infantile polycystic kidney disease), neural-tube defect, chromosomal abnormality, stuck twin, and medication use (such as indomethacin) by the mother.

▶ ANTENATAL NATURAL HISTORY

The antenatal natural history of oligohydramnios depends on the gestational age at diagnosis and the cause

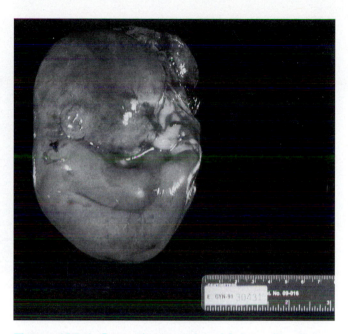

Figure 125-1. Severely constricted fetus with oligohydramnios due to bladder agenesis and a single dysplastic kidney. *(Courtesy of Dr. Joseph Semple.)*

of the oligohydramnios. Oligohydramnios accompanies a variety of serious fetal malformations, the most common being fetal renal abnormalities, and the underlying anomaly will dictate the natural history. Cardiac, skeletal, and neurologic malformations, in addition to aneuploidy and a variety of syndromic abnormalities, often coexist with the primary renal abnormality (McCurdy and Seeds 1993). Bilateral renal agenesis (Potter syndrome) is uniformly lethal because of associated pulmonary hypoplasia and renal failure (Fig. 125-1) (see Chapter 86).

The finding of significant oligohydramnios in the second trimester is associated with very high perinatal mortality (Barss et al. 1984; Bhutani et al. 1986; D'Alton et al. 1992). The combination of second-trimester oligohydramnios and elevated maternal serum α-fetoprotein (MSAFP) has an extremely poor prognosis. In one report of 21 patients with midtrimester oligohydramnios and elevated MSAFP only one infant survived (Dyer et al. 1987). Causes of perinatal loss in the setting of second trimester oligohydramnios include lethal congenital abnormalities, pulmonary hypoplasia, severe prematurity, and neonatal sepsis. Oligohydramnios in cases of chronic abruption appears to be an end-stage manifestation of severe uteroplacental insufficiency and is associated with a high incidence of intrauterine fetal death (Shenker et al. 1991).

Second-trimester oligohydramnios following preterm premature rupture of membranes (PPROM) carries a poor prognosis, with up to a 60% fetal loss rate, due mostly to pulmonary hypoplasia (Bhutani et al. 1986;

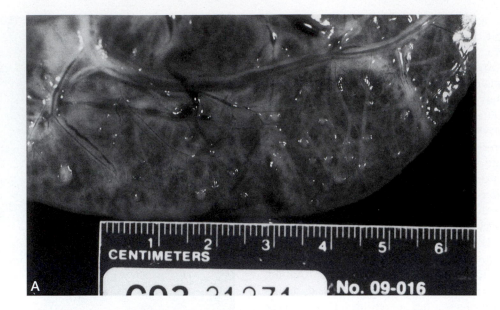

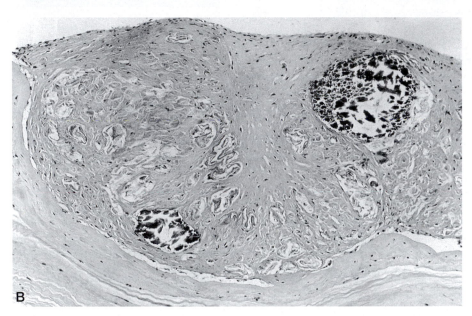

Figure 125-2. Gross (panel A) and microscopic (panel B) appearances of amnion nodosum in a fetus with oligohydramnios. *(Courtesy of Dr. Joseph Semple.)*

D'Alton et al. 1992). Sequelae of PPROM that contribute to the poor outcome include chorioamnionitis, amnion nodosum (Fig. 125-2), neonatal sepsis, neonatal pneumonia, placental abruption, and cord prolapse (Gonen et al. 1989). Neonatal outcome following PPROM can be improved by the routine administration of antibiotics, such as ampicillin and erythromycin (Mercer et al. 1997).

The combination of oligohydramnios and fetal growth restriction is associated with significantly increased perinatal morbidity and mortality rates (Chamberlain et al. 1984; Hill et al. 1983; Seeds 1984). The perinatal mortality rate ranges from 10 to 19% in these situations (Chamberlain et al. 1984). Close fetal surveillance is indicated to avoid antenatal deterioration in fetal status, and elective premature delivery may be needed.

Postmature pregnancies have increased rates of perinatal morbidity and mortality (Beischer et al. 1969). The finding of oligohydramnios in a pregnancy beyond 41 weeks of gestation identifies a subset of patients who are at significantly increased risk for adverse outcomes. There is a significantly higher risk of abnormal fetal testing, presence of fetal heart-rate decelerations during labor, meconium staining, cesarean delivery for nonreassuring fetal testing, and depressed 1- and 5-minute Apgar scores (Robson et al. 1992; Rutherford et al. 1987; Sarno et al. 1990).

Little information exists on the antenatal natural history of oligohydramnios prior to 37 weeks of gestation in the absence of intrauterine growth restriction, PPROM, or fetal anomalies. In one case–control study of pregnancies with unexplained oligohydramnios, there was a significantly higher incidence of premature delivery but no difference in overall neonatal outcomes (Garmel et al. 1997). Oligohydramnios associated with maternal hypovolemia is associated with a good perinatal outcome, and is generally reversible with hydration (Sherer et al. 1990).

▶ MANAGEMENT OF PREGNANCY

Following a diagnosis of oligohydramnios, a careful maternal history should be obtained to evaluate for illnesses such as hypertension or chronic renal disease and to assess for use of medications such as prostaglandin synthetase inhibitors. Physical examination should include a sterile speculum examination to evaluate for pooling of amniotic fluid in the vaginal vault, phenaphthazine (Nitrazine) paper analysis, and microscopic examination of a vaginal smear on a slide for the presence of ferning. The presence of oligohydramnios should prompt a thorough sonographic survey of the fetal anatomy. Visualization of the fetal anatomy may be extremely difficult in cases of severe oligohydramnios. Administration of furosemide to the mother has been advocated to improve detection of bilateral renal agenesis (Kurjak et al. 1981). Other authors have suggested that fetuses with severe growth restriction may not respond to furosemide administration secondary to decreased renal perfusion and decreased glomerular filtration rate, and therefore extreme caution should be used with this approach (Goldenberg et al. 1984).

Amnioinfusion may assist sonographic visualization of the fetus in pregnancies complicated by severe oligohydramnios. In one report of 13 pregnancies complicated by severe oligohydramnios, amnioinfusion of warmed normal saline was successfully performed in all patients and fluid for karyotype analysis was successfully obtained in 8 patients (Quetel et al. 1992). The use of amnioinfusion, together with indigocarmine–dye instillation, allowed subsequent adequate ultrasound examination in 12 of 13 patients, a correct diagnosis of ruptured membranes in 6 patients, and an antenatal diagnosis of Meckel–Gruber syndrome in one case (Quetel et al. 1992). If a structural fetal anomaly is identified, karyotyping should be performed. In cases of severe oligohydramnios prior to 24 weeks of gestation, termination of pregnancy should be discussed with the patient.

The management of pregnancies with oligohydramnios secondary to PPROM depends on the gestational age at presentation. Ruptured membranes beyond 36 to 37 weeks of gestation should be managed by prompt induction of labor to minimize infectious maternal and fetal morbidity (Hannah et al. 1996). In cases of PPROM at less than 36 to 37 weeks of gestation, expectant management is reasonable, provided there is no evidence of intrauterine infection, fetal compromise, or preterm labor. Frequent assessment in the form of daily fetal heart-rate monitoring and/or sonographic biophysical profiling is recommended. Administration of betamethasone to the mother is advocated with PPROM prior to 32 to 34 weeks of gestation to reduce complications of prematurity. Although the evidence for improving neonatal outcome is less clear than with the use of corticosteroids in patients with intact membranes, there is an additional benefit in reduction of the incidence of intraventricular hemorrhage (National Institutes of Health 1995). In cases of PPROM prior to 32 weeks of gestation, administration of antibiotics to the mother, typically ampicillin and erythromycin for 7 days, has been shown to increase the latency period prior to delivery and improves overall neonatal outcome (Mercer et al. 1997). There is no conclusive evidence to support or exclude a benefit from tocolysis in the setting of PPROM. Expectant inpatient management of PPROM is recommended from 24 to 32 weeks of gestation, provided there is reassuring maternal and fetal testing on a daily basis. In cases of PPROM from 32 to 36 weeks of gestation, evaluation of fetal lung maturity may help decide between expectant management and induction of labor.

In cases of fetal growth restriction with oligohydramnios at less than 36 to 37 weeks of gestation, careful fetal assessment is mandatory, consisting of nonstress and biophysical testing at least twice weekly. If there is absent end-diastolic flow in the fetal umbilical artery, daily fetal testing is recommended (Craigo 1994). Delivery is indicated once a gestational age of 36 to 37 weeks is reached, or if fetal testing becomes nonreassuring. In cases of oligohydramnios in the presence of an appropriately grown fetus, delivery should be considered once a gestational age of 37 weeks is reached.

The location of delivery will depend on the cause of the oligohydramnios and the gestational age at diagnosis. If a congenital abnormality is present, delivery at a tertiary-care center where appropriately trained personnel are available is recommended. In patients with PPROM, delivery location will depend on the gestational age. For patients at less than 32 weeks of gestation, delivery should occur in a tertiary-care center with a neonatal intensive care unit. The mode of delivery should be based on usual obstetric practices; there is no indication to alter the mode of delivery based solely on the presence of oligohydramnios or PPROM. However, there is an increased incidence of cesarean delivery in pregnancies complicated by oligohydramnios, regardless

of amniotic fluid volume on pregnancy outcome. Obstet Gynecol 1994;83:959–962.

Manning FA, Hill LM, Platt LD. Qualitative amniotic fluid determination by ultrasound: antepartum detection of intrauterine growth retardation. Am J Obstet Gynecol 1981;139:254–258.

McCurdy CM, Seeds JW. Oligohydramnios: problems and treatment. Semin Perinatol 1993;17:183–196.

Mercer BM, Miodovnik M, Thurnau GR, et al. Antibiotic therapy for reduction of infant morbidity after preterm premature rupture of the membranes: a randomized controlled trial. JAMA 1997;278:989–995.

Moore TR. Superiority of the four-quadrant sum over the single-deepest-pocket technique in ultrasonographic identification of abnormal amniotic fluid volumes. Am J Obstet Gynecol 1990;163:762–767.

Moore TR. Clinical evaluation of amniotic fluid volume. Semin Perinatol 1993;17:173–182.

Moore TR, Cayle JE. The amniotic fluid index in normal human pregnancy. Am J Obstet Gynecol 1990;162:1168–1173.

Nakayama DK, Glick PL, Harrison MR, et al. Experimental pulmonary hypoplasia due to oligohydramnios and its reversal by relieving thoracic compression. J Pediatr Surg 1983;18:347–353.

National Institutes of Health. Effect of corticosteroids for fetal maturation on perinatal outcomes. NIH Consensus Development Panel on the Effect of Corticosteroids for Fetal Maturation on Perinatal Outcomes. JAMA 1995;273:413–418.

Ogita S, Imanaka M, Matsumoto M, et al. Premature rupture of membranes managed with a new cervical catheter. Lancet 1984;1:1330.

Phelan JP, Ahn MO, Smith CV, et al. Amniotic fluid index measurements during pregnancy. J Reprod Med 1987;32:601–604.

Quetel TA, Mejides AA, Salman FA, et al. Amnioinfusion: an aid in the ultrasonographic evaluation of severe oligohydramnios in pregnancy. Am J Obstet Gynecol 1992;167:333–336.

Robson SC, Crawford RA, Spencer JA, et al. Intrapartum amniotic fluid index and its relationship to fetal distress. Am J Obstet Gynecol 1992;166:78–82.

Roodhooft AM, Birnholz JC, Holmes LB: Familial nature of congenital absence and severe dysgenesis of both kidneys. N Engl J Med 1984;310:1341–1345.

Rutherford SE, Phelan JP, Smith CV, et al. The four-quadrant assessment of amniotic fluid volume: an adjunct to antepartum fetal heart rate testing. Obstet Gynecol 1987;70:353–356.

Sarno AP, Ahn MO, Phelan JP: Intrapartum amniotic fluid volume at term. Association of ruptured membranes, oligohydramnios and increased fetal risk. J Reprod Med 1990;35:719–723.

Seeds JW. Impaired fetal growth: ultrasonographic evaluation and clinical management. Obstet Gynecol 1984;64:577–584.

Shenker L, Reed KL, Anderson CF, et al. Significance of oligohydramnios complicating pregnancy. Am J Obstet Gynecol 1991;164:1597–1600.

Sherer DM, Cullen JB, Thompson HO, et al. Transient oligohydramnios in a severely hypovolemic gravid woman at 35 weeks' gestation, with fluid reaccumulating immediately after intravenous maternal hydration. Am J Obstet Gynecol 1990;162:770–771.

Strong TH, Hetzler G, Paul RH. Amniotic fluid volume increase after amnioinfusion of a fixed volume. Am J Obstet Gynecol 1990;162:746–748.

CHAPTER 126

Polyhydramnios

▶ CONDITION

Polyhydramnios, also known simply as hydramnios, is a decrease in the volume of amniotic fluid. The diagnosis of polyhydramnios is most frequently made by ultrasound examination, but is often suspected by clinical examination revealing a fundal height greater than expected for gestational age. Before the advent of prenatal sonography, polyhydramnios was defined as an amniotic fluid volume of more than 2 liters. Sonographic diagnosis of polyhydramnios relies on the finding of a maximum vertical pocket of more than 8 cm (Fig. 126-1) (Chamberlain et al. 1984). However, due to the asymmetric location of the fetus within the uterus, the use of this maximum vertical pocket (MVP) technique may lead to an overestimation of the amniotic fluid volume.

The amniotic fluid index (AFI) has been described as a more reliable means of quantifying amniotic fluid volume (Phelan et al. 1987). The AFI involves the summing of the largest vertical pockets from each of the four quadrants of the uterus. A normal amniotic fluid volume is defined as an AFI of between 8 and 18 cm, while polyhydramnios is defined as an AFI of greater than 24 cm. Normal values for the AFI throughout gestation have been described based on sonographic measurements of amniotic fluid volume in 791 uncomplicated pregnancies between 16 and 42 weeks of gestation (Moore and Cayle 1990). These values are listed in Table 126-1. A reasonable working definition of polyhydramnios using current sonographic criteria is an AFI greater than the 95th percentile for the corresponding gestational age.

Amniotic fluid volume is the result of a balance between flow into and out of the amniotic cavity. In the first half of pregnancy, the majority of amniotic fluid is

▶ **TABLE 126-1.** AMNIOTIC FLUID INDEX VALUES IN NORMAL PREGNANCY

Week	No. of Patients	Amniotic Fluid Index Percentile Values				
		2.5th	5th	50th	95th	97.5th
16	32	73	79	121	185	201
17	26	77	83	127	194	211
18	17	80	87	133	202	220
19	14	83	90	137	207	225
20	25	86	93	141	212	230
21	14	88	95	143	214	233
22	14	89	97	145	216	235
23	14	90	98	146	218	237
24	23	90	98	147	219	238
25	12	89	97	147	221	240
26	11	89	97	147	223	242
27	17	85	95	146	226	245
28	25	86	94	146	228	249
29	12	84	92	145	231	254
30	17	82	90	145	234	258
31	26	79	88	144	238	263
32	25	77	86	144	242	269
33	30	74	83	143	245	274
34	31	72	81	142	248	278
35	27	70	79	140	249	279
36	39	68	77	138	249	279
37	36	66	75	135	244	275
38	27	65	73	132	239	269
39	12	64	72	127	226	255
40	64	63	71	123	214	240
41	162	63	70	116	194	216
42	30	63	69	110	175	192

Reproduced, with permission, from Moore TR, Cayle JE. The amniotic fluid index in normal human pregnancy. Am J Obstet Gynecol 1990;162:1168–1173.

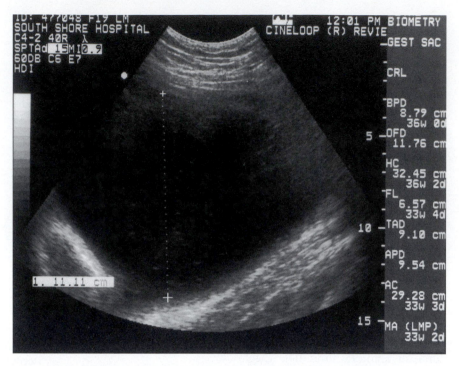

Figure 126-1. Prenatal sonographic image demonstrating a maximal vertical pocket of 11.11 cm of amniotic fluid.

a result of active transport of sodium and chloride across the amniotic membrane and fetal skin, with water moving passively in response (Brace and Resnik 1999). In the second half of pregnancy, the majority of amniotic fluid is a result of fetal micturition. Another major source of amniotic fluid is secretion from the fetus's respiratory tract. The average amniotic fluid volume is 30 ml at 10 weeks, rising to 780 ml at 32 to 35 weeks, following which time a natural decrease in volume occurs (Brace and Resnik 1999). The amniotic fluid volume is not stagnant, but is completely turned over at least once daily. Fetal urine first appears at 8 to 10 weeks of gestation, and reaches a production rate of 700 to 900 ml per day near term (Brace and Resnik 1999).

Polyhydramnios can occur because of increased production of fluid by the fetus, as in the case of hydrops, or it can be due to an obstruction to fetal swallowing, as in the case of a congenital gastrointestinal obstruction. Polyhydramnios is idiopathic in 66% of cases. Maternal diabetes mellitus accounts for 15% of cases, fetal malformations for 13%, multiple gestations for 5%, and other causes for 1% (Hill et al. 1987). However, the proportion of cases of polyhydramnios secondary to fetal malformation increases significantly as the severity of polyhydramnios increases. As the definition of polyhydramnios varies, so too does the reported incidence of associated fetal malformations. Two recent series have reported a 58 to 63% incidence of structural fetal malformations in pregnancies complicated by polyhydramnios (Damato et al. 1993; Many et al. 1996).

Fetal malformations associated with polyhydramnios include neural-tube defects (such as anencephaly), holoprosencephaly, cardiac anomalies (such as truncus arteriosus), gastrointestinal atresias or stenoses, skeletal dysplasias, neuromuscular disorders (such as myotonic dystrophy), infections (such as parvovirus), metabolic disorders (such as Gaucher disease), chromosomal abnormalities (such as trisomy 18), tumors (such as sacrococcygeal teratoma), and genetic syndromes (such as Beckwith–Wiedemann syndrome).

▶ INCIDENCE

The reported incidence of polyhydramnios varies, reflecting differences in definition. Polyhydramnios is reported in 0.1 to 3% of pregnancies when clinical methods are used to make the diagnosis (Kramer 1966). In one series of 9189 patients who had sonographic assessment of amniotic fluid volume by measuring the MVP, the overall incidence of polyhydramnios was 0.9% (Hill et al. 1987). In this study, mild polyhydramnios was diagnosed when the MVP measured between 8 and 11 cm, moderate polyhydramnios was defined as an MVP of 12 to 15 cm, and severe polyhydramnios was diagnosed when the MVP exceeded 16 cm. Mild polyhydramnios accounted for 79% of the cases, moderate polyhydramnios 16%, and severe polyhydramnios accounted for 5% (Hill et al. 1987). In another series, using an AFI cutoff of greater than 24 cm, mild polyhydramnios was diagnosed in 8% of patients (Smith et al. 1992).

▶ SONOGRAPHIC FINDINGS

Most diagnoses of polyhydramnios are now based on sonographic findings. The two most common methods of objectively measuring the amniotic fluid volume are the maximum vertical pocket (MVP) and the amniotic fluid index (AFI). The MVP involves surveying the entire uterus and measuring the depth of the deepest pocket of amniotic fluid in centimeters. Only amniotic fluid pockets free of fetal parts and umbilical cord are measured. The most commonly used cutoff for polyhydramnios using the MVP technique is a depth greater than 8 cm. The AFI involves summing the MVPs from each of the four quadrants of the uterus. In a report of sonographic AFI measurements in 197 patients, the mean AFI rose from 7 cm at 12 weeks of gestation to 20 cm at 26 weeks of gestation, and then plateaued for the remainder of gestation at approximately 16 cm (Phelan et al. 1987). The 95th percentile value for AFI at 37 weeks is 24 cm, but decreases to 19 cm at 41 weeks, reflecting the normal decrease in amniotic fluid production at term (Moore and Cayle 1990). It is important to measure the AFI with the patient supine, to orient the transducer in the maternal sagittal plane, to measure the sonographic planes perpendicular to the floor, to measure fluid pockets free from umbilical cord or fetal extremity, and to use the umbilicus and linea nigra as landmarks for dividing the uterus into four quadrants (Phelan et al. 1987).

There is no agreement in the obstetric literature as to which method of sonographic measurement of amniotic fluid volume is best. In one study comparing MVP with AFI, the correlation coefficient was 0.51, and the MVP was associated with a lower sensitivity (Moore 1990). Others have found good correlation between the MVP and AFI methods, with the MVP being better (Magann et al. 1994). In another study comparing 13 different sonographic methods of amniotic fluid volume assessment with a dye-dilution technique, the AFI underestimated the actual amniotic fluid volume by as much as 52% in cases of polyhydramnios (Dildy et al. 1992). When compared with the AFI, several of the other 12 methods of ultrasound prediction of amniotic fluid volume produced lower mean errors as compared with true amniotic fluid volume. However, the investigators concluded that the minimal improvement in accuracy offered by other ultrasound measurements was not sufficient to warrant replacement of the AFI (Dildy et al. 1992).

Sonographic assessment of polyhydramnios should include a careful survey of the fetal anatomy to rule out the presence of structural malformations. Because of the possibility of underlying fetal neuromuscular disorders, fetal swallowing, muscle tone, and fetal movement should be observed. In a study of 41 fetuses with a diagnosis of idiopathic polyhydramnios who were tested for the presence of a myotonic dystrophy mutation, 4 (9.7 %) were shown to be affected. Three of the 4 fetuses had a positive family history of myotonic dystrophy (Esplin et al. 1998).

▶ DIFFERENTIAL DIAGNOSIS

The cause of polyhydramnios is diverse, involving many maternal and fetal conditions, including those associated with immune and nonimmune hydrops fetalis. Maternal abnormalities should be considered, such as diabetes mellitus, rhesus isoimmunization, and preeclampsia resulting in the "mirror syndrome" (Ballantyne syndrome). If a multiple gestation is present, the possibility of twin-to-twin transfusion syndrome should be considered, especially if one fetus has severe oligohydramnios (stuck twin). Fetal infections associated with polyhydramnios include parvovirus, cytomegalovirus, toxoplasmosis, and syphilis. Polyhydramnios can also be seen with inborn errors of metabolism such as Gaucher disease, gangliosidoses, and mucopolysaccharidoses. Chromosomal abnormalities should also be considered, such as trisomy 18, trisomy 21, Turner syndrome, and 4p− (Wolf–Hirschhorn) syndrome.

Fetal neurologic malformations associated with polyhydramnios include anencephaly, encephalocele, meningomyelocele, holoprosencephaly, Dandy–Walker malformation, lissencephaly, and agenesis of the corpus callosum. Fetal cardiac abnormalities associated with polyhydramnios include cardiac arrhythmias, truncus arteriosus, aortic coarctation, and aortic-arch interruption. Fetal thoracic abnormalities associated with polyhydramnios include congenital cystic adenomatoid malformation (CCAM), bronchopulmonary sequestration (BPS), diaphragmatic hernia, chylothorax, and tracheal atresia. Fetal gastrointestinal malformations associated with polyhydramnios include cleft lip and palate, tracheoesophageal fistula, esophageal or intestinal atresia, omphalocele, gastroschisis, and annular pancreas. Fetal skeletal abnormalities associated with polyhydramnios include achondroplasia, osteogenesis imperfecta, hypophosphatasia, campomelic dysplasia, and thanatophoric dysplasia. Fetal neuromuscular abnormalities associated with polyhydramnios include myotonic dystrophy and arthrogryposis multiplex congenita (Bianchi and Van Marter 1994; Esplin et al. 1998). Other fetal abnormalities associated with polyhydramnios include cystic hygroma, neck masses such as cervical teratoma or goiter, sacrococcygeal teratoma, or lethal multiple pterygium syndrome.

▶ SURGICAL TREATMENT

No specific surgical treatment of the newborn is described for idiopathic polyhydramnios. However, surgical treatment may be necessary if associated structural malformations such as tracheoesophageal fistula or intestinal atresias are present.

▶ LONG-TERM OUTCOME

Long-term outcome for infants following a prenatal diagnosis of polyhydramnios depends on the gestational age at delivery and on the presence of associated structural malformations. In cases of additional malformations, the long-term outcome will primarily be dictated by the nature of the abnormality rather than by the existence of polyhydramnios.

▶ GENETICS AND RECURRENCE RISK

Recurrence of idiopathic polyhydramnios is uncommon, although case reports documenting such recurrences do exist (Sieck and Ohlsson 1984; Shimizu et al. 1988; Weissman and Zimmer 1987). In one series of 780 cases of polyhydramnios, there were 36 cases (4.6%) of recurrent polyhydramnios (Beischer et al. 1993). The risks associated with recurrent polyhydramnios include the risk of fetal malformation and premature delivery (Beischer et al. 1993). Polyhydramnios attributable to a specific genetic diagnosis may recur based on the pattern of inheritance of the condition.

REFERENCES

Ash K, Harman CR, Gritter H: TRAP sequence: successful outcome with indomethacin treatment. Obstet Gynecol 1990;76:960–962.

Beischer N, Desmedt E, Ratten G, et al. The significance of recurrent polyhydramnios. Aust NZ J Obstet Gynaecol 1993;33:25–30.

Bianchi DW, Van Marter LJ. An approach to ventilator-dependant neonates with arthrogryposis. Pediatrics 1994; 94:682–686.

Brace RA, Resnik R: Dynamics and disorders of amniotic fluid. In: Creasy RK, Resnik R, eds. Maternal-fetal medicine. 4th ed. Philadelphia: Saunders, 1999:632–643.

Brady K, Polzin WJ, Kopelman JN, et al. Risk of chromosomal abnormalities in patients with idiopathic polyhydramnios. Obstet Gynecol 1992;79:234–238.

Cabrol D, Landesman R, Muller J, et al. Treatment of polyhydramnios with prostaglandin synthetase inhibitor (indomethacin). Am J Obstet Gynecol 1987;157:422–426.

Cantor B, Tyler T, Nelson RM, et al. Oligohydramnios and transient neonatal anuria: a possible association with the maternal use of prostaglandin synthetase inhibitors. J Reprod Med 1980;24:220–223.

Carlson DE, Platt LD, Medearis AL, et al. Quantifiable polyhydramnios: diagnosis and management. Obstet Gynecol 1990;75:989–993.

Chamberlain PF, Manning FA, Morrison I, et al. Ultrasound evaluation of amniotic fluid volume. II. The relationship of increased amniotic fluid volume to perinatal outcome. Am J Obstet Gynecol 1984;150:250–254.

Csaba IF, Sulyok E, Ertl T. Relationship of maternal treatment with indomethacin to persistence of fetal circulation syndrome. J Pediatr 1978;92:484.

Damato N, Filly RA, Goldstein RB, et al. Frequency of fetal anomalies in sonographically detected polyhydramnios. J Ultrasound Med 1993;12:11–15.

De Lia JE, Kuhlmann RS, Harstad TW, et al. Fetoscopic laser ablation of placental vessels in severe previable twin-twin transfusion syndrome. Am J Obstet Gynecol 1995;172:1202–1211.

Desmedt EJ, Henry OA, Beischer NA. Polyhydramnios and associated maternal and fetal complications in singleton pregnancies. Br J Obstet Gynaecol 1990;97:1115–1122.

Dildy GA, Lira N, Moise KJ, et al. Amniotic fluid volume assessment: comparison of ultrasonographic estimates versus direct measurements with a dye-dilution technique in human pregnancy. Am J Obstet Gynecol 1992;167: 986–994.

Esplin MS, Hallam S, Farrington PF, Nelson L, Byrne J, Ward K. Myotonic dystrophy is a significant cause of idiopathic polyhydramnios. Am J Obstet Gynecol 1998; 179:974–977.

Gerson A, Roberts N, Colmorgen G, et al. Treatment of polyhydramnios with indomethacin. Am J Perinatol 1991; 8:97–98.

Greene MF, Hare JW, Krache M, et al. Prematurity among insulin requiring diabetic gravid women. Am J Obstet Gynecol 1989;161:106–111.

Hendricks SK, Conway L, Wang K, et al. Diagnosis of polyhydramnios in early gestation: indication for prenatal diagnosis? Prenat Diagn 1991;11:649–654.

Hill LM, Breckle R. Thomas ML, et al. Polyhydramnios: ultrasonically detected prevalence and neonatal outcome. Obstet Gynecol 1987;69:21–25.

Hill LM, Lazebnik N, Many A, et al. Resolving polyhydramnios: clinical significance and subsequent neonatal outcome. Ultrasound Obstet Gynecol 1995;6:421–424.

Kirshon B, Mari G, Moise KJ, et al. Effect of indomethacin on the fetal ductus arteriosus during treatment of symptomatic polyhydramnios. J Reprod Med 1990a;35:529–532.

Kirshon B, Mari G, Moise KJ. Indomethacin therapy in the treatment of symptomatic polyhydramnios. Obstet Gynecol 1990b;75:202–205.

Kramer EE. Hydramnios, oligohydramnios and fetal malformations. Clin Obstet Gynecol 1966;9:508–519.

Landy HJ, Isada NB, Larsen JW. Genetic implications of idiopathic hydramnios. Am J Obstet Gynecol 1987;157: 114–117.

Lange IR, Harman CR, Ash KM, et al. Twins with hydramnios: treating premature labor at source. Am J Obstet Gynecol 1989;160:552–557.

Magann EF, Morton ML, Nolan TE, et al. Comparative efficacy of two sonographic measurements for the detection of aberrations in the amniotic fluid volume and the effect of amniotic fluid volume on pregnancy outcome. Obstet Gynecol 1994;83:959–962.

Malas HZ, Hamlett JD. Acute recurrent polyhydramnios: management with indomethacin. Br J Obstet Gynaecol 1991;98:583–587.

Mamopoulos M, Assimakopoulos E, Reece EA, et al. Maternal indomethacin therapy in the treatment of polyhydramnios. Am J Obstet Gynecol 1990;162:1225–1229.

Many A, Lazebnik N, Hill LM. The underlying cause of polyhydramnios determines prematurity. Prenat Diagn 1996;16:55–57.

Mogilner BM, Ashkenazy M, Borenstein R, et al. Hydrops fetalis caused by maternal indomethacin treatment. Acta Obstet Gynecol Scand 1982;61:183–185.

Moise KJ. Effect of advancing gestational age on the frequency of fetal ductal constriction in association with maternal indomethacin use. Am J Obstet Gynecol 1993a; 168:1350–1353.

Moise KJ. Polyhydramnios: problems and treatment. Semin Perinatol 1993b;17:197–209.

Moore TR. The superiority of the four-quadrant sum over the single-deepest-pocket technique in ultrasonographic identification of abnormal amniotic fluid volumes. Am J Obstet Gynecol 1990;163:762–767.

Moore TR, Cayle JE. The amniotic fluid index in normal human pregnancy. Am J Obstet Gynecol 1990;162: 1168–1173.

Phelan JP, Ahn MO, Smith CV, et al. Amniotic fluid index measurements during pregnancy. J Reprod Med 1987;32: 601–604.

Phelan JP, Park YW, Ahn MO, et al. Polyhydramnios and perinatal outcome. J Perinatol 1990;10:347–350.

Queenan JT, Gadow EC. Polyhydramnios: chronic versus acute. Am J Obstet Gynecol 1970;108:349–355.

Rosen DJ, Rabinowitz R, Beyth Y, et al. Fetal urine production in normal twins and in twins with acute polyhydramnios. Fetal Diagn Ther 1990;5:57–60.

Shimizu T, Ihara Y, Kawaguchi K, et al. Human leucocyte antigen compatibility in a couple with idiopathic recurrent hydramnios. Am J Obstet Gynecol 1988;159:463–464.

Sieck UV, Ohlsson A. Fetal polyuria and hydramnios associated with Bartter's syndrome. Obstet Gynecol 1984;63: 22–24.

Simpson LL, Marx GR. Diagnosis and treatment of structural fetal cardiac abnormality and dysrhythmia. Semin Perinatol 1994;18:215–227.

Smith CV, Plambeck RD, Rayburn WF, et al. Relation of mild idiopathic polyhydramnios to perinatal outcome. Obstet Gynecol 1992;79:387–389.

Vanhaesebrouck P, Thiery M, Leroy JG, et al. Oligohydramnios, renal insufficiency, and ileal perforation in preterm infants after intrauterine exposure to indomethacin. J Pediatr 1988;113:738–743.

Weissman A, Zimmer EZ: Acute polyhydramnios recurrent in four pregnancies: a case report. J Reprod Med 1987; 32:65–66.

placenta to produce fetal hemolysis and profound fetal anemia.

The mechanism by which maternal–fetal Rh incompatibility produces immune hydrops fetalis is complex (Bowman 1999). Maternal anti-D IgG antibody attaches itself to the Rh antigen present on fetal red cells. This results in chemotaxis of phagocytes in the fetal spleen, which leads to destruction and hemolysis of fetal red cells. In response, the fetus produces more erythropoietin, which stimulates the fetal bone marrow to increase red-cell production. Eventually, marrow capacity is reached, and extramedullary erythropoiesis occurs, with fetal red-cell production in the fetal liver, spleen, kidney, adrenal glands, and intestine. Fetal hepatosplenomegaly is therefore common. Red cells produced at these sites are often immature, are nucleated, and appear in the circulation as erythroblasts. Hence the synonym erythroblastosis fetalis for immune hydrops.

The majority of cases of Rh isoimmunization lead to mild or moderate fetal or neonatal hemolytic disease. However, approximately 20 to 25% of cases result in severe hemolytic disease, with immune hydrops developing in utero (Bowman 1999). Hydrops develops in about half of these fetuses between 18 and 34 weeks of gestation, with hydrops developing in the remaining fetuses between 34 weeks and term. Hydrops most likely results from severe fetal anemia leading to extensive extramedullary erythropoiesis, with associated hepatosplenomegaly and distortion of intrahepatic architecture. This distortion results in portal and umbilical venous distortion, portal hypertension, placental edema, and placental hypoperfusion (Bowman 1999). With deteriorating hepatic synthesis, progressive hypoalbuminemia occurs, adding to the generalized edema, anasarca, and pleural and pericardial effusions. This complex mechanism leading to hydrops is probably more accurate than the theory that suggests simple congestive heart failure secondary to fetal anemia, and it also explains the inconsistent relationship that has been noted between the degree of fetal anemia and severity of hydrops (Bowman 1999).

Effective prevention programs to reduce the incidence of Rh(D) isoimmunization, using passive maternal immunization with Rh immunoglobulin, have significantly decreased the numbers of fetuses with immune hydrops. Because of the efficacy of these programs, non-Rh(D)-blood-group isoimmunization is becoming proportionately more frequent as a cause of immune hydrops. Immune hydrops secondary to ABO-blood-group incompatibility is extremely rare, as the resulting hemolytic disease is almost always mild in nature (Gilja and Shah 1988; Bowman 1999). Isoimmunization due to non-Rh(D) and non-ABO incompatibility usually occurs as a result of blood transfusions, with such atypical antibodies developing in 1 to 2% of recipients (Bowman 1999). At least 60 such atypical antibodies have been identified as potentially causing hemolytic disease of the fetus or newborn, with anti-c, anti-E, and anti-Kell antibodies being the most important causes of severe disease, including hydrops (Bowman 1990). Fetal anemia secondary to Kell isoimmunization differs from that due to Rh(D) isoimmunization, as the mechanism for anemia is most likely erythroid suppression rather than hemolysis (Vaughan et al. 1994).

▶ INCIDENCE

The risk of immune hydrops in a first Rh-sensitized pregnancy is approximately 8 to 10% (Bowman 1999). The incidence of immune hydrops has decreased significantly with the widespread use of passive immunization using Rh immunoglobulin for Rh-negative mothers at 28 weeks of gestation, following suspected fetomaternal hemorrhage, and postpartum following the delivery of an Rh-positive infant. The efficacy of this prevention program has been demonstrated by a decline in the incidence of Rh hemolytic disease of the fetus or newborn, from 65 in 10,000 births in the United States in 1960 to 10.6 in 10,000 births in 1990 (Chavez et al. 1991). The relative proportion of cases of immune hydrops secondary to non-Rh(D) atypical antibodies is increasing, as the use of Rh immunoglobulin has become widespread, with Kell isoimmunization now affecting 0.1% of all pregnancies (Caine and Mueller-Heubach 1986).

▶ SONOGRAPHIC FINDINGS

The diagnosis of hydrops is made following the detection of abnormal or increased fluid accumulation in at least two distinct fetal body cavities. Examples include pericardial effusion, pleural effusion, ascites, subcutaneous edema, cystic hygroma, polyhydramnios, and placental thickening. In general, skin thickness of at least 5 mm is required to diagnose subcutaneous edema, and a placental thickness of at least 6 cm is required to diagnose placentamegaly (Romero et al. 1988). These features do not necessarily indicate hydrops; it should be noted that skin thickening of at least 5 mm may be commonly seen in macrosomic fetuses. If abnormal fluid accumulation is confined to only one site, then the diagnosis of hydrops should not be used, and the case should be described simply in terms of the involved site, such as isolated ascites, or isolated pleural effusion.

Fetal ascites is diagnosed sonographically by the visualization of an echolucent rim encompassing the entire fetal abdomen in a transverse view. Loops of bowel and the outline of the fetal liver, spleen, bladder, and diaphragm are generally more easily seen in the presence of ascites. Pericardial effusion is diagnosed by the appearance of an echolucent rim at least 1 to 3 mm thick around both cardiac ventricles.

In general, fetal hydrops is not seen sonographically until the fetal hematocrit has fallen to below one third of its normal range. However, there is no direct relationship between actual fetal hemoglobin level and sonographic appearance or severity of hydrops. This reflects the fact that hydrops is not a result simply of high-output cardiac failure secondary to fetal anemia, but most likely reflects hepatic disruption, with the development of portal hypertension and hypoalbuminemia (Bowman 1999). The correlation between various sonographic findings and the degree of fetal anemia has been evaluated. No correlation has been found between the degree of fetal anemia and placental thickness or umbilical-vein diameter, and poor correlation has been found between fetal liver and spleen dimensions and the degree of anemia (Nicolaides et al. 1988; Roberts et al. 1989; Oepkes et al. 1993). The use of Doppler sonography to predict fetal anemia has been more successful. In one series of fetal blood sampling from 23 fetuses at risk for anemia, all anemic fetuses had a peak systolic velocity of the middle cerebral artery above the mean for gestational age (Mari et al. 1995). In another series, Doppler measurement of fetal aortic and umbilical venous flow was 90% accurate in predicting severe anemia in nonhydropic fetuses at risk (Oepkes et al. 1994). Therefore, such Doppler measurements may be useful for surveillance of hydropic fetuses following intrauterine transfusions to aid in the timing of repeat fetal blood sampling or transfusion.

▶ DIFFERENTIAL DIAGNOSIS

Following the sonographic diagnosis of hydrops, the first step is to differentiate between immune and nonimmune causes. This is easily accomplished by the performance of a maternal indirect Coombs test to screen for antibodies associated with blood-group incompatibility. Even if a maternal antibody that can be implicated in immune hydrops is detected, consideration should still be given in the differential diagnosis to the possibility of nonimmune hydrops. A detailed fetal sonographic survey of anatomy should be performed to exclude the presence of structural malformations that may also be associated with hydrops (see Chapter 128).

▶ ANTENATAL NATURAL HISTORY

No data are available on the antenatal natural history of immune hydrops managed expectantly. In general, the finding of fetal hydrops in a pregnancy complicated by Rh isoimmunization or other atypical antibodies is ominous. If left untreated, the fetus will rapidly become moribund and will most likely die in utero. Therefore, the finding of fetal hydrops in such at-risk pregnancies should be considered an emergency, and arrangements should be made promptly to either perform percutaneous umbilical blood sampling (PUBS) and possibly fetal transfusion, or immediate delivery, depending on the gestational age.

▶ MANAGEMENT OF PREGNANCY

Following the diagnosis of immune hydrops, the patient should be immediately referred to a tertiary-care center, with trained perinatologists to perform intrauterine transfusions and neonatologists to counsel parents and direct treatment of the newborn. A detailed sonographic fetal anatomy survey should be performed to quantify the severity of the hydrops and to rule out the presence of any additional structural malformations. In general, once immune hydrops has been diagnosed the prognosis for the fetus is guarded, and arrangements to perform PUBS and possible intrauterine fetal transfusion should be expedited as rapidly as possible. It should be noted, however, that this requires the assembly of an experienced multidisciplinary team, including perinatologists, sonographers, blood-bank personnel, hematology laboratory personnel, and nursing staff. The assembly of appropriate personnel can take time and is best expedited at a tertiary-care facility that has significant experience in performing fetal transfusions. If the gestational age is between 24 and 34 weeks, intramuscular betamethasone should be given to the mother to reduce the complications of prematurity in such high-risk pregnancies. If the gestational age is less than 24 weeks, the option of elective termination of the pregnancy should be discussed with the parents.

A maternal blood sample should be obtained immediately and sent to a blood bank for typing, antibody determination, and preparation of blood appropriate for fetal transfusion. The details of fetal transfusion for immune hydrops are described in the section on "Fetal Intervention." Following intrauterine transfusion, careful sonographic surveillance should be instituted, depending on the gestational age. Daily fetal testing with nonstress tests or biophysical profiles is reasonable for all potentially viable fetuses. Once there is sonographic evidence of resolution of hydrops, testing can be decreased to twice weekly. Sonographic surveillance for appropriate fetal growth should continue every 2 weeks.

Timing of delivery is variable with immune hydrops. If the fetus responds well to an initial intrauterine transfusion, repeat PUBS procedures should be scheduled at 1- to 3-week intervals, with repeat transfusions depending on changes in fetal hematocrit and the sonographic appearance of hydrops. The final PUBS is generally scheduled at 34 to 35 weeks of gestation; fetal lung maturity guides the timing of delivery. Such pregnancies should not be allowed progress beyond 37 to 38 weeks of gestation. If hydrops does not improve, or if fetal testing becomes nonreassuring despite correction of fetal anemia, premature delivery may be indicated, depending on the gestational age. It is possible that mature lecithin:sphingomyelin ratios may be obtained less frequently near term in fetuses with hydrops as compared with nonhydropic fetuses (Romero et al. 1988).

The optimal mode of delivery for the hydropic fetus is uncertain. Because of the risk of soft-tissue dystocia associated with hydrops, it is often considered safer to deliver all potentially viable fetuses with immune hydrops by cesarean section. This should minimize the chances of maternal and fetal trauma. However, there are no data to support routine cesarean delivery for immune hydrops as compared with cesarean delivery based on standard obstetric indications. A trial of labor may be reasonable in cases in which the fetal anemia has been adequately corrected, and in which the hydropic features improve. In carefully selected and monitored cases, up to 80% of fetuses with immune hydrops may successfully deliver vaginally (Bowman 1999). The optimal location of delivery should be a tertiary-care center, with the immediate availability of skilled neonatologists and other appropriate pediatric subspecialists.

▶ FETAL INTERVENTION

Immune hydrops is one of the few fetal abnormalities in which a well-established program of fetal intervention has been described. The ability to perform intrauterine fetal transfusions has revolutionized the management of Rh isoimmunization and has resulted in the survival of many fetuses that would otherwise have died from hydrops. The first step in fetal intervention for immune hydrops is to urgently schedule a PUBS procedure to document the fetal hematocrit and to perform potentially life-saving therapy.

In all cases of immune hydrops, appropriate blood for fetal transfusion should be available at the time of a scheduled PUBS procedure. The blood should be group O red cells, packed to a hematocrit of 85 to 90%, less than 4 days old, irradiated, anti-cytomegalovirus-negative, negative for the antigen to which the mother is immunized, and Kell-negative. If a previous PUBS has been performed, so that the fetal ABO blood group is known, and there is no maternal–fetal ABO incompatibility, red cells of the same ABO status as the fetus can be transfused (Bowman 1999). When the initial PUBS procedure is scheduled, appropriate blood should be available, and it should be used to prime a blood-transfusion set as the PUBS diagnostic test is being performed. This will allow for immediate transfusion as

soon as the initial fetal blood sample has been obtained, without the need to replace the needle.

The appropriate target for fetal intravascular transfusion will depend on the gestational age and fetal position. In general, the preferred target is the umbilical vein, at its placental insertion site. Sterile technique is used throughout. The mother is generally premedicated with a sedative and a prophylactic antibiotic, such as dicloxacillin. A 20-gauge spinal needle, of sufficient length to reach the target, is used to cannulate the umbilical vein under direct ultrasound guidance. The free return of blood confirms entry into the vein following removal of the needle stylet. A sample is drawn into a heparinized tuberculin syringe and sent to the hematology laboratory, which should be on standby to receive all such samples. The presence of fetal, as opposed to maternal, blood is confirmed by noting an elevated mean corpuscular volume, generally greater than 120 fl, or by alkaline denaturation. Fetal blood should also be measured for hematocrit, hemoglobin, platelet count, total bilirubin, blood type, and antibody screen. Fetal paralysis with pancuronium is generally not required in cases of hydrops, as fetal activity is often minimal. However, if fetal movement significant enough to dislodge needle access to the umbilical vein occurs, pancuronium can be injected directly into the fetal circulation.

Since the fetal hematocrit will invariably be less than 30% in cases of immune hydrops, the fetal transfusion can be started as soon as the initial fetal sample is obtained, while awaiting results of the hematocrit from the hematology laboratory. Once the initial fetal hematocrit result is available a calculation can be performed to estimate the volume of transfused blood needed to correct the fetal anemia. The volume of packed red cells to be transfused is derived using formulas that take into account the starting hematocrit, the hematocrit of transfused blood, the target hematocrit, and a correction factor for the volume of blood in the placental circulation. A commonly used formula for the volume of blood to be transfused is

$$V_T = \frac{(\text{desired final hematocrit} - \text{initial fetal hematocrit})}{(\text{donor blood hematocrit})} \times (150) \times (EFW)$$

where V_T is volume of blood transfused, 150 is a placental correction factor, and EFW is estimated fetal weight in kilograms (Kaufman and Paidas 1994).

It is generally not advised to transfuse a hydropic fetus to a final hematocrit that is either greater than 25% or greater than four times the initial hematocrit (Radunovic et al. 1992). This has been associated with fluid overload and sudden intrauterine fetal death. In cases of hydrops secondary to fetal anemia, the goal of the first intrauterine transfusion should be a hematocrit of 20 to 25%, and the transfusion should then be repeated in 48 to 72 hours to bring the final hematocrit to a level of 45 to 50%. Repeat procedures are then performed at 2- to 3-week intervals, with the last procedure being performed at 34 to 35 weeks of gestation.

Another therapeutic option for fetuses with immune hydrops is to perform a combined intravascular and intraperitoneal transfusion, with the intravascular aliquot of blood designed to provide an acute increase in fetal hematocrit and the intraperitoneal aliquot designed to provide a slower sustained increase in hematocrit. Intraperitoneal transfusion should rarely be considered an option for the hydropic fetus. If the fetus is moribund, and there is no evidence of fetal breathing, red cells placed in the intraperitoneal cavity will not be absorbed and will result in no benefit to the fetus. However, if an umbilical vessel cannot be cannulated for technical reasons, the option of intraperitoneal transfusion can be considered. If ascites is present, up to 150 ml of ascitic fluid should be drained prior to performing an intraperitoneal transfusion (Bowman 1999). This will minimize the chance of increasing the intraperitoneal pressure to a level greater than umbilical venous pressure. To do so would result in impaired return of blood to the fetal heart and subsequent fetal death. Another alternative for fetal transfusion in cases of hydrops, if an umbilical vessel cannot be cannulated, is to perform a direct fetal cardiac transfusion. However, this should be considered a method of last resort as it is associated with a significant risk of fetal death (Westgren et al. 1988).

▶ TREATMENT OF THE NEWBORN

Infants with hydrops should be delivered in a tertiary-care center, with immediate availability of a multidisciplinary neonatal resuscitation team. Most fetuses with immune hydrops should improve with successful intrauterine transfusions, so the degree of neonatal hydrops and anemia should also be improved. However, if hydrops fails to resolve with appropriate intrauterine therapy, the neonatal team should be prepared for a complex resuscitative effort. Immediate neonatal endotracheal intubation may be needed, and such intubations can be technically difficult (Carlton et al. 1989). A high-frequency ventilator and high airway-pressure settings may be needed to achieve adequate gas exchange. Paracentesis and thoracentesis, with placement of bilateral chest tubes, may also be needed to allow adequate ventilation and effective gas exchange. Placement of umbilical-artery and umbilical-vein lines may be needed to aid in the resuscitation (McMahan and Donovan 1995). Use of blood products, albumin, and diuretics may be needed to effectively maintain adequate intravascular volume without significant fluid overload or soft-tissue edema. If the neonate can be stabilized in the delivery room, transport to a neonatal intensive care unit should be arranged promptly.

Approximately 50% of neonates will require "top-up" transfusions in the neonatal intensive care unit (Saade et al. 1993). Infants should therefore be followed with weekly hematocrit and reticulocyte determinations for 4 to 6 weeks. This requirement for future transfusions may reflect persistent hypoplasia of the neonatal bone marrow, as well as the persistence of passively acquired IgG antibodies from the mother.

▶ SURGICAL TREATMENT

No surgical treatments have been described.

▶ LONG-TERM OUTCOME

Minimal data are available on the long-term follow-up of fetuses with immune hydrops. With advances in intrauterine therapy, more moribund fetuses are being rescued, and this has led to concerns regarding the long-term neurologic outcome for such infants. In one series of 38 fetuses who received intravascular transfusions for Rh isoimmunization, 35 (92%) were normal at 2 years of follow-up, and 3 had cerebral palsy, which was thought to be a result of prematurity (Doyle et al. 1993).

▶ GENETICS AND RECURRENCE RISK

The recurrence risk for immune hydrops is significant. In general, the more severe the obstetric history of Rh isoimmunization, the more likely the recurrence of severe disease in a future pregnancy. For an Rh-negative mother, if the father is homozygous for the Rh(D) allele, all of the offspring will be Rh-positive, and will therefore be at risk for severe hemolytic disease. If the father is heterozygous Rh-positive, then there is a 50:50 chance that the fetus will be Rh-positive. If the fetus is Rh-negative, the risk of hemolytic disease is zero. Preimplantation genetic diagnosis with biopsy of the eight-cell embryo is now available in cases of a heterozygous father, to predict the Rh status of a future fetus (Van den Veyver et al. 1995). However, this approach would obviously require the performance of in vitro fertilization in future pregnancies. Another less-invasive option is to perform a chorionic villus sampling or amniocentesis in future pregnancies with a heterozygous father, which would allow early prenatal diagnosis of fetal Rh and Kell status (Bennett et al. 1993).

If abnormal fluid accumulation is confined to only one site, then the diagnosis of hydrops should not be used, and the case should be described simply in terms of the involved site, such as isolated ascites or isolated pleural effusion. NIHF may initially present with an isolated fluid accumulation in one site, such as pleural effusion with congenital cystic adenomatoid malformation, but as intrathoracic pressure increases and venous return decreases, generalized hydrops may present.

Fetal ascites is diagnosed sonographically by the visualization of an echolucent rim encompassing the entire fetal abdomen in a transverse view (see Fig. 128-1). Loops of bowel and the outline of the fetal liver, spleen, bladder, and diaphragm are generally more easily seen in the presence of ascites. Pericardial effusion is diagnosed by the appearance of an echolucent rim of at least 1 to 3 mm thickness around both cardiac ventricles. Pleural effusion, which may be unilateral or bilateral, also presents as an echolucent space outlining the diaphragm.

Other sonographic features of NIHF will depend on the cause of the hydrops. A careful fetal anatomical survey, including fetal echocardiography, should be performed in all cases to detect any associated structural fetal malformations.

▶ DIFFERENTIAL DIAGNOSIS

Following the sonographic diagnosis of hydrops the first step is to differentiate between immune and nonimmune causes. This is easily accomplished by the performance of a maternal indirect Coombs test to screen for antibodies associated with blood-group incompatibility.

Following the exclusion of immune causes of hydrops, each condition listed in Table 128-1 should be considered when trying to determine the cause of NIHF. This is accomplished by a review of maternal and paternal histories, detailed fetal sonographic survey, and the use of appropriate diagnostic laboratory studies.

▶ ANTENATAL NATURAL HISTORY

The precise antenatal natural history of NIHF depends entirely on the underlying cause. The natural history of hydrops is poorly understood, so little information is available regarding prognostic factors to predict in utero progression. In general, NIHF is associated with a 75 to 90% fetal mortality rate (Romero et al. 1988). The progression of fetal signs and development reflects the underlying cause. Cases of NIHF secondary to fetal parvovirus B19 infection, for example, may result in intrauterine fetal death or may result in spontaneous resolution. By contrast, cases of NIHF associated with structural cardiac malformation almost always result in intrauterine fetal death or early neonatal death. No series are available for review describing sufficient cases of NIHF caused by each individual underlying cause, to enable accurate prediction of antenatal natural history.

▶ MANAGEMENT OF PREGNANCY

Following the sonographic detection of hydrops, the pregnant woman should be promptly referred to a tertiary-care facility, with availability of a multidisciplinary team consisting of perinatologists, neonatologists, clinical geneticists, and other pediatric subspecialists. Careful maternal and paternal histories should be obtained, to evaluate for possible health problems, family histories, or ethnic predisposition to any of the conditions listed in Table 128-1. Maternal blood work should include an indirect Coombs antibody screen, maternal blood type, Kleihauer–Betke stain, complete blood count with differential and erythrocyte indexes, hemoglobin electrophoresis, and glucose-6-phosphate dehydrogenase deficiency screen. Additional maternal blood work should include an evaluation for infectious diseases, including TORCH (toxoplasmosis, rubella, cytomegalovirus, and herpes simplex) titers, rapid plasma reagent test, and parvovirus B19 IgG and IgM titers.

A detailed fetal sonographic anatomy survey should be performed to evaluate for possible associated structural malformations. Because of the strong association between NIHF and cardiac malformations, fetal echocardiography should also be performed, with particular attention paid to possible fetal rhythm disturbances. Fetal heart-rate monitoring for 12 to 24 hours should be considered to rule out an underlying fetal arrhythmia.

Invasive testing for fetal karyotype should also be offered. This can be performed by means of amniocentesis, with the use of fluorescence in situ hybridization, to facilitate a rapid diagnosis of the common aneuploidies. However, for patients at 18 to 20 weeks of gestation or later, the preferred invasive diagnostic procedure is a fetal percutaneous umbilical blood sample (PUBS). The advantage of a PUBS is that it allows rapid determination of fetal karyotype, in addition to providing details of fetal hematocrit, platelet count, liver-function tests, hemoglobin electrophoresis, and fetal IgM specific to the various infectious causes of NIHF. In addition, it also allows the opportunity to transfuse the fetus with packed red cells immediately if profound fetal anemia is diagnosed. Amniotic fluid can be obtained at the same time as a PUBS, and may be sent for α-fetoprotein level (increased in Finnish nephrosis and sacrococcygeal teratoma), and polymerase chain reaction (PCR) testing for infectious agents. Metabolic testing can also be performed on amniotic fluid when a specific disorder is suspected.

Following the laboratory and sonographic evaluation, a diagnosis of idiopathic NIHF, or NIHF secondary to a specific condition, will be made. If a specific underlying cause has been discovered, patient counseling will be dictated by the particular abnormality. In general, the presence of hydrops together with a structural malformation, such as cardiac abnormality, is associated with a very poor prognosis. Counseling should therefore also include the possibility of elective pregnancy termination, depending on the gestational age at presentation. Patients should be counseled by a multidisciplinary team that includes a perinatologist, neonatologist, geneticist, and appropriate additional pediatric subspecialists. Options for fetal intervention to treat the underlying problem and hydrops are available and are discussed in the following section.

If expectant management of the fetus with NIHF is chosen, careful sonographic surveillance should be performed, including biophysical profiles on a frequent basis. The precise timing of fetal surveillance testing is uncertain and depends on the gestational age at presentation. If the fetus is considered viable, it may be reasonable to admit the mother and perform daily fetal testing with nonstress tests or biophysical profiles. If the hydrops appears to be resolving it would be reasonable to decrease the frequency of testing, provided that fetal testing has been reassuring to date. Repeat sonographic fetal anatomy surveys should be performed every 2 weeks to confirm appropriate fetal growth and to improve the chances of detecting an underlying structural fetal malformation.

Timing of delivery is also uncertain with NIHF. Depending on the gestational age, premature delivery may be indicated if fetal testing becomes nonreassuring. Otherwise, the most common practice is to continue expectant management until 37 weeks of gestation, or until fetal lung maturity has been confirmed by amniocentesis. It is possible that mature lecithin:sphingomyelin ratios may be less frequently obtained near term in the fetus with hydrops, as compared with nonhydropic fetuses (Romero et al. 1988). Expectant management may also be complicated by preeclampsia in up to 50% of cases, and this may necessitate immediate delivery. In addition, NIHF is frequently associated with polyhydramnios, which may precipitate preterm labor due to uterine overdistention. Periodic reduction amniocenteses may be required to prevent preterm labor and to relieve maternal discomfort from severe polyhydramnios.

The optimal mode of delivery for the hydropic fetus is uncertain, as the overall prognosis is poor regardless of the form of delivery. Because of the risk of soft-tissue dystocia associated with hydrops, it is generally advisable to deliver all potentially viable fetuses with NIHF by cesarean section. This should minimize the chances of maternal and fetal trauma. In cases in which the fetus is not expected to survive, the option of therapeutic thoracentesis or paracentesis to optimize a vaginal delivery is also reasonable. However, patients should be made aware of the extremely small likelihood of neonatal survival. The optimal location of delivery should be a tertiary-care center, with the immediate availability of skilled neonatologists and other appropriate pediatric subspecialists.

▶ FETAL INTERVENTION

The option of fetal therapy in select cases of NIHF is possible. The underlying pathology that is most amenable to prenatal therapy is fetal anemia. When a diagnostic PUBS is performed for any fetus with NIHF, immediately transfusion of packed red cells, if profound fetal anemia is diagnosed, should be available. Arrangements prior to performance of a PUBS in such cases should include preparation of group O, irradiated, packed red blood cells that are anticytomegalovirus-negative, Rh_o(D)-negative, Kell-negative, and cross-matched compatible with maternal serum. The unit of red cells should be tightly packed with a hematocrit of 85 to 90%, and a blood transfusion setup should be primed as the diagnostic PUBS is performed. This will ensure that prompt intravascular fetal transfusion can be performed as soon as a significant fetal anemia is diagnosed, and prior to withdrawal of the needle from the umbilical vein. Once a fetal hematocrit of less than 30% is detected, fetal intravascular transfusion should begin. Fetal paralysis with pancuronium is generally not required in cases of hydrops, as fetal activity is often minimal.

The volume of packed red cells to be transfused is derived using formulas that take into account the starting hematocrit, hematocrit of transfused blood, target hematocrit, and a correction factor for the volume of blood in the placental circulation. A commonly used formula for volume of blood to be transfused is

$$V_T = \frac{(\text{desired final hematocrit} - \text{initial fetal hematocrit})}{(\text{donor blood hematocrit})} \times (150) \times (EFW)$$

where V_T is volume of blood transfused, 150 is a placental correction factor, and EFW is the estimated fetal weight in kilograms (Kaufman and Paidas 1994). It is generally not advisable to transfuse a hydropic fetus to a final hematocrit that is either greater than 25% or greater than four times the initial hematocrit (Radunovic et al. 1992). This has been associated with fluid overload and sudden intrauterine fetal death. In cases of NIHF secondary to fetal anemia, the goal of the first intrauterine transfusion should be a hematocrit of 20 to 25%, and the transfusion should then be repeated in 48 to 72 hours to bring the final hematocrit to a level of 40 to 45%. For many fetuses with NIHF and anemia secondary to parvovirus B19 infection, this transfusion may be all that is needed to maintain a normal fetal hematocrit, as the initial insult to the fetal marrow is generally self-limiting. Another therapeutic option for fetuses with NIHF and anemia is to perform a combined intravascular and intraperitoneal transfusion, with the intravascular aliquot of blood designed to provide an acute increase in fetal hematocrit and the intraperitoneal aliquot designed to provide a slower sustained increase in hematocrit. To date there are no adequate series comparing these different approaches for the treatment of NIHF secondary to fetal anemia.

Other forms of fetal intervention for NIHF include medical therapy for the mother to correct fetal arrhythmias (see Chapters 44 and 54). Digoxin administration to pregnant women has been successful in the treatment of fetal arrhythmias, with resolution of hydrops in some cases (Knilans 1995).

Surgical treatment for the fetus with NIHF is also possible. Fetal thoracentesis may be performed under sonographic guidance with resolution of pleural effusions (Jones 1995). If repeat thoracenteses are needed, consideration should be given to placement of a thoracoamniotic shunt. Such procedures are likely to be beneficial only for cases of NIHF in which pleural effusions are secondary to intrinsic thoracic malformations. Other surgical procedures that can be considered for fetuses with NIHF and underlying structural malformations include open fetal surgical resection of thoracic masses or sacrococcygeal teratoma (Bullard and Harrison 1995). However, few data are available confirming whether such invasive approaches have a significant impact on fetal or neonatal outcome.

▶ TREATMENT OF THE NEWBORN

Infants with hydrops should be delivered in a tertiary-care center with immediate availability of a multidisciplinary neonatal resuscitation team. Immediate neonatal endotracheal intubation will almost certainly be needed, and such intubations can be technically difficult (Carlton et al. 1989). A high-frequency ventilator and high airway-pressure settings may be needed to achieve adequate gas exchange. Paracentesis and thoracentesis, with placement of bilateral chest tubes, may also be needed to allow adequate ventilation and effective gas exchange. Placement of umbilical-artery and umbilical-vein lines may be needed to aid in the resuscitation (McMahan and Donovan 1995). Use of blood products, albumin, and diuretics may be needed to effectively maintain adequate intravascular volume without significant fluid overload or soft-tissue edema.

If the neonate can be stabilized in the delivery room, transport to a neonatal intensive care unit should be arranged promptly. This should be followed by a thorough physical examination, with the aid of appropriate radiologic investigations and echocardiography, to confirm absence of significant structural malformation. If additional structural malformations are detected, specific therapy should be tailored to the individual abnormalities. Appropriate pediatric subspecialist consultation, including a clinical geneticist, should also be arranged.

▶ SURGICAL TREATMENT

Possible surgical treatments for fetal hydrops include fetal thoracoamniotic shunt placement for cases of NIHF associated with thoracic masses or persistent pleural effusions. Open fetal surgical resection of thoracic masses, such as congenital cystic adenomatoid malformation and bronchopulmonary sequestration, are also possible (Bullard and Harrison 1995). Open surgical resection of fetal sacrococcygeal teratoma with associated hydrops is also possible, although there are so few cases that it is currently difficult to evaluate the role of such invasive procedures.

▶ LONG-TERM OUTCOME

The prognosis for infants with hydrops depends entirely on the nature of any underlying abnormalities. The perinatal mortality rate ranges from 40 to 90%, depending on the cause, but may approach 100% in cases of NIHF associated with structural cardiac malformations (Jones 1995; Romero et al. 1988; Wilkins 1999). No long-term studies are available for counseling parents on the likely survival or morbidity if a successful neonatal resuscitation is achieved.

▶ GENETICS AND RECURRENCE RISK

A postmortem examination is indicated in all cases of NIHF that result in fetal or neonatal death. This will maximize the number of cases in which a definite underlying cause is identified and will facilitate appropriate genetic counseling and prediction of recurrence risk (Steiner 1995). Recurrence of idiopathic NIHF is rare, although case series of recurrences have been documented (Wilkins 1999). In one case series, one mother had three consecutive pregnancies complicated by recurrent idiopathic NIHF and another had two consecutive pregnancies complicated by recurrent idiopathic NIHF (Onwude et al. 1992). Patients should therefore be made aware that, while idiopathic NIHF is extremely rare, recurrences can and do occur.

REFERENCES

Arcasoy MO, Gallagher PG. Hematologic disorders and nonimmune hydrops fetalis. Semin Perinatol 1995;19:502–515.

Barron SD, Pass RF. Infectious causes of hydrops fetalis. Semin Perinatol 1995;19:493–501.

Bullard KM, Harrison MR. Before the horse is out of the barn: fetal surgery for hydrops. Semin Perinatol 1995;19:462–473.

Carbillon L, Oury JF, Guerin JM, et al. Clinical biological features of Ballantyne syndrome and the role of placental hydrops. Obstet Gynecol Surv 1997;52:310–314.

Carlton DP, McGillivray BC, Schreiber MD. Nonimmune hydrops fetalis: a multidisciplinary approach. Clin Perinatol 1989;16:839–851.

Crawford DC, Chita SK, Allan LD. Prenatal detection of congenital heart disease: factors affecting obstetric management and survival. Am J Obstet Gynecol 1988;159:352–356.

Holzgreve W, Curry CJ, Golbus MS, et al. Investigation of nonimmune hydrops fetalis. Am J Obstet Gynecol 1984;150:805–812.

Holzgreve W, Holzgreve B, Curry CJ. Nonimmune hydrops fetalis: diagnosis and management. Semin Perinatol 1985;9:52–57.

Jauniaux E, Van Maldergem L, De Munter C, et al. Nonimmune hydrops fetalis associated with genetic abnormalities. Obstet Gynecol 1990;75:568–572.

Jones DC. Nonimmune fetal hydrops: diagnosis and obstetrical management. Semin Perinatol 1995;19:447–461.

Kaufman GE, Paidas MJ. Rhesus sensitization and alloimmune thrombocytopenia. Semin Perinatol 1994;18:333–349.

Knilans TK. Cardiac abnormalities associated with hydrops fetalis. Semin Perinatol 1995;19:483–492.

Levy R, Weissman A, Blomberg G, et al. Infection by parvovirus B19 during pregnancy: a review. Obstet Gynecol Surv 1997;52:254–259.

McMahan MJ, Donovan EF. The delivery room resuscitation of the hydropic neonate. Semin Perinatol 1995;19:474–482.

Morey AL, Nicolini U, Welch CR, et al. Parvovirus B19 infection and transient fetal hydrops. Lancet 1991;337:496.

Norton ME. Nonimmune hydrops fetalis. Semin Perinatol 1994;18:321–332.

Onwude JL, Thornton JG, Mueller RH. Recurrent idiopathic non-immunologic hydrops fetalis: a report of two families, with three and two affected siblings. Br J Obstet Gynaecol 1992;99:854–856.

Radunovic N, Lockwood CJ, Alvarez M, et al. The severely anemic and hydropic isoimmune fetus: changes in fetal hematocrit associated with intrauterine death. Obstet Gynecol 1992;79:390–393.

Romero R, Pilu G, Jeanty P, et al. Nonimmune hydrops fetalis. In: Romero R, Pilu G, Jeanty P, Ghidini A, Hobbins JC, eds. Prenatal diagnosis of congenital anomalies. Norwalk, CT: Appleton & Lange, 1988:414–426.

Santolaya J, Alley D, Jaffe R, et al. Antenatal classifications of hydrops fetalis. Obstet Gynecol 1992;79:256–259.

Steiner RD. Hydrops fetalis: role of the geneticist. Semin Perinatol 1995;19:516–524.

Wilkins I. Nonimmune hydrops. In: Creasy RK, Resnik R, eds. Maternal-fetal medicine. 4th ed. Philadelphia: Saunders, 1999:769–782.

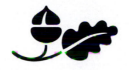

PART III

*Management of
Fetal Chromosomal
Abnormalities*

CHAPTER 129

47,XXY Karyotype (Klinefelter Syndrome)

► CONDITION

Klinefelter syndrome (47,XXY karyotype) is the spectrum of phenotypic features resulting from a sex chromosome complement that includes two or more X chromosomes and one Y chromosome (Fig. 129-1). It results from meiotic nondisjunction occurring during gametogenesis of the egg or sperm with subsequent fertilization of an XX ovum by a Y-bearing sperm, or fertilization of an X ovum by a sperm bearing both the X and Y chromosomes (Mandoki et al. 1991). There are no known predisposing factors except advanced maternal age in some, but not all, cases. The condition was first described in nine men with gynecomastia, infertility with normal Leydig cells, a normal to low 17-ketosteroid level, and a high follicle-stimulating–hormone level in the urine (Klinefelter et al. 1942; Schwartz and Root 1991). It was not until 1956 that the chromosomal basis of this abnormality was appreciated by noting the presence of the Barr body on buccal smears obtained from

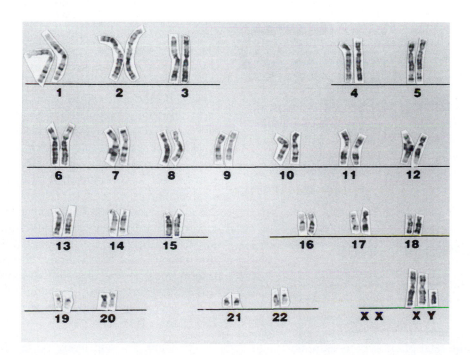

Figure 129-1. Karyotype obtained from a patient with Klinefelter syndrome, demonstrating presence of two X and one Y chromosomes. *(Courtesy of Dr. Janet Cowan.)*

affected patients, which represented the inactive extra X chromosome (Arens et al. 1988). The specific chromosomal abnormality reponsible for the disorder was not known until 1959.

The phenotype in Klinefelter syndrome is extremely variable and may be subtle. In general, affected males are identified by age-related clinical concerns. Infant patients are identified by either prenatal cytogenetic testing for advanced maternal age or by the presence of mild genital abnormalities (Schwartz and Root 1991). During school-age years, affected patients may be identified by the occurrence of learning disabilities and behavioral problems, whereas in adolescence, the clinical diagnosis is usually suspected from gynecomastia, a taller than average stature, and a possible delay in pubertal development. However, a large number of patients with Klinefelter syndrome are identified as married adults when they present during a workup for infertility (Schwartz and Root 1991).

▶ INCIDENCE

A study of 34,910 newborns performed over 13 years in Arhus, Denmark, put the incidence of Klinefelter syndrome at 1 in 576 newborn male infants (Nielsen and Wohlert 1991). 47,XXY is generally described as occurring in 1 in 500 to 1 in 800 live male births (Mandoki et al. 1991). Other variants of Klinefelter syndrome include the karyotypes 48,XXXY, which occurs in 1 in 20,000 live male births, and the karyotype 49,XXXY, which occurs in 1 in 85,000 live male births (Kleczkowska et al. 1988). For a review of the more severe clinical manifestations of 48,XXXY, the reader is referred to a study by Linden et al. (1995). In the variant Klinefelter karyotypes, it has been shown that a single parent contributes all of the extra chromosomes present.

The incidence of 47,XXY is increased in twins. In one large study of fetal karyotypes obtained at amniocentesis performed primarily for advanced maternal age, 2 cases of 47,XXY were seen in 1821 singleton fetuses. Three cases of 47,XXY were seen in 21 pairs of twins, giving an incidence of 7.1% in the twin population (Flannery et al. 1984).

▶ SONOGRAPHIC FINDINGS

No sonographic findings are characteristic for a fetus with Klinefelter syndrome. In a review of 35 cases of fetal omphalocele, one fetus had a 47,XXY karyotype, but this is probably unrelated (Gilbert and Nicolaides 1987). In general, the fetal phenotype is extremely mild and difficult to distinguish from normal.

▶ ANTENATAL NATURAL HISTORY

In cases of 47,XXY, the phenotype is not distinctly recognizable, even in fetuses studied at autopsy. In one pregnancy terminated at 20 weeks of gestation, the clinical features of Klinefelter syndrome noted in the fetus included an arm span less than its height, a minor ear abnormality, fifth-finger clinodactyly, and undescended testes (which is not unusual for a fetus at this point in gestation). Significantly, the testicular histology was normal (Flannery et al. 1984).

▶ MANAGEMENT OF PREGNANCY

Fetuses with Klinefelter syndrome are most commonly identified during amniocentesis performed for advanced maternal age, where it is the third most common chromosomal abnormality diagnosed, after trisomies 21 and 18 (Robinson et al. 1992). It is unlikely that an affected fetus will be identified on the basis of an abnormal sonographic finding. Occasionally, Klinefelter syndrome is associated with abnormalities in maternal serum screening. Reported maternal serum abnormalities include elevated levels of α-fetoprotein (Fejgin et al. 1990) and human chorionic gonadatropin (hCG) (Barnes-Kedar et al. 1993; Ben-Neriah et al. 1991).

The main concern regarding management of pregnancy is the parental decision whether to continue or terminate the pregnancy (see "Long-Term Outcome"). One of the difficulties in this area has been the ascertainment bias that exists in the medical literature, over-reporting of the more extreme phenotypic aspects of Klinefelter syndrome, and underreporting of patients who have few or no symptoms related to the condition. More recently, information has been gathered regarding developmental outcome for children who have been prenatally diagnosed with 47,XXY, and this information suggests a more considerable variability in physical and psychologic development (Robinson et al. 1992). Approximately 30 to 55% of well-informed couples opt to continue their pregnancy after an antenatal diagnosis of 47,XXY (Holmes-Siedle et al. 1987; Lancet editorial 1988; Robinson et al. 1992). More recent studies indicate that following comprehensive genetic counseling, as many as 87% of pregnancies affected by a sex chromosome abnormality are carried to term (Meschede et al. 1998). Robinson and colleagues (1992) suggest that the following information be given to prospective parents during prenatal counseling for a fetal diagnosis of 47,XXY:

1. Their son will likely be tall but phenotypically normal.

2. Puberty is usually entered normally, but testosterone supplementation therapy may be desirable after midadolescence.
3. Their son will be infertile.
4. Their son will be at risk for gynecomastia, but this will most likely be mild.
5. Their son will belong to a group of children who are at risk for developmental problems and delays in speech and neuromotor and learning abilities.
6. Due to some of the language issues, boys with 47,XXY may be shy and insecure.

However, these investigators write that a stable, nurturing, and stimulating environment will considerably enhance developmental outcome (Robinson et al. 1992).

In cases of 46,XY/47,XXY mosaicism, the prognosis is better than for the nonmosiac karyotype, with fewer developmental abnormalities and possible fertility (Robinson et al. 1992).

If the decision is made to continue the pregnancy, there is no need for a particular route of delivery. Arrangements should be made to have the parents discuss the prenatal finding of 47,XXY with a medical geneticist.

▶ FETAL INTERVENTION

There are no fetal interventions for 47,XXY.

▶ TREATMENT OF THE NEWBORN

Most newborn male infants with 47,XXY not ascertained by prenatal chromosome analysis will be missed during the neonatal period. In general, findings are normal on physical examination, although the incidence of minor congenital abnormalities may be increased as compared with siblings (Mandoki et al. 1991). Newborns with Klinefelter syndrome may have minor abnormalities of the genitalia, including cryptorchidism and hypospadias (Kleczkowska et al. 1988). A minority of infants with 47,XXY have a small penis, but penile growth occurs with local systemic testosterone treatment (Ratcliffe 1999). The mean birth weight and height for affected newborns falls well within the range of normal, although the head circumference may be and remain slightly on the small side (Ratcliffe 1999). A complete physical examination is necessary to ascertain the presence of additional congenital anomalies, but otherwise there is no indication for specific treatment during the newborn period. Exogenous testosterone therapy should not begin until around 11 to 12 years of age (Winter 1991).

▶ SURGICAL TREATMENT

Gynecomastia may be treated surgically in adolescence or adulthood. The other symptoms of Klinefelter syndrome do not require surgical treatment.

▶ LONG-TERM OUTCOME

Adult individuals with 47,XXY have a moderate increase in stature due to excessive growth of the lower extremities, resulting in a height that is greater than or equal to the arm span (Schwartz and Root 1991). The mean adult height for men with 47,XXY is at the 75th percentile (Lancet editorial 1988).

Most males enter puberty normally. Basal serum gonadotropins and response to gonadotropin-releasing hormone are normal until 12 years of age, when they rapidly elevate to reach uniformly hypergonadotropic values by age 14 (Winter 1991). With the onset of puberty, there is an initial increase in testicular volume, but during this time the seminiferous tubules undergo irregular progressive hyalinization and fibrosis, which restricts further growth beyond 2.5 cm (Rutgers 1991; Schwartz and Root 1991; Winter 1991). Patients with nonmosaic Klinefelter syndrome are invariably infertile. In a large review of 544 Belgian 47,XXY males diagnosed between 1966 and 1987, the majority (397) of affected patients were adults who were diagnosed only by an infertility workup performed for azoospermia (Kleczkowska et al. 1988). Pregnancy was achieved in the spouses of affected men by donor insemination. There is no increase in homosexual preference in males with 47,XXY (Ratcliffe 1999). Reports are appearing in the literature that indicate that successful pregnancies in the partners of affected men can also be achieved by testicular fine needle aspiration, intracytoplasmic sperm injection, and preimplatation genetic diagnosis (Reubinoff et al. 1998).

Adult men with Klinefelter syndrome demonstrate persistently low circulating testosterone and dihydrotestosterone levels, together with normal or elevated estradiol levels (Hsueh et al. 1978; Winter 1991). The increased ratio of estradiol to testosterone may play a role in the development of gynecomastia, a condition that affects 30% of XXY males (Winter 1991). Gynecomastia often regresses spontaneously, and cosmetic surgery is rarely requested (Lancet editorial 1988).

Prospective parents facing a fetal diagnosis of 47,XXY are frequently most concerned regarding the implications for developmental outcome. Individuals with 47,XXY have, in general, average to above average intelligence. In one study, 18.7% of affected individuals had an IQ of less than 90, but the scores were lowered by verbal deficits (Mandoki et al. 1991). It is now appreciated that 47,XXY males have difficulties with language production more than language comprehension (Graham et al. 1988). They may have delayed speech development, poor short-term auditory memory, and difficulties with reading and spelling (Graham et al. 1988; Lancet editorial 1988; Ratcliffe, 1999). It is recommended that special attention be paid to language development in affected males and that early referral to a speech therapist be considered. The neurocognitive problems seen are not unique to 47,XXY individuals and management is the same as that for individuals with language problems and normal chromosomes. Less than 4% of 47,XXY males are considered mildly to moderately retarded (Kleczkowska et al. 1988). The overwhelming majority of the adult patients reported in the long-term Belgian study were employed and had a normal work life, and 43% were married (Kleczkowska et al. 1988). Reports of unusual behavior such as arson are considered to be atypical due to ascertainment bias (Miller and Sulkes 1988). In a 20-year follow-up of 47,XXY males, considerable improvement in mental health, working capacity, social adjustment, and activity level was noted between the ages of 27 and 37 years (Nielsen and Pelsen 1987).

Testosterone therapy, beginning in adolescence, improves concentration, mood, social interaction, and libido and prevents osteoporosis, autoimmune disease, and the development of gynecomastia and a eunuchoid body habitus (Winter 1991).

The incidence of breast cancer is 9 in 1000 affected individuals (Evans and Crichlow 1987; Rutgers 1991). In one study of 93 males with breast cancer, 7 had 47,XXY, as ascertained by FISH analysis of surgically removed lymph nodes. This represents a 50-fold increased risk above the normal male population (Hultborn et al. 1997). 47,XXY males also have an increased risk for the development of extragonadal germ-cell tumors, including mediastinal teratocarcinoma, choriocarcinoma, and cerebral germinoma (Arens et al. 1988; Hasle et al. 1992; Rutgers 1991). It is hypothesized that these midline tumors develop in 47,XXY males because of an alteration in testicular gonadal ridge differentiation, which subsequently leads to abnormal migration of primordial germ cells from the yolk sac. Instead of advancing toward the gonads, these germ cells migrate caudally along the midline, and may undergo malignant transformation when they settle in a nonphysiologic location (Arens et al. 1988; Rutgers 1991).

▶ GENETICS AND RECURRENCE RISK

Klinefelter syndrome is due to nondisjunction occurring during meiosis. Counseling about recurrence risk should incorporate consideration of maternal age, although 50% of cases are paternal in origin. Females known to be carriers of the fragile X mutation have an increased tendency toward nondisjunction of the affected X chromosome. The incidence of the simultaneous occurrence of XXY and fragile X is 1 in 153 males with the XXY karyotype (Kleczkowska et al. 1988).

The prenatal origin of the extra X chromosome was assessed using 26 DNA probes that detected X-chromosome restriction-site polymorphisms in a total of 111 47,XXY individuals (Harvey et al. 1991). In 61 XXY males ascertained by large-scale newborn cytogenetic surveys, 27 (44%) were paternal and 34 (56%) were maternal in origin. In 41 XXY males who presented with clinical features of Klinefelter syndrome, 171 (41%) were maternal and 22 (54%) were paternal in origin. Of a group of 9 cases ascertained by amniocentesis for advanced maternal age, 4 (44%) were maternal, 4 (44%) were paternal, and 1 was unknown in origin (Harvey et al. 1991). Thirty-nine of the maternally derived cases were studied to determine the source of the nondisjunctional error. In 78% of cases it occurred during meiosis I and in 22% of cases it occurred during meiosis II. In another study, the origin of the X chromosome in 41 paternally derived cases of 47,XXY was studied using six different polymorphic genetic loci. Most cases of paternal origin were shown to result from meioses in which the X and Y chromosomes failed to recombine (Hassold and Sherman 1993).

Prenatal cytogenetic diagnosis by amniocentesis or chorionic villus sampling is recommended in subsequent pregnancies.

REFERENCES

Arens R, Marcus D, Engleberg S, Findler G, Goodman RM, Passwell JH. Cerebral germinomas and Klinefelter syndrome: a review. Cancer 1988;61:1228–1231.

Barnes-Kedar I, Amiel A, Maor O, Fejgin M. Elevated human chorionic gonadotropin levels in pregnancies with sex chromosome abnormalities. Am J Med Genet 1993;45:356–357.

Ben-Neriah Z, Anteby E, Zelikoviz B, Bach G. Increased maternal serum human chorionic gonadotropin level associated with Klinefelter's syndrome. Prenat Diagn 1991;11:923–924.

Evans DB, Crichlow RW. Carcinoma of the male breast and Klinefelter's syndrome: is there an association? CA Cancer J Clin 1987;37:246–251.

Fejgin M, Zeitune M, Amiel A, Beyth Y. Elevated maternal serum alpha-fetoprotein level and sex chromosome aneuploidy. Prenat Diagn 1990;10:414–416.

Flannery DB, Brown JA, Redwine FO, Winter P, Nance WE. Antenatally detected Klinefelter's syndrome in twins. Acta Genet Med Gemellol 1984;33:51–56.

Gilbert WM, Nicolaides KH. Fetal omphalocele: associated malformations and chromosomal defects. Obstet Gynecol 1987;70:633–635.

Graham JM, Bashir AS, Stark RE, Silbert A, Walzer S. Oral and written language abilities of XXY boys: implications for anticipatory guidance. Pediatrics 1988;81:795–806.

Harvey J, Jacobs PA, Hassold T, Pettay D. The parental origin of 47,XXY males. Birth Defects 1991;26:289–296.

Hasle H, Jacobsen BB, Asschenfeldt P, Andersen K. Mediastinal germ cell tumour associated with Klinefelter syndrome: a report of case and review of the literature. Eur J Pediatr 1992;151:735–739.

Hassold T, Sherman S. The origin of non-disjunction in humans. Chromosomes Today 1993;11:313–322.

Holmes-Siedle M, Ryyanen M, Lindenbaum RH. Parental decisions regarding termination of pregnancy following prenatal detection of a sex chromosome abnormality. Prenat Diagn 1987;7:239–244.

Hsueh WA, Hsu TH, Federman DD. Endocrine features of Klinefelter's syndrome. Medicine (Baltimore) 1978;57:447–461.

Hultborn R, Hanson C, Kopf I, Verbiene I, Warnhammar E, Weimarck A. Prevalence of Klinefelter's syndrome in male breast cancer patients. Anticancer Res 1997;17:4293–4297.

Kleczkowska A, Fryns JP, Van den Berghe H. X chromosome polysomy in the male: the Leuven experience 1966–1987. Hum Genet 1988;80:16–22.

Klinefelter HF Jr, Reifenstein EC Jr, Albright F. Syndrome characterized by gynecomastia, spermatogenesis without a-leydigism and increased excretion of follicle stimulating hormone. J Clin Endocrinol Metabol 1942;2:615–627.

Lancet editorial . Klinefelter's syndrome. Lancet 1988;1:1316–1317.

Linden MG, Bender BG, Robinson A. Sex chromosome tetrasomy and pentasomy. Pediatrics 1995;96:672–682.

Mandoki MW, Sumner GS, Hoffman RP, Riconda DL. A review of Klinefelter's syndrome in children and adolescents. J Am Acad Child Adolesc Pyschiatry 1991;30:167–172.

Meschede D, Lourwen F, Nippert I, Holzgreve W, Miny P, Horst J. Low rates of pregnancy termination for prenatally diagnosed Klinefelter syndrome and other sex chromosome polysomies. Am J Med Genet 1998;80:330–334.

Miller ME, Sulkes S. Fire-setting behavior in individuals with Klinefelter syndrome. Pediatrics 1988;82:115–117.

Nielsen J, Pelsen B. Follow-up 20 years later of 34 Klinefelter males with karyotype 47,XXY and 16 hypogonadal males with karyotype 46,XY. Hum Genet 1987;77:188–192.

Nielsen J, Wohlert M. Sex chromosome abnormalities found among 34,910 newborn children: results from a 13 year incidence study in Arhus, Denmark. Birth Defects 1991;26:209–223.

Ratclifffe S. Long-term outcome in children of sex chromosome abnormalities. Arch Dis Child 1999;80:192–195.

Reubinoff BE, Abeliovich D, Werner M, Schenker JG, Safran A, Lewin A. A birth in non-mosaic Klinefelter's syndrome after testicular fine needle aspiration, intracytoplasmic sperm injection and preimplantation genetic diagnosis. Hum Reprod 1998;13:1887–1892.

Robinson A, Bender BG, Linden MG. Prenatal diagnosis of sex chromosome abnormalities. In: Milunksy A, ed. Genetic disorders and the fetus. 3rd ed. Baltimore: John Hopkins University Press, 1992:211–239.

Rutgers JL. Advances in the pathology of intersex conditions. Hum Pathol 1991;22:884–891.

Schwartz ID, Root AW. The Klinefelter syndrome of testicular dysgenesis. Endocrinol Metab Clin North Am 1991;20:153–163.

Winter JS. Androgen therapy in Klinefelter syndrome during adolescence. Birth Defects 1991;26:235–245.

CHAPTER 130

Tetrasomy 12p (Pallister–Killian Syndrome)

► CONDITION

Tetrasomy 12p is a multiple congenital anomaly syndrome characterized by the tissue-specific presence of a marker chromosome in fibroblasts, but not lymphocytes, of affected patients. The clinical symptoms associated with this condition were first recognized in 1977, when Pallister described two adults, aged 19 and 37, who had profound retardation, severe hypotonia, coarse facial features, and pigmentary abnormalities. Both of these patients had an extra chromosome that was identified as a probable isochromosome of the short arm of chromosome 12 (Pallister et al. 1977). Independently, Teschler-Nicola and Killian reported a 3-year-old with severe mental retardation, dysmorphic facies, and sparse, dystrophic hair (Teschler-Nicola and Killian 1981). Buyse and Korf (1983) were the first to suggest that these two seemingly disparate clinical presentations actually represented different manifestations of the same syndrome. The discrepancy between the two was explained by the fact that the isochromosome 12p was demonstrable in fibroblasts but not lymphocytes from affected patients. The interesting and unique aspect of this syndrome is that mosaicism exists for the chromosomal abnormality, and diagnosis usually depends on performing a chromosome analysis on amniocytes or fibroblasts from a skin biopsy.

From the prenatal perspective, tetrasomy 12p is usually diagnosed in one of two ways: either it is a karyotype abnormality found at amniocentesis performed for advanced maternal age or it is detected when karyotyping is performed because fetal anomalies have been detected on sonography (Wilson et al. 1994). Advanced maternal age is known to be a risk factor for the development of the isochromosome 12p (Wenger et al. 1988). In a review of 30 case reports of Pallister–Killian syndrome, Wenger et al. (1988) found that the average age of the mothers of affected patients was 30 years. These authors suggested that the isochromosome 12p resulted from an abnormal division of the centromere that occurred during the first maternal meiotic division. The abnormal extra isochromosome is progressively lost in vivo during embryogenesis and in vitro during tissue culture. This hypothesis has now been proven in at least one case using molecular markers (Cormier-Daire et al. 1997).

Definitive diagnosis of tetrasomy 12p is made by karyotyping (Fig. 130-1). The extra chromosome in this syndrome was originally thought to be derived from the long arm of chromosome 21 based on similarities in the cytogenetic banding patterns between the short arm of chromosome 12 and the long arm of chromosome 21 (Zhang et al. 1989). Definitive identification of the marker chromosome as 12p was initially based on the twice-normal expression of the lactate dehydrogenase-B (LDH-B) isoenzyme, whose gene maps to chromosome 12. Normal levels of superoxide dismutase 1 (SOD-1), which maps to chromosome 21, ruled out an increased dosage effect from extra copies of chromosome 21 (Gilgenkrantz et al. 1985). More recently, fluorescence in situ hybridization (FISH) studies using DNA markers specific to the short arm of chromosome 12 have definitively identified the marker chromosome as the short arm of chromosome 12 (Butler and Dev 1995; Ohashi et al. 1993; Larramendy et al. 1993; Tejuda et al. 1992). The accurate detection of the isochromosome 12p is affected by the tissue type studied, the patient's age (fetal versus infant versus adult) and the in vitro age of the cells (Priest et al. 1992). Peripheral blood lymphocytes are continually dividing, and it has been hypothesized that

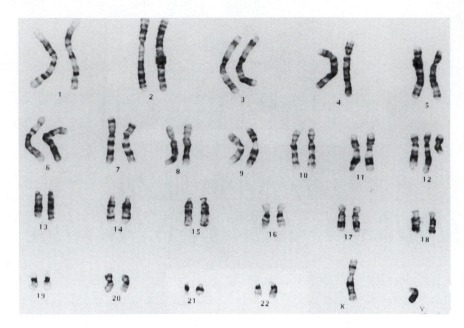

Figure 130-1. Karyotype obtained from amniocytes in an affected fetus with Pallister–Killian syndrome. Note the presence of an extra chromosome next to the normal chromosome 12 pair. *(Courtesy of Dr. Janet Cowan.)*

they lose the extra chromosome with their frequent divisions. In contrast, fibroblasts obtained from a skin biopsy normally cycle less frequently. In addition, a time-dependent in vitro selection occurs against cells that contain the isochromosome. In one study, the percentage of cells containing the marker went from 100% to 20% after only five passages in tissue culture (Speleman et al. 1991). Detection of the isochromosome 12p may be difficult in peripheral blood lymphocytes, although the marker has been seen in bone marrow aspirates obtained from newborns (Ward et al. 1988). Several authors have suggested the use of FISH analysis to detect the presence of the extra chromosome 12 short-arm interphase nuclei as opposed to metaphase chromosomes (Laramendy et al. 1993; Reeser and Wenger 1992).

▶ INCIDENCE

The incidence of Pallister–Killian syndrome or tetrasomy 12p is unknown. Tetrasomy 12p is the most frequent autosomal tetrasomy in humans (Bresson et al. 1991). The disorder is being increasingly recognized in clinical medicine.

▶ SONOGRAPHIC FINDINGS

The sonographic findings for fetuses with tetrasomy 12p are summarized in Table 130-1. The most consistent prenatal findings include polyhydramnios, short femurs, and diaphragmatic hernia (Fig. 130-2) (Priest et al. 1992;

Wilson et al. 1994). Wilson and colleagues reviewed 15 cases of tetrasomy 12p diagnosed prenatally. In six of the cases that were ascertained by amniocentesis performed for advanced maternal age, only one had fetal anomalies detected between 16 and 18 weeks of gestation. In the cases that were ascertained by the presence of fetal structural anomalies, the gestational age was more advanced, between 16 and 32 weeks (Wilson et al. 1994). The extensive range of sonographic findings described varies from normal to a large diaphragmatic hernia with shift of the heart to right side of the chest (see Chapter 38). Additional sonographic findings reported include congenital heart disease (Wilson et al. 1994) and increased cisterna magna, suggesting agenesis of the vermis or cerebellar hypoplasia (Gilgenkrantz et al. 1985; McLean et al. 1992). An additional clinical finding in fetuses with Pallister–Killian syndrome is

▶ TABLE 130-1. SONOGRAPHIC FINDINGS REPORTED IN TETRASOMY 12P

Dilated cisterna magna
Frontal bossing
Hypertelorism
Excess nuchal skin
Rhizomelic limb shortening
Postaxial polydactyly
Congenital heart disease
Diaphragmatic hernia
Cystic/dysplastic kidneys

Source: Wilson RD, Harrison K, Clarke LA, Yang SL. Tetrasomy 12p (Pallister-Killian syndrome): ultrasound indicators and confirmation by interphase FISH. Prenat Diagn 1994;14:787–792.

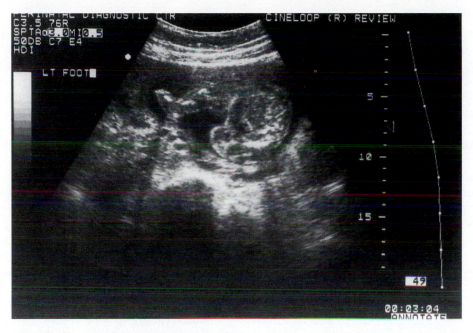

Figure 130-2. Prenatal sonographic image from a fetus with tetrasomy 12p demonstrating a shortened lower extremity.

hypertelorism. Many fetuses with tetrasomy 12p also have nuchal edema or other hydropic changes (Fig. 130-3).

▶ DIFFERENTIAL DIAGNOSIS

When isochromosome 12p is detected on an amniocentesis, it is diagnostic for Pallister–Killian syndrome.

In the setting of an unknown marker chromosome with the presence of fetal anomalies, the possible diagnosis of tetrasomy 12p must be considered. It can be confirmed with the FISH technique using chromosome-specific probes for the short arm of chromosome 12 (Mowery-Rushton et al. 1997). In the setting of a fetus with sonographic anomalies suggestive of Pallister–Killian syndrome, the differential diagnosis should also

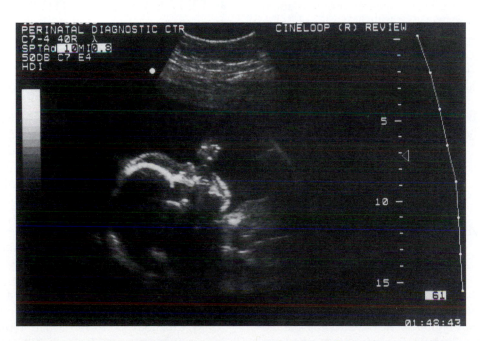

Figure 130-3. Prenatal sonographic image from the same fetus shown in Figure 130-2, demonstrating the fetal face in profile. Note the presence of frontal bossing and subcutaneous edema.

include Fryns syndrome. Both Pallister–Killian and Fryns syndromes should be considered when a prenatal diagnosis of congenital diaphragmatic hernia is made (see Chapter 38).

Fryns syndrome is a lethal condition inherited in an autosomal recessive pattern. Characteristic clinical findings during the newborn period include coarse facies, cleft palate, diaphragmatic hernia, distal digital hypoplasia, and neonatal death due to pulmonary hypoplasia. There is considerable clinical overlap between Fryns and Pallister–Killian syndromes but the terminology has often been confused. Fryns syndrome is usually lethal during the newborn period and peripheral blood chromosomes, if obtained, generally reveal a normal karyotype. In contrast, the diagnosis of Pallister–Killian syndrome is generally made in an older infant who has developmental delay and progressive coarsening of the facial features. Once the typical clinical findings of Pallister–Killian have been observed, karyotype studies generally include a skin biopsy for fibroblast culture. Thus, the two conditions may be related or contiguous on the short arm of chromosome 12. Babies who die during the neonatal period are more likely to have a diagnosis of Fryns syndrome, especially if a peripheral blood karyotype has been obtained and it is normal (Ignacio-Rodriguez et al. 1994). It has been suggested that newborn infants with clinical findings consistent with either Fryns or Pallister–Killian syndrome should have karyotypes performed on multiple tissue types to allow a correct diagnosis to be made (McPherson et al. 1993). This is important because Fryns and Pallister–Killian syndromes have different prognoses and different recurrence risks. Fryns syndrome is an autosomal recessive and Pallister–Killian syndrome (tetrasomy 12p) is considered to be a sporadic event.

▶ ANTENATAL NATURAL HISTORY

Little is known about the antenatal natural history of tetrasomy 12p. There is, however, an increased incidence of stillbirth, prematurity, and birth asphyxia associated with the condition (Schinzel 1991; Soukup and Neidich 1990).

▶ MANAGEMENT OF PREGNANCY

If polyhydramnios, short femur, and diaphragmatic hernia have been documented by prenatal sonographic examination, the diagnosis of Pallister–Killian syndrome should be considered. In this setting, an amniocentesis is more likely to be diagnostic of the chromosomal abnormality than cordocentesis, because the chromosomal abnormality is present in the majority of amniocytes but not in fetal lymphocytes (Donnenfeld et al. 1993;

Wilson et al. 1994). However, at least one case has been detected at cordocentesis (Chiesa et al. 1998). If an unknown marker chromosome is detected on amniocentesis, consideration should be given to performing FISH studies using chromosome 12p–specific probes. This is best performed in a referral cytogenetics laboratory with experience in FISH analysis.

The abnormal marker chromosome can also be recognized in samples obtained by chorionic villus biopsy. The marker has been documented in 93% of cells derived from the direct preparation (Sharland et al. 1991) and 100% of cells derived from a cultured preparation (Bernert et al. 1992). In one case, however, karyotype results from chorionic villus sampling were normal, but the infant had clinical findings of Pallister–Killian syndrome. Fibroblast cultures obtained from a skin biopsy at 1 year of age demonstrated isochromosome 12p mosaicism (Horn et al. 1995).

Once a diagnosis of tetrasomy 12p has been made, the poor prognosis for a child with this condition should be discussed with the family. If the diagnosis is made at less than 24 weeks of gestation, termination of pregnancy can be offered. Cesarean section should not be performed for fetal distress. However, if the parents desire that everything be performed for the infant, delivery in a tertiary-care hospital may be necessary because of the high frequency of associated pulmonary hypoplasia due to diaphragmatic hernia, which necessitates resuscitation by a neonatologist and treatment by a pediatric surgeon.

▶ FETAL INTERVENTION

There are no fetal interventions for tetrasomy 12p.

▶ TREATMENT OF THE NEWBORN

Because of the poor prognosis associated with this finding, resuscitation of the newborn infant with tetrasomy 12p should consist of basic supportive but not heroic measures. Recognition of the clinical features of Pallister–Killian syndrome during the newborn period is important because a normal peripheral blood karyotype does not exclude the diagnosis. To make the diagnosis in a newborn infant who did not have an amniocentesis performed prenatally, a fibroblast culture must be established from a skin biopsy (Bergoffen et al. 1993).

Newborns with tetrasomy 12p generally have a normal birth weight or they are large for gestational age. The average birth weight at term for affected infants is 3.6 kg (Reynolds et al. 1987). The typical physical findings in a newborn with Pallister–Killian syndrome include dysmorphic facies consisting of a high forehead with frontal bossing, sparse hair with bitemporal alopecia, hypertelorism, wide and flat nasal bridge, long philtrum, large mouth, short, webbed neck, supernumerary nipples, congenital heart disease, diaphragmatic hernia, proximal shortness of the upper and lower limbs, hypotonia, and imperforate anus (Reynolds et al. 1987; Schinzel 1991). In time, pigmentary abnormalities may develop. These are best diagnosed by skin examination under a Woods lamp.

Definitive diagnosis relies on the performance of chromosome studies on multiple tissues. One author has suggested performing FISH studies on easily obtained epithelial buccal mucosa (Ohashi et al. 1993).

▶ SURGICAL TREATMENT

Surgical treatment for infants with tetrasomy 12p is generally not indicated. Because of the overall poor prognosis, repair of a diaphragmatic hernia in a patient with known tetrasomy 12p is not advisable. Surgical treatment for these infants generally consists of supportive care, such as gastrostomy-tube placement to permit feeding in cases in which survival beyond the immediate neonatal period is anticipated. A diverting colostomy in infants with imperforate anus may be necessary to permit normal bowel function.

▶ LONG-TERM OUTCOME

The physical appearance of affected infants and children with tetrasomy 12p changes over time. The face becomes increasingly coarse and dysmorphic. Thick lips and a protruding tongue develop. The frontotemporal balding disappears, and hair growth becomes normal after a few years. Most affected children and adults have a generalized pigmentary dysplasia that may be evident only by Woods lamp examination. Some older patients with tetrasomy 12p are misdiagnosed as having hypomelanosis of Ito.

All patients with tetrasomy 12p are profoundly retarded. Most are completely bedridden, with flexion contractures. Almost all affected children and adults never speak or become continent and completely lack self-help skills (Schinzel 1991). The oldest reported patient is 45 years of age; thus, the chromosomal abnormality is in some cases compatible with prolonged survival.

▶ GENETICS AND RECURRENCE RISK

Tetrasomy 12p is considered to be a sporadic condition with no increased risk of recurrence (Bergoffen et al. 1993; Reynolds et al. 1987; Wenger et al. 1988). There is also no history of recurrent miscarriage in affected families.

The isochromosome 12p is generally seen in 0 to 2% of lymphocytes in a peripheral blood karyotype but 50 to 100% of fibroblasts. The marker is seen in much higher percentages of amniocytes and bone marrow cells (Schinzel 1991). Importantly, the proportion of tetrasomic cells present does not correlate with the severity of malformations, postnatal survival, or the extent of mental retardation.

For purposes of genetic counseling, the diagnosis of tetrasomy 12p can be made retrospectively on perinatal autopsy specimens in fetuses with hydrops, rhizomelic limb shortening, hypertelorism, diaphragmatic hernia, and congenital heart disease using FISH on fetal and placental tissues. This approach can be successful for diagnosis on formalin-fixed tissues (Wilson et al. 1994). Mothers who have given birth to an infant or fetus with tetrasomy 12p should be counseled that there is no increased recurrence risk. Amniocentesis is potentially indicated in a subsequent pregnancy, however, for reassurance.

REFERENCES

Bergoffen J, Punnett H, Campbell TJ, Ross AJ, Ruchelli E, Zackai EH. Diaphragmatic hernia in tetrasomy 12p mosaicism. J Pediatr 1993;122:603–606.

Bernert J, Bartels I, Gatz G, et al. Prenatal diagnosis of the Pallister-Killian mosaic aneuploidy syndrome by CVS. Am J Med Genet 1992;42:747–750.

Bresson JL, Arbez-Gindre F, Peltie J, Gouget A. Pallister-Killian mosaic tetrasomy 12p syndrome: another prenatally diagnosed case. Prenat Diagn 1991;11:271–275.

Butler MG, Dev VG. Pallister-Killian syndrome detected by fluorescence in situ hybridization. Am J Med Genet 1995;57:498–500.

Buyse ML, Korf BR. "Killian syndrome": Pallister mosaic syndrome or mosaic tetrasomy 12p? An analysis. J Clin Dysmorphol 1983;1:2–5.

Chiesa J, Hoffet M, Rousseau O, et al. Pallister–Killian syndrome [i(12p)]: first pre-natal diagnosis using cordocentesis in the second trimester confirmed by in situ hybridization. Clin Genet 1998;54:294–302.

Cormier-Daire V, LeMerrer M, Gigarel N, et al. Prezygotic origin of the isochromosome 12p in Pallister–Killian syndrome. Am J Med Genet 1998;69:166–168.

Donnenfeld AE, Campbell TJ, Byers J, Librizzi RJ, Weiner S. Tissue-specific mosaicism among fetuses with prenatally diagnosed diaphragmatic hernia. Am J Obstet Gynecol 1993;169:1017–1021.

Gilgenkrantz S, Droulle P, Schweitzer M, et al. Mosaic tetrasomy 12p. Clin Genet 1985;28:495–502.

Horn D, Majewski F, Hildebrandt B, Korner H. Pallister–Killian syndrome: normal karyotype in prenatal chorionic villi, in postnatal lymphocytes and in slowly growing epidermal cells, but mosaic tetrasomy 12p in skin fibroblasts. J Med Genet 1995;32:68–71.

Larramendy M, Heiskanen M, Wessman M, et al. Molecular cytogenetic study of patients with Pallister–Killian syndrome. Hum Genet 1993;91:121–127.

McLean S, Stanley W, Stern H, et al. Prenatal diagnosis of Pallister–Killian syndrome: resolution of cytogenetic ambiguity by use of fluorescent in situ hybridization. Prenat Diagn 1992;12:985–991.

McPherson EW, Ketterer DM, Salsburey DJ. Pallister–Killian and Fryns syndromes: nosology. Am J Med Genet 1993; 47:241–245.

Mowery-Rushton PA, Stadler MP, Kochmar SJ, McPherson E, Surti U, Hogge WA. The use of interphase FISH for prenatal diagnosis of Pallister–Killian syndrome. Prenat Diagn 1997;17:255–265.

Ohashi H, Ishikiriyama S, Fukushima Y. New diagnostic method for Pallister-Killian syndrome: detection of i(12p) in interphase nuclei of buccal mucosa by fluorescence in situ hybridization. Am J Med Genet 1993;45:123–128.

Pallister PD. The Pallister mosaic syndrome. Birth Defects 1977;13:103–110.

Priest JH, Rust JM, Fernhoff PM. Tissue specificity and stability of mosaicism in Pallister–Killian +i(12p) syndrome: relevance for prenatal diagnosis. Am J Med Genet 1992;42:820–824.

Reeser SL, Wenger SL. Failure of PHA-stimulated i(12p) lymphocytes to divide in Pallister–Killian syndrome. Am J Med Genet 1992;42:815–819.

Reynolds JF, Daniel A, Kelly TE, et al. Isochromosome 12p mosaicism: report of 11 cases. Am J Med Genet 1987;27:257–274.

Rodriguez JI, Garcia I, Alvarez J, Delicado A, Palacios J. Lethal Pallister–Killian syndrome: phenotypic similarity with Fryns syndrome. Am J Med Genet 1994;53: 176–181.

Schinzel A. Tetrasomy 12 (Pallister–Killian syndrome). J Med Genet 1991;28:122–125.

Sharland M, Hill L, Patel R, Patton M. Pallister–Killian syndrome diagnosed by chorionic villus sampling. Prenat Diagn 1991;11:477–479.

Soukup S, Neidich K. Prenatal diagnosis of Pallister–Killian syndrome. Am J Med Genet 1990;35:526–528.

Speleman F, Leroy JG, Van Roy N, et al. A further prenatal diagnosis of mosaic tetrasomy 12p. Prenat Diagn 1992; 12:529–534.

Speleman F, Leroy JG, Van Roy N, et al. Pallister–Killian syndrome: characterization of the isochromosome 12p by fluorescent in situ hybridization. Am J Med Genet 1991;41:381–387.

Tejuda MI, Uribarren A, Briones P, Vilaseca MA. A further prenatal diagnosis of mosaic tetrasomy 12p (Pallister–Killian syndrome). Prenat Diagn 1992;12:529–534.

Teschler-Nicola M, Killian W. Case report 72: mental retardation, unusual facial appearance, abnormal hair. Syndrome Ident 1981;7:6–7.

Ward BE, Hayden WM, Robinson A. Isochromosome 12p mosaicism: newborn diagnosis by direct bone marrow analysis. Am J Med Genet 1988;31:835–839.

Wenger SL, Steele MW, Yu W-D. Risk effect of maternal age in Pallister i(12p) syndrome. Clin Genet 1988;34:181–184.

Wilson RD, Harrison K, Clarke LA, Yong SL. Tetrasomy 12p (Pallister–Killian syndrome): ultrasound indicators and confirmation by interphase FISH. Prenat Diagn 1994;14: 787–792.

Zhang J, Marynen P, Devriendt K, Fryns JP, Van den Berghe H, Cassiman JJ. Molecular analysis of the isochromosome 12p in the Pallister–Killian syndrome. Hum Genet 1989;83:359–363.

CHAPTER 131
Triploidy

▶ CONDITION

Triploidy is defined as the presence of three complete sets of the normal haploid genome found in gametes. Triploidy occurs in one of three ways: (1) failure of division in meiosis 1 or 2 in the spermatocyte, resulting in an extra set of paternal chromosomes (diandry); (2) failure of division in meiosis I or II in the oocyte, resulting in an extra set of maternal chromosomes (digyny); or (3) double fertilization of a normal haploid ovum (dispermy). Using special chromosome-staining techniques, it has been shown that the extra set of chromosomes is paternal in origin in three quarters of cases (Jacobs et al. 1982). Most of the paternally derived cases are due to dispermy (Kajii and Niikawa 1977). The distribution of karyotypes seen in triploid conceptuses is 69,XXY (60%), 69,XXX (37%), and 69,XYY (3%) (Jacobs et al. 1982). The infrequent occurrence of XYY suggests that either diandry must be uncommon or that XYY carries a disadvantage for survival.

Triploid fetuses can present with a broad spectrum of phenotypic features that can range from near normalcy to multisystem involvement. McFadden and Kalousek (1991) have described two distinct fetal and placental phenotypes that appear to correlate with the parent of origin in the extra set of chromosomes. In the type I phenotype, the fetus is relatively well grown and has a proportionate head size or microcephaly. The placenta is large, with cystic changes. These cases are generally associated with diandry (Fig. 131-1). The type II phenotype predominates in the cases diagnosed after the first trimester; it consists of a markedly growth-restricted fetus with a disproportionately large head and a small, noncystic placenta (Fig. 131-2). In their series, McFadden and Kalousek were able to demonstrate that one case of type II triploidy originated from an error in maternal gametogenesis.

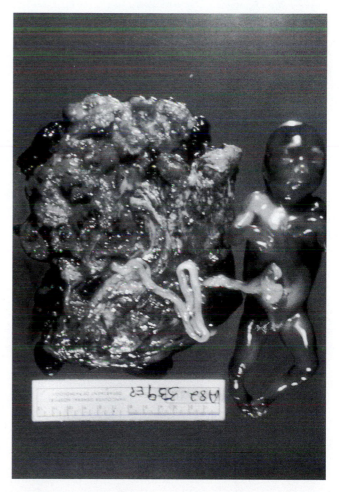

Figure 131-1. Relatively well grown fetus with large cystic placenta seen in type I triploidy. *(Reprinted from McFadden DE, Kalousek DK. Two different phenotypes of fetuses with chromosomal triploidy: correlation with parental origin of the extra haploid set. Am J Med Genet 1991;38:535–538. Copyright 1991 John Wiley & Sons. Reprinted, by permission, of John Wiley & Sons, Inc.)*

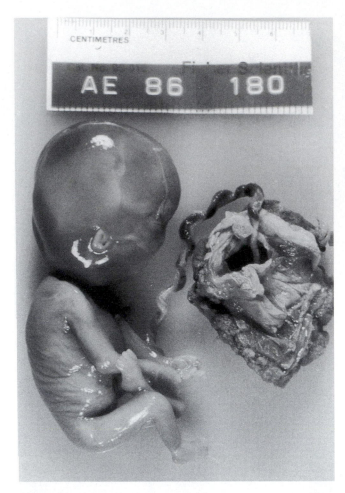

Figure 131-2. Markedly growth-restricted fetus with a disproportionately large head and a small, noncystic placenta seen in type II triploidy. *(Reprinted from McFadden DE, Kalousek DK. Two different phenotypes of fetuses with chromosomal triploidy: correlation with parental origin of the extra haploid set. Am J Med Genet 1991;38:535–538. Copyright 1991 John Wiley & Sons. Reprinted, by permission, of John Wiley & Sons, Inc.)*

▶ INCIDENCE

Human triploidy is a relatively common condition, occurring in 1 to 2 percent of all clinically recognized conceptions (Jacobs et al. 1978). Triploidy accounts for approximately 20% of spontaneous abortions due to chromosomal abnormalities (Niebuhr 1974; Wertelecki et al. 1976). After Turner syndrome (45,X), triploidy and trisomy 16 are the most common chromosomal abnormalities diagnosed in first-trimester products of conception (Lindor et al. 1992). The early pregnancy wastage is high—for each triploid infant born alive, it is estimated that 1200 are miscarried (Doshi et al. 1983).

Although triploid conceptions are very common, the live-born incidence is only 1 per 10,000 (Jacobs et al. 1982). There is no evidence for an increased risk due to advanced maternal age (Rochon and Vekemans 1990). In experimental animals, triploidy has been induced by colchicine administration, hypoxia, and heat shock (Niebuhr 1974). There is a questionable association between triploidy and delayed fertilization, due to prolonged menstrual cycles or discontinuation from oral contraceptives (Niebuhr 1974). Uchida and Freeman (1985) have described an association between preconceptual diagnostic abdominal x-ray exposure and subsequent triploid conceptuses.

▶ SONOGRAPHIC FINDINGS

No single anomaly on sonographic examination is pathognomonic of triploidy (Pircon et al. 1989a). The diagnosis of triploidy should be suspected in any pregnancy with cystic placental changes and fetal anomalies. Similarly, severe intrauterine growth restriction and a markedly increased head:body size ratio should elicit consideration of triploidy (Fig. 131-3).

Intrauterine growth restriction in triploidy has been reported as early as the first trimester (Benacerraf 1988), but the classic presentation is in the second trimester. Crane et al. (1985) have described growth curves for triploid fetuses studied on several occasions during gestation. The characteristic finding is an abnormally increased head:abdominal circumference ratio that gives the appearance of relative macrocephaly. Oligohydramnios has been reported in as many as 60% of cases (Mittal et al. 1998). Hydrocephalus is common and can be seen in the first trimester (Benacerraf 1988; Crane et al. 1985). Facial anomalies include micrognathia, microphthalmia (Wertelecki et al. 1976), a bulbous nose, and a small mouth (Bendon et al. 1988). A relatively specific finding is syndactyly of the third and fourth digits (Fig. 131-4) (Bendon et al. 1988). Approximately 25% of triploid fetuses have a neural-tube defect (Gosden et al. 1976) and 10 to 18% have associated omphaloceles or gastroschisis (Blackburn et al. 1982). Male triploid fetuses may have genital abnormalities. Ambiguous genitalia may also be due to the presence of a mosaic karyotype, with two cell lines that contain different sex chromosomes. Both polyhydramnios and oligohydramnios have been described. Other fetal findings that may be apparent sonographically include cardiac anomalies (ventricular septal defect and atrial septal defect), pulmonary hypoplasia, and renal cystic changes. It should also be noted that the absence of anomalies does not preclude a diagnosis of triploidy.

Placental abnormalities are typical of triploidy (Mittal et al. 1998). Characteristic findings include placental enlargement, hydropic changes (Wertelecki et al. 1976), a generalized hyperechoic appearance, and the presence of multiple small or a single large cyst (see Fig. 131-1) (Rubenstein et al. 1986). Abnormal

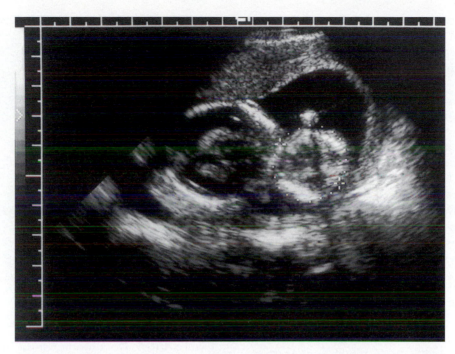

Figure 131-3. Prenatal sonographic image demonstrating increased head:body size ratio.

placental Doppler studies are also common (Jauniaux, 1999).

In cases in which triploidy is suspected, sonographic examination of the maternal ovaries may reveal the presence of associated theca lutein cysts (Meizner et al. 1991).

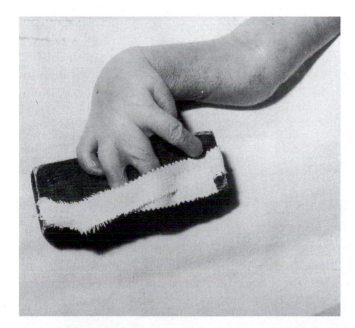

Figure 131-4. Syndactyly of the third and fourth digits seen in an infant with triploidy.

▶ DIFFERENTIAL DIAGNOSIS

The differential diagnosis includes severe intrauterine growth restriction due to uteroplacental insufficiency, infection, or other genetic syndromes. The possibility of a complete mole, with its risk for malignant change, must be excluded.

▶ ANTENATAL NATURAL HISTORY

The majority of triploid conceptions are lost during the first trimester, but one third survive beyond 15 weeks of gestation (Warburton et al. 1994). Approximately 1 in 200 ongoing pregnancies at 15 weeks involve a triploid fetus, although some of these fetuses are already dead (Hassold et al. 1980; Jacobs et al. 1982). Between 16 and 19 weeks of gestation, triploidy is found in 8.1% of all spontaneous abortions. In one study, 43% of the chromosomally abnormal fetuses lost between 16 and 19 weeks were shown to be triploid (Warburton et al. 1994).

Development of hydatidiform changes in the placenta ("partial mole") is primarily associated with the presence of two paternal sets of chromosomes (diandry or dispermy). These moles rarely undergo malignant change, as opposed to diploid moles that are not associated with a fetus.

Abnormalities in maternal serum testing are being increasingly appreciated in triploid pregnancies that survive to the second trimester. Increased maternal serum α-fetoprotein (AFP) levels have been demonstrated in several reports (Freeman et al. 1989; Pircon et al. 1989b; O'Brien et al. 1988). In most cases, amniotic fluid AFP levels have been normal unless an associated neural-tube defect is present (Freeman et al. 1989). It is important to consider triploidy in the differential diagnosis of elevated maternal serum AFP levels, as in several reported cases, the sonographic examination was within normal limits (Pircon et al. 1989a). More recently, low levels of human chorionic gonadotropin (hCG) and estriols were also shown to be associated with triploidy (Fejgin et al. 1992). It has been questioned whether this finding is due to an extra set of maternal chromosomes impairing placental function (Schmidt et al. 1994).

▶ MANAGEMENT OF PREGNANCY

Prenatal diagnosis of triploidy is important, as this condition carries serious medical risks for the mother. These risks include vaginal bleeding and severe preeclampsia (Jauniaux 1999). Prenatal recognition also prevents unnecessary cesarean delivery (Graham et al. 1989). The abnormally large cystic placenta can cause severe postpartum hemorrhage and may be retained after birth (Niebuhr 1974).

We recommend that prenatal karyotyping be performed for the following clinical situations: (1) severe intrauterine growth restriction with or without fetal anomalies documented on second-trimester sonographic examination; (2) hydatidiform placental changes noted on sonography; (3) abnormally increased maternal serum AFP levels (greater than 3.5 MoM); and (4) severe preeclampsia with fetal anomalies or hydatidiform placental changes. A full metaphase karyotype will make a definitive diagnosis and also rule out the presence of mosaicism. If a rapid diagnosis is necessary, fluorescence in situ hybridization using chromosome probes has been used on uncultured amniocytes to diagnose triploidy (Fig. 131-5) (Christensen et al. 1992; Gersen et al. 1995). Results with this technique are generally available within 48 hours. Alternatively, academic medical centers that have access to a flow-cytometry facility can send fetal blood or placental villi for DNA quantification studies (Graham et al. 1989; Thilaganathan et al. 1993; Van Oven et al. 1989). In experienced centers, a diagnosis using this method is available within a few hours.

Once the diagnosis of triploidy has been made, the poor prognosis and maternal risks should be discussed with the parents, and termination of pregnancy should be offered if the gestational age is less than 24 weeks. Early induction of labor is recommended if the diagnosis is made after 24 weeks because of the maternal

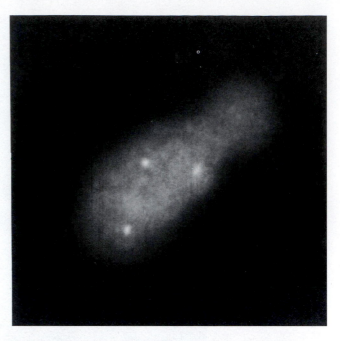

Figure 131-5. Documentation of triploidy by fluorescence in situ hybridization studies (FISH) on uncultured amniocytes. The nucleus of this cell has undergone hybridization with a chromosome-18 specific probe. The nucleus demonstrates three white dots, indicating that three copies of chromosome 18 are present. If other chromosome-specific probes were used, three dots (instead of the normal two) would be present. *(Courtesy of Dr. Brian Ward.)*

medical risks associated with continuing the pregnancy. Cesarean section is not indicated except to facilitate delivery for maternal health. Delivery in a tertiary-care center is not necessary. The advantages of delivering in a tertiary-care center are that: (1) if the infant survives postnatally, neonatal transfer will not occur; (2) when the infant dies, perinatal pathologists are available for autopsy; (3) many tertiary-care centers offer coordinated services for bereavement and genetic counseling; and (4) appropriate subspecialty referral is available for the mother if she has medical complications.

▶ FETAL INTERVENTION

There are no fetal interventions for triploidy.

▶ TREATMENT OF THE NEWBORN

Given the relative infrequency of this condition in the live-born population and the subtlety of the associated dysmorphic features, the diagnosis of triploidy in the newborn is sometimes unsuspected. The severe growth restriction usually prompts an investigation of the

▶ **TABLE 131-1.** PHENOTYPIC FEATURES OF INFANTS WITH COMPLETE TRIPLOIDY

General
    Intrauterine growth restriction
Head
    Relative macrocephaly
    Malformed, low-set ears
    Micro-ophthalmia
    Ocular coloboma
    Micrognathia
Chest
    Pulmonary hypoplasia
Cardiac
    Ventricular and atrial septal defects
Abdomen
    Omphalocele
    Renal anomalies
    Adrenal hypoplasia
    Ovarian hypoplasia
Genitalia
    Normal in females
    Anomalies in males include:
        hypospadias
        micropenis
        cryptorchidism
Extremities
    3rd and 4th digit syndactyly of the hands and/or feet
    Simian crease
    "Wine bottle" thighs
Neurologic
    Hypotonicity
    Myelomeningocoele
    Hydrocephalus

Modified from Doshi et al. 1983.

chromosomes, but results are usually not available for 3 to 7 days. The phenotypic features of infants presenting with complete triploidy are summarized in Table 131-1. The typical infant who survives postnatally has the "type II" phenotype of McFadden and Kalousek, with growth restriction, relative macrocephaly, dysplastic calvarium, ocular colobomas, cleft palate, micrognathia, hypotonicity, and genital abnormalities if male (Graham et al. 1989). Gosden and colleagues (1976) have also described an unusual appearance of the thighs due to muscular hyperplasia. They termed this physical finding "wine bottle thighs."

Hematologic abnormalities in triploid infants have also been reported. Typical findings include macrocytosis, anisocytosis, polychromasia, an increase in platelet size, and abnormalities of the granulocytes (Strobel and Brandt 1985).

Doshi and colleagues (1983) have documented pathologic findings in 43 complete and 11 mosaic triploid fetuses or infants delivered after 22 weeks of gestation. In addition to the anomalies already mentioned, they reported ovarian, adrenal, and pulmonary

hypoplasia as well as testicular Leydig-cell hyperplasia. True hermaphroditism has also been reported (Petit et al. 1992).

Importantly, the diagnosis of complete triploidy is considered lethal. There have been no survivors beyond the age of 10.5 months (Sherard et al. 1986). Newborn resuscitation and mechanical ventilation are not indicated. Warmth, nutrition, and comfort measures are recommended. Faix and colleagues (1984) have eloquently described the ethical dilemmas in a case of triploidy in which the parents insisted on employment of the full range of life-support technology. Even with their aggressive support, the infant survived for only 4 months and had marked impairment of his growth and development.

▶ **SURGICAL TREATMENT**

The lethal nature of complete triploidy precludes intervention in surgically correctable anomalies such as abdominal-wall defects. A more aggressive approach to surgically correctable lesions may be considered in cases of diploid/triploid mosaicism.

▶ **LONG-TERM OUTCOME**

The longest reported survival of an infant with triploidy is 10.5 months (Sherard et al. 1986). This male infant was small for gestational age, with a complete cleft lip and palate, digital abnormalities, and a large ventricular septal defect (Fig. 131-6). His medical problems included congestive heart failure (treated with digitalis and diuretics), seizures (treated with phenobarbital), and upper respiratory infections. He died from respiratory complications. Genotyping studies demonstrated that the extra set of chromosomes was maternal in origin. In three of the longest-surviving infants with triploidy the extra genome was also maternal (Fryns et al. 1977; Galan et al. 1991) although at least one other case was paternally derived (Niemann-Seyde et al. 1993).

In the future, we may understand the importance of the parent of origin differences in the extra chromosome set. Imprinting of certain genes may play a role.

Infants who are shown to have diploid/triploid mosaicism on their karyotype will, in general, have a milder phenotype that may permit prolonged survival to adulthood (Tantravahi et al. 1986). The majority of the patients reported have had developmental delay. Other features described in these diploid/triploid individuals include hemihypertrophy, syndactyly, ambiguous genitalia, and mild craniofacial abnormalities (Dewald et al. 1975).

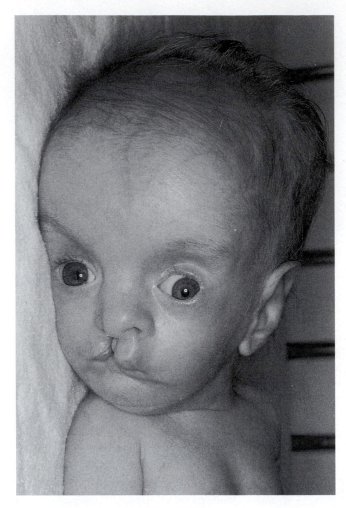

Figure 131-6. Facial appearance of a triploid male infant who survived for 10.5 months *(Reprinted from Sherard J, Bean C, Bove B, et al. Long survival in a 69,XXY triploid male. Am J Med Genet 1986;25: 307–312. Copyright © 1986 John Wiley & Sons. Reprinted, by permission, of John Wiley & Sons, Inc.)*

▶ GENETICS AND RECURRENCE RISK

The issue of whether triploidy is a random event or whether it affects future reproductive performance is currently unresolved. Three studies have suggested a slightly increased risk for other chromosomal abnormalities in future pregnancies (Boué et al. 1973; Stene et al. 1984; Uchida and Freeman 1985). We recommend prenatal cytogenetic diagnosis in subsequent pregnancies. Genetic counseling is indicated so that the family can understand the cause of the triploidy and the risk of recurrence.

REFERENCES

Benacerraf BR. Intrauterine growth retardation in the first trimester associated with triploidy. J Ultrasound Med 1988;7:153–154.

Bendon RW, Saddiqi T, Soukup S, Srivastava A. Prenatal detection of triploidy. J Pediatr 1988;112:149–153.

Blackburn WR, Miller WP, Superneau DW, Cooley NR Jr, Zellweger H, Wertelecki W. Comparative studies of infants with mosaic and complete triploidy: an analysis of 55 cases. Birth Defects 1982;18:251–274.

Boué JG, Boué A, Lazar P, Gueguen S. Outcome of pregnancies following a spontaneous abortion with chromosome abnormalities. Am J Obstet Gynecol 1973;116:806.

Christensen B, Bryndorf T, Philip J, Lundsteen C, Hansen W. Rapid prenatal diagnosis of trisomy 18 and triploidy in interphase nuclei of uncultured amniocytes by non-radioactive in situ hybridization. Prenat Diagn 1992;12: 241–250.

Crane JP, Beaver HA, Cheung SW. Antenatal untrasound findings in fetal triploidy syndrome. J Ultrasound Med 1985;4:519–524.

Dewald G, Alvarez MN, Clouier MD, Kelalis PP, Gordon H. A diploid-triploid human mosaic with cytogenetic evidence of double fertilization. Clin Genet 1975;8:149–160.

Doshi N, Surti U, Szulman AE. Morphologic anomalies in triploid liveborn fetuses. Hum Pathol 1983;14:716–723.

Faix RG, Barr M.Jr., Waterson JR. Triploidy: case report of a live-born male and an ethical dilemma. Pediatrics 1984; 74:296–298.

Fejgin M, Amiel A, Goldberger S, Barnes I, Zer T, Kohn G. Placental insufficiency as a possible cause of low maternal serum human chorionic gonadotropin and low maternal serum unconjugated estriol levels in triploidy. Am J Obstet Gynecol 1992;167:766–767.

Freeman SB, Priest JH, Macmahon WC, Fernhoff P, Elsas LJ. Prenatal ascertainment of triploidy by maternal serum alpha-fetoprotein screening. Prenat Diagn 1989;9: 339–347.

Fryns JP, van de Kerckhove A, Goddeeris P, Van den Berghe H. Unusually long survival in a case of full triploidy of maternal origin. Hum Genet 1977;38: 147–155.

Galan F, Orts F, Aguilar MS, et al. 69,XXX karyotype in a malformed liveborn female. Maternal origin of triploidy. Ann Genet 1991;34:37–39.

Gersen SL, Carelli MP, Klinger KW, Ward BE. Rapid prenatal diagnosis of 14 cases of triploidy using FISH with multiple probes. Prenat Diagn 1995;15:1–5.

Gosden CM, Wright MO, Paterson WG, Grant KA. Clinical details, cytogenetic studies, and cellular physiology of a 69,XXX fetus, with comments on the biological effect of triploidy in man. J Med Genet 1976;13:371–380.

Graham JM Jr, Rawnsley EF, Simmons GM, et al. Triploidy: pregnancy complications and clinical findings in seven cases. Prenat Diagn 1989;9:409–419.

Hassold T, Chen N, Funkhouser J, et al. A cytogenetic study of 1000 spontaneous abortions. Ann Hum Genet 1980;44: 151–178.

Jacobs PA, Angell RR, Buchanan IM, Hassold TJ, Matsuyama AM, Manuel B. The origin of human triploids. Ann Hum Genet 1978;42:49–57.

Jacobs PA, Szulman AE, Funkhouser J. Human triploidy: relationship between the parental origin of chromosomes and the development of partial mole in the placenta. Ann Hum Genet 1982;46:223–231.

Jaunniaux E. Partial moles: from postnatal to prenatal diagnosis. Placenta 1999;20:379–388.

Kajii T, Niikawa N. Origin of triploidy and tetraploidy in man: 11 cases with chromosome markers. Cytogenet Cell Genet 1977;18:109–125.

Lindor NM, Ney JA, Gaffey TA, Jenkins RB, Thibodeau SN, DeWald GW. A genetic review of complete and partial hydatidiform moles and nonmolar triploidy. Mayo Clin Proc 1992;67:791–799.

McFadden DE, Kalousek DK. Two different phenotypes of fetuses with chromosomal triploidy: correlation with parental origin of the extra haploid set. Am J Med Genet 1991;38:535–538.

Meizner I, Levy A, Vardit A, Katz M. Early prenatal ultrasonic detection of fetal triploidy syndrome. Isr J Med Sci 1991;27:92–95.

Mittal TK, Vujanic GM, Morrissey BM, Jones A. Triploidy: antenatal sonographic features with post-mortem correlation. Prenat Diagn 1998;18:1253–1262.

Niebuhr E. Triploidy in man: cytogenetical and clinical aspects. Humangenetik 1974;21:103–125.

Niemann-Seyde SC, Rehder H, Zoll B. A case of full triploidy (69,XXX) of paternal origin with unusually long survival time. Clin Genet 1993;43:79–82.

O'Brien WF, Knuppel A, Kousseff B, Sternlicht D, Nichols P. Elevated maternal serum alpha-fetoprotein in triploidy. Obstet Gynecol 1988;71:994–995.

Petit P, Moerman P, Fryns JP. Full 69,XXY triploidy and sex-reversal: a further example of true hermaphrodism associated with multiple malformations. Clin Genet 1992;41:175–177.

Pircon RA, Porto M, Towers CV, Crade M, Gocke SE. Ultrasound findings in pregnancies complicated by fetal triploidy. J Ultrasound Med 1989a;8:507–511.

Pircon RA, Towers CV, Porto M, Gocke SE, Garite TJ. Maternal serum alpha-fetoprotein and fetal triploidy. Prenat Diagn 1989b;9:701–707.

Rochon L, Vekemans MJ. Triploidy arising from a first meiotic non-disjunction in a mother carrying a reciprocal translocation. J Med Genet 1990;27:724–726.

Rubenstein JB, Swayne LC, Dise CA, Gersen SL, Schwartz JR, Risk A. Placental changes in fetal triploidy syndrome. J Ultrasound Med 1986;5:545–550.

Schmidt D, Shaffer LG, McCaskill C, Rose E, Greenberg F. Very low maternal serum chorionic gonadotropin levels in association with fetal triploidy. Am J Obstet Gynecol 1994;170:77–80.

Sherard J, Bean C, Bove B, et al. Long survival in a 69,XXY triploid male. Am J Med Genet 1986;25:307–312.

Stene J, Stene E, Mikkelse M. Risk for chromosome abnormality at amniocentesis following a child with a non-inherited chromosome aberration. Prenat Diagn 1984;4:81–95.

Strobel SL, Brandt JT. Abnormal hematologic features in a live-born female infant with triploidy. Arch Pathol Lab Med 1985;109:775–777.

Tantravahi U, Bianchi DW, Haley C, et al. Use of Y chromosome specific probes to detect low level sex chromosome mosaicism. Clin Genet 1986;29:445–448.

Thilaganathan B, Makrydimas G, Nicolaides KH. Rapid DNA quantification in the prenatal diagnosis of fetal triploidy. Br J Obstet Gynaecol 1993;100:92–94.

Uchida IA, Freeman VCP. Triploidy and chromosomes. Am J Obstet Gynecol 1985;151:65–69.

Van Oven MW, Schoots CJF, Oosterhuis JW, Keij JF, Dam-Meiring A, Huisjes HJ. The use of DNA flow cytometry in the diagnosis of triploidy in human abortions. Hum Pathol 1989;20:238–242.

Warburton D, Stein Z, Kline J, and Susser M. Chromosome abnormalities in spontaneous abortion: data from the New York City study. In: Hook EB, Porter HJ, eds. Reproductive loss. New York: Academic Press, 1994:261–287.

Wertelecki W, Graham JM Jr, Sergovich FR. The clinical syndrome of triploidy. Obstet Gynecol 1976;47:69–76.

CHAPTER 132
Trisomy 13

► CONDITION

Trisomy 13 is a constellation of congenital anomalies that results from the presence of an extra chromosome 13, either whole or translocated onto another chromosome. It is not known how the presence of the extra chromosome disrupts so many different systems during organogenesis.

Although the clinical findings of the condition were previously known, the association of the extra chromosome with the clinical syndrome was not described until 1960 (Patau et al. 1960). Synonyms for trisomy 13 include trisomy D or Patau syndrome.

► INCIDENCE

The incidence of trisomy 13 has been variously reported as 1 in 2206 to 1 in 7602 live births (Taylor et al. 1968). Most authors give the approximate incidence figure of 1 in 5000 live births (Wladimiroff et al. 1989). The incidence of trisomy 13 is equal among all races. It is thought that there are equal numbers of conceptuses of both genders. However, a slight excess of females exists at birth presumably due to a survival advantage (Jacobs et al. 1987). One case of trisomy 13 has been reported with maternal amphetamine abuse (Tsai et al. 1993).

► SONOGRAPHIC FINDINGS

Fetuses with trisomy 13 are more active in utero than comparable fetuses with trisomy 18. In addition, fetuses with trisomy 13 have a higher frequency of major congenital anomalies than fetuses with trisomy 21. The most common major abnormality seen in trisomy 13 is holoprosencephaly, which can be seen as early as 12 weeks

of gestation. Other important findings associated with trisomy 13 include an abnormal midface with hypotelorism, cleft lip or palate, and even cyclopia (see Chapter 13) (Figs. 132-1 and 132-2). Many studies have shown that there is a greatly increased incidence of congenital heart disease in fetuses affected with trisomy 13 (Wladimiroff et al. 1995). The most common cardiac defects include ventricular septal defect (VSD), hypoplastic left ventricle, or double-outlet right ventricle. Other common sonographic findings include postaxial polydactyly and echogenic or polycystic kidneys. In one study, all fetuses with trisomy 13 had one or more sonographic abnormalities or abnormal measurements present (Seoud et al. 1994).

Benacerraf et al. (1988, 1992, 1994) developed a sonographic scoring index to identify fetuses with aneuploidy. She and her co-authors gave 2 points for nuchal thickening of greater than 6 mm, 2 points for demonstration of a major structural defect, and 1 point each for a short femur, short humerus, and the presence of renal pyelectasis. This scoring system identified 2 of 2 fetuses with trisomy 13. In another report, Benacerraf and colleagues (1986) demonstrated that 6 of 6 affected fetuses with trisomy 13 had holoprosencephaly and a severely malformed face.

In the largest study of sonographic abnormalities in 33 consecutive fetuses with trisomy 13, Lehman et al. (1995) demonstrated that 91% of affected fetuses had one or more sonographically detectable abnormalities. In this study, 18 of the 33 fetuses described were at less than 20 weeks of gestation, and 15 of the affected fetuses were at greater than 20 weeks of gestation. The mean gestational age for the fetuses in the study was 20.7 weeks. Thirty of the 33 fetuses had structural abnormalities, as documented in Table 132-1. Only 3 of the fetuses had no sonographically detectable abnormalities. The most common abnormalities observed were holoprosencephaly, other central nervous system

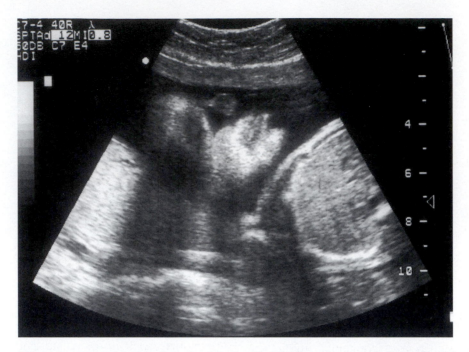

Figure 132-1. Sonographic profile of a fetus with trisomy 13 demonstrating severely abnormal midface with proboscis and absent orbit.

abnormalities, facial abnormalities, and cardiac defects (Table 132-1).

Nuchal-fold thickening is also associated with trisomy 13 (Pandya et al. 1994). In the Pandya study, 80% of fetuses with trisomy 13, 18, or 21 had a nuchal translucency of at least 3 mm. Omphalocele is also somewhat frequent in fetuses with trisomy 13. In the presence of an omphalocele, the risk of trisomy of 13 or 18 is increased by 340-fold (Snijders et al. 1995).

First trimester sonographic findings in fetuses with trisomy 13 include increased nuchal translucency measurement, decreased crown-rump length, increased fetal heart rate, holoprosencephaly, and omphalocele (Snijders et al. 1999).

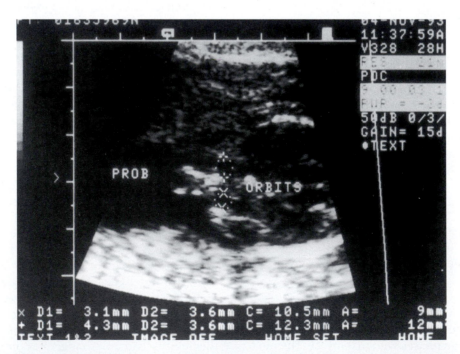

Figure 132-2. Transaxial view of fetal head indicating closely spaced orbits and a proboscis present at the same level of the orbits.

► **TABLE 132-1.** PRENATAL ULTRASOUND FINDINGS IN 33 FETUSES WITH TRISOMY 13 SYNDROME*

Sonographic Abnormality	Menstrual Age at Ultrasound Examination		
	12–20 wk (n = 18)	20–32 wk (n = 15)	Total (n = 33)
Intrauterine growth restriction[†]	4 (22)	12 (80)	16 (48)
Central nervous system and cranium			
Holoprosencephaly	4 (22)	9 (60)	13 (39)
Lateral ventricular dilation	2 (11)	1 (7)	3 (9)
Enlarged cisterna magna	2 (11)	3 (20)	5 (15)
Microcephaly[†]	0 (0)	4 (27)	4 (12)
Total	7 (39)	12 (80)	19 (58)
Face			
Cleft lip/palate*	3 (17)	9 (60)	12 (36)
Cyclopia	2 (11)	0 (0)	2 (6)
Hypoplastic face	3 (17)	7 (47)	10 (30)
Hypotelorism[†]	3 (17)	7 (47)	10 (30)
Total	6 (33)	10 (67)	16 (48)
Neck/hydrops[†]			
Nuchal thickening/cystic hygroma	6 (33)	1 (7)	7 (21)
Hydrops/lymphangiectasia	3 (17)	1 (7)	4 (12)
Total	6 (33)	2 (13)	8 (24)
Renal			
Echogenic kidneys	4 (22)	6 (40)	10 (30)
Enlarged kidneys[†]	2 (11)	6 (40)	8 (24)
Hydronephrosis	2 (11)	2 (13)	4 (12)
Total	4 (22)	7 (47)	11 (33)
Cardiac defects	8 (44)	8 (53)	16 (48)
Extremities[†]			
Polydactyly[†]	1 (6)	6 (40)	7 (21)
Club/rocker bottom feet	2 (11)	1 (7)	3 (9)
Clenched/overlapping digits[†]	0 (0)	5 (33)	5 (15)
Total	3 (17)	8 (53)	16 (48)
Abdomen			
Omphalocele	3 (17)	2 (13)	5 (15)
Bladder exstrophy	1 (6)	0 (0)	1 (3)
Echogenic bowel	2 (11)	0 (0)	2 (6)
Total	6 (33)	2 (13)	8 (24)
Other			
Echogenic chordae tendineae[†]	7 (39)	3 (20)	10 (30)
Single umbilical artery	1 (6)	7 (47)	8 (24)

*Numbers in parentheses are percentages.
[†]Statistically significant difference ($P = {<}0.05$) between frequency of detection before and after 20 menstrual weeks.

Source: Lehman CD, Nyberg DA, Winter TC, Kapur RP, Resta RG, Luthy DA. Trisomy 13 syndrome: prenatal US findings in a review of 33 cases. Radiology 1995;194:217–222.

In summary, fetuses with holoprosencephaly, cardiac abnormalities, evidence of facial clefting, and possibly polydactyly should strongly suggest a diagnosis of trisomy 13 (Twining and Zuccollo 1993).

► **DIFFERENTIAL DIAGNOSIS**

Since holoprosencephaly is one of the most commonly found malformations in trisomy 13, isolated holoprosencephaly should be considered within the differential diagnosis (see Chapter 13). Trisomy 13 is a diagnosis that can be made definitively only by karyotyping. Prior to obtaining karyotype results, however, the following diagnoses must also be considered: pseudotrisomy 13 (Cohen–Gorlin syndrome), Smith–Lemli–Opitz syndrome, and Meckel–Gruber syndrome.

Pseudotrisomy 13 syndrome has been described to encompass the triad of normal chromosomes, holoprosencephaly, and postaxial polydactyly (Seller et al.

1993). The phenotype has been expanded to include hypoplastic radii (Boles et al. 1992). The inheritance of this condition is autosomal recessive and carries a 25% risk of recurrence. Neither holoprosencephaly nor polydactyly is an obligatory manifestation of pseudotrisomy 13. Each of these anomalies is found only in 60% of affected siblings. The diagnostic criteria for this condition are a normal karyotype with either holoprosencephaly and postaxial polydactyly, or holoprosencephaly plus other major malformations without polydactyly, or postaxial polydactyly with other brain defects, such as microcephaly, hydrocephaly, or agenesis of the corpus callosum, with the presence of other malformations (Lurie and Wulfsberg 1993). Other specific organ findings can distinguish trisomy 13 from pseudotrisomy 13 in the absence of karyotyping. For example, patients with trisomy 13 have a very characteristic type of renal cystic dysplasia, whereas patients with pseudotrisomy 13 have hypoplastic kidneys but no evidence of cysts. Patients with trisomy 13 have hydronephrosis and patients with pseudotrisomy 13 have horseshoe kidneys. Scalp defects and a pathognomonic type of pancreatic fibrosis are present in patients with trisomy 13; neither of these findings is present in pseudotrisomy 13.

Another important consideration in the differential diagnosis is Meckel–Gruber syndrome. This condition was described in 1822 by Meckel and redefined by Gruber in 1934, who called the condition "dysencephalia splanchnocystica." In this condition, 100% of affected patients have polycystic kidneys, 80% have encephalocele, 70% have polydactyly, and 30% have cleft lip and palate. This condition is also inherited as an autosomal recessive (Miller 1983). In a study of 38 affected siblings, the cystic renal dysplasia was invariably present. The other findings associated with the condition, however, were less common. For example, occipital meningocele was present in only 63% of siblings and polydactyly was present in only 55% of siblings (Miller 1983). Meckel–Gruber syndrome is associated with increased levels of α-fetoprotein in the amniotic fluid.

▶ ANTENATAL NATURAL HISTORY

Trisomy 13 is associated with increased lethality in utero. For every trisomy 13 patient born alive, approximately 50 are lost prenatally as a spontaneous abortion (Jacobs et al. 1987). In one study, Jacobs and colleagues (1987) described a series of 2922 spontaneous abortuses who were karyotyped. Of these, 62 had trisomy 13. Forty-six had 47 chromosomes, consistent with a full trisomy. Sixteen had translocation trisomy 13. A similar proportion of translocation cases to full trisomy cases was seen in this study as is seen in live-born infants. Therefore, full trisomy 13 and translocation trisomy 13 are similar with respect to their effect on intrauterine mortality. In this spontaneous abortion study, trisomy 13 was shown to be the fourth most common trisomy (after trisomies 16, 21, and 22).

With regard to antenatal natural history, the mean gestational age of the fetuses with full trisomy 13 was 79.8 days and translocation trisomy 13, 82.6 days. These ages are significantly less than the fetuses with normal chromosomes who were miscarried. Only 5 of the trisomy 13 conceptuses in the study were older than 100 days of gestational age. This data suggests that specific stages in development exist in which trisomy 13 conceptuses are likely to die, but if they survive, they may survive until term.

▶ MANAGEMENT OF PREGNANCY

Fetuses with sonographic evidence of either holoprosencephaly or congenital heart disease in addition to other structural abnormalities or intrauterine growth restriction should have karyotyping performed (Fig. 132-3). Once the diagnosis of trisomy 13 has been made, the prospective parents should have the opportunity to speak with a medical geneticist regarding the implications of this diagnosis. The overall prognosis for extrauterine survival for an infant with trisomy 13 is extremely poor. In addition, there are complications for the mother when a diagnosis of trisomy 13 has been made. In particular, trisomy 13 is associated with increased risk of the mother developing preeclampsia. This was first noted by Boyd et al. (1987) who described five nulliparous women who had a fetus with trisomy 13; severe preeclampsia developed in all of the mothers. The medical records of these women were compared with four women whose first babies had trisomy 18 and seven women whose first babies had trisomy 21; preeclampsia did not develop in any of these women. A similar finding was not seen in control patients. The association between trisomy 13 and preeclampsia was later extended in a study of 25 women who gave birth to an infant with trisomy 13. These investigators showed that the incidence of preeclampsia is significantly higher when the fetus has trisomy 13 as compared with pregnancies in which the fetus has trisomy 18 or a normal karyotype (Tuohy and James 1992). This association is present in all pregnancies but more pronounced in primigravid women. This argues for a fetal factor in the pathogenesis of preeclampsia.

The current triple screen (α-fetoprotein, human chorionic gonadotropin, unconjugated estriol) does not detect fetuses with trisomy 13. A newer serum analyte, pregnancy-associated plasma protein A (PAPP-A) may be more useful in the detection of fetuses with trisomy 13. The median maternal serum PAPP-A levels are significantly lower in pregnancies that have a trisomy 13

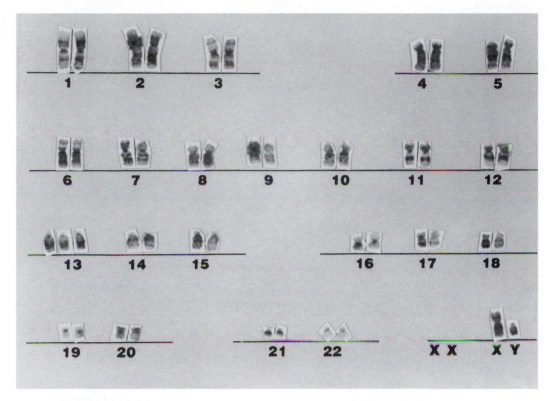

Figure 132-3. Karyotyping findings in a male fetus with trisomy 13. *(Courtesy of Dr. Janet Cowan.)*

fetus than in normal pregnancies. A level of less than 0.4 multiples of the median (MoM) detects 89% of fetuses with trisomy 13 at a calculated false positive rate of 5% (Brizot et al. 1994).

If the diagnosis of trisomy 13 is made before 24 weeks of gestation, the parents should be offered the opportunity to terminate the pregnancy. If a definite diagnosis of trisomy 13 is made after 24 weeks of gestation there is no need to deliver at a tertiary-care center, provided that the community obstetrician and pediatrician are comfortable with providing supportive care for the affected infant.

▶ FETAL INTERVENTION

There are no fetal interventions for trisomy 13.

▶ TREATMENT OF THE NEWBORN

Most infants with trisomy 13 deliver between 38 and 40 weeks of gestation, with an average birth weight of 2.48 kg (Warkany et al. 1966). The most common physical findings in live-born infants with trisomy 13 include scalp defects, which are often confused with lacerations made by fetal scalp electrodes; microcephaly with a sloping forehead; microphthalmia; cleft lip and palate;

congenital heart disease in 80 to 100% of patients; omphalocele; genital abnormalities, including cryptorchidism in all males, with micropenis in some males, and bicornuate uterus with ovarian abnormalities in most females; cystic kidneys; polydactyly, which is the most frequent external malformation of trisomy 13; and capillary hemangiomata (Hodes et al. 1978). Laboratory findings include abnormalities in the complete blood count, manifested by an increased frequency of nuclear projections in polymorphonuclear leukocytes and persistence of fetal hemoglobin. Patients who are delivered with a suspected diagnosis of trisomy 13, but without an antenatal confirmatory chromosome analysis, should have karyotyping performed. Peripheral blood leukocytes should give a definitive answer within 48 hours. If an affected infant has a life-threatening anatomic obstruction requiring surgery, fluorescence in situ hybridization (FISH) can be performed using a chromosome-13-specific probe. This study will give a tentative diagnosis of trisomy 13 within a few hours of obtaining the blood sample.

Because the few infants who survive with trisomy 13 are severely retarded, usually only comfort measures are taken. Early involvement of a medical genetics team is recommended to provide family support, to provide continuity of care if the infant is discharged to home, and to counsel about risk recurrence. Most infants with trisomy 13 die during the perinatal period.

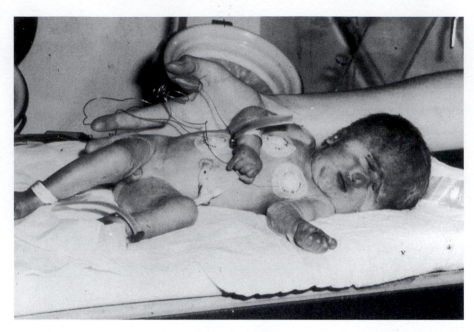

Figure 132-4. An infant with trisomy 13 with a severely abnormal midface, with bilateral microphthalmia and a single nostril.

Autopsy findings in 12 cases of trisomy 13 were described by Moerman et al. (1988). Of the 12 cases, 6 were live born, 4 were terminated electively, and 1 died in utero. The longest survival postnatally was 6 days of age. Severe craniofacial, ocular, and cerebral malformations were noted in 10 of 12 patients (Fig. 132-4). Eight of the 12 had holoprosencephaly. In all cases in which the eyes were examined, retinal dysplasia was present. The main cardiovascular anomalies were ventricular septal defect and abnormalities of the arterial valves. Four of 12 patients had complex cardiac disease, including tetralogy of Fallot or double-outlet right ventricle. Interestingly, 11 of 12 patients had malformations of the gastrointestinal tract, specifically malrotation and unfixed mesentery. A pathognomonic microscopic pancreatic dysplasia was also present. Renal cystic disease was demonstrated in most patients. Renal cysts became more prominent in number and diameter as gestational age increased. Congenital malformations of the Müllerian duct system were present in 5 of 8 affected females. The ovaries were invariably small and demonstrated ovarian dysgenesis (Moerman et al. 1988).

▶ SURGICAL TREATMENT

Surgical treatment is indicated only as a temporizing measure to allow a potentially affected infant with trisomy 13 to survive long enough to make a definitive diagnosis. Surgical treatment does not improve the overall prognosis.

▶ LONG-TERM OUTCOME

The median survival time for patients affected with trisomy 13 is 89 days (Taylor 1968). All infants who survive the perinatal period are severely retarded. Postnatal survival is inversely correlated with the severity of cardiac and brain anomalies.

Common medical problems for affected infants with trisomy 13 who survive beyond 1 month of age include feeding difficulties, gastro-eophageal reflux, poor postnatal growth, apnea, seizures, hypertension, severe developmental delay, and scoliosis.

A support organization exists for parents of long-term survivors with trisomies 13 and 18. The organization is known as S.O.F.T. (Support Organization for Trisomies 13 and 18). This organization recommends routine child care and anticipatory guidance, thorough cardiac evaluation, antibiotics prior to dental procedures if a cardiac abnormality is present, hearing evaluation, evaluation by an infant-preschool-intervention team, screening for scoliosis, and ongoing social support for families.

▶ GENETICS AND RECURRENCE RISK

Eighty percent of patients with trisomy 13 have the full trisomy due to meiotic or mitotic nondisjunction (47,XX, +13 or 47,XY +13). Twenty percent of patients have mosaicism or a translocation. The proportion of cases of translocation trisomy 13 (20 to 25%) is much higher than that seen in trisomy 21 (4%) (Jacobs et al. 1987).

The mean maternal age is increased for the full trisomies but not for translocations, although the rate of increased risk with advanced maternal age does not increase as sharply as for trisomies 18 and 21 (Schreinemachers et al. 1982).

Hassold et al. (1987) used chromosome heteromorphisms and restriction-fragment–length polymorphisms (RFLPs) to determine parental origin of the extra chromosome in 33 cases of trisomy 13. In 68% of cases, maternal meiosis I was the source of the error. This study demonstrated that pairing failure is not the primary cause of trisomy 13, as crossing over between the two nondisjoined chromosomes was detected in almost all of the cases studied. In the cases of mosaic trisomy 13, these authors demonstrated that conception began as a trisomic zygote. Subsequently, the paternal copy of chromosome 13 was lost in some cells with remaining maternal disomy due to a maternal meiosis type I error.

When the affected fetus or infant has been shown to have the full trisomy 13, the recurrence risk is 1% or the risk according to maternal age, whichever is higher. For the affected infant with a translocation, parental chromosomes should be studied. If the parents are both shown to be normal, there is less than a 1% risk of recurrence. If one parent has a balanced translocation involving chromosome 13, there is a 20% risk of a spontaneous abortion and a 5% risk of a live-born infant with trisomy 13 in subsequent pregnancies. However, if one of the parents is demonstrated to have a robertsonian translocation (a translocation between two acrocentric chromosomes that results in the loss of ribosomal material in the short arm and fusion between the two centromeres) between both copies of chromosome 13, no normal offspring are possible, and gamete donation should be considered. For parents who have had a fetus or infant with trisomy 13, prenatal diagnosis in subsequent pregnancies can be achieved by obtaining a karyotype on chorionic villus material or on amniocytes obtained at midtrimester amniocentesis.

REFERENCES

Benacerraf BR, Frigoletto FD, Greene MF. Abnormal facial features and extremities in human trisomy syndromes: prenatal US appearance. Radiology 1986;159:243–246.

Benacerraf BR, Miller WA, Frigoletto FD. Sonographic detection of fetuses with trisomy 13 and 18: accuracy and limitations. Am J Obstet Gynecol 1988;158:404–409.

Benacerraf BR, Nadel A, Bromley B. Identification of second trimester fetuses with autosomal trisomy by use of a sonographic scoring index. Radiology 1994;193:135–140.

Benacerraf BR, Neuberg D, Bromley B, Frigoletto FD. Sonographic scoring index for prenatal detection of chromosomal abnormalities. J Ultrasound Med 1992;11:449–458.

Boles RG, Teebi AS, Neilson KA, Meyn MS. Pseudo-trisomy 13 syndrome with upper limb shortness and radial hypoplasia. Am J Med Genet 1992;44:638–640.

Boyd PA, Lindenbaum RH, Redman C. Pre-eclampsia and trisomy 13: a possible association. Lancet 1987;2:325–327.

Brizot ML, Snijders JM, Bersinger NA, Kuhn P, Nicolaides KH. Maternal serum pregnancy-associated plasma protein A and fetal nuchal translucency thickness for the prediction of fetal trisomies in early pregnancy. Obstet Gynecol 1994;84:918–922.

Gruber GB, Beitrage zur frage "gekoppelter" missbildungen (akrocephalo-syndactylie und dysencephalia splanchnocystica). Beitr Pathol Anat 1934;93:459–476.

Hassold T, Jacobs PA, Leppert M, Sheldon M. Cytogenetic and molecular studies of trisomy 13. J Med Genet 1987;24:725–732.

Hodes ME, Cole J, Palmer CG, Reed T. Clinical experience with trisomies 18 and 13. J Med Genet 1978;15:48–60.

Jacobs PA, Hassold TJ, Henry A, Pettay D, Takaesu N. Trisomy 13 ascertained in a survey of spontaneous abortions. J Med Genet 1987;24:721–724.

Lehman CD, Nyberg DA, Winter TC, Kapur RP, Resta RG, Luthy DA. Trisomy 13 syndrome: prenatal US findings in a review of 33 cases. Radiology 1995;194:217–222.

Lurie IW, Wulfsberg EA. Holoprosencephaly-polydactyly syndrome: expansion of the phenotypic spectrum. Am J Med Genet 1993;47:405–409.

Meckel JF. Beschreibung Zweier durch sehr ahnliche Bildungsabweichungen entstellter Geschwister. Dtsch Arch Physiol 1822;7:99–172.

Miller WA. Case records of the Massachusetts General Hospital (Case 11-1983). N Engl J Med 1983;308:642–648.

Moerman P, Fryns JP, van der Steen K, Kleczkowska A, Lauweryns J. The pathology of trisomy 13 syndrome. Hum Genet 1988;80:349–356.

Pandya PP, Brizot ML, Kuhn P, Snijders RJM, Nicolaides KH. First trimester fetal nuchal translucency thickness and risk for trisomies. Obstet Gynecol 1994;84:420–423.

Patau K, Smith DW, Therman E, Inhorn SL, Wagner SP. Multiple congenital anomaly caused by an extra chromosome. Lancet 1960;1:790–793.

Schreinemachers DM, Cross PK, Hook EB. Rates of trisomies 21, 18, 13 and other chromosome abnormalities in about 20,000 prenatal studies compared with estimated rates in live births. Hum Genet 1982;61:318–324.

Seller MJ, Chitty LS, Dunbar H. Pseudotrisomy 13 and autosomal recessive holoprosencephaly. J Med Genet 1993;30:970–971.

Seoud MAF, Alley DC, Smith DL, Levy DL. Prenatal sonographic findings in trisomy 13, 18, 21 and 22. J Reprod Med 1994;39:781–787.

Snijders RJM, Brizot ML, Faria M, Nicolaides KH. Fetal exomphalos at 11 to 14 weeks of gestation. J Ultrasound Med 1995;14:569–574.

Snijders RJM, Sebire NJ, Nayar R, Souka A, Nicolaides KH. Increased nuchal translucency in trisomy 13 fetuses at 10–14 weeks of gestation. Am J Med Genet 1999;86:205–207.

Taylor AI. Autosomal trisomy syndromes: a detailed study of 27 cases of Edwards' syndrome and 27 cases of Patau's syndrome. J Med Genet 1968;5:227–241.

▶ **TABLE 133-1.** FREQUENCY OF ABNORMALITIES AMONG 47 FETUSES WITH TRISOMY 18 EXAMINED WITH PRENATAL SONOGRAPHY BY MENSTRUAL AGE AT DETECTION

Sonographic Abnormality	Time of Sonographic Examination*		
	14–24 Weeks (n = 29)	24–40 Weeks (n = 18)	Total Ultrasound Findings (n = 47)
Cystic hygroma or nuchal thickening	9 (31%)[†]	0 (0%)	9 (19%)
Omphalocele	5 (17%)	5 (28%)	10 (21%)
Large cisterna magna	1 (3%)	8 (44%)	9 (19%)
Cardiac defects	4 (14%)	14 (78%)	18 (38%)
Clenched hands	5 (17%)	4 (22%)	9 (19%)
Club feet or rocker-bottom feet	6 (21%)	4 (22%)	10 (21%)
Single umbilical artery	3 (10%)	3 (17%)	6 (13%)
Meningomyelocele	4 (14%)	4 (22%)	8 (17%)
Renal anomaly	5 (17%)	2 (11%)	7 (15%)
Intrauterine growth restriction	8 (28%)	16 (89%)[†]	24 (51%)

*Numbers in parentheses are percentages.
[†]Statistically significant difference ($P < 0.05$) between frequency of detection before 24 weeks versus after 24 weeks.

Source: Nyberg DA, Kramer D, Resta R, et al. Prenatal sonographic findings of trisomy 18: review of 47 cases. J Ultrasound Med 1993;2:103–113.

translucency measurement were found to be sensitive indicators for the prenatal detection of trisomy 18. A BPD:FL ratio of greater than 1.5 SD above the mean identified three of four fetuses with trisomy 18, whereas nuchal thickening identified two of four fetuses with trisomy 18 (Ginsberg et al. 1990). Combining these sonographic markers gave a positive predictive value of 1 in 47 for the detection of trisomy 18.

A variety of cranial abnormalities are seen in trisomy 18. There is an unusually shaped head with a wide occipitoparietal and narrow frontal diameter. This has been called the "strawberry sign" by Nicolaides et al. (1992). Nicolaides and colleagues hypothesized that the narrowed frontal cranium is due to hypoplasia of the face and underdevelopment of the frontal lobes. The presence of choroid plexus cysts (see Chapter 8)

▶ **TABLE 133-2.** SONOGRAPHIC MALFORMATIONS ASSOCIATED WITH TRISOMY 18

Craniofacial
    "Strawberry" calvarium
    Low-set, abnormally shaped ears
    Micrognathia
    Thickened nuchal fold or translucency
Central nervous system
    Choroid plexus cysts
    Meningomyelocele
    Enlarged cisterna magna
    Cerebellar hypoplasia
    Absence of the corpus callosum
    Microcephaly
Cardiovascular system
    Atrial septal defect
    Membranous ventricular septal defect
    Double-outlet right ventricle
    Atrioventricular canal defect
    Coarctation of the aorta
    Dextroposition of the heart
    Calcification of the chordae tendineae
    Two-vessel umbilical cord
    Pulsatile flow in umbilical vein
    Abnormal blood flow during atrial contraction

Gastrointestinal system
    Omphalocele
    Diaphragmatic hernia
    Esophageal atresia with tracheoesophageal fistula
Urogenital system
    Horseshoe kidneys
    Cystic renal dysplasia
    Hydronephrosis
    Unilateral renal agenesis
Skeletal system
    Overlapping fingers
    Limb-reduction abnormalities
    Club feet
    Rocker-bottom feet
Amniotic fluid volume
    Polyhydramnios
Intrauterine growth restriction
    Small placenta
Behavioral abnormalities

Source: Hill LM. The sonographic detection of trisomies 13, 18 and 21. Clin Obstet Gynecol 1996;39:831–850.

has elicited much debate over the association between this finding and trisomy 18. Choroid plexus cysts have been documented in 30 to 50% of fetuses with trisomy 18 (Hill 1996; Seoud et al. 1994; Snijders et al. 1994). Snijders et al. (1994) calculated a risk of trisomy 18 relative to maternal age and the number of additional sonographic abnormalities present (see Chapter 8). Another cranial sonographic finding associated with trisomy 18 is the presence of an enlarged cisterna magna due to cerebellar hypoplasia. Thurmond et al. (1989) described five fetuses with enlarged cisterna magna, which prompted a search for additional fetal anomalies. These five fetuses had a predicted biparietal diameter less than the measured biparietal diameter, and all turned out to have trisomy 18 (Thurmond et al. 1989).

Several investigators have described findings that in combination tend to predict a high risk of trisomy 18. These include the combination of polyhydramnios, abnormal hand posturing, and other major structural abnormalities (Carlson et al. 1992), and abnormalities of the fetal face and extremities (Figs. 133-1 and 133-2) (Benacerraf et al. 1986, 1988). Benacerraf and colleagues (1994) developed a scoring system to identify fetuses with trisomy 18 based on the presence of certain sonographic findings. Her group specifically looked for the presence of nuchal translucency, long-bone shortening, choroid plexus cysts, echogenic bowel, and other major anatomic defects. They prospectively evaluated 60 fetuses with various autosomal trisomies between 14 and 21 weeks of gestation and 106 normal fetuses at the same gestational age. A sonographic score of 2 or more enabled the prospective identification of trisomy 18 in 11 of 13 affected fetuses.

Although echogenic bowel is more characteristic of fetuses with trisomy 21, it has also been described in fetuses with trisomy 18 (Hamada et al. 1996). These investigators described a normal-appearing fetus during the second trimester, but echogenic bowel developed during the third trimester. They hypothesized that the mechanisms for the echogenic bowel included decreased fetal swallowing, hypoperistalsis, and a hypercellular meconium. They also noted that this fetus was intrauterine growth-restricted, which potentially caused redistribution of regional blood flow, further causing ischemia of the mesentery and the impairment of bowel motility. These abnormalities resulted in a thickened echogenic meconium.

Cardiovascular abnormalities are present in 80 to 90% of fetuses with trisomy 18. Most commonly, these include large ventricular septal defects (VSD) and double-outlet right ventricle.

Wladimiroff et al. (1989) described the antenatal sonographic markers in 16 fetuses with trisomy 18. All fetuses had a cardiac abnormality. The majority of these were due to VSDs, double-outlet right ventricle, or

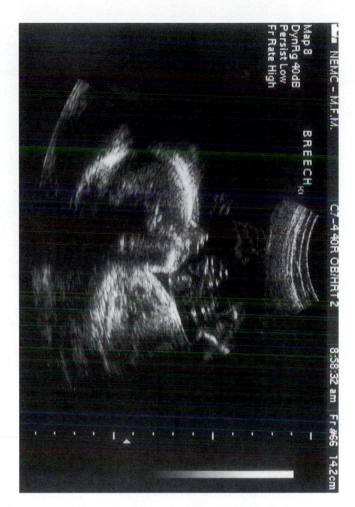

Figure 133-1. Prenatal sonographic profile of a fetus with trisomy 18. Note the micrognathia and the suggestion of a prominent occiput.

complete atrioventricular septal defect. The extracardiac structural pathology consisted of abnormal hands and feet, symmetrical IUGR, and polyhydramnios. It is thought that the increased nuchal translucency (see Chapter 34) seen in 90% of affected fetuses with trisomy 18 may be due to the cardiac abnormalities. The increased fluid collection at the back of the neck may be an early sign of congestive heart failure.

A variety of limb abnormalities are also a characteristic of trisomy 18, including the typical overlapping flexed fingers, positional abnormalities of the wrist or fingers, and rocker-bottom feet. The prenatal detection of pre-axial upper limb reduction facilitated the diagnosis of trisomy 18 in three cases (Sepulveda et al. 1995). In a report of 7 cases of fetal radial ray reduction malformations, three fetuses had trisomy 18 (Brons et al. 1990).

Single umbilical artery (see Chapter 110) is seen in 38 to 50% of fetuses with trisomy 18 (Baty et al. 1994a).

First trimester sonographic findings observed in fetuses with trisomy 18 include increased nuchal

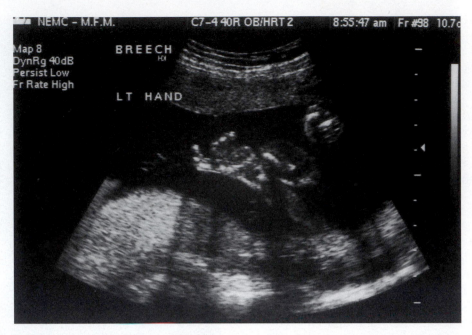

Figure 133-2. Prenatal sonographic image of same fetus shown in Figure 133-1. Note the flexed fingers, which were fixed in position, indicating the presence of camptodactyly.

translucency thickness and pulsatile blood flow in the umbilical vein (Brown et al. 1999; Sherod et al. 1997).

▶ DIFFERENTIAL DIAGNOSIS

The differential diagnosis of trisomy 18 includes Pena–Shokeir I syndrome, pseudotrisomy 18, and arthrogryposis multiplex congenita (see Chapter 102).

Pena–Shokeir I syndrome is an autosomal recessive syndrome whose hallmark features include IUGR, low-set, malformed ears, a depressed tip of the nose, small mouth, micrognathia, multiple flexion contractures, camptodactyly, rocker-bottom feet, pulmonary hypoplasia, and cryptorchidism (Muller and deJong 1986). This condition is highly lethal—30% of affected fetuses are stillborn. The prenatal sonographic findings described for this condition include polyhydramnios, scalp edema, retrognathia, feeble limb movements, flattened nasal bridge, deformed ears, flexion deformities of the extremities, small thorax, and absent fetal respiratory movements. The distinguishing features between trisomy 18 and Pena–Shokeir I syndrome are scalp edema and lung hypoplasia. Prenatal sonographic diagnosis of Pena–Shokeir I syndrome is possible only in cases of a known family history for this condition.

Pseudotrisomy 18 is a diagnosis of exclusion after a karyotype has revealed normal chromosomes. This is an autosomal recessive lethal condition that presents with micrognathia, flexion contractures of the fingers, low-set, malformed ears, and IUGR (Le Marec et al.

1981). To distinguish between pseudotrisomy 18 and trisomy 18, a normal karyotype is necessary. There are an equal number of affected females and males with pseudotrisomy 18. This differs from the excess of females seen with trisomy 18. Also, cardiac abnormalities are not characteristic of pseudotrisomy 18. Pseudotrisomy 18 is associated with consanguinity. A history of advanced maternal age is more typical for cases of trisomy 18.

The multiple flexion contractures seen in fetuses in which trisomy 18 is suspected may also be characteristic of arthrogryposis multiplex congenita (see Chapter 102). Fetuses affected with arthrogryposis may have camptodactyly, small thorax, and micrognathia.

▶ ANTENATAL NATURAL HISTORY

Trisomy 18 is highly lethal in utero. In a survey of the rates of spontaneous death of fetuses with chromosomal abnormalities detected at second-trimester amniocentesis in which the mother did not elect to terminate the pregnancy, Hook et al. (1989) determined an excess risk of 63.8% (range, 49.3 to 79.8%) of in utero death of fetuses with trisomy 18. There is significant loss of male fetuses with trisomy 18 during the second half of pregnancy (Heuther et al. 1996).

Hyett et al. (1995) studied the cardiac defects in fetuses with trisomy 18 who were identified by increased nuchal translucency measurement and were terminated between 11 and 14 weeks of gestation. There was an unusually high frequency of perimembranous

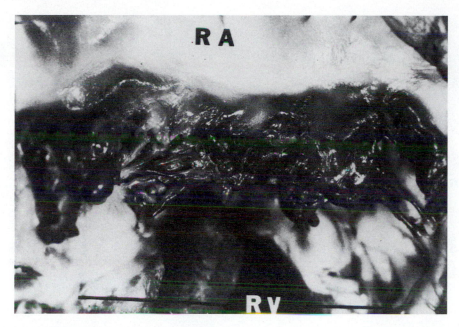

Figure 133-3. Dysplastic tricuspid valve in a 1-month-old infant with trisomy 18. The valve is thickened, gelatinous, and nodular. RA = right atrium; RV = right ventricle. *(Reprinted from Matsouka R, Misugi K, Goto A, Gilbert EF, Ando M. Congenital heart anomalies in the trisomy 18 syndrome, with reference to congenital polyvalvular disease. Am J Med Genet 1983;14:657–668. Copyright 1983 Wiley-Liss. Reprinted by permission of Wiley-Liss, Inc., a subsidiary of John Wiley & Sons, Inc.)*

ventricular septal defects and polyvalvular abnormalities, which were consistent with the developmental arrest of the cardiovascular system occurring between 6 and 8 weeks of gestation. These investigators studied 50 apparently normal fetuses and 19 fetuses with trisomy 18. All 19 had cardiac defects. A ventricular septal defect was demonstrated in 16 of 19 (84%) of fetuses, and valvular abnormalities were also seen in 84% of fetuses. Fourteen of 16 fetuses with abnormalities had more than one valve affected (Fig. 133-3). In addition, 10 of 18 fetuses studied had a hypoplastic aortic isthmus or pulmonary trunk and 6 of 18 fetuses had persistence of the left superior vena cava. It was hypothesized that hemodynamic changes due to valvular abnormalities and hypoplasia of the great vessels may be the mechanism for the increased nuchal translucency seen in trisomic fetuses (Hyett et al. 1995).

Although 80 to 85% of fetuses with trisomy 18 have a full trisomy when their amniocytes or lymphocytes are studied (Fig. 133-4), when the placenta is studied it has been documented that 5% of the fetuses have a mosaic placenta with a normal diploid cell line. The use of cytogenetic analysis has demonstrated that this diploid cell line is confined to the cytotrophoblast in viable pregnancies with trisomy 18. This suggests that a normal diploid component of the trophoblast may facilitate the prolonged intrauterine survival in cases of trisomy 18 (Harrison et al. 1993). This postzygotic loss of a trisomic chromosome in a progenitor cell of a trophoectoderm facilitates intrauterine survival of a trisomy 18 conceptus. It is placental function, therefore, that determines intrauterine survival (Kalousek et al. 1989).

▶ MANAGEMENT OF PREGNANCY

Clinical suspicion of trisomy 18 can develop because of IUGR in the third trimester or an abnormal serum screen in the second trimester. Multiple abnormalities of serum screening have been associated with a fetus with trisomy 18, including low α-fetoprotein (AFP) levels, low unconjugated estriol values, and a low β human chorionic gonadotropin (β-hCG) level. In one study, the maternal serum free β-hCG level was 0.37 multiples of the median (MoM) and the AFP level was 0.71 MoM in trisomy 18 (Spencer et al. 1983). These results were validated by Leporrier et al. (1996), who documented a low mean hCG and a mean unconjugated estriol 3 (UE3) of 0.4 MoM. With these abnormal values, the detection rate for trisomy 18 is 48% for a 0.8% false positive rate and 79% for a 3% false positive rate. Therefore, serum screening is more sensitive and specific for the detection of trisomy 18 than for trisomy 21.

Fetuses in which trisomy 18 is suspected either on the basis of abnormal serum screen or by IUGR and evidence of fetal distress should be referred to a center

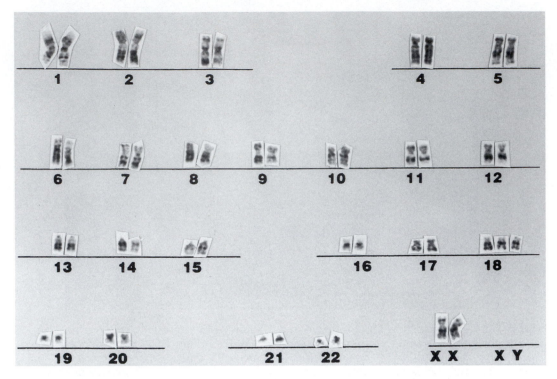

Figure 133-4. Karyotype demonstrating full trisomy 18 in a female. *(Courtesy of Dr. Janet Cowan.)*

capable of performing detailed anatomic scanning of the fetus. Furthermore, a karyotype should be performed, even when the abnormalities are detected during the third trimester. This is important because it is well documented that fetuses with trisomy 18 have an excess of post-term deliveries and fetal distress prompting emergency cesarean section. In two separate studies performed in two different countries, the incidence of cesarean delivery for fetuses with trisomy 18 was on the order of 50% (David and Glew 1980; Schneider et al. 1981). Therefore, a definitive diagnosis of a fetus with trisomy 18 may help the obstetrician and prospective parents to avoid unnecessary fetal monitoring and emergency cesarean delivery. Furthermore, antenatal knowledge that the infant has trisomy 18 will help to appropriately plan newborn resuscitation and further management.

▶ FETAL INTERVENTION

There are no fetal interventions for trisomy 18.

▶ TREATMENT OF THE NEWBORN

If the karyotype was not performed antenatally it should be performed at birth. A complete physical examination is indicated, and will demonstrate the presence of intrauterine growth restriction, a prominent occiput, and a short sternum. No single physical finding is pathognomonic for trisomy 18. The major clinical features include hypertonia, anteroposterior elongation of the skull, partial syndactyly of the toes, hypoplastic toenails, narrow chest, micrognathia, short sternum, congenital heart disease, and renal anomalies (Taylor 1968). The presence of low-arch dermal ridges, which can be seen only with a magnifying lens, is a helpful diagnostic finding, as it is generally seen in most of the fingers of affected patients with trisomy 18. Because of the delay in obtaining chromosome analysis, Marion et al. (1988) developed a bedside score for the clinical diagnosis of trisomy 18 during the immediate neonatal period. Points are given for features reported in a majority of infants with trisomy 18. The maximal attainable score is 160. In this report, in 11 patients with trisomy 18, the average score was 94.3 (range, 70 to 113). In 11 patients without trisomy 18, the average score was 41.4 (Marion et al. 1988).

Infants in whom trisomy 18 is suspected should undergo echocardiography because of the 90% incidence of congenital heart disease in affected patients. In one study of 15 autopsied cases of trisomy 18, all infants were shown to have congenital polyvalvular heart disease. Membranous VSDs were present in 87% of infants, patent ductus arteriosus (PDA) in 73%, and a high takeoff of the right coronary ostium in 80% (Matsouka et al. 1983). The most severe changes were present in the tricuspid and mitral valves with derangement of the spongiosa and fibrosa and defective elastic fibers. The heart valves are dysplastic in trisomy 18, and are noted to be thickened, gelatinous, and nodular. Other findings include long chordae tendineae and hypoplastic or absent papillary muscles (Van Praagh et al. 1989) (see Fig. 133-3). Musewe et al. (1990) reviewed the role that cardiac anomalies play in the early death seen in cases of trisomy 18. They noted that most VSDs and PDAs were large and valvular dysplasia of one or more valves was seen in 68% of cases. However, the valvular dyplasia was not associated with evidence of significant regurgitation or stenosis on Doppler studies. The cardiac anomalies most frequently encountered were not lethal. These authors suggested that an increased right ventricular volume, pulmonary hypertension, and maldevelopment of the pulmonary vasculature contributes to early death (Musewe et al. 1990).

There is a high incidence of 11 pairs of ribs in cases of trisomy 18 (Ho 1989). Because of the severity of the clinical consequences of trisomy 18 and the poor prognosis, we recommend that chromosome analysis be performed as soon as possible after birth if it was not performed antenatally. If a surgical emergency is present, consideration should be given to performing fluorescence in situ hybridization (FISH) using chromosome-18-specific probes. This will provide rapid confirmation of the clinically suspected diagnosis, and in this setting, emergency surgery should be avoided if possible (Bos et al. 1992). Major surgery is likely to inflict suffering in an infant whose life expectancy is otherwise poor.

▶ SURGICAL TREATMENT

As discussed above, surgical treatment to prolong life should be discussed with the family. In the relatively rare long-term survivors, surgical treatment may ultimately be indicated to improve their quality of life.

▶ LONG-TERM OUTCOME

In an extensive survey of 98 families with an index case of trisomy 18, Baty et al. (1984a) documented an average length of survival for males with trisomy 18 of 1.4 months and for females with trisomy 18, 9.6 months (Fig. 133-5). Many obstetricians and pediatricians mistakenly think that trisomy 18 is lethal during the newborn period. Although 55 to 65% of newborns with trisomy 18 die during the first week of life, 5 to 10% of infants are alive at 1 year of age (Root and Carey 1994).

In Baty et al.'s (1994a) study of the long-term medical outcome for infants with trisomy 18, the average neonatal hospital stay was 19.6 days, with an average number of 10.1 days on a ventilator. Eighty percent of their trisomy 18 cases went home from the hospital. Of these, 5% went home on oxygen, 12% went home on a cardiac monitor, and 44% were bottle- or breast-fed.

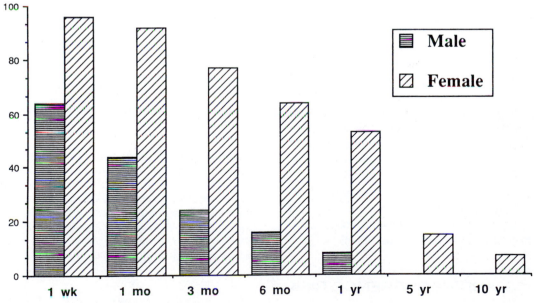

Figure 133-5. The longer-term survival of female versus male infants with trisomy 18 is clearly demonstrated in this graph. Data are based on 70 cases. *(Reprinted from Baty BJ, Blackburn BL, and Carey JC. Natural history of trisomy 18 and trisomy 13. I. Growth, physical assessment, medical histories, survival, and recurrence risk. Am J Med Genet 1994a;49:175–188. Copyright © 1994 Wiley-Liss. Reprinted, by permission, of Wiley-Liss, Inc., a subsidiary of John Wiley & Sons, Inc.)*

Nineteen percent of patients eventually required placement of a gastrostomy tube, but the average age of insertion of this tube was 8.4 months. Of long-term survivors, 17% had a known hearing loss, and of these patients, 41% eventually obtained a hearing aid. The major medical problems for long-term survivors with trisomy 18 include scoliosis, gastroesophageal reflux, hearing loss, and Wilms' tumor (Carey 1992).

Baty et al. (1994a) generated growth curves for long-term survivors with trisomy 18. These demonstrate that the weight and height curves for patients with trisomy 18 are consistently below the normal curve, except for an overlap at birth (Fig. 133-6). Long-term survivors were given immunizations in the first 6 months of life and there were no adverse complications directly attributable to the immunization.

In a related study, Baty et al. (1994b) collected developmental data on 50 individuals with trisomy 18. The developmental quotient (DQ), developmental age divided by the chronologic age, was on average 0.18. The developmental ages were studied in seven skill areas, and these differed significantly among the areas. Daily living skills and receptive language had the highest values, whereas motor and communication skill had the lowest values. During the first year of life, affected individuals with trisomy 18 achieved the following skills: following, cooing, rolling, social smile, reaching, and recognition of close adults. During the next 2 years, these individuals were able to sit unsupported, object permanence developed, and they were able to imitate actions and to recognize words. By age 4 to 6 years, affected individuals began to crawl and to follow simple commands, began helping with hygiene, and were capable of both independent playing and the use of signs. These investigators concluded that patients with trisomy 18 achieved some psychomotor maturation and continued to learn, although very slowly (Baty et al. 1994b).

In summary, the clinical history of a child with trisomy 18 is associated with apneic episodes, poor feeding, and marked failure to thrive. Management of cardiac disease is primarily medical, with administration of diuretics and digoxin (Van Dyke and Allen 1990).

The most common causes of death in individuals with trisomy 18 are cardiopulmonary arrest (68% of cases), congenital heart disease (11% of cases), and pneumonia (11% of cases) (Baty et al. 1994a).

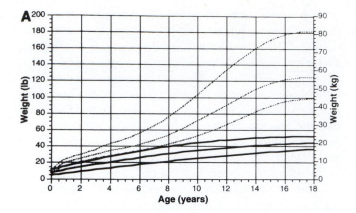

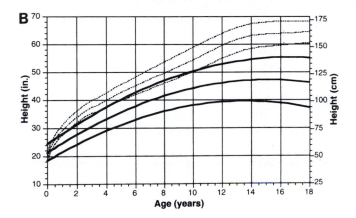

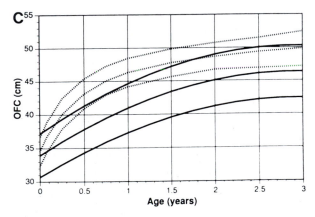

Figure 133-6. Growth curves for infants and children with trisomy 18. *(Reprinted from Baty BJ, Blackburn BL, and Carey JC. Natural history of trisomy 18 and trisomy 13. I. Growth, physical assessment, medical histories, survival, and recurrence risk. Am J Med Genet 1994a;49:175–188. Copyright © 1994 Wiley-Liss. Reprinted, by permission, of Wiley-Liss, Inc., a subsidiary of John Wiley & Sons, Inc.)*

▶ GENETICS AND RECURRENCE RISK

Trisomy 18 is due to the presence of an extra chromosome 18, which is demonstrated on karyotyping. The recurrence risk for full trisomy 18 is commonly quoted as 1% or the age-related maternal risk, whichever is higher. The data from Baty et al. (1994a) on recurrence

risk for trisomies 13 and 18 was 0.55%, based on one affected sibling from 181 subsequent pregnancies.

The origin of the extra chromosome in trisomy 18 is almost always maternal. Using molecular analysis and DNA polymorphisms, the origin of the extra chromosome was studied in 23 individuals with trisomy 18.

Twenty of 23 were informative. In 19 of 20 the extra chromosome was maternal in origin (Kupke and Müller 1989). Using DNA repeat sequences and a polymerase chain reaction–based assay, Nöthen et al. (1993) traced the parental origin in 30 cases of trisomy 18. The extra chromosome was maternal in 26 of 30 (86.7%) of cases and paternal in the remainder. When the nondisjunction resulting in trisomy 18 is due to a meiotic error, Eggerman et al. (1996) demonstrated that there was an increased number of meiosis II errors. This is somewhat different from trisomy 13 and 21, in which errors in the first meiotic division predominate.

To date, the specific region of chromosome 18 needed to produce the full phenotype of trisomy 18 has not been identified using molecular techniques (Boghosian-Sell 1994). Duplication of part of the long arm of chromosome 18 may be associated with the mental retardation seen in trisomy 18.

There is an increasing appreciation of trisomy 18 mosaicism in women who have normal intelligence but a history of amenorrhea or miscarriages (Satge et al. 1996; Uehara et al. 1996). Kohn and Shohat (1987) described a 30-year-old woman with minor dysmorphic features and normal intelligence who had karyotyping because of a history of three miscarriages. Trisomy 18 was present in 18% of her lymphocytes and 2% of her skin fibroblasts. Several patients have been diagnosed because they gave birth to a child with trisomy 18.

Prenatal diagnosis in subsequent pregnancies is by karyotyping. Prospective parents can be offered chromosome analysis on chorionic villus cells or amniocytes, which will give a definitive diagnosis in a subsequent pregnancy.

REFERENCES

Bass HN, Fox M, Wulsberg E, Sparkes RS, Crandall BF. Trisomy 18 mosaicism: clues to the diagnosis. Clin Genet 1982;22:327–330.

Baty BJ, Blackburn BL, and Carey JC. Natural history of trisomy 18 and trisomy 13. I. Growth, physical assessment, medical histories, survival, and recurrence risk. Am J Med Genet 1994a;49:175–188.

Baty BJ, Jorde LB, Blackburn BL, Carey JC. Natural history of trisomy 18 and trisomy 13. II. Psychomotor development. Am J Med Genet 1994b;49:189–194.

Benacerraf BR, Frigoletto FD, Greene MF. Abnormal facial features and extremities in human trisomy syndromes: prenatal US appearance. Radiology 1986;159:243–246.

Benacerraf B, Miller WA, Frigoletto FD. Sonographic detection of fetuses with trisomies 13 and 18: accuracy and limitations. Am J Obstet Gynecol 1988;158:404–409.

Benacerraf BR, Nadel A, Bromley B. Identification of second-trimester fetuses with autosomal trisomy by use of a sonographic scoring index. Radiology 1994;193:135–140.

Boghosian-Sell L, Mewar R, Harrison W, et al. Molecular mapping of the Edwards syndrome phenotype to two noncontiguous regions on chromosome 18. Am J Hum Genet 1994;55:476–483.

Bos AP, Broers CJM, Hazebroek FWL, et al. Avoidance of emergency surgery in newborn infants with trisomy 18. Lancet 1992;339:913–915.

Brons JTJ, Van Der Harter HJ, Van Geijn HP, et al. Prenatal ultrasonographic diagnosis of radial-ray reduction malformations. Prenat Diagn 1990;10:279–288.

Brown RN, DiLuzio L, Gomes C, Nicolaides KH. First trimester umbilical venous Doppler sonography in chromosomally normal and abnormal fetuses. J Ultrasound Med 1999;18:543–546.

Carey JC. Health supervision and anticipatory guidance for children with genetic disorders (including specific recommendations for trisomy 21, trisomy 18, and neurofibromatosis). Pediatr Clin North Am 1992;39:25–53.

Carlson DE, Platt LD, Medearis A. The ultrasound triad of fetal hydramnios, abnormal hand posturing, and any other anomaly predicts autosomal trisomy. Obstet Gynecol 1992;79:731–734.

David TJ, Glew S. Morbidity of trisomy 18 includes delivery by cesarean section. Lancet 1980;2:1295.

Droste S, Fitzsimmons J, Pascoe-Mason J, Shepard T. Growth of linear parameters in trisomy 18 fetuses. Obstet Gynecol 1990;163:158–161.

Edwards JH. A new trisomic syndrome. Lancet 1960;1:787.

Eggermann T, Nöthen MM, Eiben B, et al. Trisomy of human chromosome 18: molecular studies on parental origin and cell stage of nondisjunction. Hum Genet 1996;97:218–223.

Ginsberg N, Cadkin A, Pergament E, Verlinsky Y. Ultrasonographic detection of the second-trimester fetus with trisomy 18 and trisomy 21. Am J Obstet Gynecol 1990;163: 1186–1190.

Goldstein H, Nielsen KG. Rates and survival of individuals with trisomy 13 and 18. Clin Genet 1988;34:366–372.

Hamada, H, Okuno S, Fujiki Y, Yamada N, Sohda S, Kubo T. Echogenic fetal bowel in the third trimester associated with trisomy 18. Eur J Obstet Gynecol Reprod Biol 1996; 77:65–67.

Harrison KJ, Barrett IJ, Lomax BL, Kuchinka BD, Kalousek DK. Detection of confined placental mosaicism in trisomy 18 conceptions using interphase cytogenic analysis. Hum Genet 1993;92:353–358.

Hill LM. The sonographic detection of trisomies 13, 18, and 21. Clin Obstet Gynecol 1996;39:831–850.

Ho KN. Eleven pairs of ribs in trisomy 18. J Pediatr 1989; 113:902.

Hook EB, Topol BB, Cross PK. The natural history of cytogenetically abnormal fetuses detected at midtrimester amniocentesis which are not terminated electively: new data and estimates of the excess and relative risk of late fetal death associated with 47, +21 and some other abnormal karyotypes. Am J Hum Genet 1989;45:855–861.

Huether CA, Martin RLM, Stoppelman SM, et al. Sex ratios in fetuses and liveborn infants with autosomal aneuploidy. Am J Med Genet 1996;63:492–500.

Hyett JA, Moscoso G, Nicolaides KH. Cardiac defects in 1st-trimester fetuses with trisomy 18. Fetal Diagn Ther 1995;10:381–386.

Kalousek DK, Barrett IJ, McGillivray BC. Placental mosaicism and intrauterine survival of trisomies 13 and 18. Am J Hum Genet 1989;44:338–343.

Kohn G, Shohat M. Trisomy 18 mosaicism in an adult with normal intelligence. Am J Med Genet 1987;26:929–931.

Kupke KG, Müller U. Parental origin of the extra chromosome in trisomy 18. Am J Hum Genet 1989;45:599–605.

Le Marec B, Paty E, Roussey M, et al. La phénocopie de la trisomie 18; une maladie autosomique récessive? Arch Fr Pediatr 1981;38:253–259.

LePorrier N, Herrou M, Herlicoviez M, Leymarie P. The usefulness of hCG and unconjugated oestriol in prenatal diagnosis of trisomy 18. Br J Obstet Gynecol 1996;103:335–338.

Lynch L, Berkowitz RL. First trimester growth delay in trisomy 18. Am J Perinatol 1989;6:237–239.

Marion RW, Chitayat D, Hutcheon G, et al. Trisomy 18 score: a rapid, reliable diagnostic test for trisomy 18. J Pediatr 1988;113:45–48.

Matsouka R, Misugi K, Goto A, Gilbert EF, Ando M. Congenital heart anomalies in the trisomy 18 syndrome, with reference to congenital polyvalvular disease. Am J Med Genet 1983;14:657–668.

Muller LM, deJong G. Prenatal ultrasonographic features of the Pena–Shokeir I syndrome and the trisomy 18 syndrome. Am J Med Genet 1986;25:119–129.

Musewe NN, Alexander DJ, Teshima I, Smallhorn JF, Freedom RM. Echocardiographic evaluation of the spectrum of cardiac anomalies associated with trisomy 13 and trisomy 18. J Am Coll Cardiol 1990;15:673–677.

Nicolaides KH, Salvesen DR, Snijders RJM, et al. Strawberry-shaped skull in fetal trisomy 18. Fetal Diagn Ther 1992; 7:132–137.

Nöthen MM, Eggerman T, Erdmann J, et al. Retrospective study of the parental origin of the extra chromosome in trisomy 18 (Edwards syndrome). Hum Genet 1993;92: 347–349.

Nyberg DA, Kramer D, Resta R, et al. Prenatal sonographic findings of trisomy 18: review of 47 cases. J Ultrasound Med 1993;2:103–113.

Root S, Carey JC. Survival in trisomy 18. Am J Med Genet 1994;49:170–174.

Schneider AS, Mennutu MT, Zackai EH. High cesarean section rate in trisomy 18 births: a potential indication for late prenatal diagnosis. Am J Obstet Gynecol 1981;140:4: 367–370.

Satge D, Geneix A, Goburdhun J, et al. A history of miscarriages and mild prognathism as possible mode of presentation of mosaic trisomy 18 in women. Clin Genet 1996;50:470–473.

Seoud MA-F, Alley DC, Smith DL, Levy DL. Prenatal sonographic findings in trisomy 13, 18, 21 and 22: a review of 46 cases. J Reprod Med 1994;39:781–787.

Sepulveda W, Treadwell MC, Fisk NM. Prenatal detection of preaxial upper limb reduction in trisomy 18. Obstet Gynecol 1995;85:847–850.

Sherod C, Sebire NJ, Soares W, Snijders RJ, Nicolaides KH. Prenatal diagnosis of trisomy 18 at the 10–14 week ultrasound scan. Ultrasound Obstet Gynecol 1997;10: 387–390.

Snijders RJM, Shawa L, Nicolaides KH. Fetal choroid plexus cysts and trisomy 18: assessment of risk based on ultrasound findings and maternal age. Prenat Diagn 1994;14: 1119–1127.

Spencer K, Mallard AS, Coombes EJ, Macri JN. Prenatal screening for trisomy 18 with free β human chorionic gonadotrophin as a marker. BMJ 1993;307:1455–1458.

Taylor AI. Autosomal trisomy syndromes: a detailed study of 27 cases of Edwards' syndrome and 27 cases of Patau's syndrome. J Med Genet 1968;5:227–241.

Thurmond AS, Nelson DW, Lowensohn RI, Young WP, Davis L. Enlarged cisterna magna in trisomy 18: prenatal ultrasonographic diagnosis. Am J Obstet Gynecol 1989; 161:83–85.

Uehara S, Obara Y, Obara T, Funato T, et al. Trisomy 18 mosaicism associated with secondary amenorrhea: ratios of mosaicism in different samples and complications. Clin Genet 1996;49:91–94.

Van Dyke DC, Allen M. Clinical management considerations in long-term survivors with trisomy 18. Pediatrics 1990; 85:753–759.

Van Praagh S, Truman T, Firpo A, et al. Cardiac malformations in trisomy-18: a study of 41 postmortem cases. J Am Coll Cardiol 1989;13:7:1586–1597.

Wladimiroff JW, Stewart PA, Reuss A, Sachs ES. Cardiac and extra-cardiac anomalies as indicators for trisomies 13 and 18: a prenatal ultrasound study. Prenat Diagn 1989;9: 515–520.

Young ID, Cook JP, Metha L. Changing demography of trisomy 18. Arch Dis Child 1986;61:1035–1036.

CHAPTER 134
Trisomy 21

► CONDITION

Trisomy 21 is an abnormality due to the presence of an extra copy of chromosome 21 (Fig. 134-1). Individuals with the clinical characteristics of what we know as Down syndrome were first described by Dr. John Langdon Down in 1866. Dr. Down was a physician at the Earlswood asylum in Surrey, England. His erroneous ideas about a racial cause for Down syndrome, along with a superficial similarity in facial appearance to persons of mongoloid origin, led to the term mongolism (Cooley and Graham 1991).

The association between the clinical entity Down syndrome and an extra copy of chromosome 21 was noted in 1959 by Dr. Jerome Lejeune in Paris. Ninety-five percent of individuals with Down syndrome have

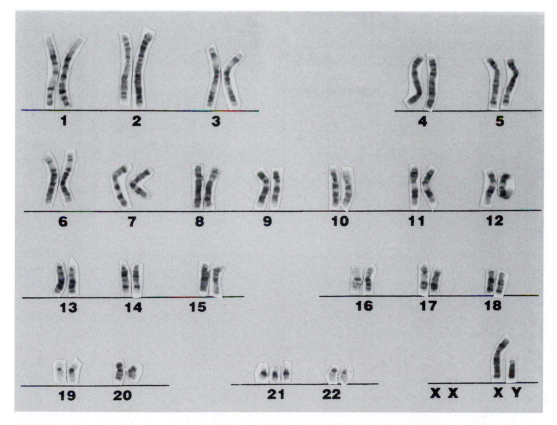

Figure 134-1. Karyotype from a male individual with Down syndrome, indicating the presence of three copies of chromosome 21. *(Courtesy of Dr. Janet Cowan.)*

three copies of chromosome 21, which results from meiotic nondisjunction of the pair of number 21 chromosomes in the formation of an egg or sperm prior to fertilization. Ninety-four percent of the time, the extra copy of the chromosome 21 is maternal in origin (Antonarakis et al. 1991). Approximately 3 to 4% of cases of Down syndrome are due to an unbalanced translocation involving chromosome 21. Fifty percent of the translocation cases occur spontaneously (de novo) and 50% are inherited from a parent with a balanced translocation. One percent of cases of Down syndrome are due to mosaicism, beginning as a trisomic conceptus with selective loss of one copy of chromosome 21 ("disomic rescue") or as mitotic nondisjunction occurring after fertilization in a specific cell line or lines.

Interestingly, a full extra copy of chromosome 21 is not needed to cause the symptoms of Down syndrome. The phenotype of Down syndrome is due to triplication of the genes expressed in a relatively small region of chromosome 21, band 21q22.

Currently, there is much interest in the noninvasive techniques of screening for Down syndrome, by both second-trimester measurement of serum proteins— α-fetoprotein (AFP), human chorionic gonadotropin (hCG) estriol, and inhibin A—as well as first-trimester serum screening, using a combination of maternal age, nuchal translucency measurement (see Chapter 34), and analysis of the serum proteins hCG and pregnancy-associated plasma protein A (PAPP-A). In theory, first-trimester screening is believed to have an 80% detection rate for Down syndrome with a 5% false positive rate (Wald and Hackshaw 1997). Fetal cells in maternal blood may eventually have a role in the diagnosis of Down syndrome due to the fact that an increased number of fetal cells cross the placenta when the fetus has trisomy 21 (Bianchi et al. 1997).

▶ INCIDENCE

The incidence of trisomy 21 is 1 in 920 live births (Krivchenia et al. 1993). The frequency of Down syndrome increases with advanced maternal age. The incidence of Down syndrome appears to be similar in all ethnic and racial groups. Published differences in the prevalence of Down syndrome according to ethnic origin are difficult to interpret owing to differences in the maternal age structure of populations and variations in completeness of reporting of affected births. Lau et al. (1998) reviewed obstetric and neonatal data on 57,742 pregnancies in an ethnic Chinese population in Hong Kong. There were 74 cases of trisomy 21 detected (for an overall incidence of 1.28 cases per 1000 deliveries). The expected and observed numbers were similar in both younger mothers and mothers older than 35 years of age.

Cuckle et al. (1991) estimated the "natural birth prevalence" of Down syndrome, which they defined as the birth prevalence that would be expected in the absence of prenatal diagnosis or induced abortion. In their study, performed in England and Wales from 1974 to 1987, the natural birth prevalence of Down syndrome increased from 12.2 in 10,000 to 13.2 in 10,000—an average of 12.6 in 10,000 births. Fourteen percent of cases of Down syndrome were avoided by prenatal diagnosis and termination of affected pregnancies. The actual birth prevalence, which reflected the utilization of prenatal diagnosis, was 10.8 in 10,000 births in this population (Cuckle et al. 1991).

▶ SONOGRAPHIC FINDINGS

Multiple-Marker Studies

The diagnosis of trisomy 21 can be made only by karyotyping fetal cells obtained by chorionic villus sampling, amniocentesis, or cordocentesis. Several authors, however, have advocated the use of a "genetic sonogram," which in addition to standard fetal biometry, seeks the presence of sonographic abnormalities such as those listed in Table 134-1. In one study of 573 high-risk pregnant women, Vintzileos et al. (1996) found that 12 of 14 fetuses with trisomy 21 had two or more sonographic markers present. When two or more abnormal sonographic markers were found in a group of pregnant women with at least a 1 in 274 risk of aneuploidy, the sensitivity was 85.7%, the specificity was 99.8%, the positive predictive value was 48%, and the negative predictive value was 99.5%. These patients were counseled that if "the results of the genetic sonogram were normal . . . the chances of having a fetus with trisomy 21 were theoretically reduced by at least 50%" (Vintzileos et al. 1996). In our practice, we counsel pregnant patients that the only definitive way of obtaining a diagnosis is to perform fetal karyotyping.

The major sonographic findings seen in fetuses with trisomy 21 are listed in Table 134-1. Many of these findings are discussed in individual chapters. In general, in cases of trisomy 21, sonographic defects tend to be more subtle than in cases of trisomies 13 or 18. These findings include nuchal edema, hydronephrosis, clinodactyly, sandal gap (wide space between first and second toes), and macroglossia (Nicolaides et al. 1992b). The frequency of major internal congenital malformations is less than with trisomies 13 or 18 (Hill 1996).

Nyberg et al. (1990) reviewed the sonographic findings in 94 consecutive fetuses with trisomy 21 over a 6-year period at a single institution. The major anomalies detected by this group included cardiac defects, duodenal atresia, cystic hygroma, omphalocele, hydrops, and hydrothorax. The anomalies detected before 20

► **TABLE 134-1.** SONOGRAPHICALLY DETECTABLE MALFORMATIONS ASSOCIATED WITH TRISOMY 21

Craniofacial
  Thickened nuchal fold
  Increased nuchal translucency measurement
  Cystic hygroma
  Protuberant tongue
Central nervous system
  Choroid plexus cysts
  Mild ventriculomegaly
Cardiovascular system
  Ventricularseptal defect
  Atrial septal defect
  Endocardial cushion defect
  Calcification of the chordae tendinae
Gastrointestinal system
  Duodenal atresia
  Echogenic bowel
  Imperforate anus
Urogenital system
  Pyelectasis
Skeletal system
  Brachycephaly with flat occiput
  Shortened long bones
  Clinodactyly
  Syndactyly
  Short, thick fingers
  Gap between 1st and 2nd toes
  Elongated ischial bones
Nonimmune hydrops
Amniotic fluid volume
  Polyhydramnios
Intrauterine growth restriction

Source: Hill LM. The sonographic detection of trisomies 13, 18, and 21. Clin Obstet Gynecol 1996;38:831–850.

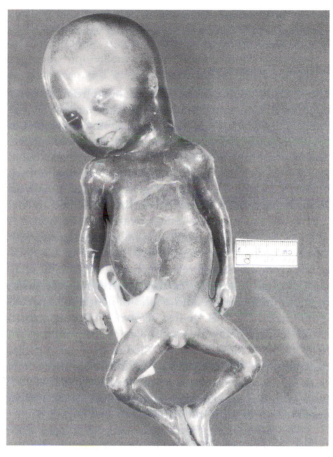

Figure 134-2. Nineteen-week-old fetus with trisomy 21. Note the relative nasal hypoplasia, small mouth, prominent tongue, and cystic hygroma. (*Courtesy of Dr. Joseph Semple.*)

weeks of gestation included cystic hygromas, nuchal thickening, and echogenic bowel (Fig. 134-2). Thirty-seven anomalies were seen in 31 fetuses; 20 anomalies in 17 fetuses were missed. These were predominantly cardiac. One or more sonographic abnormalities were observed in 33% of the fetuses with Down syndrome (Nyberg et al. 1990). More recently, Rottmensch et al. (1997) reviewed the frequency and type of abnormal sonographic findings in 187 fetuses with Down syndrome. The most commonly detected abnormalities were cystic hygroma and nuchal-fold thickness, seen in 30.5% of fetuses, followed by hydrops (9.6%), cardiac defects (7.5%), renal pyelectasis or hydronephrosis (5.9%), echogenic bowel (4.8%), and a variety of internal-organ abnormalities not typically associated with Down syndrome (16.0%). All other abnormalities had a frequency of less than 2.1%. These authors quoted a sensitivity for the sonographic detection of Down syndrome of 24.1% at less than 13 weeks of gestation and 42.6% between 14 and 23 weeks of gestation. These sensitivities were calculated on the basis of an ultrasound diagnosis without prior knowledge of the fetal karyotype. A total of 138 abnormalities were observed in 93 fetuses in this study.

Because Down syndrome features present with a variety of subtle sonographic features, Deren et al. (1998) looked at the identification of these subtle sonographic abnormalities to see if detection of Down syndrome fetuses could be improved. These authors studied clinodactyly, a dilated renal pelvis (≥ 4 mm), echogenic bowel, mild ventriculomegaly (≥ 10 to ≥ 15 mm), and a two-vessel cord. Univariate analysis revealed that all subtle anomalies except the two-vessel cord correlated with the presence of Down syndrome; however, only echogenic bowel and clinodactyly were significant in the regression analysis. In combination with standard biometry or the presence of a gross anatomic defect, searching for the presence of subtle abnormalities increased the detection rate of Down syndrome fetuses by 10%. Clinodactyly (see Chapter 103) had the highest individual sensitivity among the subtle-anomaly markers. These authors concluded that adding

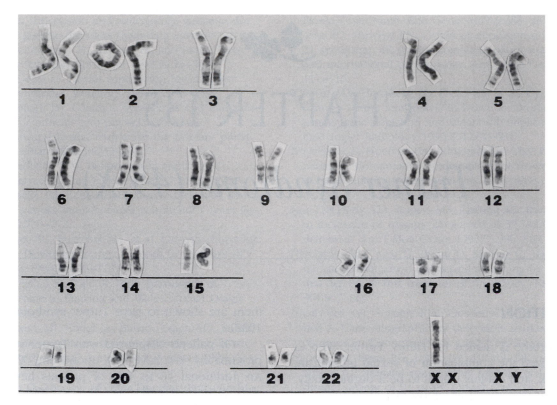

Figure 135-1. Chromosome analysis demonstrating 45,X, which is found in about half of cases of Turner syndrome. *(Courtesy of Dr. Janet Cowan.)*

resolution of a nuchal cystic hygroma and pleural effusion during the third trimester in a fetus with Turner syndrome. There was a good outcome for this case. Similarly, Chodirker et al. (1988) also described resolution of a cystic hygroma, but demonstrated the postnatal appearance of a webbed neck (pterygium colli) and

a rotated ear. Other manifestations of lymphatic malformations include transient bilateral pleural effusion, which has been demonstrated as early as the first trimester using transvaginal imaging (Shimizu et al. 1997).

The sonographic diagnosis of cystic hygroma is made by the demonstration of a thin-walled multiseptated

Figure 135-2. Septated cystic hygroma in the posterior nuchal region, as demonstrated by a fetal sonographic image. This fetus was shown to have 45,X.

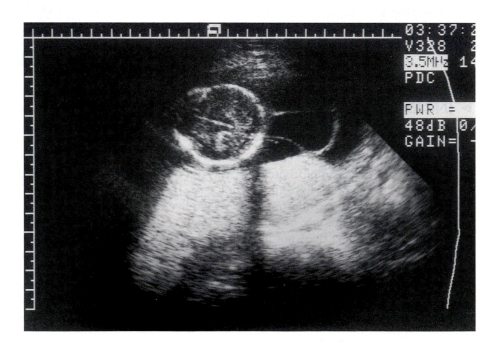

asymmetrical fluid-filled mass attached to the lateral aspect of the fetal head or neck (see Fig. 135-2). The mass is in a constant location with respect to the fetal occiput and is independent of fetal motion (Donnenfeld and Mennuti 1988; Garden et al. 1986).

A somewhat rarer presentation of the fetal lymphatic malformations seen in Turner syndrome is isolated fetal ascites. Wax et al. (1992) presented a case of massive fetal ascites and polyhydramnios detected at 32 weeks of gestation resulting from congenital intestinal lymphangiectasia. This case was later shown to be Turner syndrome.

Other manifestations of Turner syndrome may include mild intrauterine growth restriction and cardiovascular malformations. The most common cardiovascular malformations seen in Turner syndrome affect the aortic valve and include bicuspid aortic valve and coarctation of the aorta (see Chapter 46). In a Danish study of 179 female children and adults, 46 (26%) had cardiac abnormalities. Of these, 18% had aortic-valve abnormalities and 10% had coarctation of the aorta, but the majority of these were detected postnatally (Gøtzsche et al. 1994). These investigators noted that there is a decreased prevalence of cardiovascular abnormalities when the patient has mosaicism. In addition, no patient with a structural abnormality of the X chromosome had a cardiovascular malformation. Additional cardiac abnormalities described in cases of Turner syndrome include hypoplastic left heart (Natowicz and Kelley 1987) and partial anomalous pulmonary venous return (Moore 1990).

Approximately 30 to 60% of patients with Turner syndrome have a structural or positional renal anomaly (Hall et al. 1982; Hall and Gilchrist 1990). Horseshoe kidney is especially common, seen in 20% of patients with Turner syndrome. Other typical malformations include duplication of the collecting system (20% of cases) and malrotation (seen in 50% of kidneys). Renal anomalies seen in Turner syndrome rarely result in renal malfunction but may predispose to postnatal urinary tract infections.

▶ DIFFERENTIAL DIAGNOSIS

The differential diagnosis varies according to the age at presentation of symptoms. Prenatally, the lymphatic malformations predominate. The differential diagnosis for cystic hygroma includes cystic teratoma, meningocele, encephalocele, and neural-tube defect (Bluth et al. 1984). Cystic hygroma can be differentiated from neural-tube defects by the demonstration of bilateral echo-free spaces divided by septae. In addition, with a cystic hygroma there is an intact cranial vault and an intact spinal canal. Ascites and an edematous placenta can be seen in association with cystic hygroma, but is generally not seen in association with neural-tube defects or cystic teratoma.

At birth, peripheral lymphedema has the differential diagnosis of Milroy disease, and other single-gene disorders associated with lymphedema, such as lymphedema with recurrent cholestasis or lymphedema with intestinal lymphangiectasia.

Turner syndrome can be detected later in life because of short stature or amenorrhea. The differential diagnosis of short stature includes familial short stature, Noonan syndrome, dyschondrosteosis (Leri–Weill syndrome), growth hormone deficiency, and hypothyroidism (Hall et al. 1982).

Noonan syndrome can be distinguished from Turner syndrome on the basis of a normal chromosome analysis.

▶ ANTENATAL NATURAL HISTORY

Turner syndrome results from haploinsufficiency for specific genes located on the X chromosome. It is highly lethal in utero (Committee on Genetics 1995) (Fig. 135-3). It is estimated that as many as 80% of live-born infants with Turner syndrome have an additional normal cell line that permits postnatal survival (Amiel et al. 1996). In one study of four fetuses with Turner syndrome, three were phenotypically normal and one had malformations. All three that were phenotypically normal had the presence of an additional normal cell line. In the one fetus with malformations, no normal cell line could be demonstrated in any of the tissues examined (Amiel et al. 1996). In a study of 16 first-trimester fetuses with a variety of chromosomal, a monoclonal antibody was used to study the distribution syndrome of lymphatic vessels (von Kaisenberg et al. 1999). In the 3 fetuses with Turner syndrome, the vessels were hypoplastic in the upper dermis.

It is thought that the lymphatic malformations originate from hypoalbuminemia. In a study by Shepard et al. (1986), fetuses with Turner syndrome had lower albumin levels in their plasma as compared with control fetuses. These investigators postulated that early edema resulting from hypoalbuminemia may interfere with the normal development of the lymphatics. In fact, most of the congenital anomalies seen in Turner syndrome can be explained on the basis of lymphedema at critical points in development (Hall and Gilchrist 1990). Some investigators hypothesize that the lymphedema is the result of failure to open embryonic lymph channels. Pterygium colli (webbed neck) results from an in utero persistence of embryonic lymph sacs.

A correlation between neck webbing and the presence of coarctation of the aorta has been noted by Clark (1984), who postulated that large lymph channels adjacent to the aortic outflow tract misdirect blood flow to

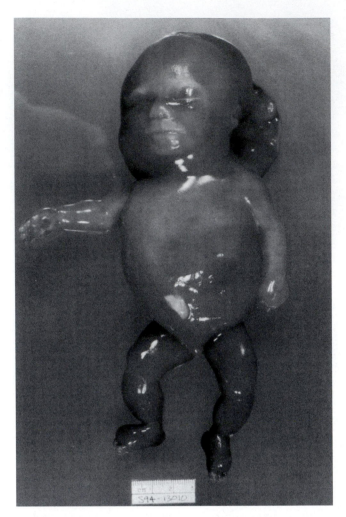

Figure 135-3. Postmortem photograph of a fetus with Turner syndrome. Note the large septated cystic hygroma, body-wall edema, and presence of pedal edema. *(Courtesy of Dr. Joseph Semple.)*

the aorta, thus producing an abnormal blood flow through the ductus arteriosus. In a study of 12 fetuses terminated between 16 and 26 weeks of gestation because of a prenatal finding of cystic hygroma or hydrops, 8 demonstrated a consistent constellation of cardiac defects. These included a small ascending aorta, relatively large pulmonary arteries that were 1.5 to 3 times the size of the aorta, a large patent ductus arteriosus, and a juxta ductal coarctation of the aorta (Lacro et al. 1988). The high incidence of left-sided flow defects among the fetuses in this study supports the hypothesis that there is a pathogenetic relationship between lymphatic obstruction and the subsequent development of congenital heart disease (see Chapter 34). In this study, lymphatic distention was demonstrated on histologic sections obtained through the base of the heart and the pulmonary hila. These data support the concept that hydrostatic pressure occurring within the jugular lymphatic sac can also distend the cardiac lymphatics (Lacro et al. 1988).

► MANAGEMENT OF PREGNANCY

In general, Turner syndrome is suspected because of the presence of an abnormal sonogram or an abnormal serum screening result. Some cases of Turner syndrome are also unexpectedly detected at amniocentesis for advanced maternal age. A unique pattern of serum screening markers is present in both hydropic and nonhydropic cases of Turner syndrome. Typically, there is a slightly reduced α-fetoprotein level, markedly reduced estriol, and increased human chorionic gonadotropin (hCG) levels in hydropic cases of Turner syndrome (Saller et al. 1992). Free β-hCG is thought to be the most effective serum marker for Turner syndrome (Laundon et al. 1996). In Laundon et al.'s study of 17 cases of Turner syndrome, the median level for the multiple of the median for free β-hCG was 4.04.

In the setting of either an abnormal sonogram or an abnormal serum screen, prospective parents should meet with a genetic counselor to discuss the indications for amniocentesis. Turner syndrome is definitively diagnosed by prenatal karyotype. Once the chromosome analysis confirms the finding of Turner syndrome, prospective parents should meet with a geneticist to discuss the long-term implications of the findings, which will differ according to the karyotype. In general, parents should know that a diagnosis of Turner syndrome implies short stature, some congenital anomalies, infertility, and some learning difficulties. However, patients with Turner syndrome have normal intelligence.

If mosaicism is present, the implications of the specific karyotype should be discussed. For example, Koeberl et al. (1995) described their experience with 12 patients diagnosed with amniocentesis for advanced maternal age or maternal serum screen and documented a fetal karyotype of 45,X/46,XX. They compared the long-term outcome for the prenatally diagnosed group with a group of 41 postnatally diagnosed girls with mosaic Turner syndrome. The patients that were diagnosed prenatally had less severe findings than the postnatal patients. These girls all had normal linear growth. Only 4 of the 12 had structural anomalies, which included atrial septal defect, ptosis, labial fusion, dysplastic kidneys, and hydrometrocolpos. None of the prenatally diagnosed group had physical findings that would have warranted karyotyping for a clinical suspicion of Turner syndrome at birth. This contrasted with the postnatally diagnosed group, who presented with a variety of congenital anomalies and short stature. These investigators suggested that most individuals with 45,X/46,XX would normally escape detection during the newborn period.

A study of 76 cases of 45,X/46,XY mosaicism was published by Chang et al. (1990). Of these patients, 95% had normal male genitalia. Four patients had significant genital anomalies, which included three cases of hypospadias and one female with clitoromegaly. The degree of amniotic fluid mosaicism did not predict the degree of genital or gonadal abnormality. It is commonly stated that patients with 45,X/46,XY are at risk for gonadoblastoma. In 11 patients who underwent gonadal biopsy, 3 had abnormal gonadal histology.

There is no indication for a cesarean section based on the diagnosis of Turner syndrome alone. The decision about whether to deliver in a tertiary-care center is made on the basis of the significance of the lymphatic malformations. If the fetus has hydrops fetalis, delivery should occur at a tertiary-care center. Similarly, if there is concern that the cystic hygroma may interfere in any way with airway management in the newborn infant, delivery should occur at a tertiary-care center. For a patient with a known karyotype, a diagnosis of Turner syndrome, but no sonographic abnormalities, delivery can safely occur in a community medical center. However, plans should be made for postnatal consultation with a pediatric cardiologist and a clinical geneticist.

▶ FETAL INTERVENTION

There are no fetal interventions for Turner syndrome.

▶ TREATMENT OF THE NEWBORN

The average birth weight of newborns with Turner syndrome is 2.8 kg (around 500 g below average) and the average length is 48 cm (2.8 cm below average) (Hall and Gilchrist 1990). Untreated infants with Turner syndrome tend to remain small, generally at the 3rd to 10th percentile for age. At birth, a complete physical examination is indicated and congenital hip dysplasia should be ruled out. We recommend consultation with a pediatric cardiologist at birth and echocardiography to rule out left-sided cardiac defects. The published percentage of individuals with Turner syndrome who have cardiovascular malformations is between 17 and 47% (Gøtzsche et al. 1994). The specific abnormalities that are greatly increased in this population of patients include aortic coarctation and bicuspid aortic valve. In a large retrospective review, Sybert (1998) demonstrated that 136 of 244 patients with Turner syndrome (56%) had cardiovascular abnormalities. Of these, 71% were structural and 29% were functional. The functional abnormalities included hypertension, mitral-valve prolapse, and conduction defects. Sybert confirmed that coarctation of the aorta and bicuspid aortic valve comprised greater than 50% of the structural abnormalities.

Eighty percent of babies with Turner syndrome are born with lymphedema. The pedal lymphedema is treated symptomatically. The cystic hygroma generally recedes, leaving folds of skin in the neck and a low hairline on the back of the neck. The protruberant ears

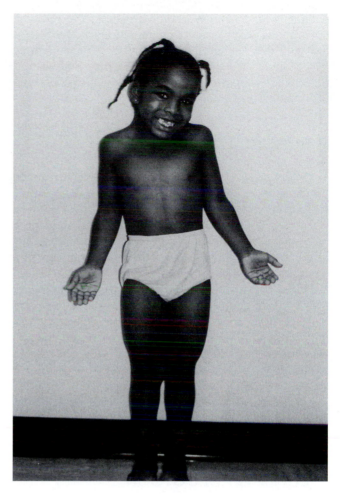

Figure 135-4. Photograph of a young girl with Turner syndrome, demonstrating the postnatal appearance of the neck webbing (Courtesy of Dr. Patricia Wheeler).

with upturned lobules are a residual manifestation of the lymphatic abnormalities that were present in utero (Fig. 135-4).

During the newborn period, an abdominal ultrasound examination is also indicated to look for the presence of renal malformations. In a postnatal study of 141 patients with Turner syndrome, Lippe et al. (1988) demonstrated renal abnormalities in 47 (33%) of patients. Ten of these patients had a horseshoe kidney, 1 had a double collecting system, 4 had complete absence of one kidney, 3 had crossed ectopia, 3 had ureteropelvic obstruction, 2 had ureterovesical obstruction, and 1 had a pelvic kidney. The 7% incidence of horseshoe kidney in patients with Turner syndrome can be compared to a prevalence of 1 in 600 normal individuals (Lippe et al. 1988).

Additional problems that can exist during the newborn period for patients with Turner syndrome include feeding difficulties due to the presence of a high arched palate and inefficient sucking and swallowing. Also, patients with Turner syndrome are subject to recurrent otitis media due to anatomic alterations at the base of the skull that change the angle of the eustachian tube.

Routine pediatric management recommendations for females with Turner syndrome have been published (Committee on Genetics 1995).

▶ SURGICAL TREATMENT

Thomson et al. (1990) described the surgical treatment for the simple neck webbing found in Turner syndrome. In four cases, they excised the excess neck skin and closed the defect to flatten the web against the side of the neck. In patients with Turner syndrome, they found that a definite band of fibrous tissue ran from the acromion to the mastoid process and was present in all cases studied. The underlying muscle and superficial layer of deep cervical fascia were noted to be normal and separate from the web. The skin anterior to the web was normal but the skin posterior to the web was freely mobile. When they biopsied the fibrous bands, they were demonstrated to consist of fibrous tissue and no other abnormalities (Thomson et al. 1990). These investigators achieved excellent cosmetic results. They recommended the lateral approach to elevate the hairline.

▶ LONG-TERM OUTCOME

The major considerations regarding long-term follow-up include treatment of short stature, cardiovascular abnormalities, including complications due to vascular malformation and hypertension, specific issues related to cognitive development, the propensity toward autoimmune disease, and issues surrounding fertility.

With regard to short stature, familial height plays a role in the ultimate height of patients affected with Turner syndrome (Hall et al. 1982). In other words, taller parents have taller daughters. For most patients with Turner syndrome, the bone age is within normal limits until ages 12 to 14 but without the influence of pubertal hormones there is no adolescent growth spurt. In a large survey taken in United States, untreated patients with Turner syndrome achieved an adult height of 143.0 cm (4 ft 8 in.). With growth hormone, patients achieved a mean height of 151.9 cm (4 ft 11.5 in.), a net gain of 8.1 cm (Saenger 1993). Growth hormone treatment should be initiated when the child's height drops below the fifth percentile of the normal female growth curve. This generally occurs between ages 2 and 5 years (Saenger 1996). Most endocrinologists recommend treatment with growth hormone until the bone age is greater than 15 years and the growth slows to less than 2 cm per year. In addition, estrogen therapy is recommended beginning at around age 14 to induce the secondary sexual characteristics. Only natural estrogens are recommended for these patients, as synthetic estrogens are incompletely metabolized. Approximately 20 to 25% of patients with Turner syndrome have spontaneous pubertal development and 2 to 5% have spontaneous onset of menstrual periods (Saenger 1996). Patients with Turner syndrome are predisposed to vascular malformations, which include intestinal telengiectasias and hemangiomas, and they have an increased incidence of ulcerative colitis and Crohn disease. The incidence of hypertension in adults with Turner syndrome is 30% (Hall et al. 1982). Individuals with Turner syndrome need to be monitored for hypertension on a lifelong basis (Sybert 1998). The risk for aortic dissection appears small, and repeated echocardiography or magnetic resonance imaging (MRI) to follow aortic-root diameters does not appear to be warranted based on available data (Sybert 1998). The majority of patients with aortic dilation have associated risk factors, such as bicuspid aortic valve or coarctation or systemic hypertension (Lin et al. 1998).

With regard to specific learning difficulties in patients with Turner syndrome, Bender et al. (1984) studied an unselected group of 16 patients with Turner syndrome. They noted a slight delay in walking and average development of language skills, but a striking deficit in perceptual organization and fine motor skills. Patients with Turner syndrome have a type of space–form blindness. They have difficulties identifying position in space, mentally rotating geometric shapes, and orienting to left–right directions. This visual–spatial impairment may be due to bilateral small volumes of the hippocampus and caudate, lenticular, and thalamic nuclei as well as parieto-occipital brain matter, as measured by MRI (Murphy et al. 1993). Importantly, intelligence is normal in Turner syndrome, unless a specific chromosomal abnormality such as a ring chromosome is present.

Other complications of Turner syndrome include otitis media, progressive sensorineural hearing loss, conductive middle ear disease (Sculerati et al. 1996), strabismus and other eye findings, such as ptosis, hypertelorism, and red–green color deficiency (Chrousos et al. 1984). Scoliosis is present in 10% of cases (Saenger 1996) and specific dermatologic abnormalities such as pigmented nevi and increased keloid formation are also characteristic. In addition, there is an increased incidence of autoimmune thyroid disease (Gruñeiro de Papendieck et al. 1987). Adult women with Turner syndrome have a high incidence of undiagnosed lipid, thyroid, and bone mineral density abnormalities (Garden et al. 1996).

Fertility issues are significant for adult patients with Turner syndrome. Several studies have performed pelvic sonography in childhood (Massarano et al. 1989; Mazzanti et al. 1997). During childhood, the ovaries can be classified as streak or nonstreak. Nonstreak ovaries retain a range of function. Patients with mosaicism have the highest percentage of detectable ovaries, as compared with patients with full monosomy 45,X (Mazzanti et al. 1997). Patients with Turner syndrome are infertile due to the ovaries consisting of fibrous streaks and an inability to ovulate. With the addition of hormonal replacement during early adolescence, patients can achieve secondary sexual characteristics and establish menses. Spontaneous pregnancy is rare, but possible. Reported cases of spontaneous pregnancy in Turner syndrome patients are associated with an increased incidence of miscarriage, perinatal fetal death, and malformations (Tarani et al 1998). Over the past few years, fertility has become possible using assisted reproductive technology and oocyte donation. In one study of 29 patients with Turner syndrome, Khastgir et al. (1997) documented 28 clinical pregnancies, including two sets of triplets. These investigators achieved a pregnancy rate of 41.2% per treatment cycle and a 17.1% implantation rate per embryo transferred. The recipient's age, specific karyotype or uterine anomaly had no influence on the treatment outcome.

▶ GENETICS AND RECURRENCE RISK

In general, Turner syndrome is considered to be a sporadic condition. It is not associated with advanced maternal age. Several studies have shown a bias for the loss of the paternal sex chromosome (Chu et al. 1994). A molecular study of 97 patients with 45,X karyotype showed that the remaining X chromosome was maternal in origin in 74% of cases (Jacobs et al. 1997).

In one study, the role of genetic imprinting was investigated. In 63 patients, 43 retained the maternal X and 20 retained the paternal X. There was a highly significant correlation between the child's height and the maternal height percentile when the X chromosome was inherited from the mother but not from the father. Similarly, there was also a strong correlation between the presence of cardiovascular abnormalities, neck webbing, and retention of the maternal X chromosome. In addition, the retention of the paternal X chromosome results in better social adjustment and superior verbal and higher-order executive function skills (Skuse et al. 1997). These recent data indicate that there is a genetic locus for social cognition, which is imprinted, and not expressed from the maternally derived X chromosome.

Patients who have Turner syndrome and have mosaicism for a small portion of the Y chromosome face a risk of gonadoblastoma. Cytogenetic analysis can fail to detect rare cells bearing a normal or structurally abnormal Y chromosome. Binder et al. (1995) screened 53 individuals with Turner syndrome for the presence of the sex-determining region Y (SRY) sequence. Of the 53 individuals, none were positive for Y-specific loci after the first round of polymerase chain reaction (PCR) but 2 were positive SRY after the second round of PCR. This indicates that the distal short arm of the Y chromosome is occasionally present. However, no cases of gonadoblastoma have been caused by low-level Y-chromosome mosaicism. These investigators did not feel that all individuals with Turner syndrome should be tested for undetected Y-chromosome sequences but that specific PCR analysis should be performed in patients with Turner syndrome who have evidence of virilization.

Patients with Turner syndrome who conceive spontaneously have a 30% chance of having a fetus with chromosomal abnormalities or congenital anomalies (Saenger 1996). Any woman with Turner syndrome who conceives spontaneously should be offered amniocentesis.

Patients who have had a previous fetus or infant with Turner syndrome may be offered chromosome analysis in a subsequent pregnancy for reassurance.

REFERENCES

Amiel A, Kidron D, Kedar I, Gaber E, Reish O, Fejgin MD. Are all phenotypically-normal Turner syndrome fetuses mosaics? Prenat Diagn 1996;16:791–795.

Bender B, Puck M, Salbenblatt J, Robinson A. Cognitive development of unselected girls with complete and partial X monosomy. Pediatrics 1984;73:175–182.

Binder G, Koch A, Wajs E, Ranke MB. Nested polymerase chain reaction study of 53 cases with Turner syndrome: is cytogenetically undetected Y mosaicism common? J Clin Endocrinol Metab 1995;80:3532–3536.

Bluth EJ, Maragos VA, Merritt CRB. Antenatal diagnosis of Turner syndrome. South Med J 1984;77:1335–1336.

Brookhyser KM, Slotnick N, Hanson FW. Third trimester resolution of cystic hygroma and pleural effusion in a fetus with Turner syndrome. Am J Perinatol 1993;10:297–299.

Chang HJ, Clark RD, Bachman H. The phenotype of 45,X/46,XY mosaicism: an analysis of 92 prenatally diagnosed cases. Am J Hum Genet 1990;46:156–167.

Chodirker BN, Harman CR, Greenberg CR. Spontaneous resolution of a cystic hygroma in a fetus with Turner syndrome. Prenat Diagn 1988;8:291–296.

Chrousos GA, Ross JL, Chrousos G, et al. Ocular findings in Turner syndrome: a prospective study. Ophthalmology 1984;91:926–928.

Chu CE, Donaldson MDC, Kelnar CJH, et al. Possible role of imprinting in the Turner phenotype. J Med Genet 1994;31:840–842.

Clark EB. Neck web and congenital heart defects: a pathogenetic association in 45 X-O Turner syndrome? Teratology 1984;29:355–361.

Cohen M, Schwartz S, Schwartz M, et al. Antenatal detection of cystic hygroma. Obstet Gynecol Surv 1989;44:481–490.

Committee on Genetics, American Academy of Pediatrics. Health supervision for children with Turner syndrome. Pediatrics 1995;96:1166–1173.

Donnenfeld AE, Mennuti MT. Sonographic findings in fetuses with common chromosome abnormalities. Clin Obstet Gynecol 1988;31:80–96.

Ford CE, Jones KW, Polani PE. A sex chromosomal anomaly in a case of gonadal dysgenesis (Turner's syndrome) Lancet 1959;1:771–713.

Garden AS, Benzie RJ, Miskin M, Gardner HA. Transactions of the forty-first annual meeting of the Society of Obstetricians and Gynaecologists of Canada. Am J Obstet Gynecol 1986;154:221–225.

Garden AS, Diver MJ, Fraser WD. Undiagnosed morbidity in adult women with Turner syndrome. Clin Endocrinol 1996;45:589–593.

Gøtzsche CO, Krag-Olsen B, Nielsen J, Sørensen KE, Kristensen BØ. Prevalence of cardiovascular malformations and association with karyotypes in Turner syndrome. Arch Dis Child 1994;71:433–436.

Gruñeiro de Papendieck L, Iorcansky S, Coco R, Rivarola MA, Bergadá C. High incidence of thyroid disturbances in 49 children with Turner syndrome. J Pediatr 1987;111:258–261.

Hall JG, Gilchrist DM. Turner syndrome and its variants. Pediatr Clin North Am 1990;37:1421–1441.

Hall JG, Sybert VP, Williamson RA, Fisher NL, Reed SD. Turner's syndrome. West J Med 1982;137:32–44.

Højberg-Gravholt C, Juul S, Weis Naeraa R, Hansen J. Prenatal and postnatal prevalence of Turner syndrome: a registry study. BMJ 1996;312:16–21.

Jacobs P, Dalton P, James R, et al. Turner syndrome: a cytogenetic and molecular study. Ann Hum Genet 1997;61:471–483.

Khastgir G, Abdalla H, Thomas A, Korea L, Latarche L, Studd J. Oocyte donation in Turner syndrome: an analysis of the factors affecting the outcome. Hum Reprod 1997;12:279–285.

Koeberl DD, McGillivray B, Sybert VP. Prenatal diagnosis of 45,X/46,XX mosaicism and 45,X: implications for postnatal outcome. Am J Hum Genet 1995;57:661–666.

Lacro RV, Jones KL, Benirschke K. Coarction of the aorta in Turner syndrome: a pathologic study of fetuses with nuchal cystic hygromas, hydrops fetalis and female genitalia. Pediatrics 1988;81:445–451.

Laundon CH, Spencer K, Macri JN, Anderson RW, Buchanan PD. Free beta hCG screening of hydropic and non-hydropic Turner syndrome pregnancies. Prenat Diagn 1996;16:853–856.

Lin AE, Lippe B, Rosenfeld RG. Further delineation of aortic dilation, dissection, and rupture in patients with Turner syndrome. Pediatrics 1998;102:e12.

Lippe B, Geffner ME, Dietrich EB, Boechat MI, Kangarloo H. Renal malformations in patients with Turner syndrome: imaging in 141 patients. Pediatrics 1988;82:852–856.

Massarano AA, Adams JA, Preece MA, Brook CGD. Ovarian ultrasound appearances in Turner syndrome. J Pediatr 1989;114:568–573.

Mazzanti L, Cacciari E, Bergamaschi R, et al. Pelvic ultrasonography in patients with Turner syndrome: age-related findings in different karyotypes. J Pediatr 1997;131:135–140.

Moore JW, Kirby WC, Rogers WM, Poth MA. Partial anomalous pulmonary venous drainage associated with 45,X Turner syndrome. Pediatrics 1990;86:273–276.

Murphy DGM, DeCarli C, Daly E, et al. X-chromosome effects on female brain: a magnetic resonance imaging study of Turner syndrome. Lancet 1993;342:1197–1200.

Natowicz M, Kelley RI. Association of Turner syndrome with hypoplastic left-heart syndrome. Am J Dis Child 1987;141:218–220.

Saenger P. Clinical review 48: the current status of diagnosis and therapeutic intervention in Turner syndrome. J Clin Endocrinol Metabol 1993;77:297–301.

Saenger P. Turner's syndrome. N Engl J Med 1996;335:1749–1754.

Saller DN, Canick JA, Schwartz S, Blitzer MG. Multiple-marker screening in pregnancies with hydropic and nonhydropic Turner syndrome. Am J Obstet Gynecol 1992;156:1021–1024.

Sculerati N, Oddoux C, Clayton M, Lim JW, Oster H. Hearing loss in Turner syndrome. Laryngoscope 1996;106:992–997.

Shepard TH, Fantel AG. Pathogenesis of congenital anomalies associated with Turner syndrome: the role of hypoalbuminemia and edema. Acta Endocrinol Suppl (Copenh) 1986;279:440–447.

Shimizu T, Hashimoto K, Shimizu M, Ozaki M, Murata Y. Bilateral pleural effusion in the first trimester: a predictor of chromosomal abnormality and embryonic death? Am J Obstet Gynecol 1997;177:470–471.

Skuse DH, James RS, Bishop DVM, et al. Evidence from Turner syndrome of an imprinted X-linked locus affecting cognitive function. Nature 1997;387:705–708.

Sybert VA. Cardiovascular malformations and complications in Turner syndrome. Pediatrics 1998;101:11.

Tarani L, Lampariello S, Raguso G, et al. Pregnancy in patients with Turner's syndrome: six new cases and review of literature. Gynecol Endocrinol 1998;12:83–87.

Thomson SJ, Tanner NSB, Mercer DM. Web neck deformity; anatomical considerations and options in surgical management. Br J Plast Surg 1990;43:94–100.

Turner HH. A syndrome of infantilism, congenital webbed neck and cubitus valgus. Endocrinology 1938;23:566–578.

von Kaisenberg CS, Nicolaides KH, Brand-Saberi B. Lymphatic vessel hypoplasia in fetuses with Turner syndrome. Hum Reprod 1999;823–826.

Wax JR, Blakemore KJ, Baser I, Stetton G. Isolated fetal ascites detected by sonography: an unusual presentation of Turner syndrome. Obstet Gynecol 1992;79:862–863.

CHAPTER 136

47,XXX Karyotype
(Triple X Syndrome, Trisomy X)

► CONDITION

The chromosome constitution 47,XXX was first described by Jacobs and colleagues (1959) in a woman of average intelligence with secondary amenorrhea. Since that time, several hundred cases have been reported in the medical literature. It is becoming increasingly clear that the phenotype of infants who are prenatally diagnosed with 47,XXX is significantly different from infants who are diagnosed by newborn screening or clinical symptomatology (Robinson et al. 1992). In general, the prenatally diagnosed infants have a more normal developmental profile. This may be due to factors unrelated to the chromosomes, such as socioeconomic status and level of parental education.

The sex chromosome aneuploidies are the most common group of abnormalities found in prenatal karyotypes, with an incidence of 1 in 250 amniocenteses (Robinson et al. 1992). Despite their frequency, sex-chromosome aneuploidy is rarely discussed in preprocedural genetic counseling. Thus, the finding of a fetal sex chromosome abnormality is usually not expected by the pregnant patient (Krone et al. 1975). This diagnosis prompts anxiety and ambivalence because, although the karyotype is abnormal, the phenotype of the affected child can be quite variable. Trisomy X can be associated with a normal outcome.

► INCIDENCE

The incidence of 47,XXX is approximately 1 in 1000 at midtrimester amniocentesis (Hook and Hamerton 1977) and 0.7 in 1000 live births (Tennes et al. 1975). These differences reflect different study populations and are not thought to reflect an increased perinatal mortality for 47,XXX fetuses. Using X-linked restriction-fragment–length polymorphisms, May et al. (1990) determined the parental origin of the extra X chromosome in 28 individuals with 47,XXX. Maternal nondisjunction was demonstrated in 26 of 28 cases. Seventy percent of these cases were due to an error in meiosis I. Thus, the etiology of trisomy X more closely resembles the autosomal trisomies. In this regard, trisomy X differs from the other sex chromosome aneuploidies in that there is a maternal age effect. Mitotic errors do not play a significant role in 47,XXX (May et al. 1990).

► SONOGRAPHIC FINDINGS

In general, there is no characteristic phenotype associated with trisomy X. The overwhelming majority of fetuses with trisomy X will have normal results on sonographic examination. The diagnosis is typically made at amniocentesis for advanced maternal age. In one study, the fetal nuchal translucency measurement was above the 95th percentile in 40% of the cases with 47,XXX, 47,XYY, or 47,XXXY (Sebire et al. 1998). In rare cases, structural abnormalities of the genitourinary tract have been described. These include bilateral renal agenesis and developmental arrest of the mesonephric and paramesonephric systems (Hogge et al. 1989); ovarian dysgenesis (Fig. 136-1), urinary-tract malformation, meconium peritonitis, and nonimmune fetal ascites (Spear and Porto 1988); exstrophy of the cloaca with unilateral renal agenesis (Lin et al. 1993); and unilateral renal agenesis, hydrometrocolpos, ovarian dysgenesis, laryngeal

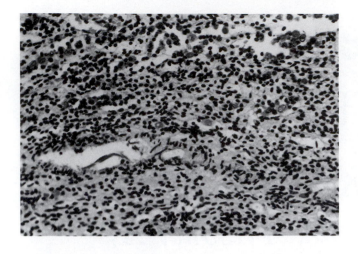

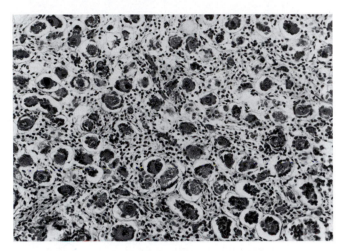

Figure 136-1. (Top) Postmortem photomicrograph of the cortex of the ovary from a fetus who spontaneously died in utero with 47,XXX. Note the relative absence of primordial follicles and germ cells. (Bottom) Comparison view of an ovary from a stillborn female fetus at 26 weeks of gestation, demonstrating numerous primordial follicles. *(Reprinted from Spear GS, Porto M. 47,XXX chromosome constitution, ovarian dysgenesis, and genitourinary malformation. Am J Med Genet 1988;29:511–515. Copyright 1988 by Wiley-Liss, Inc. Reprinted, by permission, of Wiley-Liss, Inc., a subsidiary of John Wiley & Sons, Inc.)*

atresia, pulmonary hypoplasia, and craniofacial anomalies (Hood et al. 1990). Because of the apparent clustering of cases with abnormalities in the genitourinary system, it has been suggested that the developing urogenital field may be affected by the presence of an extra X chromosome (Lin et al. 1993).

▶ DIFFERENTIAL DIAGNOSIS

When the karyotype is 47,XXX, the main consideration in the differential diagnosis is whether the abnormality

is present in all cells or in a fraction of the cells (mosaicism). A 46,XX/47,XXX mosaic karyotype will result in a significantly reduced likelihood of clinical symptoms (Robinson et al. 1992; Salbenblatt et al. 1989).

▶ ANTENATAL NATURAL HISTORY

The antenatal natural history does not differ from fetuses with a normal karyotype. If a level II sonogram was not performed at the time of the original amniocentesis, it should be offered. The parents should be counseled regarding the expectation that the remainder of the pregnancy will not be different from pregnancy with a chromosomally normal fetus.

▶ MANAGEMENT OF PREGNANCY

The main dilemma in management is the parental decision whether to continue the pregnancy (see "Long-Term Outcome"). Robinson et al. (1989, 1992) have reported their clinical experience with 530 phone consultations for a prenatal diagnosis of sex chromosome aneuploidy. In these series, 162 of the 530 consultations were reported for a diagnosis of trisomy X. Although their sample was admittedly biased in that their patient population consisted of women who elected to undergo prenatal cytogenetic diagnosis, 85% of whom were college graduates and in an upper socioeconomic class, certain trends emerged. In general, the affected patients were developing in a manner that was comparable to their normal siblings. They also had better peer relations than the previously reported group of children with sex-chromosome abnormalities (Robinson et al. 1979). In the prenatally diagnosed group of children with sex chromosome abnormalities, only 2 of 20 had intellectual quotients (IQ) as low as 90. The remainder of children were in the normal range, greater than 110. Robinson (1992) hypothesized that the improved developmental outcome was related to the supportive home environment provided by parents who knew the diagnosis and decided to continue the pregnancy. For the couples faced with a diagnosis of trisomy X in their fetus, 65% continued the pregnancy after phone consultation with Robinson's group.

▶ FETAL INTERVENTION.

There are no fetal interventions for 47,XXX karyotype.

▶ TREATMENT OF THE NEWBORN

In a study of 43 infants with trisomy X, the mean birth weight at term was 2.97 kg. There was no recognizable phenotype at birth. These infants were identified by prospective cytogenetic screening of all newborns in Denver. Their karyotype would not have been suspected from their physical examination. Congenital heart disease was diagnosed in 2 infants and congenital hip dislocation in 1. There was an increased frequency of epicanthal folds and clinodactyly (Robinson et al. 1979). The presence of minor anomalies such as these is possibly increased in 47,XXX females as compared with controls (Chudley et al. 1990).

▶ SURGICAL TREATMENT

There are no surgical treatments indicated for XXX alone.

▶ LONG-TERM OUTCOME

The most important statement regarding the long-term prognosis for a fetus with 47,XXX is that the phenotype is very variable (Linden et al. 1988; Puck et al. 1983; Tennes et al. 1975). The developmental outcome has ranged from mental retardation to college graduation (Linden et al. 1988). The general health of these children is good. Although their birth lengths are in the normal range, they become progressively taller as compared with their peers. The mean adult height of 47,XXX women is 167.9 + 7.7 cm, as compared with that in a white British control population—162.2 + 6 cm (Ogata et al. 1993). In infancy, a slight delay in neuromotor development has been noted. Salbenblatt et al. (1989) described a delay in the age of independent walking. In a prospective study of 11 girls identified at birth and followed over 22 years, Linden et al. (1988) noted that only 2 walked before the age of 12 months. At 2 years of age, they described delays in speech and language that prompted speech therapy during the preschool years. These delays are due to a specific deficits in auditory perception and in the ability to process linguistic information (Bender et al. 1983, 1989; Pennington et al. 1980).

The difficulties with verbal expression are described as the most severe of those described for the sex-chromosome abnormalities (Linden et al. 1988). It should be noted, however, that the patient population in the Linden study was derived from a postnatally diagnosed group. During the grade-school years, additional problems included clumsiness, lack of coordination, shyness, immature behavior, and poor academic performance. Sexual development is normal, with an average age of menarche of 12 years 8 months. In one fetus studied with 47,XXX, the ovary was histologically normal (Autio-Harmainen et al. 1980). Fertility and reproductive outcome is surprisingly good, with a low incidence of aneuploidy among offspring (Dewhurst

1978). One case has been reported of an individual with trisomy X, premature ovarian failure, and the presence of antithyroid and antinuclear antibodies (Michalak et al. 1983). Females with trisomy X have thicker tooth enamel than females with disomy X. This indicates that the extra X chromosome escapes inactivation to promote amelogenesis (Alvesalo et al. 1987).

In high school, 47,XXX individuals are tall, awkward, and continue to require special education. In 7 of the 11 females described by Linden et al. (1988), a psychiatric disorder or disturbance was diagnosed. An unusually high number of patients had recurrent, nonorganic abdominal pain. Again, it is important to note that these individuals were ascertained through the Denver Newborn study. This same group of young women have been described in multiple publications. The prenatally diagnosed trisomy X females have not yet reached adolescence and adulthood. Thus, it is too early to know whether their prognosis will be significantly different given the frequency of this condition in the general population. It seems likely that there are many clinically normal women who are unaware that they carry an extra X chromosome.

▶ GENETICS AND RECURRENCE RISK

Since the majority of cases are due to a maternal meiosis I error, the risk of recurrence is most strongly related to maternal age. Amniocentesis or chorionic villus sampling should be offered in a subsequent pregnancy. Theoretically, half the offspring of an individual with 47,XXX should be normal and half 47,XXX or 47,XXY. This has not been shown empirically. Scattered case reports exist of 47,XXX mothers who have had children with sex-chromosome and autosomal aneuploidies (Singer et al. 1972; Zizka et al. 1975), but most offspring are cytogenetically normal.

REFERENCES

Alvesalo L, Tammisalo E, Therman E. 47,XXX females, sex chromosomes, and tooth crown structure. Hum Genet 1987;77:345–348.

Autio-Harmainen H, Rapola J, Aula P. Fetal gonadal histology in XXXXY, XYY and XXX syndromes. Clin Genet 1980;18:1–5.

Bender B, Fry E, Pennington B, Puck M, Salbenblatt J, Robinson A. Speech and language development in 41 children with sex chromosome abnormalities. Pediatrics 1983;71:262–267.

Bender B, Fry E, Linden MG, Robinson A. Verbal and spatial processing efficiency in 32 children with sex chromosome abnormalities. Pediatr Res 1989;25:577–579.

Chudley AE, Stoeber GP, Greenberg CR. Intrauterine growth retardation and minor anomalies in 47,XXX children. Birth Defects 1990;26:267–272.

Dewhurst J. Fertility in 47,XXX and 45,X patients. J Med Genet 1978;15:132–135.

Hogge WA, Vick DJ, Schnatterly PA, MacMillan RH. Bilateral renal agenesis and Mullerian anomalies in a 47,XXX fetus. Am J Med Genet 1989;33:242–243.

Hood OJ, Hartwell EA, Shattuck KE, Rosenberg HS. Multiple congenital anomalies associated with a 47,XXX chromosome constitution. Am J Med Genet 1990;36:73–75.

Hook EB, Hamerton JL. The frequency of chromosome abnormalities detected in consecutive newborn studies—differences between studies—results by sex and severity of phenotypic involvement. In: Hook EB, Porter IH, eds. Population cytogenetics: studies in humans. New York: Academic Press, 1977:63–79.

Jacobs PA, Baikie AG, Court-Brown WM, et al. Evidence for the existence of the human "super female." Lancet 1959;2:423–425.

Krone LR, Prichard LL, Bradshaw CL, Jones OW, Peterson RM, Dixson BK. Antenatal diagnosis of an XXX female: a dilemma for genetic counseling. West J Med 1975;123:17–21.

Lin HJ, Ndiforchu F, Patell S. Exstrophy of the cloaca in a 47, XXX child: review of genitourinary malformations in triple-X patients. Am J Med Genet 1993;45:761–763.

Linden MG, Bender BG, Harmon RJ, Mrazek DA, Robinson A. 47,XXX: what is the prognosis? Pediatrics 1988;82:619–630.

May KM, Jacobs PA, Lee M, et al. The parental origin of the extra X chromosome in 47,XXX females. Am J Hum Genet 1990;46:754–761.

Michalak DP, Zacur HA, Rock JA, Woodruff JD. Autoimmunity in a patient with 47,XXX karyotype. Obstet Gynecol 1983;62:667–669.

Ogata T, Matsuo N. Sex chromosome aberrations and stature: deduction of the principal factors involved in the determination of adult height. Hum Genet 1993;91:551–562.

Pennington B, Puck M, Robinson A. Language and cognitive development in 47,XXX females followed since birth. Behav Genet 1980;10:31–41.

Puck MH, Bender BG, Borelli JB, Salbenblatt JA, Robinson A. Parents' adaptation to early diagnosis of sex chromosome anomalies. Am J Med Genet 1983;16:71–79.

Robinson A, Bender BG, Linden MG. Decisions following the intrauterine diagnosis of sex chromosome aneuploidy. Am J Med Genet 1989;34:552–554.

Robinson A, Bender BG, Linden MG. Prognosis of prenatally diagnosed children with sex chromosome aneuploidy. Am J Med Genet 1992;44:365–368.

Robinson A, Lubs HA, Nielsen J, Sorensen K. Summary of clinical findings: profiles of children with 47,XXY 47,XXX and 47,XYY karyotypes. Birth Defects 1979;15:261–266.

Salbenblatt JA, Meyers DC, Bender BG, Linden MG, Robinson A. Gross and fine motor development in 45,X and 47,XXX girls. Pediatrics 1989;84:678–682.

Sebire NJ, Snijders RJ, Brown R, Southall T, Nicolaides KH. Detection of sex chromosome abnormalities by nuchal translucency screening at 10–14 weeks. Prenat Diagn 1998;18:581–584.

Singer J, Sachdeva S, Smith GF, Hsia DYY. Triple X female and a Down's syndrome offspring. J Med Genet 1972;9:238–239.

Spear GS, Porto M. 47,XXX chromosome constitution, ovarian dysgenesis, and genitourinary malformation. Am J Med Genet 1988;29:511–515.

Tennes K, Puck M, Bryant K, Frankenburg W, Robinson A. A developmental study of girls with trisomy X. Am J Hum Genet 1975;27:71–80.

Zizka K, Balicek P, Nielsen J. XXYY son of a triple X mother. Humangenetik 1975;26:159–160.

CHAPTER 137
47,XYY Karyotype (XYY)

▶ CONDITION

The cytogenetic finding 47,XYY refers to the presence of an extra Y chromosome in the fetal cells. The extra Y chromosome is always paternal in origin and results from nondisjunction in the second meiotic division. XYY is one of the diagnoses included in the group of disorders known as sex-chromosome abnormalities. Anomalies involving the sex chromosomes are the most common abnormal findings in prenatal cytogenetic diagnosis, yet their existence is rarely discussed in pre-procedural genetic counseling. Thus, while prospective parents are reasonably prepared for a prenatal diagnosis of autosomal trisomy, the diagnosis of XYY usually comes as a surprise.

Much of the confusion regarding prognosis for males with XYY stems from studies performed in the 1960s that were highly biased by ascertainment of patients in maximum security hospitals or prisons (Price and Whatmore 1967). Fortunately, prospective longitudinal studies of newborns identified at birth do not support an increased incidence of aggression or criminality (Ratcliffe et al. 1990). As with all of the sex-chromosome abnormalities, the developmental phenotype is variable and subject to many other influences, such as parental IQ, socioeconomic status, and family stability.

▶ INCIDENCE

The incidence of 47,XYY is 1.45 in 1000 live births (Autio-Harmainen et al. 1980) and 1 in 1000 amniocenteses for advanced maternal age (Robinson et al. 1992a). The incidence is not increased among offspring of parents with advanced age. As opposed to the other sex-chromosome abnormalities, the XYY karyotype does not carry an increased chance of in utero mortality (Ferguson-Smith and Yates 1984).

▶ SONOGRAPHIC FINDINGS

There are no characteristic sonographic findings because the fetal phenotype in this condition is normal (Autio-Harmainen et al. 1980). However, in one study, the fetal nuchal translucency measurement was above the 95th percentile in 40% of the fetuses with 47,XXX, 47,XYY, or 47,XXY (Sebire et al. 1998).

▶ DIFFERENTIAL DIAGNOSIS

47,XYY is a definitive diagnosis obtained by prenatal karyotype (Fig. 137-1). Occasionally, cases of 46,XY/47,XYY mosaicism are detected, resulting from mitotic nondisjunction after fertilization. These patients are expected to have milder manifestations of the developmental abnormalities seen in this condition.

▶ ANTENATAL NATURAL HISTORY

The antenatal natural history for these fetuses does not differ from normal fetuses. A few patients with 47,XYY have been identified through abnormally increased maternal serum α-fetoprotein levels (Robinson et al. 1992a). It is unclear whether a true relationship exists between abnormalities in serum analytes and this particular chromosomal abnormality.

▶ MANAGEMENT OF PREGNANCY

The subsequent management of the pregnancy should include subspecialty referral to a clinical geneticist for parental education and counseling. No additional maternal testing is necessary other than that indicated by

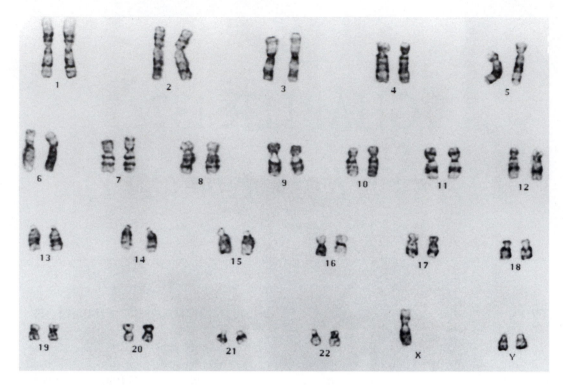

Figure 137-1. Karyotype obtained from a patient with 47,XYY demonstrating the presence of two identical Y chromosomes. *(Courtesy of Dr. Janet Cowan.)*

standard obstetric practice. There is no need for delivery at a tertiary-care center.

▶ FETAL INTERVENTION

There are no fetal interventions indicated for a 47,XXY karyotype.

▶ TREATMENT OF THE NEWBORN

The birth weights, head circumferences, and lengths of males with XYY are no different from control infants (Ratcliffe et al. 1990; Robinson et al. 1979). Although the phenotype is normal for this condition, an increased incidence of minor anomalies has been reported. In a study of 43 XYY infants identified by screening of all Denver newborns, one had congenital dislocation of the hip. Eight of the infants had one or more minor anomalies, including clinodactyly, inguinal hernia, abnormally formed ears, pectus carinatum, large or asymmetric head, strabismus, epicanthal folds, micrognathia, simian crease, and heart murmur (Robinson et al. 1979).

▶ SURGICAL TREATMENT

There are no surgical treatments indicated solely for XYY.

▶ LONG-TERM OUTCOME

XYY males tend to be tall and thin, with an average height of greater than the 75th percentile for age. This is due to an increased height velocity during childhood as compared with normal individuals (Ratcliffe et al. 1992) and affects size rather than body proportions (Varrela and Alvesalo 1985). XYY adult males achieve heights that are, on average, 13 cm taller than their fathers (Ratcliffe et al. 1990). The onset of puberty, defined as an increase in testicular volume to 4 ml or the appearance of pubic hair, occurs, on average, 6 months later than in controls (Ratcliffe et al. 1990; Robinson et al. 1992a). Testosterone production, pubertal development, and heterosexual interest have all been normal. The histology of the fetal testes in 1 case of 47,XYY was normal (Autio-Harmainen et al. 1980). The germ-cell depletion characteristic of other chromosome-abnormality syndromes is apparently rarely affected by the presence of the extra Y chromosome (Coerdt et al. 1985). XYY males have fathered normal infants. Human sperm chromosomes have been analyzed from a 47,XYY male and all of them contained only one sex chromosome. The frequencies of numerical, structural, and total abnormalities did not differ significantly from normal controls. The results of this study suggested that one Y chromosome is eliminated from the germ cells of males with XYY (Benet and Martin 1988). Despite these encouraging findings, another study reported an increased incidence of miscarriage, stillbirth, perinatal death, and chromosomally abnormal offspring in pregnancies conceived with 47,XYY men (Grass et al. 1984).

Interestingly, the presence of the extra Y chromosome affects dimensions of the palate and mandible. Palatal height and mandibular width are smaller in 47,XYY men as compared with their chromosomally normal first-degree male relatives (Laine and Alvesalo 1993). In addition, there appears to be a regulatory influence of the Y chromosome on amelogenesis that results in thicker dental enamel and larger size in the permanent teeth of 47,XYY males (Alvesalo et al. 1985).

Early development in XYY infants is essentially within normal limits. Gross motor milestones are generally first noted to be slightly delayed, with an average age of walking at 14 to 16 months. Characteristic findings include hypotonia, motor planning dysfunction, primitive reflex retention, and difficulties with bilateral coordination and visual–perceptual–motor integration. This decreased muscle tone and joint proprioception diminishes joint stability, which particularly affects the shoulder and pelvic girdles, and results in an awkward and inefficient gait (Salbenblatt et al. 1987).

In general, males with 47,XYY are not mentally retarded, but their IQs are 10 to 15 points lower than their chromosomally normal siblings (Robinson et al. 1992a). Intelligence level has a major effect on the development of psychosocial problems (Fryns 1998). Specific risks exist for mild language impairment, affecting both receptive and expressive function (Bender et al. 1983). In neurodevelopmental studies, Walzer et al. (1990) have shown that XYY males have difficulty understanding complex sentence structures, deficits in auditory memory, problems with word finding and narrative formulation, and persistent distractibility. Recommended educational intervention for 47,XYY males is no different than that for chromosomally normal children with reading and spelling difficulties. With regard to concern over the association between aggressive behavior and XYY karyotype, prospective studies of thirty-nine 47,XYY probands have not revealed marked psychiatric disturbances. However, an increased frequency of distractibility, hyperactivity, and temper tantrums have been reported (Robinson et al. 1990). The importance of a supportive family environment has been noted by Robinson et al. (1992b), who have described significant developmental differences between 47,XYY males ascertained by prenatal diagnosis versus those discovered by newborn screening. All the children in this study who were diagnosed prenatally belonged to well-educated, economically stable families. These children had fewer language deficits and learning problems, a mean IQ of 123 (range, 109 to 147), and were getting As and Bs in school (Robinson et al. 1992b)

▶ GENETICS AND RECURRENCE RISK

Although few data exist regarding the specific recurrence risk for XYY, the risk for nondisjunction involving any of the other chromosomes may be as high as 1%. Prenatal cytogenetic studies should be offered in subsequent pregnancies. Pregnant partners of 47,XYY men should also be offered prenatal karyotyping.

REFERENCES

Alvesalo L, Tammisalo E, Hakola P. Enamel thickness in 47, XYY males' permanent teeth. Ann Hum Biol 1985;12: 421–427.

Autio-Harmainen H, Rapola J, Aula P. Fetal gonadal histology in XXXXY, XYY and XXX syndromes. Clin Genet 1980;18:1–5.

Bender B, Fry E, Pennington B, Puck M, Salbenblatt J, Robinson A. Speech and language development in 41 children with sex chromosome abnormalities. Pediatrics 1983;71:262–267.

Benet J, Martin RH. Sperm chromosome complements in a 47,XYY man. Hum Genet 1988;78:313–315.

Coerdt W, Rehder H, Gaussman I, Johannison R, Gropp A. Quantitative histology of human fetal testes in chromosomal disease. Pediatr Pathol 1985;3:245–259.

Ferguson-Smith MA, Yates JRW. Maternal age specific rates for chromosome aberrations and factors influencing them: report of a collaborative European study on 52,965 amniocenteses. Prenat Diagn 1984;4:5–44.

Fryns JP. Mental status and psychosocial functioning in XYY males. Prenat Diagn 1998;18:303–304.

Grass F, McCombs J, Scott CI. Reproduction in XYY males: two new cases and implications for genetic counseling. Am J Med Genet 1984;19:553–560.

Laine T, Alvesalo L. Palatal and mandibular arch morphology in 47,XYY men and in other sex-chromosome anomalies. Arch Oral Biol 1993;38:101–105.

Price WH, Whatmore PB. Behaviour disorders and pattern of crime among XYY males identified at a maximum security hospital. BMJ 1967;1:533–536.

Ratcliffe SG, Butler GE, Jones M. Edinburgh study of growth and development of children with sex chromosome abnormalities. IV. Birth Defects Original Article Series 1990;26:1–44.

Ratcliffe SG, Pan H, McKie M. Growth during puberty in the XYY boy. Ann Hum Biol 1992;19:579–587.

Robinson A, Bender BG, Linden MG. Prenatal diagnosis of sex chromosome abnormalities. In: Milunsky A, ed. Genetic disorders and the fetus. 3rd ed. Baltimore: Johns Hopkins University Press, 1992a:211–239.

Robinson A, Bender BG, Linden MG. Prognosis of prenatally diagnosed children with sex chromosome aneuploidy. Am J Med Genet 1992b;44:365–368.

Robinson A, Bender BG, Linden MG, Salbenblatt JA. Sex chromosome aneuploidy: the Denver prospective study. Birth Defects Original Article Series 1990;26:59–115.

Robinson A, Lubs HA, Nielsen J, Sorensen K. Summary of clinical findings: profiles of children with 47,XXY,

47,XXX and 47,XYY karyotypes. Birth Defects 1979;15: 261–266.

Salbenblatt JA, Meyers DC, Bender BG, Linden MG, Robinson A. Gross and fine motor development in 47,XXY and 47,XYY males. Pediatrics 1987;80:240–244.

Sebire NJ, Snijders RA, Brown R, Southall T, Nicolaides KH. Detection of sex chromosome abnormalities by nuchal translucency screening at 10–14 weeks. Prenat Diagn 1998;18:581–584.

Varrela J, Alvesalo L. Effects of the Y chromosome on quantitative growth: an anthropometric study of 47,XYY males. Am J Phys Anthropol 1985;68:239–245.

Walzer S, Bashir AS, Silbert AR. Cognitive and behavioral factors in the learning disabilities of 47,XXY and 47,XYY boys. Birth Defects Original Article Series 1990;26:45–58.

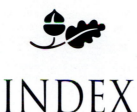

INDEX

Page numbers in *italics* denote figures; those followed by "t" denote tables.

ISBN 0-8385-2570-9

90000